59 Biodegradable Stents*

Brian Armstrong
James Zidar
Harry R. Phillips III
Richard S. Stack

Several modalities are available for the percutaneous treatment of coronary artery disease. All these modalities are limited by the development of acute complications (major dissection, abrupt closure) and restenosis. Although major dissection and closure can be effectively treated with currently available metallic stents, there are several limitations to this approach, since the incidence of subacute thrombosis with metal stents is high when used to salvage initially unsuccessful procedures.[1,2] A relatively intense level of anticoagulation is required for 4 to 6 weeks after stent placement, to decrease the incidence of stent thrombosis. This regimen poses a significant risk of bleeding and prolongs the hospitalization. Although metallic stents probably decrease the incidence of restenosis, some degree of neointimal proliferation still occurs in a significant number of cases. Given these limitations, additional modifications in stent design are desirable. An ideal stent would provide temporary support to the vessel wall to repair acute complications and allow delivery of local pharmacotherapy for the intermediate term to limit or prevent restenosis. The concept of a biode-

gradable stent is intriguing since it has the properties necessary to impact significantly in both of these areas. The concept, design, initial results of animal studies, and plans for future studies involved in the development of a clinically applicable biodegradable stent are described in this chapter.

BIODEGRADABLE STENT CONCEPT

The two ultimate goals of percutaneous coronary revascularization are to provide an adequate initial result and prevent restenosis. Neither of these goals should require the implantation of a permanent device. Major dissection and abrupt closure can be effectively treated with a perfusion balloon catheter in about 80% of cases.[3] This device is in effect a "temporary stent" allowing support to a dissection flap for several minutes to a few hours. Given this high success rate, it is likely that major dissections or episodes of abrupt closure could be successfully treated with a device that could provide support to the involved arterial segment for days to weeks. A biodegradable stent would clearly serve this function. If polymers with little thrombogenic or inflammatory activity are used to construct the biodegradable stent, the problem of subacute thrombosis (as seen

* As an inventor and developer of new technologies, Dr. Stack has U.S. patents and trademarks on biodegradable stents for which financial royalties may be received.

in currently available metal stents) should be greatly lessened.

The second problem, restenosis, occurs over a limited time frame and is unusual after 6 months.[4] There are two key components to this process; mechanical renarrowing and neointimal proliferation. Mechanical renarrowing includes acute recoil and late remodeling, both of which should be overcome if the radial (hoop) strength of the stent is adequate. Likewise, neointimal proliferation slows after 6 months. Therefore, if the mechanical support of the stent or a drug carried within the stent were present for this period of time, the problem of restenosis could potentially be resolved. After that point in time, there should be no need for a prosthetic device.

Metallic stents can successfully treat abrupt closure[5,6] and decrease the incidence of restenosis.[7] There are several limitations to metal stents, however. The continued presence of a metallic stent may provide an ongoing stimulus for vascular smooth muscle growth.[8] Also, metallic stents can cause aneurysmal dilation of the involved arterial segment.[9] The long-term consequences of these observations are unknown. One of the most significant limitations of metallic stents is their potential to cause thrombosis, requiring intensive anticoagulation for 4 to 6 weeks after initial implantation. This approach results in a prolonged hospital stay and an increased incidence of bleeding complications. Although metallic stents can be coated with heparin, the long-term benefit of this is unknown. In addition, only a limited amount of heparin can be bound to a metal stent. Moreover, other powerful pharmacologic agents could not be bound to a metal structure. These issues severely limit the use of stents composed entirely of metal as a local drug delivery device and underscore the need for a different stent design if effective drug delivery is to be possible.

MECHANISM OF ACTION

The ultimate design of a biodegradable stent must involve two steps, selecting the appropriate material for stent construction and developing a mechanical design that allows for sufficient radial strength to prevent significant recoil. The stent material chosen cannot cause significant inflammation or thrombosis (metallic stents cause some degree of local inflammatory response). It must provide adequate support to the vessel wall for several days to weeks. The breakdown products must be nontoxic. Finally, a degradable stent should produce a local vascular environment in which endothelialization can occur. Polymers have been used in vascular grafts and vascular sutures for some time and have all of the properties necessary for the development of a degradable stent. Several different polymer types have been screened for use in a biodegradable stent:

- Polylactic acid
- Polylactic-glycolic acid
- Polyglycolic acid
- Polyorthoesters
- Poly-(E-caprolactone)
- Polydihydropyrans
- Polycyanoacrylates
- Poly acetals
- Polyether urethane urea
- Silicone
- Polyethylene terephthalate

Two general types of polymers are available. Truly degradable polymers are completely resorbed over time, whereas nondegradable polymers are not significantly degraded.

The degradable polymers are desirable, but the long-term histologic reaction in humans has not yet been evaluated for any of these polymers. Polyesters such as polylactic and polyglycolic acid have many desirable features and have been used for local drug delivery.[10] Polyorthoesters have been used in the delivery of contraceptive steroids.[11] Polyglutamic acid has been used in the development of a reservoir drug delivery system. Polyanhydrides have excellent tissue compatibility and have been used in the local delivery of carmustine.[12] A polylactic acid-poly-caprolactone copolymer has been shown to carry and release argatroban successfully.[13] Several other polymer types are available, and further work is necessary to test the biocompatibility and possible utility of these polymers in the development of a biodegradable stent.

Nondegradable polymers could be employed as a coating to decrease tissue reaction to a metallic stent backbone or act as a local drug delivery platform. These polymers could be employed if they added significant radial strength to the stent design or as a local drug delivery matrix, but they would not form a truly biodegradable stent. The optimal polymer for use in a biocompatible stent is not yet known with certainty. Different animal models have led to conflicting results regarding tissue compatibility, as exemplified in studies with polyethylene terephthalate (PET) stents in porcine arteries. One group reported occlusion of the stents, whereas another group showed no significant inflammatory response (these studies are reviewed more completely below).

Other substances have been suggested as possible coatings for a stent framework. Phosphotidylcholine causes little inflammatory response.[14] Loose-fitting hydrogels of polymers have been suggested as a means of coating endovascular stents to allow drug delivery and decrease thrombogenicity, but extensive work is necessary to define the deliverability of this type of device and the incidence of polymer embolization.

The mechanical design of the stent is equally important. A larger luminal diameter is desirable in that a greater degree of neointimal proliferation would have to occur before a significant restenosis would result. The mechanical properties of a biodegradable stent would have to be such that the maximal possible lumen diameter would result after deployment. Several polymers have been shown to have sufficient radial strength to prevent significant recoil. A composite design with a nondegradable polymer on a metallic framework for additional support could also be utilized. These latter designs would not be truly degradable, but would allow a smaller amount of material to be permanently incorporated into the vessel wall while still allowing the device to be used as a drug delivery platform.

Two general design types are possible, self-expanding and balloon-expandable stents. It is not clear that a self-expanding design would have sufficient strength to allow for the maximum possible lumen diameter after deployment. Obtaining the largest possible lumen after stent deployment is important for several reasons. A larger lumen allows for improved blood flow and a decreased likelihood of thrombosis. Most importantly, if a larger lumen is achieved, a greater amount of neointimal proliferation must occur before a hemodynamically significant lesion is formed. It is by this mechanism that metallic stents probably decrease the incidence of restenosis even though a relatively increased amount of neointimal proliferation is stimulated by their placement. No conclusive evidence shows that any self-expanding stent has sufficient strength to distend the plaque sufficiently to yield the maximal acute gain possible. Therefore, a balloon-expandable stent design may prove superior. However, if a pharmacologic agent delivered locally is found to abolish neointimal proliferation completely, then a larger acute luminal gain might not be necessary, and a self-expanding design would be adequate.

ANIMAL STUDIES

Several groups have made contributions to a basic understanding of the effects of biodegradable and biocompatible polymers on vascular biology in animals. There are some fundamental differences between animal models that make generalizations difficult. In addition, there are fundamental differences in the response of coronary arteries compared with femoral or carotid arteries in any species. Moreover, proliferative and thrombotic tendencies are vastly different among pigs, dogs, and primates.

Duke Biostent Project

The first biodegradable stent model was designed by Drs. Stack and Clark at Duke University.[15] A form of poly-L-lactide (PLLA) was used to form a self-expanding mesh stent. The PLLA used was able to withstand 1,000 mmHg of pressure acutely and also had sufficient radial strength to prevent collapse due to maximal vasoconstriction in a canine femoral artery. The polymer maintained this degree of hoop strength after 30 days in a saline environment. Polymer degradation was nearly complete at 9 months and there was little inflammatory response in canine femoral arteries. Additional work showed that the stented segment had platelet aggregates and fibrin deposition by the end of the first week. At 14 days, the stent struts were covered by neointima. After 3 months, the stent remained fully expanded. By 18 months, there was nearly complete resorption of the stent material. Importantly, there was no significant inflammatory response at any time.[16,17]

This work has confirmed that a stent made of a biodegradable polymer can be successfully deployed, provide adequate radial support, and not incite an excessive thrombotic or inflammatory response. Additional design modifications are currently under way to ensure even greater strength and document the effects of the polymer in other animal models.

Mayo Clinic/Cleveland Clinic/Thoraxcenter Stent

The Mayo Clinic/Cleveland Clinic/Thoraxcenter has reported extensively on the tissue response of animals to polymeric material. Tantalum wire stents were covered with an arc of polymer occupying 90 degrees of the stent circumference. These stents were deployed in porcine coronary arteries, and the histologic response was assessed after 28 days. Stents coated with PGLA, PCL, and PHBV were used initially. In all cases, the stented arteries remained patent, but there was a significant amount of fibromuscular and inflammatory proliferation in the segment of the arterial wall adjacent to the polymer. The cellular infiltrate consisted of polymorphonuclear leukocytes, eosinophils, and mononuclear cells. Only a minimal inflammatory response was present next to the tantalum struts, except in stents with poly-orthoester, which had a significant amount of inflammation around the bare stent struts as well. There was no significant difference in response among the three polymers tested.[18] Cytotoxicity testing showed that the polymer preparations had no appreciable residual solvent remaining and that there was no direct cytotoxictity.

Nonbioabsorbable polymers have also been studied by this protocol. When polyether urethane urea, silicone, and PET were implanted in porcine coronary arteries, extensive fibromuscular and inflammatory proliferation occurred.[19] The results using PET have been disparate. At the Thoraxcenter, a self-expanding PET stent was shown to cause only minimal neointimal proliferation in porcine peripheral arteries.[20] By contrast, another group showed that self-expanding PET stents deployed in porcine coronary arteries caused an intense proliferative response that resulted in complete occlusion of the stented arterial segments in all animals.[21] In the latter study, the stents were not externally sterilized prior to placement. A recent report from Lincoff et al.[22] showed no evidence of tissue reaction in the same pig coronary model when using high molecular weight PLLA. This is the same polymer used in the Duke stent. Differences in arterial sites and polymer preparation may have accounted for some of the differences in the inflammatory responses noted above.

The Kyoto University Stent

The group at Kyoto University has developed a balloon-expandable stent made of polyglycolic acid.[23] In a canine model, thrombus was present on the stent after 3 hours. After 2 to 8 weeks, the stent was covered by neointima. This polymer had relatively rapid degradation; the fiber diameter had decreased by over 50% after 2 months.

BIODEGRADABLE STENTS AS A DRUG DELIVERY PLATFORM

Perhaps the greatest role for a biodegradable stent is as a local drug delivery device. Local delivery offers several advantages over systemic delivery. A much higher concentration of drug could be delivered to the lesion site with a local platform than could ever be attained with systemic administration. This would allow drugs with some systemic toxicity to be used safely while still providing a therapeutic drug level at the lesion site. Local delivery also allows

drug levels within the arterial media that are orders of magnitude higher than could ever be achieved with systemic administration. At these tremendous concentrations, it is possible that drugs that up to now have shown no benefit with respect to acute stent thrombosis or restenosis would be efficacious.

Several issues must be addressed when using polymers as a local drug delivery platform. The drug and polymer must be chemically compatible. The drug must be able to be absorbed into the polymer matrix or withstand the polymerization process and remain biologically active. The rate of elution of the drug from the stent must also be appropriate; if the drug disappears too rapidly, then ongoing metabolic and biochemical processes might lead to thrombosis or restenosis. The three mechanisms of release of drug from a polymer are erosion of the polymer, breaking covalent bonds between the drug and the polymer, and diffusion.

Several studies have shown that high concentrations of locally applied drugs can have a potent biologic effect. Heparin released from an ethylene-vinyl acetate copolymer placed next to the carotid artery in rats greatly inhibited smooth muscle proliferation after balloon injury.[24] In a similar experiment, dexamethasone was found to prevent proliferation when placed in a silicone polymers wrapped around the arterial adventitia.[25]

A heparin coating has been applied to self-expanding polymer stents.[26] The addition of heparin did not prevent thrombosis in a canine model. However, heparin coating significantly reduced the incidence of thrombosis when polymer-coated Palmaz-Schatz stents were placed in rabbit iliac arteries.[27] Neointimal proliferation was not decreased by the addition of heparin in this study; however, the amount of heparin incorporated into the stent was relatively small. By contrast, high-dose heparin has been shown to decrease neointima formation when a periadventitial coating was applied.[28] Recently, heparin-coated bioabsorbable stents were shown to have decreased thrombogenicity and platelet adherence when compared with noncoated stents.[29] These studies highlight the need to formulate stent and drug combinations that allow for a significant amount of local drug delivery if a significant pharmacologic effect is to result.

Dev et al.[30] showed that a polyurethane-coated stent could deliver high concentrations of forskolin and etretinate to the wall of rabbit arteries. The ratio of vessel wall to systemic levels of forskolin was 6,700, and for etretinate 950. However, the level of forskolin in the vessel wall declined dramatically within 24 hours. The same group showed that forskolin was delivered both radially and longitudinally from a polyurethane stent into the vessel wall. Moreover, forskolin delivered in this way prevented thrombosis in rabbits.[31]

Dexamethasone has been locally delivered to porcine coronary arteries using a tantalum stent coated with PLLA.[22] Dexamethasone had no impact on the extent of neointimal thickness. There was no inflammatory reaction to the PLLA in this model.

These studies demonstrate that local drug delivery via polymeric stents is possible and can produce the desired physiologic effects in some animal models. Extensive work is ongoing to define the best stent design and drug/polymer combination. Numerous antiplatelet, antithrombotic, and antiproliferative drugs may be shown to be effective.

CURRENT STATUS AND FUTURE IMPLICATIONS

Several groups are currently developing stents using both biodegradable and biocompatible polymers. Modifications of stent designs to provide the necessary hoop strength using only polymers are also under study. With design advances, biodegradable stents may provide sufficient flexibility and deliverability to expand the utility of coronary stents significantly beyond the range currently available with metallic stents. Combination (composite) stents with a metallic frame and a biodegradable or biocompatible polymer used for drug delivery are also under development. These advances will allow local delivery of antithrombotic, antiplatelet, and antiproliferative agents in pharmacologically effective doses. This ability should provide a powerful new means of preventing acute complications after percutaneous coronary interventions and should significantly decrease the incidence of restenosis. Rapid advances will certainly be made in this exciting area of interventional cardiology.

REFERENCES

1. Shaknovich A, Rocha-Singh K, Teirstein P et al. Subacute stent thrombosis in Palmaz-Schatz (PS) stents in native coronary arteries: time course, acute management and outcome. US multicenter experience, abstracted. Circulation, suppl. I. 1992;86:I-113
2. Agrawal SK, Hearn JA, Lue MW et al. Stent thrombosis and ischemic complications following coronary artery stenting, abstracted. Circulation, suppl. I. 1992; 86:I-113
3. Jackman JD, Zidar JP, Tcheng JE et al. Outcome after prolonged inflations of >20 minutes for initially unsuccessful percutaneous transluminal coronary angioplasty. Am J Cardiol 1992;69:1417
4. McBride W, Lange RA, Hills DS. Restenosis after successful coronary angioplasty: pathology and prevention. N Engl J Med 1988;318:1734
5. Roubin GS, Cannon AD, Agrawal SK et al. Intracoronary stenting for acute and threatened closure complicating percutaneous transluminal coronary angioplasty. Circulation 1992;85:916
6. Herrman HC, Buchbinder M, Clemen MW et al. Emergent use of balloon-expandable coronary stenting for failed percutaneous transluminal coronary angioplasty. Circulation 1992;86:812
7. Serruys PW, Macaya C, deJaegere P et al. Interim results of the BENESTENT trial, abstracted. Circulation, suppl. I. 1993:88:I-382
8. Santoian EC, King SB III. Intravascular stents, intimal proliferation and restenosis. J Am Coll Cardiol 1992;19:877
9. Rab ST, King SB III, Roubin GS et al. Coronary aneurysms after stent placement: a suggestion of altered vessel wall healing in the presence of anti-inflammatory agents. J Am Coll Cardiol 1991;18:1524
10. Wada R, Hyon SH, Ikada Y et al. Lactic acid oligomer microspheres containing an anticancer agent for selective lymphatic delivery. I. In vitro studies. J Bioactive Compatible Polymers 1988;3:126
11. Langer RA. New methods in drug delivery. Science 1990;249:1527
12. Brem H, Mahaley MD Jr., Vick NA et al. Interstitial chemotherapy with drug polymer implants for the treatment of recurrent gliomas. J Neurosurg 1991;74: 441
13. Wada R, Hyon S, Nakamura T et al. In vitro evaluation of sustained drug release from biodegradable elastomer. Pharm Res 1991;8:1292
14. Nordrehaug JE, Chronos N, Sigwart U. A biocompatible phosphotidylcholine coating applied to metallic stents, abstracted. J Am Coll Cardiol, suppl. A. 1994; 24:5A
15. Stack RS, Califf RM, Phillips HR III et al. Interventional cardiac catheterization at Duke University Medical Center: new interventional technology. Am J Cardiol, suppl. 2. 1988;18:3F
16. Gammon RS, Chapman GD, Agrawal GM et al. Mechanical features of the Duke biodegradable intravascular stent, abstracted. J Am Coll Cardiol, suppl. A. 1991;17:235A
17. Zidar JP, Gammon R, Chapman G et al. Short and long-term vascular tissue response in the Duke bioabsorbable stent, abstracted. J Am Coll Cardiol, suppl. A. 1993;21:439A
18. Lincoff AM, Schwartz RS, van der Giessen JW et al. Biodegradable polymers can evoke a unique inflammatory response when implanted in the coronary artery, abstracted. Circulation, suppl. I. 1992;86:I-184
19. Lincoff AM, van der Giessen WJ, Schwartz RS et al. Biodegradable and biostable polymers may both cause vigorous inflammatory responses when implanted in the porcine coronary artery, abstracted. J Am Coll Cardiol 1993;21:179A
20. van Buesekim HMM, van der Giessen JW, van Ingen Scenau D et al. Synthetic polymers as an alternative to metal in stents? In vivo and mechanical behavior of polyethylene terephthalate, abstracted. Circulation, suppl. I. 1992;86:I–731
21. Murphy JG, Schwartz RS, Edwards WD et al. Percutaneous polymeric stents in porcine coronary arteries.

Initial experience with polyethylene terephthalate stents. Circulation 1992;86:1596

22. Lincoff AM, Furst J, Ellis SG et al. Sustained local drug delivery by a novel intravascular eluting stent to prevent restenosis in the porcine coronary artery, abstracted. J Am Coll Cardiol, suppl. A. 1994;23:18A

23. Suswa T, Shiraki K, Shimizu Y. Biodegradable intracoronary stents in adult dogs. J Am Coll Cardiol, abstracted. 21:484A

24. Edelman ER, Adams DH, Karnovsky MD. Effect of controlled adventitial heparin delivery on smooth muscle cell proliferation following endothelial injury. Proc Natl Acad Sci USA 1990;87:3773

25. Ville AE, Guzman LA, Golomb G et al. Local delivery of dexamethasone for prevention of neointimal proliferation after balloon injury in the rat carotid model, abstracted. J Am Coll Cardiol, suppl. A. 21:179A

26. Bonan R, Bhat K, Lefevre T et al. Coronary artery stenting after angioplasty with self-expanding parallel wire metallic stents. Am Heart J 1991;121:1522

27. Bailey SR, Paige S, Lunn A. Heparin coating of endovascular stents decreases subacute thrombosis in a rabbit model, abstracted. Circulation, suppl. I. 1992; 86:I-186

28. Rogers C, Karnovsky M, Edelman E. Intravenous and local perivascular heparin reduce stent thrombosis and intimal hyperplasia, abstracted. Circulation, suppl. I. 1992;86:I-227

29. Zidar JP, Mohammad SF, Culp SC et al. In vitro thrombogenicity analysis of a new bioabsorbable, balloon-expandable, endovascular stent, abstracted. J Am Coll Cardiol, suppl. A. 1992;21:483A

30. Dev V, Lamber T, Sheth S et al. Kinetics of drug delivery to the arterial wall via polyurethane coated removable nitinol stent—comparative study of 2 drugs, abstracted. Circulation suppl. I. 1993;88:I–310

31. Lambert T, Dev V, Litvack F, Forrester JS, Eigler NL. Localized arterial drug delivery from a polymer coated removable metallic stent: kinetics and bioactivity of forskolin, abstracted. Circulation, suppl. I. 1993;88:I-310

Implantation of the Palmaz-Schatz Stent Without Subsequent Anticoagulation

60

Antonio Colombo
Patrick Hall

Using historical comparisons, the potential benefit of stents in decreasing the morbidity of acute closure was noted by Roubin et al.[1] Reduced restenosis rates in comparison with historical percutaneous transluminal coronary angiography (PTCA) restenosis rates have also been observed in native coronary artery lesions by Serruys et al.[2] with the Medinvent stent and by Schatz et al.[3,4] and Carrozza, et al.[5] using the Palmaz-Schatz stent. Similar observations on improved restenosis rates in vein grafts were reported by Carrozza, et al.[5] More recently, Serruys et al.[6] reported that the BENESTENT randomized trial comparing stents and angioplasty in treating de novo native coronary artery lesions also demonstrated a significant reduction in the restenosis rates in the stent treatment group (18%) versus the angioplasty group (34%).

The major limitations of increased clinical use of stents are subacute stent thrombosis and the complications associated with an aggressive anticoagulant regimen. The anticoagulant regimen has created a category of anticoagulant-related complications without eliminating subacute stent thrombosis.

Early experience at our institution with intravascular ultrasound (IVUS) evaluation after achieving an acceptable angiographic result revealed that over 80% of stents were insufficiently dilated (reported by Nakamura et al.[7] and Goldberg et al.[8]). These observations pointed to incomplete stent expansion as a primary cause of stent thrombosis rather than the inherent thrombogenicity of the metallic stent.

The hypothesis that systemic anticoagulation is not necessary following the stenting procedure when adequate stent placement and expansion are achieved was prospectively evaluated in a consecutive series of 328 patients who underwent Palmaz-Schatz intracoronary stenting. All patients that had adequate stent expansion documented by IVUS were treated with antiplatelet therapy only and did not receive anticoagulation following the stent procedure.

PATIENT POPULATION

This ongoing study was initiated on March 30, 1993. Through November 30, 1993 328 consecutive patients with 416 lesions had undergone Palmaz-Schatz intracoronary stenting. The entry criteria included (1) coronary artery disease manifested by clinical symptoms or objective evidence of myocardial ischemia either on exercise test or by nuclear scintigraphy, and (2) angiographic evidence of single or multiple vessel coronary disease with target lesion stenosis greater than 70% by visual estimates. The exclusion criteria included (1) small vessels less than 2.25 mm, and (2) angiographically critical diffuse distal disease that might compromise outflow from a stented lesion. No specific ages or ejection fraction values were used as limitations for study entry.

PRETREATMENT PROCEDURE

All patients were premedicated with aspirin (325 mg) and calcium channel blockers. During the stenting procedure, patients received a bolus of 10,000 U of heparin with additional heparin given to maintain the activated clotting times (ACT) greater than 300 seconds. Five different types of Johnson and Johnson tubular slotted stents were utilized: the Palmaz-Schatz stent, the short stent composed of one 7-mm tubular slotted segment, a 10-mm-long biliary stent, a 20-mm renal stent composed of two 10-mm segments with a central articulation, and a short (disarticulated) renal stent. A delivery system with a premounted coronary stent was used sparingly during the study (n = 7). Routine dilation or predilation was performed prior to stenting. Stents were mounted on 2.5- or 3.0-mm balloon catheters, hand crimped tightly, and deployed at 10 atm. Further dilations were performed to achieve an optimal angiographic result. Following an assessment of a good angiographic result, IVUS was performed. All subsequent treatment decisions were based on the ultrasound results in conjunction with angiographic assessment.

INTRAVASCULAR ULTRASOUND

Equipment and Measurements

Imaging was performed with a 3.9-F monorail system with a 25-MHz transducer-tipped catheter (Interpret Catheter, InterTherapy/CVIS, Sunnyvale, CA). In the last 2 months, a CVIS 2.9-F catheter was used. All images were obtained with a manual pullback system. Positioning correlations were made as necessary with fluoroscopic updates. Data were stored on 0.5″ high-resolution videotape. Quantitative measurements were performed either on-line or off-line during the procedure. After advancing the ultrasound catheter distal to the stent, images were recorded while slowly pulling the imaging catheter through the stented segment and, subsequently, into the guiding catheter. In the reference segments, measurements were performed on the vessel cross-sectional area (CSA), vessel minimal and maximal vessel diameters, lumen CSA, and lumen minimal and maximal diameters. Vessel measurements were made at the outer boundary of the echolucent media, and lumen measurements were made at the inner border of the echodense plaque. The reference artery measurements were made 2 to 3 mm on either side of the stent site to minimize the effect of balloon stretch. Intrastent lumen CSA, minimal diameter, and maximal diameter measurements were made at the tightest position within the stent. The average of the proximal and distal vessel CSA was used to reflect the vessel area of the stented segment because intense echo reverberations from the metallic struts frequently prevent measurements of the vessel dimensions within the stent.

Criteria for Optimal Stent Expansion

The intrastent dilation was considered satisfactory based on two criteria. First, there had to be adequate plaque compression achieved when the media border in the stented segment could not be identified. The quantitative measurements for adequate stent expansion evolved during the course of the study. During the initial phase, 60% of the average of the proximal and distal cross-sectional vessel area was the target area for IVUS success. With additional experience this criterion was adapted to achieve an intrastent lumen CSA equal to or larger than the distal reference lumen. Conceptually, these adjustments were made to reflect a better understanding of the overriding importance of not leaving the stent with a functional stenosis relative to the distal lumen rather than achieving a specified percent stent dilation in relation to the vessel. The unstented segments immediately adjacent to the stent were considered a part of the stent site. IVUS was also used to evaluate these nonstented segments with lesions characterized as residual plaque or dissection. Lesions with a CSA stenosis greater than 70% of the vessel area were stented or underwent additional angioplasty. Most commonly, these lesions were stented.

BALLOON DILATION STRATEGY

The initial IVUS imaging provided information on the reference vessel and lumen diameter that was helpful in choosing balloons for subsequent dilations that were within an acceptable safety margin. With increased experience, high-pressure inflations were performed with balloons that were undersized by ultrasound vessel measurements and appropriately or even slightly undersized by angiography. The final balloon dilations were performed with minimally compliant short balloons (9 mm long, Short Speedy, Schneider, Bulach, Switzerland) inflated to a maximum pressure of 15 atm or noncompliant balloons (NC Shadow, SCIMED Life Systems, Maple Grove, MN) inflated to pressures up to 20 atm. IVUS was performed after each additional balloon inflation to document whether the criteria for stent expansion were achieved.

DEFINITIONS

The following definitions are used:

Primary stenting success   successful stent deployment and achievement of an initial good angiographic result

Primary stent failure   failure to deliver the stent to the lesion site

Primary stent complications   complications during primary stenting occurring prior to the IVUS evaluation

IVUS optimization complications   complications that occurred during or following the initial ultrasound evaluation.

First step   initial IVUS evaluation (after achieving acceptable angiographic result)

Final step   final IVUS evaluation when the criteria for stent expansion was achieved

Acute stent thrombosis   stent thrombosis within 24 hours of the stent procedure

Subacute stent thrombosis   thrombosis beyond 24 hours but within 3 weeks of the stenting process

Restenosis   50% or greater diameter stenosis within or adjacent to the stent

ANGIOGRAPHIC ANALYSIS

Coronary angiograms were analyzed by an experienced angiographer not involved in the stenting procedure. The lesions were measured from an optically magnified image in a single, matched "worst" view using digital calipers (Brown and Sharp, North Kingstown, RI). The guiding catheter was used as the reference object. The diameter of the proximal and distal reference segments was averaged to give a mean reference diameter. Mean angiographic reference lumen measurements were used so as to achieve a relative correlation with the IVUS average reference vessel measurements. Reference vessel measurements, minimal lumen diameter, lesion length, and percent diameter stenosis were obtained on the baseline and final angiograms.

POSTPROCEDURE PROTOCOL AND FOLLOW-UP

If patients satisfied IVUS criteria for adequate stent expansion and the final angiogram also demonstrated a good result, no further heparin was administered and sheaths were removed in 4 to 6 hours. When procedures were performed late, heparin was infused overnight and the sheaths removed the following morning. In the first 2 months of this protocol, patients were observed in the hospital for 1 week. Subsequent to this period patients were discharged from the hospital within 2 days. Following a successful procedure, patients were treated only with antiplatelet agents. The first 252 patients received ticlopidine 250 mg PO bid for 2 months (the first 150 patients) or 1 month (subsequent 102 patients). Patients who had not received ticlopidine prior to the stent procedure also received aspirin (325 mg/d) for 3 days. The last 38 consecutive patients were treated only with aspirin 325 mg bid after a successful procedure was completed. Patients were contacted by the investigators 1 month following the stent procedure. Clinical and angiographic follow-up was performed at 4 to 6 months following the initial stent procedure.

RESULTS

The baseline characteristics of the 328 patients are shown in Table 60-1. A total of 416 lesions was treated in the following 365 vessels: left anterior descending artery in 207 (56.7%), right coronary artery in 83 (22.7%), circumflex or obtuse marginal in 49 (13.4%), saphenous vein graph in 10 (2.7%), unprotected left main in 7 (1.9%), diagonal in 6 (1.6%), and ramus intermediate in 3 (0.8%) (Fig. 60-1A). Stent sites (Fig. 60-1B) were ostial in 29 (7.0%), proximal on 156 (37.5%), midvessel in 200 (48.1%), and distal in 31 (7.4%). Stenting was performed electively in 270 (64.9%), for restenosis in 51 (12.2%), for suboptimal angioplasty result in 49 (11.8%), for dissection with acute or threatened closure in 20 (4.8%), following recanalization of a chronic total occlusion in 24 (5.8%), and for acute myocardial infarction in 2 (0.5%) lesions. The higher representation of some indications is due to their different prevalence and not to a selection bias or a policy to exclude some indications traditionally considered at a higher risk of complications. A total of 825 stents was deployed in this study population and included 399 Palmaz-Schatz stents, 387 short stents, 23 biliary stents, 4 short renal stents, and 2 renal stents. Multiple stents (defined as the placement of greater than a 15-mm length of stent) were implanted in 41% (172 of 415) of lesions, 52% (189 of 365) of vessels, and 57% (189 of 328) of patients (Fig. 60-2). The average number of stents placed per lesion was 1.5. The average number of stents deployed per patient was 1.9.

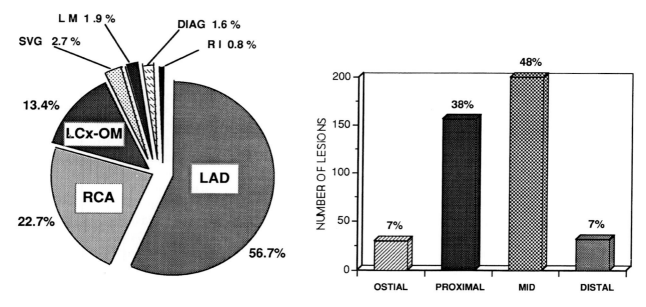

Fig. 60-1. Results of 416 lesions treated in 365 vessels. LAD, left anterior descending artery; LCx, left circumflex artery; RCA, right coronary artery; SVG, saphenous vein graft; LM, left main artery; DIAG, diagonal; RI, ramus intermediate.

Procedural Success

Primary stenting success was achieved in 316 patients (96.3%) and 402 lesions (96.6%), as seen in the flow diagram (Fig. 60-3). Primary stent failure occurred in four patients (1.2%). Two of these patients underwent elective coronary bypass, and two patients were managed medically without complication. There were 9 patients (3.5%) and 13 lesions (3.9%) that did not have IVUS performed for technical reasons, and IVUS was unsuccessful in 3 patients (5 lesions). IVUS was successfully performed in 384

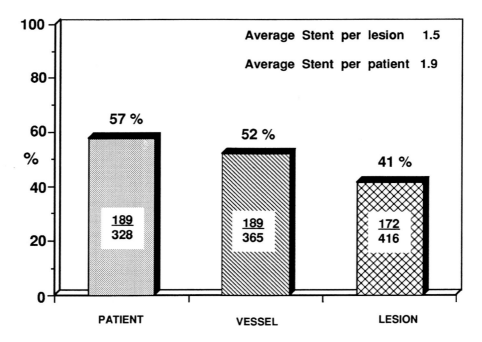

Fig. 60-2. Results of placement of multiple stents. Multiple stents are defined as deployment of greater than a 15-mm stent.

Table 60-1. Baseline Characteristics

	No.	%
Study patients	328	
Age [mean (range)]	58 ± 9	
	(31–88)	
Sex		
Male	282	86.0
Female	46	14.0
Risk factors:		
Hypercholesterolemia	159	48.5
Smoking		
Active	134	40.9
Former	44	13.4
Family history	131	39.9
Hypertension	98	29.9
Diabetes	47	14.3
Myocardial infarction		
Previous	173	52.7
Acute	2	0.5
Previous bypass	36	11.0
Previous angioplasty[a]	64	19.5
Mean % LVEF	56 ± 10	
Unstable angina	121	36.9
CCS angina class		
Class I	60	18.4
Class II	95	29.1
Class III	89	27.3
Class IV	82	25.2
No. of diseased vessels		
1	168	51.2
2	107	32.6
3	53	16.2

Abbreviations: CCS, Canadian Cardiovascular Society; LVEF, left ventricular ejection fraction.

[a] Includes prior angioplasty performed at same site and different site.

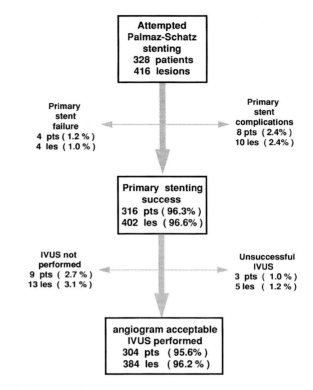

Fig. 60-3. Primary stenting success. Pts, patients; les, lesions.

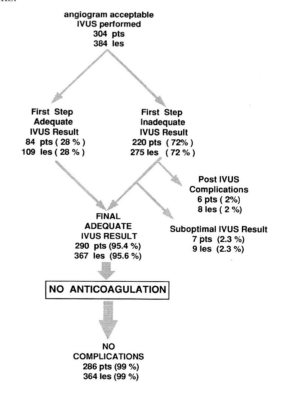

Fig. 60-4. Flow diagram showing that adequate stent expansion was achieved at the first step in 27% pf patients in 28% of lesions. Pts, patients; les, lesions.

of 402 lesions (95.6%) and 304 of 316 patients (96.2%) with successful primary stenting. As shown in Figure 60-4, adequate stent expansion was achieved at the first step in 84 of 304 patients (27%) and in 109 of 384 lesions (28%). Final adequate stent expansion was achieved in 290 of the 304 patients (95.4%) and 367 of the 384 lesions (95.6%) in which an IVUS evaluation was performed. The 290 patients who had adequate stent expansion by IVUS criteria were treated with antiplatelet medications and did not receive additional anticoagulation (heparin or Coumadin) following sheath removal. Typical examples of suboptimal stent dilation with subsequent IVUS-guided stent expansion are shown in Figures 60-5 and 60-6. As experience increased, the percentage of stents that had adequate expansion at the first step increased from 12% in the first 100 lesions to 70% in the last 100 lesions.

Thirteen patients did not have a successful IVUS result, including seven patients with a suboptimal

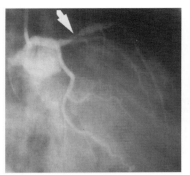
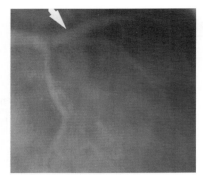
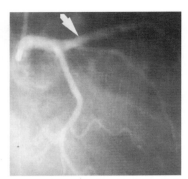

BEFORE STENT   **AFTER 4.5 MM BALLOON**   **AFTER 5.0 MM BALLOON**

AFTER 4.5 MM BALLOON
INTRASTENT: 4.9 X 4.0
AREA: 11.8
VESSEL: 5.9 X 6.3   AREA: 31.0

AFTER 5.0 MM BALLOON
INTRASTENT: 4.7 X 4.9
AREA: 18.8
VESSEL: 5.8 X 6.1   AREA: 30.2

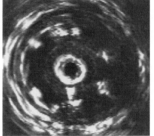

59% INCREASE IN INTRASTENT AREA

Fig. 60-5. A typical example of suboptimal stent dilation. Before stenting, after a 4.5-mm, balloon, and alter a 5.0-mm balloon.

result and six patients with complications that occurred during or following IVUS optimization. Eighteen patients (six patients with a suboptimal IVUS result, nine who did not have IVUS performed, and three patients who had an attempted but unsuccessful IVUS evaluation) were treated with conventional anticoagulation therapy and had no procedural or postprocedural complications.

Complications

Primary stent complications (Table 60-2) occurred in eight patients (2.4%) and included the following: one vessel rupture (0.2%), non-Q-wave myocardial infarction in three patients (0.9%), Q-wave myocardial infarction in three patients (0.9%), emergency coronary bypass in seven patients (2.1%), and death in one patient (0.3%). In six patients complications occurred during IVUS-guided stent dilation. One of the complications occurred during an IVUS evaluation and five occurred following the initial IVUS evaluation [three vessel ruptures (0.8%), non-Q-wave myocardial infarction in three patients (1.0%), Q-wave myocardial infarction in one patient (0.3%), emer-

gency coronary bypass in four patients (1.3%), and death in two patients (0.7%)]. Postprocedural complications are presented in Table 60-3.

One patient had an acute stent thrombosis (0.3%) with associated Q-wave myocardial infarction. This patient had had rotablation performed prior to stenting. A review of the procedural IVUS study revealed that the stent did not meet criteria for adequate stent expansion (only 35% lumen expansion and stent area smaller than distal lumen). This patient had additional IVUS-guided stent expansion without further complications. A second patient had a vessel occlusion distal to a patent stent. The complication was a result of a distal dissection that occurred during the stenting procedure. The occlusion occurred 3 hours after the stent procedure while the patient was still anticoagulated (ACT, 280 seconds). The patient had a non-Q-wave myocardial infarction and following vessel recanalization underwent emergency bypass surgery. One patient had a non-Q-wave myocardial infarction related to distal embolization from a pre-stent rotablation procedure. A repeat angiogram and IVUS study on this patient documented wide patency of the vessel and the stented segment. No subacute stent thrombosis occurred. Following the procedure,

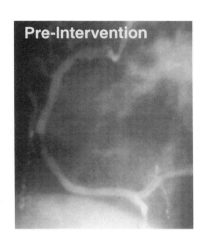

18% Increase in CSA

From higher pressure inflation

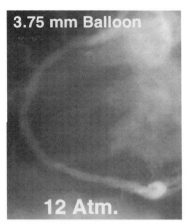

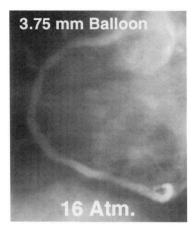

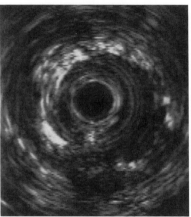

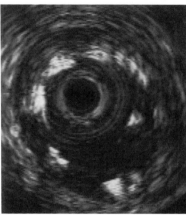

3.4 x 3.0 mm
7.1 mm²

3.3 x 3.2 mm
8.4 mm²

Fig. 60-6. A typical example of suboptimal stent dilation.

Table 60-2. Procedural Complications

	Complications[a]		
	Primary	Post-IVUS	Total
Total patient cohort	328	304[b]	328
Coronary rupture	0.2% (1/416 les.)	0.8% (3/384 les.)	1.0% (4/416 les.)
Myocardial infarction	1.8% (6)	1.3% (4)	3.0% (10)
Q-wave	0.9% (3)	0.3% (1)	1.2% (4)
Non-Q-wave	0.9% (3)	1.0% (3)	1.8% (6)
Emergency CABG	2.1% (7)	1.3% (4)	3.4% (11)
Death	0.3% (1)	0.7% (2)	0.9% (3)

Abbreviations: CABG, coronary artery bypass grafting; les., lesion.
[a] The number of patients with complications is in parentheses.
[b] Percent of complications post-IVUS was calculated based on number of patients who had an IVUS evaluation performed.

Table 60-3. Postprocedural
Complications

Complications	%
Angiographic (367 lesions)	
Acute stent thrombosis	0.3
Vessel closure[a]	0.3
Subacute stent thrombosis	0
Clinical (290 patients)	
Myocardial infarction	1.0
Q-wave	0.3
Non-Q-wave	0.6
Emergency CABG	0.3
Death	0
Vascular repair, bleeding, or hemotoma requiring transfusion	0

[a] Vessel closure distal to a patent stent.

there was one death and one vascular complication, in the same patient. This patient had an ischemic complication in the lower extremity that had the vascular sheath; and vascular surgical repair was needed. The lower extremity ischemia was recurrent and required several operations. Subsequently the patient developed renal failure from rhabdomyolysis sepsis and disseminated intravascular coagulopathy that ultimately necessitated bilateral lower extremity amputation. The patient died 17 days after the stent procedure of multiorgan failure.

Angiographic Analysis

The distribution of the stented lesions based on proximal angiographic reference lumen diameter is shown in Table 60-4. The table reveals a wide distribution of angiographic reference lumen diameters from less than 2.5 mm to larger than 4.0 mm. The proximal angiographic reference lumen diameter

Table 60-4. Proximal Angiographic
Reference Lumen Diameters
of Stent Sites

Reference Lumen Diameter (mm)	Lesions	
	%	No.
<2.5	4.8	20
2.5–2.74	8.4	35
2.75–2.99	14.0	58
3.0–3.49	41.5	173
3.5–3.99	20.7	86
>4.0	10.6	44

was less than 3.0 mm in 113 lesions (27%). The mean proximal reference lumen diameter was 3.29 ± 0.54 mm and mean distal reference lumen diameter 3.06 ± 0.57 mm. Baseline mean average reference lumen diameter was 3.18 ± 0.53 mm. The mean baseline minimum lumen diameter was 0.93 ± 0.54 mm, with a baseline percent stenosis of $70 \pm 18\%$. Median lesion length was 7.4 mm (range, 1.2 to 38.7 mm). The mean final stent diameter was 3.38 ± 0.64 mm, with a mean final percent stenosis of $-8.3 \pm 15\%$.

Intravascular Ultrasound Analysis

The lumen at the tightest point within the stent increased from 6.5 ± 2.1 mm^2 at the first step to 8.8 ± 2.5 mm^2 at the final step ($P < 0.0001$), as seen in Table 60-5. The intrastent lumen at the tightest point expanded from $49 \pm 13\%$ at the first step to $67 \pm 13\%$ at the final step ($P < 0.0001$). First-step minor stent lumen diameter increased from 2.6 ± 0.5 mm 3.1 ± 0.5 mm ($P < 0.0001$). The major IVUS diameter increased from 3.0 ± 0.5 at the first step to 3.5 ± 0.5 at the final step ($P < 0.0001$).

Restenosis

Angiographic follow-up at 4 to 6 months is available on 129 stented lesions, representing 87% of the 149 eligible lesions. Restenosis using the 50% diameter stenosis criteria was present in 15% of lesions. The restenosis rate according to the different indications for stenting were as follows; elective stenting 14% (11 of 77), stenting for restenosis 12% (2 of 16), stenting for suboptimal angioplasty result 28% (4 of 14), stenting for acute or threatened closure 28% (2 of 11), and stenting after recanalization of a chronic total occlusion 0% (0 of 11) of lesions.

DISCUSSION

Despite intensive antiplatelet and anticoagulation medication, a risk of stent thrombosis still exists in 0.4 to 3% of elective Palmaz-Schatz stent implantations. Carrozza et al.[5] report a stent thrombosis rate of 0.4% per lesion and Schatz et el.[4] noted that the stent thrombosis rate was 2.8% in a multicenter study on 247 patients. When stenting is performed for acute or threatened closure, a subacute thrombosis rate of 2% was reported by Colombo et al.[9] By contrast, Fajadet et al.[10] report a 29% thrombotic event rate following stenting for this indication. Improved experience with stenting and subsequent an-

Table 60-5. Intravascular Ultrasound Measurements (n = 384)

	Proximal Reference	Stented Site		Distal Reference
		First Step	Final Step	
Lumen				
CSA (mm^2)	8.7 ± 2.9	6.5 ± 2.1	8.8 ± 2.5^a	7.5 ± 3.2
Minor diameter (mm)	3.0 ± 0.6	2.6 ± 0.5	3.1 ± 0.5^a	2.8 ± 0.6
Major diameter (mm)	3.4 ± 0.6	3.0 ± 0.5	3.5 ± 0.5^a	3.1 ± 0.7
Vessel				
CSA (mm^2)	14.8 ± 4.1	13.6 ± 3.9^b		12.3 ± 4.6
Minor diameter (mm)	4.1 ± 0.6			3.7 ± 0.7
Major diameter (mm)	4.4 ± 0.6			4.0 ± 0.7
Lumen CSA/vessel CSA (ratio)	59 ± 15	49 ± 13	67 ± 13.0	62 ± 15

^{a} P < 0.0001 between first step and final step.
^{b} Calculated average of (the proximal and distal vessel CSA)/2.

ticoagulation management has decreased but not eliminated stent thrombosis.

The causes of thrombosis after implantation of a stainless steel stent have not been fully ascertained. Whereas stainless steel is durable and resists corrosion, the electropositivity of the metal relative to blood gives this metal an element of thrombogenicity, as reported by De Palma et al.[11] A study by Palmaz et al.[12] on [11]In-labeled platelet scans and gross inspection of stent sites in animals showed consistently less thrombus in the stent sites of animals treated with aspirin, dipyridamole, heparin, and dextran compared with control groups or groups treated with various combinations of antiplatelet and anticoagulant agents, although the finding of platelet deposition was never correlated to the clinical event of stent thrombosis. A more important factor in the low stent thrombosis rate in animals is perhaps the relative ease with which stents could be expanded in the normal or relatively undiseased animal vessels. It could be argued that the reason for the increased incidence of stent thrombosis that has been encountered in the human coronary experience is the relatively increased difficulty in consistently achieving adequate stent expansion in vessels that are severely diseased, calcified, or fibrotic.

This study demonstrates that short-term anticoagulation can be safely omitted following the stenting procedure when adequate stent expansion is achieved. Prior to the initiation of this study, preliminary work by Nakamura et al.[7] and Goldberg et al.[8] found frequent stent underexpansion. The study presented in this chapter supports this concept. The most frequent site of potential flow limitation was the lesion site within the stented segment, as evidenced by the 73% of stents that were not adequately dilated at the time of initial (first-step) IVUS imaging. When this problem was corrected, stent throm-

bosis was rare (0.3%), despite the absence of anticoagulation. The lone stent thrombosis (0.3%) occurred at a stent site that was suboptimally expanded, with slow flow related to prestent coronary rotablation. Perhaps one contribution to the low stent thrombosis rate in this study was the low number of patients stented for acute or threatened closure. Nonetheless, in the 20 patients who were stented for this indication no episodes of stent thrombosis occurred despite the absence of poststent anticoagulation treatment.

The data illustrate that IVUS is an acceptable instrument to evaluate adequate stent expansion. By study design, IVUS imaging was first performed after obtaining an acceptable angiographic result. The information obtained at the initial IVUS evaluation was used to guide further dilation if it was necessary. In a previous IVUS-guided stenting study, the mean angiographic percent stenosis was decreased from 9 ± 13 to −4 ± 12 mm with further IVUS-guided balloon dilations (P <0.0001). This corresponded to a significant increase in the stent lumen from 49 ± 10% to 65 ± 10% of the average reference vessel on IVUS evaluation. The results of the study presented in this chapter show a similar improvement in the stent lumen CSA and the intrastent diameters. Analysis of the IVUS data provides important information in evaluating the overall effect of IVUS-guided stent expansion. The percentile graph of the reference lumen and intrastent CSAs is shown in Figure 60-7. This graph demonstrates the relative stenosis that would have been left in the stented segment if no further balloon dilations were performed beyond the first step (when there was an initial acceptable angiographic result). After further dilation(s) the final stent lumen CSA roughly parallels the proximal reference lumen when the final CSA is larger than 10 mm^2. In stent segments with a final intrastent lumen CSA less than 10 mm^2, the stent

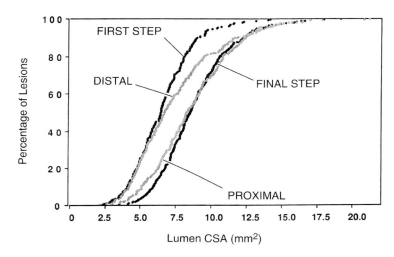

Fig. 60-7. Percentile distribution of lumen CSA's.

area is larger than the proximal and the distal lumen CSA, reflecting a slight overdilation effect. The primary reason for this overdilation effect is the criteria for IVUS success applied in the early phases of the study. After reviewing percentile distribution graphs such as that shown in Figure 60-7, the IVUS criteria was adapted, with success becoming the achievement of a final stent lumen less than or equal to the proximal reference lumen and larger than the distal lumen. This type of strategy avoids a relative stenosis at the stent site that could contribute to flow disturbances and stent thrombosis and also may decrease stent overdilation. Conceivably, by using a less aggressive method of stent dilation, the minimum safe lower limit of the therapeutic range of IVUS-guided stent expansion will be defined. The extreme lower end of the therapeutic spectrum, clinically defined by the point at which stent thrombosis becomes a problem, was not elucidated in the present study and for practical and ethical reasons may never be found.

Dilation strategies are an important part of the process of safely achieving adequate stent dilation. The primary difficulty in achieving adequate stent expansion arises from the 20 to 30% of lesions that are calcified or fibrotic and that resist dilation. A variety of different balloon inflation strategies were utilized in this study. In the first 40 lesions the strategy was to use balloons sized to the IVUS vessel diameter (oversized by angiography) without high pressures. In the subsequent 250 patients high-pressure inflations were performed with noncompliant balloons sized to the IVUS vessel diameter (angiographically oversized). In the final 100 lesions high-pressure balloon inflations were performed with noncompliant balloons that were appropriately sized to the angiographic lumen. This final approach simplifies the de-

cision process and decreases the risk of vessel dissection in unstented segments. The use of noncompliant balloon material ensures that the same balloon diameter and hence the safety margin are maintained even at high pressures up to 18 to 20 atm. A summary of the three balloon dilation strategies employed in this study is given in Table 60-6, which shows a decrease in final balloon diameter and an increase in maximal pressures despite no change in the vessel diameter. The IVUS optimization complications occurred in the first 150 lesions and were all related to balloon oversizing. Although the difference in complications between phases did not reach statistical significance, the distribution of complications shows the safety of high-pressure inflations with noncompliant balloons that are appropriately sized to the angiographic vessel diameter. This approach still yields adequate final stent expansion in over 98% of lesions and has also ensured that a higher percentage of lesions have adequate stent expansion achieved at the initial IVUS evaluation (increased from 12 to 70%), thereby decreasing procedural time.

Well-defined criteria for an angiographic successful stent expansion that would alleviate the risk of stent thrombosis and thus the need for anticoagulation have not been developed. There is a limit to visual interpretation of small percent stenosis differences on angiogram. On-line quantitative angiographic measurements may better distinguish between small lumen changes and could have a role in determining angiographic success. Careful assessment of the inflated balloon profile may provide clues as to whether a stent is adequately expanded. In our view, a mismatch between the measured balloon diameter and the subsequent angiographic lumen diameter reflects a failure in stent expansion rather than stent

Table 60-6. Balloon Diameter, Inflation Pressures, and Complications of Different Dilation Strategies (n = 384)

	Phase 1 Oversized Balloons Low Pressures (40 lesions)	Phase 2 Oversized Balloons High Pressures (250 lesions)	Phase 3 Appropriate Balloon High Pressures (96 lesions)
Mean angiographic reference lumen (mm)	3.24 ± 0.55	3.17 ± 0.54	3.14 ± 0.40^c
Balloon diameter (mm)	4.06 ± 0.63	3.88 ± 0.47	3.4 ± 0.42^a
Balloon diameter/mean angiographic reference lumen (ratio)	1.27 ± 0.20	1.24 ± 0.19	1.1 ± 0.16^a
Mean final inflation pressure (atm)	12.4 ± 2.8^b	15.2 ± 2.6	15.7 ± 3.1
Post-IVUS complications (no. of patients)	1	4	0^c

^{a} $P < 0.0001$ phase 3 compared with phase 1 or phase 2.
^{b} $P < 0.0001$ phase 1 compared with phase 2 or phase 3.
^{c} $P = $ NS.

recoil. This may point out the need for further balloon dilations with higher pressures or a larger balloon. Angiographic methods for assessing adequate stent expansion have not been prospectively evaluated. Each would have the inherent limitations of an angiographic evaluation, that of a one-dimensional assessment of result. IVUS imaging thus remains the only reliable method of definitively confirming adequate stent expansion with a degree of security that allows anticoagulation to be eliminated from the poststent medical regimen.

Antiplatelet Regimen

Ticlopidine was used in the initial 252 patients of the study presented in this chapter, with one stent thrombosis event. In 38 consecutive patients treated only with aspirin following Palmaz-Schatz stenting, no stent thromboses have occurred. Additionally, no stent thromboses have been seen in the 30 consecutive patients treated with aspirin following implantation of the Wiktor (n = 20) or Gianturco-Roubin (n = 10) stents. The lack of stent thrombosis in these 68 consecutive patients treated only with aspirin suggests that the most important variable in thrombosis prevention is adequate stent expansion rather than a specific antiplatelet agent.

Restenosis

The restenosis rate of 15% observed in the study presented in this chapter compares favorably with the 18% stent restenosis in the BENESTENT trial, as reported by Serruys, et al.[6] and the 20% restenosis rate noted by Schatz et al.[3] From these data several important points can be made: (1) this approach is

not associated with a high restenosis rate, (2) liberal use of multiple stenting is not associated with a higher restenosis rate, (3) restenosis appears to be higher in the group that has stenting performed for suboptimal angioplasty results and in the group with stenting for threatened or acute closure, (4) coronary stenting with this approach is associated with a lower restenosis rate compared with historical controls treated with conventional balloon angioplasty, and (5) other factors besides procedural aspects will be needed to reduce intimal hyperplasia and the restenosis rate further after stenting.

CONCLUSIONS AND FUTURE DIRECTIONS

This nonrandomized series of consecutive patients undergoing IVUS-guided stenting without subsequent anticoagulation presented in this chapter provides a new prospective on the future of intracoronary stenting. On the basis of these observations it is reasonable to conclude that (1) the Palmaz-Schatz stent is not thrombogenic when stent expansion is adequate, antegrade flow is brisk, and no other flow-limiting factors are present; (2) the most frequent cause of flow limitation was inadequate stent expansion; (3) anticoagulation therapy can be safely omitted following the stenting procedure when adequate stent expansion is achieved; (4) IVUS is an acceptable method of confirming adequate stent expansion; (5) IVUS and angiography provided complimentary information that allowed the poststent anticoagulation regimen to be safely eliminated; (6) adequate stent expansion can be achieved in most patients; (7) adequate stent expansion in human coronaries consistently requires high-pressure balloon dilation; and (8) the use of noncompliant balloons appropriately sized to the angiographic reference lumen diameter provides a safety margin for final high-pressure inflations of the stent. Preliminary results suggest that (1) aspirin is as effective an antiplatelet agent as ticlopidine in preventing stent thrombosis when adequate stent expansion has been achieved, and (2) the strategy utilized in this study appears to have acceptable long-term results despite the high percentage of lesions with multiple stents. Several important questions remain to be answered at present. One issue is the therapeutic range of adequate stent expansion that will allow procedures to be performed safely, while preventing stent thrombosis and optimizing the long-term effect on reducing restenosis. Another important issue is whether IVUS-guided stenting can be applied to other stents. In this regard, an IVUS-guided stent investigation has been initiated to determine if a similar approach is applicable to other types of stents (Gianturco-Roubin and Wiktor stents).

The intracoronary stent has abandoned its "friendship" with heparin and Coumadin and has acquired IVUS as a "new partner." This relationship may expand the applicability of coronary stenting in treating coronary artery disease.

REFERENCES

1. Roubin GS, Cannen AD, Agrawal SK. Intracoronary stenting for acute or threatened closure complicating percutaneous transluminal coronary angioplasty. Circulation 1992;85:916
2. Serruys PW, Strauss BN, Beatt KJ et al. Angiographic follow-up after placement of a self-expanding coronary artery stent. N Engl J Med 1991;324:13
3. Schatz RA, Goldberg SL, Leon M et al. Clinical experience with the Palmaz-Schatz coronary stent. J Am Coll Cardiol 1991;17:155B
4. Schatz RA, Baim DS, Ellis SG et al. Clinical experience with the Palmaz-Schatz coronary stent: initial results of a multicenter study. Circulation 1991;83:148
5. Carrozza JP, Kuntz RE, Levine MJ et al. Angiographic and clinical outcome of intracoronary stenting: immediate and long-term results from a large single center experience. J Am Coll Cardiol 1992;20:328
6. Serruys PW, de Jaegere P, Kiemeneij F et al. for the Benestent Study Group. A comparison of balloon expandable stent implantation with balloon angioplasty in patients with coronary artery disease. N Engl J Med 1994;331:489
7. Nakamura S, Colombo A. Gaglione S et al. Intracoronary ultrasound observations during stent implantation. Circulation 1994;89:2026
8. Goldberg SL, Colombo A, Nakamura S et al. Benefit of intracoronary ultrasound in the deployment of Palmaz-Schatz stents. J Am Coll Cardiol 1994;24:996
9. Colombo A, Goldberg SL, Almagor Y, Maiello L, Finci L. A novel strategy for stent deployment in the treatment of acute or threatened closure complicating balloon coronary angioplasty. Use of short or standard (or both) single or multiple Palmaz-Schatz stent. J Am Coll Cardiol 1993;22:1887
10. Fajadet J, Marco J, Cassagneau B, Robert G, Vandormel M. Clinical and angiographic follow-up in patients receiving a Palmaz-Schatz stent for prevention or treatment of abrupt closure after coronary angioplasty, abstracted. Eur Heart J, suppl. 1991;12:165
11. De Palma VA, Baier RE, Ford JW, Gott VL, Furuse. A. Investigation of three surface properties of several metals and their relation to blood compatibility. In Homsy C, Armeniades CD, eds: Biomaterials for Skeletal and Cardiovascular Applications. New York: Wiley, 1972:37.
12. Palmaz JC, Garcia O, Kopp DT et al. Balloon expandable intraarterial stents: effect of anticoagulation on thrombus formation, abstracted. Circulation, suppl. IV 1987;76:IV-45

61 Stenting After Bypass

S. Chiu Wong
Martin B. Leon

Gruentzig established a milestone in modern interventional cardiology with the introduction in 1977 of percutaneous balloon dilation catheters for the treatment of coronary obstructions.[1] The rapid refinement of balloon, guidewire, and guiding catheter technologies and the accumulation of operator experience in the ensuing years have resulted in a further improvement in procedural success. More recently, the superiority of balloon angioplasty [percutaneous transluminal coronary angioplasty (PTCA)] over medical treatment for symptom relief in patients with single-vessel disease has been demonstrated in the multicenter randomized Angioplasty Compared to Medicine (ACME) trial,[2] and the equivalency of balloon angioplasty to coronary artery bypass graft for long-term survival in selected patients with native multivessel disease has been shown in the Emory Angioplasty versus Surgery Trial (EAST).[3]

However, the efficacy of PTCA in the treatment of saphenous vein graft (SVG) lesions is less evident. PTCA of SVG lesions has been limited by reduced primary success, frequent periprocedural complications, and high restenosis frequency, especially in older (>4 years) vein grafts. Furthermore, repeat CABG in patients with SVG obstructions is associated with increased mortality and reduced symptom relief compared with the initial operation. These suboptimal alternatives have prompted many investigators to search for alternative catheter-based interventional techniques, including directional and extraction atherectomy, laser angioplasty, and stent implantation in an attempt to improve clinical outcomes in these patients.

The recently concluded Stent Restenosis Study (STRESS)[4] and Belgium-Netherlands Stent Study (BENESTENT)[5] trials have demonstrated that the Palmaz-Schatz stent is more effective than PTCA in reducing 6-month angiographic restenosis with improved event-free survival in the treatment of de novo lesions in native coronaries. In addition, endovascular stents have also shown promise in other clinical situations including unfavorable lesion morphologies, suboptimal PTCA results, abrupt or threatened closure, recalcitrant restenosis lesions, and treatment of SVG lesions.

In this chapter, we discuss (1) the developmental history of stents, (2) possible mechanisms to explain why stents may help to treat acute closure and prevent chronic restenosis, (3) the clinical data on various stent designs in the treatment of SVG lesions, and (4) the current limitations and future directions of stents in SVG disease.

HISTORY AND RATIONALE

The term *stent* comes from the nineteenth century British dentist Charles R. Stent, who invented a dental impression material that was later used to support the healing of skin grafts. Accordingly, any device or a scaffold that is used to maintain a patent body cavity is referred to as a stent. In 1964, Dotter first introduced the concept of an endovascular "splint"; in 1969 he reported initial experience with a spring coil stent design in an animal model[6] and subsequently (1983) studied a nitinol stent.[7] Early work by Maass et al.[8] with a spiral double-helix stainless steel spring design and by Wright et al.[9] with a zigzag pattern spring stent also helped to lay the groundwork for subsequent stent types used in clinical practice.

Despite important advances in balloon technology in the last 15 years, the frequency of abrupt vessel closure and chronic restenosis has remained unchanged. Acute closure after balloon angioplasty occurs in 4 to 7% of patients and is associated with a 5% in-hospital mortality. It is believed that acute closure results largely from plaque dissection and hemorrhage, with subsequent spasm and thrombosis at the lesion site. Therefore, stents provide a logical treatment approach by "sealing" the disrupted intimal flap and preventing subsequent vessel closure.

Angiographic restenosis occurs in about 10% of lesions during the first few days after PTCA, largely due to elastic recoil, vasospasm, platelet-fibrin thrombi deposition, or a combination of all these factors. Furthermore, chronic angiographic restenosis occurs in about 30 to 40% of patients after native coronary PTCA and in up to 70% in patients with SVG PTCA. Using intravascular ultrasound, Mintz et al.[10] noted that geometric remodeling (i.e., a late decrease in vessel cross-sectional area) accounts for about 65% of late lumen loss in patients with angiographic restenosis. By providing a mechanical support after PTCA, stents significantly reduce the amount of acute vascular recoil and prevent late vessel remodeling after dilation. In addition, detailed quantitative coronary angiographic analyses from several recent clinical studies have demonstrated that stent placement reduces restenosis frequency by achieving both a larger acute gain and final minimal lumen diameter (MLD) than PTCA.[4,5] Despite a greater late loss on follow-up angiogram, the net gain was still larger after stent implantation, resulting in a lower restenosis frequency (Fig. 61-1).

MECHANISM OF ACTION

Currently two basic stent deployment designs are under active clinical investigation:

1. Balloon-expandable stent designs make use of the plastic deformity of the metal for deployment, such that it will not change its shape once it is stretched beyond its elastic limit. Examples (Fig. 61-2A–C) of the balloon-expandable stents are the Palmaz-Schatz stent (Johnson & Johnson Interventional System [JJIS], Warren, NJ), the Flex-Stent (Cook, Bloomington, IN), and the Wiktor stent (Medtronic, San Diego, CA).
2. The spring-loaded stents consist of an elastic wire mesh that is constrained to a small diameter by a membrane or sheath at the end of a delivery catheter (Fig. 61-2D). After the stent reaches its target site, the constraining membrane is retracted and the stent will then expand radially to a predetermined diameter. An example of this type of deployment design is the Wallstent (Schneider, Minneapolis, MN).

CLINICAL ISSUES

Procedural Management

Patient Inclusion Criteria

Although the indications for stent implantation differ for various stent designs, a number of basic anatomic and clinical requirements should be fulfilled in all patients. A potential stent candidate should be a symptomatic patient with appropriately sized (3 mm or larger) target SVG with good inflow and distal

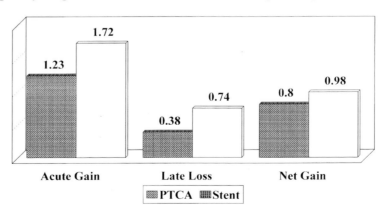

Fig. 61-1. Stent placement resulted in a larger net gain on follow-up angiogram compared with PTCA in the Stent Restenosis Study. The larger acute gain achieved at the initial procedure more than offset the greater late loss in the stent group compared with the PTCA cohort.[4]

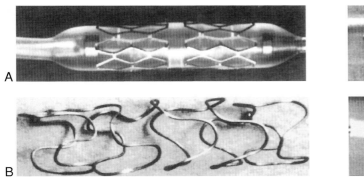 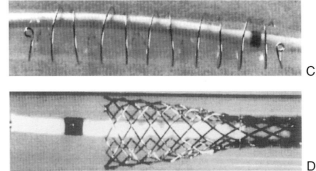

Fig. 61-2. Example of **(A)** a Palmaz-Schatz stent, **(B)** a Wiktor stent, **(C)** a Flex-Stent and **(D)** a Wallstent.

run-off beyond the target lesion. The target lesion should be free of thrombus, and distal SVG anastomotic lesions should be avoided if significant vessel size disparity exists between the SVG and the native vessel. In addition, patients were previously required to tolerate the mandated anticoagulation regimen including heparin, dextran 40, aspirin, dypyridamole, and Coumadin.

Operator Technique Issues

Selecting the appropriate guiding catheter is a critical step for a successful SVG stent deployment. For instance, in upward take-off SVGs (e.g., to circumflex), left bypass graft, hockey-stick, multipurpose, or Judkin's right guide catheters should be considered to provide optimal support.

We recommend extra-support (stiff) guidewires (0.014 or 0.018) to improve stent delivery to distal lesion sites or across tortuous proximal vessels.

If the target lesion has angiographic evidence of "friability," it may be safer to eliminate predilation if the pretreatment lesion lumen is adequate to allow safe passage of the stent delivery system, thereby avoiding unnecessary distal embolization. For the same reason, aggressive post dilatation should also be avoided in such degenerative SVGs, especially if intravascular ultrasound demonstrates good apposition of the stent against the vessel wall.

If distal embolization occurs following predilation, it is important to improve distal run-off (e.g., with intracoronary verapamil or intra-aortic balloon pump if the patient's hemodynamic condition warrants) before proceeding with actual stent deployment.

In certain lesion subsets such as aorto-ostial or fibrotic SVG lesions, we recommend the use of sequential devices such as laser angioplasty or directional atherectomy prior to stent placement (i.e., device synergy) to facilitate "optimal" stent expansion.

Clinical Management

Anticoagulation Regimen

Of the new angiplasty devices that are currently in clinical use, the conventional perioperative patient pharmacologic management is the most demanding following stent placement. The standard anticoagulation regimen dictated by previous investigation protocols included both aspirin and dipyridamole prior to the procedure and intravenous dextran 40 and heparin infusion during and immediately following the procedure. After discharge, Coumadin and dipyridamole were continued for 1 month, and aspirin was continued indefinitely. With recent advances in stent implantation strategy, including the use of ticlopidine and high-pressure adjunct balloon dilatation with or without intravascular ultrasound guidance (see Future Developments section), the anticoagulation regimen is currently under rapid evolution and simplification. Further studies are currently under way to evaluate various reduced pharmacologic regimens following "optimal" stent implantation.

Recommendations to Reduce Bleeding Complications

With the intense anticoagulation regimen that patients received after stent implantation, the frequency of bleeding complications was increased at least two- to threefold compared with PTCA. We have found the following clinical guidelines helpful for reducing these untoward bleeding events:

- Keep the activated clotting time (ACT; Hemo Tec HR) between 250 and 300 seconds intraoperatively
- Hold heparin at the end of the procedure

- Order strict bed rest for 36 to 48 hours and be liberal with sedation
- Use the reverse Trendelenberg position while patients are under strict bed rest; this will enable patients to elevate the head of the bed for comfort without bending the femoral access site
- Remove indwelling sheath promptly after the procedure when the ACT is 150 seconds or less
- Limit sheath removal to designated personnel; FemoStop may be helpful for patient comfort
- Reinitiate heparin 6 hours after hemostasis
- Keep partial thromboplastin time (PTT) between 50 and 70 seconds after stent placement and avoid wide fluctuation of PTT levels
- Initiate gastrointestinal prophylactics and stool softener as part of the standard stent regimen

Characteristics of Stent Designs and Clinical Trial Results

A number of stent designs (Table 61-1) are currently under active clinical evaluation in the treatment of SVG lesions. They include the balloon-expandable slotted tubular stent (Palmaz-Schatz stent), coil stent designs (Gianturco-Roubin and Wiktor stents), and the self-expanding wire mesh stent (Wallstent). Each stent has its own distinctive spectrum of design characteristics that confer both advantages and shortcomings for treating of SVG obstructions.

BALLOON-EXPANDABLE STENTS

Slotted Tubular Configuration: Palmaz-Schatz

Coronary Design

Of the currently available stents under clinical investigation, the Palmaz-Schatz coronary stent is the most extensively studied design for the treatment of SVG lesions in the United States. Its unique slotted tubular design is well suited for treating focal slit-like or ostial lesions, or both. Furthermore, the tendency of the stent to flare at both ends on expansion may help to entrap friable material at the target site and potentially reduce the incidence of distal embolization. On the other hand, the current coronary stent design is radiolucent, which makes precise deployment technically more challenging. Although the inclusion of the central 1-mm bridging strut greatly enhances the ease and flexibility of stent delivery, it also results in a central segment devoid of metal, which may allow plaque protrusion in certain lesion subsets (i.e., long or multiple discrete tandem lesions).

Leon et al.[11] have summarized the JJIS stent registry results on 589 consecutive patients who underwent elective Palmaz-Schatz stent placement for the treatment of symptomatic focal SVG stenoses (Fig. 61-3). Most patients were male (84%), with older SVGs (mean SVG age, 8.9 years), de novo lesions

Table 61-1. Stent Designs and Characteristics

	Balloon-Expandable				Self-Expanding
	Palmaz-Schatz Coronary	Palmaz-Schatz Biliary	Flex-Stent	Wiktor Stent	Wallstent
Stent material	Stainless steel	Stainless steel	Stainless steel	Tantalum	Stainless steel
Stent configuration	Slotted tubular	Slotted tubular	Serpentine coil	Sinusoidal coil	Wire mesh
Coil or strut thickness (mm)	0.064	0.10–0.14	0.15	0.13	0.07–0.10
Radiopacity	Poor	Good	Poor	Excellent	Poor
Stent length (mm)	15	10, 15, and 20	20	17	15–43
% Metal surface after stent expansion	10–15	10–15	10	7	15–20
Expansion range (mm)	3.0–5.0	4.0–9.0	2.0–4.0	2.0–4.5	3.0–5.5
Delivery catheter size (F)	5	4–5	4.4	4.2–5	5

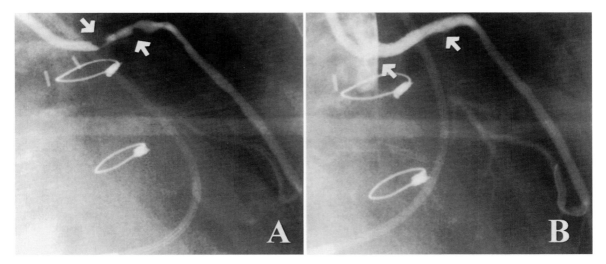

Fig. 61-3. Example of two sequential lesions in the proximal segment of an SVG to the left anterior descending artery before (**A,** *arrows*) and after (**B,** *arrows* demarcate stent site) placement of two tandem coronary Palmaz-Schatz stents.

(62%), and class 3 or 4 angina (87%). Deployment success was accomplished in 99% of lesions attempted and procedure success (successful stent deployment with no death, myocardial infarction, or CABG) was achieved in 97% of patients. After stent placement, the average lesion MLD increased from 0.7 to 3.4 mm and the average diameter stenosis decreased from 82 to 7%. Major complications occurred in 17 (2.9%) patients, including 10 (1.7%) deaths, 2 (0.3%) non-fatal Q-wave myocardial infarctions, and 5 (0.9%) urgent coronary bypass operations. Eight patients (1.4%) developed stent thrombosis. No thrombosis-related deaths occurred although three patients required bypass surgery and four patients sustained acute myocardial infarctions after stent thrombosis. Vascular and bleeding complications were frequent (15.5%), and nearly half (7.5%) required surgical intervention.

Six month follow-up angiography was obtained in 58% of eligible patients with an overall restenosis rate (≥50% diameter narrowing) of 30%. Restenosis frequency was significantly lower (18%) in patients with de novo lesions and in patients with adequate (MLD ≥ 3 mm) final stent expansion (26%). Multivariate logistic regression analysis revealed that the following factors were independent predictors for restenosis: (1) the presence of diabetes mellitus, (2) prior history of restenosis, (3) small reference vessel size, and (4) percentage of final diameter stent. The 12-month event-free survival for the entire cohort was 76.3%, and target vessel revascularization was only 13.3% (5.4% bypass surgery and 7.9% repeat angioplasty).

Pomerantz et al.[12] reported a comparative analysis on the differential impact of stent placement versus directional coronary atherectomy (DCA) in the treatment of SVG disease in 69 patients (84 lesions) treated with Palmaz-Schatz coronary stents and 28 patients (35 lesions) treated with DCA. The average SVG age (about 8 years) was comparable between the two patient cohorts. The DCA patients had a much higher prevalence of ostial (40 vs. 0%) and eccentric (61 vs. 40%) lesions. After stent placement, the lesion MLD improved from 0.9 to 3.6 mm with 0% residual diameter stenosis. With DCA, the corresponding findings were 0.9 mm, 3.5 mm and 5%. No major complications (death, emergent CABG, or Q-wave myocardial infarction) were noted in either cohort. Six-month follow-up angiography was obtained in 50 of the 64 (78%) eligible patients. Restenosis rates were similar between the two groups: 25% (8 of 35 patients) for stents and 28% (5 of 18 patients) for DCA. Despite the relatively high overall late mortality (10% at 1 year and 13% at 2 years) in these patients with pathologic aged SVGs, the 1- and 2-year event-free survivals were favorable (80% for stents and 74% for DCA) in both groups.

Biliary Design

Compared with the coronary stent, the increased strut thickness of the biliary stent confers greater radial compressive strength in exchange for decreased axial stent flexibility. The greater radial compressive strength, which potentially makes it a "better" stent for treating more rigid aorto-ostial SVG lesions, and the enhanced radiopacity permits more precise placement of the biliary stent. The

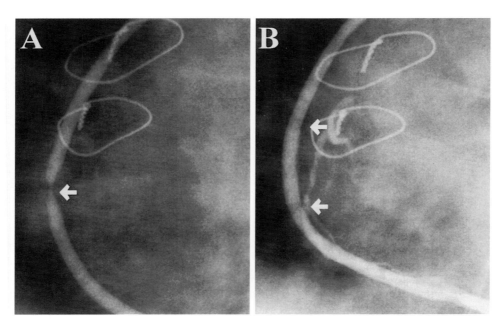

Fig. 61-4. Example of a discrete lesion in the midshaft portion of an SVG to the right coronary artery before (**A,** *arrow*) and after (**B,** *arrows* demarcate stent site) placement of a biliary Palmaz-Schatz stent.

availability of a wider assortment of stent lengths allows better matching of stent to lesion length. Finally, the expansion range (4 to 9 mm) of the biliary stent has made it more suitable for treating larger SVGs.

Application of the Palmaz-Schatz biliary stent design for the treatment of lesions in larger (≥4.5 mm) SVGs was first reported by Friedrich et al.[13] at the Beth Israel Hospital in Boston (Fig. 61-4). Piana and co-workers[14] from the same laboratory reported the immediate results and long-term outcomes using Palmaz-Schatz coronary (111 patients, 145 lesions) and biliary (44 patients, 55 lesions) stent designs in the treatment of SVG lesions. The mean patient age was 66 years, and graft age averaged 8.7 years. A history of diabetes was present in 28% of patients, and restenosis accounted for most (72%) lesions treated. After stent placement, the lesion MLD increased from 0.98 to 3.7 mm and the diameter stenosis decreased from 74 to 1%. Vascular complications were high (24%); 14% of patients required transfusion and 8.5% were treated surgically. One patient developed acute stent thrombosis and one had sudden death 6 days after the procedure. Two elective surgical coronary bypass procedures were performed, one after an unsuccessful stent deployment and the other due to recurrent angina at a nontarget site. Follow-up angiography was performed in 94 of the first 120 lesions demonstrating a restenosis (≥50% diameter stenosis) frequency of 17%. The 2-year cumulative cardiac event rate (available in 99%

of the eligible patients) was 57%, but target lesion failure rate was only 22%.

Wong et al.[15] recently reported a comparative analysis of the clinical and angiographic outcomes of 231 patients using coronary (108 patients) versus biliary (123 patients) stent designs in the treatment of SVG lesions at the Washington Hospital Center. Patients in the biliary cohort had more frequent unstable angina (93 vs. 76%) and recent (<6 weeks) myocardial infarction (30 vs. 12%). Angiographic analysis indicated that patients in the biliary cohort had a higher frequency of ostial (25 vs. 10%), de novo (72 vs. 52%), and ulcerative (31 vs. 9%) lesions than the coronary group. Biliary stent-treated lesions also had larger reference vessel diameters (3.4 vs. 3.1 mm), larger pretreatment lesion MLDs (1.3 vs. 0.8 mm), and lower residual diameter stenosis (6 vs. 14%). Both angiographic success (100% in the coronary and 98% in the biliary) and procedural success (97% in the coronary and 96% in the biliary) were similarly high in the two groups. Subacute thrombosis occurred in two (1.7%) patients in the biliary stent group and in none in the coronary stent cohort. In-hospital major complications were infrequent (2.9% for coronary stents and 1.4% for biliary stents). Access site bleeding complications remained problematic in both groups; overall, 8.4% of the patients required surgical repair and 25% of patients received blood transfusions after stent placement. The 6-month event-free survival was favorable (about 80%) in both groups, with target vessel revascularization accounting for most (90% for coronary stents and 80% for biliary stents) cardiac events.

Aorto-Ostial Lesions

Conventional balloon angioplasty of aorto-ostial (≤3 mm from aorto-ostium) SVG lesions is often associated with suboptimal results and a strikingly high (60 to 80%) restenosis rate. Stent placement provides a rigid scaffold at the aorto-ostium, which minimizes acute and chronic recoil and may provide more optimal angiographic results, thereby reducing subsequent restenosis. Wong et al.[16] reported their combined clinical experience with coronary (53 patients) and biliary (51 patients) stent placement for the treatment of aorto-ostial SVG lesions at the Washington Hospital Center and the Scripps Clinic and Research Foundation. Most patients were males (81%) with unstable angina (93%), and the average graft age was 7.4 years. Biliary stent patients had larger reference vessel diameters (3.5 vs. 3.2 mm). After stent placement, the lesion MLD increased from 0.7 to 3.1 mm (diameter stenosis decreased from 79 to 8%) in the coronary cohort and from 1.2 to 3.4 mm (diameter stenosis decreased from 67 to 5%) in the biliary group. Major complications alter stent placement were remarkably low (around 2%), with no Q-wave myocardial infarctions in either cohort; one patient in the coronary group died from procedure related causes, and one patient with subacute thrombosis in the biliary stent group underwent urgent bypass surgery. During the late follow-up period (average, 9 months), the morality rate was 6.2% (8.3% in the coronary and 4.2% in the biliary group), 2.1% of the patients had Q-wave myocardial infarction, and 6.2% had nontarget lesion revascularization procedures. Importantly, the 6-month event-free survival for these patients was quite favorable (82% in the biliary and 74% in the coronary group), although the long-term follow-up remains to be determined.

Coil Configuration

The Flex-Stent

The Flex-Stent was the first endovascular stent approved by the U.S. Food and Drug Administration for the treatment of abrupt or threatened closure of native coronaries and SVGs. Theoretically, the incomplete serpentine coil design potentially confers more flexibility in negotiating tortuous vessels, permits future intervention of the native coronary vessel after placement of the stent across an anastomotic site, and conforms better to tapering vessel size. On the other hand, the clamshell open coil configuration also renders it less suitable for the treatment of slit-like membranous or ostial lesions. Furthermore, the coils may also widen, leading to incomplete coverage of the target lesion with herniation or protrusion of friable material into the lumen, especially in larger (>4 mm) grafts.

SVG experience with the Flex-Stent has been limited. The largest experience to date, reported by Bilodeau et al.,[17] involved only 37 patients, which represented 7% of all cases in the Gianturco-Roubin Intracoronary Stent Multicenter Registry. Of the 37 lesions treated, 42% were de novo and 51% were in the ostial or proximal location. Although the Flex-Stent was intended for treatment of abrupt or threatened closure, nearly half (49%) of the stents deployed in SVGs were placed electively. No procedure-related deaths occurred, and, interestingly, all myocardial infarctions (one Q-wave and four non-Q-wave) occurred in nonelective cases. Follow-up angiography obtained in 97% of the eligible patients revealed a 35% restenosis frequency. Clinical follow-up was obtained for the entire cohort; seven (18.9%) patients underwent repeat PTCA, and three (8.1%) patients had bypass surgery, with one perioperative death. Current experience with the Flex-Stent in the treatment of SVG lesions is limited, and further clinical studies are warranted to assess its impact.

Wiktor Stent

The radiopaque tantalum wire of the Wiktor stent allows more precise stent placement. Like the Flex-Stent, the sinusoidal coil design of the Wiktor stent permits easier access to native vessels when placed across an SVG anastomotic site. Similarly, the coil design makes it less well suited for membranous or ostial lesions, and stent distortion with postdeployment instrumentation (angioscopy, intravascular ultrasound, or postdilation) may be a concern.

The Wiktor stent multicenter SVG stent registry experience was recently reported by Fortuna et al.[18] Most of the 101 study patients were male (82%) with class 3 or 4 angina (83%). Indications for stenting were elective in 59% of patients, threatened closure in 31%, acute closure in 2%, and suboptimal angioplasty results in 9%. Final stent MLD was 3.3 mm, and final diameter stenosis was 12%. Acute procedural complications included death in 1%, myocardial infarction in 3%, emergency bypass surgery in 1%, and subacute stent thrombosis in 2%. Late out-of-hospital clinical events included 6% (cardiac and noncardiac) mortality, 2% myocardial infarction, and 10% target lesion revascularization (2% elective bypass surgery and 8% repeat angioplasty). Clearly, this represents early experience, and further clinical studies are required to assess the efficacy of the stent in the treatment of SVG lesions.

SELF-EXPANDING STENTS

Wallstent

The availability of a wide array of stent lengths and diameters as well as the cross-hatched wire mesh design makes the Wallstent well suited to entrap friable SVG material. However, axial shortening on expansion may increase the technical demand for precise placement in the treatment of long tubular or ostial lesions. Clinical evaluation of the Wallstent in the treatment of SVG disease was initiated in Europe in 1986; thus far, there has been no clinical experience with this stent design in the United States.

Urban et al.[19] summarized their initial experience in 13 patients (14 vessels) in 1989 with uniform procedural success and no in-hospital complications. Follow-up (average, 7 months) angiograms obtained in 10 patients revealed a 20% restenosis (≥50% diameter stenosis) frequency. During the follow-up period, there was one death and no myocardial infarctions or repeat coronary bypass surgery.

Strauss et al.[20] reported the European multicenter Wallstent experience in 145 SVG lesions treated between 1986 and 1990. Most lesions (80%) were de novo, and 92% of stent placements were for elective indications. Importantly, unfavorable lesion subsets were preferentially treated with this stent, including long lesions and degenerative SVGs. The lesion MLD increased from 1.4 to 2.8 mm after stent implantation. After excluding 7% of those patients with early stent thrombosis, follow-up angiography (averaging 6.6 months) obtained in 82% of eligible patients showed a restenosis frequency of 34%. Over a 20-month period, the event-free survival was only 37%. Interestingly, 30% of the adverse clinical events were unrelated to the stent treatment site. Thus, although both acute angiographic findings and late restenosis outcomes appear encouraging, especially considering the very unfavorable lesion morphologies treated, the current clinical experience with this stent is limited. Further clinical trials to evaluate the efficacy of this stent design appear to be warranted.

CURRENT LIMITATIONS

Based on the favorable acute procedural results and apparently improved late clinical outcomes associated with stent implantation in SVGs (Table 61-2), many investigators believe that stents will become the preferred treatment strategy for most SVG lesions. However, current stent implantation is still associated with: (1) high (10 to 30%) access site bleeding complications due to the intense anticoagulation regimen, (2) prolonged hospitalization and increased procedural expense, and (3) infrequent but disturbing stent thrombosis with its associated morbidity.

Table 61-2. Clinical Results of Stent Placement in Saphenous Vein Graft Lesions

Stent Type	Author	No. of Lesions	Procedural Success (%)	Stent Thrombosis (%)	Major Complications[a] (%)	Angio RR (%) [F/U time in months]	EFS (%) [F/U time in months]
Palmaz-Schatz							
Coronary	Leon et al.[11]	589	97	1.4	1.7/0.3/0.9	29.7 [6.2]	81 [8.2]
	Piana et al.[14]	84	99	0	0/0/0	25 [6]	74 [24]
Biliary and coronary	Wong et al.[15]	239	95.3	1.7	1.3/0.9/0.4	NR	75 [6]
	Pomerantz et al.[12]	200	98	0.6	0.5/0/0	17 [7.1]	57 [24]
Flex-Stent	Bilodeau et al.[17]	37	NR	NR	0/2.5/0	35 [6]	73 [NR]
Wiktor	Fortuna et al.[18]	101[b]	90	2	1/3/1	NR	NR
Wallstent	Urban et al.[19]	13	100	0	0/0/0	20 [7]	70 [7]
	Strauss et al.[20]	145	NR	7	NR	39 [6.6]	37 [20]

Abbreviations: NR, not reported; F/U, follow-up; EFS, event-free survival; Angio RR, angiographic restenosis rate.
[a] Death, Q-wave myocardial infarction, CABG.
[b] Number of patients.

In addition, none of the currently available coronary stent designs are suitable for vessels larger than 4.5 mm, which are common in SVGs, and none of the currently available coronary balloons are designed with the appropriate size (>4 mm), length (e.g., 10 mm), or pressure capability (>18 atm) for optimal poststent adjunct dilation. Finally, the impact of stent placement in the treatment of aorto-ostial SVG lesions requires further clarification. Whether deployment using stronger stent designs with optimal poststent expansion, or a "device synergy" approach with initial debulking (i.e., DCA or excimer laser) followed by dilation using stents, will improve subsequent angiographic and long-term clinical results warrants further study.

FUTURE DEVELOPMENTS

Despite the aforementioned shortcomings of current stent technology, the introduction of endovascular stents has no doubt improved our ability to treat intimal dissection and reduce the frequency of restenosis in certain lesion subsets. Moreover, we should realize that both current deployment techniques and stent designs are still in early stages of development.

Recent advances in stent implantation techniques have included the use of intravascular ultrasound guidance, and high-pressure adjunct balloon dilation for optimal stent expansion (as proposed by Colombo et al.[21]) may permit reduced postprocedure anticoagulation regimens after stent implantation, which should result in a marked reduction in bleeding complications, hospital costs, and length of hospital stay. Importantly, maximizing the initial lumen area may also help to reduce further subsequent stent thrombosis and restenosis frequency.

At the Washington Hospital Center, Wong et al.[22] began patient enrollment in October 1993 for the Reduced Anticoagulation Vein Graft Stent (RAVES) study using high-pressure balloons to optimize stent expansion after deployment; the study was guided by strict intravascular ultrasound criteria (including flush stent apposition, maximal stent expansion, and stent symmetry). All postprocedural anticoagulation (dextran, heparin, and Coumadin) was discontinued

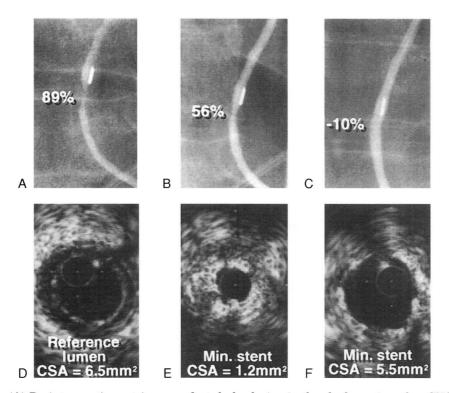

Fig. 61-5. **(A)** Preintervention angiogram of a tubular lesion in the shaft portion of an SVG to the right coronary artery. **(B)** Following stent placement, the lesion was improved from 89% diameter stenosis to 56% by quantitative coronary angiography. **(C)** After adjunct balloon dilation, diameter stenosis was further reduced to -10%. **(D)** (left to right) Corresponding intravascular ultrasound revealed a reference cross-sectional area of 6.5 mm² **(E)** The use of high-pressure adjunct balloon after deployment significantly improved the minimal cross-sectional area of the stented site from 1.2 mm² to **(F)** 5.5 mm².

after successful stent implantation, and patients were followed clinically for ischemic complications.

In the first 50 patients enrolled, no periprocedural bleeding or vascular complications and no acute or subacute stent thrombotic events were seen despite reduced anticoagulation in all successfully treated study patients. Interim quantitative coronary angiography analysis on the initial 29 study patients showed that the average diameter stenosis decreased from 61 to 16% after initial stent deployment and was further reduced to −1% after adjunct high-pressure balloon dilation. The corresponding percent area stenosis by intravascular ultrasound decreased from 69 to 28% after initial stent deployment and further decreased to −8% after adjunct balloon angioplasty (Fig. 61-5). Whether the "improved" final stent dimensions with this novel implantation technique will further lower restenosis frequency requires careful follow-up angiographic evaluation.

Comparative analysis performed more recently by Wong et al.[23] on 33 RAVES patients and 77 matched SVG patients who underwent biliary implantation with routine postoperative anticoagulation revealed a significant reduction in length of hospital stay (4 vs. 8 days), bleeding complications (3 vs. 19%), and surgical vascular repair (0 vs. 9.3%), resulting in a 38% reduction in hospital cost in the RAVES group. If similar results are achieved in a multicenter study involving a larger patient cohort, the indications for stent placement for SVG lesions with reduced antico-agulation regimen will certainly be broadened.

Finally, fixture advances in material designs will probably improve the profile and thrombogenicity and hence the safety and ease of deployment of stents in smaller (<3.0 mm) and more tortuous vessels. Indeed, heparin-coated Palmaz-Schatz stents are already being used in the ogoing BENESTENT II trial in Europe, simplifying perioperative management, reducing length of hospital stay, and minimizing stent thrombosis plus hemorrhagic complications. Similarly, future applications of genetic engineering and local delivery techniques using stents as a vehicle for drug or radiation treatment may further improve thrombotic profiles and may enhance the ability to inhibit local smooth muscle cell proliferation at the stented site. Through the joint efforts of clinical investigators, research scientists, and industry, we have little doubt that stents will become an important primary catheter-based therapy for patients with SVG pathology.

ACKNOWLEDGMENTS

This research was supported in part by a grant from the Cardiology Research Foundation and the Medlantic Research Institute.

REFERENCES

1. Gruentzig AR, Senning A, Siegenthaler WE et al. Nonoperative dilatation of coronary artery stenosis. N Engl J Med 1979;301:61–8
2. Parisi AF, Folland ED, Hartigan P. A comparison of angioplasty with medical therapy in the treatment of single-vessel coronary artery disease. N Engl J Med 1992;326:10–6.
3. Zhao XQ, Brown BG, Stewart DK et al. Arteriographic endpoints from Emory Angioplasty vs Surgery Trial, abstracted. Circulation 1993;88:I-506
4. Fischman DL, Leon MB, Baim DS et al. A randomized comparison of coronary-stent placement and balloon angioplasty in the treatment of coronary artery disease. N Engl J Med 1994;331:496–501
5. Serruys PW, de Jaegere P, Kiemeneij F et al. A comparison of balloon-expandable-stent implantation with balloon angioplasty in patients with coronary artery disease. N Engl J Med 1994;331:489–495
6. Dotter CT. Transluminally placed coilspring endarterial tube grafts, long term patency in canine popliteal artery. Invest Radiol 1969;4:329–332
7. Dotter CT, Buschmann RW, McKinney MK, Rosch J. Transluminal expandable nitinol coil stent grafting: preliminary report. Radiology 1983;147:259–260
8. Maass D, Zollikofer ChL, Largiader F, Senning A. Radiological follow-up of transluminally inserted vascular endoprostheses: an experimental study using expanding spirals. Radiology 1984;152:659–663
9. Wright KC, Wallace S, Charnsangavej C, Carrasco CH, Gianturco C. Percutaneous endovascular stents: an experimental evaluation. Radiology 1985;157:69–72
10. Mintz GS, Popma JJ, Pichard AD, et al. Arterial remodeling after coronary angioplasty: a serial intravascular ultrasound study. Circulation (in press)
11. Leon MB, Wong SC, Pichard AD. Balloon expandable stent implantation in saphenous vein grafts. pp. 111–121. In Herrmann HC, Hirshfeld JW (eds): Clinical Use of the Palmaz-Schatz Balloon-Expandable Stent. Futura, Mount Kisco, NY, 1993
12. Pomerantz RM, Kuntz RE, Carrozza JP et al. Acute and long-term outcome of narrowed saphenous venous grafts treated by endoluminal stenting and directional atherectomy. Am J Cardiol 1992;70:161–7
13. Friedrich SP, Davis SF, Kuntz R et al. Investigational use of the Palmaz-Schatz in large saphenous vein grafts. Am J Cardiol 1993;71:439–41
14. Piana RN, Moscucci M, Cohen DJ et al. Palmaz-Schatz stenting for treatment of focal vein graft stenosis: immediate results and long-term outcome. J Am Coll Cardiol 1994;23:1296–1304
15. Wong SC, Popma JJ, Pichard AD et al. A comparison of clinical and angiographic outcomes after saphenous vein graft angioplasty using coronary versus "biliary" tubular-slotted stents. Circulation 1995;91:339–50
16. Wong SC, Hong MK, Popma JJ et al. Stent placement for the treatment of aorto-ostial saphenous vein graft lesions, abstracted. J Am Coll Cardiol 1994;23:118A
17. Bilodeau L, Iyer S, Cannon AD et al. Flexible coil stent (Cook Inc.) in saphenous vein grafts: clinical and angiographic follow-up, abstracted. J Am Coll Cardiol 1992;19:264A.

18. Fortuna R, Heuser RR, Garratt KN et al. Wiktor intracoronary stent: experience in the first 101 vein graft patients, abstracted. Circulation 1993;88:I–308

19. Urban P, Sigwart U, Golf S et al. Intravascular stenting for stenosis of aortocoronary venous bypass grafts. J Am Coll Cardiol 1989;13:1085–91

20. Strauss BH, Serruys PW, Bertrand ME et al. Quantitative angiographic follow-up of the coronary Wallstent in native vessels and bypass grafts (European experience—March 1986–March 1990). Am J Cardiol 1992;69:475–81

21. Colombo A, Hall P, Almagor Y et al. Results of intravascular ultrasound guided coronary stenting without subsequent anticoagulation, abstracted. J Am Coll Cardiol 1994;23:335A

22. Wong SC, Popma J, Mintz G et al. Preliminary results from the Reduced Anticoagulation in Saphenous Vein Graft Stent (RAVES) trial. Circulation 1994;90:I-125

23. Wong SC, Popma JJ, Chuang YC et al. Economic impact of reduced anticoagulation after saphenous vein graft stent placement. J Am Coll Cardiol 1995;25:80A

24. Wong SC, Schatz RA: Developmental background and design of the Palmaz-Schatz coronary stent. pp. 3–19. In Herrmann HC, Hirshfeld JE (eds): Clinical Use of the Palmaz-Schatz Balloon-Expandable Stent. Futura, Mount Kisco, NY, 1993

62 Introduction

Cornelius Borst
Ton G. van Leeuwen

Laser angioplasty is an appealing, high-tech strategy to remove plaque by means of a percutaneous technique; the laser energy needed to vaporize plaque can be delivered effectively by glass fibers to the target site.[1,2]

To understand the 15-year history of coronary laser angioplasty, it is emphasized that laser angioplasty was initially developed for two reasons: (1) to address lesions not suited to balloon angioplasty, in particular occlusions; and (2) to replace balloon dilation by a stand-alone recanalization procedure with a reduced risk of acute complications compared with balloon angioplasty. In the first half of the 1980s, restenosis was not yet an issue. Thus the development of laser angioplasty was initially driven only by the aim to improve on the immediate result of the then current technique of balloon angioplasty. It was hypothesized that complete debulking of the obstruction is a better recanalization strategy than overstretching the atherosclerotic wall.

HISTORY AND THEORY

Continuous-Wave Laser Coupled to a Single Bare Fiber

Initially, the laser and the delivery system were determined by the availability of the argon laser (wavelengths 488 and 514 nm, visible light) and the neodymium:YAG laser (wavelength, 1064 nm, infrared), two continuous-wave lasers whose output was coupled into a single bare fiber. For lasing, the laser beam was switched on for periods ranging from 100 ms to several seconds.

In 1983, coronary laser angioplasty was introduced intraoperatively using an argon laser coupled to a bare fiber. The pioneering, albeit premature, clinical attempt and experimental studies revealed the basic limitations of the initial approach: perforation by the unguided rigid fiber with its exceedingly sharp tip, a hemodynamically inadequate channel, and thermal wall damage.

Modified Fiber Tip

To address the limitations of the bare fiber approach, modified fiber tips were developed with a blunt, atraumatic shape (1 to 2 mm in diameter). The metal laser probe (hot tip) converts light energy into heat in the metal tip. The transparent contact probe (sapphire tip) produces a combined effect of light-tissue and hot probe-tissue interaction. The mechanism of recanalization by these probes is complex and is termed *laser thermal angioplasty*.[3] A mechanical dotter effect contributes to their mechanism of action.[3,4]

Percutaneous coronary laser thermal angioplasty began in 1985,[5] but it was not pursued for long because of its high complication rate[6] and because of the promise of excimer laser ablation without adjacent tissue injury.[7,8]

Multifiber Catheters

The enhanced flexibility of multifiber catheters consisting of concentric arrays of 50- to 100-μm fibers arranged around a guidewire lumen greatly improved the safety of the laser energy delivery system because of the decreased risk of perforation by the over-the-wire tracking approach.[1]

Feedback Control of Laser Output

A sophisticated form of feedback control was initiated in the mid-1980s. If low-power diagnostic laser light, with a wavelength in the ultra-violet (UV) region, is directed through a fiber at tissue, some tissue compounds fluoresce at longer wavelengths. The fluorescent light can be picked up by the same fiber, transmitted back, and analyzed as to its spectral components. The resulting fluorescence spectrum is interpreted as a fingerprint of the tissue in contact with the fiber.[2] Subsequently, the high power, ablative laser beam, which is coupled into the same fiber is activated only if in front of the fiber plaque is recognized. If this principle is applied to each individual fiber in a flexible multifiber catheter without a guidewire channel, selective removal of all obstructive tissue, including total occlusions, is potentially feasible. This attractive treatment strategy has not yet been implemented clinically in coronary arteries.

Pulsed Laser Coronary Angioplasty

The complications of coronary laser thermal angioplasty were attributed to its thermal wall injury.[6] In 1988, pulsed excimer laser (wavelength, 308 nm, UV) coronary angioplasty was introduced clinically,[9] after in vitro experiments had demonstrated that tissue removal by the excimer laser was accompanied by minimal injury to adjacent tissue.[7,8] The lack of gross thermal injury resulted in the misnomer "cold laser angioplasty."

In 1990, holmium laser coronary angioplasty was introduced clinically.[10] The holmium-YAG laser (wavelength, 2.1 μm, infrared) is a pulsed solid-state laser that is less expensive and easier to operate and maintain than the excimer laser, which is a gas laser. For both laser systems, the laser light-tissue interaction is summarized in the next section.

It is estimated that by the start of 1995, some 15,000 coronary laser angioplasty procedures have been performed worldwide, about 90% with the excimer laser and about 10% with the holmium laser.[2] In the great majority of cases, subsequent balloon angioplasty was required to obtain a sufficiently small residual stenosis. The requirement of finishing the procedure with the balloon catheter adds to the cost of the laser intervention.

It should be noted that the impetus for the development of excimer laser angioplasty was derived from promising results of in vitro experiments in which the laser beam was delivered directly from the laser in air to the target tissue.[7,8] However, recent in vitro and in vivo experimental studies suggest that the effects of pulsed laser energy delivered by fiber or multifiber catheter to tissue under blood or saline are fundamentally different from the effects observed previously in air.[11–14]

MECHANISM OF ACTION

The conversion of laser light into heat depends on the fluence of the laser light (J/mm^2) and the absorptive properties of the tissue for the specific wavelength. In the case of continuous-wave laser ablation, heat diffusion away from the irradiated tissue causes collateral thermal damage. Fortunately, heat diffusion is a rather slow process.

In the mid-1980s, pulsed lasers were introduced (pulse duration < 1 ms) because the deposition of laser energy in such a short period prevents heat diffusion to adjacent tissue prior to evaporation of the irradiated volume. The vaporizing tissue is explosively removed, leaving a clean and cool crater. As a result, pulsed lasers have precise cutting properties and, in air, produce little thermal damage to adjacent tissue. It is assumed that collateral crater wall damage is not due to heat diffusion but only to direct absorption of nonablative laser light by the edge zone of the irradiated volume. In this model, the penetration depth of the nonablative laser light determines the thickness of the thermal damage zone.

Ablation Mechanism

Next to the conversion of the laser energy into heat (photothermal interaction), the absorption of laser light emitted by pulsed lasers may also lead to photomechanical or photochemical interaction with the irradiated tissue. Photomechanical interactions are (1) thermoelastic expansion of the heated tissue, and (2) vapor bubble formation. Thermoelastic expansion causes *stress waves,* which propagate with the speed of sound (1,500 m/sec = 1.5 mm/μs) or *shock waves,* which travel even faster. However, the major photomechanical interaction during pulsed laser ablation is tissue water vaporization, resulting in explosive removal of tissue structures and rapid *vapor bubble formation.* Vapor bubble expansion as well as shock and stress waves may contribute to the ablation mechanism of pulsed lasers. It is not known whether shock and stress waves inflict collateral tissue damage additional to the injury caused by vapor bubble expansion and implosion.

Photochemical laser-tissue interaction is, for example, molecular bond breaking by a photon of sufficiently high photon energy.

Holmium Laser Ablation

Holmium-YAG laser light (wavelength, 2.1 μm) is absorbed by water. Its penetration depth in vascular tissue and blood is approximately 400 μm. The clinical holmium laser produces 250-μs pulses at a rate of 5 Hz in trains of a few seconds to allow heat dissipation in between trains. The threshold fluence for vascular tissue ablation is about 300 mJ/mm^2/pulse. For calcifications it is higher. At a fluence of 1,000 mJ/mm^2/pulse, the estimated ablation depth per pulse is about 50 μm.

Holmium laser ablation is based on a combination of photothermal and photomechanical mechanisms: the laser light is absorbed by tissue water, which subsequently vaporizes. Vaporization amounts to explosive expansion of water. Note that 1 mm^3 of water will result in more than 1,500 mm^3 of water vapor. The water vapor can be observed in saline as a fast expanding and imploding bubble around the fiber tip (Fig. 62-1A). During ablation, bubble expansion is also present within the target tissue (Fig. 62-1B). In in vivo pig experiments, distinct dissections were

found in the aortic wall emanating from the crater (Fig. 62-2). The thickness of the necrotic zone around the crater (thermal injury) was about 360 μm. Thus the mechanism of collateral tissue damage corresponds to the mechanism of ablation.

Excimer Laser Ablation

Xenon-chloride (XeCl) excimer laser light (wavelength, 308 nm) is absorbed by lipids and nucleic acids. Its penetration depth in vascular tissue and blood is approximately 100 and 30 μm, respectively. The clinical excimer laser produces 100- to 220-ns pulses at a rate of 20 to 25 Hz (maximally 40 Hz) in trains of a few seconds to allow heat dissipation in between trains. The threshold fluence for vascular tissue ablation is about 20 mJ/mm^2/pulse. At a fluence of 50 to 60 mJ/mm^2/pulse, the ablation depth per pulse is about 3 to 4 μm. However, if the multifiber catheter is actively advanced by exerting a force of about 10 g, the catheter progresses by approximately 25 μm/pulse (J. Hamburger and G. Gijsbers, personal communication, 1995).

Whether 308-nm excimer laser ablation results in molecular bond breaking with little photothermal effects has been a matter of controversy. The precise ablation of aortic tissue in air without thermal or mechanical damage in the remaining tissue led to the hypothesis that ablation by the XeCl excimer

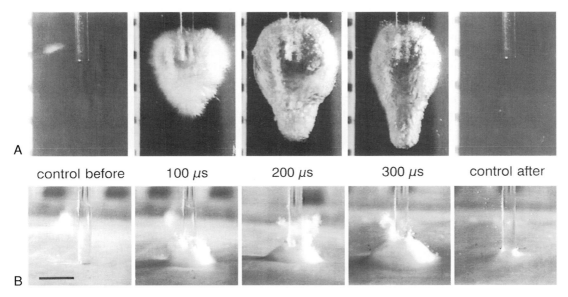

control before   100 μs   200 μs   300 μs   control after

Fig. 62-1. Photographs of the holmium laser-saline **(A)** and holmium laser-tissue **(B)** interaction before, during, and after the 500-mJ holmium laser pulse. With the 320-μm-diameter fiber tip submerged in saline **(A),** a pear-shaped water vapor bubble is formed. With the fiber tip in light contact with porcine aorta submerged in saline, a corresponding tissue elevation is observed **(B),** suggestive of bubble formation within the tissue. The average diameter of the tissue surface elevation was 2.4 mm. Scale bar = 1 mm. (From Van Leeuwen et al.,[11] with permission.)

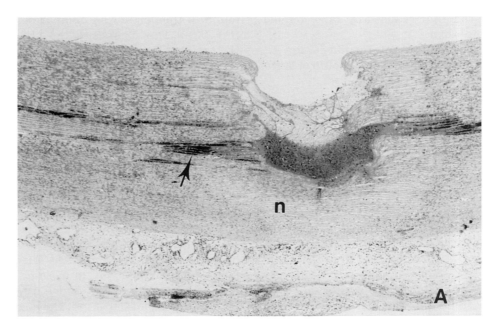

Fig. 62-2. Representative microscopic section (hematoxylin-eosin stained) of crater and adjacent wall damage after two consecutive holmium laser pulses (500 mJ/pulse, 1 Hz, 1.0-mm-diameter large aperture fiber tip) in porcine aorta after 3 days of survival ($\times$ 30). The dissections (*arrow*), which run parallel to the intimal surface, are identified by the dark staining of red blood cells. The dissections had an average diameter of 2.7 mm. Note the necrotic zone (n) at the bottom of and lateral to the crater. A, adventitia. (From Van Erven et al.[26] with permission).

laser is photochemical, (i.e., by molecular bond breaking). However, recent experimental evidence suggests that its mechanism of ablation is predominantly photothermal and photomechanical, similar to the mechanism of action of the holmium-YAG laser.[15] Furthermore, it was found that tissue ablation with the fiber tip in contact with the vessel wall submerged in saline produced frayed craters, with a necrotic zone of about 350 μm (thermal injury) and dissections similar to those observed after holmium laser ablation.[11]

UV excimer laser light is not absorbed by water, but by lipids and nucleic acids. Most of the absorbed laser light will be converted to heat, which is rapidly transferred to adjacent tissue water molecules. The instantaneous tissue water heating results in a short-lived (200 μs), fast expanding and imploding water vapor bubble (Fig. 62-3).

Delivering the excimer laser pulse in blood has a similar effect. The 308-nm laser light is well absorbed by the hemoglobin molecule, which transfers the released heat to the adjacent water molecules. Consequently, intraluminal water vapor bubble formation induces fast local expansion of the artery (*microsecond dotter effect*, Fig. 62-4). The resulting arterial wall damage reaches well beyond the penetration depth of the laser light. Intraluminal

holmium laser pulse delivery produces a similar vapor bubble and local vessel expansion (Fig. 62-4).

In conclusion, recent experimental studies suggest that the original description of excimer laser angioplasty as "cold laser" angioplasty with "minimal adjacent tissue injury" needs to be modified. Pulsed laser ablation in contact mode of tissue under blood or saline proceeds in a fundamentally different way than ablation in noncontact mode in air. In vitro, noncontact tissue ablation produces little collateral damage because tissue can be blown off on a layer-by-layer basis by each pulse. During laser angioplasty, however, the ablative surface of the catheter engages the obstruction in a blood or saline environment. Ablation results in the explosive production of a vapor bubble that cannot vent into the air. Thus, by opting for a pulsed laser, thermal collateral damage is confined at the expense of mechanical tissue damage by an explosively expanding vapor bubble.

CLINICAL IMPLICATIONS

From experimental studies a number of clinical implications may be inferred:

1. *Fluence (mJ/mm²/pulse)*. Above the fluence

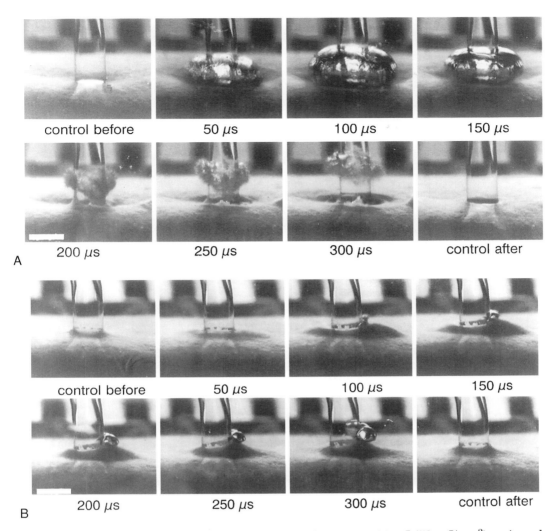

Fig. 62-3. Time-resolved photography of the interaction between a 34-mJ (53 mJ/mm²) excimer laser pulse in light contact mode **(A)** and the 900-μm-diameter fiber tip buried in porcine aorta after 15 pulses, due to force contact (0.1 N) **(B)**. Scale bar = 1 mm. (From Van Leeuwen et al.,[11] with permission.).

threshold for vascular tissue ablation, a rapidly expanding vapor bubble may be formed that exceeds the size of the catheter. In the past, some procedures may have been performed at near threshold fluence.

2. *Calcifications.* Heavily calcified lesions are ill ablated by the current laser angioplasty systems. The higher fluence required to ablate calcified plaque is not allowed by the Food and Drug Administration and would produce larger vapor bubbles.

3. *Repetition rate.* At 25- to 40-Hz pulse frequency of the excimer laser, it is likely that limited thermal collateral tissue damage is produced (approximately a 0.35-mm zone[11] because the interval between pulses is too short to allow sufficient heat dissipation.[12]

4. *Contact or noncontact.* It has been suggested that the procedure would benefit from slight retraction of the excimer laser catheter after it engaged the obstruction to allow egress of vapors.[16] However, if blood is allowed in between the catheter and the target tissue, only vapor bubbles will be created in the highly absorbing blood.

5. *Laser ablation or dotter effect?* Without close contact by active advancement of the multifiber catheter, progression per pulse drops dramatically. Since catheter progression is highly dependent on the applied advancement force, it is likely that progression is due to (a) tissue ablation, (b) advancement of the catheter, or (c) explosive vapor bubble expansion (combined dotter effects, albeit at entirely different time scales). A recent intravascular ultrasound study reported

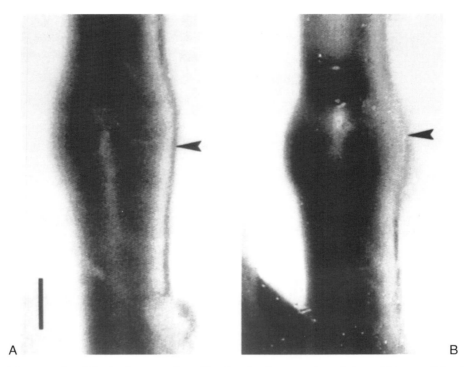

A   B

Fig. 62-4. Time-resolved flash photographs of in vivo local expansion of the rabbit carotid artery due to intraluminal bubble formation: at 200 μs after the start of a 500-mJ holmium laser pulse delivered by a 1.0-mm-large aperture tip (**A,** *arrowhead*) and at 100 μs after a 9.5-mJ excimer laser pulse delivered by a 3.5-F multifiber catheter (**B,** *arrowhead*). Scale bar = 1 mm.

that only a 9% reduction in cross-sectional plaque area was observed after excimer laser angioplasty.[17]

6. *Multiple passes.* In an excimer laser procedure, a second pass may primarily lead to hitting blood and creating vapor bubbles. If a saline flush is used, however, multiple passes may offer benefit.

7. *Fresh mural thrombus.* It is conceivable that the explosive vapor bubble expansion and implosion (bubble life time is less than 500 μs) might dislodge any fresh mural thrombus.[18]

8. *Acute complications.* Initially, the acute complications of coronary pulsed laser angioplasty were attributed to teething trouble in the development of adequately flexible, atraumatic, densely packed multifiber laser catheters. However, some of the acute complications (e.g., 22% dissections)[18] may be related to the bubble expansion and microdissections observed experimentally.[11-14]

9. *Catheter dead space and energy per pulse.* To reduce the mechanical dotter effect of the current catheters, the industry aims to reduce the dead space of the catheter by augmenting the fiber packing density. However, at constant fluence (e.g., 50 mJ/mm^2 per excimer laser pulse), reducing the dead space will increase the optically active area and hence the delivered energy per pulse. Consequently, the vapor bubble volume, which is roughly linearly dependent on pulse energy, will increase.

10. *Undersizing the catheter and the need for subsequent balloon dilation.* The incidence of dissections is positively correlated with both catheter size and energy/pulse levels.[18] According to Spectranetics (November 18, 1993), the rate of perforation is below 1% if the excimer laser catheter is more than 1.0 mm smaller than the estimated vessel size. However, if the difference between the catheter diameter and the vessel lumen diameter is 1.0 mm, or less, the perforation rate is 4.0%. If this difference is 0.5 mm or less, the perforation rate is 8.0%. It is conceivable that the progressive risk of perforation when the catheter approaches the size of the target vessel is associated with the relation between catheter size and delivered energy per pulse. At a constant fluence (e.g., 50 mJ/mm^2/pulse), increasing the catheter size is accompanied by an increase in the absolute optically active area and hence the delivered energy per

pulse. Thus, bubble size increases with catheter size. If the catheter diameter approaches the vessel diameter, expansion of the vapor bubble may cause a local expansion of the vessel wall by some 50% within 100 μs (Fig. 62-4), which may contribute to the formation of dissections and other acute complications.[11,14,15]

An alternative mechanism for the progressive risk of perforation when the catheter size approaches the artery size might be paradoxical local arterial shrinkage at the lesion site.[19]

The need to undersize the laser catheter has a consequence of major clinical importance. Since current interventions aim at a minimal residual stenosis ("bigger lumen is better"), undersizing the laser catheter may necessitate subsequent balloon angioplasty to finish the procedure. As a result, one of the two initial goals of coronary laser angioplasty has to be abandoned. It cannot be applied as a stand-alone procedure. Consequently, its acute and long-term results will always be affected by the impact of the subsequent balloon angioplasty.

11. *Saline flush during excimer laser angioplasty.* From a theoretical point of view, a saline flush would potentially reduce any complications induced by vapor bubbles arising from excimer laser pulses fired into intraluminal blood.

12. *Pulse multiplexing.* It is possible to activate only part of the fibers in a multifiber catheter. If, for example, the fibers are divided into eight sectors that are sequentially activated, for each sector a bubble is created with volume one-eighth and diameter one-half of the bubble created when all fibers are activated simultaneously. This ingenious method of reducing the bubble size may reduce complications. The clinical benefit of pulse multiplexing remains to be established.

13. *Restenosis.* Laser angioplasty was not developed to reduce coronary restenosis. The hypothesis put forward at the end of the 1980s that pulsed laser angioplasty might be of therapeutic value in this respect had and has no experimental basis.

For two reasons, it is unlikely that a substantial reduction in coronary restenosis rate will be achieved: (a) thermal injury and vapor bubble expansion and implosion may be no less of a stimulus to the vessel wall repair response than balloon angioplasty[16,20–24] and pulsed laser coronary angioplasty is not a stand-alone procedure.[18]

In the first randomized trial comparing excimer laser angioplasty (plus balloon angioplasty) with bal-

loon angioplasty in over 10-mm-long coronary lesions, both the acute and 6-month follow-up results were similar.[25]

CONCLUSIONS

By opting for a pulsed laser, thermal collateral damage is confined at the expense of mechanical tissue damage caused by an explosively expanding vapor bubble. Also, bubble size increases with catheter size. Two mechanical dotter effects are likely to contribute to the recanalization mechanism: (1) a "snowplough" effect, by active catheter advancement, and (2) a microsecond dilation effect by the expanding vapor bubble. It is clear that coronary laser angioplasty is not a stand-alone intervention, and it is unlikely that pulsed laser angioplasty will reduce coronary restenosis substantially. However, coronary laser recanalization may enable or facilitate angioplasty of otherwise contraindicated or failed lesions.

ACKNOWLEDGMENTS

C. Borst was supported by grants from the Netherlands Heart Foundation.

REFERENCES

1. Litvack F (ed). Coronary Laser Angioplasty pp. 1–276. Blackwell Scientific Publications, Boston, 1992
2. Deckelbaum LI. Cardiovascular applications of laser technology. Lasers Surg Med 1994;15:315–41
3. Verdaasdonk RM, Jansen D, Holstege FC, Borst C. Mechanism of CW Nd:YAG laser recanalization with modified fiber tips: influence of temperature and axial force on tissue penetration in vitro. Lasers Surg Med 1991;11:204–12
4. Berengoltz-Zlochin SN, Westerhof PW, Mall WPTM et al. Nd:YAG laser-assisted angioplasty in femoropopliteal artery occlusions: "hot" versus "cold" recanalization with transparent contact probe. Radiology 1992; 182:409–14
5. Sanborn TA, Faxon DP. Kellett MA, Ryan TJ. Percutaneous coronary laser thermal angioplasty. J Am Coll Cardiol 1986;1437–40
6. Linnemeier TJ, Cumberland DC, Rothbaum DA, Landin RJ, Ball MW. Human percutaneous laser-assisted coronary angioplasty: efforts to reduce spasm and thrombosis, (abstracted). J Am Coll Cardiol 1989;13: 61A
7. Grundfest WS, Litvack F, Forrester JS et al. Laser ablation of human atherosclerotic plaque without adjacent tissue injury. J Am Coll Cardiol 1985;5:929–33
8. Isner JM, Donaldson RF, Deckelbaum LI et al. The excimer laser: gross, light microscopic and ultrastructural analysis of potential advantages for use in laser

therapy of cardiovascular disease. J Am Coll Cardiol 1985;6:1102–9

9. Litvack F, Grundfest WS, Goldenberg T, Laudenslager J, Forrester JS. Percutaneous excimer laser angioplasty of aortocoronary saphenous vein grafts. J Am Coll Cardiol 1989;14:803–8

10. Geschwind HJ, Dubois-Rande JL, Murphy Chutorian D et al. Percutaneous coronary angioplasty with mid-infrared laser and a new multifiber catheter [lettter]. Lancet 1990;336:245–6

11. Van Leeuwen TG, Van Erven L, Meertens JH et al. Origin of arterial wall dissections induced by pulsed excimer and mid-infrared laser ablation in the pig. J Am Coll Cardiol 1992;19:1610–8

12. Gijsbers GHM, Sprangers RLH, Keijzer M et al. Some laser-tissue interactions in 308 nm excimer laser coronary angioplasty. J Interv Cardiol 1990;3:231–41

13. Abela GS. Abrupt closure after pulsed laser angioplasty: spasm or a "mille-feuilles" effect? J Interv Cardiol 1992;5:259–62

14. Van Leeuwen TG, Meertens JH, Velema E, Post MJ, Borst C. Intraluminal vapor bubble induced by excimer laser pulse causes microsecond arterial dilation and invagination leading to extensive wall damage in the rabbit. Circulation 1993;87:1258–63

15. Oraevsky AA, Jacques SL, Pettit GH et al. XeCl laser ablation of atherosclerotic aorta: optical properties and energy pathways. Lasers Surg Med 1992;12:585–97

16. Isner JM, Pickering JG, Mosseri M. Laser-induced dissections: pathogenesis and implications for therapy. J Am Coll Cardiol 1992;19:1619–21

17. Honye J, Mahon DJ, Nakamura S et al. Intravascular ultrasound imaging after excimer laser angioplasty. Cathet Cardiovasc Diagn 1994;32:213–22

18. Baumbach A, Bittl JA, Fleck E et al. Acute complications of excimer laser coronary angioplasty: a detailed analysis of multicenter results. J Am Coll Cardiol 1994;23:1305–13

19. Pasterkamp G, Wensing PJW, Post MJ et al. Paradoxical arterial wall shrinkage may contribute to luminal narrowing of human atherosclerotic femoral arteries. Circulation 1995;91:1444–49

20. Oomen A, Van Erven L, Vandenbroucke WVA et al. Early and late arterial healing response to catheter-induced laser, thermal, and mechanical wall damage in the rabbit. Lasers Surg Med 1990;10:363–74

21. Karsch KR, Haase KK, Wehrman M, Hassenstein S, Hanke H. Smooth muscle cell proliferation and restenosis after stand alone coronary excimer laser angioplasty. J Am Coll Cardiol 1991;17:991–4

22. Hanke H, Haase KK, Hanke S et al. Morphological changes and smooth muscle cell proliferation after experimental excimer laser treatment. Circulation 1991;83:1380–89

23. Hassenstein S, Hanke H, Kamenz J et al. Vascular injury and time course of smooth muscle cell proliferation after experimental holmium laser angioplasty. Circulation 1992;86:1575–83

24. Douek PC, Correa R, Neville R et al. Dose-dependent smooth muscle cell proliferation induced by thermal injury with pulsed infrared lasers. Circulation 1992;86:1249–56

25. Appelman YEA, Piek JJ, Strikwerda S et al. Randomised trial of excimer laser angioplasty versus balloon angioplasty for treatment of obstructive coronary artery disease. Lancet. 1996;347:79–84

26. Van Erven L, van Leewen TG, Post MJ, van der Veen MJ, Velema E, Borst C. Mid-infrared pulsed lasar ablation of the arterial wall: mechanical origin of "acoustic" wall damage and its effect on wall healing. J Thorac Vasc Surg. 1992;104:1553–9

63 Excimer Lasers

Andreas Baumbach
Karl R. Karsch

The basic concept of laser angioplasty is very attractive: Removal of atherosclerotic plaque by controlled application of light has the theoretical potential of creating a channel without the trauma to surrounding vessel wall structures that characterizes the mechanism of balloon dilation. Thus, the rational for laser angioplasty is to achieve efficient stenosis reduction with minimal traumatic side effects to the adjacent tissue. The potential benefits as compared to standard balloon dilation are (1) increased success in complicated lesions, which is due to debulking as a different mechanism of action, (2) successful angioplasty of former nondilatable lesions, (3) reduced acute vessel complications, and (4) reduced incidence of restenosis as a result of the less traumatic procedure.

The ideal laser system for angioplasty must fulfill the following criteria, most of which are met by the current excimer laser technology:

1. Absorption of light by atherosclerotic plaque
2. Efficient ablation of atherosclerotic plaque even in calcified tissue
3. Absence of thermal side effects
4. Controlled low ablation depth for a reduced risk of vessel perforation
5. Incoupling of the light into nontoxic, flexible fibers for energy transmission

MECHANISM OF ACTION

Laser is the acronym for light amplification by stimulated emission of radiation. No matter what type of amplification medium is used for the generation of coherent and monochromatic laser light, either solid, liquid, or gas, all laser systems operate by the same physical process of stimulated emission of radiation (Fig. 63-1). The laser resonator consists of an active or gain medium enclosed in a set of reflection mirrors. The medium of excimer lasers is a gas, consisting of a mixture of xenon and chloride, which in the excited state form a dimer. The acronym *excimer* stands for excited dimer. The gain medium is pumped by an external energy source that is controlled by an electronic circuit, which is responsible for the duration of the pump-pulse to the active medium. Within the resonator, the light bounces back and forth between two mirrors, stimulating more light emission from the active medium. One of the mirrors is only partially reflecting, allowing some of the laser light to exit the resonator. An optical switch inside or outside the laser cavity can further considerably reduce the pulse duration of the laser output. The laser light exiting the laser cavity is characterized by the following parameters:

1. Wavelength: XeCL excimer lasers for angioplasty emit light at a wavelength of 308 nm, which is in the ultra-violet part of the spectrum.
2. Pulse duration: The available systems of excimer lasers work with pulse durations of 120 to more than 180 nsec. The longer the pulse duration, the lower the peak energies that have to be delivered through a transmission unit (multifiber catheter) to achieve the same energy per pulse. High peak energies increase the risk of fiber damage.

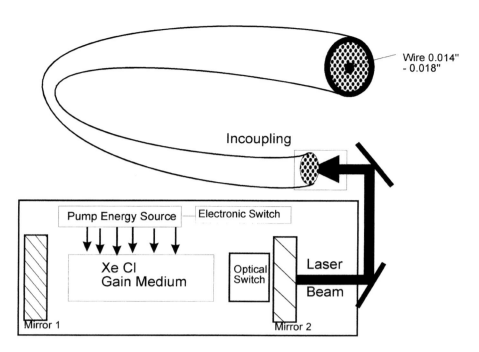

Fig. 63-1. Laser system with a multifiber catheter.

3. Energy per pulse (mJ): Energy delivered per laser pulse. This variable is included in the term:

4. Energy density: Synonym, fluence (mJ/mm²). Energy per area, which is transmitted to the tissue. The range of density applicable in coronary angioplasty is determined by the ablation threshold (no tissue removal below this threshold) and the risk of excessive side effects. The currently used densities range between 40 and 55 mJ/mm².

5. Repetition rate (Hz): Pulses per second.

The process of tissue ablation is complex. In contrast to holmium and Nd-Y AG lasers, excimer laser light is not absorbed in water. At 308 nm, the light is absorbed by tissue proteins, which leads to the breaking of molecular bonds, which then results in the transformation of tissue from the solid into the gas phase.[1] The removal of tissue is associated with little or no thermal damage to adjacent tissue.[2] However, this ablation of tissue currently is known to be associated with at least two important side effects. First, van Leeuwen et al.[3] demonstrated that a vapor bubble expands and collapses within 300 μ following the laser pulse. The bubble size is determined by the irradiation area (or tip size) and the energy per pulse. With larger catheters working at higher energy densities, the bubble size can significantly exceed the vessel size, leading to dilation and invagination of the vessel wall. Furthermore, the bubble can cause severe damage when forced to expand into the tissue,

leading to dissection. The second side effect represents probably a basic mechanism of tissue removal by laser light. Acoustic pressure waves result from absorption of laser light in tissue and blood.[4] These pressure waves can exceed 50 bars at the lateral side of the catheter tip, therefore leading to acoustic damage of adjacent tissue. The peak pressures are determined by the energy per pulse.

Tissue ablation with excimer lasers is a slow and stepwise process. The maximum ablation depth in atherosclerotic tissue is 2 to 40 μm per pulse, depending on tissue characteristics, catheter size, fluence and force applied to the tip.[5] For calcified tissue, the etch rate (tissue removal per pulse) is lower. Assuming a high ablation depth of 20 μm per pulse, ablation of a noncalcified lesion of 1-cm length will still take 500 pulses. At a standard repetition rate of 20 Hz, this will need 25 seconds of irradiation. Thus, tissue removal takes time. According to these experimental data, advancement of the laser catheter should be restricted to 0.5 mm/sec. However, some investigators propagate a fast approach to lesions, performing laser angioplasty with a fast, single-pass, and minimal (5 to 10 seconds) duration laser energy application. Given additional tissue removal by bubble and pressure wave formation, efficacy might probably be present with fast advances of the catheters. However, no experimental data exist to explain the basic mechanism of tissue removal that would support this approach. At least a partial dotter effect must be taken into consideration. It is very important to bear in mind that the effect of tissue ablation can be achieved only if the catheter tip is in contact with tissue. Irradiation in blood will result in absorption of the light by blood followed by pressure wave formation without efficient tissue removal.

LASER SYSTEMS AND CATHETER TECHNOLOGY

Clinical results have been achieved with three commercially available XeCl-excimer laser systems. The wavelength is 308 nm. All systems have adjustable repetition rates and energy densities. All systems use front-firing multifiber catheters with channels accepting standard guidewires. The systems differ, however, in laser parameters and catheter technology.

- AIS (Advanced Interventional Systems, Inc., Irvine, California)
- Long pulse duration exceeding 200 ns
- Multifiber catheters, 1.3, 1.6, 2.0, 2.2, and 2.4 mm in diameter

- Monorail systems
- Directional (eccentric) design, allowing for adjustment of the catheter to the lesion
- Spectranetics (Spectranetics, Inc., Colorado Springs, Colorado)
  - CVX 300
  - Pulse duration 135 ns
  - Multifiber catheters, 1.4, 1.7, and 2.0 mm in diameter, monorail systems
  - Eccentric catheter design, allowing for adjustment of the catheter to the lesion (Fig. 6–32)

The laser systems of AIS and Spectranetics are now combined and are distributed by Spectranetics Inc., Colorado Springs.

- Medolas (formerly, Technolas) (Medolas, Gräfelfing, Germany)
  - MAX 20
  - Pulse duration 120 ns
  - Multifiber catheters, 1.2, 1.5, 1.8, 2.1 mm in diameter, over-the-wire systems
  - Eccentric catheters and monorail system under development

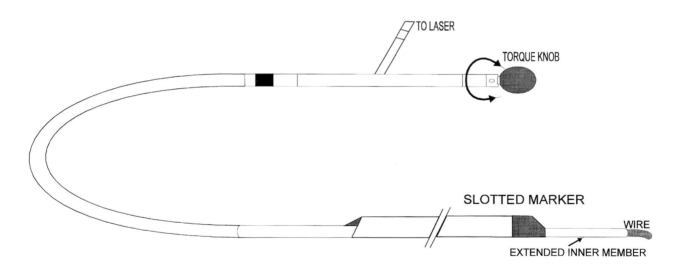

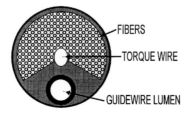

Fig. 63-2. Eccentric catheter design.

- SELCA:
- Sequential incoupling of the laser beam into 8 to 12 fiber bundles

PATIENT POPULATION

Laser angioplasty is applicable to all patients who are suitable for elective percutaneous transluminal coronary angioplasty (PTCA). Patient selection criteria are dominated by lesion morphology and vessel anatomy. Because no data that show a superior outcome of laser angioplasty are available, patients at high risk for percutaneous interventions should not be considered candidates for laser angioplasty. In particular, patients with acute ischemic events should be treated with the fastest method, which still is conventional balloon dilation.

PRETREATMENT

Patients should receive therapy with acetylsalicylic acid. As in standard PTCA, heparin is given before the intervention intravenously or intra-arterially. Some investigators advocate intravenous nitrates or calcium antagonists during the course of angioplasty to overcome the problem of vasospasm following laser angioplasty.

OPERATIVE TECHNIQUE

Laser angioplasty is performed with standard guiding catheters and standard guidewires. For small and medium laser catheter diameters, an 8-F guiding catheter is sufficient. With 2.0-mm and larger catheters, 9-F guides are recommended for proper handling of the catheter and efficient contrast injection.

Before the catheter is mounted on the guidewire, calibration must be performed. Power meters measure the laser energy at the catheter tip and adjust the output of the laser source according to the individual catheter's incoupling properties.

The laser catheter is then advanced to the target lesion. The catheter should be pushed cautiously, because its profile is larger than the conventional balloon catheters and because purely mechanical dissection of plaques is possible on the way to the target lesion. The laser tip has a radiopaque marker. Fluoroscopic guidance is necessary to obtain the optimal position. Contrast media significantly increase the pressure waves generated by laser irradiation! Before application of energy, make sure that the injected contrast medium has been washed out.

Saline Flushing

A method of saline flushing through the guiding catheter during laser irradiation is currently under investigation. By lowering the concentration of blood in front of the catheter tip, the extent of pressure wave formation may be reduced. Experimental data suggest that peak pressures are reduced by 50% in a dilution with 5% blood and 95% saline. A recently completed randomized study suggests a reduction of the incidence of dissections with saline infusion during laser angioplasty (L. Deckelbaum, personal communication).

The laser catheter is then slowly advanced into the lesion under energy delivery, applying only moderate pressure on the catheter. The laser literally bites its way through the lesion by itself. Pushing the catheter in situations without easy advancement may lead to misalignment and irradiation into the vessel wall, resulting in dissection and perforation. Irradiation should be performed in trains of 3 to 5 seconds followed by a short intermission. Always adjust the catheter coaxially by gentle pull on the guidewire. Stop irradiation if the catheter tip is directed to the vessel wall or to the branch point of a vessel.

After the laser has crossed the lesion, the catheter should be pulled back into the guide, and fluoroscopic control of the result should be obtained.

In most cases with concentric catheters, additional passes will not result in further luminal gain, because the catheter is directed through the existing channel and has no chance to reduce the lesion. However, a second pass may be beneficial, if the lesion and artery geometry suggest contact of a large catheter tip area with residual tissue. Especially with the use of eccentric catheters, allowing for adjustment of the catheter tip, additional passes can increase the lumen diameter. Note that all passes that predominantly irradiate blood result mainly in side effects and increase the risk of dissections.

Recommendations

Choice of System Parameters

Initial Energy Density

Energy density should be adjusted to the catheter size. An initial energy density of 50 mJ/mm^2 is recommended for small (1.3/1.5-mm) catheters. Large catheters (2.0 mm) should be operated at 40 mJ/mm^2 initially, because their ablation efficacy (mm^3/J) is higher.[5]

Increasing Energy Density

If no advancement of the catheter into the lesion is observed under energy application, increasing the energy density in steps of 5 mJ/mm^2 might lead to efficient ablation. The use of energy densities higher than 60 mJ/mm^2 results in increased risk of side effects, especially with the use of larger catheters and is not recommended.

Repetition Rate

A repetition rate of 20 to 25 Hz is generally recommended. Increasing the repetition rate above 25 Hz may result in accumulation of ablation products and effects. Reducing the repetition rate results in reduced ablation per time, not in reduced efficacy of the single pulse.

Catheter Size

Because the area of the catheter tip determines in part the extent of side effects, a safety margin of 1 mm between catheter diameter and vessel diameter is recommended to reduce the incidence of perforations.

Avoid

Using the laser catheter without wire guidance
Laser energy delivery into a dissection
Laser energy delivery directly at the vessel wall
Contrast injection while the laser operates
Pushing the catheter hard against resistance

MANAGMENT OF COMPLICATIONS

The majority of complications are comparable to complications seen with standard balloon dilation and warrant identical strategies. Perforations, however, are seen in 0.5 to 2% of cases. Excimer laser-induced extravasations may represent complicated dissections rather than direct holes in the artery. Therefore, in many cases perforations can be managed by balloon dilation. Long compression of the wall layers using perfusion balloon is the second choice in managment. Monitoring for pericardial effusion is mandatory; pericardial puncture might be necessary. Acute operation should be considered for patients with unappeasable extravasations.

Postoperative management and follow-up do not differ from the standard regimens for PTCA.

CLINICAL RESULTS

Apart from the reports of controlled studies, data on the results of coronary excimer laser angioplasty are available from three multicenter registries. For a summary of the results, see Table 63-1. Note that this is only a documentation of reported numbers; no effort has been made to adjust for different patient selection, definitions of success, complications, and analysis criteria.

European Registry

From January 1991 to January 1993, the clinical and angiographic data of 470 patients were included in the European Coronary Excimer Laser Angioplasty Registry.[6] Symptoms were CCS class 3 in 23%, CCS 4 in 14.7%, unstable angina in 14.7% and acute myocardial infarction in 6.6%. Of 477 treated lesions 60% were type B2, and 19% type C. The lesion was located in the left anterior descending artery in 61%, in the LCX in 16%, in the right coronary artery in 20%, in a protected left main stem in 1.3%, and in a saphenous vein graft in 2.5%.

Failure of laser angioplasty (no lesion reduction) in this intention to treat study occurred in 56 (12%) interventions. In the multivariate analysis, failure was associated with the intention to treat long segmental lesions (risk ratio [RR] 3.6, confidence Interval [CI] 2.9 to 4.4; $P = 0.0005$); segments with severe prestenotic tortuosity (RR 3.5, CI 2.4 to 4.6; $P = 0.02$); and total occlusions (RR 2.1; CI 1.4 to 2.8; $P = 0.05$). Procedural success was achieved in 89%. Individual morphologic criteria for a reduced procedural success were presence of thrombus (RR 6.4; CI 5.0 to 7.7; $P = 0.007$) and vessel calcification (RR 2.6; CI 1.9 to 3.2; $P = 0.005$). Procedural success was slightly lower in type C lesions (86%) as compared to type B2 (88%), type B1 (95%), and type A lesions (92%).

U.S. Spectranetics Registry

The U.S. registry included data on 2,131 patients treated with excimer laser coronary angioplasty. Laser success is defined as a reduction in stenosis severity of at least 20%. Procedural success is defined as a final stenosis of less than 50% without acute myocardial infarction, bypass operation, and death. In this population three generations of catheter devices are identified: An initial series with the first (approved) laser catheters (n = 921 patients), a second series with improved "metal rim" catheters (n =

Table 63-1. Success Rates and Complications of Coronary Excimer Laser Angioplasty in the Three Multicenter Registries[a]

All Patients	U.S. AIS (%)	U.S. Spectranetics (%)	European (%)
Laser success	83–86	80.1–89.6	
Procedural success	90	88.7–93.8	89
Procedural success, specific indications			
Vein grafts	92	93.7–97.4	100 (n = 12)
Ostial lesions		83.9–94.1	82
Aorto-ostial	89		
Long lesions >20 mm	87–89	88.8–90.9	83
Calcified lesions		84–85.8	80
Total occlusions	89	82.4–88.3	88
Complications			
Spasm	1.2	4.9–5.5	13.4
Dissections	13	15.6–18.8	14.7
Major dissections		4.2–5.1	4
Closure	6.5	1.4–6.3	7.8
Perforation	0.4–1.6	2.1–2.5	1.9
MI	1.7–2.3[b]	0–1.6[b]	2.1
CABG	3.4–4.0	2.1–4.8	1.9
Death	0.4–0.9	0–1.4	1.5

[a] Comparability is limited by differences in inclusion of patients, definitions, and analysis.
[b] Q-wave myocardial infarction.

1,066), and a third series with monorail catheters (N = 144). The target vessel distribution in the three series showed an increase in the treatment of saphenous vein grafts from 14% of target vessels in the first to 38.4% and 33.3% in the following series, respectively. Stand-alone PELCA was performed in 17.4%, 11.2%, and 2.8% in series 1, 2, and 3, respectively.

Laser success increased from 80.1 to 87.1% and 89.6% in the three consecutive series. Procedural success was 88.7, 91.7, and 93.8%, respectively.

An alpha cohort of lesions suitable for PELCA was identified: bypass grafts, ostial lesions, long lesions, calcified lesions, total occlusions, and failed previous PTCA. The data document a trend toward the treatment of more complex lesions, especially bypass grafts in the United States. However, procedural results improved using advanced catheter technology.

U.S. AIS Registry

Data on the first 3,000 patients and 3,592 lesions are available.[8] Laser success is defined as a reduction of stenosis severity of at least 20% with a minimum lumen diameter corresponding to the catheter size (e.g., greater 1.0 mm for the 1.6-mm catheter). The lesions were total occlusions in 10%, aorto-ostial in 14%, long (20 mm) in 20%, and they were located in a vein graft in 16%. Procedure success did not differ between the first 2,000 treated and the last 1,000

patients treated, though laser success rates did increase. Stand-alone laser angioplasty was performed in 29% in the first 2,000 and in 5% in the last 1,000 patients treated ($P < 0.001$). A significant reduction of perforations was noted in the last 1,000 patients (0.4%, compared to 1.6% in patients 1 to 2,000, $P < 0.005$). Lesion length did not influence the success rate; neither did the success rate show statistical difference for aorto-ostial lesions, vein grafts, and total occlusions.

COMPLICATIONS AND LEARNING CURVE

Data on 1,595 interventions of coronary excimer laser angioplasty in 1,521 patients were analyzed, using a merged data base from the U.S. Spectranetics and European Percutaneous Coronary Excimer Laser Angioplasty Registries.[9] Complications included dissection (22.0%), vasospasm (6.1%), filling defects (4.8%), abrupt reclosure (6.1%), embolization (2.3%), perforation (2.4%), arrhythmia (0.7%), and aneurysm formation (0.3%). Major complications were non-Q-wave myocardial infarction (2.3%). Q-wave myocardial infarction (1.0%), coronary artery bypass grafting (3.1%), and death (0.7%). Logistic regression analysis revealed a correlation between dissections and the use of larger catheter size ($P = 0.005$), high energy per pulse levels ($P = 0.0001$ for native vessels), lesion length greater than 10 mm ($P = 0.001$), and presence of a side branch ($P = 0.01$). The incidence of perforations was higher in female patients ($P = 0.004$), total occlusions ($P = 0.02$), and in the presence of a side branch ($P = 0.03$). Fatal complications were correlated to patients with multivessel disease ($P < 0.0001$), patients with acute myocardial infarction ($P = 0.0009$), and older patients (70 years, $P = 0.004$). The incidence of major complications decreased after performance of 50 laser angioplasty procedures at one institution ($P = 0.02$).

LONG-TERM RESULTS

Quantitative coronary angioplasty (QCA) analysis was performed on 114 patients of the European registry only. Restenosis (50% diameter reduction) was found in 54%. Angiographic follow-up is available on 1,187 patients of the U.S. Spectranetics registry. The restenosis rate is 44.4%. Angiographic follow-up is available on 50% of patients in the U.S. AIS registry; restenosis was seen in 54%.

CURRENT INDICATIONS

Based on registry results and comparison with historic data for PTCA, the U.S. Food and Drug Administration gave approval for coronary excimer laser angioplasty for six indications: bypass grafts, ostial lesions, long lesions, calcified lesions, total occlusions, and failed previous PTCA. Apart from the nondilatable lesion, all indications warrant randomized trials to verify superior clinical results of laser angioplasty as compared to standard PTCA.

AMRO-TRIAL

In September 1991 the Academic Medical Center (Amsterdam) and the Thoraxcenter (Rotterdam) initiated a cooperative randomized study of the efficacy of ELCA versus PTCA in the treatment of long (>10 mm) coronary stenoses or occlusions. The study included 308 patients. Laser angioplasty was followed by balloon dilatation in 98% of the laser-treated patients. The study failed to show a beneficial effect of laser treatment on acute success and on the incidence of restenosis at 6 months.[10]

COSTS

The costs that add to the standard PTCA costs are:

Laser system US $200,000–250,000
Laser catheter US $1,000–1,700

Only in stand-alone laser interventions are the costs of a balloon catheter avoided. An overall cost analysis on a per-patient basis has not yet been conducted. However, the success and complication rates do not suggest major differences in hospital stay and reinterventions as compared to conventional PTCA.

DISCUSSION

The clinical results achieved with coronary excimer laser angioplasty document the safety and feasibility of the method. The overall success rates are comparable to the results of balloon angioplasty. Possible indications for the primary use of laser angioplasty are lesions associated with a reduced success rate or high incidence of complications using conventional balloon angioplasty. However, controlled studies are warranted to document superior outcome using laser angioplasty. The incidence of restenosis is not reduced by laser angioplasty with the current technology. The registry data for restenosis are not sufficient, because the follow-up in all three registries is incomplete. However, smaller trials with a high follow-up rate confirmed restenosis rates following excimer laser angioplasty of 47% to 48%.[11]

Despite these interim results, there is an enormous potential for considerable improvements. Laser angioplasty represents a complex technology that is in the development stages. The capacity of systems with reduced pressure wave formation and with the ability to detect the target tissue await further experimental and clinical studies.

FUTURE DEVELOPMENTS

Smooth Excimer Laser Coronary Angioplasty

An innovative excimer laser system (MAX Fiberscan, Technolas, Munich, Germany) couples the laser beam sequentially into one of 8 or 12 fiber sectors of the catheter device, thus reducing the area irradiated and the amount of mass explosion per each single shot (smooth excimer laser coronary angioplasty, SELCA) (Fig. 63-3). The amounts of pressure wave formation and bubble size are considerably reduced.

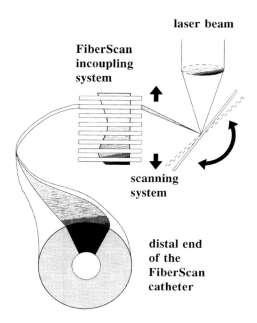

Fig. 63-3. Principle of the sequential excimer laser (SELCA).

The efficacy is similar to conventional excimer laser irradiation.[12] Initial results of human application are promising: however, the limited number of patients treated with this innovative technology does not yet allow for interpretation. The incidence of clinical complications resulting from vessel wall trauma seems to be reduced as compared to a series with conventional excimer laser angioplasty in the same institution.[13] Future trials with larger catheter size and improved catheter technology are warranted to determine the clinical value of this system and its impact on the incidence of restenosis.

Spectroscopy

A possible and promising future approach in laser technology is the use of spectroscopy as a tool to identify the target tissue.[14] Provided the ability to distinguish atherosclerotic from normal arterial tissue by their characteristic fluorescence spectra, remote spectroscopy through optical fibers can be incorporated into a "smart" laser angioplasty system. By detecting the presence of atherosclerosis, and by signaling completion of plaque ablation, fluorescence spectroscopy could guide selective laser ablation of atherosclerotic plaques. This guidance capability could result in safe and effective laser angioplasty systems.

Laser Wire

The use of a front-firing guidewire to pass total occlusions is under clinical investigation. Successful passage of occlusions that could not be passed with standard guidewires has been reported. Perforations, yet clinically insignificant, cannot be avoided.

REFERENCES

1. Srinivasan R. Ablation of polymers and biological tissue by ultraviolet lasers. Science 1986;234:559–65
2. Grundfest WS, Litvack F, Forrester JS et al. Laser ablation of human atherosclerotic plaque without adjacent tissue injury. J Am Coll Cardiol 1985;5:929–33
3. Van Leeuwen TG, Van Erven L, Meertens J, II et al. Origin of arterial wall dissections induced by pulsed excimer and mid-infrared laser ablation in the pig. J Am Coll Cardiol 1992;19:1610–8
4. Crazzolara H, Von Muench W, Rose C et al. Analysis of the acoustic response of vascular tissue irradiated by an ultraviolet laser pulse. J Appl Physics 1991;70:1847–9
5. Kvasnicka J, Nakamura F, Lange F, Geschwind HJ. Tissue ablation with excimer laser and multifiber catheter: effects of optical fiber density and fluence. J Intervent Cardiol 1992;5:263–73
6. Baumbach A, Oswald H, Kvasnicka J et al. Clinical results of coronary excimer laser angioplasty: report from the European Coronary Excimer Laser Angioplasty Registry. Eur Heart J 1994;15:89–96
7. Bittl JA, Sanborn TA, Tcheng JE et al. Clinical success, complications and restenosis rates with excimer laser coronary angioplasty. Am J Cardiol 1992;70:1533–9
8. Litvack F, Eigler NL, Margolis JR et al. Percutaneous excimer laser coronary angioplasty: results of the first consecutive 3000 patients. J Am Coll Cardiol 1994;23:323–9
9. Baumbach A, Bittl JA, Fleck E et al. Acute complications of coronary excimer laser angioplasty: a detailed analysis of multicenter results. J Am Coll Cardiol 1994;23:1305–13
10. Appelman YEA, Piek JJ, de Feyter PJ, et al. Excimer laser coronary angioplasty vs. balloon angioplasty used in long coronary lesions: The longterm results of the AMRO-trial, abstract ed. J Am Coll Cardiol 1995;25:329A
11. Karsch KR, Haase KK, Voelker W et al. Percutaneous coronary excimer laser angioplasty in patients with stable and unstable angina pectoris. Acute results and incidence of restenosis at 6 month follow-up. Circulation 1990;81:1849–59
12. Xie DY, Hassenstein Sr, Oberhoff M et al. In vitro evaluation of ablation parameters of normal and fibrous using smooth excimer laser coronary angioplasty. Lasers Surg Med 1993;13:618–24
13. Haase KK, Baumbach A, Spyridopoulos I et al. Initial clinical experience with a modified excimer laser for coronary angioplasty. Lasers Med Sci 1994;9:7–15
14. Deckelbaum, LI, Lam JK, Cabin HS et al. Discrimination of normal and atherosclerotic aorta by laser-induced fluorescence. Lasers Surg Med 1987;7:330–5

64 Holmium Lasers

Herbert J. Geschwind

The acronym laser stands for *l*ight *a*mplification by *s*timulated *e*mission of *r*adiation. The principle of laser theory was first described by Albert Einstein in 1917.[1] In 1958 Thownes and Schawlow in the United States and Prokhorov in the Soviet Union expanded on laser theory, which led to the construction of the first solid-state ruby laser in 1960 by Theodore Maiman.[2] Laser applications in medicine included ophthalmology for photocoagulation of neovascularization and tears on the retina[3] and dermatology for the treatment of pigmented lesions such as port wine stains.[4] Lasers were also used in surgical procedures, such as resection of liver tumors, to reduce bleeding. The fact that laser energy could be delivered from remote sites to areas of vascular obstruction via thin, flexible optical fibers led to the concept of arterial intervention to recanalize occluded arteries.

The earliest report on the effects of laser on atheromatous plaque in an experimental model was published in 1963 by McGuff.[5] Seventeen years later, Macruz et al.[6] showed that argon radiation could ablate calcific plaque with reduced injury on the site of application.[6] This was followed by reports by Lee et al.,[7] Abela et al.,[8] Choy et al.,[9] and Geschwind et al.[10] on the effects of various laser wavelengths on arterial tissue through various media. These preliminary experimental studies were followed by clinical applications in patients with totally occluded superficial femoral arteries by Ginsburg et al.[11] and Geschwind et al.[12] In these studies, continuous wave argon and neodymium-yttrium aluminum garnet (Nd-YAG) coupled to a single optical fiber of 0.4-mm diameter were used. The bare fiber was then replaced by a complete metal encapsulation of the distal tip leading to the "hot-tip," or laser thermal probe, system.[13] Continuous wave lasers with an emission duration of several seconds, whether delivered via bare or encapsulated fibers, resulted in a pure thermal effect with plaque vaporization and some mechanical dilation. To reduce the thermal effect, continuous wave lasers were replaced by pulsed lasers such as the ultraviolet excited dimer (excimer) laser. The stretching of the 10-ns pulse duration to 100 ns allowed greater amounts of energy to be delivered via optical fibers without destroying the coupling end of the fiber.[14]

Meanwhile, to reduce the rate of the most encountered complication, arterial wall perforation, studies were undertaken to recognize atheromatous tissue and to discriminate it from healthy tissue to focus the laser beam only on the obstructing atheromatous plaque. This was achieved using fluorescence spectroscopy.[15–17] Clinical trials have been performed first to recanalize obstructed peripheral arteries for technical and ethical reasons. Leg arteries are straight, large, and surrounded by a thick arterial wall. If perforation occurs, the clinical consequences may be mild. More space is available at the preliminary stage of technology including width and stiffness of fiber catheters. To reduce the perforation rate and increase the channel diameter created by laser irradiation, a sapphire was mounted at the laser catheter tip.[18–20] Access to coronary artery recanalization was open only when thinner, more flexible catheters were made available. Indeed, the first attempts at recanalizing coronary arteries failed and were followed by major complications including vessel wall perforation. Only when flexible, multifiber, over-the-wire guided catheters became available was it possible to apply laser technology to small, tortuous coronary vessels.[21,22]

A new method of atherectomy is now available with the main advantage of ideal fiber transmission allowing the operator to focus the high-energy tissue-ablating laser beam at the obstructing target. Many problems must be solved, however, including selection of the appropriate catheter size either to create a channel pilot through the obstruction or to debulk the artery, to avoid deleterious explosive sideeffects on the arterial wall, and to aim the beam at the diseased tissue. An avenue is open for research and development with the unique advantage of laser over mechanical atherectomy devices consisting of high energy delivery via optical technology.

RATIONALE AND MECHANISM OF ACTION

The holmium-YAG laser is a solid-state laser consisting of a rare earth, holmium, aimed at dopping an yttrium-aluminum garnet. The light is emitted at 2.1 μm of wavelength in the mid-infrared. This wavelength is not far from the optimal water absorption. The high absorption by water is considered to be an advantage, because it is the major component of all tissues, including obstructing material of the vessel lumen. The fact that this laser is a solid-state laser includes some advantages over other laser sources such as the excited dimer excimer, which is a gaseous laser, or fluid sources such as dye lasers. The reliability is higher than that of the former and the maintenance low, because no refill is needed. Indeed, gas is consumable and requires in-hospital exchanges and appropriate disposal procedures. No toxic gases are used.

The laser cavity contains a rod optically pumped with a flashlamp. The pulse rate is slow at 5 Hz, which provides adequate cooling time to minimize the potential for thermal effects. The equipment size is small and light with improved mobility. The system does not require a warm-up, alignment, or calibration period before use. Because of the solid-state technology, the system is easier to build and therefore less expensive than other lasers. An average power of 20 W is obtained with energy of 4 J/pulse maximum at a pulse length of 250 μs. The system is air cooled and self-contained and requires a single-phase 220 V/20 A circuit. The mid-infrared wavelength is readily transmitted through thin flexible silica optical fibers compatible with human coronary interventional catheters. The fibers are low-OH-fused silica fibers with a low hydroxyl content. The absorption coefficient in pure water is 30 cm^{-1}, and the depth of penetration is 333 μm. Laser energy is delivered in the free-running mode.

Tissue is removed by the two-component ablation process. In vascular obstructions, the calcified deposits are not organized but consist of salts embedded in a soft-component matrix of lipids and cross-linked proteins. The soft component is vaporized readily by laser irradiation and heated fast enough to generate superheated vapor, which rapidly expands, exerting force on the salt granules. The latter become dislodged and are accelerated out of the crater. Because the hot material is removed rapidly, much of the deposited heat is carried out of the crater before it can be transferred to the adjacent tissue via thermal diffusion. A mechanism of action similar to that observed during excimer laser irradiation may also play a major role. Fast vapor bubble expansion and implosion within the artery were observed and caused microsecond dilation and invagination after each pulse. This effect is thought to be related with the deep damage induced after irradiation on the arterial wall. The latter consisted of internal elastic lamina ruptures, dissections, and necrosis.[23] Holmium-YAG laser showed selectivity for atheroma ablation as compared with normal tissue. The mechanism is likely not to be due to preferential absorption, which is the case with dye lasers, because of the presence of carotenoid in atheromatous tissue.[24] It may be related not only to vaporization but also to liquefaction, mechanical failure, ejection of bulk material, or an explosion-like process including plasma formation or photomechanical dissolutions. Acoustic shock or pressure waves, which are thought to play a role in the ablation process, have been identified and measured.[25] We have also shown that this laser is the only one to demonstrate efficacy with the delivery tip positioned at a distance from the target.[25]

EXPERIMENTAL BACKGROUND

Early studies on arterial tissue have shown that this laser source delivered through silica optical fibers ablated calcified and noncalcified tissue in air and saline in a noncontact mode. Early in vivo healing studies in normal canine carotid arteries showed minimal chronic sequelae at 3 weeks.[26] Later studies confirmed that tissue could be ablated and that ablation thresholds depended on the amount of calcification (Fig. 64-1). Minimal thermal effect was seen in the intima and media, but a greater effect was observed in the adventitia. The thermal effect can be reduced, however, by shortening the pulse width or by limiting the total energy delivered. It was con-

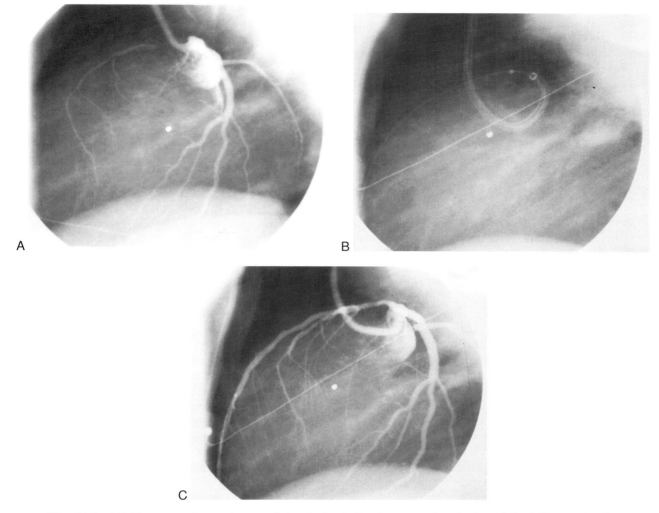

Fig. 64-1. (A) Coronary cineangiogram (lateral view) showing a total occlusion of the left anterior descending artery. **(B)** Same patient after crossing of the lesion with a 0.014″ (diameter, 1.7 mm) guidewire and positioning of the laser catheter tip against the entry of the occlusion. **(C)** Final result after laser irradiation without additional balloon dilation (laser stand-alone therapy).

cluded that controlled ablation of both normal and atherosclerotic vascular tissue can be accomplished with this wavelength.[27] Another study showed that calcific and fibrotic aortic segments could be successfully ablated and that occluded arteries in amputated legs could be recanalized without traumatic effect to the arterial wall.[28]

Cavitation bubbles could be measured during excimer, dye, or holmium-YAG laser irradiation in blood. They expanded in 75 to 250 μs and achieved varying diameters from 700 μm to 2.5 mm, depending on the energy delivered. Collapse of the bubbles also generated acoustic transients, which varied inversely with distance from the bubble center. The acoustic transients had a very high pressure ranging between 100 and 1,200 atm. They also were related to perforation,

dissection, or other unwanted tissue effects during laser angioplasty.[29] Studies from our laboratory showed that shock waves were generated by all pulsed lasers under investigation. The magnitude of shock waves was closely related to the tissue ablation efficiency with holmium-YAG. This wavelength could ablate tissue at a distance from the target in blood medium. Histology showed that all three lasers could create smooth-edged craters with minimal coagulation necrosis but that holmium-YAG as well as pulsed dye lasers ablated selectively atheroma.[30]

The mechanical effects of excimer and holmium-YAG lasers were visualized in an in vitro agar model containing lipid and calcified inclusions. Holmium-YAG laser irradiation created dissection-like explosive expansion of the inclusions, which were significantly related to the applied energy. This was not the case with excimer irradiation, the effect of which was not significant. It was concluded from these experimental studies that holmium-YAG irradiation can create target tissue dissections or perforations, whereas excimer laser ablates tissue with less traumatic effect.[31] The consequences of these laser-induced effects on the arterial wall were studied in our laboratory in normal rabbit arteries. The sites irradiated with excimer or holmium lasers via multifiber over-the-wire catheters presented with similar features consisting of shedding of the endothelium, disorganization of internal elastic lamina, localized necrosis of vascular smooth muscle cells, and fissures in the media. However, severity of lesions was greater after holmium than after excimer irradiation[32] (Plate 64-1).

In the early 1980s, it was thought that atherectomy could reduce the high restenosis rate observed after dilation resulting at least partially from vessel wall overstretching. Recent experimental studies on the long-term consequences of laser irradiation on the arterial wall failed to confirm this hypothesis. Our group has shown that 28 days after excimer or holmium laser irradiation on normal arterial rabbit wall intimal proliferation was observed. This fact was confirmed by further studies showing that after holmium irradiation, the amount of smooth muscle cells undergoing DNA synthesis in the intima was significantly increased after 7 and 14 days as well as in the medial layer along with a disruption of the internal elastic lamina. The proliferative response resulted in a significant increase of intimal thickening 6 weeks after laser ablation (Plate 64-2). This response appeared to be smaller after excimer irradiation.[33] Thus, a sufficient number of experiments have been conducted to show that pulsed holmium laser irradiation is able to ablate hard tissue with smooth-edged craters but also with deleterious side effects on the surrounding arterial wall, which may be related to fast-expanding and collapsing cavitation bubbles generating powerful shock waves.

INSTRUMENTATION

The laser source consisted of a holmium-YAG flashlamp excited pulsed laser (Eclipse 2100, Eclipse Surgical Technologies, Palo Alto, California) coupled to 1.4-, 1.5-, 1.7-, 2.0-, or more recently, 1.2-mm diameter catheters consisting of 26 to 37 optical fibers of 100 μm each or 40 to 49 fibers of 50 μm, each concentrically arranged around a 0.018″ central lumen for the passage of a conventional angioplasty guidewire. The energy delivered was 250 to 600 mJ/

pulse corresponding to a fluence of 1.0 to 1.7 J/mm^3 at a frequency of 5 Hz. The length of the catheters was 135 cm. The laser system is compact, easy to use, light enough to be transportable on wheels, and easy to store in the catheter laboratory.

OPERATIVE TECHNIQUE

A control coronary angiogram was achieved using an 8-F large lumen or 9-F guiding catheter positioned in the ostium of the target vessel via a percutaneous femoral arterial approach. The obstruction was crossed with a conventional guidewire to the distal vessel. The mutifiber catheter was then advanced over the wire against the entry of the lesion under continuous fluoroscopic control. Care was taken not to apply high pressure at the proximal end of the catheter to avoid any mechanical Dotter effect. Minimal pressure should be applied at the catheter, yet enough to maintain contact between the distal end and the ablation target. The catheter was gently advanced through the lesion with emissions of 2 or 3 seconds each to minimize the side effects of laser irradiation. After each irradiation, administration of intracoronary nitrates was recommended to prevent any spasm from occurring. After penetration of the lesion was completed, the catheter was pulled back, and control angiograms were performed to assess the effects of laser irradiation. If no significant enlargement of the obstruction could be obtained, the procedure was repeated. In case of satisfactory result with a less than 30% residual stenosis, the procedure was terminated. If a significant residual stenosis was evidenced, additional balloon angioplasty was performed. Care should also be taken to advance the laser catheter at a slow pace to allow the laser to ablate the optimal amount of obstructing tissue given the relatively low depth of penetration of each pulse.[34,35]

Pretreatment was not different from that commonly used in balloon angioplasty. Antiplatelet drugs were administered orally 24 hours before the procedure, and heparin at 10,000 U was administered before, during, and if required, 24 hours after the procedure to maintain effective anticoagulation. The arterial sheath was removed 4 to 6 or 24 hours after termination of the procedure. Patients were discharged 2 or 3 days after the procedure and kept on aspirin for at least 6 months. Follow-up consisted of clinical assessment every 2 or 3 months including exercise stress tests. In case of evidence of myocardial ischemia, repeat coronary angiography was performed. Most patients had a routine repeat angiogram at 6 months.

RESULTS

Our group presented a comparative study between excimer and holmium coronary angioplasty in 46 and 40 patients, respectively. Laser success was defined as a greater than 20% reduction in stenosis without the occurrence of a major complication such as death, myocardial infarction, or emergency coronary artery bypass graft. The success rate was lower in holmium- than in excimer-treated patients (55 vs. 72%). However, procedure success defined as less than 30% residual stenosis with laser alone or a combination of laser and dilation was higher after holmium than after excimer laser angioplsaty (98 vs. 87%). The success rate was highest in saphenous vein grafts but lower in long than in short lesions. The procedure success rate was similar in calcified and noncalcified lesions (Plate 64-3). The stand-alone laser success rate was significantly lower with holmium than with excimer laser. In terms of complications, acute closure occurred less frequently after holmium irradiation. This was also the case for dissections, which occurred in only 7% of holmium patients as compared with 28% of excimer patients.[22] A multicenter registry report showed that in 588 patients the laser success rate was 79% with a mean percent stenosis decrease from 89 to 57%, whereas clinical procedure success was achieved in 95% of lesions. Perforations occurred in 1.6%, dissections in 4.7%, thrombosis in 1.7%, death in 0.3%, myocardial infarction in 1.7%, and emergency bypass surgery in 3.1.[36] Other reports showed that holmium laser angioplasty may be an appropriate indication for thrombolysis in acute myocardial infarction and in unstable angina; a 96% procedure success rate was reported for these patients.[37]

Angiographic follow-up is now available for a significant number of patients. In our series of patients, the restenosis rate defined as greater than 50% residual stenosis was 67 and 71% for holmium and excimer, respectively. This figure was 42% in the multicenter registry and 43% in the group of patients treated for unstable angina.

Is there a special niche for laser angioplasty? Current indications include all complex lesions but, more specifically, total occlusions, provided that the guidewire can cross the obstruction before irradiation; suboptimal results after dilation; diffuse, calcified lesions; ostial lesions; saphenous vein grafts; and restenosis. Facilitation may be obtained after laser irradiation by a process that is not yet fully understood. The deleterious effect of shock waves may be in some cases beneficial, inasmuch as it may on the one hand induce damage to the arterial wall but on the other hand remodel the hard tissue of the vessel wall by splitting and fracturing calcium, thus softening tissue and increasing the wall compliance. This in turn may allow for improved results after dilation at a lower inflation pressure.

Cost-effectiveness is the major drawback of laser technology, because the source is still expensive and additional balloon angioplasty should be performed in 80% of cases. However, it may be anticipated that if improved results are obtained and more investment is made for research and development the technology may be more widely applied, thus reducing the cost of both the laser machine and the disposable.

DISCUSSION

Laser technology raised great expectations, which were followed by great disappointment.[38] This was due to the fact that this technology was unable to demonstrate any superiority over conventional balloon dilation except in few cases. However, this was the case also for other atherectomy devices, the results of which in terms of early outcome and restenosis were at least similar to those observed after dilation.

Laser angioplasty has the unique advantage of tissue ablation with a very high energy, freely transmitted via thin optical fibers. The beam may be focused on the target with improved guidance capabilities such as spectroscopic detection of diseased tissue. The multifiber catheter technology was a breakthrough in laser angioplasty because it allowed free access to the small, tortuous coronary arteries over a guidewire. However, this may not be the ultimate stage of the technology. Improved beam targetting may be anticipated using new optical devices, which may be expected to allow for smaller sized catheters to be introduced into the coronary tree. This in turn would reduce ischemia induced by obstructing devices. Presently, given the fact that with multifiber catheters the channel size is equal to that of the catheter, we are faced with the issue of debulking arteries with large catheters or creating pilot channels for subsequent dilation with small catheters. This should not be the case in the future. The side effects of pulsed laser irradiation in terms of shock waves should be reduced even though they may be beneficial in some cases, as mentioned previously. This reduction is already underway with the multiplex system, which can deliver laser energy sequentially, reducing the cavitation bubble size. However, before reducing bubble size, caution must be taken to make sure that the bubble size, expansion, and collapse are not related to ablation efficiency.

The choice of the appropriate laser source is not

yet well established. Holmium as well as excimer irradiation are effective and induce mechanical side effects on the vessel wall. It is noteworthy that a discrepancy exists between experimental data showing great damage to the wall and clinical observations which shows a reduced rate of dissections. More research should be undertaken in laser source equipment to obtain high energy delivery with small, compact, light machines. Catheter delivery should be improved and drugs made available to reduce proliferation. Only at this stage may we be able to evaluate the benefit/risk/cost ratio of pulsed laser angioplasty.

REFERENCES

1. Einstein A. Zur quantentheorie der Strahlung. Phys Z 1917;18:121–8
2. Maiman T. Stimulated optical radiation in ruby. Nature 1960;187:493–4
3. Koester CJ, Snitzer E, Campbell CJ, Rittler MC. Experimental laser retina coagulator. J Opt Soc Am 1962; 52:67
4. Apfelberg DP, Maser RM, Lash H. Argon laser treatment of cutaneous vascular abnormalities, progress report. Ann Plastic Surg 1978;1:14–8
5. Mc Guff PE, Bushnell D, Soroff HS, Deterling RA. Studies of the surgical applications of laser light. Surg Forum 1963;14:143–5
6. Macruz R, Martins JRM, Tupinamba A, Lopes EA. Therapeutic possibilities of laser beams in atheromas. Arg Brass Cardiol 1980;34:9–12
7. Lee G, Ikeda RM, Kozina J, Mason DT. Laser dissolution of coronary atherosclerotic obstruction. Am Heart J 1981;102:1074–5
8. Abela GS, Conti CR, Geiser EA, Normann S. The effect of laser radiation on atheromatous plaque: a preliminary report. Am J Cardiol 1982
9. Choy DSJ, Stertzer S, Rotterdam HL, Sharrock N. Transluminal laser catheter angioplasty. Am J Cardiol 1982;50:1206–8
10. Geschwind HJ, Boussignac G, Teisseire B et al. Laser angioplasty. Effects on coronary stenosis. Lancet 1983; 2:1334
11. Ginsburg R, Kirr DS, Guthaner P, Tohl J. Salvage of an ischemic limb by laser angioplasty: description of a new technique. Clin Cardiol 1984;7:54–8
12. Geschwind HJ, Boussignac G, Teisseire B et al. Percutaneous transluminal laser angioplasty in man. Lancet 1984;1:844
13. Sanborn TA, Faxon DP, Haudenschild CC, Ryan TJ. Experimental angioplasty: circumferential distribution of laser thermal energy with a laser probe. J Am Coll Cardiol 1985;5:934–8
14. Grundfest WS, Litvack F, Forrester J, Goldenberg T. Laser ablation of human atherosclerotic plaque without adjacent tissue injury. J Am Coll Cardiol 1985;5: 929–33
15. Deckelbaum LI, Lau JK, Cobin HS, Clubb KS. Discrimination of normal and atherosclerotic aorta by laser induced fluorescence. Lasers Surg Med 1987;7: 330–5
16. Leon MB, Lu DY, Prevosti LG, Macy W. Human arterial surface fluorescence: atherosclerotic plaque identification and effects of laser thrombus ablation. J Am Coll Cardiol 1988;12:94–102
17. Geschwind HJ, Dubois-Randé JL, Shafton E et al. Percutaneous pulsed laser-assisted balloon angioplasty guided by spectroscopy. Am Heart J 1989;117:1147–52
18. Fourrier JL, Marache P, Brunetaud JM et al. Laser recanalization of peripheral arteries by contact sapphire in man. Circulation 1986;74:II-204
19. Geschwind HJ, Blair JD, Mongkolsmai D et al. Development and experimental application of contact probe catheter for laser angioplasty. J Am Coll Cardiol 1987; 9:101–7
20. Cumberland DC, Oakley GDG, Smith GH, Taylor DI. Percutaneous laser-assisted coronary angioplasty. Lancet 1986;II:214
21. Litvack F, Grundfest W, Eigler N et al. Percutaneous excimer laser coronary angioplasty. Lancet 1989;2: 102–3
22. Geschwind HJ, Nakamura F, Kvasnicka J, Dubois-Randé JL. Excimer and Holmium YAG laser coronary angioplasty. Am Heart J 1993;125:510–22
23. van Erven L, van Leeuwen TG, Post MJ et al. Mid-infrared pulsed laser ablation of the arterial wall: mechanical origin of acoustic wall damage and its effect on wall healing. J Thorac Cardiovasc Surg 1992;104: 1053–9
24. Prince MR, Deutsch TF, Mathews-Roth MM. Preferential light absorption in atheromas in vitro. Implication for laser angioplasty. J Clin Invest 1986;78:295–302
25. Tomaru T, Geschwind HJ, Boussignac G et al. Characteristics of shock waves induced by pulsed lasers and their effects on arterial tissue: comparison of excimer, pulsed dye and Holmium-Yag lasers. Am Heart J 1992; 123:896–904
26. Aretz HT, Butterly JR, Jewell ER et al. Effects of Holmium YSGG laser irradiation on arterial tissue: preliminary results SPIE 1989;1067:127–32
27. Kopchock GE, White RA, Tabbara M et al. Holmium YAG laser ablation of vascular tissue. Lasers Surg Med 1990;10:405–13
28. Kusniec J, Scheinowitz M, Eldar M, Battler A. The effect of pulsed Holmium YAg laser on in vitro and in vivo atherosclerotic plaque. Lasers Med Science 1992; 7:455–9
29. De la Torre R, Gregory KW. Cavitation bubbles and acoustic transients may produce dissections during laser angioplasty. J Am Coll Cardiol 1992;19:48
30. Tomaru T, Geschwind HJ, Boussignac G et al. Comparison of ablation efficacy of excimer, pulsed dye and Holmium-YAG lasers relevant to shock waves. Am Heart J 1992;123:886–95
31. Asada M, Kvasnicka J, Geschwind HJ. Effects of pulsed lasers on agar model simulation of the arterial wall. Lasers Surg Med 1993;13:405–11
32. Nakamura F, Kvasnicka J, Levame M et al. Acute response of the arterial wall to pulsed laser irradiation. Lasers Surg Med 1993;13:412–20
33. Hassenstein S, Hanke H, Kamenz J et al. Vascular injury and time course of smooth muscle cell proliferation after experimental holmium laser angioplasty. Circulation 1992;86:1575–83

34. Geschwind HJ, Tomaru T, Nakamura F, Kvasnicka J. Holmium YAG laser coronary angioplasty with multi-fiber catheters. J Interven Cardiol 1991;4:171–9

35. Topaz O: Holmium laser coronary thrombolysis—a new treatment modality for revascularization in acute myocardial infarction: review. J Clin Lasers Med Surg 1992;10:427–31

36. Knopf WD, Parr KL, Moses JW et al. Multicenter reg-istry report: holmium laser angioplasty in coronary arteries. Circulation 1992;86:I.510

37. de Marchena E, Mallon S, Topaz O et al. Unstable angina treated with laser angioplasty. J Am Coll Car-diol 1993;21:196A

38. Geschwind HJ: Great expectations and disappoint-ment with laser angioplasty. Am J Cardiol 1993;72:372

65 Lasers and Balloons

J. Richard Spears

HISTORY

Incorporation of a source of electromagnetic energy within a balloon potentially greatly increases the number of basic approaches to the performance of percutaneous transluminal coronary angioplasty (PTCA). In the early 1980s, for example, I suggested the use of low-level laser radiation within a balloon to activate a photosensitive material that localized selectively within atheromatous plaques after intravenous injection[1] (Spears, U.S. Patent No. 4, 512, 762)

Hussein during this period proposed the use of laser radiation at a high power density to vaporize atheromatous lesions through a translucent balloon under angioscopic control (Hussein, U.S. Patent No. 4,470,407). Although different combinations of electromagnetic energy and a balloon might be used to produce a wide variety of tissue effects, the relevant technique that has been studied the most to date is thermal balloon angioplasty, principally, laser balloon angioplasty (LBA)[2,3] (Spears, U.S. Patent No. 4,799,479).

In industry, remodeling of polymeric materials is facilitated by the conjunctive use of heat and pressure. Although the simultaneous medical use of these two physical modalities was described in previous centuries for achieving hemostasis in wounds, bipolar electrocautery represents the first technique employing heat and pressure that gained widespread clinical use in the early part of this century. Sigel and colleagues[4] several decades ago were the first to describe the use of thermal coagulation, as delivered with an electrocautery device, to anastomose coapted vessel edges experimentally without sutures. Since that time, a great deal of interest has been shown in the use of laser energy to provide "sutureless" anastomoses.[5–7] By analogy, I posited that laser/thermal energy applied during balloon inflation could be used to prevent or to treat arterial dissections during angioplasty. Additional, perhaps more important, tissue responses to LBA were found serendipitously and include remodeling of occluding thrombus into a nonobstructive film, reduction of arterial recoil, and potentially favorable alteration of luminal surface thrombogenicity.

Preliminary clinical coronary artery studies demonstrated that LBA was effective in increasing luminal diameter and morphology when applied after conventional balloon angioplasty that resulted in a suboptimal result.[8] In contrast, when LBA was applied to a lesion immediately after an acutely successful conventional balloon angioplasty procedure, defined as a less than 50% residual stenosis, the 6-month angiographic results were not improved compared to those of a small control balloon angioplasty group.[9] The overall restenosis rate, defined as a greater than 50% stenosis on long-term follow-up angiogram, was similar for elective LBA groups and the control PTCA group. Therefore, it appeared that the procedure might be suitable primarily as a niche technology for the treatment of impending or overt acute closure induced by balloon angioplasty. A multicenter trial of the use of LBA for the treatment of acute closure that was refractory to a prolonged balloon inflation was therefore initiated. As discussed herein, LBA appeared to be an acutely effective procedure for treatment of most cases of balloon angioplasty-induced acute closure, although the angiographic restenosis rate associated with the use of the procedure in this clinical setting was relatively high.[10]

As discussed later in this chapter, two potentially important mechanisms of restenosis following LBA have been identified by our group experimentally.[11,12] A method was developed for application, during LBA, of a concentrated film of heparin mounted on the external surface of the balloon that has recently been shown to inhibit both such mechanisms experimentally. To test the hypothesis that LBA with local heparin therapy improves the safety and efficacy of angioplasty, a randomized phase II trial of the new procedure versus conventional balloon angioplasty has been designed and will be conducted following completion of a Food and Drug Administration (FDA)-approved Phase I clinical trial of the procedure with a device made in my laboratory.

RATIONALE AND MECHANISM OF ACTION

At an electron microscopic level, laser/thermal coagulation of the arterial wall experimentally results in interdigitation of fibrillary subunits of collagen across juxtaposed planes of tissue.[13] Thermal "welding" of separated tissue layers may result from other mechanisms as well,[7] but it is likely that breakage of noncovalent bonds of proteins during heating and alteration of their tertiary molecular structure, with formation of new bonds between previously separated proteins on cooling, represents one type of mechanism responsible for this effect.[14]

In a series of in vitro studies of separated and reapposed layers of human postmortem atherosclerotic aortic sections,[15-17] the relationship between temperature history and efficacy of tissue welding was defined. A continuous wave neodymium-yttrium aluminum garnet (Nd-YAG) laser operating at 1.06 μm was used for effecting tissue welding because of the known penetration depth, approximately 2 mm, at this wavelength through a variety of soft tissues. For a laser exposure duration of 20 seconds, a minimum temperature of approximately 80°C was required to fuse separated plaque-media layers of human postmortem atherosclerotic sections. The strength of the welds achieved was found to increase in a linear manner with higher peak temperatures to a maximum of approximately 150°C. At temperatures beyond the latter, vaporization of the solid, nonaqueous components of the tissue occurs. Additional in vitro studies[18,19] demonstrated the following: Repetitive fusion of layers could be performed without a reduc-

tion in the strength of the welds achieved; a tissue pressure of at least 0.5 bar facilitated tissue bonding; the tissue fusion could be performed for a variety of different types of plaque; the presence of blood between tissue layers had little effect on weld strength, in contrast to the suggestion of an early study; and exposures longer than 20 seconds produced only marginally greater weld strength.

The combination of thermal exposure over a 60°C to 100°C range during balloon inflation was found experimentally in vivo to produce a larger luminal diameter compared to the use of the same balloon without thermal exposure,[18,20] in the absence of fusion of separated tissue layers. The mechanism responsible for this observation has not been well defined, but it is likely that remodeling of connective tissue occurs under these conditions and results in a reduction of elastic recoil. Histologically, straightening of the internal elastic lamella, which normally has a ruffled appearance without intraluminal distending pressure, has been observed. In addition, loss of smooth muscle cell viability and associated loss of vasoconstrictor potential following thermal exposure may contribute to a larger luminal diameter compared to the use of distending pressure alone.

Compared to other soft tissues, thrombus strongly absorbs a variety of laser wavelengths, including 1.06 μm radiation, as a result of the presence of hemoglobin.[19] When the arterial wall is heated to 80°C to 90°C during a given Nd-YAG laser exposure, thrombus is heated to 100°C. The heat of evaporization of water prevents a significantly greater temperature rise within thrombus until the tissue is fully desiccated. In clinical practice, at the laser doses used, large occluding thrombi are probably partially dehydrated; equally important, the combination of heat and pressure is more effective than the application of pressure alone in remodeling the tissue into a nonobstructive film adherent to the luminal surface.

The results of in vitro studies suggest that, when thrombus is heated to 100°C, surface thrombogenicity on subsequent exposure to nonanticoagulated blood is reduced, very likely as a result of thermal denaturation of thrombin.[21] In contrast, a peak temperature of only 70°C was found to have no effect on the thrombogenicity of thrombus. Borst el al.[22] similarly demonstrated that in vitro platelet deposition on mechanically injured umbilical arteries was markedly reduced by prior heating of the tissue to 100°C. A subtle increase in platelet deposition was noted following tissue heating to 55°C, an observation that is similar to that in a study of burro aortic collagen.[23] The temperature dependence of tissue on its subsequent thrombogenicity is likely to be more complex in vivo, but experimental studies by Abela et al.[24] are consistent with in vitro observations.

Successful application of LBA in sealing intimal flaps and dissections, reducing arterial recoil, and remodeling thrombus in theory would acutely improve most cases when PTCA, despite full balloon inflation, produces a suboptimal result. At the time of the performance of the elective LBA clinical trials, optimism prevailed that improvement in luminal morphology with any of a variety of new angioplasty devices would translate into a significant reduction in the incidence of chronic restenosis, but the long-term results of all devices suggest that an adequate morphologic result, although a necessary prerequisite, is a poor predictor of restenosis.

INSTRUMENTATION

Laser Source

A 50-w continuous wave Nd-YAG Quantronix System 1500 Medical Laser System operating at 1.06 μm has been used for all clinical LBA studies. Although the laser cavity is cooled with a closed internal system of deionized water, a heat exchanger for maintaining a constant temperature of the coolant employs air rather than water, thereby obviating the necessity for use of an external water supply. The output of the laser is coupled to the 105-μm core of a silica fiberoptic, which is connected to the fiberoptic within the LBA catheter via a jumper cable with standard SMA fiberoptic connectors. The most important safety mechanism incorporated in the laser, which is operated under computer control, is a thermally activated shutoff device, which automatically terminates the laser exposure in the event of inadvertent fiberoptic fracture.

Laser radiation as a thermal energy source has been attractive for at least four reasons. (1) Tissue heating results from direct absorption of laser radiation by the tissue, so that within the penetration depth of the radiation, rapid temperature rises can be achieved, in comparison with indirect methods of tissue heating, such as the use of radiofrequency or microwave energy delivery, wherein the fluid contents of the balloon are heated and temperature rise in tissue occurs in large part by relatively slow thermal diffusion. Thicker neointimal flaps may therefore be amenable to treatment with a laser energy source, and, equally important, a relatively long period of thermal exposure needed with alternative energy sources (on the order of several minutes compared to 20 seconds used with the laser energy source) increases the potential for patient discomfort, myocardial ischemia, and heating of blood in contact with the balloon. (2) The axial length of tissue that is heated adjacent to the balloon can be relatively well defined, because the balloon is transparent to Nd-YAG laser radiation at 1.06 μm, and heating of the balloon and its contents occurs only by thermal diffusion from the heated tissue; by contrast, heating fluid within the balloon may produce excessive temperature rises at the proximal and distal ends of the balloon because of convection of the fluid, and heating all tissue along a balloon 2 cm in length may be excessive; loss of endothelium from thermal injury over a relatively long length may hamper its regeneration. (3) Fiberoptic transmission of laser radiation provides the greatest energy concentration per unit cross section of the delivery system, compared to alternative energy sources, thereby allowing the development of a low-profile thermal balloon catheter system. The higher tissue temperatures that also can be achieved may have utility in some cases of acute closure, should lower temperatures prove ineffective. (4) Selective absorption of laser radiation by thrombus allows greater heating, with desiccation and more effective remodeling, of this tissue compared to other tissues, unlike nonspecific heating techniques. These potential advantages may well offset the potentially increased cost of current laser energy sources compared to alternative thermal energy sources.

LBA Catheter

In studies sponsored by USCI, the LBA catheter was a 4.3-F triple-lumen device, with a separate channel for the fiberoptic in addition to the inflation/deflation and guidewire channels. The fiberoptic terminated in a helical diffusing tip for propagation of both the Nd-YAG laser radiation and a reference helium-neon (He-Ne) laser beam in an azimuthal direction. The first-generation catheter incorporated a diffusing tip that was both relatively short (<5 mm in axial length) and eccentric, while the second-generation catheter incorporated a diffusing tip that was nearly as long as the 2-cm balloon (Fig. 65-1). A gold coating at the proximal and distal ends of the balloon was therefore used in the latter to prevent potential absorption of radiation by blood. The noncompliant balloon material, polyethylene terephthalate (PET) was both transparent to 1.06 μm radiation and relatively unaffected by temperatures of 100°C.

A decremental laser power format was used in all clinical studies, because this approach was found experimentally to optimize the rate of temperature rise within arterial tissue, while minimizing the total

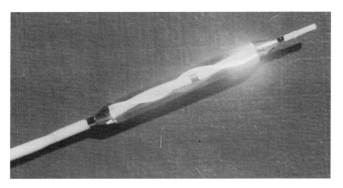

Fig. 65-1. Spears USCI LBA catheter. Within a polyethylene terephthalate (PET) balloon mounted on a 4.3-F shaft, a helical diffusing tip is used to direct continuous wave Nd-YAG laser radiation laterally about the circumference and length of the balloon. The balloon and its contents are transparent to the radiation, so that tissue heating occurs primarily by absorption of 1.06-μm radiation by the tissue.

dose administered. Laser powers, for a 3.0-mm balloon, ranged from 10 to 35 W, while the total 20-second laser dose ranged from 235 to 450 J. Peak tissue temperatures of approximately 90°C to 100°C were sought with each laser dose, although somewhat higher temperatures were probably achieved in the first group of patients, in whom the higher doses were given.

PATIENT POPULATION

The first group of LBA patients were treated electively in either a nonrandomized manner (n = 108 patients) or in a randomized trial of one of three different laser doses (n = 102 patients) versus PTCA alone (n = 33 patients). PTCA was performed initially in all patients, but in the randomized trial, a residual stenosis of less than 50% was required before randomization into the four different groups. Patients between the ages of 20 and 80 were candidates for elective LBA, as long as they were also acceptable candidates for coronary bypass surgery and did not have an exclusion criterion (left main lesion; left ventricular ejection fraction less than 30%; hemodynamic instability). Many of the patients in the nonrandomized trial were referred for LBA because of an anticipated low success rate with PTCA and therefore represented an anatomically more difficult group of patients than those in the randomized trial.

In a subsequent trial of LBA for emergency treatment of PTCA-induced acute closure, LBA was performed (n = 154 patients) only after acute closure complicating initial PTCA was refractory to a prolonged balloon inflation (at least 3 minutes and pref-

erably after longer inflations with a perfusion balloon catheter). Although exclusion criteria were similar to those of the elective trials, in practice, acute closure, including when it occurred after the patient had left the cardiac catheterization laboratory, was occasionally associated with acute transmural myocardial infarction, with associated complications such as ventricular arrhythmias, congestive heart failure, before attempted LBA reversal of the acute closure. Patients in overt cardiogenic shock were excluded from entry into the study.

PRETREATMENT

All patients were routinely premedicated with 10,000 U intravenous heparin and aspirin. Laser exposure was found to produce a variable level of substernal chest discomfort without specific analgesic premedication. Nonanesthetizing doses of fentanyl (i.e., 30 to 50 μg intravenously) given 5 minutes before LBA were found to be effective for prevention of the discomfort, which otherwise occurred usually during the last 15 seconds of the 20-second laser exposure.

OPERATIVE TECHNIQUE AND TIPS

In all cases, LBA was performed as an add-on procedure with a balloon of the same dimensions as prior PTCA, and an attempt was invariably made to achieve an optimal angiographic result with PTCA before performance of LBA. This procedure was followed to evaluate the acute efficacy of LBA, with each patient thereby serving as his or her own control. From a technical viewpoint, however, LBA can be performed during the first balloon inflation.

Immediately after positioning the LBA balloon catheter across a lesion of interest, normal saline warmed to 37°C is injected through the guide catheter to hemodilute blood during balloon inflation, thereby trapping normal saline at the origin of side branches and at the ends of the balloon, to avoid the potential for coagulation of blood at these locations. Normal saline is additionally injected through the guidewire channel during the laser exposure to prevent excessive heating of the latter, which might otherwise result in bonding of the material comprising the central channel to the guidewire.

Following a 20-second laser exposure, a period of approximately 20 seconds of continued balloon inflation allows the tissue temperature to normalize, to avoid the potential for thermal shrinkage. The total period of balloon occlusion employed during performance of LBA is therefore approximately 1 minute. Additional laser doses were given in the USCI studies if the LBA balloon length (2 cm) was insufficient to span the length of a long lesion. In a few cases, a higher laser dose was administered if the initial laser dose did not improve luminal dimensions beyond those of PTCA.

POST-LBA MANAGEMENT AND FOLLOW-UP

Patients were managed medically after LBA in a manner analogous to that following successful PTCA. In most cases, heparin was given intravenously overnight at approximately 1,000 U/hr. No additional anticoagulation, except for daily aspirin, was routinely given, including to patients in the acute closure study.

All patients were evaluated clinically at 3 and 6 months after angioplasty, and an attempt was made to obtain a coronary angiogram 6 months after the procedure. Angiography was performed earlier if indicated clinically, athough the first 15 patients treated electively were studied angiographically 1 month after the procedure as part of the protocol.

RESULTS

Complications

In the patient groups treated electively with LBA (n = 210), there were no deaths and no transmural myocardial infarctions (Table 65-1). Two patients

Table 65-1. Elective LBA (n = 210)

	n	%
Acute success rate[a]		
Initial PTCA	156	74
LBA	201	96
In-hospital complications		
Death	0	0
Q-wave myocardial infarction	4	1.9
CABG	3	1.4
Angiographic restenosis (QCA)[b]		
3- to 6-month follow-up (n = 210)	86	41
6-month follow-up alone (n = 116)	55	47

[a] Acute success rate = less than 50% residual stenosis and absence of significant in-hospital complications.

[b] Angiographic restenosis = 50% or greater diameter stenosis by computer analysis of digitized cineangiograms. The reference segment used was the greater of either the proximal or distal segment.

Abbreviations: QCA, quantitative coronary angiography.

Table 65-2. Emergent LBA for Refractory Acute Closure During PTCA (n = 154 attempts)

	n	%
Acute success rate		
Technical success rate[a]	147	96
Clinical success rate[b]	122	83
In-hospital complications		
Death		
Successful LBA	0	0
Unsuccessful LBA[c]	2	1.3
After bypass surgery	1	0.6
Device-related	0	0
Total	2	1.3
Q-wave myocardial infarction[d]	9	5.8
Bypass surgery	15	9.7
Angiographic restenosis (QCA)[e]		
6 month follow-up (n = 33)	21	64

[a] Technical success = delivery of one or more laser doses.

[b] Clinical success = less than 50% residual stenosis and no in-hospital complications (death, myocardial infarction, bypass surgery).

[c] Unsuccessful LBA = 50% or more residual stenosis.

[d] Includes myocardial infarction occurring before LBA (e.g., out-of-lab acute closure).

[e] Angiographic restenosis = more than 50% diameter stenosis by computer analysis of digitized cineangiograms.

underwent uneventful coronary bypass surgery for suboptimal angiographic results. In the group of patients (122 of the 154 patients) in whom LBA was angiographically acutely successful (<50% residual stenosis and no evidence of ischemia) in reversing PTCA-induced refractory acute closure, there were no deaths (Table 65-2). In contrast, four deaths occurred in the angiographically unsuccessful group of patients (n = 32) treated with LBA for PTCA-induced acute closure; three of the deaths occurred after emergency coronary bypass surgery.

Acute Angiographic Results

All cineangiograms were digitized and analyzed with an automated luminal edge detection algorithm for objective measurement of luminal diameter.[25,26] In the patient group treated electively with LBA in a nonrandomized manner, 29 of 102 patients had a greater than 50% stenosis after initial PTCA. A post-PTCA mean diameter stenosis in this group of 58% was reduced to a mean of 38% after LBA. The improvement in luminal dimensions was less for the group of patients with initially successful PTCA; a mean post-PTCA stenosis of 35% was reduced to a

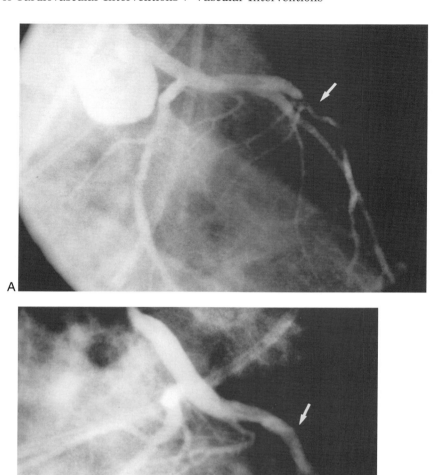

Fig. 65-2. (**A**) A severe, complex lesion in the left anterior descending coronary artery was noted (*arrow*) before PTCA. (**B**) Following PTCA, acute closure (*arrow* indicates location of 100% stump occlusion superimposed over adjacent large diagonal branch; the latter appears larger than in Fig. **A** because of the use of a smaller field size of the image intensifier) appeared to result from a severe dissection, which was further complicated by retrograde thrombus formation after use of a 20-minute inflation with a perfusion balloon catheter.   (*Figure continues*)

mean of 25% after subsequent LBA. The mean lesion severity acutely during PTCA-induced acute closure was difficult to measure, because frequent severe dissections and large intraluminal filling defects produced multiple borders and nonaxisymmetric geometry, but the post-LBA mean stenosis in this group was 36% (n = 103).

Chronic Angiographic Results

The greatest loss in luminal diameter occurred between 1 month and 6 months after the procedure.

For patients treated electively with LBA, mean percent stenosis increased from 30% at 1 month (n = 42) to 48% (n = 21) at 3 months and 52% (n = 116) at 6 months. For patients treated emergently with LBA for PTCA-induced acute closure and in whom 6-month clinical follow-up was available, mean percent stenosis increased from 39% at 1 month (n = 11) to 61% (n = 17) and 65% (n = 33) at 3 and 6 months, respectively. No statistically significant difference was found in mean percent stenosis between groups of patients treated with either one of three different

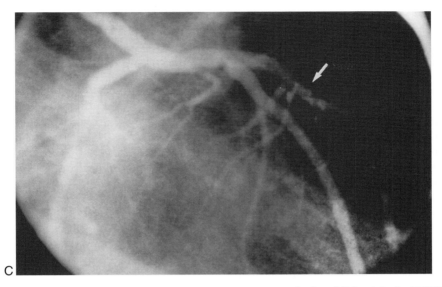

Fig. 65-2 (*continued*). **(C)** Luminal patency (arrow) was restored after LBA with the USCI device was performed in two adjacent regions within the occluded segment.

laser doses (53% for all three groups combined) or PTCA alone (45%) at the 6-month follow-up.

Angiographic restenosis, defined as greater than 50% stenosis on computer-analyzed cineangiograms obtained 6 months after the procedure, was 47% (n = 116) for patients treated electively with LBA and 64% (n = 33) for patients treated emergently with the procedure for treatment of PTCA-induced acute closure.

Follow-up Clinical Events

Of the patients randomized to LBA and followed for 6 months (n = 105), 56% were event free (no death, myocardial infarction, repeat angioplasty, or surgery) and asymptomatic 6 months after the procedure, which was similar to the 54% value found for patients randomized to PTCA alone (n = 33) at this time. In contrast, only 34% of patients treated with LBA in the nonrandomized trial were event free and asymptomatic 6 months after the procedure (n = 80). Repeat revascularization procedures (either repeat PTCA or bypass surgery) were performed in 25% of nonrandomized LBA patients, 11% of patients randomized to LBA, and 15% of patients randomized to PTCA alone. In the group of patients treated emergently with LBA for PTCA-induced acute closure, 31% required a second revascularization procedure, either repeat PTCA or bypass surgery, during a 6-month follow-up period (n = 101). Mortality during the follow-up period was 4% for the acute closure group and 1% for the randomized and nonran-

domized LBA groups. The majority of deaths occurred postoperatively following bypass surgery.

CURRENT INDICATIONS

The results of the USCI LBA trials suggest that the procedure may have utility in the treatment of acute closure complicating PTCA (Fig. 65-2). Although LBA appeared to be successful in the treatment of severe arterial dissections in approximately one-half of such cases, the success rate appeared significantly greater when thrombus or elastic recoil represented the predominant mechanisms of acute closure. Experimentally, LBA has been used to eliminate coronary vasomotor reactivity and to seal arterial perforations, but these problems have not been addressed with LBA in the clinical setting. Because of the relatively high incidence of restenosis following LBA reversal of PTCA-induced acute closure, close clinical follow-up is required, and a consideration to the use of LBA as a "bridge" procedure to semielective coronary bypass surgery should be made, particularly when the post-LBA result is suboptimal.

COSTS

Should the LBA system become commercialized, the cost of the Quantronix System 1500 Medical Laser would be approximately $125,000 (U.S.), while the unit cost of LBA catheters is anticipated to be approximately $1,000.

CURRENT OUTLOOK AND POTENTIAL DEVELOPMENTS

Despite the apparent clinical utility of LBA for the treatment of PTCA-induced acute closure, the sponsor of the initial clinical trials abandoned pursuit of additional costly studies, which would have been required for a premarket approval application, in the setting of financial difficulty following FDA-mandated withdrawal of its conventional balloon angioplasty products in the Unites States.

Recently, my colleagues and I have experimentally identified two potentially important mechanisms of restenosis after LBA. Although the magnitude of the postangioplasty diameter loss chronically is similar for LBA and conventional balloon angioplasty in a rabbit normal iliac artery model, the dominant mechanisms responsible for the diameter loss have been found to differ. Connective tissue cross-linking, which results in intramural scar contracture after LBA, was inhibited by 1 month of oral administration of β-aminopropionitrile (β-APN), a inhibitor of lysyl oxidase,[27] the extracellular enzyme responsible for cross-linking of newly synthesized collagen and elastin. As a result, the 1-month angiographic diameter loss was significantly reduced compared to controls, with no change in mean luminal diameter 6 months after the procedure (5 months after discontinuation of the drug). β-APN had no apparent effect on the diameter loss after conventional balloon angioplasty, and it is likely that arterial recoil, which may not be amenable to any type of pharmacologic treatment, represented an important mechanism for the chronic diameter loss associated with the latter. Interestingly, application of a local concentrated film of heparin during LBA, but not during conventional balloon angioplasty, was subsequently found to have a similarly beneficial effect in the same animal model. Heparin exhibits a variety of antifibrosis activities,[28–33] including inhibition of lysyl oxidase and inhibition of monocyte adhesion to the injured luminal surface, in addition to its anticoagulant and antiproliferative[34,35] effects, which may have mimicked to some extent the effect of β-APN.

In vitro studies suggest that thermal denaturation of thrombin at 100°C may reduce the thrombogenicity of thrombus,[21] but experimental in vivo studies have suggested that this tissue nevertheless retains its thrombogenic potential after LBA. The possibility exists that thermal remodeling of thrombus therefore may expose a new layer of thrombin as a potential mechanism of restenosis in some patients. Fortunately, at high concentrations, heparin effectively inhibits thrombin bound to fibrin,[36] and we have recently demonstrated that thermal energy that results in a minimum temperature response of more than 70°C in thrombus can be used to bind heparin at even higher concentrations to this tissue.[37]

An FDA-approved Phase I clinical trial of the application of LBA with a solid film of concentrated heparin (>100,000 U/g and a total dose of 3,000 U), mounted on the balloon surface and protected from premature washout with a sheath before application, has recently been completed. The trial used 3-F LBA catheter, fabricated in my laboratory, which incorporated a 7-mm long cylindric diffusing tip mounted as an integral part of the central channel (Fig. 65-3). Once the 6-month angiographic results are obtained from the Phase I trial, a Phase II trial is planned, wherein patients will be randomized to either PTCA or to LBA/local heparin applied immediately after PTCA, irrespective of the acute success of the latter. Primary end points of this study will include mean percent diameter stenosis and minimum luminal diameter on 6-month follow-up angiograms by computer analysis and cumulative event-free survival during this period of observation.

Clinical data currently are scant regarding the relationship between chronic tissue and angiographic responses and a variety of laser/thermal balloon angioplasty variables, such as the peak tissue temperature, duration of heating, axial length, tissue depth of thermal exposure, alternative laser wavelengths and energy sources, and adjunctive local and sys-

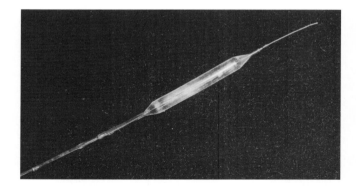

Fig. 65-3. Current-generation LBA catheter, a 3.0-F device that incorporates a diffuser with a more appropriate length (7 mm) and a cylindrically uniform pattern of continuous wave Nd-YAG laser irradiation. Heparin (3,000 U) is applied as a concentrated gel on the full surface of the body of the balloon, air-dried, and protected within a sheath before advancement of the balloon to the angioplasty site. A peak tissue temperature of 80°C to 90°C, achieved during a 20-second laser exposure, is used in conjunction with tissue pressure from the inflated balloon to simultaneously seal intimal tears, reduce arterial recoil, remodel thrombus, and enhance heparin binding to tissues, particularly pre-existing intraluminal thrombus.

temic drug regimens. The results of the proposed LBA clinical trial, in addition to those related to the use of radiofrequency or microwave radiation, may provide important insights in the next few years. Moreover, alternative applications of laser balloon angioplasty technology, such as photopolymerization[38] and photochemotherapy[39] will very likely increase the options available in the treatment of obstructive atherosclerosis.

PARTICIPATING INVESTIGATORS (USCI LBA TRIALS)

The LBA study group comprised the following investigators:

- J. Richard Spears, Harper Hospital/Wayne State University School of Medicine, Detroit, Michigan
- Vincent P. Reyes, Harper Hospital/Wayne State University School of Medicine, Detroit, Michigan
- Ronald D. Jenkins, University of Utah, Salt Lake City, Utah
- I. Nigel Sinclair, Sir Charles Gairdner Hospital, Perth, Australia
- Barry E. Hopkins, Sir Charles Gairdner Hospital, Pert, Australia
- Anthony Rickards, The National Heart Hospital, London, England
- Ulrich Sigwart, The National Heart Hospital, London, England
- Leonard Schwartz, Toronto General Hospital, Toronto, Ontario, Canada
- Harold E. Aldridge, Toronto General Hospital, Toronto, Ontario, Canada
- H. W. Thijs Plokker, St. Antonius Hospital, Nieuwegein, The Netherlands
- Wayne E. Dear, Texas Heart Institute, St. Lukes Episcopal Hospital, Houston, Texas
- James J. Ferguson, Texas Heart Institute, St. Lukes Episcopal Hospital, Houston, Texas
- Paolo Angelini, Texas Heart Institute, St. Lukes Episcopal Hospital, Houston, Texas
- Louis L. Leatherman, Texas Heart Institute, St. Lukes Episcopal Hospital, Houston, Texas
- Robert D. Safian, Beth Israel Hospital, Boston, Massachusetts
- Spencer B. King III, Emory University School of Medicine, Atlanta Georgia
- John S. Douglas, Jr., Emory University School of Medicine, Atlanta, Georgia
- Gary S. Roubin, Emory University School of Medicine, Atlanta, Georgia
- Augusto Pichard, Washington Hospital Center, Washington, DC
- Gerald Dorros, St. Luke's Hospital, Milwaukee, Wisconsin
- Marie-Claude Morice, Centre Cardiologique du Nord, Cedex, France

ACKNOWLEDGEMENT

This work was sponsored in part by NHLBI grants HL 37349 and 44683.

REFERENCES

1. Spears JR, Serur J, Shropshire D, Paulin S. Fluorescence of experimental atheromatous plaques with hematoporphyrin derivative. J Clin Invest 1983;71:395–9
2. Hiehle JF, Jr, Bourgelais D, Shapshay S et al. Nd:YAG laser fusion of human atheromatous plaque-arterial wall separations in vitro. Am J Cardiol 1985;56:953–7
3. Spears JR. PTCA restenosis: potential prevention with laser balloon angioplasty. Am J Cardiol 1987;60:61B–64B
4. Sigel B, Dunn MR. The mechanism of blood vessel closure by high frequency electrocoagulation. Surg Gynecol Obstet 1965;121:823–31
5. Jain KK, Gorisch W. Repair of small blood vessels with the Neodymium-YAG laser: a preliminary report. Surgery 1979;85:684–8
6. White RA, Abergel RP, Lyons R et al. Biological effects of laser welding on vascular healing. Lasers Surg Med 1986;6:137–141
7. Murray LW, Su L, Kopchok GE, White RA. Crosslinking of extracellular matrix proteins: a preliminary report on a possible mechanism of argon laser welding. Lasers Surg Med 1989;9:490–6
8. Spears JR, Reyes VP, Wynne J et al. Percutaneous coronary laser balloon angioplasty: initial results of a multicenter experience. J Am Coll Cardiol 1990;16:293–303
9. Spears JR, Reyes VP, Plokker HWT et al and the LBA Study Group. Laser balloon angioplasty: coronary angiographic follow-up of a multi-center trial. J Am Coll Cardiol 1990;15(2):26A
10. Spears JR, Safian RD, Douglas FS et al and the LBA Study Group. Multicenter acute and chronic results of laser balloon angioplasty for refractory abrupt closure after PTCA. Circulation 1991;84(suppl. II):II–517
11. Spears JR, Zhan H, Khurana S, et al. Modulation by β-aminoproprionitrile of vessel luminal narrowing and structural abnormalities in arterial wall collagen in a rabbit model of conventional balloon angioplasty versus laser balloon angioplasty. J Clin Invest 1995;93:1543–155
12. Spears JR, Yellayi SS, Makkar R, et al. Effects of thermal exposure on binding of heparin in vitro to the arte-

rial wall and to clot and on the chronic angiographic luminal response to local application of a heparin film during angioplasty in an in vivo rabbit model. Lasers Surg Med 1994;14:329–46

13. Schober R, Ulrich F, Sander T, et al. Laser-induced alteration of collage sbstructure allows microsurgical tissue welding. Science 1986;232:1421–2

14. Spears JR, James LM, Leonard BM et al. Plaque-media rewelding with reversible tissue optical property changes during repetitive cw Nd:YAG laser exposure. Lasers Surg Med 1988;8:477–85

15. Jenkins RD, Sinclair IN, Anand R et al. Laser balloon angioplasty: effect of tissue temperature on weld strength of human postmortem intima-media separations. Lasers Surg Med 1988;8:30–9

16. Anand RK, Sinclair IN, Jenkins RD et al. Laser balloon angioplasty: effect of constant temperature versus constant power on tissue weld strength. Lasers Surg Med 1988;8:40–4

17. Jenkins RD, Sinclair IN, Anand RK et al. Laser balloon angioplasty: effect of exposure duration on shear strength of welded layers of postmortem human aorta. Lasers Surg Med 1988;8:392–6

18. Spears JR, Sinclair IN, Jenkins RD. Laser balloon angioplasty: Experimental in vitro and in vivo studies. pp. 167–188. In Abela GS (ed): Lasers in Cardiovascular Medicine and Surgery: Fundamentals and Techniques. Kluwer Academic Publishers, Nowell, MA, 1990

19. Cheong WF, Spears JR, Welch AJ. Laser balloon angioplasty. Crit Rev Bioengin 1991;19:113–46

20. Jenkins RD, Sinclair IN, Leonard BM. Laser balloon angioplasty versus balloon angioplasty in normal rabbit illiac arteries. Lasers Surg Med 1989;9:237–47

21. Kundu SK, Ozawa T, Patel R et al. In vitro evaluation of the effect of laser irradiation on the thrombogenicity of thrombus. Thromb Res 1992;68:137–44

22. Borst C, Bos AN, Zwaginga JJ et al. Loss of blood platelet adhesion after hating native and cultured subendothelium to 100°C. Cardiovasc Res 1990;24:665–8

23. Gentry PA, Schneider MD, Miller JK. Plasma clot-promoting effect of collagen in relation to collagen-platelet interaction. Am J Vet Res 1981;42:708–15

24. Abela GS, Tomaru T, Mansour M et al. Reduced platelet deposition with laser compared to ballon angioplasty. Circulation 1990;80(suppl. II):II–254

25. Spears JR, Sandor T, Als AV. Computerized image analysis for quantitative measurement of vessel diameter from cineangiograms. Circulation 1983;68:453–61

26. Sandor T, D'Adamo A, Hanlon WB, Spears JR. High precision quantitative angiography. IEEE Trans Med Imag 1987;6:258–65

27. Tang S-S, Trackman PC, Kagan HM. Reaction of aortic lysyl oxidase with beta-aminopropionitrile. J Biol Chem 1983;258:4331–8

28. Gavriel P, Kagan HM. Inhibition by heparin of the oxidation of lysine in collagen by lysyl oxidase. Biochemistry 1988;27:2811–5

29. Frizelle S, Schwartz J, Huber SA, Leslie K. Evaluation of the effects of low molecular weight heparin on inflammation and collagen deposition in chronic coxsackievirus B3-induced myocarditis in A/J mice. Am J Pathol 1992;141:203–9

30. McPherson JM, Ledge PW, Ksander G et al. The influence of heparin on the wound healing response to collagen implants in vivo. Collagen Rel Res 1988;1:83–100

31. El Nabout R, Martin M, Remy J et al. Heparin fragments modulate the collagen phenotype of fibroblasts from radiation-induced subcutaneous fibrosis. Exp Mol Pathol 1989;51:111–122

32. Ehrlich HP, Griswold TR, Rajaratnam JBM. Studies on vascular smooth muscle cells and dermal fibroblasts in collagen matrices. Effects of heparin. Exp Cell Res 1986;164:154–62

33. Rogers C, Karnovsky MJ, Edelman ER. Heparin's inhibition of monocyte adhesion to experimentally injured arteries matches its antiproliferative effects. Circulation 1993;88(suppl. I):I–370

34. Clowes AW, Karnovsky MJ. Suppression by heparin of smooth muscle cell proliferation in injured arteries. Nature 1977;165:625–6

35. Guyton JR, Rosenberg RD, Clowes AW, Karnovsky MJ. Inhibition of rat arterial smooth muscle cell proliferation by heparin. In vivo studies with anticoagulant and nonanticoagulant heparin. Circ Res 1980;46:625–634

36. Hogg PJ, Jackson CM. Fibrin monomer protects thrombin from inactivation by heparin-antithrombin III: implications for heparin efficacy. Proc Natl Acad Sci USA 1989;86:3619–23

37. Spears JR, Yellayi SS, Makkar R et al. Effects of thermal exposure on binding of heparin in vitro to the arterial wall and to clot and on the chronic angiographic luminal response to local application of a heparin film during angioplasty in an in vivo rabbit model. Lasers Surg Med 1994;14:329–46

38. Slepian MJ, Massia SP, Sawhney A et al. Endoluminal gel paving using in situ biodegradable photopolymerized hydrogels: acute efficacy in the rabbit. Circulation 1993;88(suppl. I):I–660

39. Gregory KW, Buckley LA, Haw TE et al. Photochemotherapy using psoralen and UVA light in a porcine model of intimal hyperplasia. Circulation 1993;88(suppl. I):I–82

66 Laser Thrombolysis

Peter C. Block
Kenton Gregory

Venous and arterial thrombi can absorb a wide range of laser wavelengths within the optical spectrum. Absorption of laser energy can produce rapid, efficient vaporization and destruction of thrombus.[1–5] Therefore, lasers may be useful in the treatment of both acute or chronic thrombosis or as adjunctive therapy during mechanical recanalization of occluded vessels. The strategy for the care of patients who have been treated with lytic agents but have ongoing ischemia that is due to failure of complete thrombus removal may also include laser therapy as part of their further treatment. Though early lasers were plagued by random ablation of any tissue in the light path, the evolution of lasers and optical delivery systems now allows more specific thrombus–light interaction. Thus, lasers have the potential of rapid removal of intravascular thrombus with minimal chance of perforation or dissection.

Though thrombolytic drugs have become the mainstay of treatment for a wide range of acute and chronic thrombotic disorders, some patients fail to benefit, and many patients have contraindications to their use.[6,7] In addition, the risk of bleeding may increase the risk/benefit ratio of use of these agents, and alternative strategies need to be developed. Balloon angioplasty is commonly employed, especially in the treatment of coronary occlusion in acute myocardial infarction.[8] Though acute procedural success is high, drawbacks lie in the recurrent ischemic event rate of around 15% and restenosis rates that may range as high as 50 to 60%.[9,10] This is not surprising, because balloon dilation within a thrombosed artery

actually disrupts the luminal surface further and exposes more thrombogenic subendothelial tissue. Compression of thrombus against the vessel wall releases procoagulant factors, vasoconstrictors, mitogens, and growth factors, which may all contribute to reocclusion and restenosis rates.

Laser thrombolysis may remove thrombi without significantly damaging the underlying vessel. If adjunctive mechanical recanalization is needed, the initial removal of thrombus may reduce complication rates. Laser thrombolysis also avoids a systemic lytic state and diminishes the possibility of bleeding.

OPTICAL PROPERTIES OF THROMBUS

The optical properties of arterial and venous thrombi are variable. Any thrombus can have regions rich in red blood cells and fibrin. In fresh arterial thrombus, aggregations of platelets are present. Studies in an animal model have shown that the most significant light-absorbing molecule in thrombus is hemoglobin.[11] Transmittance and reflectance of thrombi have been measured between wavelengths of 300 and 800 nm. The absorption coefficients calculated at each wavelength and plotted against wavelength are shown in Figure 66-1. This shows the characteristic absorption spectrum of thrombus with strong absorption in the ultraviolet wave band and in the visible spectrum at 420 (Soret band), 540, and 570 nm consistent with hemoglobin absorption.[2,4] Lasers

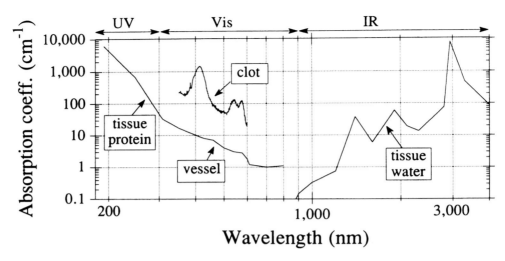

Fig. 66-1. Laser and other ablative new forms of angioplasty. Absorption spectra of arterial wall, thrombus, and water. Plots are on a log scale calculated from spectrophotometric measurements. Ultraviolet (UV), visible, and infrared (IR) wavelengths are shown. The clot is shown to have a high absorption in the visible wavelength compared to the arterial wall. (From Topol,[34] with permission.) (Spectra courtesy of Steven Jacques, Ph.D., M.D., Anderson Cancer Center.)

that emit ultraviolet or visible wavelengths at these frequencies would be likely to achieve vaporization or ablation of thrombus. Between 600 and 800 nm, absorption drops off dramatically, and light in these wavelengths is transmitted, reflected, or scattered. At higher wavelengths (1,000 to 3,000 nm), light absorption again increases in thrombi because water molecules absorb laser energy in this wave band. This supports the basis for the use of holmium-yttrium-aluminum-garnet (YAG) or erbium-YAG lasers for thrombus ablation, which emit at 2,100 and 2,940 nm, respectively.

LASER THROMBOLYSIS STUDIES

In 1983 Lee et al. reported the use of a continuous wave argon ion laser emitting light at 454 and 514 nm to vaporize a variety of thrombi using a bare-fused silica fiber to transmit the laser energy to the thrombus in vitro.[5] Later attempts to recanalize thrombosed arteries in a canine model using argon laser energy achieved recanalization, but perforation of the vessel wall by the laser light was common. Only minimal thrombus was removed, and the vessel wall was charred at the sites of laser light delivery. Such studies pointed out the limitations of continuous wave lasers as well as silica fibers, which are stiff and potentially dangerous in vivo.[12–14] Heating and vaporization of target tissues produced by continuous wave lasers also produced diffusion of thermal energy to surrounding vascular structures, re-

sulting in wide areas of thermal necrosis and injury. Vasospasm, thrombosis, and a high restenosis rate were all attributed to thermal injury.[15] In a variation, the sharp profile of the silica fiber was surrounded by a metal cap, which was heated by laser energy. Recanalization was achieved in initial animal models of thrombosis, but later human studies were unrewarding.[16,17] As an alternative, lasers emitting energy in short pulses became the delivery source of choice.[18]

PULSED LASER THROMBOLYSIS

When intense laser energy is delivered in short pulses (nanoseconds to microseconds in duration), the ablation process occurs before heat can diffuse to adjacent tissue. Therefore, lasers emitting energy in pulses less than 100 μs in duration are likely to produce little thermal injury.[7,19,20] Pulsed lasers from the ultraviolet spectrum, visible spectrum, and infrared wavelengths have been used in clinical trials of laser angioplasty. All currently used laser thrombolysis systems utilize pulsed laser sources and are summarized for comparison in Table 66-1.

THROMBOLYSIS USING EXCIMER LASER ENERGY

Excimer laser systems emit 308 nm light and can be pulsed in 100- to 200-ns pulses to remove intravascular thrombi.[21,22] Using excimer laser methods, con-

Table 66-1. Comparison of Laser Systems Used in Laser Thrombolysis

	Argon Ion	Excimer	Holmium	Pulsed Dye
Wavelenth (nm)	514	308	2100	480–577
Tissue chromophore	Hemoglobin	Protein	H_2O	Hemoglobin
Pulse duration	Continuous	100–200 ns	250 μs	1 μs
Thermal effects	+ + +	−	+	−
Selectivity	−	−	−	+
Optical delivery catheter	Single optical fiber	Fiber bundle	Fiber bundle	Flowing fluid core
Light penetration depth (μm)	100	30	300	30–100

ventional angioplasty guidewires are placed through the thrombus into the distal vessel, and the laser catheter (made up of bundles of 50 to 100 fused silica fibers circumferentially arranged around a central lumen) is advanced to the thrombus. The laser is activated at pulse energies of approximately 40 to 50 mJ/mm^2 at pulse repetition rates between 10 and 30 Hz. Thrombus can be successfully ablated using this technique.[22] However, some studies have shown high complication rates.

In a study by Estella et al.[22] using the excimer laser system, 7 of 12 patients had successful recanalization. Two had emboli, four had myocardial infarction, two had acute closure, and seven had later restenosis. Though this may raise caution in the use of excimer laser thrombolysis, refinements of excimer laser delivery systems and case selection may lead to a new indication for excimer laser thrombolysis.

THROMBOLYSIS USING THE HOLMIUM LASER

Holmium/thulium-YAG lasers produce light at a wavelength of 2,100 nm. Laser energy is delivered in 250-μs duration pulses. Because the holmium-YAG laser energy is highly absorbed by water, which has a prominent absorption peak near this wavelength (see Table 66-1) this laser can be used for thrombolysis. In addition, a solid-state crystal rather than gas or liquid is used to produce light. Because 250-μs pulses are longer than the thermal relaxation time of tissue, thermal diffusion to surrounding tissue occurs. Although excellent ablation of tissue is produced by this laser, surrounding thermal injury occurs.[23,24] Explosive vaporization of water also produces a prominent secondary cavitation-induced shock-wave effect, which can contribute to vascular damage.[25]

The holmium/thulium-YAG laser delivers energy via bundles of fused silica optical fibers. A standard percutaneous transluminal coronary angioplasty (PTCA) guidewire is first advanced through the thrombus into the distal vessel, and the laser catheter is advanced to the area of thrombus. Energy is delivered in 250- to 600-mJ/pulse energies at a repetition rate of 5 Hz. A study by Topaz et al.[26] showed an improvement in luminal dimension and a small amount of residual stenosis in all cases. No adverse procedural complications were reported. These early clinical results are promising, and further studies are awaited with interest.

SELECTIVE LASER THROMBOLYSIS

The difference in optical properties between thrombus and arterial wall can be used to minimize damage to vascular tissue and ablate thrombus selectively. The concept of selective laser photothermolysis has been used for ablation of skin lesions such as port wine stains without damaging normal skin structures nearby.[27–29] There is a large difference in optical properties between thrombi from hours to weeks of age compared to arterial or venous wall or prosthetic graft materials.[2–4] Initial studies using a new silica fiber with a rounded leading edge produced recanalization without perforation or suture disruption.[3] This study suggested that selective laser thrombolysis could be used with safety and efficacy for treatment of obstructive thrombi. A laser emitting optical radiation within the wave band of 450 to 600 nm has been developed (Palomar, 3010 flash lamp-excited pulse-dye laser; Palomar Inc., Westford, Massachusetts). This laser emits selected wavelengths by exciting fluorescent dyes and is configured to emit light at 480 nm. The light is emitted in 1- to 2-μs pulses, which is well below the 100-μs thermal relaxation time of vascular tissue. The ablation threshold for acute arterial thrombus is approximately 1.5 J/cm^2, whereas the ablation threshold for normal arterial tissue of animals and humans is nearly 150 J/cm^2. To minimize trauma to the vessel by silica fibers, a fluid core light guide can be used to

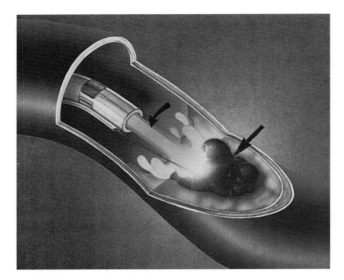

Fig. 66-2. Drawing of a fluid core laser catheter with delivery of laser energy to an arterial thrombus (*large arrow*). The catheter has a high index of refraction optical fluid core and a low index of refraction cladding so that internal reflection of light is produced. The optical core (contrast material) (*curved arrow*) flushes away intervening arterial blood. Laser energy is delivered to the thrombus without mechanical catheter contact.

channel the pulsed laser light[30,31] (Fig. 66-2). Rather than transmitting light through optical fibers, the fluid core catheter has flexibility, is inexpensive, and can transmit light through low index of refraction tubing filled with contrast material. An open-ended catheter allows the optical fluid to flow distally into the vessel, transmitting light along its path. In addition to transmitting light, the flowing contrast material flushes away blood, which minimizes absorption of light by the hemoglobin in ambient red cells. Because the light is transmitted past the end of the catheter, contact with the target is not necessary, and the clot is not disrupted by the catheter tip. Because contrast is used for transmission of light, visualization of the catheter, the target, and the distal vasculature can be performed under fluoroscopy, and the effectiveness of laser energy delivery can be observed in real time. Light is delivered to the optical catheter through a large-diameter fused silica fiber that is placed into the laser catheter via an O-ring Y adapter. The fiber is advanced in the catheter only to a point where stiffness is advantageous for pushability, leaving the more distal aspect with an open channel. This produces flexibility needed for negotiating the curves within a coronary artery and its ostial take-off from the aorta. The optical channel is 1.1 mm in diameter, producing a laser spot diameter of the same dimension. Contrast is delivered through the catheter at flow rates between 0.3 and 0.5 ml/sec by a conventional power injector. This provides adequate flow for light transmission up to 1 cm from the tip of the catheter in vitro. Then 3 to 5 ml of contrast agent are injected during a typical 5- to 10-sec burst of laser pulses. The catheter can be delivered with a standard 8-F angioplasty guiding catheter and guidewires using a monorail lumen in the distal tip of the laser catheter (Fig. 66-2).

TECHNIQUE

The laser catheter is prepared by first flushing the catheter with heparinized saline and connecting a standard Medrad injector to the injection port. Iodinated contrast agent warmed to 37°C is used. The laser fiber is connected to the laser via a screw mount, and the output is measured with an external energy meter. An initial pulse energy of 80 mJ results in a fluence at the thrombus of approximately 8 J/cm². This is above the threshold for ablation of arterial thrombus, as shown in animal studies.

The thrombolysis catheter is advanced with conventional angioplasty equipment, as mentioned. A 0.014 to 0.016″ angioplasty guidewire is used to first cross the coronary occlusion. The laser catheter is then advanced until its tip is positioned approximately 2 mm from the thrombus as shown by guiding catheter injections.

The contrast stream and laser activation is accomplished simultaneously and 5- to 10-sec rounds of laser pulses at 3 Hz are repetitively used until ablation occurs. Because contrast is injected, the laser firing produces an angiogram seen under fluoroscopy, allowing the operator to follow the amount of thrombus ablation. Usually, in the setting of acute myocardial infarction, there is also a fixed atherosclerotic obstruction present. If the residual stenosis is significant, the laser catheter should be withdrawn after thrombus has been removed and flow is re-established. The guidewire is left in place, and standard PTCA balloon angioplasty can then be accomplished via transfer techniques. Patients receive aspirin and intravenous heparin during the procedure and for 24 hours after, as is standard with most angioplasty procedures for acute myocardial infarction.

CLINICAL PILOT STUDIES

After animal studies of laser thrombolysis in acute myocardial infarction demonstrated the safety and efficacy of the technique, the initial pilot study of laser thrombolysis for acute myocardial infarction in patients who could not receive thrombolytic drugs or who failed reperfusion with thrombolysis was undertaken. Initial results from St. Vincent Hospital and Medical Center in Portland, Oregon, and St. Joseph Hospital in Atlanta, Georgia, demonstrated feasibility of thrombolysis. No perforations occurred in 20 patients, and effective thrombus removal was demonstrated in 18/20 patients. All patients needed adjunctive PTCA or directional atherectomy after thrombus removal.[32] Investigations thus far have concentrated on the treatment of acute myocardial infarction. However, subacute coronary thrombosis, postangioplasty thrombosis, coronary graft thrombosis, and other thromboses might well be treated with this technique. The developments of new catheters and lasers that will allow larger focal spots and area of laser light delivery should allow treatment of thrombus in larger vessels such as coronary artery bypass grafts.

Laser thrombolysis is feasible and may become part of the armamentarium to treat intravascular thrombosis. Its final role has yet to be established in the strategy of the treatment of thrombotic vascular disease.

REFERENCES

1. Gregory KW, Guerrero JL, Girsky M et al: Coronary artery laser thrombolysis in acute canine myocardial infarction. Circulation 1989;80:523.
2. LaMuraglia GM, Anderson RR, Parrish JA, Zhang Z, Prince MR: Selective laser ablation of venous thrombus: implications for a new approach in the treatment of pulmonary embolus. Lasers Surg Med 1988;8:486–93.
3. LaMuraglia GM, Ortu P, Fillmore D et al: Selective laser photoablation enhances thrombolytic graft recanalization. Surg Forum 1990;41:363–4.
4. LaMuraglia GM, Prince MR, Nishioka N. Optical properties of human arterial thrombus, vascular grafts and sutures: implications for selective laser thrombus ablation. IEEE J Quantum Electronics 1990;26(12):2200–6.
5. Lee G, Ikeda RM, Stobbe D et al: Effects of laser irradiation on human thrombus: demonstration of a linear dissolution-dose relation bwtween clot length and energy density. Am J Cardiol 1983;52:876–7.
6. Collen D, Topol EJ, Tiefenbrunn AJ et al: Coronary thrombolysis with recombinant human tissue-type plasminogen activator: a prospective randomized placebo-controlled trial. Circulation 1984;70:1012–27.
7. The TIMI Study group: The thrombolysis in myocardial infarction (TIMI) trial: phase I findings. N Engl J Med 1985;312:932–6.
8. O'Keefe JH, Rutherford GD, McConahay DR et al: Early and late results of coronary angioplasty without antecedent thrombolytic therapy for acute myocardial infarction. Am J Cardiol 1989;64:1221–30.
9. Grines CL, Browne KF, Vandormael M et al: Primary angioplasty in myocardial infarction (PAM) trial. Circulation 1992;86 (suppl I):1–641.
10. Hopkins J, Savage M, Zalunski A: Recurrent ischemia in the zone of prior myocardial infarction: results of coronary angioplasty of the infarct related vessel. Am Heart J 1988;115:14–19.
11. Yasuda T, Gold HK, Fallon JT et al: A canine model of coronary artery thrombosis with superimposed high grade stenosis for the investigation of re-thrombosis after thrombolysis. J Am Coll Cardiol 1989;13:1409–14.
12. Abela GS, Norman SJ, Cohen DM et al: Laser recanalization of occluded atheroscolerotic arteries in vivo and in vitro. Circulation 1985;71:403–11.
13. Choy DSJ, Stertzer S, Rotterdam HZ: Transluminal laser catheter angioplasty. Am J Cardiol 1982;50:1206–8.
14. Sanborn TA, Faxon DP, Haudenschild C et al: Experimental angioplasty: circumferential distribution of laser thermal energy with a laser probe. J Am Coll Cardiol 1985;5:934–8.
15. Douek PC, Correa R, Neville R et al: Dose dependent smooth muscle cell proliferation induced by thermal injury with pulsed infrared lasers. Circulation 1992;86:1249–56.
16. Labs JD, Caslowitz PL, Williams GM et al: Experimental treatment of thrombotic vascular occlusion. Lasers Surg Med 1991;11:363–71.
17. Tomaru T, Abela GS, Gonzales J et al: Laser recanalization of thrombosed arteries using thermal and/or modified optical probes; angiographic and angioscopic study. Angiology 1992;43:412–20.
18. Srinivasan R, Leigh W: Ablative photo-decomposition action of far-ultra-violet (193 nm) laser radiation on polyethylene terophythalate films. J Am Chem Soc 1982;104:5784–5.
19. Linkser R, Srinivasan R, Wayne JJ, Alonso DR: Far-ultra-violet laser absorption of atherosclerotic lesion. Lasers Surg Med 1984;3:201–8.
20. Anderson RR, Jaenke KF. Parrish JA: Mechanisms of selective vascular changes caused by dye lasers. Lasers Surg Med 1983;3:211–5.
21. Estella P, Bittl, JA, Landzberg JM, Ryan TJ: Intracoronary thrombus increases the risk of excimer laser coronary angioplasty. Circulation 1992;86(suppl I):654.
22. Rosenfield K, Pieczek A, Losordo DW et al: Excimer laser thrombolysis for rapid clot dissolution in lesions at high risk for embolization: a potentially useful new application for excimer laser. J Am Coll Cardiol 1992;19(suppl A):104A.
23. Stein E, Sedlacek T, Fabian RL, Nishoka NS: Acute and chronic effects of bone ablation with a pulsed holmium laser. Lasers Surg Med 1990;10:384–8.
24. Gottlob C, Kopchok GE, Peng SK et al: Holmium:YAG laser ablation of human inervertebral disc: preliminary evaluation. Lasers Surg Med 1991;12:86–91.
25. De la Torre R, Gregory KW: Cavitation bubbles and acoustic transients may produce dissections during laser angioplasty. J Am Coll Cardiol 1992;19(suppl A):48A.
26. Topaz O, Rosenbaum EA, Battista S, Peterson C, Wysham DG: Laser facilotated angioplasty and thrombolysis in acute myocardial infarction complicated by prolonged or recurrent chest pain. Cathet cardiovasc Diagn 1993;28:7–16.
27. Anderson RR, Parrish JA: Microvasculature can be se-

embolization; in addition, the deeper injury that occurs with plaque resection may be more thrombogenic in certain patients, such as those with rest pain and ischemic electrocardiographic changes.

Second, the restenosis-preventive effects of atherectomy were only modest, detectable by quantitative angiography, but not clinically, in terms of a decrease in the frequency of repeat revascularization procedures during follow-up. From these data, we have learned that the chief reason for directional atherectomy's benefit is the ability to achieve better luminal restoration than balloon angioplasty, or "the bigger, the better,"[8,9] but the luminal amelioration with atherectomy was not sufficient enough to have a clinical impact. Furthermore, there was a "price" to be paid with respect to the higher acute phase complications; increase in cost of $1,300 per patient; and in the CAVEAT I trial (only), a higher rate of late major complications (death and myocardial infarction). This latter concern of late events has not been confirmed in either the CAVEAT II or CCAT trials. Importantly, the thesis that even more aggressive atherectomy will result in a clinically meaningful improvement in restenosis avoidance is currently being tested in the Balloon versus Optimal Atherectomy Trial (BOAT). To achieve more extensive atherectomy safely, it may prove necessary to use intravascular ultrasound guidance to monitor on-line plaque versus vessel wall resection.

More than these paramount direct lessons about directional atherectomy, we have learned some essentials on how to conduct large-scale, pivotal trials of the new coronary revascularization techniques and how to use (or not use) the trials to influence clinical practice and stimulate further research. This is roughly equivalent to the transformation of some aspects of interventional cardiology from an art to a science. For example, instead of accepting strong biases emanating from a registry experience, we need to hold judgment and keep receptors open for rigorous data. Still, today, there is a widespread belief that atherectomy avoids periprocedural instability rather than engendering it. The experienced operators from CAVEAT I and II, in a real-world situation of many sites engaged in active practice, have, for now, disproved this theory. In 1993, however, in the United States alone, more than 60,000 directional atherectomy procedures were performed, representing roughly 12 to 15% of all the procedures of percutaneous coronary revascularization.

Before a similar scenario develops for other atherectomy devices, or plaque-ablative-related techniques such as atherectomy, it would be ideal to have randomized trial data available. The novelty and charm factor of a new device cannot be underestimated[10] and many will be potentially quickly and widely accepted unless there are reasons for the contrary. Ideally, we will need to have large-scale randomized trials of the rotablator, guided atherectomy, and new debulking devices completed in a timely fashion. If not, we clearly run the risk of rapid entrenchment and relative unwillingness to accept objective, clearcut data. The strident criticism of some aspects of the CAVEAT I trial,[11] for example, reflect the resistance to accept rigorously collected data as authentic and valid. These data in no way invalidate the importance of directional atherectomy as a tool for interventional cardiologists, but identify reasonable boundaries and expectations for the use of the technique, and most importantly, identify the future directions of research that are needed before this particular representative debulking technique is even more widely applied.

REFERENCES

1. Simpsom JB. How atherectomy began: a personal history. Am J Cardiol 1993;72:3E–5E
2. Baim DS, Hinohara T, Holmes D et al. for the U.S. Directional Coronary Atherectomy Investigator Group: Results of directional coronary atherectomy during multicenter preapproval testing. Am J Cardiol 1993;72:6E–11E
3. Topol EJ, Leya F, Pinkerton CA et al. on behalf of the CAVEAT Study Group: a comparison of coronary angioplasty with directional atherectomy in patients with coronary artery disease. N Engl J Med 1993;329:221–227
4. Adelman AG, Cohen EA, Kimball BP et al. A comparison of directional atherectomy with balloon angioplasty for lesions of the left anterior descending coronary artery. N Engl J Med 1993;329:228–233
5. Lincoff AM, Topol EJ. Abrupt vessel closure. pp. 207–230. In Topol EJ (ed): Textbook of Interventional Cardiology. 2nd Ed. W.B. Saunders, Philadelphia, 1994
6. Popma JJ, Califf RM, Topol EJ. Clinical trials of restenosis after coronary angioplasty. Circulation 1991;84:1426–1436
7. The CAVEAT II Investigators. The Coronary Angioplasty Versus Excisional Atherectomy Trial (CAVEAT) II: preliminary results. Circulation 1993;88(suppl. II):I-594
8. Kuntz RE, Safian RD, Carrozza JP et al. The importance of acute luminal diameter in determining restenosis after coronary atherectomy or stenting. Circulation 1992;86:1827–1835
9. Kuntz RE, Gibson CM, Nobuyoshi M, Baim DS. Generalized model of restenosis after conventional balloon angioplasty, stenting and directional atherectomy. J Am Coll Cardiol 1993;21:15–25
10. Topol EJ. Promises and pitfalls of new devices for coronary artery disease. Circulation 1991;83:689–694
11. Safian RD. Coronary atherectomy versus angioplasty. N Engl J Med 1993;329:1892

68 Directional Coronary Atherectomy

James W. Vetter
John B. Simpson

INTRODUCTION

Directional coronary atherectomy is at an evolutionary crossroads. In its current form it remains a viable alternative to other techniques such as balloon angioplasty and stenting, especially in certain anatomic situations in which it may be the treatment of choice. These include ostial left anterior descending artery (LAD) lesions, other bifurcation lesions, focal eccentric lesions, and some lesions in saphenous vein grafts. It has, however, been replaced by stents for many of the applications for which it was the best alternative to certain lesions not well treated by percutaneous transluminal coronary angioplasty in the past. It is estimated that directional coronary atherectomy is currently used in approximately 7% to 10% of coronary interventions.

The concept of selective debulking of coronary stenoses is still an attractive idea on a pathophysiologic basis, whether as a stand-alone procedure or prior to postatherectomy dilation with angioplasty or stenting. This concept has not yet been fully tested from a scientific standpoint, even with recent sophisticated studies such as the Balloon Versus Optimal Atherectomy Trial (BOAT) and the Optimal Atherectomy Restenosis Trial (OARS), chiefly because truly selective and complete removal of the atheroma is not possible with the current device. More precisely guided devices (by integrated ultrasound) have been tested in humans, and the preliminary results have been encouraging. Truly selective and more complete atheroma removal has been demonstrated using these early prototype devices. The combination of debulking of appropriate lesions followed by angioplasty or stenting to achieve maximal lumen dimensions may also improve long-term results. At this point atherectomy of appropriately selected lesions appears to be a cost-effective treatment compared with other technologies such as conventional balloon angioplasty and stents.

HISTORICAL PERSPECTIVE

The concept of removal of atheroma—*atherectomy*—was introduced by Dr. John Simpson to overcome some of the limitations of percutaneous transluminal coronary angioplasty. It was known that angioplasty provided a favorable short- and long-term result for many lesions treated by this method but that significant limitations remained. These limitations did not seem to be further diminishable as long as the mechanism was directionally uncontrolled dilation without debulking. Dr. Simpson hypothesized that by selectively removing only the diseased portion of the vessel wall a larger lumen with a smoother surface would result. A smooth surface together with minimal residual narrowing at the treatment site should result in minimal flow disturbance, thus reducing aggregation of platelets and formation of thrombus. This effect, along with a large lumen diameter at the treatment site to allow for the inevitable intimal response, could also be expected to reduce the incidence of clinically significant restenosis. Initial experience in cadaver arteries and in rabbit iliac vessels showed that atheroma could indeed be removed using a prototype directional atherectomy device. The device was then further tested in human peripheral lesions in 1985. Interestingly, even the early experience with the device suggested that the more complete the removal of atheroma, the more favorable was the short- and long-term result including a lower restenosis rate. Based on the promising peripheral experience, the coronary device was developed and first used in a patient at Sequoia Hospital (Redwood City, CA) in October of 1986; however, no tissue could be removed because of technical limitations of the early prototype device. After various modifications to the device as well as to the guiding catheters, the first successful coronary atherectomy was performed early in 1987 on a right coronary artery lesion. The device was further refined as more experience was gained; after favorable results from a 1,000-patient multicenter registry, the Simpson AtheroCath received Food and Drug Administration approval in 1990 as the first device for coronary intervention other than angioplasty.

DESCRIPTION OF THE DEVICE

The Simpson AtheroCath system includes a fully disposable catheter with a battery-powered hand-held motor drive unit. For excision of plaque, the distal end of the catheter comprises a gold-plated steel cannister with one of the walls of the cannister cut out. A low-pressure support balloon opposite the cut-out portion is inflatable to help project atheroma into the cannister. The material that collects in the cannister is then excised by manual advancement of a hardened stainless steel spinning cup-shaped blade, which, after shaving the material, packs it distally in the soft plastic nose cone, thus storing it for removal from the body. This last feature has contributed greatly to a basic understanding of the process of coronary response to injury. The material is analyzable in its intact state after removal and may be sectioned and stained or used for other studies such as in situ hybridization. The presence of thrombus, calcium, and other materials can also be determined with light microscopy study using various staining techniques. Excision of deep wall components can be reliably excluded or verified by similar examination.

CLINICAL TRIALS

In addition to the multicenter registry and other reported series including the Sequoia series, several large randomized trials and a nonrandomized study have been completed or are nearly complete. To place the results of these studies in proper perspective, it is useful to understand some of the historical background. As the procedure began to evolve at several centers simultaneously, it became apparent that great variation in technique existed. This was well demonstrated in the multicenter New Approaches to Coronary Interventions (NACI) series. Opinions varied widely about the amount of tissue that should be excised, whether postatherectomy angioplasty was safe to perform, the best size of device to use for a given artery, and other fundamental factors. At the time of the earliest large randomized trial which took place in 1991 and 1992 (the Coronary Angioplasty Versus Excisional Atherectomy Trial [CAVEAT]), it was felt by many operators that a minimal amount of material should be removed to avoid excision of deep wall components. Early reports had suggested that, at least in saphenous vein grafts, excision of deep wall components may lead to exaggerated stimulation of intimal hyperplasia, which would in turn result in an increased incidence of clinically significant restenosis. Later reports by the Beth Israel and Sequoia groups, however, had demonstrated that removal of some deep wall components was relatively common, was associated with a safe procedure, and led to a decreased incidence of restenosis. The lower restenosis rate seemed to be due to the enhanced ability of the vessel to tolerate the inevitable intimal hyperplasia simply because of large postinterventional lumen dimensions—the so-called bigger is better theory put forth by Kuntz, Baim, and others.

Despite the later reports, most CAVEAT operators still preferred to use relatively smaller devices than these two groups, and although tissue weights were not recorded, probably removed a small percentage of atheroma available for excision. This tendency, coupled with the strong discouragement for postatherectomy angioplasty (less than 5% of all patients in CAVEAT), resulted in post-treatment lumen diameters that were only minimally larger than those achieved by the angioplasty arm. Predictably, this resulted in only a modest reduction in restenosis. The Sequoia series also suggested that when too little atheroma was removed by atherectomy, use of the device without postatherectomy balloon dilation was associated with a higher rate of complications. This finding seemed to have been confirmed to some extent by the CAVEAT results. Another observation that was widely known among interventionists prior to CAVEAT was that creatine phosphokinase levels were increased after atherectomy but that these increases were generally not excessive. They also were not associated with the development of pathologic Q waves on 12-lead electrocardiograms and seemed not to have significant clinical consequences. Lastly, these so-called creatine phosphokinase bumps did not seem to be comparable to spontaneously occurring non-Q-wave myocardial infarctions in that rates of subsequent myocardial infarction or sudden death did not seem to be higher than expected. Nevertheless, this subject was heatedly debated during CAVEAT and remains controversial. The Beth Israel group and others have continued to study this interesting phenomenon, the cause of which is not yet clear. One of the major criticisms of CAVEAT, then, was that the way directional atherectomy was performed was suboptimal, although it was in line with the current thinking of many of the operators.

This conclusion prompted a group of experienced operators to design a study using more contemporary methods of performing the procedure. The focus of the study was maximal post-treatment lumen diameter and could include postdirectional atherectomy angioplasty if necessary. Postatherectomy angioplasty was not discouraged, since it was felt that this was a safe way to achieve an even larger postatherectomy minimum lumen diameter. The prerandomized trial known as OARS could include ultrasound; however, the randomized trial known as BOAT was to use "optimal" directional atherectomy followed by balloon angioplasty but without ultrasound guidance. This last restriction was to make the procedure as "mainstream" as possible since it was anticipated that many operators would not routinely use ultrasound in their laboratories.

The acute results of these two trials have demonstrated that they have met a very important early objective—the achievement of a large lumen diameter without increased risk of complications. Placing the acute results into models developed by the Beth Israel group from observations of a wide variety of interventional studies (including CAVEAT, various stent studies, and their own series) would predict a favorably lower restenosis rate than that found with conventional balloon angioplasty. This theoretical conclusion is based on the relatively larger lumen diameter after treatment (2.8 mm) and the low residual stenosis (less than 15%) compared with the angioplasty arm of the BOAT study. Interestingly, however, even with the low residual stenoses seen in both OARS and BOAT trials, it is apparent from ultrasound imaging that the so-called optimal atherectomy achieved in these studies may indeed be far from truly optimal. Ultrasound imaging reported by Mintz, Yock, Fitzgerald, and co-workers has shown that on average 60% of the plaque burden remains, even after relatively aggressive atherectomy, as in the OARS study. The basic reason for this finding is that angiographic guidance of directional atherectomy is known to be relatively imprecise, especially when compared with on-line ultrasound guidance. This limitation had been known for several years and led to the conception by Yock and co-workers of a device with integrated real-time ultrasound guidance. This device would enable the operator to excise the atheroma much more precisely while avoiding deep cuts into the media and adventitia layers of the vessel wall. An integrated device has been successfully developed by Devices for Vascular Intervention and has been used in humans by Ribeiro, Yock, and Vetter. The findings of this preliminary series are being reported by Yock, Fitzgerald, and co-workers and demonstrate that even with the early devices, far fewer cuts are necessary to achieve little residual stenosis. In addition, even though these first procedures were purposely done conservatively, only 30% of the atheroma burden remained at the treatment site. Equally importantly, only a very small amount of media was seen (in one specimen), and no adventitia was excised. These very encouraging preliminary results await further studies with refined devices.

OTHER LIMITATIONS

Well-described limitations for directional atherectomy include heavily calcified lesions as well as excessively tortuous and noncompliant vessels. The procedure is known to be complex and requires a high degree of expertise for its safe use. The large guiding catheters that are required to perform the procedure require skill and great care in use. These factors, along with the risk of perforation due to potential deep wall cuts, have led to the characterization of directional atherectomy as a "niche" procedure, best suited for only a few highly specific indications. These indications usually comprise focal, noncalcified or minimally calcified eccentric lesions and lesions located in the ostium of the LAD as well as other bifurcation sites.

CURRENT INDICATIONS

Indications for use of directional atherectomy naturally vary based on a particular operator's experience, comfort level with the procedure, and personal bias. Some operators, for example, feel that the procedure is highly useful for salvaging unfavorable angioplasty results when elastic recoil or limited dissections are the mechanisms responsible for angioplasty failure. Others feel the procedure is indicated for restenosis lesions, since it is known to be safer in these types of lesions and can yield a relatively large post-treatment lumen diameter. Still others feel it is indicated mainly for ostial LAD, protected left main, and bifurcation lesions, as well as focal vein graft lesions and bulky eccentric lesions. Some operators, on the other hand, see little useful application for the procedure in the age of stents, although others see directional atherectomy as a more cost-effective device compared with stents for certain lesion subsets. Yet another perspective comes from the interventional scientists curious about the potentially favorable effects of atheroma removal. They feel that the basic concept of selective and more complete removal of the diseased material from the vessel wall has still not been tested adequately and therefore the real benefits could be as yet largely unrealized.

FUTURE DIRECTIONS

Among those scientists who believe that it is worthwhile to explore potential benefits of atherectomy, two divergent tacks are being taken. One involves various degrees of atheroma removal with the device, followed by stenting ("debulk, then stent") as a way to improve both short- and long-term results over those achievable by either device alone ("bigger is better"). The other major tack involves use of various configurations of integrated devices such as the guided directional coronary atherectomy catheter (ultrasound device envisioned by Yock and others). In addition to these ideas for the future of directional coronary atherectomy, incremental technical improvements in the current device itself are also under way. These include incorporation of a flexible housing (for tortuous, noncompliant vessels) and use of a hardened cutter within the device (for fibrocalcific and calcific lesions).

SUMMARY

Directional coronary atherectomy remains a viable alternative in the treatment of selected coronary lesions. In addition to being a safe and predictable therapeutic modality, it remains a powerful biopsy tool, able to contribute to the understanding of the mechanism of atheroma formation and vessel response to various forms of injury and intervention. Interesting associations continue to emerge in the literature, such as the frequent isolation of *Chlamydia pneumoniae* from restenosis specimens, and these findings are made possible by retrieval of tissue with the device. Incremental technical improvements to minimize its current limitations may expand its role as a therapeutic device. More extensive

developments such as the integration of ultrasound may have a more profound effect if they enable the device to remove atheroma more completely and more selectively.

SUGGESTED READINGS

Annex BH, Denning SM, Channon KM et al. Differential expression of tissue factor protein in directional atherectomy specimens from patients with stable and unstable coronary syndromes. Circulation 1995;91:619–622

Arbustini E, De Servi S, Bramucci E et al. Comparison of coronary lesions obtained by directional coronary atherectomy in unstable angina, stable angina, and restenosis after either atherectomy or angioplasty. Am J Cardiol 1995;75:675–682

Baim DS, Hinohara T, Holmes D et al. Results of directional coronary atherectomy during multicenter pre-approval testing. Am J Cardiol 1993;72:6E–11E

Baim DS, Kent KM, King SB. Evaluating new devices: acute (in-hospital) results from the new approaches to coronary intervention registry. Circulation 1994;89:471–481

Baim DS, Kuntz RE. Directional coronary atherectomy: how much luminal enlargement is optimal? Am J Cardiol 1993;72:65E–70E

Baim DS, Whitlow PL. The future of directional coronary atherectomy. Am J Cardiol 1993;72:108E

Boehrer JD, Ellis SG, Pieper K et al. Directional atherectomy versus balloon angioplasty for coronary ostial and nonostial left anterior descending coronary artery lesions: results from a randomized multicenter trial. The CAVEAT-1 investigators. Coronary Angioplasty Versus Excisional Atherectomy Trial. J Am Coll Cardiol 1995;25:1380–1386

Campbell LA, O'Brien ER, Cappuccio AL et al. Detection of *Chlamydia pneumoniae* TWAR in human coronary atherectomy tissues. J Infect Dis 1995;172:585–588

Cohen DJ, Breall JA, Ho KKL et al. Economics of elective coronary revascularization: comparison of costs and charges for conventional angioplasty, atherectomy, stenting, and bypass surgery. J Am Coll Cardiol 1993;22:1052–1059

Dick RJ, Popma JJ, Muller DW et al. In-hospital costs associated with new percutaneous coronary devices. Am J Cardiol 1991;68:879

DiSciascio G, Cowley MJ, Goudreau E et al. Histopathologic correlates of unstable ischemic syndromes in patients undergoing directional coronary atherectomy: in vivo evidence of thrombosis, ulceration, and inflammation. Am Heart J 1994;128:419–426

Escaned J, van Suylen RJ, MacLeod DC et al. Histologic characteristics of tissue excised during directional coronary atherectomy in stable and unstable angina pectoris. Am J Cardiol 1993;71:1442–1447

Flugelman MY, Virmani R, Correa R et al. Smooth muscle cell abundance and fibroblast growth factors in coronary lesions of patients with nonfatal unstable angina. A clue to the mechanism of transformation from the stable to the unstable clinical state. Circulation 1993;88:2493–2500

Gordon P, Kugelmass A, Cohen D et al. Balloon postdilatation can safely improve the results of successful (but suboptimal) directional coronary atherectomy. Am J Cardiol 1993;72:71–79

Hillis LD. Efficacy and safety of coronary balloon angioplasty and directional atherectomy (editorial; comment). Circulation 1990;82:305–307

Hinohara T, Robertson G, Selmon M et al. Directional coronary atherectomy. J Invas Cardiol 1990;2:217–226

Hinohara T, Robertson G, Selmon M et al. Restenosis after directional coronary atherectomy. J Am Coll Cardiol 1992;20:623–632

Hinohara T, Rowe MH, Robertson GC et al. Effect of lesion characteristics on outcome of directional coronary atherectomy. J Am Coll Cardiol 1991;17:1112–1120

Hofling B, Welsch U, Heimerl J et al. Analysis of atherectomy specimens. Am J Cardiol 1993;71:96E–107E

Kugelmas AD, Cohen DJ, Moscucci M et al. Elevation of the creatine kinase myocardial isoform following otherwise successful directional coronary atherectomy and coronary stenting. Am J Cardiol 1994;74:748–754

Kuntz RE, Baim DS. Defining coronary restenosis: newer clinical and angiographic paradigms. Circulation 1993; 88:1310–1323

MacLeod DC, de Jong M, Umans VA et al. Directional atherectomy combining basic research and intervention. Am Heart J 1993;125:1748–1759

MacLeod DC, Strauss BH, de Jong M et al. Proliferation and extracellular matrix synthesis of smooth muscle cells cultured from human coronary atherosclerotic and restenotic lesions. J Am Coll Cardiol 1994;23:59–65

Miller M, Kuntz R, Friedrich S et al. Frequency and consequences of intimal hyperplasia in specimens retrieved by directional atherectomy of native primary coronary artery stenoses and subsequent restenoses. Am J Cardiol 1993;71:652–658

O'Brien ER, Garvin MR, Stewart DK et al. The importance of the vasa vasorum to cellular proliferation in human coronary atherectomy specimens. Circulation 1993;88: 3331

Popma JJ, Mintz GS, Satler LF et al. Clinical and angiographic outcome after directional coronary atherectomy: a qualitative and quantitative analysis using coronary arteriography and intravascular ultrasound. Am J Cardiol 1993;72:55E–64E.

Safian RD, Gelbfish JS, Erny RE et al. Coronary atherectomy: clinical, angiographic, and histologic findings and observations regarding potential mechanisms. Circulation 1990;82:69

Simonton CA. Lesion-specific technique considerations in directional coronary atherectomy. Cathet Cardiovasc Diagn 1993;29:131–135

Simpson JB. How atherectomy began: a personal history. Am J Cardiol 1993;72:3E–5E

Strauss BH, Umans VA, van Suylen RJ et al. Directional atherectomy for treatment of restenosis within coronary stents: clinical, angiographic and histologic results. J Am Coll Cardiol 1992;20:1465–1473

Strikwerda S, Umans V, van der Linden MM et al. Percutaneous directional atherectomy for discrete coronary lesions in cardiac transplant patients. Am Heart J 1992; 123:1686–1690

Topol EJ, Leya F, Pinkerton CA et al. Comparison of directional atherectomy with coronary angioplasty in patients with coronary artery disease. N Engl J Med 1993; 329:221–227.

Umans VA, Baptista J, di Mario C et al. Angiographic ultrasonic and angioscopic assessment of the coronary artery wall and luminaria configuration after directional atherectomy: the mechanism revisited. Am Heart J 1995;130:217–227

Waller BF, Johnson DE, Schnitt SJ et al. Histologic analysis of directional coronary atherectomy samples. Am J Cardiol 1993;72:80E–87E

Wilcox JN. Molecular biology: insight into the causes and prevention of restenosis after arterial intervention. Am J Cardiol 1993;72:88E–95E

Yock P, Yock C, Ribeiro E et al. Use of GDCA: initial human experience, abstract ed. Am Heart J (in press)

the widespread use of directional atherectomy to treat lesions that could be treated by angioplasty, at least in native vessels. With cognizance of the higher rate of complications, a judicious approach to the use of atherectomy in selected native vessels and vein grafts can be advocated.

Like most randomized trials, the CAVEAT project raised many new questions. For example, the clinical significance of the excess of non-Q-wave myocardial infarction, largely a product of blinded central adjudication, needs to be further investigated. However, the question asked by most, and in particular by converts to the bigger-is-better hypothesis, is whether a larger initial lumen following more aggressive atherectomy or angioplasty, or atherectomy with routine adjunctive angioplasty would reduce restenosis and reduce cumulative clinical end points. It may be that true directional atherectomy guided by on-line intravascular ultrasound would best maximize plaque resection while minimizing medial and adventitial trauma, and so minimizing the chance of procedural complications. Such questions cannot be answered by single-center or multicenter registries but will form the basis of future randomized trials.

ACKNOWLEDGMENTS

The authors gratefully acknowledge the contributions of all the study investigators, study nurses, and co-ordinating center personnel involved in the successful completion of the CAVEAT project. In particular, we thank Lisa Berdan, Gordon Keeler, and Karen Pieper at the Duke Co-ordinating Center for their assistance.

REFERENCES

1. US Directional Coronary Atherectomy Investigator Group. Directional coronary atherectomy: multicenter experience. Circulation 1990;82(suppl.):III-71
2. Hinohara T, Rowe MH, Robertson GC et al. Effect of lesion characteristics on outcome of directional coronary atherectomy. J Am Coll Cardiol 1991;17:1112–20
3. Popma JJ, Topol EJ, Hinohara T et al for the US Directional Atherectomy Investigator Group. Abrupt vessel closure after directional coronary atherectomy. J Am Coll Cardiol 1992;19:1372–9
4. Baim DS, Hinohara T, Holmes D et al. Results of directional coronary atherectomy during multicenter pre-approval testing. Am J Cardiol 1993;72:6E–11E
5. Topol EJ, Leya F, Pinkerton CA et al. A comparison of directional atherectomy with coronary angioplasty in patients with coronary artery disease. N Engl J Med 1993;329:221–7
6. Berdan LG, Califf RM for the CAVEAT Investigators. Restenosis: does the six month angiogram tell the story? CAVEAT one year followup. Circulation 1993;88(suppl.):I-595
7. Elliott JM, Berdan LG, Holmes DR et al. for the CAVEAT Study Investigators. One year follow-up in the Coronary Angioplasty Versus Excisional Atherectomy Trial (CAVEAT I). Circulation 1995;91:2158–66
8. Holmes DR, Topol EJ, Califf RM et al. A multicenter, randomized trial of coronary angioplasty versus directional atherectomy for patients with saphenous vein bypass graft lesions. Circulation 1995;91:1966–74
9. Adelman AG, Cohen EA, Kimball BP et al. A comparison of directional atherectomy with balloon angioplasty for lesions of the left anterior descending coronary artery. N Engl J Med 1993;329:228–33
10. Kuntz RE, Foley DP, Keeler GP et al for the CAVEAT Investigators. Relationship of acute luminal gain to late loss following directional atherectomy or balloon angioplasty in CAVEAT. Circulation 1993;88(suppl.II):I-495
11. Ellis SG, Umans VA, Whitlow PL et al on behalf of the CAVEAT Investigators. Angiographic restenosis in CAVEAT is determined by the acute result (not the device used to obtain it). Circulation 1993:88(suppl.):I-495
12. Boehrer JD, Ellis SG, Keeler GP et al. Differential benefit of directional atherectomy over angioplasty for left anterior descending in proximal, *non-ostial lesions:* results from CAVEAT. J Am Coll Cardiol 1994;(suppl.):386A
13. Whitlow P, Grassman E for the CAVEAT Investigators. The Coronary Angioplasty Versus Excisional Atherectomy Trial (CAVEAT): lesion morphology and outcome. Circulation 1993;88(suppl.):I-546
14. Abdelmeguid AE, Sapp SK, Ellis SG. Significance of mild transient creatine kinase release after coronary interventions. Circulation 1993;88(suppl.):I-299
15. Berdan LG, Holmes DR, Keeler G et al for the CAVEAT II Investigators. High event rate in patients with saphenous vein grafts undergoing percutaneous coronary interventions: CAVEAT II one year followup. Circulation 1994;90(suppl.):I-63
16. Lincoff AM, Keeler GP, Debowey D, Topol EJ, for the CAVEAT Study Group. Is clinical site variability an important determinant of outcome following percutaneous revascularization with new technology? Insights from CAVEAT. Circulation 1993;88(suppl.):I-653
17. Cohen EA, Kimball BP, Sykora K, Adelman AG. Lumen narrowing after atherectomy is proportionally greater than after PTCA. Circulation 1993;88(suppl.):I-546
18. Kuntz RE, Gibson CM, Nobuyoshi M, Baim DS. Generalized model of restenosis after conventional balloon angioplasty, stenting and directional atherectomy. J Am Coll Cardiol 1993;21:15–25

70 The Transluminal Extraction-Endarterectomy Catheter

Brigitta C. Brott
Michael H. Sketch, Jr.
Richard S. Stack

Percutaneous transluminal coronary balloon angioplasty (PTCA) has progressed over the past 15 years into being frequently the procedure of choice for patients with single-vessel and multivessel coronary artery disease, as well as for many with coronary artery bypass grafts. Although balloon technology continues to improve, the abrupt occlusion rate following PTCA is 6.8%, and there remains a 30 to 50% incidence of restenosis within 6 months of successful balloon dilation.[1,2] To overcome these limitations, an array of new devices has been developed, including stents, lasers, and atherectomy catheters. Three atherectomy devices have been developed: the directional coronary atherectomy catheter (Devices for Vascular Intervention, Inc., Redwood City, California), the Rotablator (Heart Technology, Inc., Bellevue, Washington), and the transluminal extraction-endarterectomy catheter (TEC) device. Each catheter has its own potential niche in the treatment of coronary lesions.

The TEC device is a percutaneous motor-driven device that can excise and aspirate plaque and thrombus. It was invented by InterVentional Technologies, Inc. (San Diego, California), and developed at Duke University Medical Center. The TEC device was approved by the U.S. Food and Drug Administration in May 1989 for use in peripheral arteries and in May 1993 for use in coronary arteries and saphenous vein bypass grafts.

HISTORICAL DEVELOPMENT

Initial evaluation of the TEC device was performed in human cadaveric normal and atherosclerotic arteries and in in vivo canine arteries.[3,4] In the normal arterial segments, histologic analysis revealed focal intimal disruption with occasional excision limited to less than 25% of the media. TEC atherectomy successfully removed atherosclerotic plaque in all of the diseased arteries. The depth of plaque resection was primarily limited to the media, although there was occasional disruption of the external elastic lamina. No evidence of dissections or perforations was found. The resected material consisted of a mixture of collagen, modified smooth muscle cells, elastic tissue, and cholesterol crystals, and ranged in size from 0.1 to 2.8 mm in maximum dimension. Building on the foundation of these experimental studies, clinical investigation of the TEC was begun in peripheral arteries in December 1987 and in coronary arteries in July 1988.

THE TEC DEVICE

The TEC device is a motor-driven hollow flexible torque tube with a distal cutter head that consists of two stainless steel blades (Fig. 70-1).[5,6] At the tip of the conical head is a small lumen for passage of

71 Rotational Ablation

David C. Auth

HISTORY

The Rotablator rotational ablation system developed and manufactured by Heart Technology, Inc. (Redmond, Washington) is a unique primary treatment device that originated from the search for a solution to the limitations of conventional balloon angioplasty, in particular the less than optimal results with percutaneous transluminal coronary angioplasty (PTCA) in treating unfavorable lesions, that is, calcified, eccentric, tortuous lesions. Furthermore, the higher success and decreased complications with rotational ablation in these types of lesions have expanded the indications of percutaneous revascularization, offering an alternative treatment modality to patients otherwise facing the certainty of bypass surgery. Finally, the Rotablator device is a tool to investigate whether debulking or dilation is a more effective method for increasing luminal diameter of a vessel and for decreasing the signals for restenosis.

In the early development of the Rotablator system, several design prototypes were evaluated, leading to the most important fundamental changes—the elimination of suction evacuation of debris fragments and the incorporation of a guidewire. The resulting device design, with its air turbine and diamond-coated burr, has greater flexibility and is capable of high rotational speeds with low torque, which facilitates a reduction in the size of particles "sanded" away during the ablation procedure. The Rotablator rotational ablation system has been extensively tested in animal and human clinical investigations.[1–5]

SYSTEM DESCRIPTION

Primary components of the Rotablator system are the advancer, guidewire, wireClip, and control console (Fig. 71-1). The Rotablator advancer houses an air turbine, which spins the elliptic-shaped burr at speeds up to 190,000 revolutions per minute (rpm). The burr is coated with 5 to 10-μm diamond microcrystals on the distal portion (Fig. 71-2). The burr is attached to a flexible drive shaft inside a Teflon sheath through which saline is infused to lubricate the drive and turbine as well as to aid in washing away microparticulate from the ablation.

The drive shaft and burr are independently advanced over a specially designed 0.009" (0.23-mm) guidewire, which has a formable 0.017" platinum spring tip. The Heart Technology, Inc., wireClip torquing tool should be attached to the guidewire when it is loaded into the burr and advancer. In addition to torquing and placement of the wire, the wireClip is used to prevent the guidewire from spinning when the advancer is activated during the exchange procedure.

The advancer is interfaced to the console, which controls the rotational speed of the burr by regulating the supply of compressed gas to the air turbine. The rotation per minute of the spinning burr are continuously displayed on a digital readout. Depressing the foot pedal initiates high-speed rotation of the burr (150,000 to 190,000 rpm) and activates an air brake locking mechanism in the advancer, which prevents the guidewire from spinning while the burr is rotating. For low rotation speeds (60,000 to 90,000 rpm) to facilitate the exchange procedure, the Dynaglide button on the foot pedal is depressed.

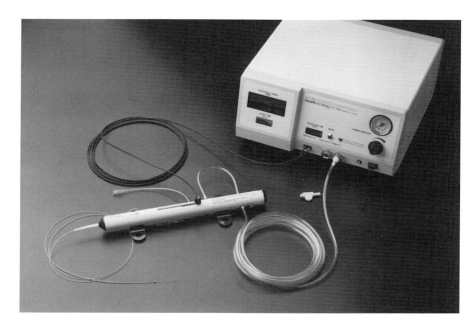

Fig. 71-1. Rotablator rotational ablation system.

RATIONALE AND MECHANISMS OF ACTION

Rather than fracturing plaque, the Rotablator system uses a high-speed burr covered with diamond microcrystals to remove the occlusive material and restore luminal patency. The crystals pulverize fibrous, calcified, or fatty atherosclerotic tissue into particles that are smaller than red blood cells. These tissue particles are then disposed of naturally by the body's reticuloendothelial system.

Two major physical principles make the Rotablator system effective in the treatment of coronary artery lesions: differential cutting and orthogonal displacement of friction.

Differential Cutting

The Rotablator system works on the principle of differential cutting. This same principle is used in orthopedic cast saws that can cut through a rigid inelastic plaster cast without harming the elastic skin underneath. Inelastic materials such as plaque are unable to move out of the way of the diamond-coated cutting surface of the high-speed burr, but elastic

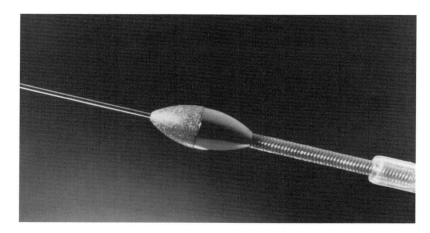

Fig. 71-2. Rotablator diamond-coated burr.

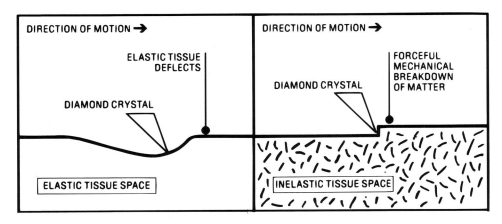

Fig. 71-3. Principle of differential cutting **(A)** Elastic tissue is able to deflect out of the way. **(B)** Inelastic tissue is unable to deflect out of the way.

materials such as normal vessel walls deflect and are not ablated (Fig. 71-3).

Orthogonal Displacement of Friction

Orthogonal displacement of friction is a principle of physics referring to the change, or displacement, in the effective friction in one direction between two adjacent sliding surfaces. Friction normally occurs between sliding surfaces in contact and opposes the relative motion between them. However, when the available friction is used up by a significant sliding motion in one direction, then little friction is available at 90 degrees to the sliding motion direction. This principle is easily demonstrated by pulling a cork out of a bottle. If the cork is twisted as it is pulled, the frictional force is reduced and the cork is more easily removed.

The principle of orthogonal displacement of friction is particularly useful when advancing the Rotablator device through distal arteries and tortuous anatomy because it dramatically reduces the longitudinal friction when the system is operating in excess of a few thousand rotations per minute. When the Rotablator burr spins at 60,000 rpm or greater, the longitudinal friction vector is virtually eliminated.

PATIENT SELECTION

Percutaneous rotational ablation with the Rotablator system, either as a sole therapy or with adjunctive balloon angioplasty, is indicated in patients with coronary artery disease who are acceptable candidates for bypass surgery.

The preferred treatment subgroups for Rotablator rotational ablation include calcified lesions; long lesions (<25 mm); eccentric lesions; restenotic lesions; distal lesions; lesions in small, tortuous vessels; and lesions undilatable or uncrossable with balloon angioplasty. Any lesion to be treated with rotational ablation must be crossable with the Rotablator guidewire.

Treatment with the Rotablator system is contraindicated in saphenous vein graft lesions, in the presence of intracoronary thrombus, and angiographic evidence of dissections or intimal flaps. Further, hemodynamic performance must be considered if the area subtended by the treatment vessel is one of the only remaining functional regions of myocardium.

PROCEDURAL REVIEW

The following is a basic overview of the recommended technique employed during the Heart Technology, Inc., multicenter clinical studies with the Rotablator rotational ablation system.

Patients are premedicated with 325 mg of aspirin orally and calcium channel blockers. Immediately before arrival in the catherization laboratory patients receive diazepam and diphenhydramine orally. Intravenous heparin (10,000 to 15,000 U) is given during the procedure and additional heparin administered to maintain the activated clotting time at greater than 300 seconds. All patients are adequately hydrated before the procedure to allow for increased vasodilation.

Depending on the reference segment of the vessel to be treated, the sheath and guiding catheter that will accommodate the largest burr required to accomplish the procedure are selected. The guiding catheter should have side holes, and its inside diameter should exceed the largest burr diameter by a minimum of .004" to provide adequate clearance of the burr as it is advanced.

With the appropriate sheath inserted, a temporary pacemaker is advanced into the right ventricular apex in patients undergoing ablation of the right coronary artery or dominant left circumflex vessel (that was due to the high incidence of transient atrioventricular block). In certain circumstances, such as collateralized right coronary arteries and proximal left anterior descending arteries it is not infrequent that pacing is required. In those situations, the temporary pacemaker is placed.

During the procedure, patients are treated with a continuous infusion of intravenous nitroglycerin. Intracoronary nitroglycerin and calcium channel blockers should be available in the event of coronary vasospasm.

Once the guiding catheter is manipulated and seated into the ostium of the target vessel, a bare .009" guidewire (which is not preloaded into the Rotablator system) is advanced across the stenosis into the distal vessel, allowing adequate distal clearance of the platinum spring tip from the lesion site. The Rotablator device is then advanced over the wire, using standard angioplasty techniques, and positioned proximal to the lesion. The burr should not be spinning while advancing through the guide catheter, because this may cause ablation of the Teflon coating of the guide.

When choosing the appropriate burr size for the rotational ablation procedure, the "stepped technique" is recommended in which the lesion is treated with a small burr first, followed by incrementally larger burrs to ultimately reach a 0.75–0.85 burr/artery ratio. This technique allows for optimal plaque abrasion, presents less plaque burden to the microcirculation, and reduces the risk of torsional dissection. If it is not possible to achieve a 0.75–0.85 burr/artery ratio with the Rotablator alone, complementary low-pressure balloon inflations (1 atm or less) should be used.

The burr is activated by depressing the foot pedal switch and is advanced using the independent advancer knob over a distance of 7 cm. Turbine air pressure is adjusted on the console, allowing for high-speed rotation of the burr over the normal operating range (150,000 to 190,000 rpm depending on the burr size).

With the burr positioned proximal to the lesion, the speed is readjusted to set the optimum rotational speed for ablation. The optimum rotational speed for 1.25- to 2.0-mm Rotablator burrs is 180,000 rpm, and 160,000 rpm for 2.15- to 2.5-mm burrs. To ensure complete debulking and maximum lumen size relative to burr diameter and small particle size, the burr should be advanced slowly, allowing a decrease of no more than 5,000 rpm. Slow and steady advancement of the burr is further aided by audible feedback from the spinning burr as well as tactile and visual cues such as the absence of darting.

Removal of the burr through the guiding catheter is facilitated by orthogonal displacement of friction and low-speed (60,000 to 90,000 rpm) rotation. The back of the burr is smooth (no diamond microchips) and, therefore, has no ablative effect on the vessel wall or guiding catheter when retracted. The brake defeat is employed to allow the advancer drive shaft and burr to be moved along the guidewire. The guidewire is then immobilized with the wireClip, preventing the now-free guidewire from spinning.

COMPLICATIONS

Vasospasm

Occasionally, intense vasospasm along the artery follows treatment; this frequently can be treated with small boluses of intracoronary nitroglycerin. When this does not alleviate the vasospasm after several minutes, low-pressure (1 to 3 atm) balloon inflations at the site have been beneficial in mechanically breaking the spasm. Intracoronary injections of calcium channel blockers may also be considered to relieve vasospasm.

No/Slow Flow

No or slow flow has been seen in a small subset of patients undergoing high-speed rotational ablation. Slow flow is an attenuation of flow from TIMI-3 to TIMI-2 to TIMI-1 flow. No flow is defined as the complete attenuation of flow to TIMI-0. Both of these events likely reflect the amount of plaque burden distributed into the distal microcirculation and its ability or capacity to handle and clear those microparticles. Appropriate Rotablator technique such as the stepped burr approach may impact the amount of plaque burden in the distal bed and reduce the incidence of the slow-flow phenomenon.

If no or slow flow does occur and is not resolved within a few minutes, be certain that the blood pressure is adequate for coronary blood flow by infusing fluids and intracoronary nitroglycerin. If flow continues to be compromised, a balloon catheter at low-pressure inflations (1 atm) distal and at the lesion site should be employed.

Bradycardia

Bradycardia is a common occurrence in patients undergoing treatment of the right coronary artery or dominant left circumflex artery. Therefore, the routine placement of a temporary pacemaker in the right ventricular apex is appropriate in these patients.

POSTPROCEDURE MANAGEMENT

Postprocedure, the patient is maintained on intravenous nitroglycerin, and fluids (usually saline) are infused.

It is not uncommon that, despite a coronary angiogram that demonstrates an excellent result with TIMI-3 flow and patency of all the arterial branches, the patient has persistent chest pain and electrocardiographic abnormalities including ST elevation or depression. The general pattern is that the pain diminishes and is relieved with normalization of the S-T wave segments within the first 20-minutes after the procedure.

It is recommended that the patient be monitored in a telemetry setting overnight. In addition to intravenous nitroglycerin and fluids, medications consist of aspirin and calcium channel blockers. Intravascular sheaths can be maintained overnight, but, based on the angiographic result, this can be left to the discretion of the operator.

The issue of anticoagulation is not without controversy. In uncomplicated cases, heparin overnight is usually adequate. If there is evidence of dissection or thrombus, 48 to 72 hours may be beneficial and, in patients with excessively long lesions or total occlusions, 72 hours should be considered.

RESULTS

Clinical studies for the Rotablator system in coronary use were begun in 1988. The Heart Technology, Inc., multicenter investigator registry included 2,736 procedures (3,424 lesions) from a number of leading medical centers in the United States and Europe. In June 1993 Heart Technology received U.S. Food and Drug Administration approval to market the Rotablator system for use in coronary arteries.

Primary success was defined as a greater than 50% luminal diameter with at least a 20% reduction in overall stenosis and no major complications, with or without complementary or adjunctive balloon angioplasty. Primary success with the Rotablator proce-

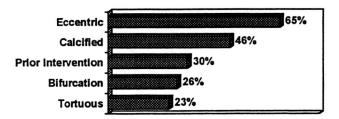

Fig. 71-4. Complex lesion characteristics.

dure alone was 83% and increased to 95% with the use of adjunctive balloon angioplasty.

Angiographic complications included a perforation rate of 0.7%, acute occlusion of 4.0%, and a dissection rate of 13.7%. Major clinical complications include myocardial infarction in 1.1%, emergency coronary artery bypass graft surgery in 2.5%, and mortality in 1.0%. The low rate of complications was achieved despite the complexity of the lesions treated. (Fig. 71-4).

COSTS

The reusable Rotablator system control console has a U.S. list price of $7,500. The single-use Rotablator advancer unit has a U.S. list price of $1,095. Both the type A and type C guidewires available from Heart Technology have a U.S. list price of $750 per set of five wires. The Heart Technology wireClip torquer has a U.S. list price of $50 per set of five.

DISCUSSION

Current Outlook

Since the completion of the multicenter trials, a large number of interventional cardiologists have been trained in Heart Technology's 2-day physician training program. To date, Heart Technology, Inc., has certified more than 1700 interventional cardiologists from over 1600 U.S. hospital centers in the use of the Rotablator rotational ablation system. Physicians from approximately 250 international hospital centers have also been trained since the device's international release.

Future Development

During its 13-year development, the Rotablator rotational ablation system has been tested in animal models, human cadaver tissue, and clinically evaluated. In the near future, Heart Technology will invest

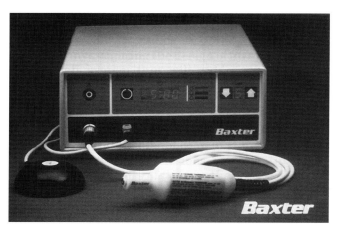

Fig. 72-1. The generator. Settings for energy time are available in minutes (5:00) and power (5 depicted here). There is a foot switch, and the main cable leads to the hand-held transducer, where the 19.5-kHz alternating current is converted to mechanical oscillations.

RATIONALE

The mechanisms of action of therapeutic ultrasound appear to be as follows:

1. As previously mentioned, hard plaque elements are selectively disrupted and fragmented by the longitudinal vibration. The probe will pass through porcelain but does not damage the finger when abutted against it.
2. The probe's oscillation causes rapid formation and implosion of microbubbles. This acoustic cavita-

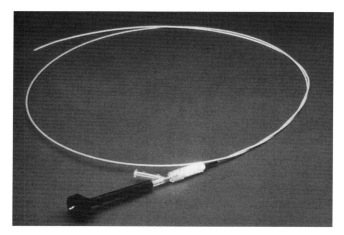

Fig. 72-2. The ultrasound catheter. The black connector, connected to the proximal end of the wave guide, screws into the transducer. The wire connector provides a saline flash around the wave guide, through to the catheter tip. The wave guide terminates in the probe tip. The probe has a guidewire lumen 25 cm long for rapid exchange.

tion is maximal at the interface between materials of different acoustic impedance. It is probably the mechanism of ultrasound dissolution of thrombus.
3. The local temperature could rise, causing a thermal effect, but in practice this is prevented by constant irrigation of saline around the probe tip, the wave guide being enclosed in a catheter, terminating just behind the probe (Fig. 72-2).

EXPERIMENTAL RESULTS

Much experimental work, using in vitro arterial specimens and in vivo canine models of both peripheral and coronary arteries, has been performed. This research has shown the following:

1. Total occlusions can be recanalized with little or no ultrasound induced damage to normal vessel wall, and with no sign of spasm or embolization.[1]
2. Ultrasound imaging, far from causing spasm, is vasorelaxant and antispasmodic. This is a time- and power-dependent effect (an increasing effect seen after 30 and 60 seconds of exposure) but is independent of the presence of endothelium. It may be due to breaking down of actin–actin bonds.[1]
3. Acute thrombus is dissolved with, again, minimal or no effects on normal vessel wall. Ninety percent of particles produced are less than 10 μm in diameter, and significant distal embolization has not been seen.[2,3]
4. Vessel wall compliance, for example, to balloon dilation, is increased.[1]

PERIPHERAL CLINICAL EXPERIENCE

The safety of therapeutic ultrasound during percutaneous angioplasty of total occlusions in the femoral/popliteal segment was confirmed. Dissection or perforation did sometimes occur using the probe as a recanalization device without a guidewire,[4] but this was related to the (then) considerable stiffness of the wave guide rather than the ultrasound energy itself. There was no instance of thrombosis, clinically or angiographically apparent embolism, or spasm in 45 patients. Technical developments included a more flexible over-the-wire device allowing prolonged exposure, for example, application of energy for 1 min/cm of lesion; the results suggested that compliance to subsequent balloon dilation was indeed, as had been suggested experimentally, enhanced.

THE CORONARY SYSTEM

Eventually, a system of sufficient flexibility to allow percutaneous coronary application was developed[5] and was first used clinically in 1993. The prototype coronary probe had a tip of 1.7-mm diameter and was ensheathed in a catheter of 4.6-F diameter. The catheter has a through lumen, the tip of which has two side holes and lies just behind the probe (see Fig. 72-2). There is a through lumen for flushing of saline, which is in practice given at 10 ml/min via an angiographic pump during energy application. The probe itself has a guidewire lumen, continuing through the catheter for 25 cm, thus allowing rapid exchange as with balloon catheters. The system is compatible with conventional percutaneous transluminal coronary angioplasty (PTCA) wires up to 0.018″ diameter; in practice we routinely use 0.014″ wires (Fig. 72-3.) This early system, though certainly suitable

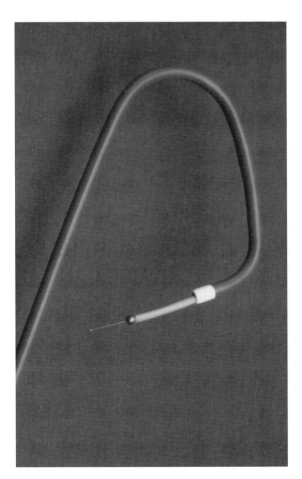

Fig. 72-3. The distal end of the ultrasound catheter, showing the probe tip, which oscillates during application of energy. The 0.014″ guidewire passing through the probe tip is seen, and the whole has been introduced through a left Judkins guide catheter.

for percutaneous coronary intervention, was quite stiff, reminiscent of balloon catheters of over a decade ago. The later version, comprising a 1.2-mm probe with a more flexible wave guide while providing more energy transmission, allowed use in less favorable anatomy (though very tortuous segments or angles still cannot be negotiated) and the lower profile facilitated crossing of severe lesions. The system is compatible with standard 8-F (or even 7-F large-lumen) guide catheters, and though Judkins shapes are often used, those providing better support, such as Amplatz, Voda, or Champ configurations, are chosen more often than in conventional angioplasty.

TECHNIQUE

Most procedures have been with the ultrasound catheter over a wire; we have recently used it as a recanalization device (see following discussion). Once the lesion has been crossed with the PTCA guidewire, the ultrasound catheter is advanced over it to the lesion. Though friction has not really been a problem, this is reduced during advancement and subsequent withdrawal if power is applied. The probe is abutted onto the lesion with gentle forward pressure and power applied; a characteristic of ultrasound, which is unusual in powered intracoronary devices, is that delivery is measured in minutes rather than seconds. As the experimental data suggest an additive effect with time, we have subjected many lesions to a total of 10 minutes of energy, without any sign of adverse effects. The probe gradually advances through the lesion with a combination of ultrasound energy and forward pressure, but we do try to minimize the Dotter effect by giving the probe time to advance. If there are features of ischemia because the lesion is occluded by the presence of the catheter, it is withdrawn into the guide catheter for a while. Even if the lesion is traversed quickly, we continue application of energy within it (moving the probe slowly back and forth in the case of long lesions), so almost all have had 5 or 10 minutes of exposure. Even if the lesion cannot be crossed with the probe, energy is still applied for the requisite time while the probe is being abutted onto the lesion because much (and perhaps the most important portion) of the lesion is still being exposed to the ultrasound energy. We have performed adjunctive balloon dilation in all cases, because a definitive lumen has never been produced by the ultrasound probe alone. We inflate the chosen balloon (usually 3 mm) in 0.5-atm steps every 15 seconds, because we are particularly interested in the "stenosis resolution" or "yield" pressure of the lesions

We have been impressed by the relative lack of complications and the angiographically good cosmetic results in long lesions, suggesting that ultrasound exposure before balloon injury does modify the lesion and render it more amenable, even if convincing evidence, or indeed usefulness, of actual debulking is relatively lacking. Any doubts that the ultrasound was affecting the plaque were dispelled by intraoperative experience in the Royal Perth Hospital (with colleagues Eccleston, Hodge and Cumpston); plaque elements sprayed freely from the arteriotomy site during application of energy but happily consisted of only small particles when examined. Further evidence was provided by experience during PTCA in Sheffield, in which the mean yield or stenosis resolution pressure was 2.9 atm in lesions after ultrasound exposure compared to 5.0 atm in a matched group undergoing conventional PTCA alone. There were several anecdotal cases in the multicenter experience of balloon-resistant lesions being rendered amenable by ultrasound, confirming the experimental findings of the ability of ultrasound to enhance vessel wall compliance.

Whether treatment of thrombus in clinical angioplasty is facilitated by ultrasound, as abundantly suggested by in vitro and animal experiments, is not clear. There has been favorable experience in the setting of acute myocardial infarction (particularly in Hamburg) and occasional examples where thrombus appears to have been ablated (see Fig. 72-5), but further experience, including a trial in recently thrombosed grafts, is needed.

As previously mentioned, there has been recent interest in using the ultrasound probe to recanalize chronic total occlusions. So far, these have been with reasonably favorable anatomy, when a conventional attempt was deemed appropriate but in which the consistency of the occlusion was found to be resistant. At first we tried ultrasound only when sustained attempts with progressively stiffer wires, supported by a Tracker catheter, and then the Magnum 021 system, had failed, but now the study centers have agreed on a compromise protocol in which attempts with an Advanced Cardiovascular System, (ACS) intermediate wire or equivalent are made; an attempt with ultrasound is then allowed.

Is restenosis any less after ultrasound-assisted angioplasty? It would probably be a surprise if it was; there are conflicting data at present. In the CRUSADE data base, angiographic restenosis (>50% diameter stenosis on quantitative coronary angiography) was 49% in 71 patients who had reached the routine 6-month angiogram point, whereas in Sheffield the rate in 46 patients, by the same criterion, is 30%. This may in part be due to simpler lesions being treated in the initial feasibility stage in the Sheffield center—time and further experience will tell. At least there is no particular suggestion of any increased vessel wall response after ultrasound exposure.

What of the future? In the near term, the particular niches mentioned are being further investigated by the multicenter group, including the CRUSADE centers, Milan (with a particular interest in total occlusions), and Royal Perth Hospital (with a particular interest in thrombosed grafts). The threshold for using ultrasound in a given patient or situation can be lower than with many new devices because of the simplicity of the equipment, the technique, and because it is so remarkably well tolerated. Technical advances continue; more flexible wave guides capable of carrying more energy are being developed and a transducer-tipped catheter, which would obviate the need for the energy to be transmitted throughout the catheter length and thus allow much greater flexibility, is technically feasible. Other applications for therapeutic ultrasound are being tried: these include intraoperative ablation of disease, the use of ultrasound to enhance local drug delivery, and even the treatment of arrhythmias.

REFERENCES

1. Steffen W, Siegel RJ. Ultrasound angioplasty—a review. J. Intervent Cardiol 1993;6(1):77–88
2. Hartnell GE, Saxton JM, Friedel SE et al. Ultrasonic thrombus ablation: in vitro assessment of novel device for intracoronary use. J Intervent Cardiol 1993;6(1):69–76
3. Steffen W, Fishbein MC, Luo H et al. High intensity, low frequency catheter-delivered ultrasound dissolution of occlusive coronary artery thrombi: an in vitro and in vivo study. J am Coll Cardiol 1994;24:1571–9
4. Siegel RJ, Gaines P, Crew JR, Cumberland DC. Clinical trial of percutaneous peripheral ultrasound angioplasty. J Am Coll Cardiol 1993;22:480–8
5. Siegel R, Gunn J, Ahsan A et al. Use of therapeutic ultrasound in percutaneous coronary angioplasty: experimental in vitro studies and initial clinical experience. Circulation 1994;89:1587–92
6. Ultrasonic angioplasty for chronic total coronary artery occlusion. Lancet 1994;344:1225
7. Hamm CW, Bertrand ME, de Scheerder I for the CRUSADE Investigators. Initial multicenter experience with therapeutic ultrasonic coronary angioplasty in patients. J Am Coll Cardiol 1995; Feb(Suppl):268A

73 Aortic Coarctation

P. Syamasundar Rao

Aortic coarctation may be present as a congenital malformation or may develop following surgery for native aortic coarctation or interrupted aortic arch. Until now, surgical treatment has been the only management option. Since the availability of balloon angioplasty, many groups of workers are considering this technique as a preferred option for the management of coarctation. In this chapter, I discuss balloon angioplasty of native aortic coarctations and postoperative recoarctations. A brief discussion of balloon therapy of other types of aortic obstruction is included. Limited experience with stents in managing coarctation is also reviewed.

NATIVE COARCTATION OF THE AORTA

Coarctation of the aorta may be defined as a congenital cardiac anomaly consisting of a constricted aortic segment comprising localized medial thickening with some infolding of the media and superimposed intimal tissue. The coarcted segment may be discrete, or a long segment of the aorta is narrowed; the former is more common. The classic coarctation is located in the thoracic aorta distal to the origin of the left subclavian artery, at about the level of the ductal structure. Rarely, the coarctation may be present in the lower thoracic or abdominal aorta. Varying degrees of hypoplasia of the isthmus and transverse aortic arch are present in the majority of coarctation patients. The most commonly associated defects are patent ductus arteriosus, ventricular septal defect, and aortic stenosis. The younger the infant

presents, the more likely that there is a significant associated defect. The prevalence of coarctation may vary between 5 and 8% of all congenital heart defects.

Neonates and infants with significant associated defects and occasionally those without associated defects may present with signs of heart failure or failure to thrive. Rapid deterioration of the infants with symptoms of low cardiac output can be seen and may be associated with rapid spontaneous closure of the ductus arteriosus. Children beyond infancy usually are asymptomatic; an occasional child may complain of pain or weakness in legs. Most often, the coarctation is detected because of a murmur or hypertension detected on routine examination.

Neonates and infants may have signs of heart failure including tachypnea, dyspnea, tachycardia, hepatomegaly, rales in the lung fields, and rarely, presacral and periorbital edema. When the infant is in heart failure, all pulses are diminished. Following treatment of heart failure, prominent brachial pulses with weak or nonpalpable femoral arterial pulses may be discerned. Blood pressure differential between arms and legs (>20 mmHg) may be appreciated. Auscultatory findings of associated aortic stenosis or ventricular septal defect may be heard. With isolated coarctation, there may either be a nonspecific ejection murmur or no murmur.

In older children, adolescents, and adults, a clinical diagnosis of aortic coarctation is best made by simultaneous palpation of femoral and brachial pulses; the femoral pulses are absent or decreased and delayed when compared with brachial pulses. Blood pressure in both arms and one leg must be determined; a pressure difference of more than 20

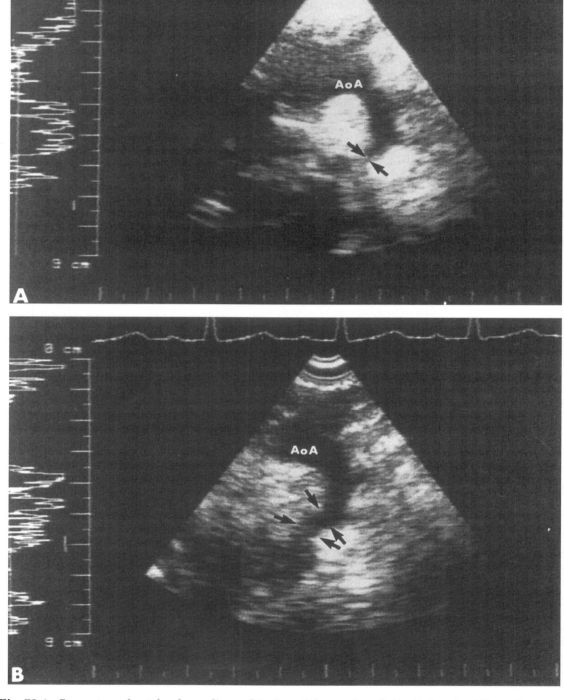

Fig. 73-1. Suprasternal notch echocardiographic view of the aortic arch (AoA) showing **(A)** aortic coarctation (*two arrows*). The same view following balloon angioplasty **(B)** shows much wider coarctation site (*four arrows*). (From Rao,[12] with permission.)

mmHg in favor of the arms may be considered evidence for aortic coarctation. Increased left ventricular impulse, a thrill in the suprasternal notch, ejection systolic click of the associated bicuspid aortic valve, and a nonspecific ejection systolic murmur may be detected.

Two-dimensional echocardiographic imaging usually shows coarctation in suprasternal notch views (Fig. 73-1 and 73-2). Increased Doppler flow velocity in the descending aorta with extension of the flow throughout the diastole by continuous wave Doppler (Fig. 73-2) are present. Instantaneous peak pressure gradients can be calculated using a modified Bernoulli equation, although the calculated gradients usually are overestimates[1] of catheter measured peak-to-peak gradients.

Cardiac catheterization and selective cineangiography, although not required for diagnosis, are helpful in demonstrating the anatomic nature of the aortic obstruction, assessing the extent of collateral circulation, determining the presence and severity of associated lesions, and more recently as a prerequisite before balloon angioplasty. A peak-to-peak systolic pressure gradient more than 20 mmHg (Fig. 73-3) is generally considered as evidence for significant coarctation. Aortography will demonstrate (Figs. 73-4 and 73-5) the coarctation.

In infants with congestive heart failure, the initial management consists of anticongestive medications, followed by relief of aortic obstruction. Infants with shock-like syndrome and those with metabolic acidosis may be benefited by intravenous prostaglandin E$_1$

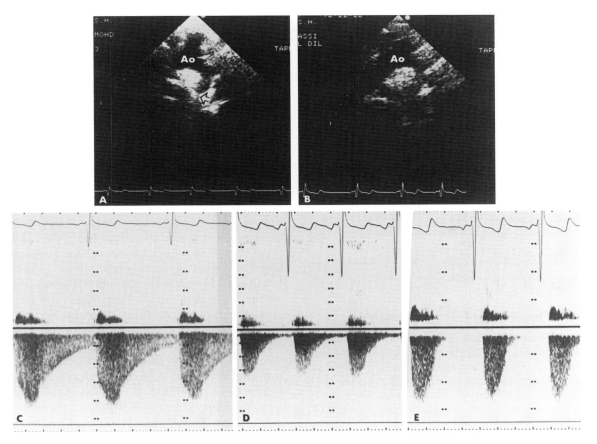

Fig. 73-2. Selected frames from two-dimensional echocardiogram from the suprasternal notch before **(A)** and immediately after **(B)** balloon angioplasty of aortic coarctation. The aorta (Ao) is shown with severe coarctation (*arrow*) in Fig. A, which improved markedly in the postangioplasty echocardiogram **(B).** Continuous wave Doppler flow velocity recordings from the suprasternal notch view directing the ultrasound beam toward the descending aorta before **(C),** immediately after **(D),** and 6 months following **(E)** balloon angioplasty. Note the high peak Doppler flow velocities with pandiastolic flow in Fig. C. The peak Doppler flow velocity fell immediately following balloon angioplasty **(D),** which decreased further on follow-up **(E).** Also note that the Doppler flow velocity, which was pandiastolic before balloon angioplasty **(C),** was present only in early diastole immediately angioplasty **(D).** At follow-up **(E),** there appears to be only systolic Doppler flow in the descending aorta. (From Rao,[53] with permission.)

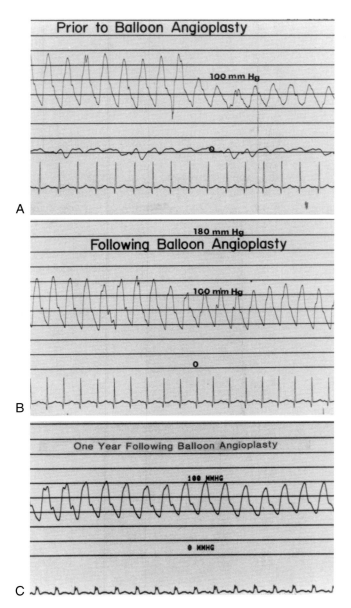

Fig. 73-3. Pressure pullback tracings across the site of aortic coarctation before **(A)**, immediately after **(B)**, and 1 year following **(C)** balloon angioplasty. Note the peak-to-peak systolic gradient across the coarctation site **(A)**, which improved immediately after balloon angioplasty **(B)**, and this gradient reduction persisted at follow-up **(C)**. (From Rao et al.,[54] with permission.)

infusion (0.05 to 0.1 μg/kg/min) because of its ductal dilating effect. We do not ordinarily administer prostaglandins if balloon angioplasty is contemplated. If hypertension is the problem, it is advisable to relieve aortic obstruction promptly rather than to treat hypertension with antihypertensive medications.

Relief of aortic obstruction can be achieved by surgical therapy and balloon angioplasty. Since the initial descriptions of balloon angioplasty of neonatal postmortem native coarctation[2] and postsurgical recoarctation,[3] a large number of investigators reported their experiences with balloon angioplasty of native aortic coarctation and consider this treatment option an effective alternative to surgical therapy.

Indications

The indications for balloon coarctation angioplasty are hypertension or congestive heart failure, which are very similar to indications for surgery. Although there is some concern with regard to development of aneurysms[4,5] following balloon angioplasty of native coarctations, a general consensus is emerging that these coarctations should be balloon dilated. This is particularly true in the neonate and small infant because of high morbidity and mortality as well as the high recurrence rate following surgery. Balloon dilation of coarctation of the aorta appears to offer a relatively safe and effective alternative to surgical repair in neonates and young infants. With angioplasty, operative intervention may be avoided entirely or at least be postponed until an older age and large size when surgical results are much better with regard to operative mortality and recoarctation. Should recurrence occur following angioplasty, or should aneurysm form at the site of dilation, the infant could undergo surgical resection at a later date when not as acutely ill.

With regard to older children with native coarctation, because of concern for developing aneurysm, the general recommendation has been that this procedure should probably be performed at selected centers with expertise in this lesion, and its general use by all should await longer follow-up results and reports of follow-up on a larger number of patients. It is worthwhile noting differences in the evolution of recommendation for balloon angioplasty for native versus recoarctation. Balloon dilation of postoperative recoarctations has been recommended[6] as the therapy of choice; this recommendation was made before the availability of data on immediate results in a significant number of patients and before the availability of any follow-up results. In contradistinction, balloon angioplasty for native coarctation was not recommended,[7] despite the availability of convincing data.[8] This type of recommendation is based in part on the speculation that the scar tissue in recoarctation may prevent progression of aneurysms, once they develop. Now that more data are available, the immediate results of balloon angioplasty in recoarctation appear good with significant reduction in gradient across the coarctation. However, the follow-up data are scanty. The availabledata with regard

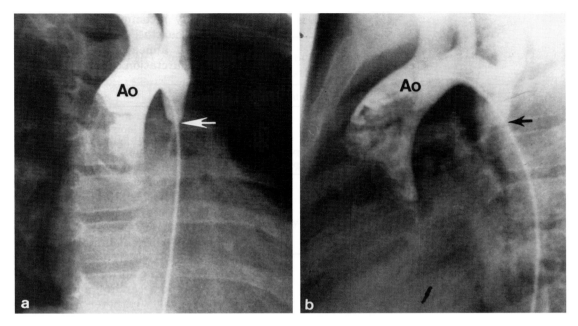

Fig. 73-4. Selected cineangiographic frames from an aortogram in posteroanterior **(A)** and lateral **(B)** views demonstrating aortic coarctation (*arrow*). Ao, aorta. (From Rao,[52] with permission.)

to recurrence and aneurysmal formation in postoperative recoarctations are tabulated elsewhere[9] and compared with that associated with native aortic coarctations. Although the number of patients with follow-up catheterization after balloon angioplasty of postoperative recoarctation is not large, it can be seen (Table 73-1) that neither the recurrence rate nor the rate of aneurysmal formation following balloon angioplasty of postoperative recoarctation is significantly different ($P > 0.1$) from that seen with native coarctations. In addition, when mortality and complication rates of balloon angioplasty in both groups were compared,[10] they were very similar (Table 73-2). Therefore, it is hard to justify balloon angioplasty

Table 73-1. Follow-up Cardiac Catheterization and Angiographic Results of Balloon Angioplasty Postoperative Recoarctations and Native Aortic Coarctations

| Authors[b] | Recoarctations | | | | | Native Coarctations | | | | |
	No. With FU	Rec[a] No.	Rec[a] %	Aneurysm No.	Aneurysm %	No. With FU	Rec[a] No.	Rec[a] %	Aneurysm No.	Aneurysm %
Lock et al.	1	1	100	1	0	—	—		—	
Finaley et al.	1	0	0	0	0	—	—		—	
Lababidi et al.	4	0	0	0	0	13	5	38	0	0
Allen et al.	6	0	0	0	0	1	0	0	0	0
Marvin et al.	—	—		—		11	—		6	55
Wren et al.	—	—		—		14	2	14	1	17
Cooper et al.	—	—		—		7	3	43	3	43
Beekman et al.	—	—		—		14	4	29	1	7
Saul et al.	5	2	40	2	40	—	—		—	
Morrow et al.	—	—		—		10	1	10	2	20
Rao	3	0	0	0	0	20	3	15	0	0
Total	20	3	15	3	15	90	18	20	13	14

[a] Recoarctation is defined as grdient in excess of 30 mmHg.
[b] See Rao[9] for sources.
Abbreviations: FU, Follow-up; rec, recurrent coarctation.
(Modified from Rao,[9] with permission.)

at the level of the diaphragm, as measured from a frozen video recording. I usually choose a balloon that is midway between the size of the aortic isthmus (or transverse aortic arch) and the size of the descending aorta at the level of diaphragm. If adequate relief of obstruction (pressure gradient reduction to <20 mmHg and angiographic improvement) is not achieved, a balloon as large as the diameter of the descending aorta at the level of diaphragm is chosen for additional dilation.[12,15]

Other technical details that are important in preventing complications are (1) heparinization of the patient with 100 U/kg. I usually give heparin before introducing the balloon angioplasty catheter. If facilities are available, activated clotting times should be measured every 30 minutes and maintained between 225 and 250 seconds. The heparin effect is neither reversed nor continued after the procedure. It is important to administer adequate doses of heparin to prevent thromboembolism. (2) Pressure of balloon inflation should be monitored, and attempts are made not to exceed that stated by the manufacturer; this is to prevent balloon rupture and its adverse effect.[16] (3) It is highly important that a catheter or a guidewire not be manipulated over the site of freshly dilated coarctation. A guidewire should always be left in place across the coarctation segment, and all angiographic and balloon dilation catheters should be exchanged over the guidewire. (4) Balloon size should be carefully chosen (see preceding discussion) to prevent aneurysm. (5) The tip of the J-shaped guidewire should be positioned in the proximal ascending aorta during balloon inflation so as to prevent inadvertent straightening of the catheter, which may cause injury to the aortic wall.

Mechanism of Angioplasty

Intimal and medial tears following dilation of human aortic coarctation were observed by several workers[12] as well as by our group. Indeed, the data from Suarez de Lezo et al.,[17] suggest that there is less gradient at follow-up in patients with intimal tears immediately after angioplasty than those without intimal tears. Thus, the mechanism of relief of aortic obstruction is by tearing of intima and media.

Results

Acute Results

While the initial experience showed poor results,[18] subsequent reports on balloon angioplasty appear encouraging, and the results have been detailed elsewhere.[12,19,20] Reduction of pressure gradient across the coarctation and increase in the size of the coarcted segment are observed in all age groups (Fig. 73-7). In our recently reported experience with 67 consecutive native coarctations, the peak-to-peak systolic pressure gradient across aortic coarctation decreased (P >0.001) from 46 ± 17 (mean ± SD) to 11 ± 9 mmHg, and the coarcted aortic segment diameter increased (p <0.001) from 3.5 ± 1.8 to 7.6 ± 3.1 mm following balloon angioplasty.

Improvement in pressure gradient (see Fig. 73-3) and in echocardiographic (see Fig. 73-1 and 73-2), Doppler (see Fig. 73-2), and angiographic (Fig. 73-5 and 73-8) appearance are seen. Even the collateral vessels diminish promptly, as illustrated in Figure

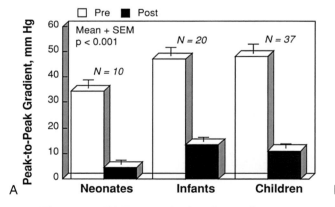
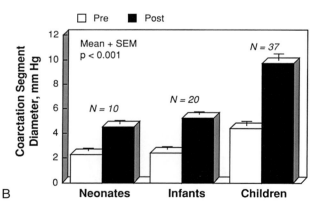

Fig. 73-7. (A) Bar graph of peak systolic pressure gradients (mmHg) across the aortic coarctation before (Pre) and following (Post) balloon angioplasty in neonates (<30 days), infants (1 to 12 months), and children (1 to 15 years). Note the significant (P <0.001) decrease in pressure gradient in each subgroup. Mean + standard error of mean (SEM) are marked. N indicates the number of subjects in each subgroup. **(B)** Bar graph depicting change in the diameter of the coarcted aortic segment (millimeters) following balloon angioplasty. Note the significant (P <0.001) increase in the diameter of the coarcted aortic segment in each subgroup. (From Rao,[52] with permission.)

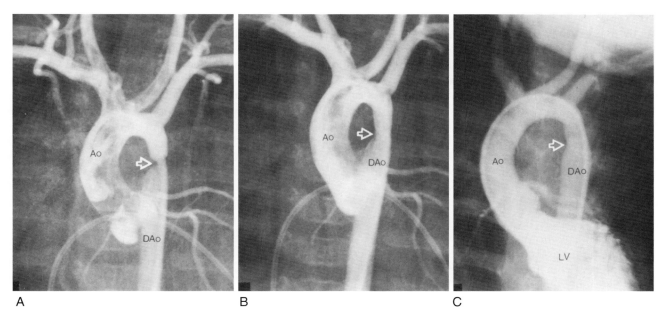

A   B   C

Fig. 73-8. Selected cine frames from angiograms before **(A),** immediately following **(B),** and 1 year after **(C)** balloon angioplasty. Note that the coarcted aortic segment (*arrow*) improved markedly after angioplasty **(B),** which remains wide open at follow-up **(C).** Ao, aorta; DAo, descending aorta; LV, left ventricle. (From Rao,[52] with permission.)

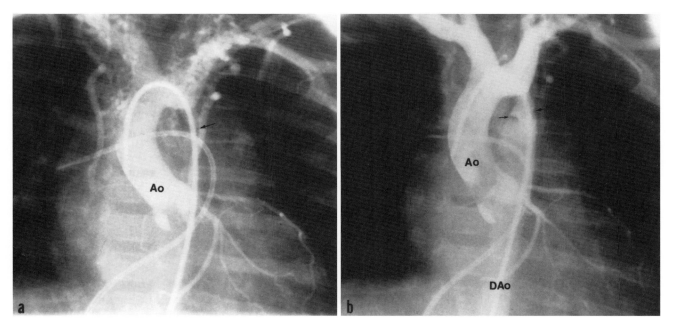

Fig. 73-9. (A) A selected cineangiographic frame from a posteroanterior view of an aortogram before balloon angioplasty showing aortic coarctation (*arrow*) and a large number of collateral vessels. **(B)** Immediately following balloon angioplasty, the aortogram shows marked decrease in collateral vessels. Both Figs. A and B were obtained at a similar phase of cineangiogram. In Fig. B, the sites of dilated coarctation segment (*lateral arrow*) and an intimal tear (*medial arrow*) are also shown. Also, note a greater opacification of the descending aorta (DAo) in Fig. B than in A. Ao, aorta. (From Rao,[12] with permission.)

73-9. The femoral pulses, which had been either absent or markedly reduced and delayed (when compared to brachial pulses) become palpable with increased pulse volume after balloon angioplasty. The infants who were in heart failure improved, as did their hypertension. The infants who were ventilator dependent were weaned off of the ventilator support and were extubated. Most infants (beyond neonate period) and children are discharged from the hospital within 24 hours after balloon angioplasty. None of our patients required immediate surgical intervention.

Intermediate-Term Follow-up

Several investigators have reported 1- to 2-year follow-up results; some of these have been reviewed previously[12,19] and these studies suggest continued improvement. From our own study,[20] 60 patients (58 catheterization, 2 clinical) were followed. The residual gradients at 14 ± 11 (mean $\pm$ SD) months following angioplasty remained low at 16 ± 15 mmHg. These gradients continue to be lower ($P <0.001$) than those before angioplasty (46 ± 17 mmHg) and are slightly higher (p <0.05) than the gradients (11 ± 9 mmHg) immediately following angioplasty (Fig. 73-10). Angiographically measured coarctation seg-

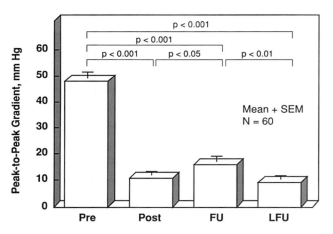

Fig. 73-10. Bar graph showing immediate and follow-up results after balloon angioplasty of aortic coarctation. Peak-to-peak systolic pressure gradients across the coarctation in mmHg (mean + SEM) are shown. Note the significant ($P <0.001$) drop in the gradient following angioplasty (Pre, before, vs. Post, immediately following). The gradient increases ($P <0.05$) slightly at a mean follow-up of 15 months (range, 4 to 56 months). However, these values are lower ($P <.0001$) than before angioplasty. At late follow-up (LFU), 6 months to 9 years (median 5 years) following balloon angioplasty, the blood pressure-measured arm–leg peak pressure difference is lower than catheterization-measured peak gradients before ($P <0.001$) balloon angioplasty and those obtained at intermediate-term follow-up ($P <0.01$). (From Rao,[52] with permission.)

ments remained wide. Improvement may be demonstrated by Doppler (see Fig. 73-2E), pressure gradient (see Fig. 73-3), and angiographic (see Fig. 73-8) data. Only a modest increase in (11 ± 9 vs. 16 ± 15 mmHg, $P <0.05$) was seen in peak gradients for the group as a whole, but when individual patient values were examined, 15 (25%) of the 60 patients had evidence for recoarctation, defined as a peak-to-peak systolic pressure gradient in excess of 20 mmHg. The incidence of recoarctation is higher in neonates (5 [83%] of 6; $P <0.01$) and in infants (7 [39%] of 18; $P = 0.011$) than in children (3 [8%] of 36). Ten of these children underwent repeat balloon angioplasty, and their gradients were reduced ($P <0.001$) from 39 ± 11 mmHg to 10 ± 6 mmHg. Early in our experience, 2 patients underwent surgical resection with good result. The final 3 children had no discrete narrowing and had no hypertension, and therefore no intervention was recommended. Aneurysms developed in 3 (5%) of 58 who underwent follow-up catheterization and angioplasty; 1 of these patients required surgical excision of the aneurysm and the other 2 were followed clinically.

Long-Term Follow-up

Data are scanty on long-term follow-up after balloon angioplasty of native coarctation.[20,21] Despite the problems of recoarctation and aneurysms, some requiring repeat intervention at intermediate-term follow-up, the long-term follow-up results (5 to 9 years) appear encouraging, in that there was minimal incidence of late recoarctation and no late aneurysm formation. Event-free survival curves (Fig. 73-11) following initial balloon angioplasty suggest that the event-free rates are better ($P <0.001$) for children than for infants and neonates. In the majority of children, the arm blood pressure remained normal, and blood pressure determined gradient between arms and legs remained low (see Fig. 73-10).

Applicability to Adult Patients

Although balloon angioplasty of aortic coarctation has most frequently been used in neonates, infants, and children, it can be used in adult patients as well. Lababidi et al.[22] and Attia and Lababidi[23] reported their experience with balloon dilation of native coarctation in eight consecutive adults, aged 19 to 30 years (25 ± 5 years). The systolic pressure gradient across the coarctation was reduced from 48 ± 19 mmHg to 7 ± 5 mmHg. The size of the coarcted segment increased from 6.8 ± 2.2 mm to 15.2 ± 5.0 mm. No complications were encountered. Clinical and echo Doppler follow-up 1 year after the procedure re-

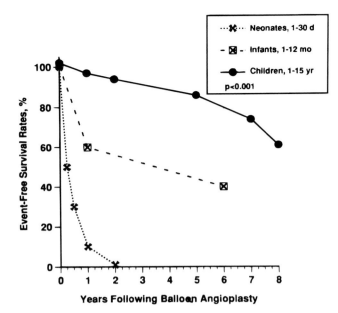

Fig. 73-11. Actuarial event-free survival curves of neonates (<30 days), infants (1 to 12 months), and children (1 to 15 years) undergoing balloon angioplasty for treatment of aortic coarctation. Note that event-free survival rates are better for the children group than for the neonatal and infant groups. (From Rao,[52] with permission.)

vealed good result with no more than 15 mmHg peak systolic blood pressure difference, measured by cuff, between arms and legs. They concluded that results in young adults are similar to those observed in children; balloon angioplasty should be considered as an option to surgical intervention; and follow-up studies (longer than 1 year) are required. Other reports followed, which are tabulated in (Table 73-3). Based on this review, it appears that aortic perforation during the procedure and aneurysmal formation at follow-up are also seen in adults. In addition, intimal dissection that persisted at 6-month follow-up was seen in one patient. Therefore, it is prudent to (1) avoid manipulation of tips of the catheters and guidewires in the region of freshly dilated coarctation; (2) choose an appropriate-sized balloon (no larger than the diameter of the descending aorta at the level of the diaphragm); and (3) monitor for development of aneurysms and, if found, closely follow the progression of aneurysms by repeated angiography or magnetic resonance imaging.

Complications

Complications during and immediately after balloon angioplasty have been remarkably minimal. Blood loss requiring transfusion has been reported, but

more recently, the availability of better designed catheter/guidewire exchange systems has diminished blood loss and the need for transfusion. Femoral artery thrombosis requiring heparin, urokinase (or streptokinase), or thrombectomy has been reported.[24] Use of smaller catheters and low-profile balloons may reduce the arterial complication rate. Though rare, cerebrovascular accidents, transmural tears with or without vessel wall perforation, balloon rupture at high inflation pressure, reopening of the ductal structure, prolongation of QT interval, and hypertension with a forme fruste postcoarctotomy syndrome have been reported following balloon angioplasty. Deaths associated with balloon angioplasty of aortic coarctation have been reported; these were either related to vessel wall rupture, ventricular fibrillation, additional surgery, or severity of associated heart defects. All deaths were in the infant group, and to the best of my knowledge, no deaths have been reported in children.[12] Meticulous attention to the details of the technique (as described), use of appropriate diameter and length of the balloon, low-profile balloon catheters, avoiding extremely high inflation pressures, and short inflation/deflation cycles may prevent or reduce complications.

Complications at follow-up include restenosis, aneurysm formation, and femoral artery occlusion. The issues related to restenosis and aneurysms are discussed in later sections of this chapter. Detailed studies from our group revealed that while indices of arterial insufficiency at rest are marginally lower (P = 0.06 to 0.07) in balloon than in arterial catheterization and control groups, these was no evidence for lower limb growth retardation.[25]

Comparison Between Surgical and Balloon Therapy

Data comparing surgical intervention with balloon angioplasty procedure are scanty. In an attempt to compare safety and efficacy of balloon angioplasty with surgical correction of aortic coarctation, we scrutinized 49 papers (published 1980 to 1991) reporting on results of surgery in infants 1 year of age or younger and 9 papers reporting on the results of balloon angioplasty and compared them.[12,19] These data revealed that recoarctation rates are similar, while mortality rates are slightly higher in the surgical than in the balloon angioplasty series. Similar comparison of results in children older than 1 year also revealed identical findings.[12,19]

Shaddy and associates[26] prospectively randomized 36 patients, aged 3 to 10 years to either balloon angioplasty (20 patients) or surgery (16 patients) and found similar immediate pressure gradient relief in

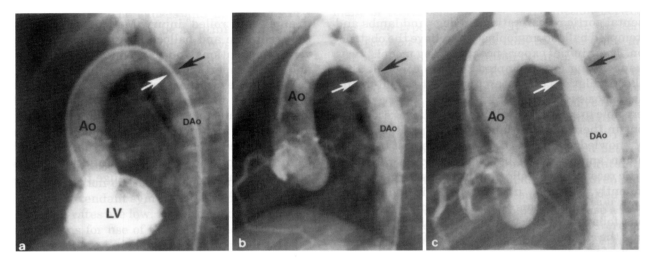

Fig. 73-14. (A) Left ventricular (LV) cineangiogram in a lateral view showing severe aortic recoarctation (*arrow*) in a child who previously underwent resection and end-to-end anastomosis. Note improvement immediately following **(B)** and 1 year after **(C),** balloon angioplasty demonstrated by aortic (Ao) root angiography (*arrows*). DAo, descending aorta. (From Rao,[36] with permission.)

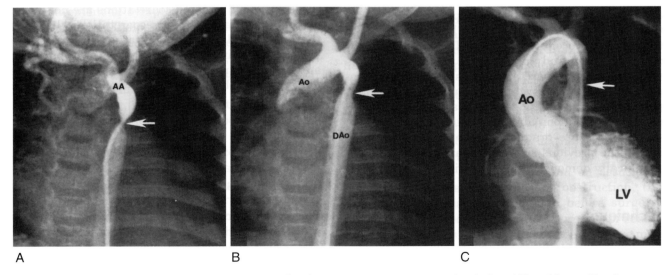

Fig. 73-15. Aortic arch (AA) cineangiographic frames in posteroanterior view before **(A)** and immediately after **(B)** balloon angioplasty of aortic recoarctation that developed (*arrow*) following surgical repair of aortic coarctation by a subclavian flap angioplasty. **(B)** Note significant improvement after angioplasty. **(C)** Left ventricular (LV) angiography 1 year following balloon dilation revealed excellent results. Also note marked improvement in collateral vessels both immediately after **(B)** and 12 months following **(C)** balloon angioplasty. Ao, aorta; DAo, descending aorta. (From Rao,[36] with permission.)

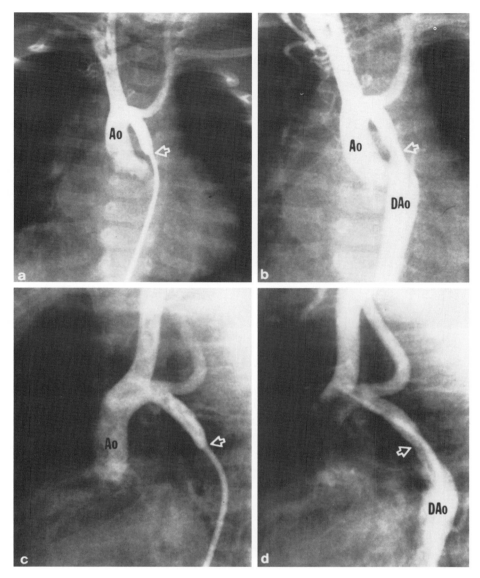

Fig. 73-16. Selected frames from aortic arch cineangiography in posteroanterior **(A & B)** and lateral **(C & D)** views before **(A & C)** and immediately following **(B & D)** balloon angioplasty in a child who developed recoarctation after repair of an interrupted aortic arch with a subclavian artery turndown procedure. Note the complete obstruction to blood flow **(A & C)** before angioplasty (*arrows*) with improvement in flow to the descending aorta (DAo) and an increase in coarcted segment size **(B & D)** following angioplasty (*arrows*). Ao, aorta. (From Rao,[36] with permission.)

Follow-up Results

A limited number of studies have been reported. These and our patients are tabulated (Table 73-4). Of the 76 patients in whom follow-up data are available, 19 (25%) had significant restenosis at follow-up. Aneurysms were found in 7 (9%) of 76 patients. Follow-up information on a larger number of patients for a longer duration of follow-up may be necessary before one can be certain of the long-term favorable effects of balloon angioplasty of postoperative recoarctation.

Complications

In the VACA Registry involving 200 patients, five (2.5%) deaths were reported following balloon angioplasty,[42] and this death rate is higher than that seen with native coarctations (0.7%, 1 of 141), also reported by VACA Registry,[43] although this difference did not attain statistical significance (*P* is between 0.05 and 0.1). Other significant complications reported by the registry included balloon rupture (9.5%), femoral artery complications (8.5%), post-

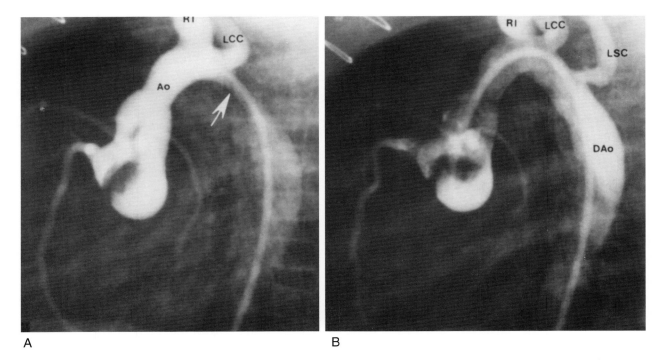

Fig. 73-17. Selected cineangiographic frames from lateral view before and immediately after balloon angioplasty of severe coarctation that developed within weeks of surgery for interrupted aortic arch. Note the markedly narrowed tubular narrowing (*white arrow*) **(A),** which became wide open after balloon angioplasty **(B).** The left subclavian artery (LSC), which is not opacified in Fig. A is well visualized in Fig. B. Ao, aorta; LCC, left common carotid artery; RI, right innominate artery.

coarctotomy syndrome (2%), and neurologic event (1.5%).

Causes of Restenosis

As stated in the previous section (see Table 73-4), a 9 to 80% restenosis rate is reported; the average for the entire group of 76 patients with follow-up data was 25% (19 of 76). Anjos et al.[44] found a 42% recurrence rate at a mean follow-up of 1.8 years. They examined several factors and found that aortic arch diameter and ratio of balloon/aortic diameter at the level of the diaphragm were significantly smaller in the poor result group. The high prevalence of a smaller aortic arch in the poor result group is similar to that found with recoarctation after balloon dilation of native coarctation.[28]

Aneurysms

Development of aneurysms at follow-up is another complication that needs to be addressed. The incidence of this complication appears to be 9% (see Table 73-4), similar to that seen following balloon angioplasty of native coarctation (see Table 73-1). It has previously been thought that circumferential

scar tissue at the recoarctation site following previous surgical repair may prevent formation of aneurysms, and if formed, prevent their rupture.[7,42] Such a hypothesis may not be tenable, at least in some patients; in the VACA Registry,[42] little scar tissue was observed surrounding a previous surgical repair site in a patient with aortic rupture following balloon angioplasty. Because the number of patients studied is small, the true incidence of aneurysms after balloon dilation of recoarctation is not known. In addition, reports of "aneurysms" without any intervention[45] and following surgery without balloon intervention[35] make the evaluation of aneurysms and the establishing of a causal relationship between the aneurysmal bulge and a procedure (surgery or balloon angioplasty) difficult. Careful review of angiograms (in multiple projection) performed before surgery or balloon angioplasty and their comparison with postdilation studies are necessary to detect "new aneurysms," presumably related to the procedure. Once detected, careful follow-up studies such as nuclear magnetic resonance or angiography are highly recommended to document the natural history of such aneurysms. For further discussion on aneurysms, see the preceding section dealing with native aortic coarctations.

Table 73-4. Follow-up Results of Balloon Angioplasty of Postoperative Recoarctations

Authors[a]	Year	No. of Patients Followed	Duration of Follow-Up, Months, mean ± SD (range)	Follow-Up Gradients, mmHg (range)	Aneurysm (%)	Restenosis[b] (%)	Comments
Lock et al.	1983	3	3.4 ± 2.9 (0.25–6.0)	15 ± 13 (5–30)	0	1 (33)	—
Lababidi	1984	4	—	10 ± 6 (5–18)	0	0	Duration of follow-up not given
Allen et al.	1986	6	7 ± 2 (4–11)	7 ± 8 (0–20)	0	1 (17)	Femoral artery occlusion at follow-up
Lorber et al.	1986	5	12 ± 12 (2–30)	24 ± 17 (0–45)	0	4 (80)	Repeat BA in 2
Saul et al.	1987	5	—	24 ± 22 (3–50)	2 (40)	2 (40)	Repeat BA in 2
Cooper et al.	1989	21	12 ± 8 (2–24)	12 ± 9	3 (14)[c]	3 (14)	Repeat BA in 3
Anjos et al[d]	1992	26	22 ± 22 (2–80)	—	2 (8)	11 (42)	Follow-up mean gradients for the entire group were not given; repeat BA in 3; surgery in 5
Rao	1993	11	30 ± 16 (8–42)	6 ± 6 (0–21)	0	1 (9)[e]	Femoral artery occlusion in 1
Totals		76		—	7 (9)	19 (25)	

[a] See Rao[39] for sources.
[b] Restenosis is defined as peak-to-peak gradient >20 mmHg.
[c] Includes 1 aneurysm that developed immediately after BA.
[d] Includes Lorber's cases previously reported, and therefore, the latter are excluded from totals.
[e] The gradient was across the hypoplastic aortic arch and not across the dilated aortic coarctation.
(Modified from Rao et al.,[39] with permission.)

Comparison With Surgery

The operative mortality rate for the second operation for recoarctation following initial surgical repair of aortic coarctation is high and varied from 0 to 33%.[36] The mortality rate following balloon angioplasty of aortic coarctations varied from 0 to 2.5%[42] and compares favorably with the operative mortality following a second surgery cited earlier.[36] Recoarctation rates following a second operation for postsurgical recoarctation are also high and varied from 6 to 30%,[19,36] and these recoarctation rates appear comparable to those reported (25%, 19 of 76; see Table 73-4) for balloon angioplasty for postoperative recoarctation. However, there are limitations to comparing the surgical data with balloon angioplasty data because of the small number of balloon angioplasty patients available for follow-up, the shorter duration of follow-up, and the possible inaccuracy of comparing older surgical studies with current balloon angioplasty. Nonetheless, there are advantages to balloon therapy, namely, avoidance of intubation, anesthesia, repeat thoracotomy, possible bleeding while isolating the recoarcted segment, risk of spinal cord injury, and stay in the intensive care unit. In addition, shorter duration of hospitalization and less expense are advantages of balloon angioplasty.

Summary and Conclusions

Since the first human application of balloon angioplasty of the postoperative aortic recoarctation in 1982 by Singer and his associates,[3] this technique has been used extensively by many other workers. Balloon dilation of aortic recoarctation is second to only valvar pulmonic stenosis with regard to the acceptability by cardiologists. Immediate results seem excellent with an acceptable complication rate. The results and risks appear comparable to those seen with repeat surgical intervention. Follow-up results are available in only a limited number of patients, with recurrence and aneurysm formation rates of 25 and 9%, respectively. These and arterial complication rates are likely to diminish because of progressive improvement of the balloon catheter technology and a greater understanding by cardiologists of the angioplasty technique.

Most cardiologists agree that balloon angioplasty is the treatment of choice for management of aortic recoarctations. A peak-to-peak systolic pressure gradient across the operative site in excess of 20 mmHg with angiographic demonstration of discrete narrowing is an indication for balloon dilation. Use of heparin, appropriate choice of balloon diameter, and avoidance of manipulation of the tips of the catheters/guidewires in the vicinity of freshly dilated coarctation are important technical features of balloon angioplasty. Periodic evaluation for evidence of renarrowing and aneurysms is necessary; these may be performed by clinical, echo Doppler, nuclear magnetic resonance, and angiographic studies.

OTHER STENOTIC LESIONS OF THE AORTA

Congenital and acquired lesions of the aorta, including atherosclerotic obstructions and Takayasu's disease, can be balloon dilated,[12] resulting in decreased pressure gradient, increased distal perfusion, and reduced proximal hypertension. The technique of balloon angioplasty, selection of balloon size, and other technical issues are similar to those described for native and postsurgical aortic coarctations. Follow-up results for these lesions are scanty and are needed.

INTRAVASCULAR STENTS

Implantation of intervascular stents for relieving obstructive atherosclerotic peripheral vascular disease has been well established. Application of similar technology to treat coronary artery lesions, branch pulmonary artery stenosis, and systemic venous obstruction followed. There is limited experience with the use of stents in the treatment of aortic coarctation.[46,47]

Both experimental and clinical data support the view that the stents, once implanted, are covered with smooth neointimal tissue similar to that observed following their implantation in iliac arteries and pulmonary arteries. Branch vessels that arise perpendicular to aortic axis remain patent after stent deployment. It has also been shown, in experimental animal models, that stents can be redilated, to keep up with somatic growth.[48,49]

Indications

The indications for placement of stents are not well-defined at this time. At the present time, based on limited experience, the indications are hypoplasia of isthmus and tortuous coarctation with malalignment of the proximal with distal aortic segment,

which are difficult to treat surgically.[47] Recurrent aortic coarctations or a small aneurysm following previous surgery or balloon angioplasty may be another indication for stent placement. Generally, balloon angioplasty is performed initially, and stents are implanted if balloon angioplasty is unsuccessful.

Technique

Stents

Stents Balloon-expandable Palmaz-Schatz stents (Johnson & Johnson, Warren, New Jersey) are the most commonly used stents for relief of aortic obstruction. Self-expandable Z stent (Gianturco-Cook Instruments) and wall stent (Medinvent-Schneider) have been used for other congenital heart defects. Their use for treatment of aortic coarctation, however, is limited.[46]

Procedure

Initially, a diagnostic catheterization is performed percutaneously, and pressure and angiographic data are evaluated for consideration of stent deployment. Conventional balloon angioplasty is performed initially, and if this is unsuccessful, stent implantation is performed. Initial balloon angioplasty provides the advantage of evaluating whether the stenotic lesion can be stretched. However, partial opening of the stenotic lesion may increase the chances of dislodgment and distal migration of the stent.

We recommend administering heparin (see preceding section entitled "Native Coarctation of the Aorta"), while other workers[47] do not. Angiographic frames showing good visualization of the stenotic sites are selected and frozen. Appropriate land marks (ribs, sternal wires, or right heart catheter) are selected for positioning the stent.

An 8-F long sheath is inserted, and it's tip is positioned proximal to the site of obstruction. We use an 8-mm diameter Olbert balloon catheter, because it can be inserted through an 8-F sheath, and the balloon fabric is such that it holds the stent without dislodgment. The Palmaz stent is mounted and crimped over a 40-mm-long balloon; the stent is placed in the middle of balloon between the two markers. A 0.035″ guidewire is left in place within balloon during crimping. The balloon catheter, with the stent mounted on it, is advanced over an extra-stiff Amplatz 0.035″ J-tip guidewire (the tip positioned in the ascending aorta) but within the sheath. Care is taken to avoid stent dislodgment during its passage through the valve of the sheath. The distal end of the stent is positioned 5 to 6 mm past the stenotic lesion. Because of the balloon inflation characteristics, the stent will move proximally, and therefore, the distal end of the stent is placed beyond the stenotic lesion.[50] Also, it is important that the distal end of the stent is a few millimeters distal to the origin of the left common carotid artery. The sheath is withdrawn into the descending aorta, proximal to the balloon, while the guidewire and stent-mounted balloon catheter are held in place. After the correct position of the stent is verified relative to the frozen angiographic frames and landmarks, the balloon is inflated; the pressure of inflation should not exceed the manufacturers' recommended burst pressure. The stent opens up and is deployed within the aorta. A second balloon inflation is usually performed with repositioning of the balloon, if necessary. The balloon catheter is removed, leaving the guidewire and the sheath in place. Then, a balloon with a diameter equal to the descending aortic diameter at the level of diaphragm is positioned within the stent and the stent redilated. Remember that the stent becomes shorter as its diameter increase, and this factor should be considered in initial positioning of the stent. Aortography to visualize residual obstruction, if any, and pressure fullback tracings across the opened-up coarcted aortic segment are obtained to evaluate the results of stent placement. There is no consensus with regard to anticoagulation following stent deployment. We recommend 5 to 10 mg/kg/day of aspirin for a 6-week period.

Results

The reported experience with stent implantation for treatment of aortic coarctation is limited to a few case reports[46,51] and a small clinical series consisting of 10 patients.[47] In the majority of patients, balloon-expandable Palmaz stents have been used. Despite marginal results in the initially reported experience,[51] results in the subsequent reports[46,47] are encouraging. In the 10 patients reported by Suarez de Lezo,[47] the peak-to-peak systolic pressure gradient across the narrowed aortic segments decreased from 43 ± 12 to 2 ± 3 mmHg after stent deployment. Angiographic stenosis has either disappeared (in 7 patients) or markedly reduced (in 3 patients); the ratio of diameter of the isthmus/descending aorta at the level of diaphragm improved from 0.65 ± 0.14 to 1.0 ± 0.08 ($P < 0.01$) following stent placement. The side branches of the aorta remained patent. At a mean follow-up of 4.4 ± 2.5 months, the blood pressures were normal without detectable peak instantaneous Doppler gradients.

Complications

Loss of femoral artery pulse (20%) and disruption of the aortic wall (10%) requiring a placement of a second stent have been reported.[47]

Conclusions/Comments

Although experience is limited, the stents appear to be useful adjuncts to balloon angioplasty in the management of patients with isthmic hypoplasia and tortuous coarcted segments. They may also have an effective role in the treatment of aortic disruptions/aneurysms following previous balloon or surgical therapy. Because of the need for inserting large sheaths into the femoral artery for stent delivery, the arterial compromise may be significant. The latter is likely to improve with miniaturization of stent-delivery systems. Implantation of stents in older children and adults in whom the aortic size has attained adult size may not be problematic, although such a procedure in infants and young children whose aorta will grow with time may pose a problem unless the stents can be redilated. Feasibility of redilation has been shown in animal models[48,49] but remains to be demonstrated in human subjects. Biodegradable stents, when they become available, may resolve this issue. Deployment of stents produces a noncompliant and nonpulsatile aortic segment. It remains to be seen whether such an aortic segment will have an adverse effect on blood pressure regulation. With these reservations in mind, it is prudent to reserve aortic implantation of stents for patients in whom there are no other effective and safe alternative methods of management.

ACKNOWLEDGMENT

I thank Lela Trotter for her assistance in the preparation of the manuscript.

REFERENCES

1. Rao PS, Carey P. Doppler ultrasound in the prediction of pressure gradients across aortic coarctation. Am Heart J 1989;118:229–307
2. Sos T, Sniderman K, Rettek-Sos B et al. Percutaneous transluminal dilatation of coarctation of thoracic aorta post mortem. Lancet 1979;2:970–1
3. Singer MI, Rowen M, Dorsey TJ. Transluminal aortic balloon angioplasty for coarctation of the aorta in the newborn. Am Heart J 1982;103:131–2
4. Cooper RS, Ritter SB, Rothe WB et al. Angioplasty for

coarctation of the aorta: long-term results. Circulation 1987;75:600–4

5. Brandt B, III, Marvin WJ, Jr, Rose EF et al. Surgical treatment of coarctation of the aorta after balloon angioplasty. J Thorac Cardiovasc Surg 1987;94:715–9

6. Lock JE, Keane JF, Fellows KE. The use of catheter intervention procedures for congenital heart disease. Editorial. J Am Coll Cardiol 1986;7:1420–3

7. Lock JE. Now that we can dilate, should we? Editorial. Am J Cardiol 1984;54:1360

8. Lababidi Z, Daskalopoulos DA, Stoeckle H, Jr. Transluminal balloon coarctation angioplasty: experience with 27 patients. Am J Cardiol 1984;54:1288–91

9. Rao PS. Which aortic coarctations should we balloon-dilate? Editorial. Am Heart J 1989;117:787–9

10. Rao PS. Balloon angioplasty of native coarctation. Letter. Am J Cardiol 1990;66:1401

11. Rao PS. Technique of balloon valvuloplasty/angioplasty. pp. 29–44. In Rao PS (ed): Transcatheter Therapy in Pediatric Cardiology. Wiley-Liss, New York, 1993 pp. 29–44.

12. Rao PS. Balloon angioplasty of native aortic coarctation. pp. 153–196. In Rao PS (ed): Transcatheter Therapy in Pediatric Cardiology. Wiley-Liss, New York, 1993 pp. 153–196.

13. Wren C, Peart J, Bain H et al. Balloon dilatation of unoperated aortic coarctation: immediate results and one year follow-up. Br Heart J 1987;58:369–73

14. Rao PS, Wilson AD, Brazy J. Transumbilical balloon angioplasty for the neonate with aortic coarctation. Am Heart J 1992;124:1622–4

15. Rao PS. Balloon angioplasty of native aortic coarctation. Letter. J Am Coll Cardiol 1992;20:756–7

16. Rao PS. Fatal aortic rupture during balloon dilatation of recoarctation. Letter. Br Heart J 1991;66:406–7

17. Suarez de Lezo J, Sancho M, Pan M et al. Angiographic follow-up after balloon angioplasty for coarctation of the aorta. J Am Coll Cardiol 1989;13:689–95

18. Lock JE, Bass JL, Amplatz K et al. Balloon dilation angioplasty of aortic coarctations in infants and children. Circulation 1983;68:109–16

19. Rao PS, Chopra PS. Role of balloon angioplasty in the treatment of aortic coarctation. Ann Thoracic Surg 1991;52:621–31

20. Rao PS, Galal O, Wilson AD. Balloon angioplasty of native aortic coarctation in infants and children: long-term results, abstracted. Europ Heart J 1994;15:263

21. Lababidi Z. Percutaneous balloon coarctation angioplasty: long-term results. J Intervent Cardiol 1992;5:57–62

22. Lababidi Z, Madigan N, Wu J et al. Balloon angioplasty in an adult. Am J Cardiol 1982;53:350–1

23. Attia JM, Lababidi ZA. Early results of balloon angioplasty of native coarctations in young adults. Am J Cardiol 1988;61:930–1

24. Rothman A. Arterial complications of interventional cardiac catheterization in patients with congenital heart disease. Editorial. Circulation, 1990;82:1868–71

25. Reddy SCB, Lee HY, Pie T, Rao PS. Arterial insufficiency and limb growth retardation following transfemoral artery balloon dilatations, abstracted. Circulation 1995;92:I–310.

26. Shaddy RE, Boucek MM, Sturtevant JE et al. Comparison of angioplasty and surgery for unoperated coarctation of the aorta. Circulation 1993;87:793–9

27. Rao PS, Chopra PS, Koscik R et al. Surgical versus balloon therapy for aortic coarctation in infants ≤3 months old. J Am Coll Cardiol 1994;23:1479–83

28. Rao PS, Thapar MK, Kutayli F et al. Causes of recoarctation after balloon angioplasty of unoperated aortic coarctation. J Am Coll Cardiol 1989;13:109–15

29. Beekman RH, Rocchini AP, Dick M, II et al. Percutaneous balloon angioplasty for native coarctation of the aorta. J Am Coll Cardiol 1987;10:1078–84

30. Rao PS, Koscik R. Validation of risk factors in predicting recoarctation after initially successful balloon angioplasty for native aortic coarctation. Am Heart J 1995;130:116–21

31. Rao PS, Carey P. Remodeling of the aorta after successful balloon coarctation angioplasty. J Am Coll Cardiol 1989;14:1312–7

32. Fontes VF, Esteves CA, Brago SLM et al. It is valid to dilate native aortic coarctation with a balloon catheter. Int J Cardiol 1990;27:311–6

33. Isner JM, Donaldson RF, Fulton D et al. Cystic medial necrosis in coarctation of the aorta: a potential factor contributing to adverse consequences observed after percutaneous balloon angioplasty of coarctation sites. Circulation 1987;75:689–95

34. Parks WJ, Ngo TD, Plauth WH et al. Incidence of aneurysm formation after Dacron patch aortoplasty repair for coarctation of the aorta: long-term results and assessment utilizing magnetic resonance angiography with three-dimensional surface rendering. J Am Coll Cardiol 1995;26:266–71

35. Pinzon JL, Burrows PE, Benson LN et al. Repair of coarctation of the aorta in children: postoperative morphology. Radiology 1991;180:199–203

36. Rao PS. Balloon angioplasty for aortic recoarctation following previous surgery. pp. 197–212. Rao PS(ed): In Transcatheter Therapy in Pediatric Cardiology. Wiley-Liss, New York, 1993

37. Castaneda-Zuniga WR, Lock JE, Vlodaver Z et al. Transluminal dilatation of coarctation of the abnormal aorta: an experimental study in dogs. Radiology 1982;143:693–7

38. Lock JE, Niemi T, Burke BA et al. Transcutaneous angioplasty of experimental aortic coarctation. Circulation 1982;66:1280–6

39. Rao PS, Wilson AD, Chopra PS. Immediate and follow-up results of balloon angioplasty of postoperative recoarctation in infants and children. Am Heart J 1990;120:1315–20

40. Rao PS. Aortic rupture following balloon angioplasty of aortic coarctation. Editorial. Am Heart J 1993;125:1205–6

41. Rao PS. Pseudoaneurysm following balloon angioplasty? Letter. Catheter Cardiovasc Diagn 1991;23:150–3

42. Hellenbrand WE, Allen HD, Golinko RJ et al. Balloon angioplasty for aortic recoarctation: results of Valvuloplasty and Angioplasty of Congenital Anomalies Registry. Am J Cardiol 1990;65:793–7

43. Tynan M, Finley JP, Fontes V et al. Balloon angioplasty for the treatment of native coarctation: results of Valvuloplasty and Angioplasty of Congenital Anomalies Registry. Am J Cardiol 1990;65:790–2

44. Anjos R, Qureshi SA, Rosenthal E et al. Determinants of hemodynamic results of balloon dilation of aortic recoarctation. Am Cardiol 1992;69:665–71

45. Parik SR, Hurwitz RA, Hubbard JE et al. Preoperative

and postoperative "aneurysm" associated with coarctation of the aorta. J Am Coll Cardiol 1991;17:1367–72

46. Redington AN, Hayes AM, Ho SY. Transcatheter stent implantation to treat aortic coarctation in infancy. Br Heart J 1993;69:80–2

47. Suarez de Lezo J, Pan M, Romero M et al. Balloon-expandable stent repair of severe coarctation of the aorta. Am Heart J 1995;129:1002–8

48. Gifka RG, Vick W, III, O'Laughlin MP. Balloon expandable intravascular stents: aortic implantation and late further dilation in growing minipigs. Am Heart J 1993;126:979–84

49. Morrow WR, Palmaz J, Tio FO et al. Re-expansion of balloon-expandable stents after growth. J Am Coll Cardiol 1993;22:2007–13

50. Bjarnason H, Hunter DW, Ferral H. Placement of the Palmaz stent with use of a 8-F introducer sheath and Olbert balloons. J Vas Intervent Radiol 1993;4:435–9

51. O'Laughlin MP, Perry SB, Lock JE et al. Use of endovascular stents in congenital heart disease. Circulation 1991;83:1923–39

52. Rao PS. Coarctation of the aorta. Semin Nephrol 1995;15:87–105

53. Rao PS. Value of echo-Doppler studies in the evaluation of the results of balloon angioplasty of aortic coarctation. J Cardiovasc Ultrasonogr 1988;7:215–20

54. Rao PS, Najjar HN, Mardini MK, et al. Balloon angioplasty for coarctation of the aorta: immediate and long-term results. Am Heart J 1988;115:657–65

74 Transluminal Therapy of Abdominal Aortic Aneurysm

Julio C. Palmaz

BACKGROUND

Abdominal aortic aneurysm (AAA) is the 13th leading cause of death in the United States, accounting for approximately 15,000 casualties per year. The incidence at autopsy studies averages 4%, and it has strong predominance in white men. This incidence seems to be increasing during the past few decades, either because of increased awareness or aging of the patient population or both.

The cause of AAA remains unknown, but multiple causative factors have been recognized. Smoking and hypertension are common in these patients, but constitutional defects such as abnormal proteolysis or structural defects in the vascular wall matrix seem to be necessary for the expression of the disease. It is unclear whether or not there is a genetic component in AAA, but inheritance seems to influence the development of the disease.[1] Untreated AAA mortality is excessively high. From 27 to 50% of patients with a ruptured AAA die before surgery, and of those who do not, 42 to 80% die in the perioperative period.[2] Elective repair of AAA carries a mortality risk of 3 to 14%, depending on surgical experience, type of facilities, and coexisting risks.

Patients with AAA share many risk factors with patients with widespread atherosclerosis. Myocardial dysfunction, pulmonary and renal insufficiency, and prior abdominal operations are some of the factors that significantly increase the operative risk. Attempts at decreasing the physiologic impact of the standard aneurysm resection were attempted in the past by nonresective techniques such as aneurysmal exclusion by iliac artery occlusion followed by axillobyfemoral bypass. It is uncertain, however, whether these techniques are effective in protecting against aneurysmal rupture. More recently, new efforts to treat patients who are at high risk for abdominal operation have focused on endoluminal or transluminal techniques. These techniques involve the placement of bypass material within the lumen of the aneurysmal sac via the femoral approach and are the subject of this chapter.

Historical Background of Endoluminal Bypass

Early attempts at endoluminal repair of vessels can be found in the work of Robert Abbe,[3] who reported repairs of vessels in animals with the aid of glass tubes. Blakemore et al.[4] used metallic tubes as coupling devices to establish continuity in injured vessels. A more recent example of this concept may be found in the sutureless aortic graft (Meadox Medicals, Oakland, New Jersey), which is usually applied for the treatment of dissecting aneurysms of the thoracic aorta.[5]

The first report attempting to combine x-ray-guided, transcatheter techniques and an intraluminal bypass device was by Balko et al.[6] This device consists of a wire stent coated with polyurethane. On extrusion from a delivery catheter, the spring-loaded tube opens up to a diameter a few times larger than the delivery catheter to bridge a portion of a vessel. Lawrence et al.[7] had a similar idea that combined a self-expanding stent and thin Dacron. At the University of Texas Health Science Center at San Antonio, this principle was furthered by combining Palmaz balloon-expandable stents affixed to the end of bypass Dacron prosthesis.[8] Later, a new approach was tried in our laboratories based on long balloon-expandable stents covered in their entire length by thin-walled, polytetrafluoroethylene (PTFE).[9]

More recently, other devices combining metallic fixation devices and Dacron conduits have been the subject of clinical evaluation. These are the EVT (Endovascular Technologies, Menlo Park, Califonia)[10] and a device described by Chuter et al.,[11] a combination of self-expanding stents and a bifurcated Dacron bypass. An additional device, consisting of a conduit of Dacron fibers and titanium wire, was reported by Picquet et al.[12]

The Animal Model of Abdominal Aortic Aneurysm

Almost as important as the development of a practical endoluminal bypass is the creation of a realistic and relevant abdominal aneurysmal model. Of the many animal models proposed,[8,14–16] only a few are adequate for the evaluation of endovascular bypass techniques. Among the limitations are (1) small aneurysmal size forcing miniaturization of the experimental equipment below practical limits. A similar consideration also applies to the access vessels, because when they are too small they are prone to spasm and thrombosis, and the resulting incidence of access site complications is unrealistically high. (2) Excessive thrombogenicity of the aneurysmal sac such as seen after interposition of a fusiform Dacron sac is another limitation.[8] This model has the advantage of yielding uniform aneurysms, both in size and shape. This allows for reproducible testing of the endovascular device, but it thromboses quite easily after the endovascular bypass is established. This is due to the inherent thrombogenicity of Dacron, the lack of endothelialization over its luminal surface, and the absence of side branches providing an outflow to the excluded aneurysmal lumen. An additional disadvantage of this model is its tendency to shrink as the Dacron sac becomes embedded in fibrous tissue. This causes aneurysmal shortening and kinking of the endovascular conduit with possible failure. Additionally, this model does not adequately mimic the human aneurysm in its tendency to grow and eventually rupture.

We favor the canine model of AAA created by placing a patch of autologous tissue in the anterior abdominal wall. Dogs are adequate for this purpose because, unlike sheep and pigs, they have large arteries relative to their body size. A convenient abdominal aneurysm model results from incising the anterior aortic wall longitudinally followed by placement of a leaf-shaped patch of autologous tissue. This can be procured from a segment of inferior vena cava or abdominal fascia; prefer the latter. Abdominal fascia is strong and easy to suture, it partially endothelializes, and it tends to expand with time. The aneurysmal shape is generally saccular, and its diameter usually exceeds 3 cm for a 45 to 60-pound dog. The advantages include the preservation of lumbar and inferior mesenteric arteries and persistent patency of the aneurysm despite the formation of laminar thrombus on the part of its circumference. Its tendency to grow with time and its autologous nature are obvious advantages because they provide some of the challenges encountered in human AAA.

STRATEGIES FOR THE DEVELOPMENT OF ENDOVASCULAR BYPASS TECHNIQUES

One of the most relevant issues in deciding on the material to use in the construction of endovascular devices is the biocompatibility of the materials and their mechanical endurance. Despite the fact that computer projection studies and accelerated tests may provide a rough estimate of material performance in the long-term, the critical nature of this application requires actual time testing in vivo. This entails a very long period of animal and clinical trials before safety and efficacy may be proved. One alternative is the combined or modified use of materials and devices whose performance is already proven and whose use in clinical applications has been time honored. This is true for Dacron and PTFE used as bypass conduits as well as for stainless steel alloys employed in the construction of endovascular stents. It is not surprising, therefore, that most of the endovascular bypass devices in trials today combine these materials in one way or another.

The timing for development of these techniques is opportune because recent refinements in catheterization materials and imaging techniques have made available many of the ancillary equipment components without which this novel therapy would be impossible. Several manufacturers (Cook, Inc., Bloomington, Indiana; Angiomed, Karlsrue, Germany; Applied Vascular, Laguna Hills, California) provide plastic sheaths with hemostatic valves that can be fashioned as delivery systems or device carriers.

Acceptable diameters for endovascular sheaths range from 18 to 22 outer diameter. Adequate lengths range from 35 to 50 cm. Diameters larger than 22 F would preclude use in the majority of patients. Diameters 16 F and smaller may allow percutaneous introduction. The new silicone, multiplane hemostatic valves are very effective to prevent blood loss within diameters ranging from that of a guidewire to the maximum diameter allowed by the valve opening. Thin-walled sheaths have a lower profile but kink easily. Thick-walled sheaths have good push and torque ability but are more rigid and tend to damage the iliac vessels. Thin walled sheaths with embedded metal braid incorporated in the thickness of the plastic material may be ideal for this purpose. Large balloon angioplasty catheters needed for devices dependent on balloon-expandable stents need to be available in diameters ranging from 15 to 30 mm. Because the larger the balloon diameter, the lower its pressure burst limit, the construction of balloons used for this application is critical. The balloon-deflated profile must be as low as possible, while its burst limit should be no less than 6 atm for a balloon 25 mm in diameter. The ends of the balloon must be tapered to allow unimpeded withdrawal from the sheath. The shaft should be not larger than 9 F. Smaller shaft sizes allow overall lower system profile but prolong the inflation–deflation time as the balloon channel becomes smaller. Also, manipulation may be compromised with smaller balloon shafts. A shaft tapered at the balloon site is the best compromise.

The overall size of the device mounted in its delivery system depends on the wall thickness of the stent or fixation device, the graft material, and the folded balloon, if the system uses one. The ratio of expanded to unexpanded diameter determines the device's ability to be introduced and successfully deployed at the target site. A ratio less than 4 is unacceptable and larger than 6 is desirable. This determines that the device's outer diameter should be 6 mm or less in its unexpanded or folded diameter to be clinically useful. Guidewires used for the delivery of cardiovascular devices should be not shorter than 180 cm, should be as rigid as possible, and should have a diameter of 0.035″. Larger diameter wires would limit the choice of catheterization equipment used.

Imaging of the AAA before endovascular bypass is critical because it provides essential information for the choice of length and diameter of the bypass device, size and configuration of the access vessels, patent side branches, presence of mural thrombus, and so on. Because a discrepancy of up to 25% may exist in the assessed measurements between angiography after correction for magnification, computed tomography (CT), and ultrasound, it is best to evaluate the aneurysm with a single, reliable imaging modality.

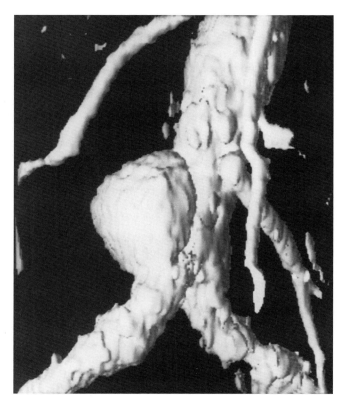

Fig. 74-1. Surface-rendered, three-dimensional reconstruction of 1.5-mm spiral CT sections following bolus contrast injection in a single breath-hold. A saccular aneurysm is seen, projecting to the right of the distal abdominal aorta and extending partially into the right iliac artery.

This is conveniently provided by spiral CT with three-dimensional reconstructions for rotational views of the aneurysm (Fig. 74-1). If the image acquisition can be obtained in a single breath-hold after bolus intravenous contrast injection, the measurements can be quite accurate.

Imaging during the placement of the device must be of the state-of-the-art quality. The roentgenographic equipment must have a large heat capacity tube, multiple field image intensifier, instant replay of digital images obtained at a rate of at least three images per second, and flexible positioning like that of x-ray tube and image intensifier mounted on a C-arm. Endovascular ultrasound may be useful for this technique but may result in increased cost, manipulation, and overall procedure time.

In general, if this technique is to benefit those who cannot undergo surgery and eventually become an alternative for those who can, it must be proven safe and effective. Cost-effectiveness, usually absent in most new techniques, will probably not be part of endoluminal bypass procedures. An inventory of devices of multiple sizes and configurations and all the ancillary catheterization materials is likely to be expensive. A possible way to decrease the cost of these materials is to design a device that would fit all sizes and to seek the use of inexpensive sheaths, balloons, catheter, and guidewires already available rather than to resort to customized equipment.

CLINICAL ASSESSMENT: STUDY GOALS

Like any other new therapeutic modality, endoluminal bypass of AAA initially will be applied to patients who represent a worst-case scenario; therefore stringent conditions will be imposed to evaluate both safety and efficacy. From the ethical point of view, selection of patients in whom the operative risk is high seems justified because of the inherent potential benefit of a technique that does not require extensive surgery. Some devices require iliac arteries of large diameter and relatively straight course to allow the use of their large introducer systems. This entails an extensive search for the "ideal" patient with the right clinical and anatomic circumstances. All the endoluminal devices require an infrarenal neck. This is a portion of the aorta below the renal arteries of relatively normal diameter and at least 10 mm in length. A "neck" above the bifurcation would be ideal for straight tube bypass placement, but such anatomy is definitely unusual. A neck below the renals and above the bifurcation is present in only 12% of all aneurysms, while an additional 34% includes those with an infrarenal neck but no distal neck (J. Allenberg, University of Heidelberg, 1994, personal communication). This suggests that if this technique were to be applied liberally, it could be used in approximately half of the patients eligible for treatment.

Unlike surgical endoaneurysmorrhaphy, placement of an endoluminal bypass entails leaving the aneurysmal wall intact in the lumen outside the bypass conduit. The long-term fate of the aneurysm and its contents is not known, particularly, whether the protection against aneurysmal growth and rupture provided by the endoluminal bypass depends on complete thrombosis of the aneurysmal lumen. Conceivably, the presence of the bypass conduit would attenuate the pulse pressure on the aneurysmal wall so that enlargement and rupture would not occur even if a "leak" is present. A leak represents circulating blood escaping the lumen of the bypass into the excluded aneurysmal lumen. Typically, a side branch of the aneurysm such as a lumbar vessel maintains persistence of the leak. The limited experience available suggests that such leaks tend to decrease in size

with time, to a size commensurate with the vessel that provides its outflow. Despite their unknown significance, leaks must be considered a technical failure to exclude the aneurysm and recorded as such. An important study goal is the serial imaging of bypassed aneurysms to follow-up diameter, fate of the leaks, and rate of aneurysmal rupture. Serial imaging should also provide information about integrity of the anchoring devices and bypass material as well as potential enlargement of the aortoiliac segments not covered by the device. Although serial ultrasound may provide useful information, spiral CT may be the ideal imaging modality for follow-up purposes.

TECHNICAL ASPECTS OF ENDOVASCULAR BYPASS

The procedure is performed in the angiographic laboratory by interventionalists, surgeons, and anesthesiologists working as a team. The patient is placed under general gaseous anesthesia after surgical preparation of the skin of abdomen and both groins, setup of standard monitoring procedures, and placement of a catheter in the abdominal aorta through the left brachial artery.

One or both common femoral arteries are dissected free, depending on whether a straight or a bifurcated bypass is to be placed. In case of a straight tube, the side with the least degree of iliac artery tortuousity or narrowing is chosen.

Following placement of vascular loops on the common femoral artery, a transverse arteriotomy is performed, and a suture is placed on the proximal edge

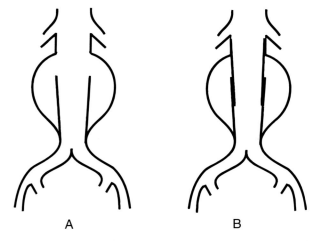

Fig. 74-2. Schematic representation of an AAA not involving the aortic bifurcation. **(A)** The distal stent graft is positioned first. **(B)** The second one is overlapped as needed to cover the infrarenal "neck."

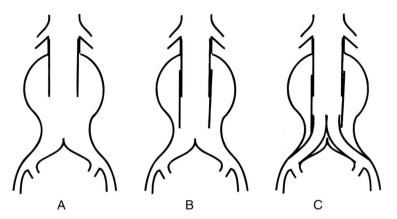

Fig. 74-3. **(A)** Schematic representation of an AAA involving the aortic bifurcation. The proximal stent graft is positioned first. **(B)** This is followed by a second one, overlapped as much as necessary so that the distal end is within 1 to 2 cm above the bifurcation. **(C)** Two iliac stent grafts are placed "kissing" in the midline. These overlap the distal stent graft by 1/3 to 1/2 of their total length.

to facilitate introduction of the delivery sheath. First, a guidewire is placed over a short straight catheter and positioned in the thoracic aorta. The delivery sheath with the stent–graft combination crimped over a balloon is advanced over the wire and posi-

tioned in the distal aorta. If the length of the aneurysm requires two stent grafts, the distal one is placed first (Fig. 74-2). During balloon inflation, care is taken to avoid expanding the balloon in the proximal iliac artery to prevent rupture. This is accom-

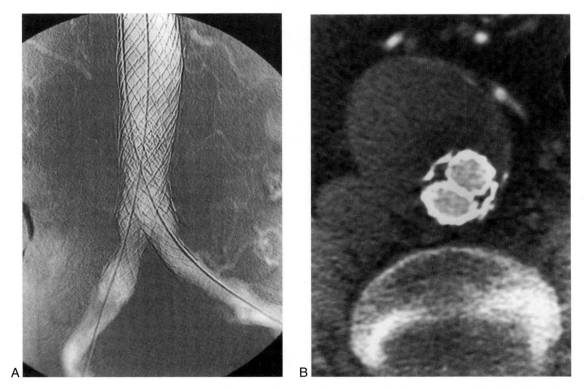

Fig. 74-4. **(A)** Completion aortogram after transluminal bypass of the AAA depicted in Fig. 74-1. Two overlapping stent grafts were used proximally, and two "kissing" stent grafts were used to reconstruct the aortic bifurcation. **(B)** Spiral CT section at the prosthetic bifurcation 24 hours following transluminal bypass. Intravenous bolus injection of contrast material shows patency of the iliac stent graft lumen and thrombosis of the excluded aortic lumen.

plished by using coaxial tubing over the shaft of the balloon catheter. The distal end of the tubing abuts against the distal end of the stent to avoid dislodgment from the balloon during withdrawal of the sheath, and it prevents expansion of the tapered portion of the balloon.

Following placement of the distal stent graft, the proximal one is deployed with a degree of overlap that depends on the patient's anatomy. This is established by contrast injection through the brachial catheter and serial, digital recording. During balloon inflation, great care is taken to correct the stent graft position as it is deployed. Because the stent shortens approximately 20% at full expansion, corrections must be done during deployment, depending where the stent anchors first. Shortening occurs toward the anchored end of the stent. This coaxial or "stacked" placement of the stent grafts allows for intraoperative sizing of the total tube length and in case of miscalculation or misposition, an additional coaxial stent graft may be placed using the same technique.

If a leak into the aneurysmal sac is detected on the control angiogram, a larger balloon is inflated in the stent graft to achieve a good seal.

Aneurysmal aortic bifurcations require a bypass with an inverted Y configuration (Fig. 74-3). This entails bilateral femoral arteriotomies because the bifurcated conduit is created by simultaneous deployment of "kissing" stent grafts. These may also be "stacked" by adding additional units to conform to the desired length. The diameter of the balloons needed to deploy the kissing stent grafts must be calculated according to the following formula:

$$d = (\sqrt{A/\pi}) \times 2$$

where A is the area of the conduit at the distal aorta and d is the individual kissing stent diameter. Following simultaneous deployment of the iliac stent grafts, the elastic recoil of the aortic stent graft presses the iliac stents together, flattening their surface at the point of contact (Fig. 74-4B). However, the small spaces remaining between the kissing stent grafts may be a source of a leak if side branches provide outflow. Most commonly, the iliac stent grafts must be tapered, because the diameter of the iliac vessels is usually smaller than the proximal diameter, as calculated. Heparin is administered before introduction of the first stent graft and as needed during the procedure. Broad-spectrum antibiotics are administered intravenously during the procedure as well.

REFERENCES

1. Reilly JM, Tilson MD. Incidence and etiology of abdominal aortic aneurysm. Surg Clin North Am 1989; 69:705–9
2. Quill DS, Colgan MP, Sumner DS. Ultrasonic screening for the detection of abdominal aortic aneurysm. Surg Clin North Am 1989;69:713–20
3. Abbe R. The surgery of the hand. Trans NY Acad Med 1994;10:639–62
4. Blakemore AH, Lord SW, Stefko PL. The severed primary artery in the war-wounded: a nonsuture method of bridging arterial defects. Surgery 1992;12:488
5. Ablaza SGG, Ghosh SC, Grana VP. Use of a ringed intraluminal graft in the surgical treatment of dissecting aneurysms of the thoracic aorta. J Thorac Cardiovasc Surg 1978;76:390–6
6. Balko A, Piasecki GJ, Shah DM et al. Transfemoral placement of intraluminal polyurethane prosthesis for abdominal aortic aneurysm. J Surg Res 1986;40:305–9
7. Lawrence DD, Charsangavej C, Wright KC et al. Percutaneous endovascular graft: experimental evaluation. Radiology 1987;163:357–60
8. Laborde JC, Parodi JC, Clem MF et al. Intraluminal bypass of abdominal aortic aneurysm: feasibility study. Radiology 1992;184:185–90
9. Palmaz JC. Research initiative in vascular disease. Bethesda, MD, March 25, 1994
10. Moore WS. Transfemoral endovascular repair of abdominal aortic aneurysm using the endovascular graft system device. Vascular and Endovascular Surgical Techniques. In Greenhalgh RM (ed): WB Saunders, Philadelphia, 1994
11. Chuter TAM, Green RM, Ouriel K et al. Transfemoral endovascular aortic graft placement. J Vasc Surg 1993;18:185–97
12. Picquet P, Rolland PH, Bartoli JM et al. Tantalum-Dacron coknit stent for endovascular treatment of aortic aneurysms: a preliminary experimental study. J Vasc Surg 1994;19:698–706
13. Anidjar S, Salzman JL, Lagneso P et al. Elastase-induced experimental aneurysms in rats. Circulation 1990;82:973–81
14. Boudghene F, Anidjar S, Allsire E et al. Endovascular grafting in elastase-induced experimental aortic aneurysm in dogs: Feasibility and preliminary results. J Vasc Intervent Radiol 1993;4:497–504
15. White JV. In vivo aneurysm formation in the rabbit after topical adventitial elastolysis. Research initiatives in vascular disease Bethesda, MD, March 26, 1994
16. Mirich D, Wright KC, Wallace S et al. Percutaneously placed endovascular grafts for aortic aneurysms: feasibility study. Radiology 1989;170:1033–7

75 Aneurysms, False Aneurysms, and Arteriovenous Fistulas

Juan Carlos Parodi

This chapter describes the development of an endovascular treatment for abdominal aortic aneurysms (AAA), arteriovenous (AV) fistulae, and arterial false aneurysms. Initial results of treatment for dissecting aneurysms and thoracic aneurysms are also analyzed.

The diagnosis of AAA has been established with increasing frequency during the past two decades.[1] This observation is probably related to aging in the population, as well as to extensive use of ultrasonography and computerized tomographic (CT) scanning for different pathologies. Although AAAs may occasionally cause distal embolization, rupture remains the most common and deadly complication. Elective replacement with a synthetic graft has proved to be the most appropriate method to prevent AAA rupture for nearly 40 years, and at respected medical centers, it has been associated with a postoperative mortality of less than 5%.[2] Nonfatal complications occur with some regularity irrespective of the setting in which the operation is performed. Vascular surgeons are increasingly encountering older patients with severe co-morbid conditions. This can increase operative morbidity and may even elevate mortality of aortic surgery to a figure in excess of 60%.[3]

It seems inevitable that every vascular surgeon will, with some frequency, encounter patients who represent a prohibitive risk for conventional graft replacement, yet alternative forms of treatment (such as axillofemoral bypass in conjunction with induced AAA thrombosis) have generally been abandoned despite preliminary reports of their initial success.[4]

In 1976, we began to develop a plan for endovascular treatment of AAA based on the fundamental principles of aortic replacement. We developed two prototypes, the first a self-expandable metal cage with a zigzag configuration covered by a nylon fabric and the second a Silastic bag with a cylindrical lumen. We eventually abandoned both of these prototypes because of the discouraging results we had in animal experiences, but we reinitiated our project in 1988 using balloon-expandable stents.

Our current approach is predicated on the concept that stents may be used in place of sutures to secure the proximal and distal ends of a fabric graft extending the length of the AAA. In AV fistulae and false aneurysms, a covered balloon-expandable stent has been used. A tubular Dacron or polytetrafluoroethylene (PTFE) graft or a segment of autologous deep vein have been used to cover stents. Experimental study had shown that stents could replace surgical suture and could act as friction seals to fix ends of the graft to the vessel wall. These friction seals were developed by transluminal graft stent combination by suturing a modified Palmaz stent to the partially overlapping ends of a tubular, knitted Dacron graft. This was done so that the stent expansion would press the graft against the aortic wall, creating a watertight seal. Placing of the stent-graft assembly was planned to be done by actually mounting the assembly on a large balloon catheter. This would be placed under fluoroscopy through an 18-F sheath (inner diameter) introduced through a femoral arteriotomy (Fig. 75-1).

This chapter details the endoluminal treatment of 92 patients: 78 AAAs (in 1 patient an AAA and a common iliac aneurysm were treated simultaneously; an infrarenal dissection with aneurysmal dila-

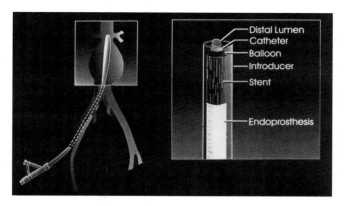

Fig. 75-1. Graft-stent combination is mounted on valvuloplasty balloon and placed under fluoroscopy through sheath introduced by femoral arteriotomy.

tion is also included in this group), 1 thoracic-abdominal aneurysm, 1 ascending aortic dissection, 7 post-traumatic AV fistulas, 1 infected false aneurysm of the common femoral artery, and 4 false aneurysms (axillary artery, common carotid artery, internal and carotid artery, and subclavian artery).

MATERIALS AND METHODS

Graft-Stent Device

A Teflon 18-F (inner diameter) sheath, 45 cm in length with a hemostatic valve closure in the operator end contains the balloon catheter, consisting of a 9-F polyethylene shaft and one or two nylon balloons, 3.5 cm in length, and either 30, 25, or 16 mm in diameter. The assembly contains one or two balloon-expandable stents (in case of two balloons, either two aortic stents or an aortic and an iliac stent). A thin-walled, crimped, knitted Dacron graft was sutured to the stents, overlapping one-half of the length of the stent (Fig. 75-2).

The stent is made of annealed stainless steel, 316L, because this alloy has been widely used in a variety of prosthetic applications. Corrosion of implanted metal pieces usually occurs at sites of cracks and crevices on the metal surface. Therefore, the surface of metal stents must be uniform. The balloon-expandable stent is made as a single piece to avoid motion between parts. Micromotion between metal surfaces disrupts protective oxide films, allowing the area to corrode rapidly.

The graft is a thin-walled (0.2 mm) weft-knitted graft with compliant ends (45%) to allow expansion of the stent. Diameters of the grafts are 18 and 20 mm when tubular grafts are applied and 18 and 8 mm when tapered grafts for the aortoiliac position

are needed. For thoracic aorta application, a 25-mm diameter graft was utilized.

The balloon catheter we currently use (Balt, Paris, France) is constructed of nylon and has some degree of compliance. This compliance allow us to use only two balloon sizes (25 and 30 mm in diameter). For aortoiliac grafting either a double balloon (25 and 12 mm in diameter) or two independent balloons are used. When AV fistulas or false aneurysms were treated, a covered stent was constructed by covering the stent with an expandable Dacron graft or a pre-expanded PTFE graft. On two occasions the stent was covered with autogenous vein because of concerns about infection. The only case of false aneurysm of the internal carotid artery was treated by a vein-covered stent with the rationale of providing a less thrombogenic surface.

Procedure

Under local or epidural anesthesia the patient is prepared and draped as for a standard AAA resection.[5] In the two cases in which the thoracic aneurysm was treated, general anesthesia was utilized. A small in-

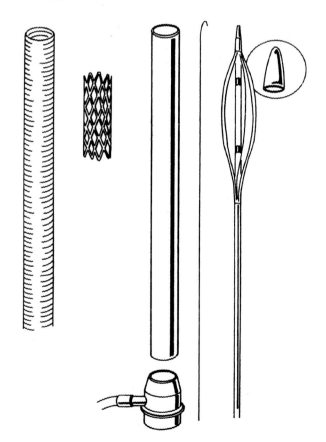

Fig. 75-2. The elements comprising the endovascular device.

cision is developed over the chosen common femoral artery; usually the straighter and wider artery is selected for access. A soft-tip guidewire is advanced in the aorta up to the level of the diaphragm. Over the wire a pigtail diagnostic catheter is placed inside the lumen of the aorta with the tip located proximal to the renal arteries. The first injection of 30 ml of contrast media is given. The pigtail catheter has radiopaque marks engraved on its surface every 2 cm to facilitate lengths and diameter measurements using quantitative angiography.

With previously obtained images (angiogram and CT scan) and the new angiogram, target areas are defined. They could be the proximal neck of the aneurysm and distal cuff if this latter exists, or the common iliac artery if the distal cuff is absent. The preloaded sheath containing the stent and graft mounted on a balloon is placed inside the lumen of the aneurysm under fluoroscopic guidance. Once in place, the sheath is removed and the cranial balloon

is inflated with a diluted solution of ionic contrast media and saline. (We discarded the nonionic contrast media because of the potential problem of crystallization.) The balloon is kept inflated for 1 minute and then gently deflated. Before proceeding with balloon inflation, the main blood pressure is dropped using nitroglycerin solution. Pressure is kept at 70 mmHg during balloon inflation. The size of the balloon is selected beforehand according to the diameter of the neck of the aneurysm measured by the previous angiogram and CT scan.

After securing the proximal stent, the second stent is placed. In some cases in which a double balloon device is used, the second balloon (either aortic or iliac) is positioned at the appropriate level and inflated deploying the second stent. A final angiogram is performed. If an aortoiliac graft is placed, the procedure ends with a femorofemoral bypass and balloon or stent occlusion of the contralateral common iliac artery (Fig. 75-3).

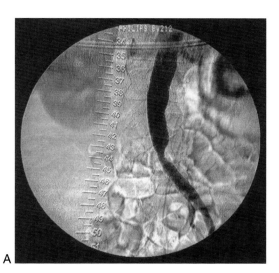

A

Fig. 75-3. (A) Aortoiliac graft in place. **(B)** Balloon occlusion of the contralateral iliac artery. **(C)** Femorofemoral bypass.

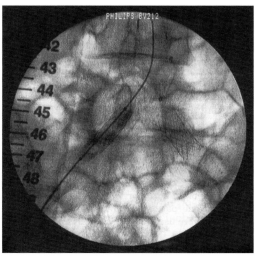

B

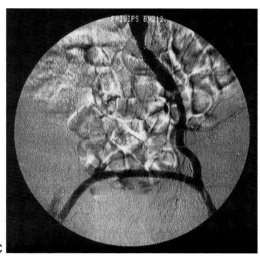

C

One patient developed a distal aortic dilation 18 months after the initial procedure. The distal stent was placed too distally of the aortic bifurcation and in contact with mural thrombus and not with normal aortic wall. The complication was corrected by adding a short segment of graft and performing a surgical anastomosis between the old graft and the aortic bifurcation. The patient recovered uneventfully. Four patients who had only the proximal stent deployed developed a distal reflux with shrinkage of the graft 8, 18, 24, and 29 months, respectively, after the procedure. Two had an additional procedure to correct this complication (insertion of a covered stent at the distal end) sealing the leak completely in one. The second patient was left with a minimal leak since it was impossible with our current resources to obtain the expected result. One patient is ready to have additional treatment, and the fourth declined further procedures.

One patient who had had an aortoiliac graft implanted 2 years before developed a distal leak. The iliac artery in which the distal stent was implanted was aneurysmal, and the stent was anchored at the point of a ring of normal caliber in the middle of the common iliac artery. The aneurysm increased in size, and the leak was created. An attempt to seal the leak failed.

Two patients with aortoaortic grafts with two stents developed a distal leak after 12 and 16 months, for unexplained reasons. Two patients died 13 and 24 months, respectively, after the procedure affected carcinomas of the colon. An additional patient died after being admitted to the clinic because of cardiac failure and respiratory insufficiency 8 months after the initial procedure. Two patients died of cardiac insufficiency 6 and 7 months after the procedure. One patient with proximal leak (failure) died of a ruptured AAA 2 months after the unsuccessful procedure. One patient who had a late failure 16 months after the procedure (distal leak after an aortoaortic graft) sustained a ruptured aneurysm and died. One patient was readmitted to the clinic 3 months after the initial procedure with a pulmonary edema and was discharged after 1 week. One patient developed a subdural hematoma 3 months after the initial treatment. He did well after the hematoma was surgically drained. The hematoma was probably caused by a small trauma since our patients did not receive specific medication after the treatment, not even antiplatelet drugs.

Sixty-two percent of the patients from the initial group and 80% of the initially successful group of patients had good results after the primary procedure until the last clinical visit or until the moment of their death caused by an unrelated cause.

Only one patient with an aortoiliac procedure had a late failure (distal reflux into the aneurysmal sac). Initial results of aortoiliac procedures were inferior when compared with aortoaortic procedures due to the larger profile of the introducer needed for its deployment, which generated inconveniences with access. However, late results were more favorable with the aortoiliac procedure. Most of the complications were correctable by additional endoluminal procedures.

Arteriovenous Fistulae

Six patients were treated using this procedure. In the first patient a subclavian AV fistula developed after a gunshot wound sustained 2 years before the consultation. As a consequence of this high-output AV fistula, the patient developed congestive heart failure. Under local anesthesia a covered palmaz iliac stent was inserted, closing the abnormal communication. The stent was covered with a knitted Dacron graft. A 12-mm-diameter balloon was used to deploy the stent-graft device. The patient had a favorable outcome.

The second patient had a common iliac-inferior vena cava fistula, caused by an accident during laparoscopic surgery. A percutaneous stent-graft was applied from the ipsilateral common femoral artery. The third patient was referred to us to resolve an AV fistula between the abdominal aorta and the inferior vein cava. The patient had sustained a gunshot wound several months before and had had four surgical attempts to treat multiple lesions in the abdomen including the AV fistula. The last attempt was unsuccessful and ended with a cardiac arrest after an exsanguination in an attempt to close the communication. The inferior vena cava was ligated and the procedure concluded after reanimation of the patient with large volumes of whole blood. The patient was transferred to our clinic and treated a few days later with an endoluminal procedure performed under local anesthesia. A 3.5-cm covered stent was deployed, covering the communication and effectively interrupting the flow through the fistula. The patient was discharged the next day. An additional patient who was admitted because of an aortocava fistula was treated successfully in the same way.

The sixth patient treated for an AV fistula was a young woman who had been attacked in her store and received a gunshot wound in her right thigh. An AV fistula between the superficial femoral artery and vein was diagnosed. A covered stent was applied at the site of the fistula percutaneously using a 14-F sheath applied anterogradely through the common femoral artery.

Infected Femoral False Aneurysm

A patient was admitted with an infected false aneurysm of the common femoral artery caused by a coronary stenting procedure performed 10 days before. The patient suffered from renal insufficiency and unstable angina. A stent covered with autologous vein was deployed through the superficial femoral artery. Expansion of the false aneurysm subsided, and the cavity was debrided and drained.

A 30-year-old man who sustained a gunshot wound in the right supraclavicular region developed an AV fistula between the subclavian artery and vein and a false aneurysm of the thyrocervical branch of the subclavian artery. A detachable balloon occluded the false aneurysm of the branch and a Dacron-covered stent occluded the abnormal communication between the artery and vein.

A 20-year old man was admitted to the clinic with a false aneurysm of the common carotid artery near its take-off from the innominate trunk. The patient had the acquired immunodeficiency syndrome. A covered stent using autologous vein was deployed, covering the orifice of the carotid artery.

The last vascular trauma case we treated was a 38-year-old patient who had sustained a neck trauma in the past and developed a false aneurysm at the level of the base of the skull (probably related to a carotid dissection). The patient had had five episodes of cerebral ischemia with resulting cerebral infarcts depicted in the CT scan. The last two episodes of cerebral ischemia had occurred during oral anticoagulation treatment. The patient was treated using a vein-covered palmaz stent. He had no further episodes of cerebral ischemia, and the false aneurysm was effectively excluded.

All the procedures used to treat trauma cases were successful. Two patients were treated for common iliac aneurysms, and one patient had an AAA treated simultaneously. Both procedures were successful in the short and long term.

Secondary Procedures

When the endoluminal treatment failed either initially or after variable periods of time after an initially successful procedure (usually signs of incomplete sealing of the graft were the indicators of failure). Secondary procedures were considered to solve the problem. Needless to say, because of the prohibitive risk of a standard surgical treatment, in many cases if the initial endoluminal treatment could not be completed, the procedure was abandoned, leaving the patient in the same situation as

before treatment. Exceptions were one patient in whom the stent-graft was mispositioned (which resulted in occlusion of both iliac arteries) and a second patient in whom the device migrated caudally because of incomplete deployment of the stent. Both patients were operated on immediately.

An additional patient who had a distal reflux a few months after the primary procedure required surgical insertion of a graft, which was anastomosed to the initial graft placed endoluminally and then sutured to the distal aorta.

One patient had an unsuccessful endoluminal procedure. A proximal leak could not be repaired endoluminally. Because of the prohibitive risk, an operation was not performed. He sustained a ruptured aneurysm 2 months later and underwent surgery. During surgery he sustained a cardiac arrest shortly after laparotomy was performed. It is important to note that the area in which the stent was placed could not be clamped. Since the proximal stent was deployed flush to the renal ostia, clamping was performed at the supraceliac area and then a balloon inflated at the level of the neck, releasing the supraceliac clamp. Another comment should be made regarding sutures in the presence of metal stents. Suture in contact with metal can rupture immediately or as a result of friction after some time. Thus it is not advisable, to suture a graft at the level of the stent. There are two ways to overcome this problem. One is to remove the stent. If the stent was deployed recently (less than 2 weeks) it is possible to compress the stent, reducing its diameter, and then to remove it. If the stent was inserted weeks or months before, trying to remove it is not recommended since the wall of the artery will become severely damaged. Facing this dilemma, we believe that it is advisable to place a second stent graft inside the first.

All other secondary procedures were endoluminal, not surgical procedures.

DISCUSSION

After 80 procedures for treating aneurysms and 12 for other applications (AV fistulas and false aneurysms), some preliminary conclusions may be formed. The procedure is feasible and when successfully applied has the great attraction of simplicity. The application of covered stents in trauma cases appears to be one of the main applications of this method since it transforms a complicated and potentially dangerous procedure into a simple and safe one. Stenosis can be defined as the only potential complication in the long term. In the near future stent grafts could eventually be used in acute injuries of the vessel, both in civil or war conditions to stop blood loss temporarily or definitively. This procedure can be combined with endovascular control of bleeding of secondary branches using detachable balloons, coils, occluding stents, or injection of fluids that become solid inside the body when body temperature is reached. This procedure proved useful in injuries of vessels such as the subclavian artery that represent a real challenge even to the experienced surgeon. More problems arose when treating aortic aneurysms than those that could be predicted initially. The procedure is simple in theory, but several details should be taken care of before moving ahead with widespread use.

Reliable Measurements

Measurement of diameters and lengths is crucial. We learned with great effort how to obtain reliable data by using enhanced CT scans, quantitative angiography, three-dimensional reconstruction using magnetic resonance imaging (MRI) or CT scans, intraluminal measurement, and some geometric calculations. Understanding that elongation occurs as dilation of the aorta develops and also that elongation occurs in different planes allowed us to calculate more accurately the actual length of the artery. Using a diagnostic catheter with radiopaque marks helps in obtaining length and diameter measurements. However, one factor that should be considered to prevent misinterpretation of the data obtained is parallax. Parallax is a result of the dispersion of the x-ray beams. As soon as the beams are released from the source of radiation, they are not completely parallel, which makes measurements performed at the periphery of the x-ray screen distorted. Error in measuring aneurysmal length caused by parallax can be in excess of 3 cm. Another cause of error in measuring length using a catheter is that the location of the catheter inside the lumen depends on the morphology of the lumen and does not always occupy the center of the lumen. As a matter of fact, a catheter will seat in the shortest way inside the lumen. The graft to be used is not linear like the catheter, since it has some volume and a diameter not less than 18 mm. Location of the catheter inside the lumen of the aneurysm is also influenced by the presence of angles, a catheter is semirigid; thus it does not duplicate the shape of the curves. As a result, in very tortuous aneurysms, the axial length is underestimated when measured using a catheter with radiopaque marks. One simple maneuver to prevent or diminish error from parallax is to use only the center of the screen for measurements, using either a radiopaque ruler or a diagnostic catheter with marks.

We developed a simple software program based on the pythagorean theorem to overcome the problem of measuring lengths in tortuous aneurysms. The unknown side of the triangle is the hypotenuse. The triangle is formed as follows: one side is the distance between slices of the CT scan (usually 0.5 to 1 cm); the second side, forming a 90-degree angle with the former, is the distance between the center of the lumen of the two adjacent slices; the third side is the actual axis of the lumen, it opposes to the right angle, and for this reason it is considered the hypotenuse.

Vertical measurement in the presence of elongation is incorrect since it does not count the extra length provoked by elongation. Making CT scan studies with slices every 5 mm and measuring displacement of the axis of the lumen is all that is needed. As was described above, two of the three sides of a triangle are known. One side is the distance between slices (5 or 10 mm) and the second is the distance between two consecutive center points of the aneurysmal lumen. When no change in the vertical axis occurs, this side is equivalent to 0. Then the distance between two consecutive slices is simply the interval between slices (5 mm or 1 cm). On the other hand, when the axis varies, the second side has a value. This figure should be included in the pythagorean equation and its square added to the square of the slice length. The square root of the sum is the actual distance between two center points of the lumen of the aneurysm. Adding the distances between consecutive slices results in the length of the selected section of the axis.

At this point we know that we need a hologram rather than a three-dimensional reconstruction shown on a two-dimension screen. Measurement is accomplished between the lower renal artery and the aortic bifurcation. As in surgery, we prefer to cover the whole length between these two sites with a stent graft. A problem arises, however, when the cut is made oblique to the axis of the AAA, since tortuosity makes the axis of the aneurysm not parallel to the axis of the body. When the artery bends and the slice is taken perpendicular to the body axis, the shape of the slice is not circular but oval, being the actual diameter the smaller. When this oval figure is obtained, it is not possible, (by this method alone) to determine which is the center of the slice. Additional data are necessary.

A simpler method of measurement involves using the spiral CT scan. The three-dimensions image is developed, and the segment between the more distal renal artery and the aortic bifurcation is divided into

10 equal segments. The image is rotated 360 degrees, and the maximum length of each segment measured in any of the images of rotation is considered the actual length. The sum of the maximum length of all 10 segments is equivalent to the actual length of the artery.

It appears that the final answer in regard to measurement will come from computer image processing using three-dimensional reconstruction of spiral CT or MRI scans and probably a simulation program of insertion of a stent-graft device. In the mean time we prefer to overestimate the length instead of underestimate it since excess graft can be accommodated by the accordion mechanism allowed by the crimping of the graft. If kinking results, it could be solved by inserting an inner stent at that level, as has occurred in our experience.

Access Problems

Narrow, stenotic, and tortuous iliac arteries were responsible for certain difficulties. The rigid stent and the large diameter of the sheath needed for implantation represented a drawback from the beginning. We overcame some of these problems by modifying the device and using different maneuvers during the procedure.

Reducing the diameter of the sheath to 18 F was a remarkable advance toward the ideal device. The use of an extrastiff wire, the pull-down maneuver, and sometimes implantation of a temporary conduit on the common iliac artery were also useful resources to overcome some of the problems. The pull-down maneuver consists of dissecting free the common femoral and external iliac arteries by simply lifting up the inguinal ligament and using blunt dissection to reach the iliac bifurcation from the groin. Small branches should be divided between suture ligatures. When the arteries are free and the artery has been gently pulled toward the patient's feet, the tortuous artery becomes straighter, making introduction of the sheath possible.

Study of morphologic changes in aneurysms for several years has revealed that in the initial stages almost all aneurysms have a proximal neck and distal cuff of more than 2 cm. In the second stage, the distal cuff becomes shorter. In the third stage the distal cuff tends to disappear, whereas the proximal neck becomes shorter, but still longer than 2 cm. After this stage we found that elongation takes place, which creates tortuosity. Usually the distal curve opposes to the proximal one. This results in a configuration by which if the convexity of the proximal neck is to the left, the distal cuff curves to the right, leav-ing the right iliac artery straight and the left with the tendency to produce a right angle. These findings dictate that in some groups of patients a tubular graft is appropriate. When the distal aortic cuff is not present, an aortobiiliac graft must be used, as advocated by Chuter.[6] Additionally, when the angle between the iliac arteries becomes larger than 90 degrees, an aortoiliac graft should be used and femorofemoral bypass placed.

We foresee that the three systems available will be applicable in patients harboring AAA. Small and medium-sized AAA will benefit from an aortoaortic system and large aneurysms from aortobiiliac or aortoiliac systems with the addition of a femorofemoral bypass and exclusion of the contralateral common iliac artery. We believe, at this stage, that endoluminal treatment of AAA will be applicable in patients with large or symptomatic aneurysms in whom the standard surgical graft replacement represents a prohibitive operative risk. For those patients the best solution will be the aortoiliac procedure, since most of them have tortuous and often aneurysmatic iliac arteries. Frequently the axis of both common iliac arteries defines an angle in excess of 100 degrees, making the placement of a bifurcated graft impossible.

The issue of arterial dilation should be addressed. We still do not know what will be the impact of a stent embedded in the vessel wall in terms of prevention of future dilation. In the mean time we have elected to treat high-risk patients with large or symptomatic aneurysms. We believe that only well-controlled limited trials involving young patients with small aneurysms should be conducted because of the uncertain long-term results of endoluminal treatment for AAA.

Anchoring Mechanism

Because of their high radial force, balloon-expandable stents appear to be the ideal device for anchoring. This is probably true for the time of implant and shortly after. The diameter of arteries increases with time and in addition the effect of a stent producing an internal radial force would produce further dilation.

We had one case of stent migration when the stent was incompletely deployed. Intraluminal ultrasound will be the ideal way to check the completeness of stent deployment. In this regard the pioneer work of Rodney White[7] indicates that intraluminal ultrasound should be almost mandatory as a completion study after finishing a stent-graft implantation. In our modest experience with this method, abnormalities were found with intraluminal ultrasound that were not detected with digital angiogram. As predicated by White, ultrasound real-time imaging during stent deployment will probably be a requirement in the future to obtain reliable results. The ultrasound probe can be placed in one of the lumens of the balloon catheter and positioned at the level of the balloon. In our opinion this will be one of the most striking new developments to improve the endoluminal technique for treating AAA.

In regard to the use of a modification of the J & J stent as an anchoring system, it should be said that clinical results utilizing the J & J stent in occlusive disease cannot be compared with the reaction of the arterial tissue in this new application. Arteries in patients with AAA are usually dilated, not stenotic, and the arterial wall is often thinner than that of the normal arteries and much thinner than the atherosclerotic artery. We do not know the reaction of the thin-walled artery, and it also should be emphasized that this segment of the artery with normal or nearly normal diameter displays some biochemical changes (such as enhanced activity of elastase and collagenase) that make the situation more unpredictable. Probably the next generation of stents will have an intermediate radial force, which will be enough to anchor the graft properly but while not producing dilation of the artery.

We have performed experiments in pigs using an extraperitoneal laparoscopic approach and placing a tape around the aorta close to the renal arteries to create an external banding and prevent dilation of the artery. The tape is a polyethylene mesh with wide interstices to avoid decubitus when compressing the arterial wall when the stent is inside. The extraperitoneal laparoscopic approach does not seem to be difficult and will perhaps represent a step forward in eventually treat young patients with a long life expectancy harboring AAA without the compromise of the stent-graft attachment caused by arterial dilation.

Microembolization

We consider microembolization the most important and feared problem with this procedure. Whereas we were able to resolve almost all problems, microembolization as a complication occurred four times in our experience; three of the four cases resulted in death and in the remaining case discrete microembolization of the right foot was successfully treated with intra-arterial administration of prostaglandin E_1. The two cases that resulted in massive microembolization were technically difficult procedures in patients with large aneurysms. In one of them visceral ischemia was found in the postmortem examination: technical problems had occurred during the procedure in relation to inappropriate balloon sizing. The third case of occurred again after a complex situation created by a technical balloon failure. The patient died suddenly 48 hours after the procedure. Postmortem examination disclosed visceral embolization. The mild, reversible case of microembolization occurred on the side of implantation of an occluding stent after an aortoiliac graft implantation with the addition of a femorofemoral bypass and was caused by incomplete deployment of the stent.

When we reviewed our cases of embolization, it appeared clear that large and tortuous aneurysms pose an increased potential incidence of embolization probably caused by the following:

1. When advancing the guidewire from the femoral artery into the aorta and then into the proximal neck, the operator will negotiate it inside a large and tortuous chamber coated with friable material. Sometimes it is very difficult to get the guidewire inside the proximal neck, since from within the cavity of the aneurysm, the orifice of the proximal neck is very often small. Such maneuvers could eventually cause dislodgment of particles of the laminated thrombus. Thus it is advisable in cases of large aneurysms with wide lumens to insert the guidewire percutaneously from the brachial artery.
2. Very often miscalculation of the length of the aneurysm created the necessity to change the device or use complementary procedures such as implanting a third covered stent to increase the length of the device or cover a leak. The more intravascular manipulation we perform the greater is the risk for dislodgment of particles from the aortic wall.

Preventing Microembolization

The following measures can be taken to prevent microembolization:

1. In cases of large aneurysms with large lumens, the soft-tip guidewire should be introduced from the brachial artery distalwise and recovered from the common femoral artery that has been chosen in advance.
2. Care should be taken to measure the length and diameters of the arteries precisely and to perform a simple, well-planned procedure.
3. After successfully treating patients who were admitted because of spontaneous visceral and distal embolization, we can state that even in the pres-

ence of friable thrombus in the lumen of the AAA, endoluminal treatment can be performed safely.

Future Improvements

It is clear that the development of an endovascular treatment for AAAs represents a new and different challenge for the medical industry. We foresee the future in terms of the ideal device to be utilized in endoluminal treatment of aneurysms as the following.

Anchoring Mechanism

The balloon-expandable stent we are using seems to be the ideal way to obtain a dependable fixation of the graft. A computer projection study of the stress load to the stent struts during the foreseeable life span of an average patient suggested that the fatigue limit of the stent will not be approached. A flexible stent will be needed to negotiate tortuous iliac arteries. Hooks are probably not needed and are dangerous.

Self-expandable, spring-loaded stents are, in general, weaker in terms of radial force and also would not accommodate irregular lumens. Besides, if they are made of multiple parts, micromotion between metal surfaces disrupts protective oxide films, allowing the area to corrode rapidly and leading to mechanical failure. One should keep in mind that this device should stay intact for the life span of the patient.

Self-expandable, spring-loaded stents made of nitinol with thermal memory deserve an independent comment. In these stents a combination of two forces exists that when interacting create a stronger force. Radial force in self-expandable stents depends on the strength and diameter of the wire, among other characteristics. If, in addition to this mechanism, a second force generated by thermal memory of the metal produces a secondary expansion of the stent as soon as the given temperature is reached, the final hoop stress will be almost comparable with a strong, one-piece, balloon-expandable stent.

Graft

Either Dacron or PTFE could be used. A thin wall is needed for crimping in the case of Dacron or stretchability if PTFE is used. Crimping is needed to obtain a kink-resistant graft.

Balloons

Balloons should be partially compliant, scratch-resistant, reinforced to prevent rupture, and wrapped in such a way that rotation will not take place or at least should not be significant. A rigid, noncompliant balloon could be an inconvenience in dealing with patients with irregular lumens, in whom gaps between the stent and arterial wall could generate thrombus and leaks between the graft and arterial lumen.

Preprocedure Studies

Studies should include CT scans (slices every 5 mm or less and three-dimensional reconstruction) and angiography. Spiral CT scan, when available, would represent a significant advantage. MR angiography with additional software could be the procedure of choice in the future.

Studies During the Procedure

A high-resolution fluoroscopy is needed during the procedure. Road mapping seems advantageous. Intravascular ultrasound proved highly useful to assess the completeness of stent deployment. We used this imaging technique in two instances. The second time it allowed us to detect and resolve a graft fold in the iliac artery that was missed in the arteriogram.

In the near future it will be possible to complete the procedure without using x-rays. MRI and ultrasound could eventually cover all needs (providing that new developments now being researched are completed) without irradiating the patient and the attending staff.

Some Doubts and Problems

We still have some basic doubts about the procedure we are proposing. Long-term stent-graft interaction is one of our main concerns. Stent edges could cause damage to the graft through direct mechanical action or through material fatigue. Since the stent and the graft are covered by tissue in a few weeks, the potential impact of this possible damage will probably be without clinical importance. What is unquestionable is that the device should be designed to last a lifetime, accomplishing aneurysm exclusion and keeping the flow through it.

A second main concern is the tissue reaction after endovascular treatment of AAA. It is known that both the composition and mechanical properties of AAAs are different from those of nonaneurysmal aortas.[8] The aneurysms are stiffer, and the volume fractions of collagen and ground substance are increased, whereas the volume fractions of elastin and muscle are decreased in aneurysms. Changes in diameter of the neck of the aneurysm after stent implantation are not known to occur. Intimal hyperplasia develops regularly over the stent, and some atrophy of the media and reaction of the adventitia is expected after stent implantation. These changes and also the presence of the stent itself, forming part of the architecture of the arterial wall, will probably keep dilation from diminishing the tension of the wall.

It should be emphasized that watertight sealing between the arterial wall and the stent-graft unit should be obtained from the very first. Lack of leak into the aneurysmal sac when injecting contrast media should not be considered as a primary success. Graft and stent in contact with thrombus can seal temporarily, but not for long. The thrombus dissolves and a leak can appear in a few weeks or months. Endovascular ultrasound or CT scanning with contrast media can reaveal definitively the completeness of stent deployment. Both ends of the graft should be in contact and sealed with the arterial wall and not with the thrombus to consider the result acceptable. X-ray images during procedures should be interpreted through a reconstruction of the actual aneurysm based on CT images taken in small slices (5 mm or less). A clear definition on where the thrombus starts and ends will allow stents to be placed in the appropriate site.

Spontaneous embolization is the second most common and most important spontaneous complication of AAAs. Embolization takes place when the thrombus becomes friable and the mural thrombus suffers a dissection. Usually microthombi migrate to the extremities and also, in a retrograde fashion, to the visceral arteries, mainly the renal arteries. In our experience these very sick patients can be treated endoluminally. Provided that great care is taken to prevent rupture and damage of this friable material while the procedure is performed, thrombus can be effectively excluded, interrupting the shower of microemboli. We treated three patients affected by spontaneous microembolization with this method, using intra-arterial prostaglandin E_1 injection to control distal tissue damage.[9]

The relationship between a stented graft and microembolization deserves a special comment. Microembolization is the most dreaded complication in the use of stented grafts for endoluminal treatment of AAAs. On the other hand, endoluminal exclusion of AAAs is an emerging tool to treat microembolization from aneurysms. At first glance, it seems unreasonable to use a therapy for a condition that can be caused by the proposed technique. The explanation is that aneurysms that embolize spontaneously are usually small. Small aneurysms have straight iliac arteries, and aneurysms are usually nontortuous. Conversely, aneurysms that caused microembolization during endoluminal treatment were, in our experience, very large and tortuous. Iliac arteries were elongated. All these characteristics created technical difficulties in performing endoluminal exclusion of the aneurysm. In 50 such procedures, massive microembolization occurred in 3 (3.7%) and mild unilateral microembolization in one (1.2%).

In spite of our encouraging results, we are aware of the necessity to perform controlled trials with enough patients followed for a long period before introducing endoluminal treatment into clinical practice. In the mean time, experience should be concentrated in a few centers with appropriate equipment and a skillful group of surgeons and interventional radiologists or cardiologists with experience in interventional vascular procedures.

Caution should be used in forming definitive conclusions, since we are finding new abnormalities among our group of patients as much as 3 years after performing what we considered a successful procedure. Before this procedure can be offered to the medical community as an alternative treatment for AAA, clear, unremarkable long-term experience should be available.

Regarding other applications of the stent-graft combination, treatment of AV fistulae appears to be a simple and effective application of the principle. It will save time and will prevent bleeding and peripheral nerve injuries. Treatment of false aneurysms in nonaccessible places is also a promising application, since this represents vascular trauma. Arterial dissections (mostly aortic) will probably be efficiently treated endoluminally by interrupting the flow caused by intimal tearing. One of our cases showed how promising this approach could be. The development of an "internal bypass" after balloon dilation is an appealing idea in view of the failure of balloon dilation in long stenoses or occlusions. In theory, isolating the inner surface of the treated artery will eventually prevent interaction between the damaged intima and the circulating elements and blood substances. Our initial experience with treating thoracic aneurysms (one resulting from a type A dissection and the second from a thoracoabdominal aneurysm with no compromise of the visceral arteries) indicates that the procedure is simpler than treating AAA and is highly promising.

REFERENCES

1. Melton NJ, Bickerstaff LK, Hollier LH et al. Changing incidence of abdominal aortic aneurysms: a population based study. Am J Epidemiol 1984;120:379–86

2. Brown OW, Hollier LH, Pairolero PC et al. Abdominal aortic aneurysm and coronary artery disease: a reassessment. Arch Surg 1981;116:1484–8

3. McCombs RP, Roberts B. Acute renal failure after resection of abdominal aortic aneurysm. Surg Gynecol Obstet 1979;148:175–9

4. Karmody AL, Leather RP, Goldman M et al. The current position of non-resection treatment for abdominal aortic aneurysms. Surgery 1983;94:591–7

5. Parodi JC, Palmaz JC, Barone HD. Transfemoral intraluminal graft implantation for abdominal aortic aneurysms. Ann Vasc Surg 1991;5:491–9

6. Chuter T. Bifurcated endovascular graft insertion for abdominal aortic aneurysms. p. 92. In Greenhalgh RM (ed): Vascular and Endovascular Surgical Techniques. WB Saunders, Philadelphia, 1991

7. Cavaye DM, White RA. Intraluminal ultrasound and the management of peripheral vascular disease. pp. 137–156. In: Advances in Vascular Surgery Vol. 1. Mosby-Year Book, St. Louis, 1993

8. He CM, Roach MR. The composition and mechanical properties of abdominal aortic aneurysms. J Vasc Surg 1994;20:6–13

9. Parodi J. Use of intra-arterial injection of prostagandin E1 in the blue toe syndrome. In Yao J. (ed): (in press)

Self-Expanding Intraluminal Grafts in Treatment of Abdominal Aortic Aneurysm

76

Carlos E. Ruiz
He Ping Zhang

Abdominal aortic aneurysm (AAA) is a serious peripheral arterial disorder that mainly affects the elderly. The prevalence has been estimated to be between 3 and 6% among those age over 65. Approximately 100,000 AAAs are diagnosed each year in the United States. The cause of death is due to rupture of the aneurysm with a mortality rate of up to 90%. Surgery is currently the only recognized effective treatment for AAA; however, it carries substantial morbidity and mortality. In recent years, more than 40,000 aortic reconstructions have been performed annually in the United States, and the demand for AAA repair is expected to increase as our population ages. Therefore, a nonsurgical alternative to AAA repair is attractive; particularly, it would reduce the risk of AAA rupture as well as the morbidity and mortality associated with surgical repair.

Percutaneous implantation of a graft to bridge an aneurysm may provide an alternative solution for surgical reconstruction in patients with AAA. Previous studies have reported several AAA-excluding devices, including a polyurethane-coated expandable stent, a Dacron-wrapped Gianturco stent, and a weft-knit Dacron tube with balloon-expandable stents, to treat AAA in animal models.[1-4] Although these grafts can exclude aneurysms after their expansion, certain complications, such as graft thrombosis and ischemia of the important organs resulting from covering major arterial branches, were encountered. These complications were most likely related to the design of the devices.

In an attempt to overcome these complications, we have developed a self-expandable endovascular graft (Schneider U.S. Stent Division, Minneapolis, Minnesota), which can be implanted percutaneously, and we tested it by placing it in dogs with surgically created AAA. We evaluated the feasibility, safety, and efficacy of the graft and its immediate and later effects in treatment of AAA in the canine model.

GRAFT CONSTRUCTION

The graft was a self-expandable, stainless-steel, woven-mesh endovascular prosthesis with a delivery system. It was constrained by a removable plastic sleeve, and as the sleeve was withdrawn, the device returned to its original, unconstrained size, anchoring it against the vessel wall. Two types of grafts were used in the study (Table 76-1). One type was a stent covered with porous polyurethane (Fig. 76-1A), and the other one was a plain stent (Fig. 76-1B). The graft was constrained in an elongated configuration on a unistep delivery system. Three covered grafts and five uncovered grafts were used in the trial.

CREATION OF AAA MODEL

This study included eight mongrel dogs weighing 18 to 24 kg. Creation of AAA was performed in each dog under general anesthesia. After incising of the skin layer, a piece of fascia muscularis tissue about 3 to 3.5 cm long by 2 to 2.5 cm wide was taken. After the retro-

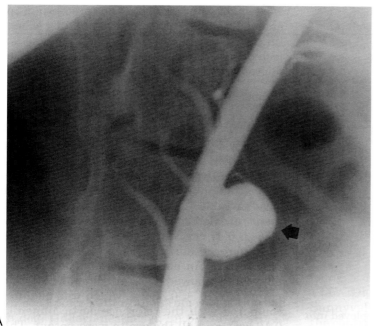

A

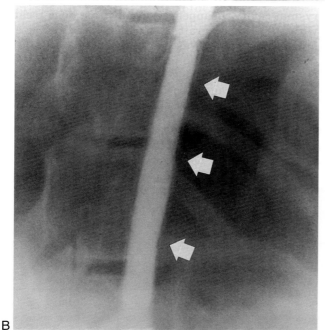

B

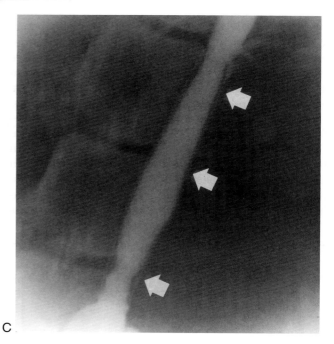

C

Fig. 76-3. Aortogram showing the abdominal aortic aneurysm before and after placement of the covered graft and follow-up in dog 7. **(A)** The saccular aneurysm (*arrow*) 8 weeks after surgical creation. **(B)** Immediate after-placement of the covered graft (*arrows*). The graft was fully expanded, the aneurysm was completely excluded, and flow through the arterial branches was restricted. **(C)** Patent graft (*arrows*) at 4 weeks' follow-up with no angiographic evidence of aneurysm.

diameter of the grafted aortic lumen was essentially the same as immediately after graft implantation. The aortograms showed that all the grafts were patent with vigorous flow through the grafted section of the aorta. The cavity of the aneurysm could not be visualized in four dogs (two with covered stents and two with uncovered stents) (see Fig. 76-3C). Some cavitary filling with contrast was observed in dog 5, who had received an uncovered stent, but the size of the aneurysmal cavity was significantly reduced as compared to the size before and immediate after

graft implantation (see Fig. 76-4C). Importantly, the major arterial branches that had been bridged by the uncovered grafts were widely open with unrestricted flow (Fig. 76-5). Dog 3, who had received a covered graft, developed paraplegia secondary to a spinal cord infarction 48 hours after graft placement. This animal was euthanized 2½ weeks later because of decubitus ulcer formation. A premortem aortogram indicated that the section of the aorta with graft was completely occluded with only very limited aortic flow from collateral arteries distal to the graft.

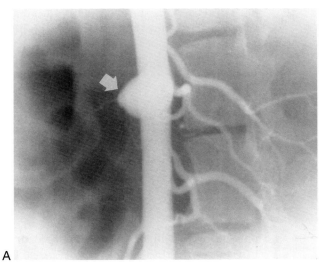

A

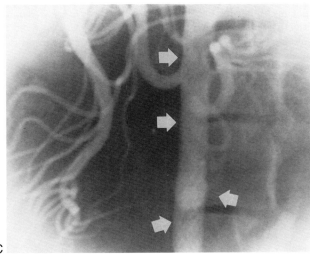

Fig. 76-4. Aortogram showing the abdominal aortic aneurysm before and after placement of the uncovered graft and follow-up in dog 5. **(A)** The saccular aneurysm (*arrow*) 8 weeks after surgical creation. **(B)** Immediate after-placement of the uncovered graft (*small arrows*). The residual aneurysm was observed, but the size was significantly reduced (*large arrow*), and flow through the arterial branches was maintained. **(C)** Patent graft (*left arrows*) at 4 weeks' follow-up. The size of the residual aneurysm was further reduced (*right arrow*).

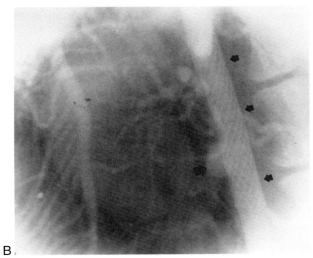

B

C

GROSS AND HISTOPATHOLOGIC EXAMINATION

No migration of the graft was noted in the dogs. Two dogs (dogs 1 and 2) were killed shortly after the graft placements. Both showed a fully expanded, patent graft across the site of the aneurysm with no clot. Dog 3, who had angiographic evidence of thrombosis, was found to have thrombus filling the entire lumen of the graft as well as the cavity of the aneurysm. In the remaining 5 dogs, all grafts were patent with no visible clot in the lumen. The grafts were either totally or partially surfaced with neointima (Plate 76-1A). The cavities of the saccular aneurysms were essentially completely filled with clot, while the fusiform aneurysms showed adherence of the graft to the aortic wall with contraction of the aortic aneurysm diameter but without thrombosis. In dog 5, who showed angiographic evidence of a small residual an-

eurysm, the graft wires were covered by neointima around the edges of the aneurysm, and the cavity was partially filled with clot. In two dogs in whom the uncovered grafts had been intentionally placed across the major arteries, these arteries were wildly patent with no evidence of obstruction by neointima (Plate 76-1B).

The covered grafts showed fibroblastic and histiocytic permeation of the coating fabric by light microscopy, with patchy chronic inflammation and variable endothelialization of the surface. A fibroblastic reaction was focally present in the intima beneath the graft. Some areas showed fibroplasia of the intimal surface as well, with a thin layer of adherent thrombus. Dog 3, with thrombosis of a covered graft, showed focal necrosis of the inner aortic wall, apparently secondary to the thrombosis. Histologic study of reaction associated with the uncovered graft showed a mild histiocytic and giant cell reaction to

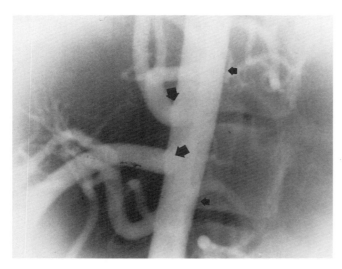

Fig. 76-5. Aortogram showing unrestricted flow through superior and inferior mesenteric arteries (*large arrows*) bridged by uncovered graft (*small arrows*) in dog 8 at 4 weeks' follow-up. No angiographic evidence of the residual aneurysm was found.

the bare wires, with a thin overlying layer of neointima composed largely of myofibroblastic-type cells and little reaction in the underlying aorta. The clot in the aneurysms typically showed peripheral organization, as would be expected.

Scanning electron microscopy showed the neointimal surface to be covered by cells with the appearance of fibroblasts, with variably sized islands of endothelial cells partially covering the fibroblasts. The covered grafts appeared in general to have more endothelialization of their surface (Fig. 76-6) than the uncovered grafts.

DISCUSSION

Aortic abdominal aneurysmectomy has been the only effective treatment to prevent rupture of AAA and to save life when rupture occurs. However, it is a major operation, and a number of specific postoperative complications may occur. Patients with advanced age or with underlying systemic disease are particularly at high risk to undergo surgical repair. Furthermore, the estimation of direct cost for AAA repair is 2.3 billion per year in the United States. Thus, AAA imposes a considerable economic burden on already strained health-care resources.

Unfortunately, the refinement and further simplification of surgical techniques in AAA repair seems unlikely at present. On the other hand, a nonsurgical alternative with implantation of an AAA-excluding device has been tested in animal experimental studies. This alternative may have less morbidity and mortality and may potentially reduce the cost for treatment of AAA as well.

Table 76-3 highlights the features of AAA-excluding devices used in previous studies. All these grafts were able to exclude aneurysm after graft deploy-

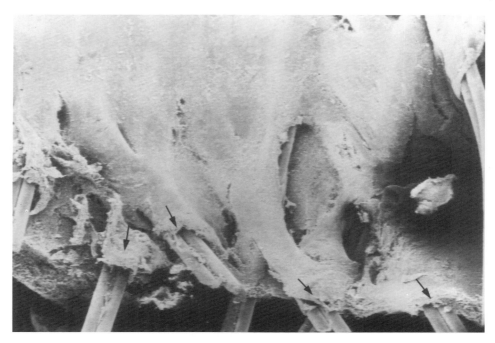

Fig. 76-6. Scanning electron microscopy. The wires of the covered graft were surfaced by neoendothelia (arrows) ($\times 51$).

Table 76-3. Endovascular Grafts to Treat AAA From Previous Studies

Author	Animal	Features of Grafts	Delivery Catheter	Immediate Results	Follow-up Results
Balko, et al.[1]	3 Sheep	Graft consisted of biomedical grade elastomeric polyurethane with a Nitinol or stainless steel frame	15F	Successfully excluded aneurysms	Not available
Lawrence et al.[2]	6 Dogs	Graft constructed by wrapping a Dacron cylinder around the Gianturco expandable metallic stent; full expanded size of 10 mm in diameter	11 F	Successfully excluded aneurysms	Patent grafts except for one dog; graft covered by neointima; infarction of the kidney with branch arteries in 2 dogs resulting from graft covering these arteries
Mirich et al.[3]	6 Dogs	Modified Gianturco stent covered with porous nylon; full expanded size of 11–12 mm in diameter	12 F	Successfully excluded aneurysms; incomplete expansion of the caudal end of the graft in one dog	Patent grafts and side branches in 5 dogs; cephalad migration of graft in one dog resulted in thrombus formation and occlusion of renal arteries
Laborde et al.[4]	8 Dogs	Graft consisted of a weft-knit Dacron tube with balloon-expandable stents attached at both ends; expanded size of 10 mm in diameter	14 F	Excluded aneurysms, but 2 grafts were twisted, resulting in early thrombosis and complete occlusion	Irregularities of Dacron graft in 4 dogs; neointima covered the stent portion of luminal surface of the grafts

ment. The graft developed by Balko et al.[1] had one significant disadvantage. Because the graft is covered by Nitinol, which has potential premature expansion inside of catheter, it requires constant clod saline irrigation during insertion. In addition, the large delivery catheter (15 F) required has also limited its application.

Lawrence et al.[2] developed an expandable Gianturco stent covered with Dacron. However, because of the nonexpandable nature of a Dacron covering, as well as its tendency to wrinkle, there was substantial concern about its long-term promotion of thrombosis and fibrogenesis, with eventual narrowing of the lumen. Furthermore, the side branches were occluded in the part of the device that was covered by the Dacron.

Mirich et al.[3] modified the Gianturco stent, which was covered by porous nylon material, to allow stretching and to maintain patency of the side atrial branches where covered by the graft. Except for one dog, no evidence of graft migration or luminal narrowing was found. Although arterial branches covered by the graft were maintained on angiography, microscopic examination revealed that neointima was on the fabric strands across the side branch orifices of the dogs, with evidence of renal ischemia in one dog, which indicated that these vessels may eventually be occluded.

More recently, Laborde et al.[4] developed a weft-knit Dacron tube with balloon-expandable stents. Two dogs had graft early occlusion caused by torsion of the graft as a result of defective folding of the graft inside the delivery sheath. At follow-up, the remaining six dogs had patent grafts but four of them had evidence of kinking of the graft that was due to shrinkage of the artificial aneurysm. Histopathologic study found that endothelialization was complete on the stents and partial on the artificial aneurysms.

One important disadvantage associated with these AAA-excluding devices is that all required quite a large delivery system. Although the delivery catheter used in our study is relatively small as compared with previous studies—12 F with a covered graft and 10 F with an uncovered graft—it is still fairly large, and further refinements are needed.

We have demonstrated two types of grafts in treatment of AAA. Except for one dog in which the graft was occluded, no complications associated with the graft were encountered. The two graft types have slightly different features and may, therefore, have potentially different clinical applications. The covered graft may be useful for emergency treatment of ruptured and acutely expanding AAAs, because it can seal off the leaking aneurysms immediately on deployment of the graft, stopping bleeding more completely than the uncovered graft, as a result of its fabric coat. However, it cannot be allowed to bridge the entrance of any major arterial branch, because it would also interrupt blood flow through that artery. Fortunately, most human AAAs are harbored below the renal arteries, and it would not be necessary to bridge these arteries with covered graft.

On the other hand, the uncovered graft may be potentially useful for elective therapy of stable AAAs, because the device not only can significantly reduce the size of the aneurysm immediately after its deployment but also can maintain the origins of the branch arteries. In the two dogs in which the uncovered grafts were placed across major arterial branches, those branches were widely patent, maintaining unrestricted blood flow. Although the opening of the aneurysmal cavity was not completely surfaced with neointima in two of the three dogs receiving an uncovered graft, a thin layer of neointima was on the wires of the grafts, which may eventually seal off the opening. This unique aspect of the uncovered graft may improve the long-term safety of this type of treatment for AAA. Importantly, because uncovered graft can substantially reduce the size of aneurysm, it indicates that the likelihood of AAA rupture be minimized because a strong correlation has been demonstrated between aneurysm size and the likelihood of rupture.

The mechanism of closure of the saccular aneurysms by the uncovered graft likely is by reduction of blood flow in the aneurysm cavity secondary to the shear forces introduced by the wires that cross the aneurysm opening. This is suggested by the nearly complete exclusion of contrast from the aneurysm cavity immediately after placement of the graft. The mechanism of shrinkage of the fusiform aneurysms is less clear. However, the almost immediate reduction in the angiographically demonstrated diameter of the aorta in the region of the aneurysm in two of the three dogs with fusiform aneurysms suggests that the shear forces introduced by the graft wires may redirect blood flow back toward the lumen and away from the dilated aortic walls, allowing for healing and contraction of the dilated aorta. The one case in which the diameter was slightly greater immediately after graft placement appears to be due to placement of a relatively large stent in a fairly small dog, which resulted in some initial stretching of the aorta. This case, however, later showed normalization of the aortic diameter within 4 weeks of follow-up. The obliteration of the aneurysms in all cases appears to be due to the presence of the graft, and not to spontaneous thrombosis, because angiography demonstrated immediate changes in the effective size of the aorta after graft placement. Furthermore, the aortogram before graft placement showed that

the size of the aneurysms appeared to be larger rather than reduced from the original created size in the initial 8 weeks after aneurysm creation—a period designed to serve as a control for any possible spontaneous healing, regression, or thrombosis of the aneurysms.

One important issue that should be considered, however, is that shape and configuration of surgically created AAA in the animal model are not close to the most common AAA in humans; in particular, the opening of the aneurysmal cavity is much smaller in dog than in human AAAs. It is uncertain whether neointimal surfacing of an uncovered graft would be as rapid and complete in these large aneurysms as it was in this animal study. Further studies are indicated in this regard.

Placement of the device is straightforward and feasible and appears to be safe. We did not encounter any difficulty in either positioning or deploying the graft. However, one must be sure that the graft is in the correct position before withdrawing the covering sheath for deployment, because it is not retrievable once deployed. Also, the renal and major branch arteries must not be bridged with a covered graft, otherwise kidney or other visceral damage will almost certainly ensue.

Two issues are critical for the success of endovascular graft placement: minimal thrombosis and rapid endothelialization. Palmaz et al.[5,6] have demonstrated absence of thrombosis over a long period after aortic graft placements. This suggests that anticoagulation may not be necessary following arterial graft placements, particularly in the aorta, because it is unlikely to have thrombus formation in the aortic lumen, which is due to the vigorous blood flow. However, Schatz[7] pointed out that without adequate anticoagulation, metallic stents, regardless of design and configuration, have an inherent thrombogenic effect. In our study, the graft in dog 3 was completely occluded by thrombus, which may be prevented by administering anticoagulant. Similar graft thrombosis has been reported by others[3]; we feel that anticoagulation may be important and is required for graft placement even in the aorta. Further studies are warranted to clarify this important issue.

Although infection and colonization of the area with graft did not occur in our study, this possibility must be given serious consideration. Prophylactic antibiotics are recommended for a short period following graft placement. Once the graft is completely covered with neoendothelium, the likelihood of the infection as well as thrombosis may be minimized.

Our study documents the feasibility of percutaneous placement of an endovascular graft in the treatment of AAA in an animal model. The immediate and short-term follow-up results are encouraging. However, longer follow-up and a larger sample size are necessary to establish both the long-term efficacy and safety of this procedure. If this AAA-excluding device can be proven safe and effective for humans as well, it has the potential for substantially reducing the morbidity and mortality associated with AAA.

REFERENCE

1. Balko A, Piasecki GJ, Shah DM et al. Transfemoral placement of intraluminal polyurethane prosthesis for abdominal aortic aneurysm. J Surg Res 1986;40:305–9

2. Lawrence DD, Charnsangavej C, Wright KC et al. Percutaneous endovascular graft: experimental evaluation. Radiology 1987;163:357–60

3. Mirich D, Wright KC, Wallace S et al. Percutaneously placed endovascular grafts for aortic aneurysms: feasibility study. Radiology 1989;170:1033–7

4. Laborde JC, Parodi JC, Clem MF et al. Intraluminal bypass of abdominal aortic aneurysm: feasibility study. Radiology 1992;184:185–90

5. Palmaz JC, Windeler SA, Garcia F et al. Atherosclerotic rabbit aortas: expandable intraluminal grafting. *Radiology*, 1986;160:723–726

6. Palmaz JC, Sibbitt RR, Tio FO et al. Expandable intraluminal vascular graft: a feasibility study. *Surgery*, 1986;99:199–205

7. Schatz RA. A view of vascular stents. *Circulation*. 1989; 79:445–462

77 Endovascular Treatment for Iliac Disease

H. Rousseau
F. Joffre
P. Tregant
R. Aziza
T. Oya
F. Blain

The nonsurgical treatment of atheromatous iliac vessels was initially described by Charles Dotter and MP Judkins in 1964.[1] Since then, because of the easy access to the aortoiliac anatomic region by a simple retrograde femoral artery puncture, and because of the frequency of atheromatous lesions at this level, this region has become a preferred site for percutaneous transluminal angioplasty (PTA).[2–25]

Even though the long-term results are less favorable than for surgery, angioplasty should be part of the therapeutic arsenal in the treatment of iliac lesions. As compared to surgery, its advantages are multiple: a safe, simple, less aggressive method, necessitating a short hospitalization. In the case of recurrence, it may be repeated without compromising a subsequent surgical intervention. Finally, it may be performed as a complement to a surgical bypass.

In addition to balloon angioplasty for simple iliac stenosis, recent technological progress, dominated by vascular endoprostheses, has broadened the indications, as well as permitted the treatment of complex lesions, particularly iliac obstruction.

PRINCIPLES OF THE TECHNIQUE

Approach

The homolateral retrograde femoral puncture of the iliac axis to be treated is the approach most used for treating an iliac PTA.

A contralateral approach is technically possible but necessitates the crossing of the aortic bifurcation and, thus, may be the origin of contralateral or homolateral embolus migration. This approach may be used if an arteriography is done at the same time by a contralateral puncture to avoid a second puncture or to treat a distal iliac lesion. This approach is also used frequently in the case of homolateral retrograde recanalization failure. It is thus possible, after contralateral recanalization, to catch the guidewire by a homolateral approach, using different techniques (Dormia probes).[26]

Axillary and brachial vessels are rarely used, which is due to a more frequent local complication rate and to the technical difficulties often encountered with these approaches.

In the absence of a pulse, a retrograde femoral

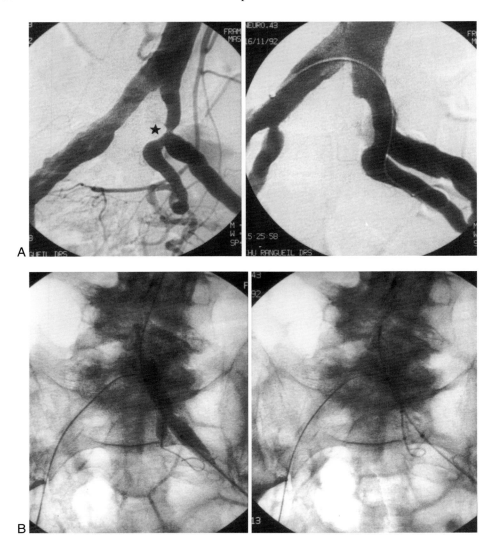

Fig. 77-1. **(A)** A 41-year-old man with left lower extremity claudication. Diagnostic angiography revealed a short stenosis of the left common iliac artery, Society of Cardiovascular Interventional Radiology (SCVIR) lesion category 2. An internal iliac artery stenosis was also present (*). **(B)** Dilation was performed using the "kissing balloon" technique with simultaneous inflation of bilateral balloons (from a retrograde approach, PTA of the internal iliac artery lesion was performed at the same time). The lesions responded well to angioplasty with only minimal residual narrowing and no residual hemodynamic pressure gradient.

puncture may be realized under radioscopic control after contralateral contrast injection. One may also be aided through radioscopy, by parietal calcifications, or by sonographic or Doppler exploration. For lesions situated at the aortoiliac bifurcation or at the hypogastric artery ostia, dilation may be realized by kissing, using two simultaneously filled balloons, after a bilateral approach of the iliac vessels[13,19,20]. (Fig. 77-1).

Dilation

Once the stenosis has been traversed by a guidewire, the dilation is achieved with a balloon catheter, the diameter of which is adapted to the adjacent proximal and distal arterial diameters considered normal. If the totality of the vascular axis to be treated is pathologic, the choice of catheter is made as a function of the contralateral artery diameter. As a rule, the dilation is achieved using a catheter whose diameter is equal to or slightly greater than that of the artery (+1 mm).

The dilation is achieved, with a mean duration of 1 minute, under radioscopic and manometric control, at a pressure of about 6 atm, sometimes greater in the case of residual stenosis. At this time, semicompliant catheters are available, which, as a function of the pressure exercised at the catheter's interior, can discretely increase its diameter and thus progressively adapt itself to the residual stenosis.[27]

Result Checking

Two parameters are verified: the morphologic result and the hemodynamic result.

Ideally, angiographic control images in the two orthogonal planes better permit the visualization of parietal anomalies secondary to the dilation. Finally, it is essential to verify the runoff after dilation to eliminate a distal obstruction that is due to embolic migration.

For many, the measure of transstenotic pressure gradients remains a determinant factor of postangioplastic success. A result is considered satisfactory when the residual stenosis is inferior to 30% and the transstenotic pressure gradient is inferior to 15 mmHg at basal conditions or inferior to 20 mmHg after a pharmacologically induced hyperemia.[28] In addition, a satisfactory result implies the absence of an obstructive dissection with the same hemodynamic criteria.

Direct guidance and real-time monitoring of interventional procedures will become possible with new endovascular imaging (angioscopy and ultrasound). Fiberoptic angioscopy has some potential advantages in application to intravascular imaging. The imaging field for the angioscopes is three-dimensional in a forward direction, so that inspection of lesions can be performed without having to cross with the catheter. However, the potential use of angioscopy as a guiding modality for endovascular therapies appears to be relatively limited by the need to clear the blood of the lumen by a flushing system.

Intravascular ultrasound can both characterize the diseased vessel and confirm the effect of angioplasty, thus allowing for treatment of the complications and hopefully improving the long-term outcome. The major advantage of ultrasound catheters is their ability to image through blood without the need for a flushing system (Fig. 77-2).

Associated Anticoagulant Treatment

Treatment with anticoagulants in conjunction with PTA currently remains controversial. The anticoagulant protocol used most is platelet antiaggregants for 48 hours before the angioplasty, and for the following 6 months, and in situ heparin injection (3 to 5,000 IU) after breaching the obstruction. Intravenous heparin is most often continued for 24 hours after the angioplasty (TPT = 2 × control).

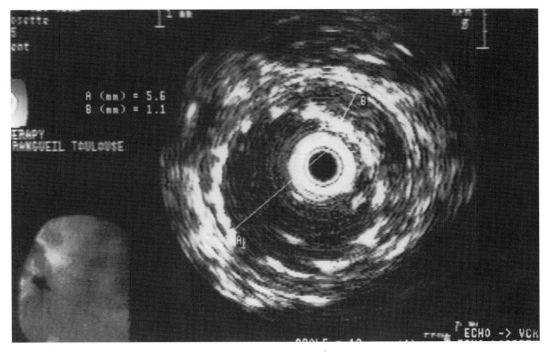

Fig. 77-2. With intravascular ultrasound, one can directly measure the cross-sectional area of a stented vessel **(A)** as well as establish the relationship of the stent to adjacent structures. **(B)** Atheroma compressed by the stent.

Treatment of Iliac Occlusions

For treatment of recent occlusions (<7 days), use of fibrinolytics should be considered before dilation. These, by lysis of the thrombotic portion of the obstruction, permit visualization of the stenosis, which is sometimes short and easily treated by dilation.[29–32] The delay of action (between 4 and 24 hours), the cost, and the fact that the efficacy and the absence of migration are not guaranteed have led certain teams to opt for an alternative course of action. Excluding acute ischemia, which rarely occurs in isolated iliac obstructions, the patient is treated secondarily (after 1 month), by immediate placement of an endoprosthesis, before dilation, to avoid distal migration, with fixation of the endovascular emboligenic material. This technique seems to decrease significantly the rate of distal emboli.[33–35]

In the treatment of chronic occlusions, three alternatives may be considered: (1) Equally use fibrinolytics, but the chance of success is diminished, with the aforementioned inconveniences; (2) dilation as a first choice, with prosthesis placement if the result is insufficient[36–46] (Fig. 77-3); (3) prosthesis placement as a first choice to avoid distal migration, as mentioned previously.[33–35] This last technique implies the systematic use of an endoprosthesis, whereas nearly 30% of obstructions treated by simple dilation do not need it. Furthermore, this method poses the problem of positioning the autoexpansive prostheses, because of their shortening after dilation.

Other Endovascular Treatment

Beside the classic balloon angioplasty, other endoluminal revascularization techniques are used. They can be schematically divided into three groups: fibrinolytics, mechanical treatment, and vascular endoprostheses.

Fibrinolytics are used essentially in iliac occlusions and embolic migration after iliac angioplasty. The interest and the inconvenience of fibrinolytics have been described. The use of these products for treating distal emboli seems to be less justified at this time. We prefer using thromboaspiration catheters, whose efficacy is more rapid and more certain, regardless of the nature of the embolus, thrombus, or atheromatous plaque.

Other mechanical revascularization devices (laser,

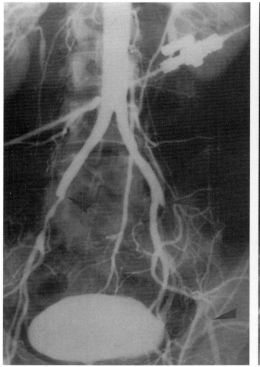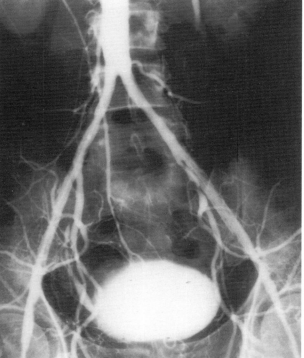

Fig. 77-3. (A) A patient presenting with a 6-month history of severe bilateral lower extremity claudication. Complete occlusion of the external iliac arteries with reconstitution of the femoral artery were present (arrow head). **(B)** After balloon dilation, marked improvement in lumen caliber and resolution of the transtenotic gradient were observed. The patient did well at 4-year follow-up.

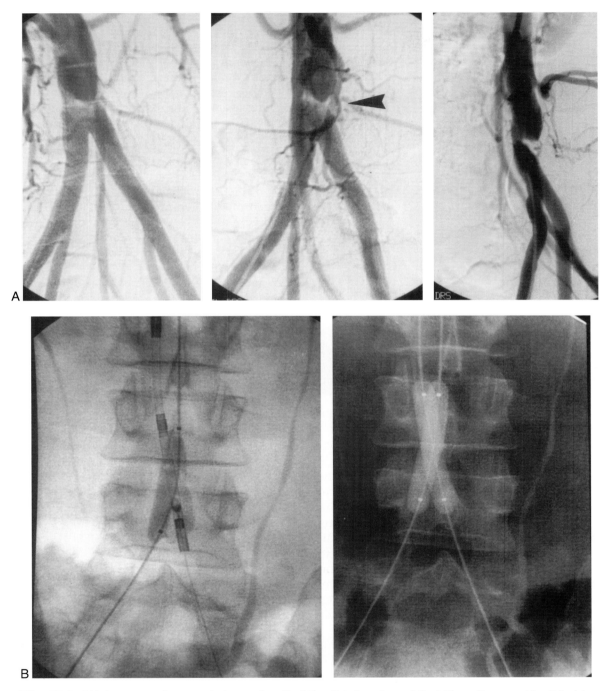

Fig. 77-4. **(A)** An eccentric stenosis (*arrowhead*) of the distal aorta and its bifurcation was identified in this patient with symptoms of bilateral lower extremity claudication. **(B)** Dilation and atherectomy with the Simpson atherectomy device were performed using the "kissing balloon" technique with simultaneous inflation of bilateral balloons and atherectomy. (*Figure continues.*)

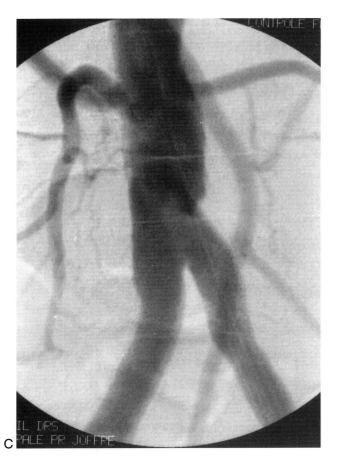

Fig. 77-4. (*Continued*). **(C)** After, marked improvement in the lumen caliber is seen. The patient did well at 1-year follow-up.

atherotomes, or atherectomes) are little used at the iliac level, because, regardless of the functional mechanism employed, they create a channel within the obstruction corresponding to the catheter's size, which is insufficient for the iliac vessels. For sufficient results, large-diameter catheters would have to be employed, thus causing more frequent local complications. The only actual indication is the use of the Simpson catheter for treating certain ulcerated lesions (Fig. 77-4)[47–49] as well as for restenoses inside endoprostheses.[44]

The role of vascular endoprostheses is evident for the treatment of angioplasty complications (Fig. 77-5). Three types of prostheses are currently used:

1. The autoexpansive Wallstent prosthesis, made of stainless steel filaments, braided and nonwelded, presenting a great flexibility: This prosthesis has two disadvantages: its low radiopacity and its retraction of about 30% during its placement.[33–35,42–45,49]

2. Two balloon-expandable prostheses: (a) The Strecker prosthesis, made from knitted tantalum wires. This flexible prosthesis, very radiopaque, presents an electronegative charge at its surface, which makes it theoretically less thrombogenic. Its rather weak radial force renders it relatively unstable after positioning.[50] (b) The Palmaz prosthesis is rigid and made from stainless steel. It has two disadvantages: Its length is limited to 3 cm (several prostheses are necessary for treating long lesions), and its rigidity, which prevents its clearing prominent vascular curves, as well as its crossover placement.[41,51–54]

Other prostheses are currently being evaluated: (1) nitinol autoexpansive prostheses (memory-formed metal), Memotherm (Angiomed) and Cragg (Mintec), and (2) balloon-expandable prostheses, Viktor (Meadox) and the Cordis prosthesis. These prostheses are at the clinical experimentation phase of their evaluation.

Whatever type of prosthesis used, the indications are essentially represented by immediate technical failures after PTA, whether they are obstructive dissections or hemodynamically significant residual stenoses. Another principal indication for prosthesis is in cases of long iliac obstructions, as mentioned previously.[33–35]

RESULTS

To analyze and compare published results of the different treatment modalities in arteriopathies, vascular surgical and radiologic committee directives were recently published.[55] Technical results should first be differentiated from clinical results, and results immediately after dilation should be differentiated from short-term (first-month) and long-term results. One should indicate primary patency (defined as patency obtained after the first dilation without a complementary act) and secondary patency (obtained after complementary intervention). These results should be expressed in a cumulative patency as a function of time, following actuarial curves.

From a clinical point of view, the evaluation of the benefits of angioplasty should take into account not only the decrease in claudication as seen in walking tests but equally the objective parameters, represented by the systolic pressure index—arm/ankle, or arm/thigh in the case of associated femoral occlusion.

Unfortunately, only a few recent studies respect these criteria, rendering the analysis of older publications (radiologic or surgical) difficult.

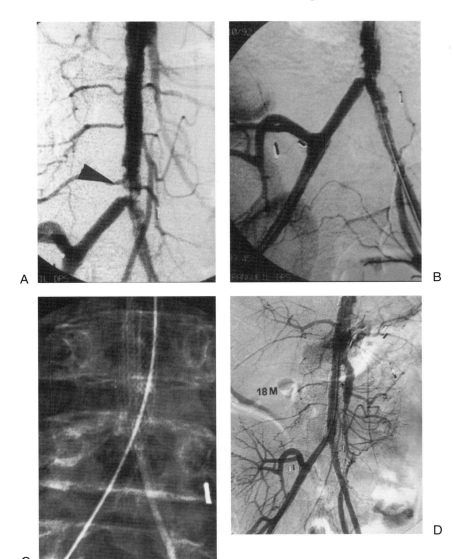

Fig. 77-5. A 22-year-old woman presenting with bilateral claudication and hypertension after renal transplantation. **(A)** Diagnostic aortogram demonstrating diffuse atherosclerotic disease involving distal aorta and bifurcation (*arrowhead*). A 28-mm transstenotic gradient was present. **(B)** Following PTA of the distal aorta and its bifurcation, residual gradients were present. **(C)** Two "kissing" endoprostheses were implanted simultaneously. Immediate and late angiographic controls show the perfect regularity of the arterial walls. **(D)** Follow-up angiography at 18 months demonstrated the patency of the stents.

Immediate Results

Success Rate

Of 6,620 iliac PTAs analyzed by Rholl and Van Breda, the mean technical success rate is 92% (73 to 100%).[24] The results are appreciably the same for primitive or external iliac arteries.

The clinical results are better when a good distal vessel bed exists and when the symptomatology is that of claudication (94%, as opposed to 91% in the cases of critical ischemia).[18] Diabetes, on the other hand, does not seem to play a determinant role.

Clinical results observed after dilation of iliac recanalization are less favorable (between 40 and 78%).[36,38] They are better when the lesion is short and when only the primitive iliac artery is concerned.[38] These results, however, were observed with the older technical methods. At present, and particularly because of the use of hydrophilic guides and vascular endoprostheses, these results are much better.[33]

Complications[7–24,56]

The amputation rate is 0.1%. The mortality rate after angioplasty is 0.2%. Most often this is due to myocardial infarction occurring immediately after the angioplasty. This is, in fact, the evidence of the diffuse nature of atheromatous lesions throughout the organism. It emphasizes the importance of a cardiac, as well as neurologic, workup of these polyvascular patients, before any peripheral therapy.

Technical failures are essentially represented by the failure of recanalization, which is between 1.4

and 5.5%.[14,23] This rate is greater for the treatment of iliac obstructions and is proportional to the length of the obstruction. At present, however, these failures are less frequent, which is again due to the use of hydrophilic guides and vascular prostheses.

Two types of complications should be distinguished: those that are due to the angioplasty itself and those inherent in any arterial puncture.

Angioplasty Site Complications

The Complications at the angioplasty site are dominated by dissections and residual stenoses.

Dissections. One should distinguish between banal linear dissections, observed by Roth et al.[57] in more than 60% of cases after noncomplicated dilations, and true obstructive dissections with hemodynamic repercussions, which should be considered complications and treated as such. In such a case, a second dilation is performed with the same balloon at a weak pressure for 3 to 4 minutes, to reapply the walls of the dissection. In case of failure, an endoprostheses is placed.

Residal Stenoses. To be significant, residual stenoses should be greater than 30% and lead to hemodynamic compromise, according to the aforementioned criteria. There, again, dilation with greater pressure is attempted, sometimes completed by a prosthesis.

Embolic Migrations. Observed in 1.6% of cases, embolic migrations most often occur in the homolateral member but may be observed contralaterally when the lesion is at the iliac bifurcation. These emboli are most often thrombotic material but may be atherosclerotic. Currently, these are treated essentially by thromboaspiration, technically simple, of low cost, and immediately effective regardless of the nature of the embolus. As described earlier, these migrations most often occur during recanalizations (3 to 20% of cases).[33,34,36,38]

Arterial Rupture. Arterial rupture is observed in 0.2% of cases, essentially during recanalizations (3% of cases for Colapinto et al.).[38] It is a major complication of angioplasty and should be urgently treated by prolonged dilation at low pressure to plug the perforation[58] (Fig. 77-6). When this is ineffective, placement of a covered endoprosthesis should allow the exclusion of this zone from the parietal perforation.

Puncture Site Complications

Complications at the puncture site are dominated by hematomas and are observed in 2.9% of cases. Other complications are false aneurysms (0.5%) and acute thrombosis (1.9%).

In synthesis, a mean rate of complication of 8.1% (2 to 21%) is seen, of which 2.7% are considered major, and 1.2% necessitate a surgical intervention. This rate tends to decrease as a result of the evolution of the material, better adapted to percutaneous angioplasty, and to improved care of these complications by the interventional radiologist.

Late Results

Late results show great variability between the different series published. This is due to the different result criteria (clinical and hemodynamic results), different appreciation of immediate technical failure, as well as other associated therapy necessary for secondary permeability.

PTA Results

As described in the literature, in 6,564 iliac dilations, at 1, 3, and 5 years, a permeability rate of 91% (63 to 100,) 80% (58 to 95,) and 72% (32 to 92,) was respectively observed.[24] Secondary failure was due to either restenosis, observed most often within the first 6 months, or to the natural course of the atheromatous disease.

Long-term results depend on several factors: (1) The site: The common iliac artery seems more favorable than the external iliac artery (60 vs. 47% at 5 years). (2) The presence of a good distal vascular bed seems equally to be a positive factor. (3) The clinical presentation: the results are better in the context of claudication than in severe ischemia. (4) Finally, the post dilation angiographic findings (absence of residual stenosis or obstructive dissection) are a factor.

Endoprosthetic Results

Endoprosthetic results are equally of interest, especially because the majority are placed following an ineffective angioplasty.

A multicenter study of therapy with the Palmaz prosthesis[53] showed an early clinical success rate of 99%; 91 and 84% at 1 and 2 years, respectively. At 43 months, however, the clinical success rate was no more than 69%, for a permeability of 92%; this was related to the disease evolution independent of the initially treated lesion.

With the Wallstent prosthesis, similar results were observed with early, 1- and 2-year permeability at 99, 95, and 88%, respectively.[34,44,45]

Several studies have shown that in the treatment of iliac occlusions comparable results are obtained, if primary failure of recanalization is excluded.[33,34,41]

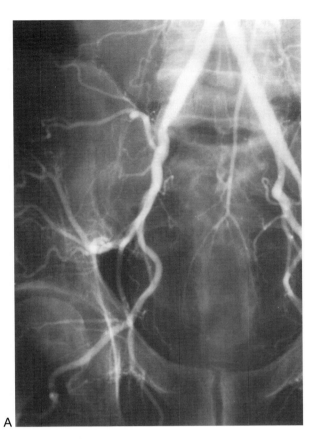

A

Fig. 77-6. (A) From a contralateral approach, PTA of this right external iliac artery lesion was performed, resulting in marked improvement in the lumen. **(B)** Following dilation, the patient experienced severe pelvic pain. Imaging revealed no extravasation of contrast from the dilation site, but an eccentric compression of the bladder was seen indicating vascular rupture. **(C)** Reinflation of the angioplasty balloon resulted in tamponade of the rupture site avoiding emergency surgical repair. (*Figure continues.*)

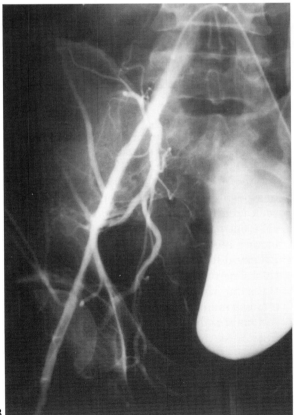

B

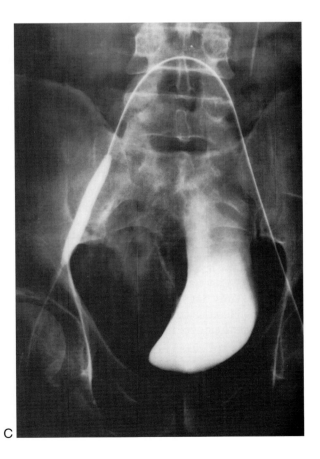

C

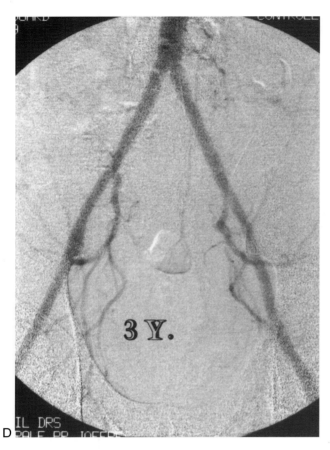

Fig. 77-6 (*Continued*). (**D**) The patient continued to do well 3 years post-PTA.

Emboli, however, are more frequent (between 4.7% and 17%), but the majority are treated percutaneously by thromboaspiration techniques.[33]

The most recent results of a randomized study in 247 patients by Richter et al.,[54] comparing PTA to endoprostheses in the treatment of iliac lesions, showed immediate success in 98% of prostheses and 91% for PTA. The 5-year cumulative permeability rates, confirmed by angiography, are, respectively, 94 and 65% for prosthesis and PTA. These results lead to the reflection that long-term results should improve if endoprostheses were used systematically for treatment of iliac lesions. This is difficult to envisage for economic reasons. Unfortunately, the actual progress of this study does not as yet allow for identifying the group of lesions that may or may not benefit from an endoprosthesis as a first choice.

DISCUSSION

In light of these results, one may better evaluate which are the better indications for an iliac angioplasty. These indications depend on a battery of clinical and anatomoradiologic arguments.

1. The real clinical effect of an iliac lesion, in the context of eventual associated vascular lesions, should be evaluated. The hemodynamic effect of a lesion should be quantified locally by systolic indexes, at rest and during effort. The functional evaluation of the lesion should be associated with a general workup of the polyvascular patient.

2. The angiographic aspect of the lesion is equally fundamental (Table 77-1): A short, concentric stenosis represents the ideal anatomic indication.[57] Segmented common or external iliac occlusions have become an indication for endovascular treatment, particularly with the advent of endoprostheses. Inversely, a long recanalization of the entire iliac axes is often achievable, but it is technically more delicate and presents a greater risk of complications, thus questioning its indication versus a surgical revascularization technique. The presence of parietal calcifications is not a contraindication, but the presence of an endoluminal calcified deposit compromises the effectiveness of dilation. These calcifications may be the source of rupture of the angioplasty balloon during the dilation (Table 77-1).

As a function of these angiographic parameters and of the clinical context, these indications may be qualified as simple, delicate, and those that lend themselves to discussion.

The simple case corresponds to an isolated, short, proximal, concentric, and noncalcified stenosis in a patient presenting with claudication associated with a good distal bed. In the presence of critical ischemia, the goal is the preservation of the leg and the indications for dilation should be large.

The controversial cases are represented by the following:

- Stenosis responsible for functional symptoms only during intense effort in athletic subjects: Dilation may be justified in young patients, if their physical capacity has been sufficiently limited for them to seek treatment, after well-followed medical treatment has failed, and after the risk factors have been eliminated.
- Bilateral lesions with unilateral claudication: One may propose either a dilation at the same time of the different lesions, or a subsequent dilation of the contralateral lesions if they become symptomatic, after initial treatment of the most significant lesion.
- Restenoses: These may be dilated with a success rate equal to primary dilation.
- Emboligenic lesions responsible for "blue toe syndromes:" These may be successfully

Table 77-1. The Guidelines for Iliac PTA Established by the Society of Cardiovascular and Interventional Radiology[59]

Category	Description	Guidelines
1	Stenoses <3 cm, concentric, noncalcified	Best indication for PTA
2	Stenoses 3–5 cm, concentric, noncalcified Stenoses <3 cm, eccentric, calcified	Well suited for PTA; includes lesions followed by distal bypass
3	Stenoses 5–10 cm	Amenable to PTA; moderate chance of success versus surgery
	Chronic occlusions <5 cm	PTA may be performed in patients with high surgical risk or lack of surgical material
4	1. Stenoses >10 cm 2. Chronic occlusions >5 cm, after thrombolysis 3. Extensive bilateral 4. Stenoses associated with aneurysms or other lesions requiring surgery	PTA has limited role, low technical success, poor long-term benefit PTA only when no surgical options or in very high-risk patients

treated by placement of a prosthesis before dilation[46] or by an atherectomy,[47] without risk of further emboli.

The more controversial cases are those with extended iliac artery lesions, particularly those with occlusions and complex stenoses (ostial lesions). The therapeutic choice should be made after a medicoradiosurgical assessment, to evaluate the risks, advantages, and disadvantages of each method. This should be adapted to the patient's clinical presentation and general clinical status, as well as to the status of the proximal and distal vessels.

Dilation or Surgery?

Two surgical interventions are currently employed at this site: endarterectomy and, especially, aortoiliac bypass.

It is difficult to compare the results of angioplasties with those of surgery, because these two therapeutic techniques do not address the same form of disease; surgery is indicated for more extensive disease. Moreover, analysis of results, as often seen in the literature, excludes those patients in whom angioplasty was a technical failure. Finally, these retrospective studies do not take into account the most recent technical progress of each of these therapeutic methods.

As reviewed by Brothers and Greenfield[60] in 1990, the long-term results of aortoiliac reconstructions show (1) for aortoiliac endarterectomy, a perioperative mortality between 1 and 16%, a primary permeability between 55 and 93% at 5 years, and between 48 and 76% at 10 years; (2) for aortoiliac bypass, a

mortality rate between 0 and 17.5%, with permeability rates between 62.4 and 95%, and between 62 and 82% at 5 and 10 years, respectively.

Few randomized prospective studies comparing angioplasty and surgery have been published. The study by Wolf et al.[61] concerns lesions accessible to angioplasty, situated at the iliac level or distal to it, in patients presenting essentially with claudication. This comparison shows that average annual mortality was higher in the bypass group, that primary success favored the bypass group, and that limb salvages favored the PTA group (the differences were not statistically significant). At 4 years, however, no difference was found between the two groups in terms of permeability, amputations, or patient survival.

The retrospective study by Doubilet and Abrams,[62] comparing the effectiveness of the (2) treatment modalities over 5 years, concludes, "By treating focalized lesions (all sites included) with primary angioplasty, followed by surgery in the case of failure, we should save 352 lives, conserve 5600 permeable members, and, thus, decrease the number of complications by 297."[62]

When economic considerations become a growing concern in health-care policy, the comparison between angioplasty and surgery should be evaluated with this in mind. Doubilet and Abrams[62] showed that at 5 years, the cost of surgery (including the hospitalization as well as income lost by the patients as a result of work stoppage) is 5.4 times greater than for dilation. The authors concluded that angioplasty as first-line therapy would lead to a savings of $81.9 millions.

These results have led to a certain therapeutic consensus regarding iliac artery lesions, as previously described. Dilation and surgery should be seen more as complementary than competitive. Dilation may be associated with surgical revascularization, either by associating dilation with femoropopliteal or distal bypass, or by associating iliac dilation with a crossing bypass for treating a contralateral obstruction.[63-66] Angioplasty may be used to treat surgical complications, particularly secondary stenoses after bypass surgery.

CONCLUSION

Because of the high percentage of clinical success associated with a low complication rate, angioplasty should currently be proposed as first-choice treatment for simple iliac lesions. Even though the long-term success rate is lower than after surgery, recurrences are easily accessible to a second PTA, without risking the prognosis of the member, which is the opposite for obstructions of surgical bypasses. The new endovascular technical devices, particularly vascular endoprostheses, have allowed expansion of the indications to include complex lesions and obstructions. These advances permit equal management of the complications inherent in this type of treatment, whether local (residual stenoses or obstructive dissections) or distant (emboli).

These encouraging results can be obtained only by a proper evaluation and technical mastery of these new endovascular procedures. Finally, the long-term effectiveness of these therapeutic modalities depends on a good knowledge of the pathology and the indications as well as on active consultation among the different vascular disciplines.

REFERENCES

1. Dotter CT, Judkins MP. Transluminal treatment of arteriosclerotic obstruction: description of a new technic and a preliminary report of its application. Circulation 1964;30:654
2. Gruntzig A, Kumpe DA. Technique of percutaneous transluminal angioplasty with the Gruntzig balloon catheter. AJR Am J Roentgenol 1979;132:547
3. Van Andel GJ. Transluminal iliac angioplasty: long term results. Radiology 1980;135:607
4. Colapinto RF, Harries Jones EP, Johnston KW. Percutaneous transluminal dilatation and recanalization in the treatment of peripheral vascular disease. Radiology 1980;135:583
5. Motarjeme A, Keifer JW, Zuska AJ. Percutaneous transluminal angioplasty of the iliac arteries: 66 experiences. AJR Am J Roentgenol 1980;135:937
6. Waltman AC. Percutaneous transluminal angioplasty: iliac and deep femoral arteries. AJR Am J Roentgenol 1980;135:921
7. Spence RK, Freiman DB, Gatenby R. Long-term results of transluminal angioplasty of the iliac and femoral arteries. Arch Surg 1981;116:1377
8. Van Andel GJ. Long-term results of iliac and femoral angioplasty. Ann Radiol 1981;24:365
9. Kadir S, White RI, Kaufman SL. Long-term results of aortoiliac angioplasty. Surgery 1982;94:10
10. Zeitler E, Richter EI, Roth FJ, Schoop W. Results of percutaneous transluminal angioplasty. Radiology 1983;146:57
11. Gallino A, Mahler F, Probst P, Nachbur B. Percutaneous transluminal angioplasty of the arteries of the lower limbs: a 5 year follow-up. Circulation 1984;70:619
12. Katzen BT. Percutaneous transluminal angioplasty for arterial disease of the lower extremities. AJR Am J Roentgenol 1984;142:23
13. Tegtmeyer CJ, Kellum CD, Kron IL, Mentzer RM. Percutaneous transluminal angioplasty in the region of the aortic bifurcation. Radiology 1985;157:661
14. Van Andel GJ, Van Erp WF, Krepel VM, Breslau PJ. Percutaneous transluminal dilatation of the iliac artery: long-term results. Radiology 1985;156:321
15. Jeans WD, Danton RM, Baird RN, Horrocks M. A comparison of the costs of vascular surgery and balloon dilatation in lower limb ischaemic disease. Br J Radiol 1986;59:453
16. Gardiner GA, Meyerovitz MF, Stokes KR. Complications of transluminal angioplasty. Radiology 1986;159:201
17. Blankensteijn JD, Van Broonhoven TJ, Lampmann L. Role of percutaneous transluminal angioplasty in aorto-iliac reconstruction. J Cardiovasc Surg 1986;27:466
18. Johnston KW, Rae M, Hogg Johnston SA. 5-year results of a prospective study of percutaneous transluminal angioplasty. Ann Surg 1987;206:403
19. Morag B, Rubinstein Z, Kessler A. Percutaneous transluminal angioplasty of the distal abdominal aorta and its bifurcation. Cardiovasc Intervent Radiol 1987;12:1
20. Belli AM, Hemingway AP, Cumberland DC, Welsh CL. Percutaneous transluminal angioplasty of the distal abdominal aorta. Eur J Vasc Surg 1989;3:449
21. Becker GJ. Noncoronary angioplasty. Radiology 1989;170:921
22. Wilson SE, Sheppard B. Results of percutaneous transluminal angioplasty for peripheral vascular occlusive disease. Ann Vasc Surg 1990;4:94
23. Stokes KR, Strunk HM, Campbell DR. Five-year results of iliac and femoropopliteal angioplasty in diabetic patients. Radiology 1990;174:977
24. Rholl KS, Van Breda A. Percutaneous intervention for aortoiliac disease. pp. 433-6. In Strandness DE, van Breda A (eds): Vascular Diseases: Surgical and Interventional Therapy. Churchill Livingstone, New York, 1994
25. Johnston KW. Factors that influence the outcome of aortoiliac and femoropopliteal percutaneous transluminal angioplasty. Endovasc Surg 1992;72:843
26. Kashdan BJ, Trost DW, Jagust MB. Retrograde approach for contralateral iliac and infrainguinal percutaneous transluminal angioplasty: experience in 100 patients. J Vasc Intervent Radiol 1992;3:515

27. Matsumoto AH, Barth KH, Selby JB, Tegtmeyer CJ. Peripheral angioplasty balloon technology. Cardiovasc Intervent Radiol 1993;16:135

28. Kaufman SI, Barth KH. Hemodynamic measurements in the evaluation and follow-up of transluminal angioplasty of the iliac and femoral arteries. Radiology 1982;142:329

29. McNamara TO, Bomberger RA. Factors affecting initial and 6 month patency rates after intraarterial thrombolysis with high dose urokinase. Am J Surg 1986;152:709

30. Van Breda A, Katzen BT, Deutsch AS. Urokinase versus streptokinase in local thrombolysis. Radiology 1987;165:109

31. McNamara TO. Thrombolysis as an alternative initial therapy for the acutely ischemia lower limb. Semin Vasc Surg 1992;5:89

32. Bookstein JJ, Valji K. Pulse-spray pharmacomechanical thrombolysis. Cardiovasc Intervent Radiol 1992; 15:228

33. Rousseau H, George P, Elias A et al. Iliac occlusions: respective role of the new endovascular technique. Balloon angioplasty vs. stents. Presented at the 16th World Congress of the International Union of Angiology, Paris, September, 13–18, 1992

34. Vorwerk D, Gunther RW. Stent placement in iliac arterial lesions: three years of clinical experience with the wallstent. Cardiovasc Intervent Radiol 1992;15:285

35. Long AL, Page PE, Raynaud AC. Percutaneous iliac artery stent: angiographic long-term followup. Radiology 1991;180:771

36. Ring EJ, Freiman DB, McLean GK, Schwaarz W. Percutaneous recanalization of common iliac artery occlusions: an unacceptable complication rate? AJR Am J Roentgenol 1982;139:587

37. Pilla TJ, Peterson GJ, Tantana S. Percutaneous recanalization of iliac artery occlusions: an alternative to surgery in the high risk patient. AJR Am J Roentgenol 1984;143:313

38. Colapinto RF, Stronell RD, Johnston WK. Transluminal angioplasty of complete iliac obstructions. AJR Am J Roentgenol 1982;146:859

39. Daniell SJN, Dacie JE, Lumley JSP. Is percutaneous transluminal angioplasty for common iliac occlusion a safe procedure? J Vasc Intervent Radiol 1987;2:89

40. Ginsburg R, Thorpe P, Bowles CR. Pull-through approach to percutaneous angioplasty of totally occluded common iliac arteries. Radiology 1989;172:111

41. Rees CR, Palmaz JC, Garcia O. Angioplasty and stenting of completing occluded iliac arteries. Radiology 1989;172:953

42. Gunther RW, Vorwerk D, Bohndorf K. Iliac and femoral artery stenoses and occlusions: treatment with intravascular stents. Radiology 1989;172:725

43. Vorwerk D, Guenther RW. Mechanical revascularization of occluded iliac arteries with use of self-expandable endoprosthesis. Radiology 1990;175:411

44. Zollikofer CL, Antonucci F, Pfyffer M. Arterial stent placement with use of the wallstent: midterm results of clinical experience. Radiology 1991;179:449

45. Raillat C, Rousseau H, Joffre F, Roux D. Treatment of iliac artery stenoses with the wallstent endoprosthesis. AJR Am J Roentgenol 1990;154:613

46. Rousseau H, Joffre F, Raillat C et al. Iliac artery endo-

prosthesis: radiologic and histologic findings after 2 years. AJR Am J Roentgenol 1989;153:1075

47. Dolmatch BL, Rholl KS, Moskowitz LB. Blue toe syndrome: treatment with percutaneous atherectomy. Radiology 1989;172:799

48. Clugston RA, Eisenhauer AC, Matthews RV. Atherectomy of the distal aorta using a "kissing-balloon" technique for the treatment of blue toe syndrome. AJR Am J Roentgenol 1992;159:125

49. Kim D, Gianturco LE, Porter DH. Peripheral directional atherectomy: 4-year experience. Radiology 1992;183:773

50. Strecker EP, Liermann D, Barth KH, Hellmut RD. Expandable tubular stents for treatment of arterial occlusive diseases: experimental and clinical results. Radiology 1990;175:97

51. Palmaz JC, Garcia OJ, Schatz RA. Placement of balloon-expandable intraluminal stents in iliac arteries: first 171 procedures. Radiology 1990;174:969

52. Becker GJ, Palmaz JC, Res CR. Angioplasty induced dissections in human iliac arteries: management with Palmaz balloon-expandable intraluminal stents. Radiology 1990;176:31

53. Palmaz JC, Laborde JC, Rivera FJ. Stenting of the iliac areries with the palmaz stent: experience from a multicenter trial. Cardiovasc Intervent Radiol 1992; 15:291

54. Richter G, Roeren T, Brado M, Noeldge C. Further update of the randomized trial: iliac stent placement versus PTA—morphology, clinical success rates, and failure analysis, abstracted. Society of Cardiovascular and Interventional Radiology, Annual Meeting, New Orleans, LA, 1993

55. Rutherford RB, Becker GJ. Standards for evaluating and reporting the results of surgical and percutaneous therapy for peripheral arterial disease. J Vasc Intervent Radiol 1991;2:169

56. Belli AM, Cumberland DC, Knox AM. The complication reate of percutaneous peripheral balloon angioplasty. Clin Radiol 1990;41:380

57. Roth FJ, Cappius G, Fingerhut E. Radiological pattern at and after angioplasty. pp. 73. In Dotter CT, Gruntzig A et al (eds): Percutaneous Transluminal Angioplasty. Springer-Verlag, Berlin, 1983

58. Joseph N, Levy E, Lipman S. Angioplasty-related iliac artery rupture: treatment by temporary balloon occlusion. Cardiovasc Intervent Radiol 1987;10:276

59. Guidelines for percutaneous transluminal angioplasty. Standards of Practice Committee of the Society of Cardiovascular and Interventional Radiology. Radiology 1990;177:619

60. Brothers TE, Greenfield LJ. Long-term results of aortoiliac reconstruction. J Vasc Intervent Radiol 1990;1:49

61. Wolf GL, Wilson SE, Cross AP, Deupree RH. Surgery or balloon angioplasty for peripheral vascular disease: a randomized clinical trial. J Vasc Intervent Radiol 1993;4:639

62. Doubilet P, Abrams HL. The cost of underutilization. Percutaneous transluminal angioplasty for peripheral vascular disease. N Engl J Med 1984;310:95

63. Zeitler E, Raithel D, Gailer H. PTA combined with surgical vascular operations in iliac and femoral obstruction. Ann Radiol 1987;30:142

64. Griffith CDM, Harrison JD, Gregson RHS. Transluminal iliac angioplasty with distal bypass surgery in pa-

Renovascular Hypertension

The prevalence of renovascular hypertension is about 1 to 5% in all patients with this condition depending on the survey; it is caused by the renin angiotensin mechanism set in motion by unilateral or bilateral renal ischemia. Since renal artery stenosis is well suited to PTRA, a screening method for these

In older patients with severe hypertension and evolving renal failure or pulmonary edema, screening for renal artery stenosis may be indicated. However, it is not often possible to improve renal function by PTRA because of generalized atherosclerosis, renal artery occlusions, aortic aneurysms, impaired vascular ac-

tients with critical limb ischaemia. J R Coll Surg Edinb 1989;34:253

65. Brewster DC, Cambria RP, Darling RC. Long-term results of combined iliac balloon angioplasty and distal surgical revascularization. Ann Surg 1989;210:324

66. Walker PJ, Harris JP, May J. Combined percutaneous transluminal angioplasty and extraanatomic bypass for symptomatic unilateral iliac artery occlusion with contralateral iliac artery stenosis. Ann Vasc Surg 1991;5:209

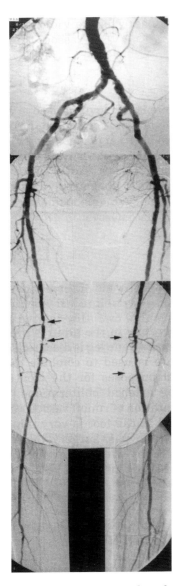

Fig. 79-1. Aortoiliac leg arteriography after catheterization from the brachial artery. Irregular stenoses in the SFA on both legs.

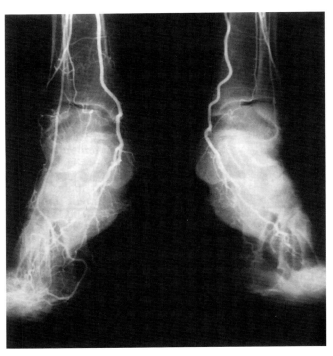

Fig. 79-2. Ankle and foot arteries demonstrating patency of the posterior tibial artery and the left plantar artery. Occlusion of the left anterior tibial artery and of the distal plantar artery with collateral circulation through the dorsal pedal artery, with hypervascularity at the distal foot are seen in a diabetic man with gangrene in the right foot.

Additional information can be achieved by control of the pain-free walking distance, by oscillography at rest and after exercise, and by measurement of the ABI after stress.

Having determined the clinical situation, the angiographic technique must be chosen.

Among the different risk factors for arteriosclerosis (smoking, diabetes, hypertension, hypercholesterinemia) in peripheral occlusive vascular disease, cigarette smoking and diabetes are the most important.

Arteriosclerotic obstructions, single and multiple stenoses, as well as occlusions mainly are located in Hunter's channel of the SFA (Fig. 79-3) and are often symmetric on both thighs (Fig. 79-1).

More uncommon are isolated popliteal artery stenoses, common femoral artery obliterations, or obliterations in the proximal part of the SFA. Before interventional radiologic treatment, the determination of calcifications (Fig. 79-4) and collateral pathways is necessary. Before vascular surgery, it is important to have precise information on the condition of the run-in and run off vessels, to prevent early reocclusion. Therefore, oblique projections in bifurcational arteries, for example, in the iliac or femoral bifurcation, complement anteroposterior one-plane angiography. Additional needle angiography may be needed.

DIABETIC VASCULAR DISEASE

In patients with a history of diabetes of several years, the most common obliterations in macroangiopathy are occlusions of the tibiofibular and foot arteries (Fig. 79-5) as well as stenoses of the deep femoral artery.[9] Avascular obliterations of foot arteries and hypervascular obliterations occur in patients with diabetic gangrene. The SFA and the iliac arteries are mainly normal in diabetic patients.

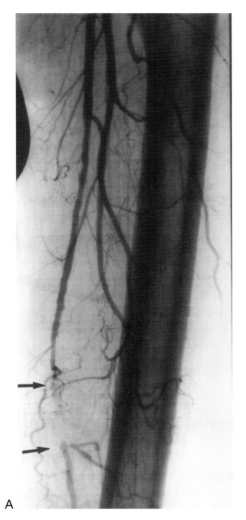 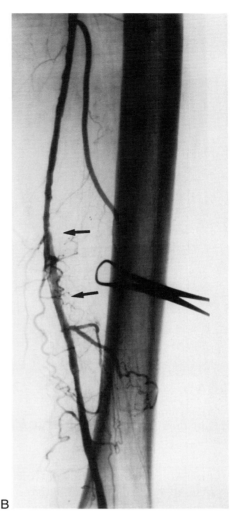

A   B

Fig. 79-3. **(A)** Antegrade angiography of the thigh arteries demonstrate a segmental SFA occlusion in Hunter's channel, 5 cm in length, and partially calcified plaque, proximally. Collateral circulation from the deep femoral artery to the distal femoral artery. **(B)** Angiography after PTA shows residual stenoses but reduced collateral circulation.

The most important collateral vessels are the deep femoral arteries for the thigh, the sural arteries for the popliteal artery, and the peroneal artery for the lower leg at the ankle.

BUERGER'S DISEASE

In addition to peripheral occlusive vascular disease, mainly resulting from arteriosclerosis, endangiitis or thromboangiitis obliterans (Buerger/Winniwarter's disease) play an important role. About 2 to 5% of patients with peripheral vascular disease in Europe suffer from this inflammatory disease, which can be observed mainly in men younger than 45 years of age.[10]

In these patients, obliterations are located mainly in the posterior tibial or anterior tibial artery, and typical collateral pathways along the vasa vasorum of the posterior tibial artery can be observed (Fig. 79-6).

The most common signs[1,11,12] of thromboangiitis obliterans in angiography are as follows:

- The iliac arteries and the superficial femoral artery are normal.
- The tibioperoneal arteries show segmental occlusions at several locations.
- Corkscrew-like collateral arteries along the vasa vasorum, mainly in the posterior tibial artery.[10,12]
- Claudications are not mainly in the calf but in the foot (instep claudication).

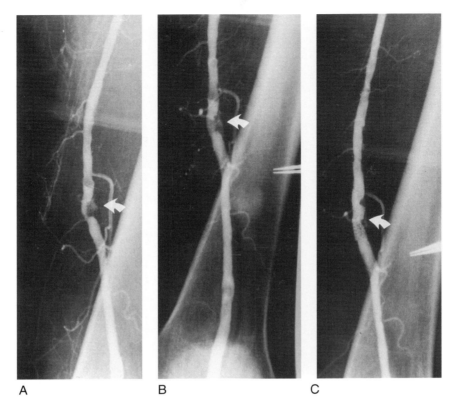

A   B   C

Fig. 79-4. (A) Asymmetric stenosis in the distal SFA with calcified plaque. **(B)** Angiography after Simpson atherectomy showing residual stenosis. **(C)** Control angiography after application of a Strecker stent, 4 cm in length.

In most cases inflammatory symptoms of phlebitis saltans or migrans are also in the patients' history. These patients are heavy smokers, and in several cases there was also an adverse social background.

POPLITEAL ANEURYSMS

The popliteal aneurysm, or femoropopliteal aneurysmatic disease, is the second most common arterial aneurysm and can be bilateral or unilateral.[13–15] Typical clinical complications are thrombosis of the aneurysm or peripheral embolization. In all cases, palpation and auscultation of the popliteal fossa are necessary, and the primary diagnosis can be established with ultrasound, computed tomography, or angiography. A popliteal occlusion can always be a thrombosed aneurysm. Because of the ectasia and dilation of the femoropopliteal artery, the inflow vessel of the iliac arteries, and the turbulence in the aneurysmal sack in these cases, DSA provides much better chances for clear docmentation of the extent of the aneurysm than conventional angiography. In the past, documentation of aneurysms has always shown the need for more than one angiography be-

cause the flow and turbulence need a long time exposure before clear visualization and also because of the run off vessels and the aneurysm in its total extent (Fig. 79-7).

POPLITEAL ARTERY ENTRAPMENT

As a result of atypical insertion of the gastrocnemius muscle or hypertrophy of the soleus muscle, the popliteal artery can be compressed at the time of plantar flexion.[15,16] The clinically symptomatic patients are mainly young men over 20 years of age, and on angiography, the popliteal artery is compressed at rest, from anterior to dorsal lateral or medial. The differential diagnosis in patients with popliteal artery occlusion therefore must include consideration of embolus, aneurysm, and popliteal compression syndrome. In patients with dislocation of the popliteal artery with asymmetric stenoses, popliteal artery entrapment as well as cystic degeneration of the adventitia can be present. Therefore, not only angiography but also ultrasound or computed tomography are necessary before vascular surgery.

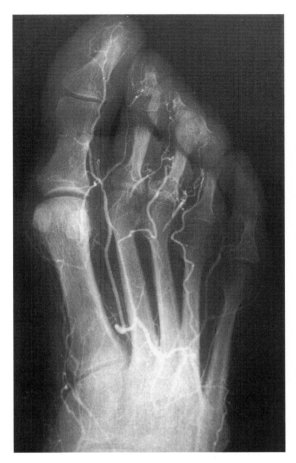

Fig. 79-5. Foot angiography in a patient with diabetic gangrene demonstrates multiple digital artery occlusions, as well as an occlusion of the plantar artery. Avascular diabetic macroangiopathy.

CYSTIC ADVENTITIA DEGENERATION

Cystic adventitia degeneration is a very rare disease that can cause clinical symptoms such as popliteal stenosis and popliteal occlusion.[17] An endovascular treatment is not successful here, and neither is thrombolysis nor angioplasty. Surgical repair with excision of the cyst in the arterial wall is the classic treatment of this disease.

TREATMENT OF FEMOROPLITEAL ARTERY OBLITERATIONS

The four different types of treatment are

1. Vascular surgery

2. Interventional radiology with angioplasty, local thrombolysis, and their modifications
3. Systemic thrombolysis
4. Exercise and medication

The classic treatment of femoropopliteal obliterations in patients with claudication is exercise, whereas in patients with critical limb ischemia having rest pain and gangrene, the classic treatment is bypass surgery. Former types of treatment such as sympathectomy have become less important,[7] but in all cases with local necrosis and gangrene, local therapy in combination with antibiotics is one part of the treatment.[13] The second, but most important, part of treatment in all stages of peripheral occlusive vascular disease is percutaneous transluminal angioplasty (PTA) to improve the peripheral vascular flow.[5,18–24]

Vascular surgery is used mainly as femoropopliteal bypass surgery in various modifications. The preferred bypass material is the saphenous vein.[15,25] Local thrombendarterectomy is less important, but in the groin, the deep femoral artery "profunda patch plastique" is successful in several patients.

INTERVENTIONAL RADIOLOGY

The approach for interventional treatment can use the percutaneous access from the groin of the ipsilateral side, from the groin of the contralateral side, and after puncture of the popliteal artery in a retrograde or orthograde direction.[21,24]

After puncture with the Seldinger or Cournand needle or any of their modifications, a sheath is placed in the groin over a guidewire. With the help of a sheath with a sidearm for injection of contrast medium and pharmaceutical drugs—under fluoroscopic control, using image intensifier systems, mainly digital angiography—PTA is a very reliable treatment of limited trauma to the inner arterial wall, initiated by Charles Dotter and Melvin Judkins in 1964.[18]

While dilation with the bouginage technique[26] and recanalization with guidewires and simple catheters are the basics of treatment, dilation with balloon catheters according to Grüntzig and Hopff[27] has improved percutaneous techniques. The benefit of balloon angioplasty is a reduced complication rate at the puncture site (hematomas, bleedings, and early rethrombosis), and it also has provided the possibility of treating arteries with a diameter larger than the catheter itself, thus enabling the dilation.[5,19]

The mechanism of dilation is very complex,[19] and the success depends on

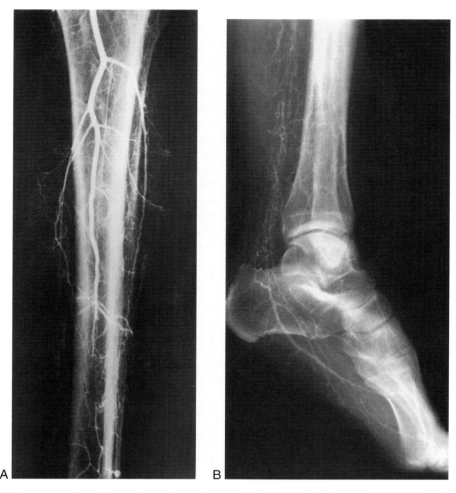

Fig. 79-6. Tibioperoneal peripheral vascular disease. **(A & B)** Occlusions of all tibial arteries, direct corkscrew-like collaterals along the posterior tibial artery. Patient's age, location, history, and angiography indicating endangiitis (Buerger's disease).

- Rupture of intimal and medial layers
- Stretching of the arterial wall
- Compression of parts of the media and organized thrombus

Dilation is also affected by several influences of the vasa vasorum in the adventitia and restoration by formation of a new intima, like a fibrotic scar. Depending on the vessel diameter, the scar caused by the smooth muscle cells that produce intimal hyperplasia is highly important. The clinical situation has shown that intimal hyperplasia in iliac arteries with a diameter of about 8 mm is less important than in small arteries.[21] Therefore, restenoses occur very seldom in iliac arteries, and the long-term patency is very high. In contrast, in distal SFA obliterations, the restenosis rate that is due to intimal hyperplasia is higher, especially in long-segment stenoses (Fig. 79-8) with atherosclerotic plaque. Reobliterations in

the first postprocedure days are mainly thrombi. Restenoses within 3 to 6 months very often can be identified histologically as intimal hyperplasia, but stenoses or occlusions that occur later are again arteriosclerotic.

TECHNIQUE OF PTA IN THE SFA AND POPLITEAL ARTERIES

After antegrade puncture and introduction of a sheath, 5,000 IU of heparin are injected. To start, an angiography for localization of all significant obliterations is necessary. After that, stenoses and occlusions are recanalized using a guidewire and a catheter. Stenoses are crossed best with slippery guidewires, either straight or with a curved tip, followed by a Cobra catheter.

After successful guiding of all lesions, the pilot

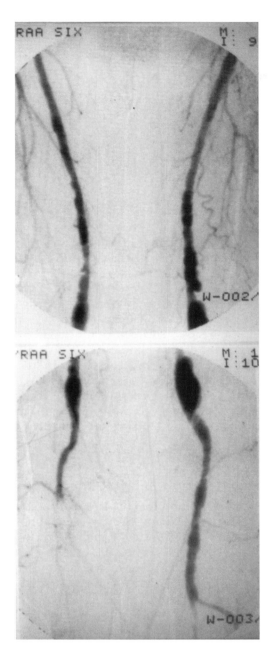

Fig. 79-7. Digital subtraction angiography in a patient with bilateral popliteal artery aneurysms with peripheral embolization in the right tibioperoneal artery.

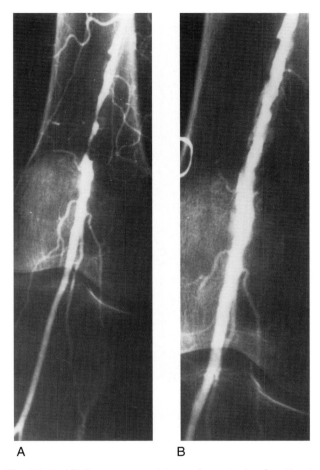

A B

Fig. 79-8. **(A)** Long-segment irregular arteriosclerotic stenosis in the femoropopliteal artery with irregularities in the proximal SFA. The patient has gangrene in the foot. **(B)** Control angiography after angioplasty with the Dotter-Grüntzig balloon angioplasty.

catheter is exchanged for a balloon catheter of the selected balloon diameter and length over a more rigid guidewire. In the SFA artery, mainly balloon catheters with a diameter of 6 mm are used, with a length between 2 and 8 cm. In the popliteal artery, mainly 5- to 6-mm diameter balloons are used, with a length of 4 cm or longer.

Tibiofibular artery obliterations (Fig. 79-9) are recanalized with a guidewire. Small balloon catheters

are preferred such as Schwarten's balloon[28] or the on-the-wire balloon, such as the Tegwire catheter[29] or the SOS viper catheters[30] with a soft tip and a more rigid shaft. After successful recanalization and dilation, a control angiography is necessary to assess the outcome and to indicate additional types of medicamentous treatment or the need of stent application.

SPECIAL DEVICES

Additional techniques, in cases where the recanalization with guidewire and catheter failed, are rotating catheters, low-rotating devices,[31] high-rotating devices,[32] or the Rotablator.[33,34] Localized stenoses can also be treated by atherectomy.[35,36]

These mechanical devices can help to recanalize the vascular system, especially in cases with multiple stenoses and a small residual lumen. Even today,

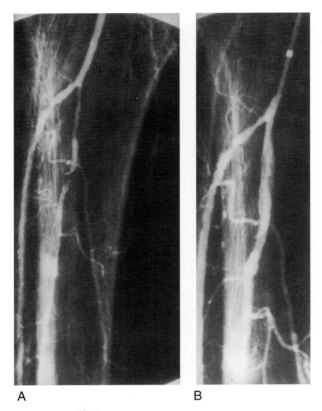

Fig. 79-9. The same patient as in Fig. 79-8. **(A)** Long-segment stenosis of the tibioperoneal trunk, proximal occlusion of the peroneal artery, long-segment stenosis, and atherosclerosis of the posterior tibial artery. **(B)** Control angiography after recanalization and balloon angioplasty.

in patients with long-segment occlusions, from the beginning, the best type of treatment is a femoropopliteal bypass—provided that the runoff situation is good; in patients with femoropopliteal occlusions with critical limb ischemia and at risk of total leg amputation, a femorocrural or femoropedal bypass is best.[15,17,37] In case of simple lesions in the popliteal and lower leg arteries, PTA can be used as a primary method of choice—but with a few restrictions—to prevent more severe complications and to spare the patient a higher risk.[11,20,24,38] Laser-assisted angioplasty has been used for several years, and as some studies have shown,[39,40] in some cases the primary success rate is increased by 10 to 20%. The long-term results, however, are not better than after balloon angioplasty.[40,41] Therefore, with increasing experience and modern guidewires, laser-assisted angioplasty is superfluous. In about 80% the guidewire plus balloon catheter technique (Dotter/Grüntzig procedure) is successful.[20,21,42]

By contrast, the percutaneous application of stents or endoprostheses[43–46] is of interest and successful in patients with long-segment occlusions and contraindications to vascular surgery, or in patients with dissection or collapsing artery, to control the complications of angioplasty. The long-term results of stent treatment in the SFA and popliteal arteries are not as good as in iliac arteries. Here, it is only a second-choice method.

COMPLEMENTARY MEDICAMENTOUS TREATMENT

After every successful recanalization and angioplasty, the same type of follow-up treatment as after percutaneous transluminal coronary angioplasty or PTA of the iliac arteries is important. At the time of the procedure, anticoagulation is necessary, followed by 2 or 3 days of heparinization. Afterward, aggregation inhibitors and, in severe cases with critical limb ischemia, anticoagulation for patients with partial thrombin time below 25% can be indicated. Statistically significant double-blind studies have not given preference to one of the different types in long-term treatment, neither anticoagulation ("Marcumar", "Warfarin"), nor aggregation inhibitors (acetylsalicylic acid). The restenosis rate with both types of treatment varies between 20% and 50% after 1 year.

RESULTS

The results of interventional radiologic treatments can be defined by a summary of several publications, which like my own experience show better primary success and long-term results in patients with claudication than in patients with critical limb ischemia. Also, the results were better in nondiabetic than in diabetic patients. Among diabetics, those receiving oral medication had inferior results compared with those receiving insulin and its modifications.

REFERENCES

1. Henninges D, Zeitler E. Die Angiographie bei der Differenzierung der arteriellen Verschlußkrankheit. Verh Dtsch Ges Inn Med 1979;85:1408–11
2. Allen EV, Brown GE. Thrombo-angiitis obliterans. Ann Intern Med 1928;1:535–57
3. Fontaine R, Kim M, Kieny R. Die chirurgische Behandlung der peripheren Durchblutungsstörungen. Helv Chir Acta 1954;21:499–515
4. Greenwood LH, Hallett JW, Jr et al. The angiographic evaluation of lower-extremity arterial disease in the young adult. Cardiovasc Intervent Radiol 1985;8:183–6

5. Zeitler E, Grüntzig A, Schoop W (eds). Percutaneous Vascular Recanalization. Springer-Verlag, New York, 1978

6. Cachovan M. A Critique of the Fontaine Classification. In: Critical Ischemia, Vol. 1, pp. 7–9. 1991

7. European Working Group on Critical Leg Ischemia. Second European Consensus Document on Chronic Critical Leg Ischemia. Circulation 1991;84(suppl. 4): 1–26

8. Rutherford RB, Becker GJ. Standards for evaluation and reporting the results of surgical and percutaneous therapy for peripheral arterial disease. J Vasc Intervent Radiol 1991;2:169–74

9. Zeitler E. Angiographische Röntgendiagnose bei diabetischer Makroangiopathie. pp. 28–136. In Alexander K, Cachovan M (eds): Diabetische Angiopathien. Witzstrock, Baden-Baden, Germany, 1977

10. Diehm C, Schäfer M. Das Buerger-Syndrom (Thromboangiitis obliterans). Springer-Verlag, Berlin, Germany, 1993

11. Capek P, MacLean GK, Berkowitz HD. Femoropopliteal angioplasty: factors influencing long-term success. Circulation 1991;83(suppl. 1):170–80

12. Hagen B, Lohse S. Clinical and radiologic aspects of Buerger's disease. Cardiovasc Intervent Radiol 1984; 7:283–93

13. Heberer G, Rau G, Schoop W. Angiologie, Begr v. M. Ratschow. Thieme, Stuttgart, Germany, 1974

14. Sandmann W, Kniemeyer HW (eds). Aneurysmen der großen Arterien. Huber, Bern, Switzerland, 1991

15. Vollmar J. Rekonstruktive Chirurgie der Arterien. Thieme, Stuttgart, Germany, 1975

16. Alexander K. Angiologie. Urban and Schwarzenberg, Berlin, 1994

17. Bollinger A. Funktionelle Angiologie. Lehrbuch und Atlas. Thieme, Stuttgart, Germany, 1979

18. Dotter CT, Judkins MP. Transluminal treatment of arteriosclerotic obstruction. Description of a new technique and a preliminary report of its application. Circulation 1964;30:654–70

19. Dotter CT, Grüntzig AR, Schoop W, Zeitler E. Percutaneous transluminal angioplasty. Springer-Verlag, New York, 1983

20. Morgenstern BR, Getrajdman GI, Laffey KJ et al. Total occlusion of the femoropopliteal artery: high technical success rate of conventional balloon angioplasty. Radiology 1989;172:937–40

21. Roth FJ et al. Perkutane Gefäßrekanalisation. pp. 20–43. In Günther RW, Thelen M (eds): Interventionelle Radiologie. Thieme, Stuttgart, Germany, 1988

22. Schneider E, Grüntzig A, Bollinger A. Die perkutane transluminale Angioplastie (PTA) in den Stadien III und IV der peripheren arteriellen Verschlußkrankheiten. VASA 1982;11:336–341

23. Zeitler E, Schoop W, Zahnow W. The treatment of occlusive arterial disease by transluminal catheter angioplasty. Radiology 1971;99:19–26

24. Zeitler E. Percutaneous transluminal angioplasty of the femorotibial arteries. In Dondelinger RF, Rossi P, Kurdziel JC, Wallace S (eds): Interventional Radiology. Thieme New York, 1990

25. Kunlin J. Le traitement de l'artérite oblitérante par la greffe veineuse. Arch Med Coeur 1949;42:371

26. Van Andel GJ. Transluminal angioplasty according to Dotter-Judkins. Radiol Clin North Am 1975;44:228

27. Grüntzig A, Hopff H. Perkutane Rekanalisation chronischer arterieller Verschlüsse mit einem neuen Dilatationskatheter. Dtsch Med Wochenschr 1974;99: 2502–5

28. Schwarten DE. Clinical and anatomical considerations for nonoperative therapy in tibial disease and the results of angioplasty. Eur J Vasc Surg 1991;4: 149–52

29. Tegtmeyer CJ, Hartwell GD, Selby JB et al. Results and complications of angioplasty in aortoiliac disease. Circulation 1991;83(suppl. 1):153–60

30. Sos T. Tibial angioplasty. Presented at Nürnberger Tage für Radiologische Diagnostik '94, Nuremberg, Germany, 1994

31. Vallbracht C. Wiedereröffnung chronischer Arterienverschlüsse. Z Kardiol 1991;80(suppl. 9):95–102

32. Kensey K, Zeitler E, Reed M, Feith F. The Kensey catheter. pp. 116–122. In Zeitler E, Seyferth W (eds): Pros and Cons in PTA and Auxiliary Methods. Springer-Verlag, New York, 1989

33. Henry M, Amor M, Ethevenot G, Henry J. Percutaneous peripheral rotational ablation using the Rotablator. Presented at the 3rd International Course, Nancy, France, 1992

34. Warth DC, Buchbinder M, William ON et al. Rotational ablation using the Rotablator for angiographically unfavorable lesions, abstracted. J Am Coll Cardiol 1991;17(suppl. A):125

35. Schwarten DE, Katzen BT, Simpson JB et al. Simpson catheter for percutaneous transluminal removal of atheroma. Am J Roentgenol 1988;150:799–801

36. Simpson JB, Selmon MR, Robertson GC et al. Transluminal atherectomy for occlusive peripheral vascular disease. Am J Cardiol 1988;61:96–101

37. Kappert A. Lehrbuch und Atlas der Angiologie. 12. Auflage, Switzerland, 1984

38. Johnston KW. Femoral and popliteal arteries: reanalysis of results of balloon angioplasty. Radiology 1992; 183:767–71

39. Lammer J, Pilger E, Karnel F et al. Femoropopliteal laser recanalization. A multicenter study. Radiology 1990;30:45–9

40. Lammer J, Pilger E, Karnel F et al. Laser angioplasty results of a prospective multicenter-study at 3-year follow-up. Radiology 1991;178:335–7

41. Zeitler E, Seyferth W (eds). Pros and Cons in PTA and Auxiliary Methods. Springer-Verlag, New York, 1989

42. Becker GJ, Katzen BT, Dake MD. Noncoronary angioplasty. Radiology 1989;170:921–40

43. Liermann D. Stents. Thieme, New York, 1995

44. Palmaz JC, Richter GM, Noeldge G et al. Die intraluminale Stent-Implantation nach Palmaz. Radiologe 1987;27:560–3

45. Strecker EP, Schneider B, Wolf HRD et al. Flexible, percutaneously insertable, balloon-expandable arterial prosthesis. pp. 179–187. In Zeitler E, Seyferth W (eds): Pros and Cons in PTA and Auxiliary Methods. Springer-Verlag, New York, 1989

46. Zeitler E. The Future of the Stents. In Liermann D: Stents. Thieme, New York, 1995;401–403

80 Percutaneous Interventions for the Arteries Below the Knee

Gerald Dorros
Michael R. Jaff

Revascularization of the distal popliteal or tibioperoneal vessels for patients suffering claudication, ischemic rest pain, nonhealing ulcer(s), or gangrene can be successfully managed with balloon angioplasty or alternative or adjunctive percutaneous procedures.[1-4] Stenotic and occlusive disease of the distal popliteal and tibial arteries that is due to arteriosclerosis obliterans poses an interesting challenge to the vascular specialist. The surgical approach to this problem has been less than satisfying, with popliteal-tibial, tibio-tibial, and tibioperoneal bypass grafts offering inadequate long-term patency rates. However, the majority of primary care physicians, vascular surgeons, and cardiovascular interventionists do not understand that the clinical presentation caused by anatomic pathology can be effectively, safely, and successfully managed with balloons, thrombolytic agents, atherectomy devices, and stents.

INDICATIONS

Previously, percutaneous interventions were used in below-knee vessels for limb salvage, nonhealing wounds, or gangrene.[2,4] Recent publications, however, have supported its use in chronic limb ischemia (Fig. 80-1) as well as claudication[1,3] (Fig. 80-2). Angioplasty is better suited for more focal disease, while rotational ablation with or without adjunctive balloon angioplasty is meritorious in more diffuse disease (Fig. 80-3). In addition, percutaneous interventions appear to provide a better alternative than surgery in patients with concomitant medical problems (e.g., prior coronary atherosclerosis or cerebrovascular disease). Furthermore, diffuse disease (>5 cm in length) may not be a contraindication to angioplasty, because the percutaneous intervention has an excellent initial success rate with long, low-profile balloons, which may be sufficient to permit relief of rest pain or healing of the ulcer or nonhealing wound.

METHODOLOGY

The medical history, including identification of those patients with diabetes mellitus, helps determine indications and coexistent medical illness before intervention. Physical examination—including elevation dependency testing along with palpation of pulses, examination of the skin for trophic changes, ultrasound visualization, the ankle-brachial index, contrast arteriography, and magnetic resonance angiography—enables assessment of the clinical and anatomic situation. Diagnostic angiograms, extending from the infrarenal aorta or aortic bifurcation to the toes, enable planning of a successful interventional strategy.

The antegrade cannulation of the superficial femoral artery can often be accomplished by simple angiographic techniques. The common femoral artery is palpated. Local anesthesia is placed 1 to 2 cm above the inguinal ligament, and an arterial needle without an obturator is inserted at a 30-degree angle with

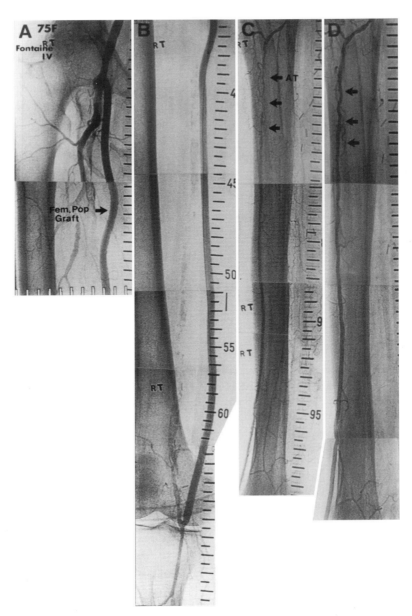

Fig. 80-1. A 75-year-old woman, following recent myocardial revascularization surgery with a nonhealing vein graft donor graff. Femoral popliteal grafting was performed 3 weeks following myocardial revascularization surgery to permit wound healing. The wound failed to close. The patient was referred for intervention. **(A & B)** The patent femoral popliteal graft (fern-pop graft). **(C)** The anterior tibial (AT) artery with a severe proximal narrowing, and the occluded posterior tibial and peroneal arteries. **(D)** The results of balloon angioplasty. The balloon catheter had been introduced via the contralateral approach and then traversed the length of the femoral popliteal graft to get to the anterior tibial artery. The wound healed in 3 weeks.

the skin, pointed toward the point of femoral artery palpation, and is slowly inserted. Once the arterial pulsation is transmitted to the needle, the needle is slowly advanced into the artery, perforating the anterior wall only. Blood is withdrawn into the syringe; an 0.035″ steerable, Wholey wire (ACS, Mountainview, California) is advanced into the superficial

or common femoral artery. The wire position is checked fluoroscopically, and if it is in the superficial femoral artery, a 6-F arterial sheath is advanced into the artery. Heparin (3,000 to 5,000 U) is administered.

The ease of antegrade superficial femoral cannulation may not be so facile, and a few points may make

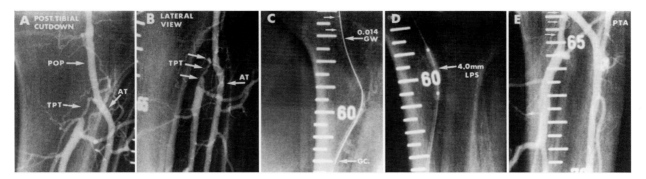

Fig. 80-2. (A) The angiogram shows patent popliteal (POP) and anterior tibial(AT) arteries and an apparent recanalized tibioperoneal trunk (TPT). **(B)** However, recanalization of the tibioperoneal trunk had not occurred, as seen on the lateral angiogram (*arrows*). Antegrade attempts to enter the tibioperoneal trunk were unsuccessful. **(C)** A posterior tibial cut-down enabled the 0.014″ guidewire to retrogradely traverse the occlusion and allow passage of a coronary angioplasty catheter (GC). **(D)** Balloon angioplasty was performed with a 4.0-mm coronary angioplasty catheter. **(E)** Angioplasty demonstrated recanalization of the tibioperoneal trunk.

the procedure easier and successful. First, the anatomy and potential anatomic variations of the common femoral, circumflex femoral, deep femoral (profunda femoralis), and superficial femoral arteries may create difficulty in just isolating the superficial femoral artery. The angulated views, especially the caudal angulated oblique views, will separate the vessels and allow the steerable guide to be directed toward the appropriate vessel. However, if during cannulation, the profunda femoris artery is entered, and passage of the guidewire confirms this on fluoroscopic visualization, then a 4- or 5-F dilator is inserted over the wire, into the vessel. This prevents bleeding from the puncture site and, also in conjunction with the caudal view, permits visualization of the profunda. When contrast is injected through the dilator, it will retrogradely fill the superficial femoral artery and allow needle entry into the visualized target. The use of contrast, oblique views, and careful planning can make the cannulation easier and prevent the problems of subsequent hematoma formation.

Arterial cannulation is primarily attained ipsilaterally and permits device passage antegradely

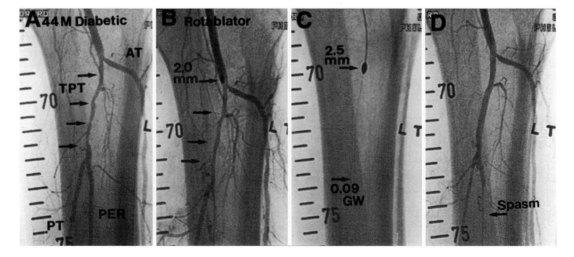

Fig. 80-3. A 44-year-old diabetic man, Fontaine Class III with rest pain. **(A)** The angiogram shows a patent anterior tibial (AT) artery and severely narrowed tibioperoneal trunk (TPT). The peroneal (PER) and the posterior tibial (PT) arteries are patent. **(B & C)** Rotational ablation with **(B)** a 2.0-mm burr and **(C)** a 2.5-mm burr over the 0.09″ guidewire (GW). **(D)** Recanalization of the tibioperoneal trunk with distal vessel (peroneal and posterior tibial) spasm, which resolved spontaneously (within 15 minutes) following the procedure.

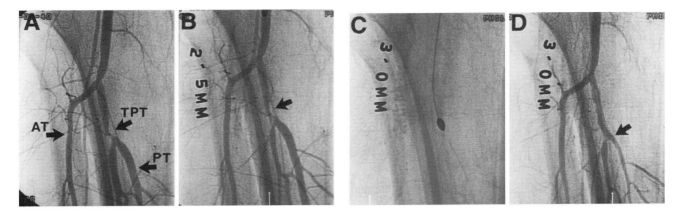

Fig. 80-4. (A) Preinterventional angiogram. **(B)** Angiogram following a 2.5-mm rotational ablation. **(C)** 3-mm burr. **(D)** Final angiogram without need for balloon angioplasty. AT, anterior tibial: TPT, tibioperoneal trunk; PT, posterial tibial artery.

through the superficial femoral, popliteal, and tibioperoneal vessels. Contrast injection, through the arterial sheath, allows for accurate device positioning across the lesion. Distal popliteal and proximal tibioperoneal disease can be also approached contralaterally (Fig. 80-1) using a 6- to 8-F coronary angioplasty guide catheter that has been positioned in the superficial femoral or popliteal artery; this technique enables contrast injection and passage of the balloon angioplasty catheters. In addition, once the devices

are removed, and despite use of anticoagulation, only the nonintervened arterial side is compressed to obtain hemostasis. If the ipsilateral approach must be used because the balloon catheters are not of sufficient length, or if an atherectomy device or stent is required, then contrast injections through the guide catheter, which had been retracted into the common femoral artery, will enable more facile antegrade arterial cannulation.

The medications used are relatively few. Heparin

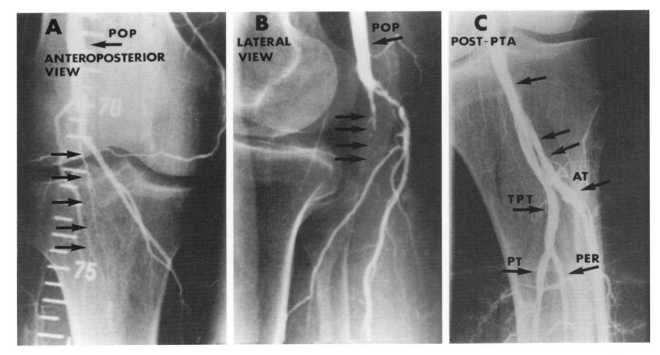

Fig. 80-5. (A & B) An occluded distal popliteal artery visualized in **(A)** the anteroposterior view and **(B)** the lateral view. **(C)** Following balloon angioplasty with recanalization of the anterior tibial and posterior tibial artery. AT, anterior tibial: TPT, tibioperoneal trunk: PT, posterior tibial: PER, peroneal.

is administered in 3,000- to 5,000-U dosages with an additional 2,500 U given if the procedure lasts more than 1 hour. Nifedipine (10 mg) is given before entry into the catheterization laboratory. Intra-arterial nitroglycerin or verapamil are given only in problem situations.

The equipment needed to accomplish tibioperoneal angioplasty is easy to obtain and is readily available. The arterial sheath (6 F) is usually 40 cm long, so that contrast can be injected from the sheath side-arm and provide adequate visualization (Daig Corporation, Minneapolis, Minnesota). The balloon catheter systems are usually between 3 and 4 F, are similar to coronary angioplasty equipment, are coated to make them more slippery, and vary in balloon size (1.5 to 6.0 mm in diameter, and from 2 to 10 cm in length). The guidewires are all steerable and usually vary in diameter (0.014″, 0.018″, and 0.025″), are composed of stainless steel or nitinol, and may have a hydrophilic coating. These products can be obtained from a multiplicity of vendors (including Meditech, Boston Scientific Corporation, Natick, Massachusetts; Microvena Corporation, White Bear Lake, Minnesota; Cordis Corporation, Miami, Florida; Schneider Corporation, Minneapolis, Minnesota). The Rotoblator traverses a 0.09″ stainless steel guidewire and requires a larger arterial sheath for burrs greater than 2.0 mm (Heart Technology, Inc., Bellevue, Washington).

Angioplasty results have been clearly and dramatically helped by the use of soft, steerable wires; low-profile, trackable, coated balloons; as well as long (10 cm) and longer (35 to 40 cm) balloons. Rotational ablation (Rotablator), often coincident with intravascular ultrasound, has enabled stenotic vessels to be recanalized without any adjunctive balloon angioplasty (Fig. 80-4), leaving a smooth vessel wall, which results in nonturbulent, laminar blood flow. The major difficulty is that the 3.0-mm burr requires a 9-F arterial sheath.

RESULTS

The outcome of 398 patients (272 male, 126 female; average age of 67 years) with acute stenosis or occlusion was successful in 369/398 cases (276/286 [97%] stenoses and 55/82 [67%] occlusions). The presence of prior bypass surgery did not adversely affect the procedural outcome (252/276 [91%] without and 117/122 [96%] with prior vascular surgery). Angioplasty of the tibioperoneal vessels was associated with more proximal lesions that required intervention, with

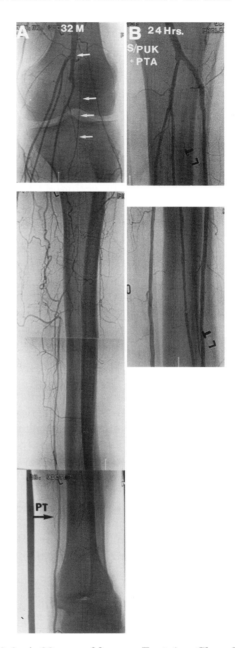

Fig. 80-6. A 32-year-old man, Fontaine Class III, with critical limb ischemia. **(A)** Occlusion of the popliteal and tibioperoneal vessels. **(B)** Following 24 hours of urokinase infusion (s/p UK) and subsequent balloon angioplasty, all three tibioperoneal vessels were recanalized.

nearly 68% having superficial femoral or popliteal disease.

The indications for intervention (predominant symptom) was claudication in 82%, impending limb loss (Fontaine Class IV) in 10%, and as a means of improving outflow in the other 8%. Percutaneous transluminal angioplasty was accompanied by thrombolysis in 10% and rotational ablation in 12% of cases. Complications were encountered in 94 patients (24%) and included contrast-induced renal failure (4%), distal embolization (3%), and emergency peripheral vascular surgery (2%) of cases. At hospital discharge, 93% of patients were clinically improved, 4% were unchanged, and 3% were worse.

The procedural outcome of stenotic lesions, focal and diffuse, is successful in more than 97% of cases, with few associated significant complications. The lower success of recanalizing occluded tibioperoneal vessels (67%) as compared to the stenotic vessels (>97%) has been directly influenced by our concerted attempt to avoid creating a significant perforation, tear, or rupture which would place the patient at risk for a compartmental syndrome; the surgical treatment, fasciotomy, has significant associated morbidity. However, the use of prolonged, thrombolytic (urokinase) infusions, hydrophilic wires, and rotational ablation has increased our success rate in occluded tibioperoneal vessels today to more than 85% (Fig. 80-5 and 80-6), without increasing our complication rates.

The small stents (balloon-expandable, tubular stainless steel, and balloon-expandable, flexible, serpentine, stainless steel stents), as well as prolonged balloon inflations (30 to 60 minutes), have enabled the nightmare of a tear to be successfully managed in almost all instances. In addition, when the distal popliteal or tibioperoneal occlusion cannot be crossed antegradely, the interventionist, in conjunction with the vascular surgeon, can achieve recanalization by direct exposure and cannulation of the ankle vessel (dorsalis pedis or posterior tibial artery) and then by retrogradely traversing the occlusion.

SUMMARY

Percutaneous transluminal angioplasty, catheter-directed thrombolytic therapy, hydrophilic guidewires, prolonged balloon inflation, rotational ablation, and stainless steel stents have enabled the tibioperoneal vessels to undergo revascularization with outstanding immediate and clinical success, a low complication rate, and without the need for emergency surgery or amputation. Revascularization of the tibioperoneal vessels can prevent amputation in critical limb ischemia, improvement in, or elimination of, claudication, and as a complement to peripheral vascular surgical bypass, to improve immediate outflow or to overcome outflow obstruction that subsequently arose because of disease progression. Revascularization of the tibioperoneal vessels can prevent amputation, improve the patient's quality of life, and be a significant complement to peripheral vascular surgery.

REFERENCES

1. Dorros G, Lewin RF. Jamnadas P, Mathiak LM. Below-the-knee angioplasty: tibioperoneal vessels, the acute outcome. Cather Cardiovasc Diagn 1990;19:170–8
2. Saab MH, Smith DC, Aka PK et al. Percutaneous transluminal angioplasty of tibial arteries for limb salvage. Cardiovasc Intervent Radiol 1992;15:211–26
3. Schwarten DE, Cutcliff WC. Arterial occlusive disease below the knee: treatment with percutaneous transluminal angioplasty performed with low-profile catheters and steerable guidewires. Radiology 1988;169:71–4
4. Dorros G, Hall P, Prince C. Successful limb salvage after recanalization of an occluded infrapopliteal artery utilizing a balloon expandable (Palmaz-Schatz) stent. Cath Cardiovascular Diagn 1993;28:83–8

81 Carotid Artery

Gerald Dorros

In the United States stroke is the third leading cause of death, and approximately 500,000 Americans suffer new strokes each year. Roughly one-third of those people with acute thrombotic strokes die within 30 days of its onset, and between 150,000 and 200,000 people in the United States die annually from a stroke. Furthermore, stroke ranks as a leading cause of long-term physical and intellectual disability. Thus, since a stroke may be the result of ischemia produced by arterial blood flow obstruction, methodologies that can relieve these impediments may have a significant impact on the incidence of stroke.

The recently released results of large prospective randomized trials have helped to clarify several issues concerning the value of carotid endarterectomy for prevention of ischemic stroke. The North American Symptomatic Carotid Endarterectomy Trial (NASCET)[1] enrolled a large number of *symptomatic,* generally healthy patients who were randomized to either medical treatment (including aspirin and risk factor modification) or the best medical treatment plus carotid endarterectomy. These trials revealed the following findings:

1. Patients with a carotid diameter stenosis of 70% or more had a significantly reduced risk of stroke. In the NASCET trial the cumulative ipsilateral stroke rate at 2 years was 26% for those in the medical group and 9% for those in the surgical group. This 17% absolute reduction in the surgical group is a 65% relative risk reduction favoring surgery.
2. No difference was found between medically and surgically treated patients when stenosis severity was less than 30%.

3. The value of carotid endarterectomy for patients with 30 to 69% stenosis remains unknown.
4. The NASCET trial demonstrated that for patients with symptomatic carotid stenosis between 70 and 99% endarterectomy was far superior to medical management in reducing the risk of stroke

The Asymptomatic Carotid Atherosclerosis Study (ACAS),[2] a randomized prospective clinical trial, enrolled patients if they were 40 to 79 years of age, had a life expectancy of at least 5 years, and had at least 60% carotid stenosis near the bifurcation of the common or internal carotid artery; the objective was to determine if surgical revascularization (carotid endarterectomy) would reduce the overall 5-year risk of ipsilateral stroke in asymptomatic patients. A total of 1,662 patients was randomized to either medical management or surgery. The aggregate risk of stroke over 5 years was 4.8% for the surgical group and 10.6% for the medical group. The study found that carotid endarterectomy was beneficial, with an absolute reduction of 5.8% in the risk of the primary end point (fatal and nonfatal ipsilateral stroke) within 5 years.

The natural history of carotid artery disease[3] has demonstrated that (1) bruits and stenoses are important markers of atherosclerosis, (2) ultrasound techniques can measure and follow carotid artery lesions, (3) more severe stenoses correlated with higher probability of serious stroke, (4) stenoses progress and frequently occlude without symptoms, and (5) symptoms are more common when the artery is occluded.

Carotid endarterectomy has been proved to be an effective treatment of carotid obstructive lesions. Patients who survive surgery without neurologic morbidity have a decreased frequency of subsequent neurologic deficits (transient or permanent) compared with medically managed patients. However, the disparity in the results of carotid endarterectomy has remained significant and reflects the patient population, patient selection, surgical experience and skill, modifications of surgical and anesthesia techniques, and the neurologic status of the patient prior to surgery. The morbidity and mortality risks of carotid endarterectomy, like other surgical procedures requiring general or even local anesthesia, are increased by advanced age (>70 years) and co-morbidity (e.g., severe obstructive pulmonary disease, chronic renal failure, hemorrhagic diathesis, and severe, advanced atherosclerotic heart disease). Specific technical and anatomic operative problems can make a particular surgical procedure more hazardous, [e.g., simultaneous bilateral carotid endarterectomy, unilateral carotid endarterectomy combined with coronary bypass surgery, endarterectomized vessel with a suture line narrowing (restenosis), vessel occlusion, or a severe narrowing or occlusion of the other extracranial major vessels, especially the contralateral internal carotid, and intracranial lesions (which could inhibit blood flow to the circle of Willis)].

Percutaneous transluminal coronary angioplasty (PTCA) and stent-supported angioplasty have been used extensively as alternatives to surgical revascularization in both peripheral and coronary atherosclerotic vascular disease. Significant but less extensive experience exists with PTCA or stent use (or both) in the supra-aortic arteries including the carotid and vertebral arteries. In a review of over 700 supra-aortic artery PTCAs, the success rate was 95% and the care of major complications was 0.5%, with no deaths; 338 of these procedures were in the carotid, vertebral, or innominate arteries. Within their series of 105 symptomatic patients, Kachel et al.[4] found only 35 stenoses of the internal carotid artery and 15 stenoses of the vertebral artery; the remaining lesions involved the external carotid, common carotid, innominate, or subclavian arteries. The success rate was 95.2%, with no major complications. In our carotid angioplasty series, I reported on 42 lesions 8 of which had stent placement. The angioplasties were complicated by four procedural neurologic deficits (two transient ischemic attacks, one reversible ischemic neurologic deficit, and one cerebrovascular accident producing a mortality). All patients were discharged with clinical improvement at follow-up the incidence of restenosis in nonstented patients appeared to approximate 20% and was much less than 20% in patients with stented vessels. However,

the restenosis rate for carotid vessels appears to be consistent with that of other similarly sized vessels. Large vessels, such as the iliacs and proximal femoral arteries, have low restenosis rates, especially after stent placement. Therefore, one would expect the carotid arteries, which typically range in size from 4 to 10 mm, with most being 5 to 8 mm in diameter, to have relatively low restenosis rates (10 to 15%). However, problems with flaps and potential vessel closure would have a serious clinical impact; the recent BENESTENT II coronary stent data (with a low restenosis rate of approximately 11%) make stent-supported angioplasty a potentially good alternative to balloon angioplasty because of its predictability. A large lumen may be maintained, acute closure is precluded, the procedure requires only aspirin afterward, and stent placement is easy.

Since the current treatment for carotid stenosis is endarterectomy, PTCA or stent support angioplasty must be shown to have a comparable or lower complication rate than endarterectomy to be considered a viable therapeutic alternative. Morbidity and mortality rates for carotid endarterectomy, as has been discussed, range from 2 to 18%.

Balloon or stent-supported angioplasty offers several potential advantages over carotid endarterectomy: local anesthesia allowing continuous monitoring of neurologic status, treatment of lesions inaccessible to surgery (e.g., a stenosis originating at the carotid bulb and extending into the siphon), reduced patient discomfort, a percutaneous procedure with the potential to be done on an outpatient basis, shorter hospital stay, reduced cost, and possibly a significantly lower morbidity and mortality. Endovascular therapy may be particularly well suited for patients with symptomatic carotid disease who have severe coronary artery disease and a high morbidity and mortality with carotid endarterectomy.

Carotid balloon or stent-supported angioplasty has not yet been definitively demonstrated to be equivalent yet alone the treatment of choice. First, a prospective, observational study must be performed to obtain data on endovascular, high risk, surgical patients with a stenosis of 70% or more as part of the study. This multisite, multidisciplinary study must collect data to assess the procedure and would primarily involve stent-supported angioplasty. The study should have several unique features, as follows

1. Strict, well-defined inclusion and exclusion criteria: *patients with severe stenotic carotid lesions (70% diameter stenosis) who should have one of the following:*
   a. Documented progression of carotid obstructive

disease substantiated by physical examination or invasive or noninvasive studies

b. Recurrent neurologic deficits, presumably related to a lesion producing ipsilateral cerebral ischemic symptoms

c. Partial or complete resolution of a stroke-related neurologic deficit, with an ipsilateral lesion

d. High risk for carotid surgery because of advanced age, co-morbidity, bleeding disorders, poor anesthesia risk, severe triple-vessel coronary disease, or left main coronary involvement

e. A restenosed vessel after carotid endarterectomy

f. An occluded internal carotid artery, narrowed ipsilateral external carotid artery, ipsilateral ischemia-related cerebral ischemic symptoms, and candidacy for temporal to middle central artery bypass

g. Fibromuscular dysplasia

h. A carotid stenosis of 70% or more using the NASCET and ACAS methodology

2. Standardized diagnostic imaging before and after the procedure

3. A quantitative stroke scale evaluation performed before and after intervention by an independent neurologist

4. Long-term clinical and diagnostic imaging follow-up

5. The involvement of clinicians with extensive expertise in cerebrovascular and cardiovascular disease and angioplasty and the ability to assess whether this pilot study provides sufficient information to allow initiation of a randomized trial of stent-supported angioplasty versus carotid endarterectomy.

Presently, stent-supported carotid angioplasty appears to be the most promising technique for revascularization of the stenotic extracranial vessels and may compare well with surgery. In addition, the predictability of stent revascularization, its future ability to incorporate coverings within or over the stent to prevent distal embolization, and the presence of a memory to resume its desired shape after external compression all predict a bright future for this technique. However, only time and carefully randomized trials comparing endovascular reconstruction to carotid endarterectomy patients will reveal the answer.

REFERENCES

1. North American Symptomatic Carotid Endarterectomy Trial Collaborators. Beneficial effect of carotid endarterectomy in symptomatic patients with high-grade carotid stenosis. N Engl J Med 1991;325:445–53

2. The Asymptomatic Carotid Atherosclerosis Study Group. Study design for randomized prospective trial of carotid endarterectomy for asymptomatic atherosclerosis. Stroke 1989;20:844–9

3. Caplan LR. Carotid artery disease. N Engl J Med 1986;315:868–86

4. Kachel R, Endert G, Basche S, Grossmann K, Glaser FH. Percutaneous transluminal angioplasty (dilatation) of carotid, vertebral, and innominate stenoses. Cardiovasc Intervent Radiol 1987;10:142–6

82 Subclavian Arteries and Veins

Reiner Kachel

Diseases of the arteries and veins of the upper extremity are rare and diagnosed relatively late compared to angiopathy of the lower extremity. The main pathologic entities encountered are stenosing changes of the subclavian artery or brachiocephalic trunk and obstructed runoff in the region of the subclavian vein or innominate vein. Possible causes follow:

1. Constriction of the artery or vein from outside by parts of the musculoskeletal system, tumors, inflammatory processes, and cicatricial formations
2. Obliterating arteriosclerotic or inflammatory angiopathy
3. Thrombosis or embolism

Whereas surgical intervention is essential in arterial or venous compression from outside (thoracic outlet syndrome or Paget-von-Schroetter syndrome), interventional radiologic procedures such as percutaneous transluminal angioplasty (PTA) and local thrombolysis have become increasingly established in the management of obliterating arteriosclerotic and inflammatory diseases and thromboembolism. Arteriosclerosis is the most common cause of obliterative disease of the subclavian artery. Inflammatory diseases such as Takayasu's arteritis—a chronic inflammatory arteriopathy of unknown etiology involving the aorta and the main arteries departing from it—are very rare.

The only procedures previously available for the treatment of obliterative arterial disease of the subclavian artery were corrective, vascular surgical procedures such as direct thromboendarterectomy, by-pass surgery, or resection of the affected segments of the vessel with reimplantation into the aortic arch or common carotid artery.

The introduction of PTA by Charles T. Dotter and M. P. Judkins in 1964[1] and the development of the double-lumen balloon dilation catheter by Andreas Grüntzig and H. Hopff in 1974[2] opened up new, previously unimaginable avenues in the treatment of obliterative arterial disease. Within the last few years, this new method has become established in the treatment of circulatory disorders of the pelvic and leg arteries, the coronary arteries, the renal arteries, and the visceral arteries and is already used as a routine procedure in many hospitals.

PTA of the supra-aortic vessels, on the other hand, remained a controversial procedure for quite a long time, apparently because the risk of embolization to the brain was overestimated. Proposals for the treatment of supra-aortic vascular stenoses were first made by Mathias in 1977.[3] The scientific work of Mathias,[4] Kachel,[5,6] Theron,[7] Motarjeme et al.,[8] McNamara,[9] and Vitek[10] demonstrated that the use of PTA is also feasible in the region of the brachiocephalic arteries without an unjustifiably high risk. This chapter presents our results and previously internationally published results of PTA in obliteration of the subclavian artery.

CLINICAL FEATURES OF OCCLUSIVE DISEASE OF THE SUBCLAVIAN ARTERY AND VEIN

Arteriosclerotic or inflammatory obliteration of the subclavian artery occurs mainly in the first segment between its origin at the aorta and the orifice of the vertebral artery or in the brachiocephalic trunk. It leads to hypoperfusion of the upper extremity or to additional vertebrobasilar circulatory disturbances in the event of vertebrobasilar collateral formation. Consequently, the most common symptoms in stenosing subclavian changes are those of brachial and vertebrobasilar insufficiency. The severity of brachial insufficiency (arm claudication) is graded in four stages corresponding to Fontaine's stages in peripheral arterial occlusive disease.

- *Stage I:* The absence of clinical symptoms even on heavy loading of the arms and demonstration of asymptomatic subclavian bruit, differences in the pulse and blood pressure between both arms, and verified arterial stenosis
- *Stage II:* Work-dependent, intermittent clinical symptoms such as pain, weakness, myasthenia, paraesthesias, sensation of cold, arm claudication, and so on, and verifiable differences in the pulse and blood pressure between the both arms
- *Stage III:* Clinical symptoms as in stage II even at rest
- *Stage IV:* Rest pain and trophic changes in the skin of the fingers, but mainly at the fingertips

In the presence of high-grade stenoses or occlusions in the first segment of the subclavian artery or brachiocephalic trunk, the arm is supplied via arterial collaterals of the vertebrobasilar system, which results in a phenomenon to which Fisher[11] gave the name "subclavian steal syndrome" in 1961. The subclavian steal syndrome leads to neurologic symptoms such as vertigo, dizziness, disturbances of vision (amaurosis fugax, flickering, double vision etc.), ataxia, and sudden, transient loss of tonicity of the extremity muscles (drop attacks). Vertebrobasilar insufficiency is likewise divided into four stages (stage I, asymptomatic stage; stage II, transient neurologic symptoms, stage III, progressive neurologic symptoms; stage IV, permanent neurologic deficits).

Around 5 to 10% of patients with subclavian occlusive disease also display symptoms of coronary artery disease. Coronary subclavian steal via the coronary and internal mammary artery is the most common cause of the anginal syndrome (Fig. 82-1).

Obliteration of the subclavian vein is caused primarily by thrombosis (the Paget-von Schroetter syndrome), which leads to considerable obstruction. Clinical symptoms are a feeling of heaviness, livid discoloration, and pronounced swelling of the affected arm. Pain of varying severity also occurs.

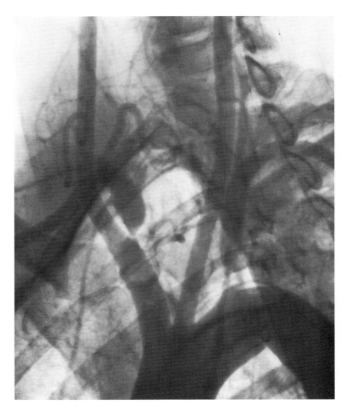

Fig. 82-1. High-grade stenoses of the left and right subclavian artery with subclavian steal and coronary-mammary steal on the right (no antegrade perfusion of the right vertebral artery, retrograde perfusion of the right internal mammary artery).

PERCUTANEOUS TRANSLUMINAL ANGIOPLASTY AND THROMBOLYSIS

Pretherapeutic Examination Techniques

The following examination techniques should be employed before any decision regarding therapy is taken in patients with suspected stenosing changes of the subclavian artery or brachiocephalic trunk:

- Cliniconeurologic examination including separate measurement of the blood pressure in both arms
- Doppler sonography
- Pulse oscillography
- Conventional or digital subtraction angiography
- Intra-arterial pressure measurement

Documentation of the relevant case history and a thorough clinical examination are both extremely important, and special value must also be attached to accurate documentation of the pulse status, vascular auscultation, separate measurement of the blood pressure in both arms, and Doppler sonography. If the brachial symptoms are accompanied by neurologic symptoms in the form of vertebrobasilar or cerebrovascular insufficiency, it will also be necessary to perform cerebral computerized tomography and cerebral magnetic resonance imaging for assessment of morphologic cerebral changes and to use nuclear medical methods (single photon emission computed tomography, positron emission tomography) or to measure cerebral perfusion by magnetic resonance imaging for evaluation of disturbances of vertebrobasilar or cerebrovascular perfusion. These noninvasive diagnostic procedures are followed by angiographic visualization of the brachiocephalic arteries. Selective demonstration of the supra-aortic arteries must be performed if the supra-aortic vascular situation cannot be unequivocally clarified by brachiocephalic angiography. If stenosing arterial changes are demonstrated, the use of intra-arterial pressure measurements and intravascular ultrasound tomography (IVUS) are of great help in deciding whether PTA is indicated. Fresh thrombotic deposits—which are difficult to diagnose with angiography or sonography—are readily demonstrable by means of [111]Indium platelet scintigraphy.[12] Angiographic clarification by means of arm–shoulder venography is required immediately if there is clinical suspicion of a fresh thrombosis of the subclavian vein. If the angiogram is positive, treatment by local thrombolysis should be instituted.

Patient Preparation

Patients must be first be informed about their illness, the currently available therapeutic procedures, the results of treatment, and possible complications. Patients must fast on the day of the operation. Sedatives should be given only to very anxious patients. Before PTA is commenced, the clotting parameters and blood group must be determined, conserved blood made ready, and venous access ensured for the infusion of electrolyte solution.

Instruments

The following materials are required for PTA of stenosis or occlusion of the subclavian artery:

- Seldinger initial puncture needle
- Teflon-coated straight guidewire, 0.024 to 0.032″

- Introducer sheath set 6 F (Teflon sheath, vessel dilator, Tuohy-Borst Adaptor)
- Diagnostic catheter 5 F (Simmons catheter,
- Head-hunter catheter, Judkins right catheter, multipurpose catheter, cerebral catheter with a tapered tip, Berenstein catheter)
- Terumo guidewire, 0.032″
- Overlong Teflon-coated guidewire (length, 250 cm)
- Balloon dilation catheter (2.5-F percutaneous transluminal coronary angiography catheter and 5-F dilation catheter: working length, 120 cm; catheter tip, 5 mm; balloon length, 20 mm, balloon diameter, 4 to 14 mm; pressure capacity, 8 to 12 atm)
- Injection syringe with pressure manometer 10-ml and 20-ml injection syringes
- IVUS catheter for intravascular sonography

Technical Performance of PTA and Thrombolysis

The patient is first given a local anesthetic, after which an inguinal or axillary catheter introducer sheath is inserted. General brachiocephalic angiography is then performed in at least two projections simultaneously (right anterior oblique, left anterior oblique) with a 5- or 6-F diagnostic catheter—if at all possible, using the intra-arterial digital subtraction technique—to confirm the suspected diagnosis, to locate the stenosis exactly, and to rule out fresh changes (ulceration, thrombotic deposits, occlusions, etc.). This is followed by probing of the stenosis under image-intensified television fluoroscopic control and introduction of an overlong, straight guidewire (length, 200 to 250 cm) into the poststenotic region of the stenosed vessel and replacement of the diagnostic catheter with a Grüntzig balloon catheter via the guidewire. After the dilation segment has been positioned in the stenosis, the balloon is inflated manually by means of a 10-ml injection syringe and a pressure manometer using a contrast medium-water mixture in the proportion 1:1 at pressures between 800 and 1,200 kPa (8 to 12 atm), depending on the type of catheter being used. In general, two to four dilations, each lasting 20 to 120 seconds, are required to expand the stenosis. I achieved better morphologic and functional results using dilation times of 60 to 120 seconds. The diameter of balloon to be used is 6 to 14 mm depending on the diameter of the vessel. It is advisable to use a diameter that corresponds to the diame-

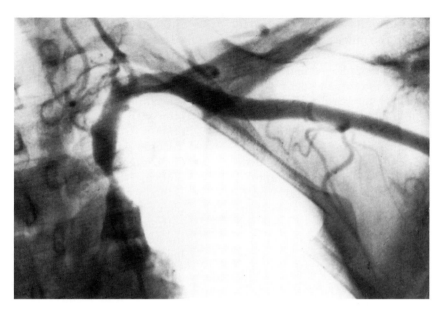

Fig. 82-2. High-grade stenosis of the left proximal subclavian artery with subclavian steal.

ter of the healthy vessel as measured prestenotically or post-stenotically in a segment of the artery not changed by the disease. The balloon should be no longer than 2 cm in the case of short or circular stenoses. Longer balloons are required only in the case of long stenoses, and they should then be 1 cm longer than the stenosis itself. High-grade stenoses might sometimes require successive dilation first with a 2.5-F coronary dilation catheter to 3- to 4-mm diameter and then with an 5-F dilation catheter and a balloon with a diameter of 6 to 15 mm. Intra-arterial heparin-

ization with 100 U heparin/1 kg body weight must always be performed before dilation. Transaxillary or transbrachial access must be chosen if the stenosed region of the subclavian artery or brachiocephalic trunk cannot be accessed transfemorally. Because the axillary or brachial artery cannot usually be palpated in high-grade subclavian stenosis, I recommend transaxillary or transbrachial puncture under sonographic control. After successful dilation, the result must be documented by angiography and intra-arterial blood pressure measurement (Figs. 82-2 to 82-6).

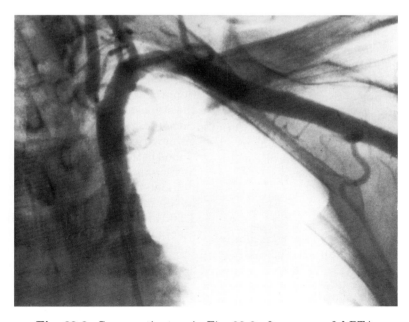

Fig. 82-3. Same patient as in Fig. 82-2 after successful PTA.

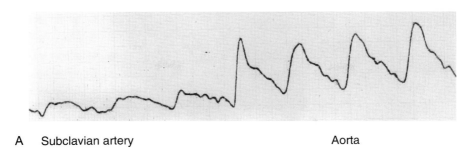

A   Subclavian artery   Aorta

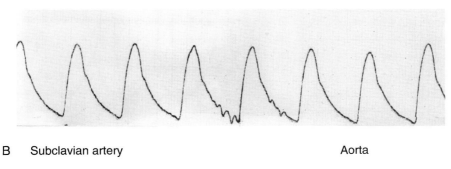

B   Subclavian artery   Aorta

Fig. 82-4. Intra-arterial blood pressure measurement in the subclavian artery and the aorta with high-grade pressure gradient before **(A)** and after **(B)** PTA.

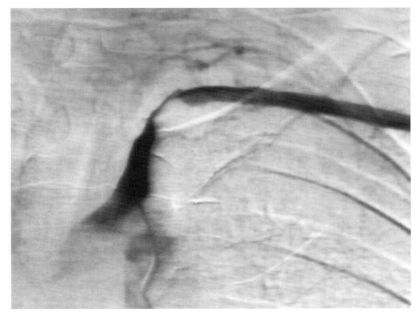

Fig. 82-5. Long proximal subclavian artery stenosis with subclavian steal.

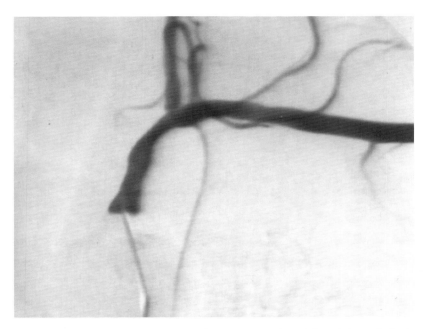

Fig. 82-6. Same patient as in Fig. 82-5 with situation after PTA of the subclavian artery.

Based on my own positive experience, I recommend not only pre- and post-therapeutic intra-arterial blood pressure measurements but also the performance of intravascular ultrasound tomography to assess the morphology of the vessel wall (intimal lesions, intimal flaps, dissections, intramural haematomas, etc.). If these methods demonstrate PTA-induced dissection, a stent must be implanted to avoid embolic or thrombotic complications. In my experience, self-expanding and balloon-expanded stents produce equally good results.

In occlusion of the subclavian artery, the artery is first probed with a diagnostic catheter. A straight Terumo wire is introduced carefully through this catheter using rotating movements. After the guidewire has passed the occlusion and is lying demonstrably within the lumen, a straight 5-F diagnostic catheter is advanced through the occlusion. The Terumo wire is then replaced by an overlong, Teflon-coated guidewire, which remains in situ, and the diagnostic catheter is exchanged over it for a dilation balloon catheter. After the balloon segment has been positioned in the occlusion, recanalization is performed with pressures between 10 and 12 atm for 60 to 120 seconds. To prevent early occlusions, the author implants arterial stents following recanalization.

It sometimes proves impossible to probe older occlusions of the subclavian artery via the transfemoral route. Experience shows that recanalization can nevertheless be performed in more than 50% of these cases using a retrograde, transaxillary approach.[4,9] In many cases, however, the guidewire ends up not in the center of the still-open proximal subclavian "stump"—the ideal situation—but, as a result of being advanced subintimally because of the curvature of the vessel, more to the side of the lumen. This eccentric recanalization consistently results in reocclusion owing to a "valve effect" of the open central vascular stump immediately after recanalization and withdrawal of the balloon catheter. In all these cases, I completed recanalization successfully by implanting an endovascular prosthesis (stent) (Figs. 82-7 to 82-11).

Follow-up treatment is generally performed with platelet-aggregation inhibitors. Based on our excellent experiences, we recommend heparinization for a period of 2 to 3 days with 20,000 to 25,000 U heparin/24 hrs and overlapping oral therapy with anticoagulants (Marcumar) from the second day. The anticoagulant therapy should be continued for at least 6 months with appropriate monitoring of the Quick value. Platelet aggregation inhibitors (acetylsalicylic acid) should be prescribed if the transaxillary procedure was used or if oral anticoagulants are contraindicated.

The dilation catheter is removed after successful PTA, but the Teflon sheath with the Borst adaptor is left in place for another 24 hours to allow selective vascular catheterization with angiographic clarification and local thrombolysis treatment or redilation in the event of complications (early occlusions or embolization).

Immediately after PTA, the patient's blood pressure, foot and arm pulses, and pressure dressing should be checked first at half-hourly and then at hourly intervals. Even after successful dilation or re-canalization, I check on the dilated vascular region and the puncture site by scintigraphy with a gamma camera after 30 minutes and 24 and 48 hours to detect any incipient thrombotic deposition even before the occurrence of clinical symptoms and to institute local thrombolysis. With this in view, the patient's own platelets are radioactively labeled with [111]-indium pertechnetate before PTA.[12]

Acute ischemic symptoms with pain, loss of pulse, pallor, and sensation of cold are frequently caused by fresh thrombosis or embolism or by thrombosis or embolism based on existing stenosis. The actual cause in such cases can be diagnosed only by selective intra-arterial digital subtraction angiography (DSA) or conventional angiography.

Acute arterial embolism should be treated by vascular surgery with embolectomy. Local thrombolysis is the treatment of first choice in acute arterial thrombosis with or without demonstrable stenosing arteriopathy. I start the procedure by infiltrating the thrombus with the thrombolytic urokinase (other au-

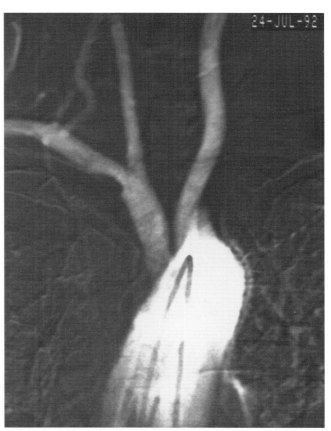

Fig. 82-8. Same patient as in Fig. 82-7 after successful PTA of the innominate and left common carotid artery.

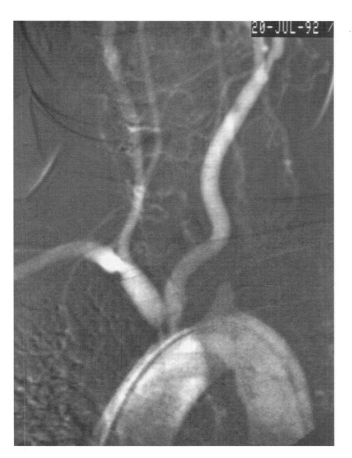

Fig. 82-7. High-grade stenosis of the innominate and left common carotid artery and an occlusion of the left subclavian artery.

thors prefer rtPA). The use of a thrombolysis guide-wire with side holes introduced through a diagnostic catheter is helpful. The thrombolytic agent is injected into the thrombus manually under pressure (jet phenomenon via side holes, which is pulse spray thrombolysis). Then 20,000 U urokinase are administered as bolus injections at intervals of 10 minutes over a period of 50 to 60 minutes, followed by infusion of the thrombolytic agent by injection pump in a dose of 100,000 to 200,000 U urokinase over 2 hours. Heparinization with 1,000 U heparin per hour is required during the thrombolysis procedure to prevent rethrombosing or thrombotic deposits in the catheter. Angiography should be performed at intervals of 30 minutes to determine when the infusion should be terminated, that is, when the thrombus is just about completely dissolved. Follow-up treatment with infusions of heparin corresponding to that after successful PTA is required to prevent rethrombosis.

Again as after PTA, successful thrombolysis must also be followed by long-term treatment with platelet aggregation inhibitors or oral anticoagulants over at least 6 months. If, after successful thrombolysis, arterial stenosing is found to be one of the causes of

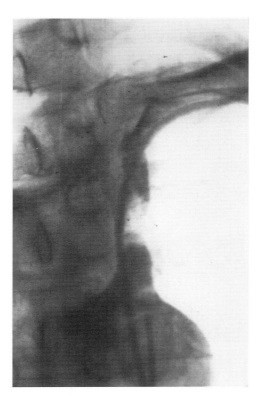

Fig. 82-9. Same patient as Figs. 82-7 and 82-8 after recanalization of the subclavian artery occlusion with "valve effect" after deflation of the balloon with reocclusion.

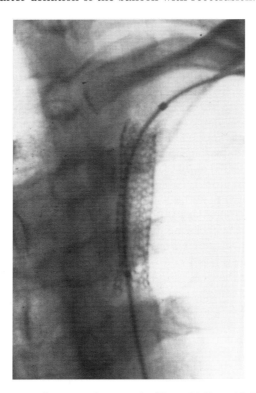

Fig. 82-10. Same patient as in Figs. 82-7 to 82-9 after stent application.

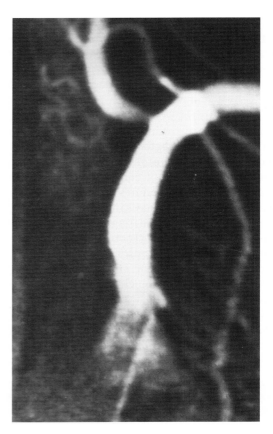

Fig. 82-11. Same patient as in Figs. 82-7 to 82-9 after successful stent application.

the thrombosis, the stenosis must then be eliminated by PTA, as described.

The results of PTA should be followed up at intervals of 6 to 12 months by means of clinical examination with vascular auscultation, exact documentation of the pulse status, and, if at all possible, ultrasound-supported blood pressure measurements and Doppler sonographic studies. If symptoms recur or objective signs of restenosing are seen, the noninvasive diagnostic measures must be followed by angiography after the situation has been explained to the patient and the patient has agreed to and has been prepared for repeat PTA. This is then performed in the same session if angiography reveals hemodynamically effective restenosis.

If venous obliteration is present, venography of the arm and shoulder is performed for further clarification of the situation. As in thrombotic changes in the arterial system, I prefer local to systemic thrombolysis on demonstration of a thrombotic occlusion. The thrombolytic should, if possible, be delivered into the thrombus itself. The technical procedure and dosage of the thrombolytic correspond to those in arterial thrombosis, the only difference being that the lysis catheter is introduced over a Terumo guidewire with a flexible tip. The result of thrombolysis must be documented by angiography.

Results

I have performed PTA in a total of more than 300 patients presenting with supra-aortic vascular obliteration. PTA of stenosis of the subclavian artery and brachiocephalic trunk was employed in 94 patients with symptoms of brachial or vertebrobasilar insufficiency. Percutaneous transluminal recanalization was attempted in another 24 patients presenting with occlusion of the subclavian artery.

Dilation of subclavian stenosis succeeded in all patients, whereas recanalization of occlusion of the artery was successful in 17 of 24. The occlusion was overcome transfemorally in only 7 patients; transaxillary access was required in the other 17. In all these cases, the axillary artery was punctured under ultrasound control because the artery could not be palpated. Of 6 patients with occlusion of the subclavian artery, a stent was implanted transfemorally in 3 and via transaxillary access in 3. The primary success rate in this patient population was 100% in the case of stenosis and only 71% in the case of occlusions of the subclavian artery.

In three patients, a fresh post-stenotic thrombosis with complete occlusion of the subclavian artery was diagnosed in addition to the stenosis. Management in these cases consisted of local thrombolysis followed by PTA. No complications were observed (Figs. 82-12 and 82-13).

During the total of 118 procedures involving the subclavian artery and brachiocephalic trunk, minor complications were observed in only two patients. They consisted of after-bleeding from the puncture site with extensive hematomas (one axillary and one inguinal), which, however, healed completely under conservative therapy with no sequelae. No nerve damage or other permanent injury was observed. No embolization to the brain or the digital arteries occurred.

To date, the international literature reports 1,018 cases of successful PTA in the region of the subclavian artery. My results and the previously published results are summarized in Table 82-1.[4,7–10,13–15]

Against expectation, the complication rate is relatively low, 3 to 5% according to the literature. No deaths have so far been reported, and serious complications (two permanent neurologic deficits and one amputation of the limb) have been observed in only three cases. Further details are provided in Table 82-2.

Follow-up

Follow-up in the study population reported here was done at intervals of 6 to 12 months over a period of 6 to 149 months; the mean follow-up period was 79 months. During this period, restenosis with recurrence of symptoms occurred in only two patients after 6 and 12 months. Both patients had presented with heavily calcified stenosis of the subclavian artery, and PTA had caused pronounced dissection in

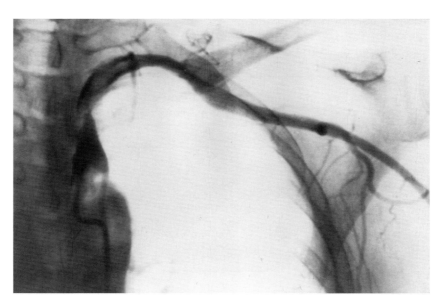

Fig. 82-12. High-grade stenosis of the left subclavian artery with 20-mm long post-stenotic fresh thrombosis without antegrade perfusion of the vertebral artery.

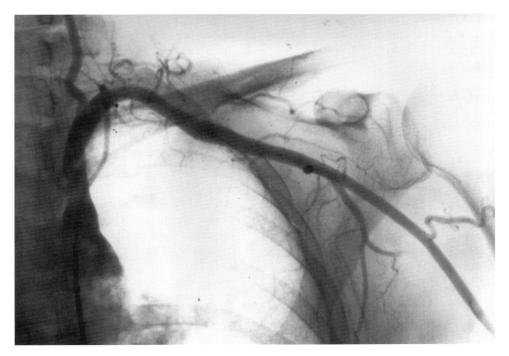

Fig. 82-13. Same patient as in Fig. 82-12 after successful local thrombolysis and PTA.

the dilated region of the vessel. One patient was redilated and has now remained asymptomatic for more than 10 years (Figs. 82-14 and 82-15). The second patient opted for surgical correction in the form of a carotid-subclavian bypass; unfortunately, thrombotic occlusion rendered the bypass nonfunctional after 12 months.

DISCUSSION

While many centers already use transluminal angioplasty as a routine procedure in the region of the pelvic and leg arteries, the renal arteries, and the coronary arteries, its use in the region of the brachiocephalic arteries is relatively rare. The objections raised to its use in this region follow:

1. Increased risk of embolism, which is due to detached plaque material
2. Intimal lesions with secondary thrombus formation and the risk of embolization to the digital and cerebral arteries

Experience to date shows these objections to be groundless.[3,7,16] The risk of embolization to the vertebrobasilar vascular region is extremely low even

	Personal Results (%)	Published Results (%)
Angioplasties	118	1,018
Localization		
Left	99 (83.9%)	805 (79.1%)
Right	19 (16.1%)	213 (20.9%)
Brachial symptoms	118 (100%)	743 (73%)
Neurologic symptoms	83 (70.3%)	662 (65%)
Subclavian steal	95 (80.5%)	789 (77.5%)
Coronary steal	9 (7.6%)	—
Primary success	111 (94.1%)	953 (93.5%)
Complications	2 (1.7%)	27 (2.7%)
Morbidity	0 (0%)	3 (0.3%)
Long-term success	112/118 (95%)	80–95% (—)
Follow-up (months)	79 (—)	13–50 (—)

Table 82-1. Personal and Published Results of 1,018 Angioplasties of Subclavian Artery

Table 82-2. Complications of 1,018 Angioplasties of Subclavian Artery (Personal and Published Results)

Complications	Personal Data (%)	Published Data (%)
Complications of puncture		
Thrombosis of femoral artery		2 (0.2%)
Thrombosis of axillary artery		2 (0.2%)
Stenosis of brachial artery		1 (0.1%)
Temporary median nerve palsy		1 (0.1%)
Hematoma		
Inguinal	1 (0.8%)	3 (0.3%)
Axillary	1 (0.8%)	1 (0.1%)
Complications of angioplasty		
Dissections of subclavian artery		1 (0.1%)
False aneurysm		1 (0.1%)
Thrombosis of subclavian artery		2 (0.2%) 1 Bypass
Thrombosis of iliac artery		1 (0.1%) Bypass
Embolisms of fingers		6 (0.6%)
Embolisms of arm		2 (0.2%)
Amputation of arm		1 (0.1%)
Transient ischemic attacks		2 (0.2%)
Stroke		2 (0.2%)
Total	2/118 (1.7%)	28/1,1018 (2.8%)

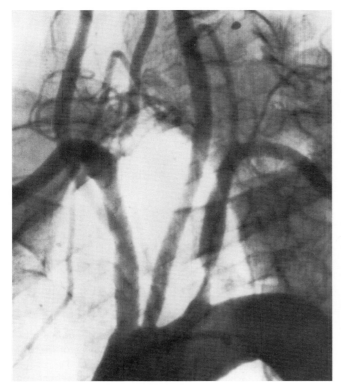

Fig. 82-14. High-grade stenosis of the left subclavian artery and subclavian steal (no antegrade perfusion of the left vertebral artery).

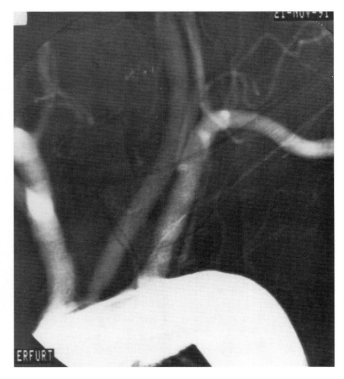

Fig. 82-15. Same patient as in Fig. 82-14. Control angiography 11 years after PTA of the left subclavian artery without restenosis.

in the case of high-grade stenosis and occlusion in the first segment of the subclavian artery before the orifice of the vertebral artery. This conclusion is based on the angiographic studies by Ringelstein and Zeumer,[17] which showed that, in high-grade stenosis or occlusion of the subclavian artery with the subclavian steal syndrome, a reversed flow into the vertebral artery does not occur until 20 seconds to 20 minutes or longer despite equalization of the pre- and post-stenotic pressure difference by PTA. This observation was extremely helpful, because embolization to the vertebrobasilar vascular system is virtually ruled out by the delayed mechanism of reversed blood flow into the vertebral artery. Embolization to the digital arteries is likewise extremely rare and, when it does occur, leads to clinical symptoms in only a few cases.[4,9,10,13]

The numerous procedures currently employed in vascular surgery (thromboendarterectomy, various bypass operations, subclavian–carotid transposition, ligature of the vertebral artery, etc.) are burdened with complication rates of up to 13%, consisting mainly of nerve lesions with pareses, chylothorax, lymph fistulae, hemorrhagic complications, suture aneurysms, early thrombotic occlusion, and infections. Intrathoracic intervention has now been largely abandoned in favor of extrathoracic vascular reconstruction. Subclavian-carotid transposition and carotidosubclavian bypass have been popular just recently. Although the complication rate of vascular surgery has fallen substantially in the last few years, damage to nerves with pareses is still reported by almost all authors.

Because literature reports are unanimous in claiming a primary success rate of more than 92% for PTA, and the available early and long-term results are comparable to or better than those of corrective vascular surgical procedures, PTA constitutes an alternative to surgery in symptomatic stenosis or occlusion of the subclavian artery. Based on the unexpectedly low complication rate of 3 to 5% minor events with no mortality and a reported morbidity of 0.3%, I consider PTA to be the method of first choice in the treatment of patients with symptomatic stenosis or occlusion of the subclavian artery, particularly because the stress placed on the patients is many times lower than with corrective surgical procedures.[4,8,9,13,15] Despite the relatively unfavorable success rate of around 60% in older thrombotic occlusion of the subclavian artery, an attempt at percutaneous transluminal recanalization is justified as a primary treatment modality, because no reports have been published of complications occurring in unsuccessful recanalization. Furthermore, unsuccessful PTA in occlusion of the subclavian artery does

not place the patient or the vascular surgeon at a disadvantage on subsequent corrective treatment in the form of subclavian-carotid transposition or carotidosubclavian bypass.

PTA displays the following advantages over corrective vascular surgical procedures:

1. Minimal stress on the frequently multimorbid patients with concomitant pulmonary and cardiac disease, multivessel disease, etc.
2. Simple technical performance of PTA.
3. Beneficial use of PTA in one session in cases of multivessel disease (Figs. 82-16 to 82-18).
4. Greater cost-effectiveness than vascular surgery as a result of the low cost of the procedure and shorter hospital stay.
5. Postoperative restenosis after subclavian–carotid

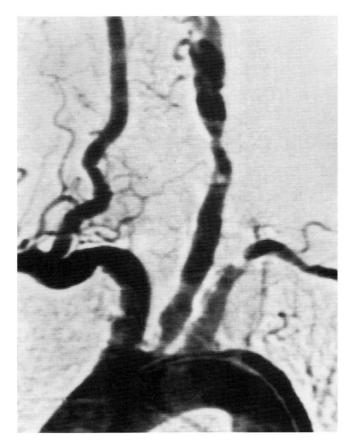

Fig. 82-16. A 59-year-old woman with occlusion of the right iliac artery, multiple high-grade stenoses of the left iliac arteries, after PTA of both renal arteries and carotidendarterectomy twice on the left internal carotid artery and transient ischemic attacks. Brachiocephalic angiogram with occlusion of the right common and internal carotid artery, high-grade restenosis after carotidendarterectomy and high-grade stenosis at origin of the left common carotid artery and the proximal left subclavian artery.

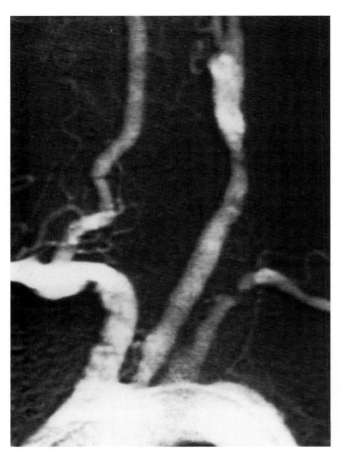

Fig. 82-17. Same patient as Fig. 82-16 after PTA of the carotid restenosis and the stenosis at the origin of the left common carotid artery.

transposition or carotidosubclavian bypass is technically simple to correct by PTA, a method burdened with fewer complications than the vascular surgical procedures.

6. Restenosis after PTA can be eliminated by repeat PTA with few complications and a lasting effect.

7. High-grade stenosis or occlusion that cannot be catheterized and in which PTA as an attempt must be discontinued (approximately 58%) can be successfully treated by vascular surgery without any disadvantage to the patient or surgeon.

The reported complication rate of 3 to 5% minor events and 0.3% morbidity is a further advantage of PTA.[9,13,15] The feared complication of embolism in the circulation of the arm occurred in only 7 cases, the only clinical manifestation in 6 being transient ischemia of a finger that did not require treatment. The other patient suffered complications with distal arterial occlusion necessitating amputation of the limb after technically successful dilation.[13-15] Two of three serious complications described in the litera-

ture in connection with PTA of the subclavian artery were permanent hemipareses in the vascular region of the contralateral carotid artery, which occurred after successful PTA during follow-up angiography with a pigtail catheter and which, strictly speaking, cannot be attributed to the actual procedure of PTA.[4,14]

The indications for PTA are the same as those for vascular surgery. Only high-grade stenosis with narrowing of the lumen of more than 75% and occlusion of the subclavian artery leading to clinical symptoms with signs of brachial, vertebrobasilar insufficiency, or symptoms of coronary steal syndrome should ever be treated. A secondary indication is that of providing inflow to extra-anatomic grafts, such as axillofemoral grafts or internal mammary-coronary grafts.

In view of the numerous advantages over corrective vascular surgical procedures, the primary success rates of more than 93%, and the similarly good long-term results with freedom from complaints or

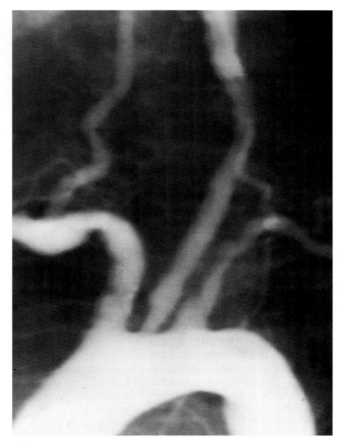

Fig. 82-18. Same patient as Fig. 82-16 and 82-17 after successful PTA of three stenoses in one session (stenosis at origin of the left common carotid artery, restenosis after carotidendarterectomy, and proximal subclavian artery stenosis).

distinct improvement of complaints in more than 90% of patients, PTA of stenosis or occlusion of the subclavian artery must be regarded as the treatment of first choice. The combined use of local thrombolysis and PTA is to be recommended in the presence of additional thrombotic complications. Acute embolic occlusion of the subclavian artery without additional stenosing is extremely rare and is an absolute indication for surgical embolectomy.[4,5,10]

The combination of local thrombolysis and PTA is indicated in the presence of stenosis and thrombotic occlusion because the vascular constriction cannot be eliminated by embolectomy. The combined use of embolectomy and PTA via the surgical access is also possible and, in my view, preferred to a two-session procedure (embolectomy followed by PTA) as long as the necessary equipment is available (an efficient fluoroscope in the operating theater).

Basing on my results previously published results, I suggest that PTA is indicated in symptomatic stenosis primarily when the following morphologic situations are present:

1. High-grade stenosis (more than 75% narrowing of the lumen)
2. Smooth-walled stenosis without ulceration, thrombotic deposits, or marked mural calcification
3. Short or circular stenosis
4. No constriction of the artery from the outside by space-occupying processes or scarring

PTA can be particularly successful and beneficial in patients with multivessel involvement or an increased surgical risk that is due to severe concomitant cardiac and pulmonary disease. Ulcerated and heavily calcified as well as long stenosis of the subclavian artery can likewise be dilated without a significant increase of the risk. In these cases, however, experience shows that a stent must also be implanted—particularly in the case of long and calcified stenosis—because PTA can cause dissection, which in turn can lead to early occlusion. The implantation of stents can prevent early occlusion or embolization to the periphery.

Not even thrombotic deposits constitute a contraindication to PTA. To prevent embolism, the deposits should be eliminated by local thrombolysis before PTA is performed.

Constriction of the artery from the outside by tumors, scarring, or costoclavicular narrowness (the thoracic outlet syndrome) cannot be eliminated by PTA and requires surgical correction.

An important condition for the performance of PTA in the region of the brachiocephalic arteries is a team consisting of interventional radiologist, angiologist, neurologist, and vascular surgeon, who together decide whether conservative, vascular surgical, or interventional radiologic therapy is indicated. Moreover, the equipment required must be state of the art, and the physician performing PTA must have adequate experience with the catheterization and PTA of other vascular regions.

The use of laser angioplasty is unlikely to improve the results of PTA in the region of the subclavian artery in future, because it has failed to produce convincing results in other vascular regions despite a succession of new and further developments in laser technology.

REFERENCES

1. Dotter CT, Judkins MP. Transluminal treatment of arteriosclerotic obstruction: description of a new technique and a preliminary report of its application. Circulation 1964;30:654–70
2. Grüntzig A, Hopf H. Perkutane Rekanalisation chronischer arterieller Verschlüsse mit einem neuen Dilatationskatheter. Dtsch Med Wochenschr 1974;99:2502–5
3. Mathias K. Ein neuartiges Kathetersystem zur perkutanen Angioplastie von Karotisstenosen. Fortschr Med 1977;95:1007–11
4. Mathias K. Percutaneous transluminal angioplasty of the supraaortic arteries. pp. 546–83. In Dondelinger RF, Rossi P, Kurdziel JC, Wallace S (eds): Interventional Radiology. Georg-Thieme-Verlag, New York 1990
5. Kachel R. Angioplasty of neck and intercranial vessels. pp. 127–132. In Kadir S (ed): Current Practice of Interventional Radiology. BC Decker, Philadelphia 1991
6. Kachel R. Endovascular treatment of carotid and vertebral arteries. pp. 112–9. In Bernstein EF, Callow AD, Nicolaides AN, Shifrin EG (eds): Cerebral Revascularisation. Med-Orion, 1993
7. Theron J, Melancon D, Ethier R. "Pre"-subclavian steal syndromes and their treatment by angioplasty: hemodynamic classification of subclavian artery stenoses. Neuroradiology 1985;27:265–70
8. Motarjeme A, Keifer JW, Zuska AJ, Nabawi P. Percutaneous transluminal angioplasty for treatment of subclavian steal. Radiology 1985;155:611–3
9. Mc Namara ThO. Angioplasty of stenoses of the proximal upper extremity and cranial vessels. pp. 261–71. In Kadir S (ed): Current Practice of Interventional Radiology. BC Decker, Philadelphia, 1991
10. Vitek JJ. Subclavian artery angioplasty at the origin of the vertebral artery. Radiology 1989;170:407–9
11. Fisher CM. A new syndrome—"the subclavian steal." N Engl J Med 1961;265:912–3
12. Kachel R, Endert G, Reiß Zimmermann GU et al. 111-Indium-Thombozytenszintigraphie und perkutane Dilatation (Angioplastik) von supra-aortalen Gefäßstenosen. Fortschr Röntgenstr 1986;145:336–9
13. Düber C, Klose KJ, Kopp H, Schmiedt W. Percutaneous transluminal angioplasty for occlusion of the subclavian artery: short- and long-term results. Cardiovasc Intervent Radiol 1992;15:205–10

14. Millaire A, Trinca M, Marache P et al. Subclavian angioplasty immediate and late results in 50 patients. Cathet Cardiovasc Diagn 1993;29(1):8–17

15. Romanowski CA, Fairlie NC, Procker AE, Cumberland DC. Percutaneous transluminal angioplasty of the subclavian and axillary arteries: initial results and long-term follow-up. Clin Radiol 1992; 46:104–7

16. Kachel R, Basche St, Großmann K, Endler S. Percutaneous transluminal angioplasty (PTA) of supra-aortic arteries especially the internal carotid artery. Neuroradiology 1991;33:191–4

17. Ringelstein EB, Zeumer H. Delayed reversal of vertebral artery flow following percutaneous transluminal angioplasty for subclavian steal. Neuroradiology 1984; 26:189–98

83 Pulmonary Arteries and Veins

Andrew Redington

Intravascular stenting was first described as early as 1969.[1] Transluminally placed coil-spring devices placed in the popliteal artery of dogs were shown to have reasonable long-term patency. Other devices were tested experimentally in the early 1980s,[2–4] but the first clinical experience was published as recently as 1987[5]; since then, the utility of peripheral arterial and coronary arterial stent implantation has become established, and the use of stents in adults with acquired cardiovascular disease has become commonplace. The use of stents in patients with congenital heart disease is also increasingly reported. Stenting of pulmonary arterial stenoses for lesions resistant to standard balloon dilation in older children and young adults is now the treatment of choice. The indications for the use of stents are widening and include stenosed veins and operative pathways, aortopulmonary collaterals, the right ventricular outflow tract, some cases of coarctation, and pulmonary venous stenosis, the latter of which is briefly discussed in this chapter.

RATIONALE AND MECHANISM OF ACTION

Pulmonary arterial and venous stenoses can be naturally occurring, but such patients are relatively rare. More commonly, dilation of postoperative stenoses is required. This is particularly the case for pulmonary arterial stenosis, in patients following surgery for tetralogy of Fallot, pulmonary atresia, and so on. A significant proportion of these patients will benefit from standard or high-pressure balloon dilation without the need for intravascular stenting. Nonetheless, 30 to 40% will have an inadequate response to balloon dilation despite complete relief of stenosis during dilation of the balloon. These dynamic stenoses, expandable but not dilatable, are those best suited to intravascular stenting.

INSTRUMENTATION

Two main types of stents are used in the treatment of congenital heart disease. Most frequently, a balloon-expandable stent (Johnson & Johnson) has been used.[6] This stent, originally designed for intracoronary and peripheral vascular stenoses has been adapted for use in the pulmonary vascular tree. The following sizes are now available: small, dilatable up to 6 mm; medium, dilatable up to 13 mm; and large, dilatable up to 20 mm. The stents are dilated well beyond recommended diameters to improve the utility of the device. One must be aware, however, that considerable shortening occurs when these devices are overdilated, and there is a risk of fracture at the extremes.

Less commonly used are the self-expanding stents[5,7] (Wallstents, Schneider). The mechanism of deployment and action is identical to the intracoronary version and the advantages of these stents when used in the pulmonary arteries are similar. The relatively small delivery system, relatively longer length, and longitudinal flexibility means that these stents have specific indications and can be placed in areas where balloon-expandable stents would either be suboptimal or impossible to deploy.

INDICATIONS AND PATIENT SELECTION

Any pulmonary arterial or pulmonary venous stenosis that is expandable by balloon dilation but that recoils on deflation of the balloon or restenoses after a previous dilation may be considered for intravascular stent placement. It is clearly futile to place a stent across a non dilatable lesion. Naturally occurring pulmonary arterial and venous stenosis is rare, and these lesions respond least well to both balloon dilation and stent placement. Nonetheless, those with discrete, dilatable, lesions may be suitable. The vast majority of patients in this category will be postoperative. In general, calcified stenoses will rarely respond to balloon dilation and thus will fail to respond to intravascular stenting, but all other lesions are potentially stentable. However, very proximal lesions, close to the pulmonary valve, and very distal lesions (where stent implantation in a stenotic lesion may lead to an occlusion of an adjacent branch of the vascular tree) may be less suitable.

Postoperative pulmonary venous stenosis is usually in the setting of a previously repaired anomalous pulmonary venous drainage. Obstruction of the anastomotic line, for example, after repair of supracardiac total anomalous pulmonary venous drainage (TAPVC), may be difficult to stent because of the short length between individual pulmonary veins and the left atrium. Discrete stenosis of the individual veins themselves is much more amenable to stent placement.

Choice of Device

Balloon-Expandable Stents (Prototype, Palmaz Stent; Johnson & Johnson)

Balloon-expandable stents are mounted on relatively large balloons and carried through relatively large sheaths. Most of the published literature describes the use of this type of stent, and they have several advantages. They are re-expandable (so that redilation to keep pace with growth is possible) and durable (thus maintaining patency in vessels with very resistant stenoses). Redilation of intravascular stents has been described. The ultimate diameter is rarely as great as that predicted from balloon size, but nonetheless some additional enlargement can usually be obtained. Balloon-expandable stents can be mounted on high-pressure balloons. Thus, resistant stenoses requiring high-pressure balloons can be treated with these devices.

Self-Expanding Stents (Prototype, Wallstents; Schneider)

Unlike the balloon-expandable stents, self-expanding stents have a lower collapse pressure. The radial force that these devices exert varies depending on length, diameter, and so on but is in the order of 4 to 6 atmo. Thus, stenoses requiring high-pressure balloon dilation (8 to 20 atmo) may not be suitable for self-expanding stents. The other major disadvantage of this type of stent is that they cannot be over-dilated. Thus, the maximum deployed size cannot be exceeded, and so these stents are not suitable for patients in whom expansion concomitant with somatic growth is required. It remains to be seen whether an over-size self-expanding stent can be placed in a much smaller vessel and subsequently redilated. Early unpublished results of such a strategy suggest that the potential for this is limited.

There are several advantages to the Wallstent delivery system, however. It is generally smaller than the equivalent balloon-expandable system, it has longitudinal flexibility both during and after deployment in the vessels. Stents are also available in long sizes, obviating the need for multiple overlapping balloon-expandable stents in diffusely stenotic vessels or vessels with multiple stenoses. Indeed, it may be possible to deploy these stents when balloon-expandable stents cannot be used.

OPERATIVE TECHNIQUE AND TIPS

Pulmonary Arterial Stenosis

The prestent evaluation of any patient must involve prior angiography in multiple views to display the anatomy of the vessel and its stenosis to its maximum advantage. Balloon dilation with the same make and size of balloon that is going to be used for stent deployment is the method of choice. This enables the operator to assess the possibility of displacement, stripping, or recoil during subsequent stent placement. If a stable balloon dilation procedure can be performed, then subsequent stent placement is rarely complicated or hazardous. To facilitate reassessment after initial balloon dilation, a second angiographic catheter placed from the contralateral groin may be helpful. This enables maintenance of the position of the wire and the balloon during the procedure. It will subsequently allow careful evaluation of the position of the stent before its deployment. A second venous access may also be required if there is bilateral stenosis, particularly at the origin of each pulmonary artery. A second wire and balloon will be required to protect the contralateral stenosis during stent placement in the target pulmonary artery.

Deployment of balloon-expandable stents does not necessarily require the use of a high-pressure balloon system. The operator, however, must be confident of the balloon technology in use, because rupture of the balloon during deployment considerably complicates stent placement. The usable length of the balloon must exceed the length of the stent by at least 5 mm at each end (Fig. 83-1). A balloon system with a small shaft size is clearly an advantage but also may be disadvantagous if the stent is not stable on the balloon after crimping. Hand crimping is the method of choice, but care must be taken not to perforate the balloon during mounting. The stent and balloon is delivered over the wire, through a guiding vascular sheath. For the medium-sized Johnson and Johnson stent, a 7- or 8-F sheath is required, and an 11- or 12-F sheath is ideal for use of the largest stents (Fig. 83-2). The tip of the sheath is placed well beyond the stenosed area in the first instance. The balloon and stent system must be observed as it is passed through the sheath. This is because longitudinal stent movement along the balloon may occur when negotiating acute bends within the sheath. Several strategies overcome displacement of the stent during its passage through the sheath; a gentle bend in the stent as it is placed on the balloon sometimes helps tracking through an awkward bend. Alternatively, while the stent is gripped or protected with a small piece of smaller sheath material, the balloon can be slightly inflated proximally and distally so as to anchor the stent in the middle of the balloon before passage through the sheath (this technique also ensures that both proximal and distal parts of the balloon will inflate during subsequent balloon inflation, thus avoiding stripping backwards or forwards over the balloon during inflation). The final alternative, and most usually preferred, is to insert the sheath

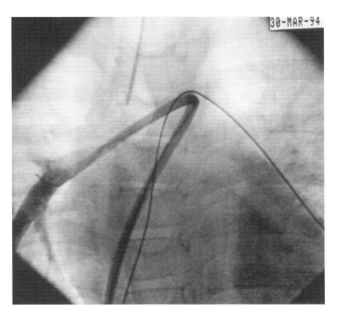

Fig. 83-2. Stenting of a proximal stenosis in the right pulmonary artery. An 11-F transseptal sheath has been passed over a superstiff guidewire into the distal pulmonary artery.

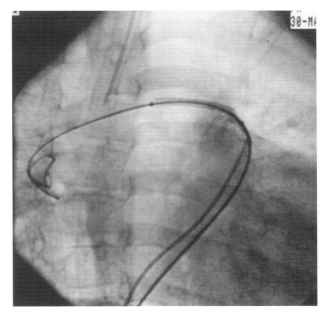

Fig. 83-3. The balloon-mounted stent has been passed through the sheath to the point of pulmonary arterial stenosis. The sheath has been withdrawn to leave the sheath and balloon in position. The sheath, however, remains in the outflow tract to provide additional support to avoid movement during balloon inflation. Note also how the floppy tip of the superstiff guidewire is looped in the distal pulmonary artery, again to maintain stability.

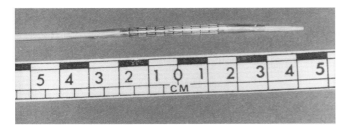

Fig. 83-1. A balloon-mounted stent. This has been hand-crimped onto a standard balloon catheter. It is important that an adequate length of balloon extends beyond the proximal and distal ends of the stent.

system into the inferior caval vein, removing the dilator at this stage. The balloon system is then delivered through the sheath such that the tip of the balloon catheter forms the tip of the stent, balloon, and sheath system. This is then advanced together across the stenosis, making displacement of the stent far less likely. This latter technique can be performed only when the stenosed segment itself is quite large, however.

It is clearly imperative to use a very stiff guiding wire. The floppy tip of, for example, an Amplatz superstiff guidewire, or Schneider backup wire should be placed in the distalmost part of the pulmo-

nary artery to be dilated. Ideally, a loop is formed so that the maximum length of the stiffest part of the guidewire is across the stenosis (Fig. 83-3). This will aid all of the preceding techniques.

Once the stent is across the stenotic area, the guiding sheath is withdrawn far enough proximally so that the proximal part of the balloon can inflate normally. It is unwise to withdraw the sheath too far, because it provides additional support within the intracardiac course of the system, wire, and delivery system. The position of the stent before deployment can be checked using additional angiography if required (Fig. 83-3). Stent deployment is performed by

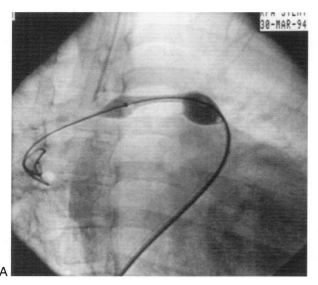
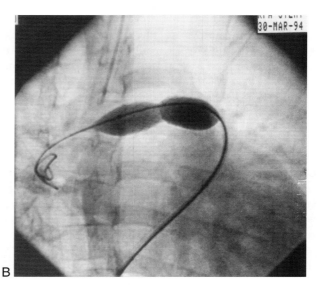

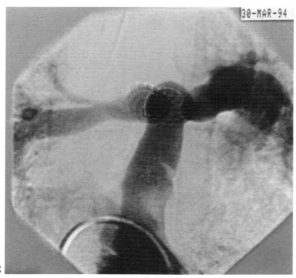

Fig. 83-4. (A) The balloon is inflated with a 50:50 saline/contrast mixture. It is important that both ends of the balloon inflate simultaneously. **(B)** The balloon during inflation. **(C)** The result of balloon inflation. A subtotal occlusion of the right pulmonary artery at its origin has been almost completely relieved. A small residual waste occurred at the point of maximal narrowing.

rapid balloon dilation using 25:75 contrast/saline mixture (Figs. 83-4). This is best done by a second or third operator while the rest of the system is maintained in rigid position at the groin and at the overlap points of sheath, balloon, and wire. One or more balloon dilations may be required. Occasionally, a smaller balloon is used for initial dilation, followed by larger balloons to further dilate the stent in situ.

MANAGEMENT OF DISASTERS

Despite the careful precautions described, potential disasters can happen during stent deployment. Balloon perforation by the stent, during deployment, is the most frequent. Thankfully, the balloon rarely ruptures before partial deployment of the stent. It is usually therefore possible to remove the balloon and reinflate a second balloon within the stent without hazard. Great care must be taken to ensure that the balloon is not snagged by one of the sharp points of the stent. If this is the case, then advancement of the guiding sheath with gentle withdrawal of the balloon usually maintains stent position. If this is not possible, the second catheter access can be used. Placement of a large sheath against the proximal end of the stent, through the contralateral groin, anchors it as the balloon catheter is withdrawn from the stent. Finally, a second balloon can be advanced through the second sheath, fully dilated within the stent, and at the same time the first balloon is withdrawn from the sheath.

Stent displacement during deployment has also been reported (Figs. 83-5). It may be possible to "catch" the malpositioned stent by reinflating the balloon within the stent and carefully repositioning it across the stenosis. Alternatively, the same technique can be used to remove the stent from the pulmonary artery to the right atrium and then deploy the stent in the superior or inferior caval vein. Although this is unsatisfactory, it is clearly preferred to cardiopulmonary bypass for removal of the errant stent. It is difficult to remove a partially inflated stent using a transcatheter snare. Snaring, crushing, and removal through a very large intravascular sheath have been reported, but these are the least satisfactory options.

SELF-EXPANDING STENTS

The technique of delivering self-expanding stents has already been described for coronary arterial stenoses.[5,7] The same procedure is followed in pulmonary arterial and venous stenoses.[9] Once again, a

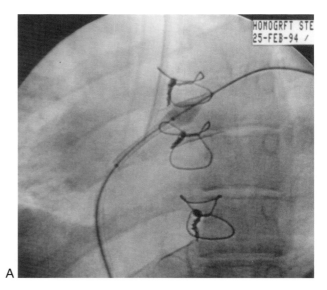

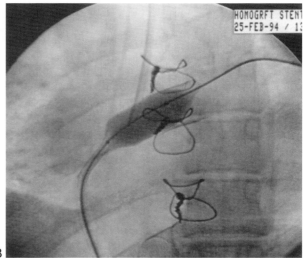

Fig. 83-5. (A&B) Stent implantation in a Fontan anastomosis. A self-expanding stent has been placed previously. Note how inflation of the balloon leads to inflation of the distal part only. With further inflation, the stent is stripped back toward the sheath. In this case, the balloon was deflated, withdrawn through the stent, and the stent was advanced into the stenosis and subsequent balloon dilation led to a satisfactory position (see text for details).

stable wire position is required, but no delivery sheath is necessary. The system is deployed over the wire (Figs. 83-6 and 83-7), and it is possible to begin to deploy the stent far distally to the stenotic area. When approximately 50% of the stent has been exposed from behind the rolling membrane, the distal part of the stent is brought toward the area of stenosis by traction on the delivery system. Once an adequate position has been maintained, the remainder of the stent can be opened. This ensures perfect

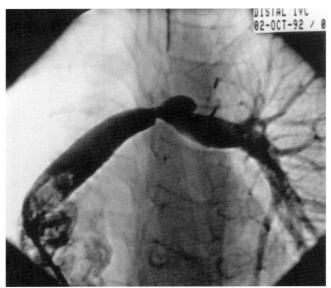

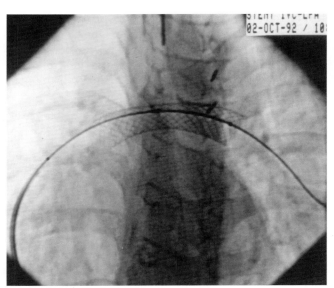

Fig. 83-6. A stenosed inferior cava to pulmonary artery anastomosis after balloon dilation. This is a balloon-expandable but resistant stenosis, and so a self-expanding stent was placed.

Fig. 83-7. This shows the self-expanding stent in position immediately after deployment (see Fig. 53-6). The delivery system can be seen across the stenosis (marked by the radiopaque markers). The rolling membrane (just proximal to the most proximal radiopaque marker) has been withdrawn completely. Note how the stent molds to the shape of the vessel.

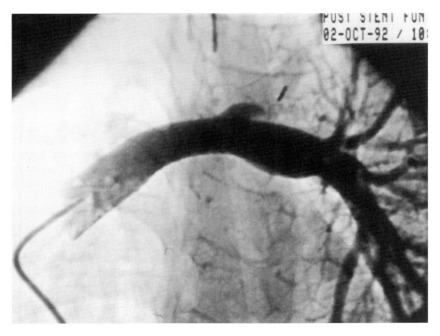

Fig. 83-8. Postimplantation angiogram (see Fig. 83-6). Complete relief of the stenosis was achieved.

placement of the stent across the stenosis (Figs. 83-8). It is always easier to withdraw a partially deployed stent (whether balloon-expandable or self-expanding) than to advance it.

POST PROCEDURAL MANAGEMENT

No special precautions or treatment are required after stent placement in most pulmonary arterial stenoses. It is our policy to anticoagulate all patients with cavopulmonary or Fontan-like connections, and so stent placement in these circulations does not necessitate any change in management. Because of the increased likelihood of thrombosis in these circulations, careful regulation of anticoagulation is clearly desirable under these circumstances.

RESULTS: SHORT AND LONG-TERM FOLLOW-UP

Pulmonary Arterial Stenosis

Relatively few data are available concerning the use of self-expanding stents, and these are confined to short-term follow-up only. Balloon-expandable stents have been available longer. The early results are very encouraging. In the North American collaborative study, the largest published so far, the incidence of adverse events was low, and the early effectiveness of the technique was established.[8] With correct selection, complete relief, or at least, adequate relief is obtained in most expandable lesions. The midterm results are equally encouraging.[10] Redilation of some of these stents has been performed with mixed results (Figs. 83-9). Restenosis, intimal proliferation, thrombosis, and unforeseen events were remarkably infrequent, however.

Pulmonary Venous Stenosis

The results for native pulmonary venous stenosis are almost directly contradictory to those for pulmonary arterial stenosis. Whereas balloon dilation and stenting of pulmonary arterial stenosis is a highly successful technique that has rapidly gained almost universal approval, the results for balloon dilation and subsequent stenting of pulmonary venous stenosis remain depressing (Figs. 83-10 and 83-11). Stent implantation at the time of surgery has also been performed (Fig. 83-12) when access or patient size has been a problem. No very large series have been con-

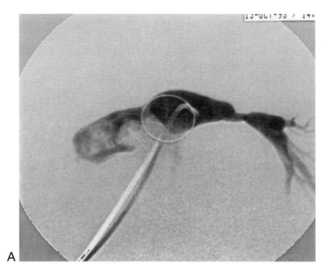

A

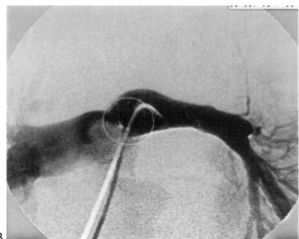

B

Fig. 83-9. (A&B) Digital subtraction angiogram of severe distal stenosis of the left pulmonary artery after balloon dilation. Placement of a medium-sized Johnson & Johnson stent completely relieves the stenosis. The main pulmonary artery diameter is only 8 mm, however. Redilation will be required in the future to keep pace with somatic growth (see text for details).

ducted because of the rarity of native pulmonary venous stenosis. Restenosis that is due to either thrombosis or intimal overgrowth is common, and very few successful results have been achieved. Postoperative pulmonary venous stenosis is more amenable to stent placement, as one may imagine. Again, relatively few patients with relatively little long-term data are available, but anecdotal reports from all the large groups performing such interventions suggest that for those with discrete postoperative stenoses there is a role for stent placement if surgery is undesirable.

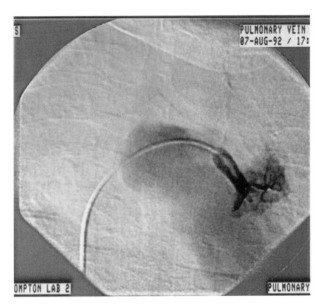

Fig. 83-10. Selective left lower pulmonary venous injection. A severe stenosis is present at its entry point with the left atrium.

COSTS

The costs of stent placement are relatively modest by comparison with, for example, umbrella occlusion techniques. Both balloon-expandable and self-expandable stents cost in the order of $600 to $700. The additional cost of balloons, sheaths, wires, and

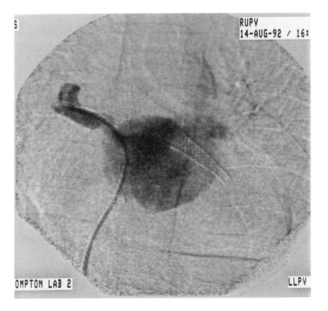

Fig. 83-11. A self-expanding stent has been placed across the stenosis and at follow-up was patent. However, further stenoses of the right and left upper pulmonary veins progressed (see Fig. 83-12).

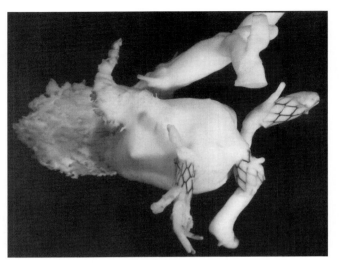

Fig. 83-12. Postmortem silastic cast taken from the patient described in Fig. 83-10 and 83-11. Balloon-expandable stents have been placed in the mouth of each of the pulmonary veins, intraoperatively. Although the stenosis was relieved, this patient died of pulmonary hypertensive crisis 2 days after the procedure.

so on must be taken into account, however. Another important factor will be the use of multiple stents. It is sometimes necessary to dovetail two or three self-expanding stents completely to relieve a diffusely stenotic pulmonary artery in an adult. A single long self-expanding stent may be more satisfactory under these circumstances (particularly after the Fontan procedure), and this will considerably decrease the overall cost of the procedure.

DISCUSSION

Pulmonary arterial stenting using balloon-expandable stents has rapidly become an accepted part of the armamentarium of pediatric and adult interventional cardiologists. Many lesions are amenable to intravascular stenting.[11-15] Some questions remain unanswered regarding redilation, and so on, but the midterm results are encouraging. A measure of the utility of these techniques is the enthusiasm with which surgeons have welcomed them as an alternative to reoperation! The role of self-expanding stents is limited. They may be particularly useful in diffusely stenotic or tortuous pulmonary arterial and venous stenoses.

REFERENCES

1. Dotter CT. Transluminally placed coil spring endarterial tube grafts: long-term patency in canine femoral artery. Invest Radiol 1969;4:329–32

2. Dotter CT, Bushmann RW, McKinney MK, Rosch J. Transluminar expandable Nitonol coil stent grafting: preliminary report. Radiology 1983;147:259–60

3. Wright KC, Wallace S, Chanarnsangavej C et al. Percutaneous endovascular stents: an experimental evaluation. Radiology 1985;156:69–72

4. Palmaz JC, Windeler SA, Garcia F et al. Athroslerotic rabbit aortas: expandable intraluminar grafting. Radiology 1986;160:723–6

5. Sigwart U, Puel J, Mirkovitch V et al. Intravascular stents to prevent occlusion and restenosis alter transluminal angioplasty.

6. Palmaz JC, Ladborde JC, Rivera FF et al. Stenting of the iliac arteries with the Palmaz stent: experience from a multicentre trial. Cardiosvac Intervent Radiol 1992;15:291–7

7. Goy JJ, Sigwart U, Vogt P et al. Long-term follow up of the first 56 patients treated with intracoronary self-expanding stents (the Lausanne experience). Am J Cardiol 1991;67:269–72

8. O'Laughlin MP, Perry SB, Lock JE, Mullins CE. Use of endovascular stents in congenital heart disease. Circulation 1991;83:1923–39

9. Redington AN, Weil J, Somerville J. Self-expanding stents in congenital heart disease. Br Heart J 1994; 72:378–83

10. O'Laughlin MP, Slack MC, Grifka RG et al. Implantation and intermediate-term follow up of stents in congenital heart disease. Circulation 1993;88(2):605–14

11. Ruiz CE, Gamra H, Zhang HP et al. Stenting of the ductus arteries as a bridge to cardiac transplantation in infants with the hypoplastic left heart syndrome. N Engl J Med 1993;328:1605–8

12. Gibbs JL, Wren C, Watterson KG et al. Stenting of the arterial duct combined with banding of the pulmonary arteries and atrial septectomy or septostomy: a new approach to palliation for the hypoplastic left heart syndrome. Br Heart J 1993;69:551–6

13. Gibbs JL, Rothman MT, Rees MR et al. Stenting of the arterial duct: a new approach to palliation for pulmonary atresia. Br Heart J 1992;67:240–6

14. Redington AN, Hayes AM, Ho SY. Transcatheter stent implantation to treat aortic coarctation in infancy. Br Heart J 1993;69:80–3

15. Hoskin MC, Benson LN, Nakanishi T et al. Intravascular stent prosthesis for right ventricular outflow tract obstruction. J Am Coll Cardiol 1992;20:373–80

84 Cerebral Vessels

Robert D.G. Ferguson
John G. Ferguson

HISTORY

Cerebral percutaneous transluminal angioplasty (CPTA) refers to therapeutic balloon dilation of a vessel located between the aorta and cerebral end arteries (arterioles). In this vascular territory, the most commonly treated vessels are the following:

- Innominate
- Subclavian (prevertebral)
- Common carotid
- Internal carotid
- External carotid
- Vertebral
- Basilar
- Anterior cerebral
- Middle cerebral
- Posterior cerebral

Angioplasty of the innominate, subclavian, proximal vertebral, (Fig. 84-1) and common carotid arteries has been referred to as brachiocephalic percutaneous transluminal angioplasty (PTA) in previous publications. This term has generally not been applied to treatment of internal carotid artery or distal vertebral lesions (Fig. 84-2). The term brachiocephalic PTA is not used in this discussion, because it excludes the intracranial arteries and includes arteries that do not have the brain as an end organ; that is, the subclavian artery distal to the vertebral and the axillary arteries.

CPTA has become synonymous with high-pressure inflation, using non-elastomer balloons for treatment of structural vaso-occlusive disease that is due primarily to atherosclerosis. Low-pressure angioplasty with elastomer balloons, for treatment of subarachnoid hemorrhage-induced vasospasm, has been performed successfully for over a decade. These procedures differ in the nature of the target lesion, as well as the technology and techniques used. This discussion focuses on the use of angioplasty in the treatment of structural vascular occlusive lesions, particularly those that are due to atherosclerosis. See Eskridge[1] for a detailed discussion of percutaneous intervention in the treatment of vasospasm that is due to subarachnoid hemorrhage.

Kerber and colleagues[2] performed the first human carotid artery dilations in 1980 and demonstrated that atherosclerotic lesions of the common carotid artery could be dilated without necessarily provoking symptomatic atherothromboembolism. Later that year, Mullan et al.[3] reported the first human internal carotid artery dilation. Angioplasty of this nonatherosclerotic, weblike lesion resulted in immediate disappearance of the patient's complaint of a pulsating noise in the ear and a vibration (thrill) in the neck.

Several case series have since been reported and have demonstrated the feasibility of performing cerebral angioplasty for treatment of structural occlusive disease, in several hundred mostly symptomatic patients.[4–8] However, there are no reports of definitive comparative CPTA studies. Moreover, the data concerning systematic angiographic follow-up are

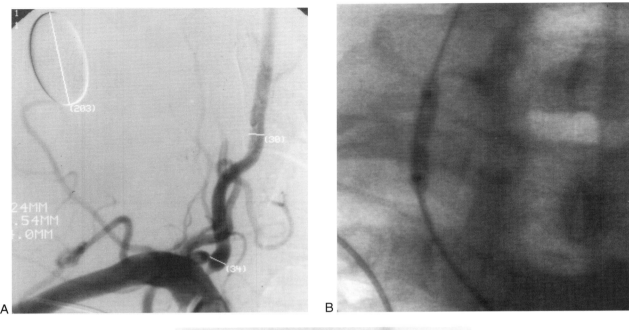

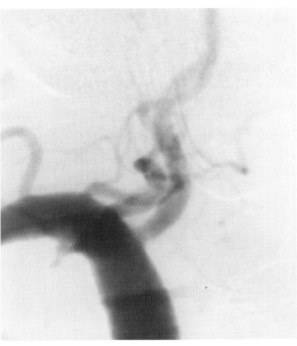

Fig. 84-1. A 64-year-old man with episodic left facial weakness. **(A)** Initial angiogram shows a 72% stenosis at the right vertebral artery origin. Using a quarter as a standard of measurement, the post-stenotic segment was measured as 4 mm in diameter. **(B)** A partially inflated 4 × 20-mm balloon across the stenosis. **(C)** Final angiogram shows residual 19% stenosis following angioplasty.

sparse. Hence, the clinical effectiveness and therapeutic role of cerebral angioplasty need to be defined, before widespread implementation can be justified.

The Carotid and Vertebral Artery Transluminal Angioplasty Study (CAVATAS) (M. Brown, principal investigator, 1994, personal communication) in England is attempting to compare surgery and angioplasty for treatment of carotid and vertebral occlusive lesions. The largest, prospective experience to date comes from the The North American Cerebral Percutaneous Transluminal Angioplasty Register (NACPTAR).

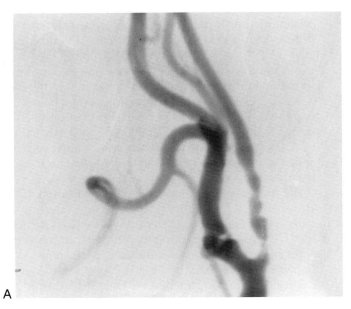
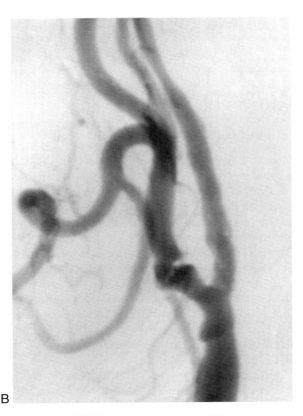

A   B

Fig. 84-2. (A) A 65-year-old man with postendarterectomy restenosis. **(B)** Postangioplasty carotid angiography shows improved luminal diameter following dilation with a 4-mm × 4-cm balloon catheter.

Taken together, these studies demonstrate that, in selected patients, cerebral angioplasty can effect a marked change in the degree of stenosis of atherosclerotic target lesions, with an incidence of complications similar to that observed in other vascular territories during the early stages of angioplasty development.

RATIONALE AND MECHANISM OF ACTION

There are several reasons for doing CPTA. First, it is designed to increase the cross-sectional area of the target vessel at a point of narrowing. The concomitant increase in flow reserve may protect against hemodynamic (low-flow) stroke, while the increase in cross-sectional area may forestall hemodynamically critical narrowing. Second, long-term remodeling after PTA may favorably alter rheology and permit restoration of endothelial integrity, thereby improving target segment function while reducing thrombus-promoting turbulence. It is hypothesized that achieving these goals may minimize or prevent cerebral ischemia and infarction, in patients who are at

risk for large-vessel thrombotic occlusion and plaque-derived thromboembolism.

No reliable morphologic data are available concerning the mechanism of successful angioplasty in human cerebral arteries. Until such evidence is available, it seems likely, given the similarities in the arteries and the atherosclerotic processes within them, that the mechanism of successful PTA in the cerebral arteries is similar to that in other vascular territories of similar size; that is, endothelial denudation with cracking and splitting of the target plaque, along with stretching of the adjacent media and adventitia leading to aneurysmal dilation of the target segment, with an attendant increase in cross-sectional area.[9]

INSTRUMENTATION

No devices have a Food and Drug Administration (FDA)-approved indication for cerebral angioplasty. Several major device manufacturers and pharmaceutical companies are pursuing device approval for specific neurovascular indications. Currently, extracranial angioplasty typically employs 5-F angioplasty systems of the type used in the peripheral circulation, while intracranial lesions are treated using 3 F or smaller systems more typical of those used in the coronary circulation.

PATIENT POPULATION

Patient Selection

Patient eligibility is based on clinical and angiographic criteria. Almost all of our patients have had a history of either transient or, less often, fixed neurologic deficits. Patients with fixed neurologic deficits are considered for CPTA if viable tissue is present in the compromised vascular territory. Most patients have been nonsurgical candidates with hemodynamically significant lesions. The majority of cases involve a single target lesion. The incremental cost/benefit ratio of multivessel CPTA is unknown. Therefore, we perform multivessel angioplasty only in the presence of a strong indication for complete revascularization, and we stage multiple-vessel CPTA at 1- to 2-week intervals.

Initially, the Memphis Vascular Research Foundation protocol required a stenosis greater than or equal to 70% to qualify for CPTA. However, we are reassessing the concept of hemodynamic significance. Traditionally, the critical determinant of a lesion's significance has been reduction in arterial diameter, at the point of maximum stenosis, to 70% of the unaffected, adjacent, proximal arterial segment. We suspect that a lesion's potential for flow disruption, in addition to volumetric flow restriction, is important in the pathogenesis of cerebral thromboembolism. In particular, flow disruption may create a hypercoagulable microenvironment at the site of a plaque, thereby promoting in situ thrombosis, clot fragmentation, and distal embolization. The frequent observation of small stenoses after thrombolysis in acute myocardial infarction,[10] as well as the results of a recent randomized controlled trial by the investigators of the Asymptomatic Carotid Atherosclerosis Study (ACAS)[11] lend credence to this hypothesis. In addition to improving lumen caliber, CPTA of stenoses that are less than 70% may, in the long term, improve the structural and functional integrity of the target segment.

PRETREATMENT

Preangioplasty Pharmacotherapy

It can be difficult discriminate atheroma-associated thrombus at angiography in many patients. Because of the risk of clot fragmentation with distal emboliza-

tion, we use an aggressive approach to treat plaque-associated thrombus. Hence, we consider an irregular plaque contour presumptive evidence for lesion-associated thrombus (Fig. 84-3). Although unproven, we believe that this indicant justifies pre-CPTA fibrinolytic infusion at the site of the lesion, unless there is evidence of cerebral infarction, in the distribution of the target artery within the prior month. When so indicated, we infuse 250,000 U of urokinase over 1 hour and reassess. A definite change in target lesion appearance suggests thrombus and prompts continued infusion until lesion appearance stabilizes or the quantitative fibrinogen level drops below 100 mg/dl. We have not observed significant bleeding complications with this approach, and we believe that the benefits outweigh the risks; however, prospective comparative studies are needed to confirm this thesis.

All patients are pretreated with 325-mg aspirin. In cases of aspirin intolerance, ticlopidine may be substituted; however, it should be started 5 days before CPTA. Before passing a catheter into the target artery, systemic anticoagulation is initiated with heparin sulfate, usually 5000 U, in a bolus. We use calcium channel antagonists to treat intraprocedural hypertension or vasospasm of the target vessels. We routinely perform angioplasty under local anesthesia with sedation. However, we obtain anesthesiology assistance for sedation and general anesthesia standby in most cases of intracranial angioplasty. We routinely pretreat patients undergoing carotid bulb CPTA with intravenous atropine, to prevent profound bradycardia or asystole. We do not use a prophylactic pacemaker for CPTA without stenting; however, until additional data are available, prophylactic pacing may be justified when inserting a stent in the carotid bulb. We obtain surgical backup, with neurosurgery or vascular surgery, depending on the location of the target lesion. All patients are evaluated by a clinical neuroscientist before angioplasty to record baseline neurologic status, and all patients undergo either computed tomographic (CT) or magnetic resonance imaging (MRI) scanning of the brain before initiating treatment, to document prior brain injury, and to detect co-morbidity such as aneurysms or arteriovenous malformations that could alter the therapeutic approach.

OPERATIVE TECHNIQUE AND TIPS

All patients undergo automated blood pressure monitoring, pulse oximetry, and systematic serial neurologic checks. A baseline diagnostic angiogram is per-

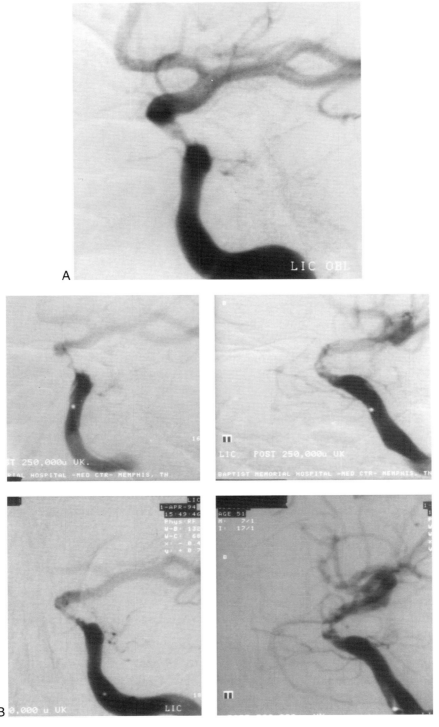

Fig. 84-3. A 51-year-old man with left cerebral Transient Ischemic Attacks (TIAs). **(A)** Pretherapy left internal carotid arteriogram shows 81% stenosis of the cavernous left internal carotid artery and absence of opthalmic artery. **(B)** Left internal carotid arteriogram (top left, anteroposterior (AP) and top right, lateral) after local intra-arterial infusion of 250,000 U of urokinase, showing early thrombolysis and clot reformation. After 500,000 U of urokinase **(B)** (bottom left, AP, and bottom right, lateral), there is progressive thrombolysis and improvement in luminal diameter. *Figure continues.*

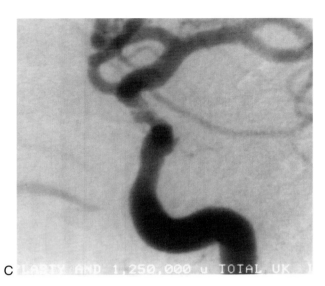
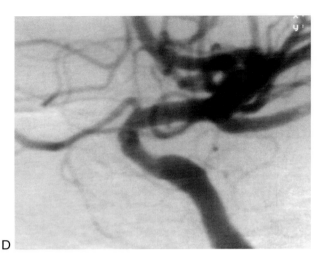

Fig. 84-3. (*continued*) **(C & D)** Final carotid arteriogram following local infusion of 1,250,000 U of urokinase and angioplasty, with a 3 × 15-mm balloon catheter showing a 39% residual stenosis. Note the recanalization of the opthalmic artery.

formed to look for thrombus and to determine the target vessel diameter.

The native vessel diameter is estimated from the angiogram, taking magnification into account. In general, we select a balloon that approximates the estimated native diameter. In some cases, oversized balloons are required to achieve an adequate angiographic result. However, we do not use balloons that exceed the estimated diameter by more than 120% or 1 mm. As noted previously, if there is evidence for intravascular thrombus, local intra-arterial fibrinolytic infusion is initiated. This is done by placing a catheter adjacent to the thrombus and administering 250,000 IU of urokinase by continuous infusion, for 1 hour. The infusion is then terminated unless there is a change in the degree or contour of the stenosis. Otherwise, the infusion is continued at the same rate until no further change is noted. In our experience, this regimen has no significant effect on fibrinogen levels, unless the infusion is continued for several hours. If higher doses of urokinase are given, the quantitative fibrinogen level is monitored at hourly intervals. The diagnostic catheter is then exchanged for the balloon catheter. The catheter is positioned across the stenosis, and the balloon is inflated (usually to the maximum rated pressure). The choice of inflation time relates primarily to the location of the lesion. Inflation times vary from a few seconds to 2 minutes. Generally speaking, we use the shortest inflation times (as brief as 5 seconds) in intracranial lesions, where important branches with little potential for collateral reconstitution may be occluded during balloon inflation, for example, the basilar artery. After balloon deflation, an angiogram is performed. In the event of an unsatisfactory technical result (e.g., >30% residual stenosis), repeat angioplasty may be performed with the same balloon or with a larger balloon, as specified above. Following the final balloon inflation, we typically keep the patient in the angiography suite for a period of 20 to 30 minutes, following which, we do a final angiogram of the target site and distal (intracranial) vascular bed, to exclude the possibility of subclinical cerebral embolization.

COMPLICATIONS AND THEIR TREATMENT

Vasospasm may be encountered before or after angioplasty. It almost invariably resolves with standard doses of sublingual nitroglycerin and Nifedipine, or slowly administered intra-arterial papavarine (30 to 60 mg; concentration, 3 to 6 mg/ml).

All patients who experience new or worsening clinical neurologic deficits are given oxygen, 4 L by nasal prongs and, except in cases of intracranial hemorrhage, volume expansion and vasopressors to maintain cerebral perfusion pressure. Atropine is used to treat sinus bradycardia provoked by dilation of lesions in the carotid bulb. Nifedipine is effective in cases of intraprocedural systemic hypertension. The threshold for treating hypertension varies according to the presence and timing of cerebral injury, the use

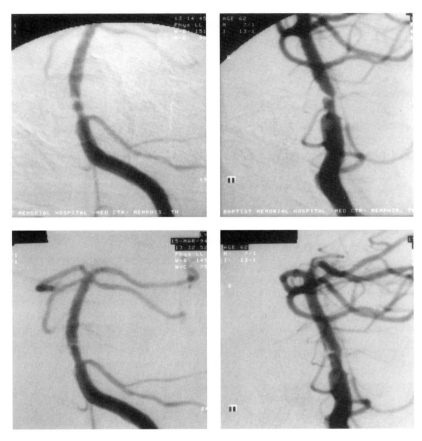

Fig. 84-4. A 62-year-old man with intermittent left facial, right arm, and right leg weakness while on coumadin, persantine, and aspirin therapy. Initial angiography of the basilar artery in the anteroposterior (AP) **(A)** and lateral **(B)** projections showed a midbasilar stenosis of 81%. **(C & D)** Images obtained following angioplasty with a 2.5 × 20-mm balloon catheter and 618,000 U of intra-arterial urokinase show improved caliber and flow. A focal residual stenosis of 45% and a post-stenotic intimal cleft is noted.

of adjunctive fibrinolytic therapy, and the presence of co-morbidity that predisposes hemorrhage.

Site-specific fibrinolysis is a form of neurovascular rescue for thrombotic or thromboembolic angioplasty complications (Fig. 84-4). Whenever intravascular thrombus is suspected following angioplasty, we immediately initiate local, site-specific fibrinolytic infusion. Urokinase is administered by hand injection using short pulses or infused continuously at a rate of up to 10,000 U/min, through a microcatheter positioned as close as possible to the target thrombus. A baseline quantitative fibrinogen is drawn when local intra-arterial fibrinolytic therapy is initiated, and it is repeated every hour to assess the systemic effects of therapy. Systemic anticoagulation with heparin is used to maintain clotting times two to three times the laboratory control value. Serial angiographic injections and neurologic evaluations are done to detect manifestations of intracranial hemorrhage. In the absence of hemorrhagic complications, fibrino-

lytic infusion is continued until the angiographic findings that formed the basis for initiating fibrinolytic therapy resolve or excessive fibrinogen depletion occurs; that is, the quantitative fibrinogen drops below 100 mg/dl.

Surgery is rarely required. Intracranial surgical embolectomy is a heroic measure. It is seldom remedial in cerebral embolism of insoluble particulate material secondary to plaque fragmentation. Interarterial bypass may be indicated in extracranial arterial dissection without embolization because tissue viability is usually prolonged by collateral flow. Acute occlusion of the target vessel, resulting from dissection, may be treated by placing a temporary stenting catheter, or a permanent implantable stent, to restore perfusion (see following discussion).

Acute neurologic decompensation is usually related to structural damage which leads to vaso-occlusion caused by thrombus or arterial dissection. Occasionally, however, transient neurologic dysfunction is due to cerebral hypoperfusion produced by balloon inflation, in which case, balloon deflation is corrective.

In cases of vessel rupture, control of bleeding is paramount. Remedial therapy includes reversal of anticoagulation with protamine and temporary or permanent therapeutic occlusion of the target vessel at the site of rupture using neurointerventional embolotherapy.[12] Depending on lesion location, it may be possible to avoid sacrificing the damaged vessel by means of a stent.

POSTOPERATIVE MANAGEMENT

Following angioplasty, the patient is transferred to an intensive care unit, ordinarily the neurologic intensive care unit. A follow-up CT or MRI scan is performed after 24 hours to look for subclinical, ischemic cerebral damage. Systemic anticoagulation may be (1) reversed with protamine, (2) continued for 18 to 48 hours, (3) re-initiated after a pause to remove the catheter or sheath, or (4) continued indefinitely by means of Coumadin. The regimen of choice depends on several factors. For example, we continue systemic anticoagulation for at least 24 hours, in all patients who require postdilation fibrinolytic therapy for in situ thrombosis. Sustained heparinization is used in angioplasty of intracranial vessels because our experience suggests a significant increase in the rate of in situ thrombosis in these vessels. Patients with intra- or extracranial lesions that have an irregular lumen or intimal flap following angioplasty are anticoagulated for up to 5 days, depending on the degree of luminal irregularity and intimal tearing. Patients who are hypercoagulable are maintained on heparin, followed by Coumadin for weeks and in some instances months. We use low-molecular-weight dextran, as an alternative to heparin, in cases of heparin toxicity. All patients are indefinitely maintained on platelet antiaggregates, usually aspirin. The patient is counseled on personal habits and lifestyles that may increase the risk for recurrent ischemic neurologic events. Particular emphasis is placed on abstinence from tobacco products and control of systemic blood pressure.

FOLLOW-UP

We repeat conventional arteriography at 6 to 12 months. When the patient or referring clinician refuses this form of follow-up, we use duplex sonography or MR angiography. Duplex sonography and MR angiography are accurate in detecting restenosis for most lesions distal to the common carotid artery, but they have variable reliability for more proximal lesions. We attempt to obtain clinical follow-up at 3 to 6 months, and again at 1 year.

SHORT AND LONG-TERM RESULTS

Despite the time elapsed since the first reported cerebral angioplasty, reliable data concerning its therapeutic effectiveness are scarce. In particular, no comparative studies have assessed its benefits relative to therapeutic alternatives. Little can be concluded based on the retrospective series of cases that comprise the bulk of patients reported to date. The only prospective data derived from a protocol-based multicenter study with inclusion/exclusion criteria and a primary hypothesis were reported in preliminary form in 1993. That report comprises 113 angioplasties in 102 symptomatic nonsurgical patients. The average stenosis pre-CPTA was 80%. The average stenosis immediately postangioplasty was 30%, yielding a mean difference of 50%. Major complications included death, which occurred in 2 of 113 angioplasties, and stroke, which occurred in an additional 8 angioplasties, resulting in a combined major complication rate of 8.8%.

There are no definitive reports concerning the long-term results of CPTA. It appears that patients who have a successful cerebral angioplasty do well for several months; however, this notion is based on uncontrolled, retrospective data with incomplete patient follow-up. There is a general belief that the restenosis rate is similar to that observed in angioplasty of vessels of similar caliber in other vascular territories. NACPTAR data are currently being analyzed to assess this proposition; however, definitive comparative studies with long-term follow-up are required to establish CPTA's therapeutic role and durability.

CURRENT INDICATIONS

Nonbrachiocephalic CPTA should be attempted only by multidisciplinary teams, with formal training in the anatomy, pathophysiology, prognosis, and treatment of occlusive cerebrovascular disease. Until definitive therapeutic studies are published and accepted by the medical community, nonbrachiocephalic CPTA should be performed under the auspices of an Institutional Review Board approved investigational protocol, except under extraordinary circumstances. While CPTA has been used primarily in symptomatic nonsurgical patients with quantitatively significant stenoses, who have failed medical therapy, recent studies[13,14] have prompted re-evaluation of whether a preliminary trial of medical therapy is mandatory. Also, the concept of hemodynamic significance is changing. While the final report of the ACAS[11] has yet to be published in a peer-reviewed journal, the National Institute of Neurological Disorders and Stroke (NINDS) advisory regarding the trial, suggests an elevated stroke risk for stenoses less than 70%, as well as the benefit of internal carotid artery revascularization in asymptomatic patients.

COSTS

No reliable estimates have been made of the relative cost of CPTA and surgery for lesions that are amenable to both approaches. Projections concerning relative long-term costs are pointless because no reliable data are available concerning reintervention and late clinical follow-up. If CPTA is clinically effective it could reduce short-term costs such as those related to anesthesia and length of hospital stay, as well as blood typing, screening, and transfusion.

DISCUSSION (CURRENT OUTLOOK AND POTENTIAL DEVELOPMENTS)

Cerebral Protection Strategies

The greatest impediment to cerebral angioplasty is the fear of embolic complications caused by plaque disruption.[4,15] Though the incidence of clinically significant embolism has been lower than anticipated, a practicable system or technique that reduces the probability or consequences of distal embolization would be indispensable. Proposed systems include those advocated by Theron,[16] Ferguson,[17] and Koike.[18] While elements of these methods are theoretically appealing, they have practical limitations,[17] and there is no compelling evidence establishing their efficacy.

Perfusion Devices

Perfusion devices are a form of mechanical cerebral protection designed to reduce the risk of hypoperfusion injury that is associated with temporary flow arrest during balloon inflation.[4] This form of protection uses extracorporeal bypass with autologous, heparinized arterial blood injected through the angioplasty catheter. It is assumed that the system delivers enough oxygen, to prevent permanent ischemic damage resulting from balloon-induced hypoperfusion. This practice has not been widely adopted due to the fact that balloon-associated hypoperfusion is short lived and therefore, unlikely to cause permanent neuronal damage. The role of this technique in preserving cerebral perfusion, in CPTA complicated by abrupt arterial occlusion, has not been investigated.

Stenting Catheters and Implantable Stents

Evidence from randomized trials indicates that coronary stenting, in adequately sized arteries, is associated with better initial results and a lower rate of restenosis than angioplasty alone.[19,20] Moreover, in the hands of some operators, stent implantation is successful in as high as 95% of cases.[21,22] These observations have led to speculation about the possible use of primary stenting in the cerebral circulation. Primary stenting in selected patients warrants further study. Anecdotal experience suggests a better initial technical result in some cerebrovascular occlusive lesions, that is, increased postprocedure diameter, which is regarded as the most important determinant of long-term success/patency. In addition, stents may prevent or reduce the incidence of distal embolization, associated with plaque fragmentation and secondary thromboembolism, from thrombus-laden ulcers. These theoretical advantages have stimulated interest in developing a protocol to evaluate primary stenting for the treatment of cerebrovascular occlusive disease.

The use of stents for vascular rescue following dissection or intraplaque hemorrhage is less controversial. Of several methods proposed to treat immediate occlusion complicating cerebral angioplasty, stenting appears to be the most promising; however, the practical limitations of current stent-delivery systems restrict this form of therapy. When occlusion secondary to dissection complicates CPTA, and stenting is unfeasible, the simplest approach involves reinflation of the balloon to appose the intimal flap, while maintaining systemic anticoagulation. This is done for an extended period of time, usually at a lower pressure than that used for angioplasty. This maneuver can provoke ischemia because it prevents translesional blood flow; if it is unsuccessful, a stenting catheter can be used as an internal conduit. The stenting catheter provides temporary restoration of blood flow until surgical correction is possible.

Direct Angioplasty in Acute Thromboembolic Occlusion

The use of intracranial CPTA has been restricted, until now, to the treatment of luminal narrowing as a consequence of plaque or cerebral vasospasm. Direct angioplasty for thromboembolic occlusion has not been studied in the cerebral circulation due to concerns about the possibility of clot propagation into vital perforating or cortical branches. Recently, however, we have, in a single case, successfully performed angioplasty as the initial maneuver to restore flow in acute middle cerebral artery thromboembolic occlusion. Further study is warranted to evaluate angioplasty's role in the treatment of hyperacute stroke.

REFERENCES

1. Eskridge JM, Newell DW, Pendelton GA. Transluminal angioplasty for treatment of vasospasm. Neurosurg Clin North Am 1990;321–33
2. Kerber CW, Cromwell LD, Leohden OL. Catheter dilatation of proximal stenosis during distal bifurcation endarterectomy. Am J Neuroradiol 1980;1:348–9
3. Mullan S, Duda EE, Patro NAS. Some examples of balloon technology in neurosurgery. J Neurosurg 1980;52:321–9
4. Tsai FY, Matovich V, Hieshima G et al. Percutaneous angioplasty of the carotid artery. Am J Neuroradiol 1986;7:349–58
5. Becker G, Katzen B, Dake M. Noncoronary angioplasty. Radiology 1989;170:921–40
6. Kachel R, Basche S, Heerklotz I et al. Percutaneous transluminal angioplasty (PTA) of supra-aortic arteries especially the internal carotid artery. Neuroradiology 1991;33:191–4
7. Theron J. Angioplasty of brachiocephalic vessels. pp. 167–80. In Vinuela F, Halbach VV, Dion JE (eds): Interventional Neuroradiology: Endovascular Therapy of the Central Nervous System. New York, Raven Press, 1992
8. Munari LM, Belloni G, Perretti A et al. Carotid percutaneous angioplasty. Neurol Res 1992;4(suppl.):156–8
9. Landau C, Lange RA, Hillis LD. Percutaneous transluminal angioplasty. N Engl J Med 1994;330:981–93
10. Fuster V, Badimon L, Badimon JJ, Chesebro JH. The Pathogenesis of coronary artery disease and the acute coronary syndromes. Part 1. N Engl J Med 1992;326:242–50
11. Investigators of the Asymptomatic Carotid Atherosclerosis Study (ACAS). Clinical Advisory on Carotid Endarterectomy for Patients with Asymptomatic Carotid Artery Stenosis. National Institute of Neurological Disorders and Stroke Clinical Alert, September 30, 1994
12. Philips CD, Ferguson RDG. The contribution of interventional neuroradiology in selected vascular lesions of the head and neck. Adv Plast Reconstr Surg 1989; 8
13. European Carotid Surgery Trialists' Collaborative Group: MRC European Surgery Trial Interim results for symptomatic patients with severe (70 to 99%) or with mild (0% to 29%) carotid stenosis. Lancet 1991; 337:1235–43
14. North American Symptomatic Carotid Endarterectomy Trial Collaborators. Beneficial effect of carotid endarterectomy in symptomatic patients with high grade carotid stenosis. N Engl J Med 1991;325:445–53
15. Imparato AM, Rilez TS, Ecorstein F. The carotid bifurcation plaque: pathologic findings associated with cerebral ischemia. Stroke 1979;10:238–245
16. Theron J, Courtheoux P, Alachkar F, Maiza D. New triple coaxial catheter system for carotid angioplasty with cerebral protection. Am J Neuroradiol 1990;11:869–74
17. Ferguson R. Getting it right the first time. Am J Neuroradiol 1990;11:875–7
18. Koike T, Minakawa T, Abe H et al. PTA of supra-aortic arteries with temporary balloon occlusion to avoid distal embolism. Neurol Med Chir (Tokyo) 1992;32:140–7
19. Serruys PW, de Jaegere P, Kiemeneij F et al. A comparison of balloon-expandable-stent implantation with balloon angioplasty in patients with coronary artery disease. Benestent Study Group. Engl J Med 1994;331:489–95
20. Fischman DL, Leon MB, Baim DS et al. A randomized comparison of coronary-stent placement and balloon angioplasty in the treatment of coronary artery disease. Stent Restenosis Study Investigators. N Eng J Med 1994; 331:496–501
21. Haude M, Erbel R, Hafner G et al. Multicenter results after coronary implantation of balloon-expandable Plamaz-Shatz stents. Z Cardiol 1993;82:77–86
22. George BS, Voorhes WD, III, Roubin GS et al. Multicenter investigation of coronary stenting to treat acute or threatened closure after percutaneous transluminal angioplasty; clinical and angiographic outcome. J Am Coll Cardiol 1993;22:135–43

85 Endoluminal Treatment of Venous Stenoses

F. Joffre
H. Rousseau
P. Tregant

In the treatment of vascular affections, percutaneous endoluminal techniques, in particular percutaneous transluminal angioplasty (PTA), have been applied principally in arterial pathology, frequently neglecting venous pathology. Several reasons may explain this neglect.

- Venous pathology is more unusual and is less threatening for the patient.
- The different histopathologic nature of the lesions may have explained the poor results of balloon angioplasty in the treatment of these lesions.

The development of metallic endoprostheses has led to a reconsideration of the endoluminal treatment of venous lesions and to proposal of use of these methods in certain indications, particularly for the treatment of arteriovenous fistula for dialysis (AVFD) obstructions and for the treatment of large venous trunk obstructions (superior and inferior vena cava and their principal afferent branches).

ENDOLUMINAL TREATMENT OF OBSTRUCTIVE LESIONS OF AVFD

The quality of life and the survival, of renal-insufficiency patients depend largely on the correct functioning of their AVFD. Punctured more than 150 times per year by large trocars, and submitted to an intense hemodynamic flow, AVFD may lead to complications, resulting in the loss of venous access, imposing the creation of a secondary AVFD, and thus diminishing the possibility of further AVFD. The objective of endoluminal treatment in this case is to maximize the preservation of these AVFD.

Transluminal Angioplasty of AVFD Stenoses

The risk of acute thrombosis and the loss of vascular access impose a rapid and efficacious treatment of these stenoses. A precise morphologic evaluation by angiography is necessary before any therapeutic choice is made.[1] The stenosis is found either at the arteriovenous anastomosis or at the venous component of the fistula.

Technique[2,3]

The vascular approach is achieved by a retrograde puncture for distal lesions or an anterograde puncture for proximal lesions. When edema is present, sonography may be used to guide the puncture. After opacification, the balloon caliber is chosen.

A 5-F balloon catheter, 3 to 4 cm long and 6 to 12 mm in diameter, depending on the case, is used. The balloon should sustain an elevated pressure, greater than 15 atm.[4] Insufflation should be prolonged (1 to 2 minutes) with heparin protection (3,000 U in situ). This may be painful, and thus, perivenous local anesthesia in the dilation zone is necessary. Frequently, a residual stenosis persists on the balloon, leading to a repeated dilation using a catheter with a greater caliber as well as higher pressure and for a duration of 2 to 3 minutes.

If the control angiogram shows significant parietal damage, a prolonged dilation to remodel the vascular lumen is performed. After catheter removal, prolonged compression is necessary. Except in cases for which immediate hemodialysis following the procedure is essential, the intervention may be performed on an outpatient basis.

Results

Complications are rare. In 1 to 2% of cases, rupture at the dilation site with contrast material leakage may be encountered. Most frequently, this resolves after compression, but sometimes, a pseudo-aneurysm forms, and surgical repair is indicated. Infectious complications are generally prevented by routine aseptic measures. Thrombus formation is exceptional.

Immediate results are satisfactory (Figs. 85-1 and 85-2) in 70 to 90% of cases, depending on the series. Long-term results are poor, because only 45% of treated vessels are patent at 1 year and only 12% at 2 years. The delay of restenosis is variable, occurring between 2 months and 2 years, but seemingly constant in the same patient. These stenoses may benefit from repeated balloon angioplasties, which have the advantage of maintaining the venous structures without a surgical intervention. Long-term results depend on the type of lesion treated. Stenoses that are long, greater than 3 cm, respond poorly to PTA. In addition, distal lesions recur more easily than proximal ones.

Indications

The indications depend on the type of lesion. Anastomotic stenoses should be treated only when the flow is insufficient for appropriate dialysis, and in the presence of an important risk for thrombosis formation. These stenoses, often angulated, may be difficult to dilate, and surgical repair may be preferred in such cases. Proximal stenoses of the venous side, on the other hand, are excellent indications for PTA.

Endoprostheses and AVFD Stenoses

Endoprostheses and AVFD stenoses complete the endoluminal treatment possibilities and, thus, improve PTA results[5,6] (Fig. 85-3).

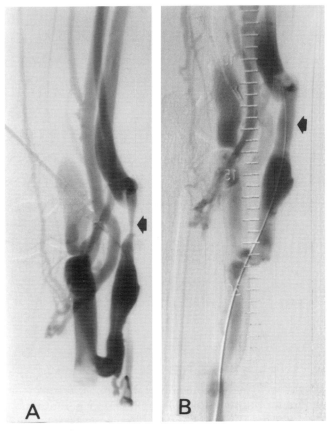

Fig. 85-1. Endoluminal treatment of an AVDF stenosis. **(A)** Tight stenosis of the venous segment of a Cimmino-Brescia AVDF (*arrow*). **(B)** Good result immediately after PTA (*arrow*).

Technique

The principal types of available stents for this purpose are Gianturco, Palmaz, Strecker, and Wallstent, each having their advantages and their drawbacks.[7-10] According to the literature, the Wallstent endoprosthesis has been the most used.[11] The implantation technique is the same as for the PTA. The diameter is chosen as a function of the opacification, taking into account the x-ray magnification: To avoid secondary displacement, a 1-mm greater diameter than the true lumen of the vessel is necessary. In the case of a long lesion, several endoprostheses may be inserted end to end, with a slight overlapping. Vascular access should not, however, be prevented by the presence of the endoprosthesis; the puncture through it is impossible. The endoprosthesis is placed under in situ heparin cover (3 to 5,000 U).

Results

The initial success rate is near 100% in most reported series, with absence of residual stenosis, disappearance of symptoms, and continued normal hemodi-

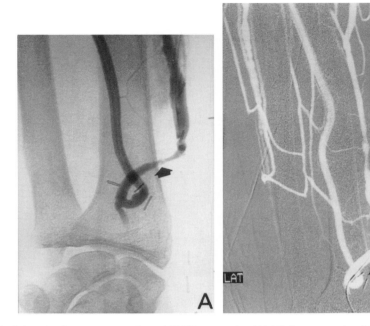

Fig. 85-2. Endoluminal treatment of an AVDF stenosis. **(A)** Tight stenosis of the venous segment of a Cimmino-Brescia AVDF (*arrow*). **(B)** Good result immediately after PTA (*arrow*).

alysis. The complication rate is greater than in PTA alone, with a risk of acute thrombosis in 8% of cases, despite the use of in situ heparin. This complication most often is due to inadequate implantation and may be treated by in situ thrombolysis and the placement of a new endoprosthesis as a complement. Other complications are exceptional.

Angiographic follow-up shows the appearance of intimal hyperplasia inside the stent. This hyperplasia leads to restenosis in most of the cases; but this occurs with a variable delay, from 3 months to 3 years. Primary patency is 50% at 1 year. These restenoses, however, are accessible to a second endoluminal intervention (a simple PTA, an atherectomy of the Simpson type or placement of a new stent). Secondary patency, thus obtained, is 82% at 1 year, 79% at 2 years, and 71% at 3 years. The best results are obtained when the vein is of large caliber.[6]

Indications[7,11]

Endoprostheses have two main advantages:

- The immediate success rate is 100%, and dialysis may thus be undertaken instantly.
- Despite the risk of restenosis, the reintervention rate is reduced by 7 as compared to PTA alone. Its use, however, cannot be systematic, given its much

greater cost, as well as a higher percentage of possible complications.

Endoprostheses may not be used at the puncture zone. They should be reserved for stenoses resistant to balloon PTA, for large dissections and obstructions, and repeated restenoses within a short interval, less than 3 months.

Endoluminal Treatment of Acute Obstructions of AVFD

Acute obstruction by thrombosis is a major complication that should be rapidly diagnosed and treated to conserve vascular access in hemodialyzed patients.[12] It is most often secondary to a resistant stenosis, unknown or neglected, or occurring during a sudden fall in blood pressure. Percutaneous treatment should, most often, treat the thrombosis, then, if possible, reduce the responsible stenosis (see Fig. 85-3).

The method of treatment of these stenoses has already been discussed. The treatment of acute thrombosis relies on in situ fibrinolysis. Most fibrinolytic protocols use urokinase. This treatment is administered after having eliminated the classic contraindications of thrombolysis (recent surgery, previous stroke, hemorrhage) and after checking of correct hemostatic parameters. After puncture, the guide is brought in contact with the clot, traversing it to ob-

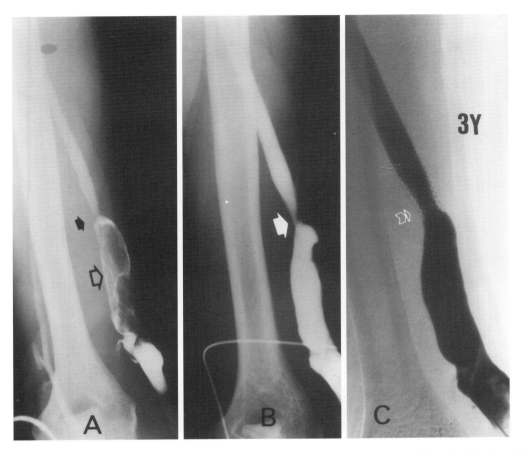

Fig. 85-3. Endoluminal treatment of an AVDF stenosis. **(A)** Acute thrombosis of a vein distal to AVDF (*arrow*) that is due to a tight stenosis (*black arrow*). **(B)** Result after thrombolysis. **(C)** Control 3 years after stenting of the AVDF stenosis (*white arrow*).

tain better contact between the drug and the clot. The catheter presents lateral holes for a length of 5 to 10 cm, permitting the injection of urokinase under pressure into the clot. After injecting a starting dose of 75,000 to 100,000 U of urokinase, the in situ fibrinolysis is then administered at a rate of 30,000 to 40,000 U/h by an electric syringe. The catheter is progressively advanced during the treatment into the clot to obtain total lysis. Prophylactic antibiotic therapy is systematically added. After 3 to 4 hours, control generally shows total lysis of the thrombus, if the treatment was begun early. If few thrombotic fragments persist, adherent to the wall, their disappearance by natural lysis is probable. Treatment of the responsible lesion is then realized by PTA or by endoprosthesis placement.

Recently, other techniques have supplemented the therapeutic methods for acute thrombosis:

- Thromboaspiration permits clot removal, on condition that it is of small quantity, and that there is no blood flow. This may be associated with thrombolysis. A large-diameter catheter (8 to 9 F) is used with a large lumen; which, when brought into contact with the thrombus, allows the aspiration and removal of thrombotic fragments.
- Other methods are in the course of evaluation: mechanical thrombolyzer and rheolytic thrombolyzer.

Conclusion

Endoluminal methods may be used largely for maintaining the permeability of vascular access in patients undergoing periodic hemodialysis. Even if the long-term patency results are poor, the combination of the different percutaneous methods and their eventual repetition permit the circumvention of the multiple surgical interventions that patients had to undergo previously. The low morbidity, simplicity, and noninvasive nature of these procedures permit their realization on an outpatient basis.

ENDOLUMINAL TREATMENT IN OBSTRUCTIVE LESIONS OF THE LARGE VENOUS TRUNKS

Until recently, stenotic lesions of the large venous trunks (inferior and superior vena cava and their afferent branches) rarely have been treated using endoluminal techniques. The development of endoprostheses has changed this situation and now permits an elegant therapeutic solution for clinical problems that are frequently difficult to manage and treat.

The most common lesions concern the superior vena cava system and may be dramatic in the case of sudden onset of superior vena cava syndrome.[13] These patients present, in fact, with stenoses of the superior vena cava or its branches, which evolve progressively but may be complicated rapidly by an acute thrombosis. The most frequent cause is malignant pathology, dominated by pulmonary cancer with mediastinal extension (75 to 90% of cases.) In these situations, radiotherapy or chemotherapy are not immediately effective and may not be repeated. Despite a relatively short survival rate, endoprosthesis placement allows for a simple and unaggressive treatment, giving the patient acceptable comfort, in particular, suppressing the violent headaches secondary to venous stasis. Benign stenoses may be encountered (postradiation fibrosis, aortic aneurysm compression, stenoses distal to AVFD).

The lesions of the inferior vena cava are less frequent. Most often, they are due to compression by tumors or retroperitoneal fibrosis, usually malignant. A particular cause should be noted, corresponding to stenoses of the distal end of the inferior vena cava associated stenoses of the hepatic veins in the context of the Budd-Chiari syndrome.

In all cases, the misdiagnosis leads to a complete occlusion of the venous system, thus leading to more

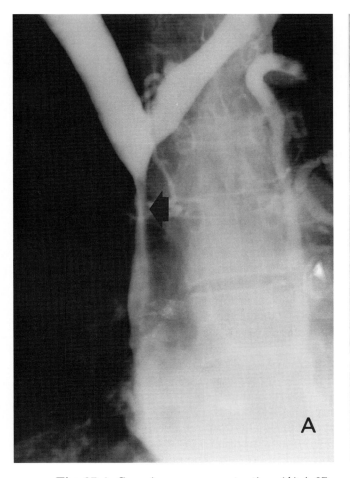
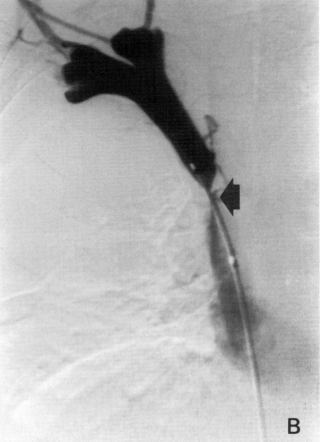

Fig. 85-4. Superior vena cava stenting. **(A)** A 67-year-old woman with caval syndrome that is probably due to mediastinal fibrosis after radiotherapy for mammary tumor. The front view of inferior vena cava phlebography shows a regular tight stenosis of the superior vena cava (*arrow*). **(B)** Control after balloon PTA showing a persisting stenosis. (*Figure continues.*)

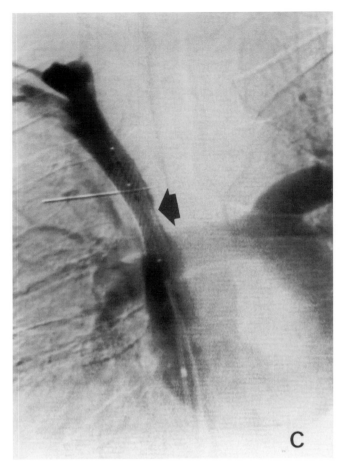 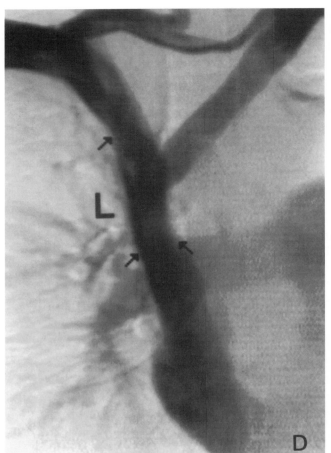

Fig. 85-4 (*Continued*). **(C)** Immediate result after stenting (*arrow*). **(D)** Excellent patency 1 year after the placement of the stent.

difficulties for endoluminal treatment and impossibility in some cases.

Technique

A multiplane (front and lateral view) angiographic exploration of the caval system is necessary for correctly appreciating the vascular diameter and the exact topography of the lesions, especially in relation to the bifurcations. In the case of a total occlusion, presumably related to a recent thrombus, in situ fibrinolysis should be initially realized as described previously. The lesion is then crossed using a metallic guidewire. A hydrophilic guidewire is particularly useful in cases of total occlusion. Failure to cross the lesion is possible, leading to another vascular approach. Passage of the stenosis by the catheter may be difficult, which may lead to using the "pull-through" technique with a double puncture (brachial and femoral veins) and external recuperation of the guidewire at the femoral region, with a basket-type probe. This technique allows for the stabilization of the guide and facilitates catheter progression. A rigid guide should be employed. The following step consists of dilating the lesion with a balloon (sometimes two kissing balloons for the superior or inferior vena cava) and using high pressure (greater than 12 bars) for at least 2 minutes.

Given the elastic and resistant nature of these lesions, endoprosthetic placement is practically constant.[14,15]

Three types of endoprostheses have been used by different groups for treating these lesions: the Wallstent endoprosthesis,[10] the Gianturco endoprosthesis,[14] and the Palmaz endoprosthesis.[9] The type chosen should be of a sufficient diameter (10 to 30 mm) and greater than 10% of the venous diameter to avoid migration. The endoprosthesis should also present a radial force sufficient for resisting against the parietal pressure. A long endoprosthesis should be selected, to ensure its stabilization, particularly in diaphragmatic stenoses. In cases of a long stenosis, endoprostheses may be placed end to end, with a slight overlapping.

In the literature, the Gianturco endoprosthesis has been most widely used, particularly for the large-caliber veins.[8] Because of its poor stability, however, there is a tendency to replace it with the Wallstent type, whose autoexpandability prevents its migration, as well as adapting to sinuous veins by its flexibility. This prosthesis, nevertheless, has the disadvantage of having a low radiopacity.[16]

The Palmaz endoprosthesis, because of its rigidity, may be preferred in the case of a highly resistant stenosis, but its short length limits its use.

The endoprosthesis is released by a 7- to 9-F catheter, depending on the model, at the level of the lesion, which has been carefully located. In the case of the autoexpandable type (Wallstent), its opening may be accelerated by a second dilation inside the prosthesis. The intervention is realized with an in situ injection of 5,000 U of heparin.

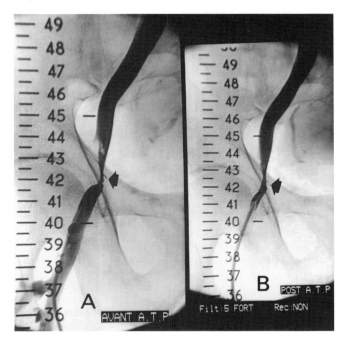

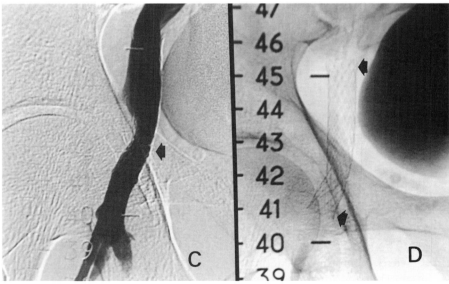

Fig. 85-5. External iliac vein stenting. **(A)** Stenosis of the external iliac vein *(arrow)* secondary to extrinsic fibrosis that is due to surgical treatment of eventration with a plastic plaque. **(B)** Result after balloon PTA with absence of effect. **(C)** Excellent patency after stent placement *(arrow)* **(D)** The Wallstent-type endoprosthesis in place *(arrow).*

Results

Whatever type of endoprosthesis is used, the results are practically identical.[16] The results are immediately satisfactory in almost 100% of cases, on condition that the lesion could be crossed. Collateral circulation—facial, upper or lower member edema—decreases, as well as the clinical symptoms. Immediate failure is exceptional and is due to endoprosthetic migration or misplacement, which is manifested by a recurrence or aggravation of symptoms secondary to acute thrombosis. The patient should be re-treated by in situ thrombolysis and by a second stent insertion. Complications are rare, occurring in less than 1% of cases (bacteremia, puncture site hematoma, endoprosthetic migration).

Long-term patency depends on etiology and duration of patient survival. In cases of malignant lesions, the large majority of patients die, with a patent stent. In some cases of slow evolutivity, restenosis by tumor proliferation may sometimes occur. A new treatment can eventually be proposed.

In cases of benign lesions, the patency rate is difficult to evaluate, given the low number of reported cases (Figs. 85-4 and 85-5). Restenosis by intimal hyperplasia, at the extremities or the center of the prosthesis, may occur rapidly within 2 to 3 months or after a greater delay (1 to 2 years.) A new endoluminal treatment can then be envisaged. The particular case of Budd-Chiari syndrome should be discussed because certain lesions (diaphragm) react favorably to PTA and do not always necessitate an endoprosthesis.

Indications

More than 100 patients presenting with occlusive lesions of the large venous trunks have been reported in the literature.[8] The treatment of superior vena cava syndrome secondary to neoplasia appears justified because of its associated morbidity and because it is life-threatening. This simple and fast treatment allows patients to indisputably improve their quality of life, even if the survival duration is short. These endoprostheses may be placed on an emergency basis in cases of acute obstruction and before radiotherapy.

The treatment in the case of benign obstruction is more controversial, given that long-term restenosis is unavoidable and justifies repeated treatments. The prevention of acute thrombosis, however, which may be catastrophic, justifies managing these patients by endoluminal treatment.

CONCLUSION

Venous lesions have been neglected for a long time by interventional radiology. Their natural course is, in fact, different from that of arterial lesions. PTA may be efficient during several months. Endoprosthetic use represents a certain, but not definitive, progress. Most patients, with the exception of those with neoplastic stenoses, for which treatment is palliative, will have to submit to several endoluminal interventions to maintain patency permeability of their venous system. This is, nevertheless, indispensable to avoid an acute thrombosis, which may be dramatic.

These results, however, must be compared with surgical treatment, which is particularly associated with consequences, and frequently is impossible, especially in cases of lesions of the large veins of the superior and inferior caval systems.

REFERENCES

1. Gilula IA, Staple TW, Anderson CB, Anderson LS. Venous angiography of hemodialysis fistulae. Radiology 1975;115:555
2. Daniell SJN, Dacie JE. Percutaneous transluminal angioplasty of brachiocephalic vein stenoses in patients with dialysis shunts. Radiology 1988;169:280–1
3. Heidler R, Zeitler E, Gessler U. Percutaneous transluminal dilatation of stenosis behind av-fistulas in hemodialysis patients. p. 142. In: Percutaneous Vascular Recanalization. Springer-Verlag, New York, 1978
4. Glanz S, Gordon DH, Butt KMH et al. Stenotic lesions in dialysis access fistulas: treatment by transluminal angioplasty using high-pressure balloons. Radiology 1985;156:236
5. Quinn SF, Schuman ES, Hall L et al. Venous stenoses in patients who undergo hemodialysis: treatment with self-expandable endovascular stents. Radiology 1992;183:499–504
6. Turmel-Rodrigues J, Pengloan J, Blanchier D et al. Insufficient dialysis shunts: improved long-term patency rates with close hemodynamic monitoring, repeated percutaneous balloon angioplasty, and stent placement. Radiology 1993;187:273–8
7. Antonucci F, Salomonowitz E, Stuckmann G et al. Placement of venous stents: clinical experience with a self-expanding prosthesis. Radiology 1992;183:493–7
8. Irving JD, Dondelinger RF, Reidy JF et al. Gianturco self-expanding stents: clinical experience in the vena cava and large veins. Cardiovasc Intervent Radiol 1992;15:328–33
9. Palmaz J, Sibbit RR, Reuter SR. Expandable intraluminal graft: a preliminary study. Radiology 1985;156:73–7
10. Rousseau H, Puel J, Joffre F. Self-expanding endovascular prosthesis: an experimental study. Radiology 1987;164:709–14
11. Rousseau H, Morfaux V, Joffre F et al. Treatment of haemodialysis arterio-venous fistula stenosis by per-

cutaneous implantation of new intravascular stent. J Intervent Radiol 1989;4:161–7

12. Caruana RJ, Raja RR, Zeit RM. Thrombotic complications of indwelling central catheters used for chronic hemodialysis. Am J Kidney Dis 1987;9:497–501

13. Lokich JJ, Goodman R. Superior vena caval syndrome: clinical management. JAMA 1975;231:58–61

14. Rosch J, Uchida BT, Hall LD et al. Gianturco-Rösch expandable Z-stents in the treatment of superior vena cava syndrome. Cardiovasc Intervent Radiol 1992;15: 319–27

15. Zollikofer CI, Antonucci F, Struckmann G et al. Use of the wallstent in the venous system including hemodialysis-related stenoses. Cardiovasc Intervent Radiol 1992;15:334–41

16. Zollikofer CL, Largiader I, Bruhlmann WF et al. Endovascular stenting of veins and grafts: preliminary clinical experience. Radiology 1988;167:707–12

Ventral Septal Defect and Other Intracardiac Shunt Closures

86

Andrew Redington

HISTORY

Transcatheter closure of extracardiac shunts (e.g, Patent Ductus Arteriosus [PDA], aortopulmonary collaterals, etc.) has a long history and is now part of accepted clinical practice. The history of transcatheter closure of intracardiac shunt is much shorter, and to some extent the various techniques remain experimental. The first series using an umbrella-like system to close atrial septal defects was reported in 1976.[1] Successful closure was achieved in 5 of 10 patients, but the device was large and delivery complex. It was not until the late 1980s that the use of potentially clinically useful devices were reported. Several devices are in development, but to date, the Food and Drug Administration (FDA) has not fully approved any of these devices for routine clinical use. Thus, any procedures performed should be part of an experimental protocol with fully informed patient and institutional approval.

RATIONALE AND MECHANISM OF ACTION

The reasons for pursuing transcatheter techniques for closure of intracardiac defects are clear. Surgical closure requires median sternotomy and cardiopulmonary bypass, and particularly in patients who have undergone previous surgery, the avoidance of surgical morbidity and mortality are major potential benefits.

All of these devices follow a broad pattern. There is an occluding disk of fabric, supported by a metal framework of some sort, and a counteroccluding portion, which lies on the other side of the septal structure being closed. Because the atrial septum is a relatively thin structure, some degree of enforced apposition of the distal and proximal occluding devices is required. This has been achieved using a variety of techniques.

INSTRUMENTATION

Although clinical experience is limited with all of the devices described in this section, we will concentrate on the three most commonly used.

1. The clamshell device[2]
2. Modified Rashkind umbrella[3]
3. Sideris buttoned occluder device[4]

The Clamshell

The clamshell device evolved from the Rashkind double umbrella duct-occluding device. The concept is similar. There are counteroccluding Dacron fabric disks, each mounted on hinged and sprung metal supporting arms. The key difference is the additional hinge point in each of the arms of the occluder and counteroccluder. This ensures circumferential apposition and thus makes residual leak and embolization less likely. The delivery system (11 F) and technique of the deployment follow the broad principles of delivery of the Rashkind umbrella device. The size of the device ranges from 17 to 45 mm.

Modified Rashkind Umbrella

The modified Rashkind umbrella and lock clamshell device has limited applications because of the relatively small size of the currently available Rashkind devices. The unmodified umbrella device does not achieve circumferential apposition and so would be unstable in some defects. This is overcome by placing a gentle bend in each of the arms of both the proximal and distal umbrellas (Fig. 86-1), so that when the device is fully deployed, arms and material overlap with potential apposition of the umbrellas themselves. The technique of deployment is identical to that for the arterial duct, although occasionally downsizing of the delivery system (see following discussion) is required to reduce the overall sheath size in smaller patients.

The Sideris Buttoned Occluder Device

The Sideris buttoned occluder device uses the same general principle, but its key difference is that the occluding and counteroccluding elements are initially separate and are joined during the process of deployment. The occluder is a square of fabric mounted between a crossing metal support. The single-span counteroccluder has a perforated latex central portion through which the button of the occluding device is drawn (Fig. 86-2). Both occluder and counteroccluder are passed longitudinally through the delivery sheath, which significantly reduces the necessary sheath size. Device diameters range from 17 to 50 mm, and the delivery sheath required ranges from 5 to 8 F.

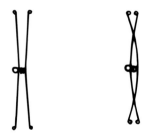

Fig. 86-1. (A & B) Modification of the standard Rashkind double umbrella device by placing a gentle bend in each of the arms. This produces overlapping when in the deployed state. This enables circumferential apposition so that there is stability in thin-walled structures such as the atrial septum. (From Redington and Rigby,[3] with permission.)

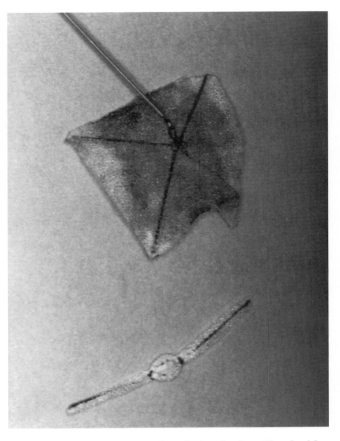

Fig. 86-2. Sideris buttoned occluder device. The double-spanned distal occluder can be seen attached to its delivery system. Note the button marked with a radiopaque marker. On the right is the single-spanned counteroccluding device.

INDICATIONS AND PATIENT SELECTION

All of these devices have been used primarily to close naturally occurring and iatrogenic atrial septal defects. They have all, to a greater or lesser extent, also found a role in the closure of the ventricular septal defects. The clamshell and modified ductal device have also been used to close unusual intracardiac shunts such as perivalvular leaks, sinus of valsalva aneurysm, and so on, but experience is limited.

Atrial Septal Defects

Naturally occurring secundum atrial septal defects are by definition defects in the floor of the oval fossa. They can, however, excavate toward the superior and inferior caval veins, coronary sinus, and posterior wall of the aorta. It is this extension from the confines of the oval fossa itself that makes some secundum atrial septal defects unsuitable for transcatheter closure. Careful evaluation by transthoracic cross-sectional echocardiography will identify some defects that are either too large (over 25 mm), or whose margins make transcatheter closure unfavorable. The final arbiter, however, must be transesophageal echocardiography. This technique allows full delineation of the extent of the atrial septal defect. It is a crucial part of the preprocedural evaluation as well as being fundamental to the success of the procedure itself, which without transesophageal echocardiographic guidance would be difficult to perform. Primum atrial septal defects, coronary sinus, or sinus venosus atrial septal defects cannot be considered for transcatheter closure. This is because of their proximity to other important intracardiac structures that would make device closure hazardous.

Iatrogenic interatrial communications are generally smaller than naturally occurring secondary defects. The most common form is the surgically created fenestration in the intra-atrial baffle at the time of the fenestrated Fontan procedure. The indications and rationale for this procedure are beyond the scope of this chapter, but closure of these defects can easily be achieved using any of the devices described previously.

Ventricular Septal Defect

The indications for transcatheter closure of ventricular septal defects are even more limited than that for the atrial septal defects. This is because of their proximity to important structures within the heart.

Muscular defects, ideally those placed in the apical trabecular portion, are most suitable for device closure. This is because they are generally the most difficult to close surgically (sometimes requiring left ventriculotomy) and because they are well away from atrioventricular valve and semilunar valve structure. Multiple defects may require more than one device, and this needs to be borne in mind when deciding the timing and sequence of closure (see following discussion).

Perimembranous Defects

By contrast to muscular defects, all perimembranous ventricular septal defects are (by definition) close to atrioventricular and semilunar valve structures. Only a very small proportion of these defects will be suitable for transcatheter closure. Perimembranous outlet defects, particularly those close to the aortic valve, are not suitable. Thus, only perimembranous inlet and trabecular defects can be considered, and only those defects in which there is well-developed tricuspid valve tissue aneurysm, into which the distal umbrella can be placed, should be considered. Once again, transesophageal echocardiographic screening is mandatory both for preprocedural selection and intraprocedural evaluation, before release of the device. This should be considered only after exclusion of snaring of atrioventricular valve tissue or tensor apparatus and interference with semilunar valve tissue.

Postoperative ventricular septal defects may be difficult to close using transcatheter techniques. This is because the orientation and position of the surgical patch material make crossing the residual defect difficult and reduce the chances of complete closure following deployment. Nonetheless, relatively small defects, particularly at the posterior and inferior margins of the defect, can be considered for closure. Superior defects, which often lie beneath the aortic, pulmonary, or mitral valves, are rarely suitable for transcatheter closure.

Other Lesions

A small number of patients with paraprosthetic leak,[5] fistulae, and sinus of valsalva aneurysm[6] have had their defect closed using the clamshell or modified Rashkind device. Each patient must be considered on their own merits, and detailed indications cannot be given, for obvious reasons. Once again, the major consideration must be the proximity of the defect to important structures such as the prosthesis itself, valve tissue apparatus, and coronary arteries.

OPERATIVE TECHNIQUE AND TIPS

Atrial Septal Defect

Iatrogenic interatrial communications are usually of known size and the appropriate device size can therefore be easily selected. In general, the diameter of the device should be approximately 220 to 250% of the largest diameter of the defect. The assessment of the defect size is particularly crucial when closing naturally occurring atrial septal defects. Echocardiographic assessment is notoriously inaccurate when compared to the stretched diameter measured by balloon during the procedure. It is the latter measurement that is the most important when selecting the appropriate-sized device. Balloon sizing can be performed with any of the commercially available spherical balloon-tipped catheters (Baxter-Edwards Laboratories, Cordis, etc.). The balloon is inflated with 5 to 20 ml of saline contrast mix and brought gently toward the atrial septum. Gentle traction is applied during balloon deflation, and the residual volume is noted at the point where the balloon passes through the atrial septum. The size of the stretched diameter of the atrial septum can either be measured from the transesophageal echocardiogram of the balloon as it passes through the septum, from the angiogram of the same, or more usually directly after the balloon has been removed and reinflated to its previously known volume. The radius of the device must be at least 110% of the stretched diameter to avoid device prolapse or embolization. Subsequent deployment of the device follows the same broad principles no matter which type is being used. A stiff guidewire (035 to 038″) is placed distally in the left upper or middle pulmonary vein. The delivery sheath is passed over this. It is essential to purge the sheath and delivery system to avoid air embolism. It is our practice to fully heparinize the patient and whenever possible to maintain a continuous heparinized flush through the delivery sheath during deployment. With each of the devices, the distal occluding element is passed out of the sheath into the left atrium and withdrawn toward the atrial septum under transesophageal echocardiographic and fluoroscopic control. It is important that the distal occluder lies in the approximate plane of the atrial septum so as to avoid prolapse of the arms through the defect itself (Plates 86-1 and 86-2). This is less of a problem with the buttoned occluding device, because it can more easily be maneuvered within the atrium itself. For the clamshell and modified umbrella, particular care has to be taken when shaping the delivery sheath. This has to be individualized according to the size of the patient, and if incorrect, it is better to remove the sheath and start again (an exchange wire can be passed along the withdrawn device to maintain vascular access) than to continue with an inappropriately shaped sheath. Deployment of the proximal occluder of the clamshell and umbrella device is straightforward and is achieved by simply withdrawing the sheath over the delivery system. Deployment of the counteroccluder of the buttoned device is more complicated. This is passed over the delivery system and pushed toward the occluder using a separate catheter. It is attached to the occluder by pulling the button through the latex membrane of the counteroc-

cluder. Thus, each of these devices has a left atrial and right atrial portion. Transesophageal echocardiography will establish whether positioning is adequate, and if there is uncertainty, the procedure should be revised. It should be noted that considerable movement may sometimes occur, particularly during the release of the clamshell and umbrella devices. This should be expected, and often leads to improved echocardiographic appearances, particularly in regard to residual shunting.

Ventricular Septal Defect

Although the basic technique of deployment in treating ventricular septal defects is similar to that for atrial septal defects (Figs. 86-3 to 86-8 and Plate 86-3), there are one or two key differences in assessment and approach. Balloon sizing of perimembranous defects is very difficult to achieve, and so transesophageal echocardiographic estimate must be relied on. The most important difference, however, is the technique of crossing the defect. Perimembranous ventricular septal defects can usually be crossed antegradely using a simple femoral venous approach. Catheters with a "right coronary" curve are particularly useful for steering through the defects under these circumstances. It is more difficult to cross apical muscular defects in this way. Passage across

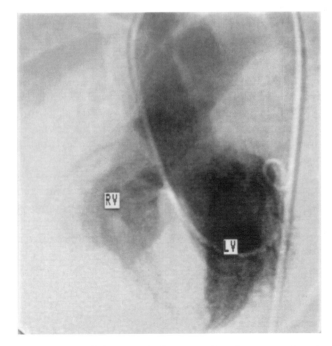

Fig. 86-3. A left ventriculogram showing a moderate-sized perimembranous ventricular septal defect.

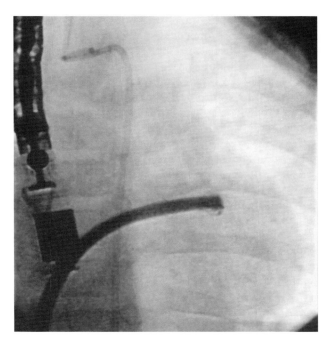

Fig. 86-4. The ventricular septal defect has been traversed antegradely, and the 11-F sheath is in the left ventricle. Note the transesophageal echo probe that was used for precise positioning at the time of deployment.

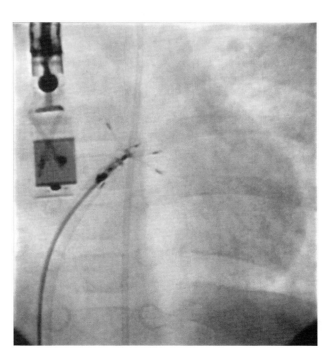

Fig. 86-6. The distal umbrella has been opened and is being withdrawn to the site of the ventricular septal defect.

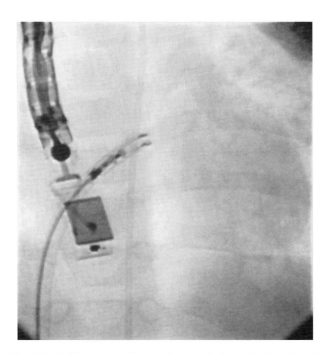

Fig. 86-5. The umbrella is advanced through the sheath.

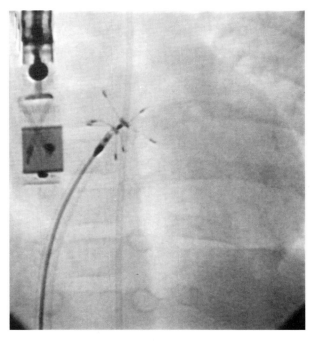

Fig. 86-7. The transseptal sheath is withdrawn, and the proximal umbrella is opened on the right ventricular aspect of the ventricular septal defect.

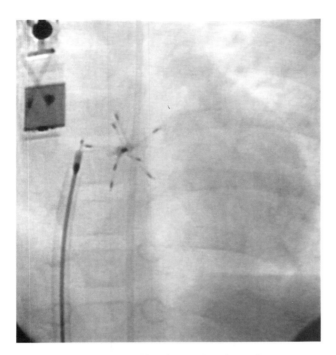

Fig. 86-8. The device is released.

these defects is greatly facilitated from the internal jugular route. Some muscular ventricular septal defects and many postoperative defects require a transarterial retrograde approach (Fig. 86-9). It is clearly impractical to deploy the device via this route, so an arteriovenous circuit needs to be established. After the ventricular septal defect has been crossed retrogradely, the wire is placed in the right atrium or pulmonary artery. This is snared by the antegrade venous catheter and is withdrawn to provide an arteriovenous circuit. The delivery sheath can then be passed antegradely transvenously through the defect and the device deployed. Once again, very careful attention to adequately purging catheters and sheaths is necessary to avoid systemic embolization. Precise placement of the device and assessment of its position can be confirmed with precision only by transesophageal echocardiography and should be considered a mandatory part of these procedures. Particular attention should be paid to the possibility of entrapment of atrioventricular valve tissue and tensor apparatus or interference with semilunar valve function. This should be established beyond doubt before release of the device.

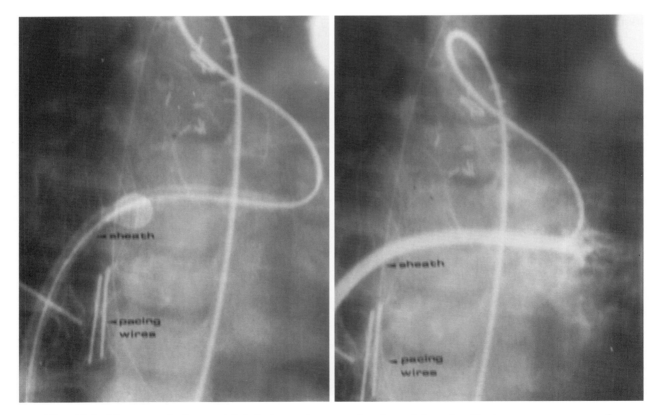

Fig. 86-9. Most ventricular septal defects can be crossed antegradely using the transvenous approach. In this case, a retrograde arterial passage was required. An arteriovenous circuit is established by snaring a wire in the right atrium, right ventricle, or pulmonary artery. The delivery sheath can then be passed antegradely using the transvenous route.

POSTPROCEDURAL MANAGEMENT

It is our practice to maintain electrocardiographic monitoring for 24 hours after transcatheter closure of ventricular septal defects. Anticoagulation is not required following ventricular septal defect closure, but for atrial septal defect closure, 24 hours of systemic heparinization during the institution of formal anticoagulation has been our routine. No scientific data support this, however. Discharge on the first or second postprocedural day is the norm.

RESULTS: SHORT AND LONG-TERM FOLLOW-UP

Atrial Septal Defect

The midterm results of atrial septal defect closure using the clamshell device have recently been published. Small residual shunts occur in approximately 20%, but these are rarely of hemodynamic significance. This device, however, is currently unavailable because of unexpected fracture of the metal arms of the device. This has not caused major clinical sequelae, but the device is being redesigned to prevent this complication.

The midterm results of the use of the modified umbrella device in 16 defects have also recently been published.[7] Because of the limitations in size, this device has only infrequently been used in naturally occurring defects, but it clearly has a role in selected cases and for closure of the surgically created fenestration in the modified Fontan procedures. No arm fractures have been seen, but clearly, this device is subject to less stresses than the larger clamshell devices. There have been similarly encouraging midterm results with the buttoned occluder device. Complete closure can be achieved in approximately 80%, and the morbidity is low.[8] One or two serious embolic complications have occurred, however (personal communication), and the design of the delivery system of this device in particular is being modified to prevent this. The other early complication that is being made less frequent by design modification is that of unbuttoning of the device. This necessitates snaring and removal of the device, and only on rare occasions has surgical removal been required.

Ventricular Septal Defect

Transcatheter closure of muscular ventricular septal defects is clearly feasible and may offer an alternative in those cases where surgical closure would be difficult. Again, published clinical experience is limited, but transcatheter closure appears to be superior to intraoperative device closure of these defects. Whether or not it is reasonable to perform transcatheter closure of straightforward muscular defects before debanding of the pulmonary artery, for example, is a difficult question to answer and will depend on the institutional experience. These lesions can be simply closed by the surgeon with little increase in overall morbidity and only brief extension of the period of cardiopulmonary bypass.

Even less information is available regarding transcatheter closure of perimembranous ventricular septal defect. Early complications include embolization of the device to the pulmonary artery and on one occasion to the left ventricular outflow tract. Transient hemolysis has occurred in two patients, and perforation of an aortic valve leaflet has occurred in one. Overall, uncomplicated closure of perimembranous ventricular septal defect was achieved in only 8 of 22 carefully selected cases in whom it was attempted.[9] Therefore, at this time, transcatheter closure of perimembranous ventricular septal defect must remain part of an experimental protocol, and the exact indications are yet to be described.

COSTS

The costs of these devices vary from country to country, and the overall cost of the technique clearly depends on many factors, not the least of which is the number of devices deployed. In general the overall financial cost of these procedures, when cardiopulmonary bypass has been avoided, will be significantly less than that of the surgical alternative. Once again, however, an institutional approach must be taken toward the cost–benefit analysis of these procedures. It is probable, but by no means certain, that the cost of these devices and delivery systems will reduce as their clinical application becomes more widespread.

DISCUSSION

It seems likely that in the next decade transcatheter closure of secundum atrial septal defect will become part of accepted clinical practice. The role of these devices in closure of ventricular septal defects and other intracardiac communications is less certain. While the avoidance of the morbidity and mortality of cardiopulmonary bypass, median stenotomy, and cardiopulmonary bypass is a laudible goal, it should not be forgotten that the surgical alternative to most of these techniques is extremely satisfactory. It is only by these standards that the utility of transcatheter techniques can be judged.

REFERENCES

1. Mills NL, King TD. Nonoperative closure of left-to-right shunts. J Thorac Cardiovasc Surg 1976;72:371–8
2. Lock JE, Hellenbrand WE, Laston L et al. Clamshell umbrella closure of atrial septal defects: Initial experience. Circulation 1989;80(suppl.2):592
3. Redington AN, Rigby ML. Novel uses of the Rashkind ductal umbrella in adults and children with congenital heart disease. Br Heart J 1993;69:47–51
4. Sideris EB, Sideris SE, Thanopoulos BD et al. Transvenous atrial septal defect occlusion by the "buttoned" device. Am J Cardiol 1990;66:1524–6
5. Hourihan M, Perry SB, Mandell VS et al. Transcatheter umbrella closure of valvular and paravalvular leaks. J Am Coll Cardiol 1992;6:131–7
6. Cullen S, Somerville J, Redington AN. Transcatheter closure of a ruptured aneurysm of the sinus of valsalva. Br Heart J 1994;71:479–80
7. Redington AN, Rigby ML. Transcatheter closure of interatrial communication with a modified umbrella device. Br Heart J 1994;92:392–7
8. Rao PS, Wilson AD, Levy JM et al. Role of "buttoned" double-disc device in the management of atrial septal defects. Am Heart J 1992;123:191–200
9. Rigby ML, Redington AN. Primary transcatheter umbrella closure of perimembranous ventricular septal defect. Br Heart J 1994;72:368–71

87 Transcatheter Closure of the Persistent Arterial Duct

Rajiv Chaturvedi
Andrew Redington

HISTORY

Almost 30 years after Gross and Hubbard's first surgical duct ligation, Porstmann in 1967 reported duct closure by retrograde arterial delivery of a foam plug.

Most persistent ducts, however, are detected in young children, whose small arteries preclude the use of bulky devices like the Porstmann plug. It was the development and evolution of the Rashkind double umbrella from its first presentation in 1979 to its current form that has resulted in the majority of persistent ducts, in European centers at least, being closed by catheter techniques.

Although a burgeoning number of devices are available for duct closure, there is substantial clinical experience only with the Rashkind double umbrella. They should all be regarded as experimental and requiring institutional approval and informed consent.

RATIONALE AND MECHANISM OF ACTION

Surgical duct ligation is well established as an effective procedure with a mortality rate of less than 1%, but there are advantages to transcatheter duct occlusion:

1. Avoidance of a thoracotomy and its sequelae, for example, a scar, postoperative pain, and hospitalization for about 5 days.

2. Avoidance of a general anesthetic in centers that perform the procedure with sedation only.
3. Avoidance of the occasional requirement for cardiopulmonary bypass in some heavily calcified adult ducts.
4. Potentially cheaper. This is certainly true if coils are used, but it is a contentious issue for the Rashkind umbrella.[1]

All methods rely on partial/total occlusion of the duct and induction of intraluminal thrombosis. The most commonly used coils have Dacron fibers to encourage thrombosis. Umbrella devices have foam occluder and counteroccluder faces that straddle the duct and obstruct flow.

INSTRUMENTATION

There are three main categories of devices:

1. Foam plugs (e.g., Porstmann plug, the Botalloccluder)
2. Double-disk devices (Rashkind double umbrella, Sideris buttoned occluder)
3. Coils (Gianturco spring coils, duct occlud, detachable coils)

Foam Plugs

The Porstmann plug required large arterial sheaths and, although mainly used in adults, still had a significant arterial injury rate. The Porstmann plug is not commercially available, but a modified version is used in China. The Botalloccluder is a conical foam plug mounted on a stainless steel frame that is attached to and released from the delivery catheter by a screw mechanism. There are four plug sizes 8- to 14-mm diameter, but these require large 10- to 16-F introducer sheaths. Although it is delivered by a transvenous route and a relatively large series with good results[2] has been published, the fear of vascular injury has restricted its use to Eastern Europe. Foam plugs will not be discussed further.

Double-Disk Devices

The occluder and counteroccluder disks consist of foam stretched on a metal frame. These devices have a relatively rigid delivery system and are deployed through a long sheath that allows a venous approach to be used in virtually all patients. The Rashkind double umbrella is available in two sizes, 12- or 17-mm diameter. The arms are collapsed for delivery and spring open on release. The front-loading technique[3] allows smaller introducer sheaths to be used, 6 F instead of 8 F for the 12-mm device and 9 F (or 8 F with difficulty) instead of 11 F for the 17-mm device.

The Sideris adjustable buttoned occluder has an X-shaped frame of two wires that can be folded to lie parallel to each other, allowing use of a smaller introducer sheath. The counteroccluder is rhomboid in shape and has a central rubber "buttonhole." The Sideris duct device has an 8-mm button loop with two knots ("buttons") rather than the 2-mm single button loop of the atrial septal defect (ASD) device. This enables the counteroccluder to be locked in position either 8 or 4 mm from the occluder by pushing the buttonhole through the first or second button. Sideris duct devices are available in 15- to 20-mm sizes and require a 7-F introducer sheath.

Coils

Coils are made of stainless steel or platinum with attached Dacron fibers to encourage thrombosis. Gianturco coils are preloaded in extended form in cylinders and passed into the lumen of a standard catheter using a 0.038″ wire. Once released from the constraint of the cylinder, they reform a coil of the stated helical diameter. For a given helical diameter, a longer extended length will result in more loops being formed on extrusion from the cylinder. Coils come in a wide range of external diameters, helical diameters, and lengths and can be delivered using a 4-F or 5-F catheter.

Detachable coils are of the same basic stainless steel and Dacron fiber design but are attached and released by a screw mechanism. This allows loop formation and exact placement before release, increasing the accuracy of positioning and decreasing the the risk of embolization. Detachable coils of helical diameters 3 to 5 mm, 8 mm, and 10 mm are available and can be deployed by a 5-F catheter.

INDICATIONS AND PATIENT SELECTION

Current accepted clinical practice is to recommend closure of all persistent arterial ducts, independent of the method used. In Campbell's[4] 1968 analysis of the natural history of the persistent arterial duct, he estimated that of people who survive the high 20 to 40% mortality in infancy, a mortality of 0.5% each year occurs in the first two decades, rising to about 4% each year after the fourth decade. By 60 years of age, 50 to 70% will have died, and the duct will have closed in 20%. Death was due to bacterial endarteritis (45%) and heart failure (30%).

With Doppler echocardiography, it is possible to demonstrate ducts that will never produce heart failure and may not even have a murmur. The rationale for closure of these "silent" ducts is the avoidance of bacterial endarteritis, although the true risk of infective endarteritis in these ducts with tiny shunts is unknown. Similarly, the risk of endarteritis in the presence of a residual shunt around a duct device is unknown, although in most institutions, leaks after previous transcatheter closure undergo repeat intervention.

In most centers with access to the devices (they are not uniformly available), transcatheter duct occlusion is the method of choice, and surgical ligation is reserved for cases of failed transcatheter occlusion (very large ducts, window-type ducts) or as a rescue procedure (combined ligation and retrieval of an embolized device). The 17-mm Rashkind umbrella should be used for ducts of 4 to 8-mm diameter and with caution in children less than 10 kg, because of the risk of left pulmonary artery stenosis. The 12-mm Rashkind umbrella is used in ducts less than 4 mm in diameter, but these are increasingly being closed with coils that are simple to use and much cheaper.

OPERATIVE TECHNIQUE AND TIPS

Rashkind Double Umbrella

The duct anatomy and minimal diameter are defined by a lateral aortogram using a 4-F pigtail catheter and are calibrated with a 6-F (5-mm) multipurpose catheter transvenously placed in the main pulmo-

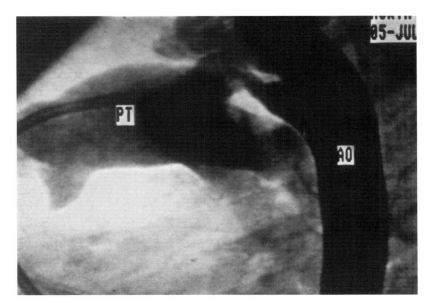

Fig. 87-1. The lateral aortogram profiles the arterial duct.

nary artery (Fig. 87-1). The narrowest part of the duct usually lies between the anterior and posterior tracheal borders. With increased experience, a solely transvenous approach can be used, and the aortogram can be performed by advancing the multipurpose catheter into the descending aorta. The multipurpose catheter is passed through the duct into the aorta, and a 0.035″ exchange-length wire is placed in the abdominal aorta. The long sheath may require partial straightening in hot water before placing it across the duct over the wire. The umbrella is loaded into the pod, purged, inverted into the sheath, and advanced to the tricuspid valve. The folded umbrella is then advanced out of the pod into the sheath toward the tip of the sheath. The sheath is withdrawn so that its tip is free in the descending aorta. The umbrella is then advanced until the distal arms are fully open. The sheath–distal umbrella is withdrawn into the duct, taking care to avoid independent movement of the sheath. When the distal umbrella is fixed in the aortic ampulla, the sheath is then withdrawn to deploy the proximal umbrella in the pulmonary artery (Fig. 87-2). The device is then released. At this stage it is important to ensure complete release of the device, because there is often some tethering to the fabric. If in doubt, the sheath should be readvanced to the device, untethering it from the device without displacement.

Closure Using the Sideris Button Occluder

The steps up to and including placing a long 7-F sheath across the duct on an exchange wire are as for the Rashkind device. The Sideris occluder is folded and positioned in the sheath, and a 7-F endhole catheter is advanced along the exchange wire, pushing the occluder in front of it. The occluder is opened in the aorta by withdrawing the sheath and is pulled up to the aortic end of duct. The counteroccluder is then advanced to the pulmonary artery side of the duct, and the button of the occluder is pulled through the buttonhole of the counteroccluder by gently exerting traction on the occluder against the duct while advancing the counteroccluder with the long sheath. It is released by holding the device in place with the long sheath and pulling one end of the nylon strand, which attaches the occluder to the delivery wire.

Coils

Coils can be used to close small native ducts less than 4 mm and residual ducts after surgical ligation or previous device implantation. The helical diameter of the coil should be twice the minimum angiographic duct diameter, and the coil length should allow formation of three to four loops.

Gianturco coils are deployed using either an antegrade venous route or more usually a retrograde arterial route. The duct is crossed using a 6-F nontapered catheter, the coil is loaded into and advanced up the catheter with a guidewire until one or two loops of the coil are in the pulmonary artery or aortic ampulla. Using the lateral aortogram as reference and the tracheal shadow as a landmark, the catheter is pulled back until the coil loop is resisted by the

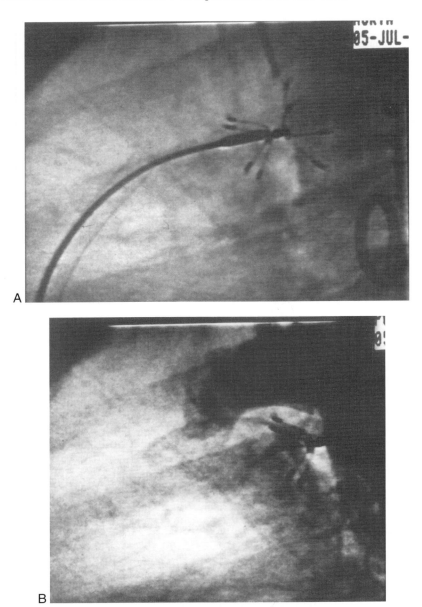

Fig. 87-2. The Rashkind double umbrella. **(A)** The device positioned in the duct still attached to the delivery wire. **(B)** The lateral aortogram after device release demonstrating duct closure.

pulmonary artery end of the duct, and then the catheter is slowly pulled back into the aorta while the coil is advanced. With release, the coil should form at least two further loops on the opposite side of the duct. Duct-occlud devices are deployed through a 4- or 5-F custom-built delivery catheter.[5] The process of delivery is identical to that of detachable coils (see following discussion), but it has a different release mechanism (Fig. 87-3).

Detachable coils can be deployed by the transvenous route because there is complete control of the coil during placement, and so there is much less risk of systemic embolism. For the very small duct, however, a transarterial route may be technically more straightforward. The coil cartridge is screwed onto the delivery wire, and the straightening mandril is advanced until it reaches the tip of the coil, and it should be maintained in this position until the coil is extruded from the catheter. With a 4- or 5-F nontapered end-hole catheter across the duct, the coil is advanced, and the straightening mandril is withdrawn until two loops are formed in the

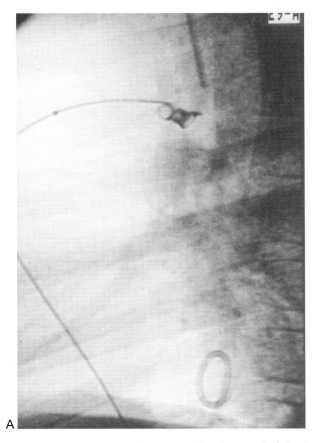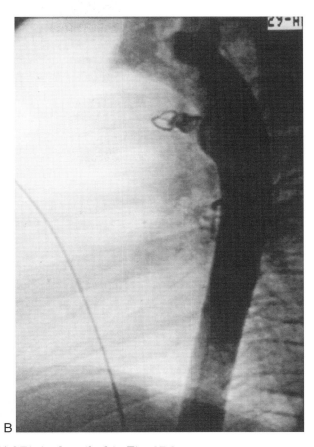

Fig. 87-3. The duct-occlud device. **(A&B)** As described in Fig. 87-2.

aorta. The whole assembly is withdrawn until the loops are held up in the ampulla. The mandril is withdrawn proximal to the coil attachment point, then the delivery wire is withdrawn to form the remaining loops in the main pulmonary artery. Once the coil position is satisfactory, the delivery wire is rotated counter clockwise to release the coil (Fig 87-4).

POST PROCEDURAL MANAGEMENT

Patients can be discharged on the same or next day depending on recovery from sedation/anesthesia. Antibiotic prophylaxis is continued for 6 months to allow endothelialization of the device. If there is a residual murmur or Doppler-detectable flow on routine scanning at 6-month follow-up, then antibiotic prophylaxis is continued.

RESULTS

Transcatheter persistent arterial duct occlusion still remains an experimental procedure. All large series refer to the Rashkind double umbrella and at present include the learning curve experience of each center.

Rashkind Umbrella

The four largest series report on a total of more than 1,200 patients treated with the Rashkind umbrella.[1,6-8] The end point for success in all but one series[1] was loss of flow on Doppler echocardiography. A second device is required in 5 to 10% of patients,[6-8] and Hoskings et al.[7] found residual shunting on Doppler echocardiography present in 38% at 1 year, 18% at 2 years, and 8% at 40 months. Main complications are device embolization, device-induced hemolysis, and potential for left pulmonary artery stenosis. Embolization occurs in 2 to 3% of patients, and

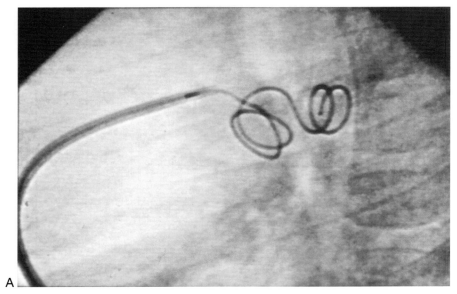

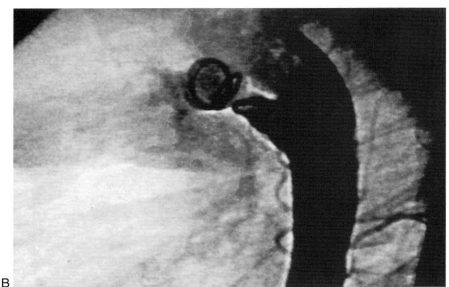

Fig. 87-4. The detachable coil. **(A&B)** As described in Fig. 87-2.

hemolysis in about 0.5%. Hemolysis can be treated either by device removal or by closing the residual leak.[9,10] In children less than 10 kg, Nykanen et al.[10] found that about 10% had accelerated flow into the left pulmonary artery, and one 8.7-kg child required removal of a 17-mm device. The European Registry reported two early deaths of 686 patients treated; none of the other series reported any deaths. Postprocedural anemia requiring transfusion is virtually never a problem now, with greater experience and the use of a hemostatic valve on the long sheath. The Rashkind umbrella has also been used with success in adults, including five with calcified ducts with no complications.[11]

Sideris Buttoned Occluder

Rao et al.[12] reported on 14 patients weighing 7.2 to 19 kg whose ducts were closed with 15- to 20-mm buttoned occluders. No complications were reported, and 14% had residual shunting at 24 months' follow-up.

Coils

Moore et al.[13] treated 30 patients weighing 8.1 to 42.2 kg with ducts less than 3.0 mm on angiography with Gianturco spring coils. Two thirds of these ducts were clinically apparent. In one patient, two coils embolized into the left pulmonary artery and could not be retrieved. The 29 others had successful deployment of coils, and two of these required 2 coils. There was 93% closure by 6 months. Lloyd et al.[14] reported similar results at the expense of a higher embolization rate (about 8%), but these occurred at the very start of the series. A wholly antegrade transvenous approach was used in a series of 33 patients weighing 2.3 to 64 kg, with a median duct diameter of 2.8 mm.[15] Eighteen of 33 patients had multiple coils,[1,6,9,15] 31 had complete closure, and there were no embolic complications. No series on detachable coil duct closure has been reported.

COSTS

The cost of transcatheter persistent arterial duct occlusion depends on the device and protocol used by each institution. The procedure is cheaper if done on an outpatient basis with sedation only. The greatest clinical experience is with the Rashkind double umbrella; however, it is also the most expensive device available. Many ducts that are suitable for closure with the 12-mm umbrella can be closed by coils at less than one tenth of the cost with at least equal efficacy.

DISCUSSION

In many institutions, transcatheter duct occlusion has become the treatment of choice. This has been due to a combination of enthusiasm for the procedure by cardiologists but also a genuine wish by parents to avoid prolonged hospitalization and a thoracotomy scar for their child. With cheaper devices in the future, transcatheter duct occlusion likely will also be demonstrated to be more economical than surgical ligation.

The best indication for duct occlusion is the presence of a hemodynamically significant left-to-right shunt. In terms of a public health measure, the utility and cost-effectiveness of occluding, surgically or by catheterization, clinically "silent" ducts remains to be demonstrated. In the modern era of widespread antibiotic prophylaxis against bacteremia and dramatically improved outcomes for bacterial endocar-

ditis, there must be some degree of diminishing returns.

REFERENCES

1. Gray DT, Fyler DC, Walker AM et al for the Patent Ductus Arteriosus Closure Comparative Study Group. Clinical outcome and costs of transcatheter as compared with surgical closure of patent ductus arteriosus. N Engl J Med 1993;329:1517–23
2. Verin VE, Saveliev SV, Kolody SM, Prokubovski VI. Results of transcatheter closure of the patent ductus arteriosus with the Botalloccluder. J Am Coll Cardiol 1993;22:1509–14
3. Perry SB, Lock JE. Front-loading of the double-umbrella devices, a new technique for umbrella delivery for closing cardiovascular defects. Am J Cardiol 1992; 70:917–20
4. Campbell M. Natural history of persistent ductus arteriosus. Br Heart J 1968;30:4–13
5. Tometzki AJP, Houston AB, Redington AN et al. Closure of Blalock-Taussig shunts using a new detachable coil device. Br Heart J 1995;73:383–4
6. Anonymous. Transcatheter occlusion of persistent arterial duct. Report of the European Registry. Lancet 1992;340:1062–6
7. Hosking MCK, Benson LN, Musewe N et al. Transcatheter occlusion of the persistently patent ductus arteriosus, forty month follow-up and prevalence. Circulation 1991;84:2313–7
8. Ali Khan MA, Al Youssef S, Mullins CE, Sawyer WB. Experience with 205 procedures of transcatheter closure of the ductus arteriosus in 182 patients, with special reference to residual shunts and long-term follow-up. J Thorac Cardiovasc Surg 1995;104:1721–7
9. Gatzoulis MA, Rigby ML, Redington AN. Umbrella occlusion of persistent arterial duct in children under two years. Br Heart J 1994;72:364–7
10. Nykanen DG, Hayes AM, Benson LN, Freedom RM. Transcatheter patent ductus arteriosus occlusion: application in the small child. J Am Coll Cardiol 1994; 23:1666–70
11. Schenk MH, O'Laughlin MP, Rokey R et al. Transcatheter occlusion of patent ductus arteriosus in adults. Am J Cardiol 1993;72:591–5
12. Rao PS, Sideris EB, Haddad J et al. Transcatheter occlusion of patent ductus arteriosus with adjustable buttoned device, initial clinical experience. Circulation 1993;88:1119–26
13. Moore JW, George L, Kirkpatrick SE et al. Percutaneous closure of the small patent ductus arteriosus using occluding spring coils. J Am Coll Cardiol 1994;23: 759–65
14. Lloyd TR, Fedderly R, Mendelsohn AM et al. Transcatheter occlusion of patent ductus arteriosus with Gianturco coils. Circulation 1993;88:1412–20
15. Hijazi ZM, Geggel RL. Results of anterograde transcatheter closure of patent ductus arteriosus using multiple Gianturco coils. Am J Cardiol 1994;74:925–9

88 Technical Evaluation of Metallic Stents in TIPS

P. Rossi
L. Broglia
M. Rossi
P. Ricci
F. Arata
S. Abbondanza

The transjugular intrahepatic portal-systemic shunt (TIPS) is a feasible and effective method in decompressing the portal system and preventing variceal hemorrage.[1]

It was first suggested by Rösch[2] in 1969, but despite the improvements developed by Colapinto,[3] it remained only a clinical possibility for a long time, because it was compromised by the early occlusion of the intrahepatic tract.

In 1989 the introduction of expandable metallic stents was a turning point and allowed Richter[4] to successfully use TIPS in humans. Since then, TIPS has become a safe and effective nonoperative procedure for portal decompression.

Depending on the experience of the authors, both balloon- and self-expanding stents have been widely described in the litterature as effective for TIPS, with satisfactory long term-result, ranging from 2 to 6 years of follow-up.[5]

In fact, stent selection is one of the most important factors to achieve the success in TIPS procedure and it should take into account both the anatomy of the patient and the physical characteristics of the stent, including the length, the diameter, and the flexibility of the stent. Expecially with self-expanding stents, the elasticity, radial force, mesh profile, and the delivery system which differ among stents, has to be known by the radiologist for proper selection.[6,7]

However, as reported by the literature a certain preference for self-expanding stents exists among different authors, which could be the consequence of the various aspects of the stent, not the least of which is their easier deployment.[8,9]

Among the stents currently available in Europe and successfully used in the TIPS procedure, we report here the most important features of the more largely used balloon- and self-expanding stents.

BALLOON EXPANDABLE STENTS

Palmaz Stent

The Palmaz stent (Johnson & Johnson, Warren, New Jersey) consists of a single segment, tubular stainless steel mesh, with a wall thickness of 0.15 mm. The stents used in the TIPS procedure are 3 or 4 cm in length and can be dilated to the desired diameter from 8 to 12 mm, depending on the balloon size used for delivery, because it cannot expand by itself.[5] However, if needed, it can be increased in diameter even several months after deployment. When expanded, it is approximately 13% the surface area.[10] The Palmaz stent is a high-hoop strength stent,[11] has no longitudinal flexibility, is completely nonelastic and, if deformed, retains its shape completely. Since it is available in a 3 cm length, at least two or three stents are required to cover the whole intrahepatic tract, which increases the duration and the cost of the procedure.

Because its stiffness it cannot adapt to curved paths and angulation of the stent can occur, expecially when more than one stent is required.

Tantalum-Strecker Stents

Tantalum-Strecker stents (Meditech, Boston Scientific, Watertown, Massachusetts) designed in a cylindrical shape and made of a single metallic tantalum filament, 0.13 mm in diameter. It is knitted in a series of loosely connected loops[10,12] and mounted on a 5-F ultrathin balloon catheter. It is fixed by thin silicone sleeves at both ends of the balloon to avoid the displacement of the stent on the balloon during introduction, especially along curved tracts. This anchoring device also permits easy release of the stent upon full expansion. The stent is produced in different diameters (from 4 to 11 mm), and length (from 2 to 6 cm); however, in performing the TIPS procedure, the most adequate size is 9 to 11 mm in diameter and 4 to 6 cm in length. Overstretching the stent by 1 to 2 mm is also possible with an oversized balloon, if a larger diameter is needed. It is highly radiopaque, and undergoes a minimal shortening during expansion, which allows for a precise positioning. It is flexible and soft and, after expansion, can be compressed. When fully expanded, it occupies 30% of the surface area.[9]

SELF-EXPANDING STENTS

Wallstent

The Wallstent (Medinvent, Zurich, Switzerland) consists of a tubular mesh of woven steel monofilaments, with a wire diameter of 0.12 mm and a varying diameter of 8 to 10 mm (Fig. 88-1). The unconstrained length of the stent can be selected according to what is required. The length of the stent, however, varies considerably, with considerable shortening as it dilates.

Another peculiarity of the Wallstent is its longitudinal flexibility, which adapts itself to curved paths over 70° to 80°, expanding itself even when heavily bended or curved. The edges of the stent, which are made of cut tubular woven monofilaments, are spiky, representing a sort of anchoring device, this can be considered a disadvantage, since these spikes may penetrate structures.[13,14]

The prosthesis comes with a 7-F introducer system, with three radiopaque markers for precise localization of its release. This stent, in fact, is poorly radiopaque, especially in obese subjects or when ascites is present, therefore, its fluoroscopic identification is uncertain, even with the best equipment.

Nitinol Strecker Stent

The Nitinol Strecker stent (Boston Scientific, Watertown, Massachusetts) is made of a 0.13-mm thick nickel-titanium alloy wire (Ellastoy), knitted into a cylindrically-shaped flexible mesh with looped ends (Fig. 88-2). When expanded, it is approximately 30% of the surface area, like the Tantalum-Strecker stent.[6,8,15] The 10-F delivery system is comprised of an introducer shaft with three radiopaque markers, one at the proximal end, one in the middle, and one at the distal end, and a cover sheath which releases the stent upon retraction. The distance between the distal and the middle marker represents the actual

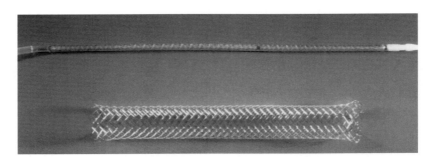

Fig. 88-1. Wallstent: the top the introducing system is shown. The image shows a fully expanded Wallstent, cut in a cylindrical shape and with spiky edges.

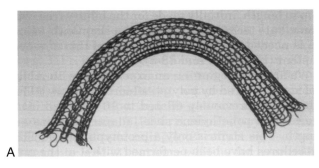

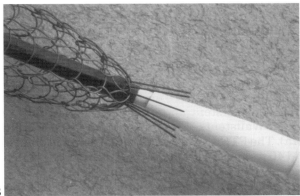

Fig. 88-2. (A) Nitinol Strecker stent fully expanded: It is knitted into a cylindrical flexible mesh with looped ends at both its extremities. (B) Nitinol Strecker stent kept in position by the six-prongs anchoring system.

length of the stent after release. Radiopacity of the stent is very low, therefore it is mandatory to rely on the three radiopaque markers of the delivery system.

The distal end is provided with an anchoring system that consists of six prongs, which should prevent the shortening of the distal end of the stent after deployment; however, as the stent fully expands to its original diameter, shortening (0.5 to 1 cm) can occur.[12] Because of its looped ends, in case of disloca-

tion or misplacement, it can be removed easily with a loop technique or grasping forceps, or it could be reentered during angiographic controls. Its radial force is good and full expansion of the stent is achieved in 24 to 48 hours.

Memotherm

The Memotherm (Angiomed, Karlsruhe, Germany) is a nitinol plate with memory metal properties, which means that the stent finally reaches its predetermined diameter in an expansion time of at least 5 minutes.[16] The romboid openings are laser cut and the plate soldered to form a tubular structure. To improve longitudinal flexibility, horizontal cuts are made, separating the apices of the romboid windows. The final result is very similar to the aspect of a Palmaz stent when fully open.

The delivery device is a 10-F introducer, with a gun at the terminal end. Delivery is very easy and precise because of the stent radiopacity; the stent does not retract, a sharp shooting deployment can, therefore, be performed.

The hoop strength of this stent and the surface area are probably similar to the Palmaz stent, approximately 13%.[9]

It has a very low profile, but it does not perform too well in curved paths of 60° to 80°; they tend to angulate, thus decreasing their lumen.

Gianturco/Rösch "Z" Stent

The Gianturco/Rösch "Z" stent (Cook, Inc., Bloomingtoon, Indiana) consists of a stainless steel wire bent into a zigzag pattern and soldered at the end to form a closed circle (Fig. 88-3). The stent is 6 to 7.5 cm long and consists of four to five 1.5-cm-long stent

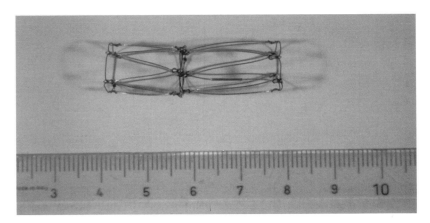

Fig. 88-3. Gianturco-Rosh "Z" stent.

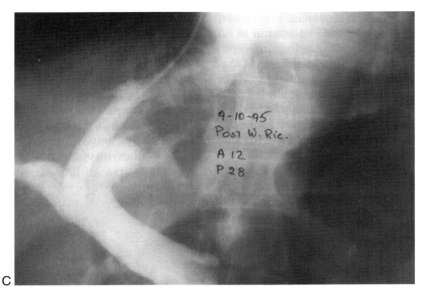

Fig. 88-5. (*Continued*).

controls with US Color-Doppler imaging, endoscopy and angiography at 5 days. Thereafter, clinical evaluation and US Color-Doppler examination took place at 30 days and at 3 to 6, and 12 to 24 months. Angiographic controls after 5 days, 3 to 6 months, and 12 to 24 months have been performed both in asymptomatic and symptomatic patients, to assess the validity of other noninvasive modality in the evaluation of stent patency.

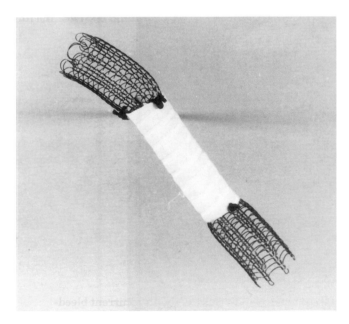

Fig. 88-6. Prototype: Nitinol stent covered by a 6-mm PTFE membrane, predilated to 10 mm in diameter. The narrowing in the covered portion of the stent suggests that a pre-dilation to 12 mm should be more appropriate.

However, since we have obtained a good correspondence between US Color-Doppler imaging and angiographic examinations with an overall sensitivity of 89%, a specificity of 93%, and an overall accuracy of 91% in evaluating shunt malfunctions, we prefer to limit angiography only to patients with echographic evidence of shunt malfunctioning.

The results of our angiographic controls are as shown in Table 88-2 and our clinical results can be found in Table 88-3. In our experience, we have observed no significant differences in results between Wallstents and Nitinol Strecker stents which we have used in the majority of our cases.

We cannot offer any opinion about the other available stents because of our lack of experience with these type of stents.[5,10,17] However, we believe that all of the stents now available on the market can offer technical and immediate good results in the TIPS procedure but long-term patency is compromised by possible early thrombosis within the stent or intimal hyperplasia. Usually, these stent-related complications respond well to balloon dilation and only in a few cases does another stent have to be placed. Some authors suggest that repeated balloon dilation appears to stabilize growth of pseudointimal tissue in the tract and appears to decrease recurrence of stenosis.[17] Considering this aspect, patients have to be submitted to continous controls, expecially with US Color-Doppler imaging to detect stent abnormality, either before clinical evidence of increased portal pressure, and to recanalize the shunt promptly.

On the basis of our experience, we suggest a close follow-up, with controls, every 3 to 6 months, to guar-

Table 88-1. Experience with Nitinol Strecker and Wallstent Stents

Technical Aspects	Nitinol Strecker	Wallstents
Success	100%	100%
Deployment	Easy	Easy
Caliber of the introducer	10 F	7 F
Malpositioning	None	1 (1.3%)
Dislodgement	3 (6%)	None
Removal	Easy (1 case)	Very difficult (1 case)
Shortening of the stent	1 (1.3%)	1 (2%)
Incomplete expansion (48 hrs)	5 (10%)	3 (4%)
Stent angulation	None	None

Table 88-2. Results of Angiographic Controls

Controls	Nitinol Strecker	Wallstents
5-day Angiograms	35	58
Partial thrombosis of the stent	6/35 (17%)	7/58% (12%)
Obstruction of the shunt	1/35 (3%)	5/58 (8.6%)
1–6 Months Angiograms	23	32
Stent stenosis	7/23 (30%)	8/32 (25%)
Hepatic vein stenosis	None	2/32 (6%)
Obstruction of the shunt	1/23 (4%)	2/32 (6%)
6–24 Months Angiograms	7	15
Stent stenosis	4/7 (57%)	8/15 (53%)
Hepatic vein stenosis	1/7 (14%)	1/15 (6%)
Obstruction of the shunt	1/7 (14%)	1/15 (6%)

antee what is called the "assisted patency" of the stent.

A recent study, performed to evaluate neointima formation of Nitinol Strecker stents and Wallstents, showed a more pronounced neointima formation in Nitinol stents than in Wallstents. However, the authors have concluded that this difference is too insignificant to be relevant to patency of large vessels.[20]

In the future we hope to overcome these problems using covered stents, which have low profile, porosity of the material, and an easy delivery system. However, preliminary experience is reported only with animals, with good results using PTFE, compared with uncovered stents[19] and Dacron covered stents.[18]

Of course, covered stents in humans will require an higher technical ability especially in deploying the stent correctly, to avoid complications.

On the basis of the reported study, covered stents should improve shunt patency, but should be approached with extreme caution.

REFERENCES

1. Coldwell DM, Ring EJ, Rees CR et al. Multicenter investigation of the role of Transjugular Intrahepatic Portosystemic Shunt in management of Portosystemic Shunt in management of portal hypertension. Radiology 1995;196:335–40
2. Rosch J, Hanafee WN, Snow H. Transjugular portal venography and radiologic portacaval shunt: an experimental study. Radiology 1969;92:1112–4
3. Colapinto RF, Stronell RD, Birch SJ et al. Creation of an intrahepatic portosystemic shunt with a Gruentzig balloon catheter. Can Med Assoc J 1982;126:267–8
4. Richter GM, Noeldge G, Palmaz JC et al. Transjugular intrahepatic portacaval stent shunt:preliminary clinical results. Radiology 1990;174:1027–30

Table 88-3. Clinical Results

	Nitinol Strecker	Wallstents
New episodes of encephalopathy	11/50 (22%)	11/76 (14%)
Rebleeding	4/48 (8%)	4/76 (5%)
Ascites resolution	4/7 (72%)	9/12 (75%)
Ascites improvement	2/7 (28%)	3/12 (25%)
30-day mortality	5/42 (12%)	10/63 (16%)
Late mortality	3/37 (8%)	8/53 (15%)

5. Richter GM, Noeldge G, Roeren T, Kauffmann GW, Palmaz JC. TIPS: concepts and results. pp. 139 to 147. In Liermann PD (ed): Stents—State of the Art and Future Developments. Boston Scientific, Boston, 1995

6. Rossi P, Maccioni F, Broglia L, Ricci P. Nitinol Strecker stents in TIPS. pp. 162–6. In Liermann PD (ed). Stents—State of the Art and Future Developments. Boston Scientific, Boston, 1995

7. Rossi P, Maccioni F, Bezzi M, Broglia L. TIPS: technical aspects and clinical results. HIT Angiography Interven Radiol Topics 1994;9:1–17

8. Flueckiger F, Sternthal H, Klein GE et al. Strength, elasticity and plasticity of expandable metal stents: in vitro studies with three types of stress. JVIR 1994;5: 745–50

9. Fontaine A, Spigos DG, Eaton G et al. Stent induced intimal hyperplasia: are there fundamental differences between flexible and rigid stent designs? J Vasc Interv Radiol 1994;5:739–44

10. Maynar M, Cabrera J, Gorriz E et al. Transjugular intrahepatic portacaval shunt. JVIR,1993;4:63

11. Dake MD, Grant OW, Saltiel F et al. Comparison of balloon expandable stents: can they resists arterial vasoconstrictor forces. JVIR 1993;4:20–1

12. Rossi P, Maynar M, Bezzi M et al. Nitinol and tantalum Strecker in TIPS. In Conn HO, Pelmos JC, Rosch J and Rossle M (eds). TIPS: Transjugular Intrahepatic Portal-Systemic Stent-Shunts. Conn, MD (in press)

13. Rousseau H, Vinel JP, Bilbao JI et al. Transjugular Intrahepatic portosystemic shunts, using the Wallstent prosthesis: a follow-up study. JVIR 1994;17: 7–11

14. La Berge JM, Ring EJ, Gordon RL et al. Creation of transjugular intrahepatic portosystemic shunts with the Wallstent endoprosthesis: result in 100 patients. Radiology 1993;187:413–20

15. Bezzi M, Orsi F, Salvatori FM, Maccioni F, Rossi P. Self-expandable Nitinol stent for the management of biliary obstruction: long-term clinical results. JVIR 1994;5:287–93

16. Liermann D, Berkefeld J, Grosso M, Kollath J. Memory alloy endoprostheses and TIPS: initial results. pp. 167–176 In Liermann PD (ed) Stents—State of the Art and Future Developments Boston Scientific, Boston 1995

17. Rosch J, Barton RE, Petersen BD et al. TIPS with Self-expandable Z-stent. pp. 153–161. In Liermann PD (ed): Stents—State of the Art and Future Developments. Boston Scientific, Boston, 1995

18. Rousseau H. TIPS. presented at "Strategie terapeutiche dell'ipertensione portale: ruolo della TIPS". Torino October 6–8, 1995

19. Nishimine K, Saxon RR, Kichikawa K et al. Improved Transjugular Intrahepatic Portosystemic Shunt patency with PTFE-covered stent-graft: Experimental results in swine Radiology 1995;196:341–7

20. Shurmann K, Vorwerk D, Kulish A et al. Experimental arterial stent placement. Comparison of a new Nitinol stent and Wallstent. Invest Radiol 1995;30:412–20

89 Pelvic Shunts

E. Zeitler

The vascular supply of the pelvic organs in women and men differs, according to specific biologic functions.[1–6] In men, there is only the internal pudendal artery supplying the penis and the prostate—where arteriovenous (AV) malformations are unlikely to occur except as post-traumatic lesions—and the testicular artery—which has practically never been involved either in arteriosclerosis or in AV shunts. The female pelvic organs, in contrast, do have a distinct vascular supply. The uterine artery and the ovarian artery both are well-developed vessels with the ability of higher perfusion of the end organ, as required especially in pregnancy.

One distinguishes between acquired and congenital AV shunts. Acquired shunts result from either trauma or surgery and for other various reasons.[3,7,8]

Traumatic shunts are mainly solitary lesions of relatively large calibers. They are characterized by direct communication between the so-called "high- and low-pressure systems," without the involvement of organ and terminal vascular systems, respectively. The sign of an AV shunt is decreased total resistance in the affected artery, which impairs the neighboring organ arteries and leads to morphologic changes in the draining vein. The elevated blood volume causes an increasing stress to the heart and, as a consequence, to the entire cardiovascular system.[9] An AV shunt can be described as a "leak" in the circulation of the organism. The abrupt increase of pressure in the venous part of the AV fistula prevents the outflow of blood from the drained territory. In cases of acute, acquired fistulas of large calibers, shock may occur as a result of hypovolemia.[7] If this rare occurrence does not happen, the circulation adapts to the situation, and the entire circulating blood volume increases.

The sequelae of a severe AV shunt in the long run are caused by the chronic volume stress to the heart, which may result in hypertension and myocardial insufficiency.[2,9] In moderate shunt volumes in pelvic and leg arteries, a latency period of several years often occurs between the formation of a shunt and the manifestation of cardiac symptoms. At pelvic and leg arteries, the shunt volume can be assessed by color-coded duplex sonography and by comparison with the healthy side. A more precise determination, however, is possible with nuclear medicine methods.[10,11]

The arterial pressure in the supplying arteries decreases, which leads to an arterioarterial pressure gradient in the region of the shunt arteries. In congenital AV shunts or after surgical creation of an AV shunt, flow is still present in the runoff artery distal to the AV shunt.[9] The shunt can also be supplied by collateral arteries. Therefore, the multiple supplying arteries of an AV shunt have to be considered in planning the appropriate therapy.

Although the existence and location of an AV shunt can be determined noninvasively with auscultation and ultrasound Doppler technique, the morphologic situation must be assessed precisely before any therapeutic intervention. Arteriography in at least two projections, possibly using balloon occlusion arteriography, can help in making the decision. Surgically created AV shunts are mainly AV communications between the common femoral artery and the femoral vein, following surgical or interventional removal of a thrombus in the pelvic veins. This mainly serves

Handbook of
CARDIOVASCULAR
INTERVENTIONS

Handbook of

CARDIOVASCULAR INTERVENTIONS

EDITED BY

ULRICH SIGWART, M.D.

Professor
Department of Medicine
University of Dusseldorf
Dusseldorf, Germany
Director
Department of Invasive Cardiology
Imperial College Royal Brompton Hospital
London, United Kingdom

MICHEL BERTRAND, M.D.

Professor
Division of Cardiology
Department of Medicine
University of Lille II
Chairman
Department of Cardiology
Cardiology Hospital
Lille, France

PATRICK W. SERRUYS, M.D., PH.D.

Professor
Department of Interventional Cardiology
Erasmus University
Research Director
Catheterization Laboratory
Thoraxcenter
Dijkzigt University Hospital
Rotterdam, The Netherlands

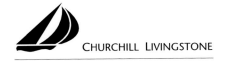

CHURCHILL LIVINGSTONE

New York, Edinburgh, London, Madrid, Melbourne, San Francisco, Tokyo

CHURCHILL LIVINGSTONE

Medical Division of Pearson Professional Limited

Distributed in the United States of America by Churchill Livingstone Inc., 650 Avenue of the Americas, New York, N.Y. 10011, and by associated companies, branches, and representatives throughout the world.

First published 1996

ISBN 0 443 07970 6

British Library Cataloguing in Publication Data
A catalogue record for this book is available from the British Library

Library of Congress Cataloging in Publication Data
A catalog record for this book is available from the Library of Congress

Acquisitions Editor: **Lucy Gardner**
Assistant Editor: **Jennifer Hardy**
Production Editor: **Colleen Quinn**
Production Supervisor: **Laura Mosberg Cohen**
Cover Design: **Jeannette Jacobs**

Printed in the United States of America

Contributors

S. ABBONDANZA, M.D.
Resident, Diagnostic Radiology, Department of Radiology, University of Trieste, Trieste, Italy

F. ARATA, M.D.
Resident, Diagnostic Radiology, Department of Radiology, University of Rome "La Sapienza," Rome, Italy

BRIAN ARMSTRONG, M.D.
Attending Physician, Department of Cardiology, Holston Valley Hospital and Medical Center, Kingsport, Tennessee

DAVID C. AUTH, PH.D., P.E.
Affiliate Professor, Department of Bioengineering, University of Washington School of Medicine, Seattle, Washington; Consultant, Boston Scientific Corporation, Natick, Massachusetts

BOAZ AVITALL, M.D., Ph.D.
Associate Professor and Director, Clinical and Research Cardiac Electrophysiology Laboratories, Department of Medicine, University of Illinois College of Medicine, Chicago, Illinois

R. AZIZA, M.D.
Consultant, Department of Radiology, Radiology Service, Toulouse, France

JOZEF BARTUNEK, M.D.
Clinical Research Fellow, Cardiovascular Center, OLV Hospital, Aalst, Belgium

ANDREAS BAUMBACH, M.D.
Division of Cardiology, Department of Medicine, University of Tubingen, Tubingen, Germany

IRIS BAUMGARTNER, M.D.
Staff, Angiology Division, Department of Medicine, University of Bern, Inselspital, Bern, Switzerland

JACQUES BERLAND, M.D.
Associate Professor, Department of Cardiology, University of Rouen; Chief, Unit of Cardiology Interventions, Department of Cardiology, Saint-Hilaire Clinic, Rouen, France

MICHEL BERTRAND, M.D.
Professor, Division of Cardiology, Department of Medicine, University of Lille II; Chairman, Department of Cardiology, Cardiology Hospital, Lille, France

RAFAEL BEYAR, M.D., D.Sc.
Professor and Head, Heart System Research Center, Department of Biomedical Engineering, Technion-Israel Institute of Technology; Head, Division of Invasive Cardiology, Department of Cardiology, Rambam Medical Center, Haifa, Israel

F. BLAIN, M.D.
Chief of Clinic, Department of Radiology, Toulouse University—Rangueil, Toulouse, France; Radiologist, Department of Interventional and Diagnostic Imaging, Clinique D'Occitanie, Muret, France

PETER C. BLOCK, M.D.
Professor, Department of Biomedical Science and Engineering, Oregon Graduate Institute of Science and Technology; Associate Director, Heart Institute, St. Vincent Hospital and Medical Center, Portland, Oregon

MARTIN BORGGREFE, M.D.
Associate Professor, Department of Cardiology and Angiology, University of Munster; Consultant Cardiologist, Department of Cardiology, Hospital of the Westfalische Wilhelms University and Institute for Arteriosclerosis Research, Munster, Germany

CORNELIUS BORST, M.D.
Professor, Department of Cardiology, Heart Lung Institute, Utrecht University; Physician, Heart and Lung Institute, Utrecht University Hospital, Utrecht, The Netherlands

JEFFREY A. BREALL, M.D. Ph.D.
Assistant Professor, Division of Cardiology, Department of Medicine, Georgetown University School of Medicine; Associate Director, Cardiac Catheterization Laboratory, Division of Cardiology, Department of Medicine, Georgetown University Hospital, Washington, DC

GÜNTER BREITHARDT, M.D.
Professor, Department of Cardiology and Angiology, University of Munster; Head, Department of Cardiology and Angiology, Hospital of the Westfalische Wilhelms University and Institute for Arteriosclerosis Research, Munster, Germany

L. BROGLIA, M.D.
Resident, Diagnostic Radiology, Department of Radiology, University of Rome, "La Sapienza," Rome, Italy

BRIGITTA C. BROTT, M.D.
Assistant Professor, Division of Cardiology, Department of Medicine, Vanderbilt University School of Medicine; Cardiologist, Veterans Affairs Medical Center, Nashville, Tennessee

PEDRO BRUGADA, M.D.
Professor, Department of Cardiology, Cardiovascular Research and Teaching Institute; Cardiologist, Cardiovascular Center, OLV Hospital, Aalst, Belgium

C. E. BULLER, M.D.
Associate Professor, Department of Medicine, University of British Columbia Faculty of Medicine; Research Director, Division of Cardiology, Vancouver Hospital and Health Sciences Centre, Vancouver, British Columbia, Canada

CHARLES N. S. CHAN, M.B., M.R.C.P.
Consultant Cardiologist and Director, Cardiac Catheterization Laboratories, Department of Cardiology, Singapore Heart Centre/Singapore General Hospital, Singapore

RAJIV CHATURVEDI, M.D.
Lecturer, Department of Paediatrics, Royal Brompton Hospital, Imperial College, London, United Kingdom

ANTONIO COLOMBO, M.D.
Director, Cardiac Catheterization Laboratory, Department of Cardiology, Columbus Hospital, Milan, Italy; Director, Investigational Angioplasty, Department of Cardiology, Lenox Hill Hospital, New York, New York

B. CORMIER, M.D.
Cardiologist and Head, Echocardiographic Laboratory, Department of Cardiology, Tenon Hospital, Paris, France

ALAIN CRIBIER, M.D.
Professor, Department of Cardiology, University of Rouen; Director, Catheterization Laboratory, Department of Cardiology, Charles Nicolle Hospital, Rouen, France

DAVID CUMBERLAND, M.D.
Professor, Interventional Cardiology, Department of Cardiac Sciences, University of Sheffield; Interventional Cardiologist, Clinical Sciences Centre, Northern General Hospital, Sheffield, United Kingdom

NICOLAS DANCHIN, M.D.
Professor, Department of Cardiology, CHU of Nancy, Nancy, France; Head, Department of Cardiology A, Hospital of Brabois, Vandoeuvre-les-Nancy, France

BERNARD DE BRUYNE, M.D., PH.D.
Co-Director, Cardiovascular Center, OLV Hospital, Aalst, Belgium

PIM J. DE FEYTER, M.D.
Director, Catheterization Laboratory, Department of Cardiology, Thoraxcenter, Dijkzigt University Hospital, Rotterdam, The Netherlands

ANTHONY C. DE FRANCO, M.D.
Assistant Professor, Department of Internal Medicine, Ohio State University College of Medicine, Columbus, Ohio; Interventional Cardiologist, Department of Cardiology, Cleveland Clinic Foundation, Cleveland, Ohio

PETER P. DE JAEGERE, M.D., Ph.D.
Cardiologist, Department of Cardiology, Thoraxcenter Dijkzigt University Hospital, Rotterdam, The Netherlands

VISHVA DEV, M.D.
Associate Professor, University of California, Los Angeles, UCLA School of Medicine; Director, Catheterization and Interventional Cardiology, Department of Cardiology, Veterans Affairs Medical Center, Los Angeles, California

DAI-DO DO, M.D.
Staff, Angiology Division, Department of Medicine, University of Bern, Inselspital, Bern, Switzerland

THOMAS J. DONOHUE, M.D.
Assistant Professor, Department of Internal Medicine, Saint Louis University School of Medicine; Attending Physician, Cardiac Catheterization Laboratory, Saint Louis University Hospital, St. Louis, Missouri

GERALD DORROS, M.D.
Medical Director, William Dorros Isadore Feuer Interventional Cardiovascular Disease Foundation; Cardiovascular Interventionist, Milwaukee Heart and Vascular Clinic and St. Luke's Medical Center, Milwaukee, Wisconsin

JOHN S. DOUGLAS, JR., M.D.
Associate Professor, Division of Cardiology, Andreas Gruentzig Cardiovascular Center, Emory Heart Center, Department of Medicine, Emory University School of Medicine; Co-Director, Cardiovascular Laboratory, Emory University Hospital, Atlanta, Georgia

NEAL EIGLER, M.D.
Associate Professor, Department of Cardiology, University of California, Los Angeles, UCLA School of Medicine; Co-Director, Cardiovascular Intervention Center, Department of Cardiology, Cedars-Sinai Medical Center, Los Angeles, California

JOHN M. ELLIOTT, M.B.
Senior Lecturer, Department of Cardiology, Christchurch School of Medicine, Christchurch, New Zealand

STEPHEN G. ELLIS, M.D.
Professor, Department of Medicine, Ohio State University College of Medicine, Columbus, Ohio; Director, Sones Cardiac Catheterization Laboratories, Cleveland Clinic Foundation, Cleveland, Ohio

HÅKAN EMANUELSSON, M.D.
Associate Professor, Department of Cardiology, Heart and Lung Institution, University of Göteborg; Director, Division of Cardiology, Sahigrenska Hospital, Göteborg, Sweden

JEAN-CHRISTIAN FARCOT, M.D.
Professor, Department of Cardiology, College of Medicine of the Hospitals of Paris; Adjoint Professor, Department of Cardiology, University of Paris—West, Paris, France; Practitioner, Cardiology Service, Ambroise Pare Hospital, Boulogne-sur-Seine, France

DAVID P. FAXON, M.D.
Professor, Division of Cardiology, Department of Medicine, University of Southern California School of Medicine; Chief, Division of Cardiology, Los Angeles County and University of Southern California Medical Center, Los Angeles, California

JOHN G. FERGUSON, M.D.
Director, Clinical Epidemiology, Memphis Vascular Research Foundation, Memphis, Tennessee

ROBERT D. G. FERGUSON, M.D.
Director, Memphis Vascular Research Foundation, Memphis, Tennessee

PETER J. FITZGERALD, M.D., Ph.D.
Assistant Professor, Division of Cardiovascular Medicine, Co-Director, Center for Research in Cardiovascular Interventions, Department of Medicine, Stanford University School of Medicine, Stanford, California

JAMES S. FORRESTER, M.D.
Professor, Department of Medicine, and George Burns and Gracie Allen Professor, Department of Cardiology, University of California, Los Angeles, UCLA School of Medicine; Director, Cardiovascular Research Institute, Cedars-Sinai Medical Center, Los Angeles, California

BERNARD J. GERSH, M.D.
W. Proctor Harvey Teaching Professor of Cardiology, Chief, Division of Cardiology, Department of Medicine, Georgetown University School of Medicine, Washington, DC

HERBERT J. GESCHWIND, M.D.
Professor, Departments of Physiology and Physics, Faculty of Science, University of Paris XII; Director, Cardiac Catheterization Laboratory and Interventional Cardiology Unit, Henri Mondor University Hospital, Créteil, France

SIMON GIBBS, M.D.
Senior Lecturer, Department of Cardiac Medicine, National Heart and Lung Institute, Imperial College School of Science, Technology, and Medicine; Consultant Cardiologist, Department of Cardiology, Royal Brompton Hospital, London, United Kingdom

KENTON GREGORY, M.D.
Assistant Professor, Division of Cardiology, Department of Medicine, Oregon Health Sciences University School of Medicine; Director, Oregon Medical Laser Center, St. Vincent Hospital and Medical Center, Portland, Oregon

JULIAN GUNN, M.D.
Lecturer, Department of Cardiac Sciences, University of Sheffield; Senior Registrar, Clinical Sciences Centre, Northern General Hospital, Sheffield, United Kingdom

JÜRGEN HAASE, M.D., Ph.D.
Cardiologist, Department of Cardiology, Heart Center and Red Cross Hospital, Frankfurt, Germany

PATRICK HALL, M.D.
Interventional Cardiologist, Arizona Heart Institute, Phoenix, Arizona

NAOYA HAMASAKI, M.D.
Assistant Director, Department of Cardiology, Kokura Memorial Hospital, Kitakyushu, Japan

JAAP N. HAMBURGER, M.D.
Director, Laser Laboratory, Department of Interventional Cardiology, Thoraxcenter, Dijkzigt University Hospital, Rotterdam, The Netherlands

JOHN C. HARRINGTON, M.D.
Director, Cardiac Catheterization Laboratory, Naval Medical Center, San Diego, California

GUY R. HEYNDRICKX, M.D., Ph.D.
Co-Director, Cardiovascular Center, OLV Hospital, Aalst, Belgium

GERHARD HINDRICKS, M.D.
Department of Cardiology and Angiology, University of Munster; Hospital of the Westfalische Wilhelms University and Institute for Arteriosclerosis Research, Munster, Germany

DAVID HO, M.D., Ph.D., F.R.A.C.P.
Associate Professor of Medicine, Cardiology Division, The University of Hong Kong, Hong Kong; Director, Interventional Cardiology and Cardiac Catheterization Laboratories, Department of Medicine, Queen Mary Hospital, Hong Kong

BERTHOLD HÖFLING, M.D.
Professor, Department of Medicine, Klinikum Großhadern, Ludwig-Maximilians University, Munich, Germany

MANFRED HOFMANN, M.D.
Cardiologist, Department of Cardiology, Heart Center and Red Cross Hospital, Frankfurt, Germany

DAVID R. HOLMES, JR., M.D.
Professor of Medicine, Mayo Medical School; Director, Adult Cardiac Catheterization Laboratory, Mayo Clinic and Mayo Foundation, Rochester, Minnesota

TANYA Y. HUEHNS, M.R.C.P.
Lecturer, Department of Medicine, Klinikum Großhadern, Ludwig-Maximilians University, Munich, Germany

JEFFREY M. ISNER, M.D.
Professor, Department of Medicine and Radiology, Tufts University School of Medicine; Chief, Cardiovascular Research, Department of Medicine and Cardiology, St. Elizabeth's Hospital, Boston, Massachusetts

B. IUNG, M.D.
Cardiologist, Department of Cardiology, Tenon Hospital, Paris, France

MICHAEL R. JAFF, D.O.
Peripheral Vascular Specialist, Milwaukee Heart and Vascular Clinic and St. Luke's Medical Center, Milwaukee, Wisconsin

F. JOFFRE, M.D.
Professor, Department of Radiology, Paul Sabatier University—Rangueil Hospital University; Head, Department of Radiology, Radiology Service, Toulouse, France

SATOSHI KABURAGI, M.D.
Associate Director, Department of Cardiology, Kokura Memorial Hospital, Kitakyushu, Japan

REINER KACHEL, M.D.
Professor, Department of Diagnostic Radiology, Medical School of University of Erfurt; Head, Neuroradiology and MRI, Department of Diagnostic Radiology, University of Erfurt Hospital, Erfurt, Germany

JOEL K. KAHN, M.D.
Assistant Professor, Department of Internal Medicine, Wayne State University School of Medicine, Detroit, Michigan; Interventional Cardiologist, Department of Medicine, William Beaumont Hospital, Royal Oak, Michigan

KARL R. KARSCH, M.D.
Professor, Department of Cardiology, Eberhard-Karls-University, Tubingen, Germany

MORTON J. KERN, M.D.
Professor, Department of Internal Medicine, Saint Louis University School of Medicine; Director, J. G. Mudd Cardiac Catheterization Laboratory, Saint Louis University Hospital, St. Louis, Missouri

M. MUSA KHAN, M.D.
Fellow in Cardiology, Department of Medicine, Baylor College of Medicine; Cardiology Fellow, Department of Cardiology, The Methodist Hospital, Houston, Texas

MEHRAN KHORSANDI, M.D.
Assistant Professor, Department of Cardiology, University of California, Los Angeles, UCLA School of Medicine; Attending Physician, Cardiology, Cedars-Sinai Medical Center, Los Angeles, California

T. KIMURA, M.D.
Assistant Director, Department of Cardiology, Kokura Memorial Hospital, Kitakyushu, Japan

MILAN KOTHARI, M.D.
Clinical Fellow, Department of Cardiology, University of Rouen; Department of Cardiology, Charles Nicolle Hospital, Rouen, France

HANS KOTTKAMP, M.D.
Department of Cardiology and Angiology, University of Munster; Hospital of the Westfalische Wilhelms University and Institute for Arteriosclerosis Research, Munster, Germany

JOEL KUPFER, M.D.
Associate Professor, Department of Cardiology, University of California, Los Angeles, UCLA School of Medicine; Co-Director, Cardiac Noninvasive Laboratory, Department of Cardiology, Cedars-Sinai Medical Center, Los Angeles, California

STANLEY K. LAU, M.D.
Consultant, Chandra Cardiovascular Consultants, Sioux City, Iowa

MARTIN B. LEON, M.D.
Associate Professor, Division of Cardiology, Department of Internal Medicine, Georgetown University Medical Center, Division of Cardiology, Department of Internal Medicine, Washington Hospital Center, Washington, DC

BRICE LETAC, M.D.
Professor, Department of Cardiology, University of Rouen; Head, Department of Cardiology, Charles Nicolle Hospital, Rouen, France

DAVID T. LINKER, M.D.
Associate Professor, Department of Medicine, University of Washington School of Medicine; Associate Director of Echocardiography, Division of Cardiology, University Medical Center, Seattle, Washington

FRANK LITVACK, M.D.
Associate Professor, Department of Cardiology, University of California, Los Angeles, UCLA School of Medicine; Co-Director, Cardiovascular Intervention Center, Department of Cardiology, Cedars-Sinai Medical Center, Los Angeles, California

FELIX MAHLER, M.D.
Professor, Angiology Division, Department of Internal Medicine, University of Bern, Inselspital, Bern, Switzerland

KEN MAHRER, M.D.
Staff, Department of Cardiology, Virginia Mason Medical Center, Seattle, Washington

RAYMOND G. McKAY, M.D.
Associate Professor, Department of Medicine, University of Connecticut School of Medicine, Farmington, Connecticut; Director, Cardiac Laboratory, Department of Medicine, Hartford Hospital, Hartford, Connecticut

BERNHARD MEIER, M.D.
Professor and Head, Department of Cardiology, University Hospital, Bern, Switzerland

DAVID MOLITERNO, M.D.
Department of Medicine, Vanderbilt University School of Medicine, Nashville, Tennessee

MARIE-ANGÈLE MOREL, B.Sc.
Staff, Catheterization Laboratory, Thoraxcenter, Dijkzigt University Hospital, Rotterdam, The Netherlands

DOUGLASS A. MORRISON, M.D.
Professor, Division of Cardiology, Department of Medicine, University of Colorado School of Medicine; Director, Cardiac Catheterization Laboratory, Acting Chief, Department of Cardiology, Veteran's Affairs Medical Center, Denver, Colorado

M. MOSCOVICH, M.D.
Professor, Department of Medicine, University of British Columbia Faculty of Medicine; Director, Cardiac Catheterization Laboratory, Department of Cardiology, Vancouver Hospital and Health Sciences Centre, Vancouver, British Columbia, Canada

RICHARD MYLER, M.D.
Professor, Department of Medicine, University of California, San Francisco, School of Medicine, San Francisco, California; Medical Director, San Francisco Heart Institute, Daly City, California

PAUL NELLENS, M.D.
Cardiovascular Research and Teaching Institute; Cardiovascular Center, OLV Hospital, Aalst, Belgium

STEVEN E. NISSEN, M.D.
Professor, Division of Cardiology, Department of Internal Medicine, Ohio State University College of Medicine, Columbus, Ohio; Director, Coronary Intensive Care Unit, Vice-Chairman, Department of Cardiology, Cleveland Clinic Foundation, Cleveland, Ohio

HENRY NITA, M.D.
Department of Surgical Sciences, University of Sheffield; Clinical Sciences Centre, Northern General Hospital, Sheffield, United Kingdom

M. NOBUYOSHI, M.D.
Vice Medical Director, Kokura Memorial Hospital, Kitakyushu, Japan

HIDEYUKI NOSAKA, M.D.
Assistant Director, Department of Cardiology, Kokura Memorial Hospital, Kitakyushu, Japan

E. MAGNUS OHMAN, M.D.
Assistant Professor, Division of Cardiology, Department of Medicine, Duke University School of Medicine; Coordinator, Clinical Trials in Interventional Cardiology, Division of Cardiology, Department of Medicine, Duke University Hospital, Durham, North Carolina

JAMES M. O'MEARA
Director, Cardiac Imaging Laboratory, Cardiac Catheterization Laboratory, Ochsner Medical Institution, New Orleans, Louisiana

WILLIAM W. O'NEILL, M.D.
Director, Cardiology Division, William Beaumont Hospital, Royal Oak, Michigan

T. OYA, M.D.
Assistant Professor, Department of Radiology, Nippon Medical School, Sendagi, Tokyo, Japan; Director, Department of Diagnostic and Interventional Radiology, Nissan Tamagawa Hospital, Seta, Tokyo, Japan

JULIO C. PALMAZ, M.D.
Stewart R. Reuter Professor, Cardiovascular Section, Department of Radiology, University of Texas Medical School at San Antonio; Chief, Cardiovascular and Special Interventional Radiology, University Health System, San Antonio, Texas

JUAN CARLOS PARODI, M.D.
Adjunct Associate Professor, Division of Surgical Sciences, Bowman Gray School of Medicine of Wake Forest University, Winston-Salem, North Carolina; Director, Fundacion; Chief, Department of Vascular Surgery, Instituto Cardiovascular de Buenos Aires, Buenos Aires, Argentina

DUŠAN PAVČNIK, M.D., Ph.D.
Research Professor of Interventional Therapy, Department of Radiology, Dotter Interventional Institute, Oregon Health Sciences University School of Medicine, Portland, Oregon

I. M. PENN, M.D.
Associate Professor, Department of Medicine, University of British Colombia Faculty of Medicine; Director, Interventional Cardiology, Division of Cardiology, Vancouver Hospital and Health Sciences Centre, Vancouver, British Columbia, Canada

KIRK L. PETERSON, M.D.
Perlman Professor of Cardiology, Department of Medicine, University of California, San Diego, School of Medicine, San Diego, California

HARRY R. PHILLIPS III, M.D., F.A.C.C.
Associate Professor, Division of Cardiology, Department of Medicine, Duke University School of Medicine; Co-Director, Interventional Cardiovascular Program, Department of Cardiology, Duke University Hospital, Durham, North Carolina

NICO H. J. PIJLS, M.D., Ph.D.
Department of Cardiology, Catharina Hospital, Eindhoven, The Netherlands

WOLFGANG PREUSLER, M.D.
Cardiologist and Head, Department of Cardiology, Heart Center and Red Cross Hospital, Frankfurt, Germany

ALBERT E. RAIZNER, M.D.
Professor, Department of Medicine, Baylor College of Medicine; Director, Cardiac Catheterization Laboratories, Department of Cardiology, The Methodist Hospital, Houston, Texas

P. SYAMASUNDAR RAO, M.D.
Professor, Division of Pediatric Cardiology, Department of Pediatrics, University of Wisconsin Medical School, Madison, Wisconsin, and Saint Louis University School of Medicine, St. Louis, Missouri; Director, Division of Pediatric Cardiology, Department of Pediatrics, Cardinal Glennon Children's Hospital, St. Louis, Missouri

S. G. RAY, M.D.
Senior Interventional Cardiology Fellow, Division of Cardiology, Vancouver Hospital and Health Sciences Centre, Vancouver, British Columbia, Canada

ANDREW REDINGTON, M.D.
Consultant Cardiologist, Department of Paediatrics, Royal Brompton Hospital, Imperial College, London, United Kingdom

NICOLAUS REIFART, M.D.
Professor, Department of Medicine, Johann-Wolfgang Goethe University; Head, Department of Cardiology, Heart Center and Red Cross Hospital, Frankfurt, Germany

D. R. RICCI
Professor, Department of Medicine, University of British Columbia Faculty of Medicine; Head, Division of Cardiology, Vancouver Hospital and Health Sciences Centre, Vancouver, British Colombia, Canada

P. RICCI, M.D.
Assistant Professor, Department of Radiology, University of Rome "La Sapienza," Rome, Italy

KENNETH J. ROSENFIELD, M.D.
Assistant Professor, Department of Medicine, Tufts University School of Medicine; Interventional Cardiologist, Department of Cardiology, St. Elizabeth's Hospital, Boston, Massachusetts

M. ROSSI, M.D.
Assistant Professor, Department of Radiology, University of Rome "La Sapienza," Rome, Italy

P. ROSSI, M.D.
Professor, Department of Radiology, University of Rome "La Sapienza," Rome, Italy

GARY ROUBIN, M.D., Ph.D.
Professor, Departments of Medicine and Radiology, University of Alabama School of Medicine; Director, Interventional Cardiology and Adult Cardiac Catheterization Laboratories, University of Alabama, Birmingham, Alabama

H. ROUSSEAU, M.D.
Professor, Department of Radiology, Paul Sabatier University—Rangueil University; Head, Cardiovascular Radiology Section, Department of Radiology, Radiology Service, Toulouse, France

CARLOS E. RUIZ, M.D., Ph.D.
Professor, Division of Cardiology, Department of Medicine, and Professor, Department of Pediatrics, Loma Linda University School of Medicine; Director, Cardiovascular Laboratories, Division of Cardiology, Loma Linda University Medical Center and Children's Hospital, Loma Linda, California

RICHARD A. SCHATZ, M.D.
Research Director, Cardiovascular Interventions, Department of Cardiology, Scripps Clinic and Research Foundation, La Jolla, California

FRANZ SCHWARZ, M.D.
Professor, Department of Medicine, Ruprecht Karls University, Heidelberg; Department of Cardiology, Heart Center and Red Cross Hospital, Frankfurt, Germany

PATRICK W. SERRUYS, M.D., PH.D.
Professor, Department of Interventional Cardiology, Eramus University; Research Director, Catheterization Laboratory, Thoraxcenter, Dijkzigt University Hospital, Rotterdam, The Netherlands

IAN SHEARER, M.D.
Perfusionist Chief, Department of Perfusion Services, Duke University Hospital, Durham, North Carolina

ROBERT SIEGEL, M.D.
Professor, Department of Medicine, University of California, Los Angeles, UCLA School of Medicine; Director, Cardiac Noninvasive Laboratory, Cedars-Sinai Medical Center, Los Angeles, California

ULRICH SIGWART, M.D.
Professor, Department of Medicine, University of Dusseldorf, Dusseldorf, Germany; Director, Department of Invasive Cardiology, Royal Brompton Hospital, Imperial College, London, United Kingdom

JOHN B. SIMPSON, M.D.
Staff Cardiologist, Department of Cardiovascular Medicne, Sequoia Hospital, Redwood City, California

MICHAEL H. SKETCH, JR., M.D.
Assistant Professor, Division of Cardiology, Department of Medicine, Duke University School of Medicine; Director, Adult Cardiac Catheterization Laboratories, Division of Cardiology, Department of Medicine, Duke University Hospital, Durham, North Carolina

J. RICHARD SPEARS, M.D.
Professor, Division of Cardiology, Department of Internal Medicine, Wayne State University School of Medicine; Director, Cardiac Laser Laboratory, Departments of Medicine and Cardiology, Harper Hospital, Detroit, Michigan

RICHARD S. STACK, M.D.
Associate Professor, Department of Medicine, Duke University School of Medicine; Director, Interventional Cardiovascular Program, Duke University Hospital, Durham, North Carolina

CHRISTODOULOS STEFANADIS, M.D., F.A.C.C., F.E.S.C.
Associate Professor, Department of Cardiology, University of Athens School of Medicine; Chief, Coronary Care Unit, Department of Cardiology, Hippokration Hospital, Athens, Greece

HANS STÖRGER, M.D.
Cardiologist and Head, Department of Cardiology, Heart Center and Red Cross Hospital, Frankfurt, Germany

JEAN-FRANÇOIS TANGUAY, M.D.
Department of Cardiology, Montreal Heart Institute, Montreal, Quebec, Canada

ERIC J. TOPOL, M.D.
Chairman, Department of Cardiology, Director, J. J. Jacobs Center for Thrombosis and Vascular Biology, Cleveland Clinic Foundation, Cleveland, Ohio

PAVLOS TOUTOUZAS, M.D., F.A.C.C., F.E.S.C.
Professor and Chairman, Department of Cardiology, University of Athens School of Medicine; Chief, Department of Cardiology, Hippokration Hospital, Athens, Greece

P. TREGANT, M.D.
Consultant, Department of Radiology, Radiology Service, Toulouse, France

JÜRGEN TRILLER, M.D.
Professor, Institute for Diagnostic Radiology, University of Bern, Inselspital, Bern, Switerland

E. MURAT TUZCU, M.D.
Associate Professor, Division of Cardiology, Department of Internal Medicine, Ohio State University College of Medicine, Columbus, Ohio; Staff Cardiologist, Cleveland Clinic Foundation, Cleveland, Ohio

A. VAHANIAN, M.D.
Professor, Department of Cardiology, Faculty of Medicine Paris VI; Chief, Department of Cardiology, Tenon Hospital, Paris, France

CHRISTIAN VALLBRACHT, M.D.
Associate Professor, Department of Medicine, J. W. Goethe University, Frankfurt, Germany; Head, Department of Cardiology and Angiology, Centre for Cardiovascular Diseases, Rotenburg, Germany

MICHÈL VANDORMAEL, M.D.
Director, Department of Cardiology, Saint-Jean Clinic, Brussels, Belgium

TON G. VAN LEEUWEN, Ph.D.
Assistant Professor, Interuniversity Cardiology Institute of the Netherlands, Royal Dutch Academy of Science; Physician, Department of Cardiology, Heart Lung Institute, Utrecht University Hospital, Utrecht, The Netherlands

JAMES VETTER, M.D.
Staff Cardiologist, Department of Cardiovascular Medicine, Sequoia Hospital, Redwood City, California

ROBERT A. VOGEL, M.D.
Head, Division of Cardiology and Herbert Berger Professor, Department of Medicine, University of Maryland School of Medicine; Head, Division of Cardiology, University Hospital, Baltimore, Maryland

M. C. VROLIX, M.D.
Director, Department of Invasive Cardiology, Saint Janshospital, Genk, Belgium

CHRISTOPHER J. WHITE, M.D.
Director, Invasive Cardiology, Healthcare International, Glasglow, Scotland

S. CHIU WONG, M.D.
Assistant Professor, Department of Internal Medicine, Cornell University Medical College, New York, New York; Director, Cardiovascular Interventions, Department of Internal Medicine, New York Hospital Medical Center of Queens, Flushing, New York

PAUL G. YOCK, M.D.
Associate Professor, Division of Cardiovascular Medicine; Director, Center for Research in Cardiovascular Interventions, Department of Medicine, Stanford University School of Medicine, Stanford, California

E. ZEITLER, M.D.
Professor, Department of Medicine, University of Erlangen-Nuremburg; Director, Institute of Diagnostic and Interventional Radiology, Teaching Hospital of Nuremburg-Nord (Emer), Nuremburg, Germany

HE PING ZHANG, M.D.
Senior Cardiovascular Research Associate, Division of Cardiology, Department of Medicine, Loma Linda University School of Medicine; Senior Cardiovascular Research Associate, White Memorial Medical Center, Loma Linda, California

JAMES ZIDAR, M.D.
Assistant Professor, Division of Cardiology, Department of Medicine, Duke University School of Medicine; Cardiologist, Duke University Hospital, Durham, North Carolina

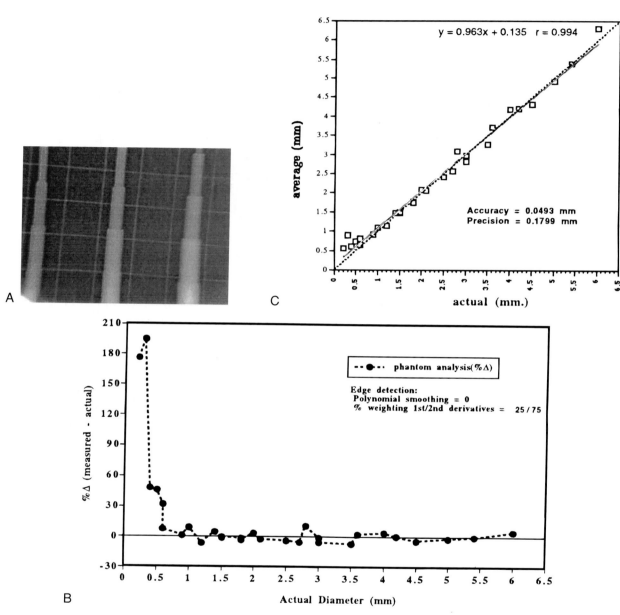

Fig. 1-3. (A) Precision-bored, contrast-filled conduits for validation of quantitative coronary angiography edge recognition algorithms. **(B)** Plot of actual diameter of contrast-filled phantom conduit versus the percentage difference between the measured and actual diameter for conduits between 0.3 and 6.0 mm in diameter. **(C)** Regression plot of actual (*horizontal axis*) versus average measured diameter (*vertical axis*) for series of contrast-filled phantom conduits. Note the high correlation and relatively favorable calculated values for accuracy and precision.

pathophysiology associated with atherosclerotic obstruction. Significant progress has been made in utilizing the kinetics of contrast wash-in and washout through the coronary artery tree and the myocardium to assess coronary flow reserve. Initial efforts involved use of sequential end-diastolic frames following a proximal contrast injection to quantify the arrival time of contrast in the more distal tributaries of the artery. However, such methods suffered from

a relatively low temporal resolution and variability in the profile of contrast injection. Use of impulse response analysis, based upon a lagged normal density model of the input (epicardial) and output (microcirculation) of the coronary arterial tree, has proven to show better correlation with independent measures of myocardial blood flow and coronary reserve measurements.[10] Recently, Eigler and colleagues[11] applied this same technique to patients

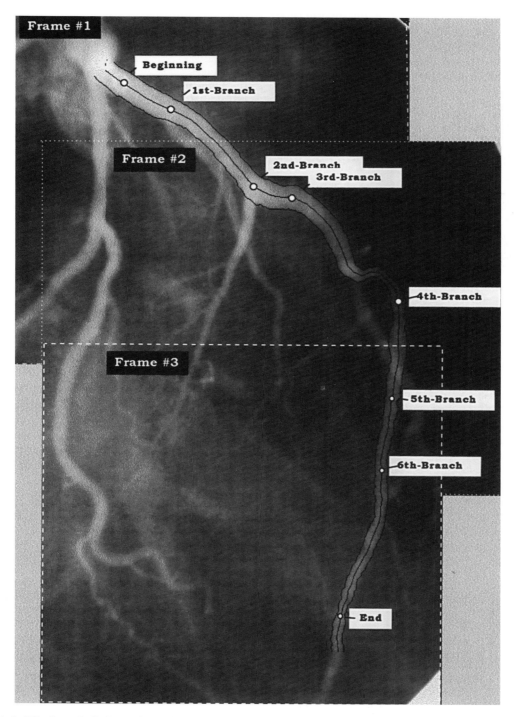

Fig. 1-4. Display of whole analyzable artery for quantitation of a diameter function over multiple contiguous segments of a given coronary artery. Frames are superimposed by autocorrelation. Branch points are utilized as fiducial points between the beginning and end of the function. See text for details.

during coronary balloon angioplasty and demonstrated significant improvement in an index (Tmicro-1) of the regional mean transit time for the microcirculatory compartment after successful balloon angioplasty of an upstream lesion. The technique requires a single, hand-injected bolus of contrast material without any pharmacologic interventions.

NEW RADIOGRAPHIC CONTRAST AGENTS IN ANGIOCARDIOGRAPHY

In the performance of cardiac angiography, injection of iodinated contrast is essential for delineation of the anatomic relation of an individual cardiac structure to its neighbors, demonstration of intracardiac shunts, assessment of the motion of ventricular and atrial chambers throughout the cardiac cycle, and for evaluation of the severity of pathoanatomic changes in the lumen of the coronary and pulmonary vessels. Conventional iodinated, high-osmolar contrast agents, used since the 1950's, are solutions of sodium or meglumine salts (diatrozoate with or without citrate) that have two osmotically active particles for every three iodine atoms (Table 1-3). Such solutions have an osmolality that is approximately 5.8 times that of plasma and cause significant hemodynamic, electrophysiologic, and clinical side effects. Nevertheless, they are optimally radiopaque, enhance diagnostic images, and for many years their clinical benefit outweighed their risk and side effects. Low-osmolar nonionic contrast agents were developed, primarily in Europe in the 1980s and first approved for use in the United States in 1985 (Table 1-3). These agents are widely acknowledged to reduce the most common nonsevere side effects such as nausea, vomiting, heat sensation, urticaria, and itching (Table 1-4). However, significant controversy has developed over the benefit of such agents in relation to their much higher cost. Also, issues have recently been raised as to differing effects on the coagulation

Table 1-4. Incidence of the Common Side Effects with Ionic and Nonionic Iodinated Contrast Agents

Side Effect	Ionic (%)	Nonionic (%)
Nausea	4.6	1.0
Vomiting	1.8	0.4
Heat sensation	2.3	0.9
Urticaria	3.2	0.5
Itching	3.0	0.5

(From Katayama et al.,[12] with permission.)

system. These issues have become ever more relevant to the cardiologist as increasing catheterization procedures are performed for therapeutic reasons.

Specific Attributes of High-Osmolar, Ionic Contrast Agents

For many years high-osmolar, ionic contrast agents (osmolality of approximately 1,600 to 2,000 mOsm/kg) have been noted to have hemodynamic and electrophysiologic effects during their administration. With these agents two osmotically active particles are given for every three iodine atoms. All of this class have a negative inotropic effect on the myocardium as evidenced by a depression of peak dP/dt. Moreover, the osmotic load of the usual dose (24 to 60 ml over 3 seconds) causes expansion of the circulating blood volume and an increase in the left ventricular end-diastolic volume and pressure. At the same time these agents are vasodilators and cause a drop in both systemic and coronary arterial vascular resistance. These vasodilatory effects are transient and disappear in approximately 60 seconds after administration of the contrast agent.

Electrophysiologic perturbations are also prominent in the pharmacologic effects of high-osmolar, ionic contrast agents. Injection of one of these agents into the coronary artery that supplies the sinoatrial node causes a distinct depression of sinus automatic-

Table 1-3. Commonly Used Iodinated Contrast Agents in Angiocardiography

Product Category	Proprietary Name	Generic Constituent	Calcium Chelation	Anticoagulant Effect
High osmolar, ionic	Renografin-76	Diatrozoate and citrate	(+)	(+ + +)
High osmolar, ionic	Hypaque-76	Diatrozoate only	(−)	(+ + +)
Low osmolar, ionic	Hexabrix	Ioxaglate	(−)	(+ + +)
Low osmolar, nonionic	Isovue	Iopamidol	(−)	(+)
Low osmolar, nonionic	Omnipaque	Iohexol	(−)	(+)
Low osmolar, nonionic	Optiray	Ioversol	(−)	(+)

Color Plates

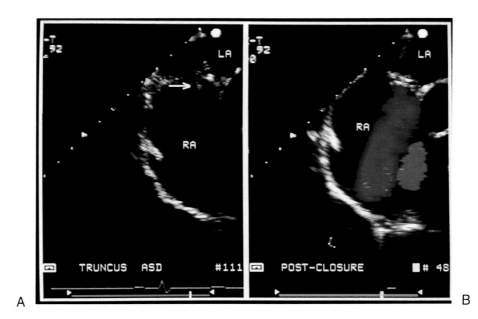

A   B

Plate 86-2.

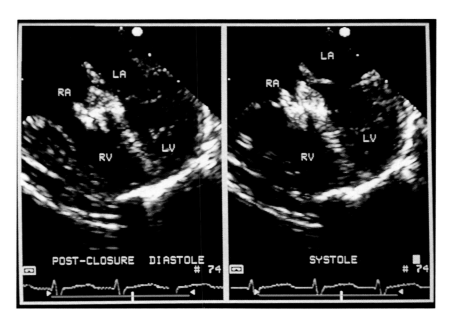

Plate 86-3.

Plate 86-2. (A) The modified umbrella device being pulled into the defect. **(B)** The device after deployment. Note how closely opposed the proximal and sital umbrellas are. Complete closure is seen.

Plate 86-3. Transesophageal echo from the same case in Figs. 86-3 to 86-8. Note the position of the distal and proximal umbrellas. There is no interference with the tricuspid or mitral valve function. Complete closure was achieved.

ity that is transient and reversed by vagolytic maneuvers or drugs. Similarly, when contrast is injected into the coronary artery supplying the atrioventricular node, there is a depression of conductivity manifested by increasing A-V nodal block (first, second, or third degree) that is again transient. Preadministration of atropine significantly protects against this response. There are also notable effects on repolarization associated with injection of these agents. The Q-T interval on the electrocardiogram is prolonged irrespective of the route of administration. With coronary artery injections, there are also prominent, yet transitory, ST-T wave changes, reflecting effects on myocardial repolarization.

Depression of renal function, manifested by a transient reduction in the creatinine clearance and elevation of both the serum blood urea nitrogen and creatinine, has been noted for many years with these agents. A severe contrast-induced nephropathy, associated with acute tubular necrosis, can be a serious complication of patients with preexistent renal disease (e.g., those with serum creatinine greater than 2.2 mg%) and in those patients with diabetic nephrosclerosis.

Specific Attributes of Low-Osmolar, Ionic and Nonionic Contrast Agents

Low-osmolar contrast agents exhibit the same radiopacity as high-osmolar agents yet their osmolalities are in the range of 600 to 900 mOsm/kg. The nonionic monomers (e.g., iopamidol) in this group have eliminated the sodium and meglumine ions, yet maintained three iodine atoms per molecule. All the members of this class have less negative inotropic effect on the myocardium, are less potent vasodilators, and exhibit less effect on the left ventricular end-diastolic volume and pressure. They also have much less potential for causing a sinus bradycardia and atrioventricular block during selective coronary angiography.

Effects of Contrast Agents on the Coagulation System

All contrast agents are known to have an anticoagulant effect manifest by their ability to prolong the activated partial thromboplastin time. This property appears to be independent of the osmolar state; however, ionic, as compared to nonionic, agents appear to be more potent anticoagulants (Table 1-3). As compared to nonionic agents, ionic agents demonstrate greater prolongation of the activated partial throm-

boplastin time and show greater inhibition of clot formation in glass or plastic syringes.

There appear to be some differences in platelet activation between high- and low-osmolar contrast agents. A study by Chronos and associates[13] used immunolabeling and flow cytometry to assess in vitro the effects of various contrast agents on platelet activation. Control blood, mixed with saline, demonstrated approximately 2% platelet activation. Hexabrix, an ionic, low-osmolar agent, activated 3% of platelets, an insignificant value compared to the control blood. However, Omnipaque, a nonionic, low-osmolar agent showed 60–80% platelet activation by 1 minute. These ex vivo observations would suggest that the nonionic agents as compared to ionic agents, irrespective of osmolarity, have a strong propensity to cause platelet activation, the earliest step in arterial thrombotic occlusion. In separate analyses, these same authors reported that blood drawn from patients pretreated with aspirin and heparin, and subsequently exposed in vitro to Omnipaque, showed significant platelet activation, while Hexabrix showed no change from control.

SUMMARY

Over the last decades refinements and automation in the design and technology of radiographic equipment have provided consistently improved angiographic cardiac images for the interventional cardiologist. Moreover, improved television scanning, x-ray tube shielding, and filtering techniques have served to reduce radiation exposure for both patient and cardiac angiographic suite personnel. Nevertheless, the significant radiation exposure inherent in the field of interventional cardiology mandates frugal activation of the x-ray tube during any given procedure.

New image processing and storage techniques have allowed immediate review and quantitation of contrast injections. Digital processing has eventuated in sensitive new approaches to the identification of abnormal pathophysiologic processes. Finally, the development of new angiographic contrast agents, although expensive, has reduced complications related to their use.

Although now a relatively old technique, cardiac angiography will likely remain an indispensable diagnostic tool for the practice of interventional cardiology.

REFERENCES

1. Johns PC, Renaud L. Radiation risk associated with PTCA. Primary Cardiol 1994;20:27–31
2. Pattee JL, Johns PC, Chambers RJ. Radiation risk

to patients from transluminal coronary angioplasty. J Am Coll Cardiol 1993;22:1044–1051

3. International Commission on Radiological Protection Publication 60. 1990 Recommendations of the International Commission on Radiological Protection. Oxford: Pergamon Press; 1991:24, Table 4

4. Renaud L. A 5-year follow-up of the radiation exposure to in-room personnel during cardiac catheterization. Health Phys 1992;62:10–15

5. den Boer A, de Feyter PJ, Hummel WA, et al. Reduction of radiation exposure while maintaining high-quality fluoroscopic images during interventional cardiology using novel x-ray tube technology with extra beam filtering. Circulation 1994;89:2710–2714

6. Sheehan FH, Bolson EL, Dodge HT, et al. Advantages and applications of the centerline method for characterizing regional ventricular function. Circulation 1986;74:293–305

7. Gibson CM, Safian RD. Limitations of cineangiography: impact of new technologies for image processing and quantitation. Trends Cardiovasc Med 1992;2:156–60

8. Brown BG, Bolson E, Frimer M, Dodge HT. Quantitative coronary arteriography: estimation of dimensions, hemodynamic resistance, and atheroma mass of coronary artery lesions using the arteriogram and digital computation. Circulation 1977;55:329–337

9. Penny WF, Rockman H, Long J, et al. Heterogeneity of vasomotor response to acetylcholine along the human coronary artery. J Am Coll Cardiol 1995;25:1046–1055

10. Eigler NL, Pfaff JM, Zeiher AM, et al. Digital angiographic impulse response analysis of regional myocardial perfusion: linearity, reproducibility, accuracy, and comparison with conventional indicator dilution curve parameters in phantom and canine models. Circ Res 1989;64:853–866

11. Schuhlen H, Eigler NL, Zeiher AM, et al. Digital angiographic assessment of the physiological changes to the regional microcirculation induced by successful coronary angioplasty. Circulation 1994;90:163–171

12. Katayama H, Yamaguchi K, Kozuka T et al. Adverse reactions to ionic and nonionic contrast media: a report from The Japanese Committee on the Safety of Contrast Media. Radiology 1990;175:621–628

13. Chronos NAF, Goodall AH, Wilson DJ, et al. Profound platelet degranulation is an important side effect of some types of contrast media used in interventional cardiology. Circulation 1993;88(Part I):2035–2044

2 Intravascular Ultrasound: Physics and Equipment

David T. Linker

HISTORY

Although the clinical application of intravascular ultrasound is relatively new, the concepts date back to the beginning of ultrasound in cardiac diagnosis. In the 1950s, Cieszynski[1] was the first to report using a catheter-mounted transducer to measure chamber dimensions in dogs. The first real-time cross-sectional intravascular imaging catheter was developed by Bom and colleagues[2] and reported in 1972. At the time, transthoracic ultrasonic imaging was gaining popularity, and an invasive method did not seem as attractive.

The explosion of intravascular interventions in the late 1970s provided the motivation for developing intravascular imaging devices, and several groups started or revived activities in the field during the middle 1980s. In 1988, Yock and coworkers[3] presented the first in vivo results of the use of this new generation of intravascular imaging devices. Since then, better and smaller catheter have been produced, along with advances in the clinical and research applications of these techniques. For a more detailed review of the history of intravascular ultrasound development, see Tobis and Yock[4] or Bom and colleagues.[5]

RATIONALE AND MECHANISM OF ACTION

Three major features distinguish intravascular ultrasound from other forms of vascular imaging, and each of these features results in both advantages and disadvantages: (1) the technique is invasive, (2) it provides real-time imaging, and (3) the imaging is cross-sectional. In many ways, these characteristics overlap, providing a basis for discussing the motivation and physical principles involved in intravascular imaging.

Invasive Technique

Intravascular ultrasound is invasive, with all of the obvious disadvantages that this entails. The advantage, however, is that we are able to bring the ultrasound transducer very close to the structures we wish to image, which allows us to use a very high frequency, resulting in very high resolution. This results in a "cascade" of consequences, most of which are favorable (Table 2-1). In general, all ultrasound imaging is a balance between resolution and penetration. Resolution is in large part related to the

Table 2-1. Consequences of Using an Invasive Technique	
Change	Consequence
Short transducer to tissue distance	Less attenuation of ultrasound signal
Less attenuation of ultrasound signal	Higher frequencies can be used
Higher ultrasound frequencies	Higher resolution of tissue
	Blood contrast more prominent

transducer frequency, although this is modified by the size and shape of the transducer and characteristics of the ultrasound instrument. If all other factors are equal, a higher transducer frequency would result in proportionally higher resolution. If this were the only factor to consider, we would always use the highest frequency we could design and construct for highest resolution.

The limitation is that the penetration of ultrasound into tissue is inversely related to frequency. High frequencies tend to penetrate tissue more poorly than lower frequencies, limiting the depth to which we can conduct the examination. This is similar (but opposite in its frequency dependency) to the phenomenon of beam hardening in x-ray imaging. The most extreme form of this frequency dependency is in the case of blood, which has a 16-fold increase in backscattering efficiency for a doubling of the frequency.[6] This is the reason that blood is so easily visible on intravascular ultrasound images using frequencies equal to or over 30 MHz.

Because of the problem of ultrasound penetration with higher frequencies, we must balance the depth to which we can image, which is improved by lowering the transducer frequency, against the resolution, which is improved by raising the transducer frequency. We can improve the depth to some degree by the technique of *time-gain compensation,* which adjusts the gain to different (usually higher) levels at greater depths to compensate for the decreased signal strength. This is done by changing the gain at different times after the ultrasound pulse has been transmitted, since the time between transmission of the pulse and reception corresponds to the depth; hence the term time-gain compensation. Because intravascular ultrasound is invasive, we are able to accept very short penetration distances of only a few centimeters, and therefore are able to increase the transducer frequency to 20 MHz and beyond for intraarterial imaging, allowing resolution in the range of 100 μm or less.

As we reduce the size of the transducer-catheter combination to enter smaller vessels, we must increase the transducer frequency to even maintain the same angular resolution. This is because the diameter of the transducer also influences the resolution directly, so that a reduction in diameter results in a reduction in resolution, unless we also raise the frequency of the transducer at the same time.

For certain applications we need a greater ultrasound penetration depth, for example, imaging in the great arteries and intracardiac imaging, where important structures can be located several centimeters from the catheter. In these cases, the same principles apply, requiring us to decrease the frequency of the transducer to 10 to 15 MHz to obtain adequate penetration of the ultrasound beam—even through blood. As a result, the diameter of the transducer, and therefore the catheter, must be increased. Catheters for these applications are typically 7 F (2.3 mm in diameter) or larger versus intraarterial catheters, which are now as small as 2.9 F (less than 1 mm in diameter).

Real-Time Imaging

The ability to view images at the same time as they are being created is an obvious advantage, both for on-line guidance of the imaging process itself and for being able to provide immediate information to guide interventions. The disadvantage of real-time imaging is less apparent, that is, we have very limited possibilities for image processing and improvement. Magnetic resonance imaging, and some computed tomography techniques are based on averaging of images acquired over a period of time. This permits considerable noise reduction, which is not available to the same degree in ultrasound imaging.

Limited image averaging is available on many ultrasound instruments, in the form of real-time frame averaging, which is sometimes called frame averaging, temporal filtering, temporal averaging, time averaging, or persistence, among other terms. This technique allows a weighted average of several images (frames) to be displayed on the screen in real time. For structures that move very little during the imaging, such as peripheral arteries, this can provide an improvement of the image quality. For arteries with motion, such as the coronaries, too much temporal averaging can cause a blurring of the image. Systems with this feature can usually be adjusted to obtain the optimal balance between blurring and noise.

This form of real-time filtering is different from "off-line" postprocessing, which is performed on a computer after digitizing the image to enhance certain features for teaching purposes. Off-line processing creates pictures different from those seen by the user during performance of the study, while the temporal filtering described is applied to the images presented to the operator during the examination.

Cross-Sectional Imaging

Perhaps the most important characteristic of intravascular ultrasound is that it produces a cross-sectional image of the artery and the contents of the stenosis. Angiography, by comparison, gives a projected image of the shadow of the lumen, filled with contrast. Fiberoptic angioscopy shows the inside surface of the vessel. A cross-sectional image gives us accurate luminal dimensions, and displays the contents of the atherosclerosis causing the stenosis. As a result, intravascular ultrasound is more sensitive than angiography in detecting the atherosclerotic process.[7] Angiography relies on luminal narrowing to detect disease, but in the early stages of the atherosclerotic process, there is often a compensatory dilation of the adventitia, so that luminal narrowing occurs only after a large amount of atherosclerotic material develops, filling up 40% to 50% of the lumen.[8]

We are also able to identify some of the contents of stenotic lesions, although the correlation is not perfect[9] because the physics of ultrasound limits identification.[6,10] We should be aware of two effects in particular. Increasing frequency leads to greater scattering from fibrous tissue, approaching that of calcified tissue,[6,10,11] so that one should probably not identify tissues as calcium-containing unless there is also shadowing, regardless of the brightness of the echoes. Also, the angle dependency of arterial tissues when examined at these frequencies may cause dramatic changes in the strength of the backscattered signal,[12] which can complicate identification of arterial structures[13] or even obscure them.[14]

The direction of the beam also has an effect. When the ultrasonic pulse travels from a less echogenic structure (dark) to a more echogenic structure (bright), the intensity transition in the returning echo occurs at the correct place. If the pulse goes from a more echogenic structure to a less echogenic structure, however, the intensity transition is delayed, due to the length of the transmitted pulse. This means that measurements of dark structures, such as the muscular media, can be underestimated due

to the "bleeding" of the bright intima, especially if there is significant hyperplasia of the intima. Table 2-2 summarizes the correlations between appearance and possible interpretation. Some correlations between the content of stenotic lesions and the results of intravascular interventions[15,16] suggest that the shape of the lesion, as well as contents, such as calcium, can effect the likelihood of dissection.

The disadvantage of cross-sectional imaging is that we do not see a complete overview of the arterial circulation of interest in a "map" format. Angiography is far superior in this respect.

INSTRUMENTATION

Ultrasound

The requirements for the instrument used for intravascular ultrasound are similar in most ways to those for a general ultrasound instrument. The generation of the ultrasound pulses, reception, processing, and display are practically identical. The only significant differences in these stages have to do with the frequency, which is much higher for intravascular ultrasound (10–40 MHz compared to 2–10 MHz), and the shape of the display. Since an intravascular ultrasound system creates a cross-sectional view of the artery, it has a circular display, rather than the familiar sector display of other cardiac ultrasound systems.

The control of the ultrasound beam direction is significantly different, however, since all intravascular ultrasound systems have either a mechanically rotating system, or an electronically steered synthetic aperture, both described later in this section. These two types of systems are similar in concept, but significantly different in practice from mechanical and phased-array transducers used in conventional ul-

Table 2-2. Image Observations and Possible Interpretations

Finding	Interpretation	Look for or Check
Bright echo	Fibrous tissue	
	Perpendicular beam	Angle relative to transducer
	Calcification	Shadowing
Uniform speckle in lumen	Flowing blood	Varies with cardiac cycle
	Stagnant blood	Little cyclic variation
	Thrombus	Little cyclic variation
Shadowing	Calcium	Bright echo
	Total reflection	Surface causing reflection
Defect in artery wall	Dissection/rupture	Blood flow in defect
	Lipid "lake"	Fibrous cap, echoes present distally
	Gain too low (dropout)	Gain settings

trasound. Most intravascular ultrasound instruments are specifically built for this purpose or are modified versions of conventional ultrasound machines. Some have remote control devices, so that the operator can control the instrument from the sterile field.

Some manufacturers have created "combined" instruments that can be used as both an intravascular ultrasound machine and as a full-featured conventional ultrasound machine. This can be accomplished without any loss of image quality for either mode of use. There may be some disadvantage in size and ease of use compared to a dedicated machine, however. For laboratories where the number of intravascular ultrasound studies and conventional ultrasound examinations is low, this may be an attractive option.

Catheter Operation

To produce a cross-sectional image, the ultrasound pulses must be transmitted in a given direction, and the returning ultrasound received from the same direction, and the whole process repeated in a sequence of different directions until a cross section can be built up using interpolation. For convenience, the direction involved in transmission and reception is called a beam.

The design of the catheter depends on the method used for steering these beams—mechanical or electronic (Fig. 2-1 and Table 2-3).

Mechanical Beam Steering

All mechanical systems rely on physical rotation to direct the beam in various directions, but this can be accomplished in two different ways: The transducer is rotated directly or the transducer is pointed at a mirror that is rotated. At first, these two methods may appear to be almost identical, and the added complexity of a mirror unnecessary. The reason for adopting the mirror technique is that the image is distorted in the area adjacent to the transducer itself, due to (1) the vibrations generated during transmission of the pulse, called the ring-down artifact, and (2) the lack of focus, called the near-field artifact (Fig. 2-2). The ring-down artifact results because the same transducer is used to generate the transmitted ultrasound pulse and receive the returning signal. When the transducer is excited to create the pulse, it "rings," much like a damped bell, thereby producing a signal that overwhelms any received signal for the period immediately after the transmission of the pulse. The near-field artifact which extends farther

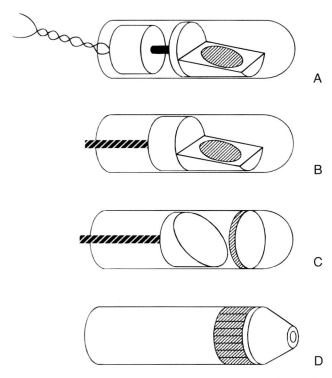

Fig. 2-1. Three fundamental design decisions can be made in making an intravascular ultrasound catheter. The first is whether the system will use mechanical beam steering (**A**) to (**C**), or electronic (**D**). The second is whether the rotational motion of a mechanical system is provided by a micromotor (**A**) or by a cable (**B**) + (**C**). Finally, the mechanical system may either have a rotating transducer design (**B**) or a rotating mirror design (**C**). A micromotor-rotating mirror design is also possible, but is not shown here. The transducers are indicated by crosshatching.

from the transducer face, results from interference of the wavefronts when the distance to the object being imaged is very different for different parts of the transducer face. This problem is similar to trying to focus near the surface of an optical lens if the lens was not designed for this type of work.

There is always a region near the transducer that gives poorer quality, or no imaging. By adopting a rotating mirror design, these regions are "buried" inside the catheter itself, but at the cost of greater complexity of design. A rotating transducer design partially buries these artifacts, and a synthetic aperture (discussed later), with the transducers on the surface of the catheter, must deal with both of the artifacts. For each catheter design, this is a tradeoff that must be evaluated.

The second way in which mechanical systems differ from one another is how the mechanical energy is transmitted to the tip of the catheter to rotate the mirror or transducer. The simplest way, concep-

Table 2-3. Consequences of Catheter Design Choices

Choice	Consequences/Choice	Secondary Consequences
Electronic beam steering	No moving parts	Always uniform imaging Easier to make flexible
	Transducers on surface	Ring-down and near-field artifacts
	Less resolution	
Mechanical beam steering	Rotating cable	Nonuniform rotation can be a problem
	Micromotor	Uniform rotation Difficult to make in smallest sizes
	Rotating mirror	Near-field and ring-down reduced
	Rotating transducer	Ring-down artifact reduced Near-field still a problem Simpler design than rotating mirror

tually, is to have a small electric motor embedded in the tip of the catheter (Fig. 2-1A). The problem with this technique is that the design of such a motor is extremely challenging. In spite of this, one research group has already designed, built, and tested such a catheter system for intravascular applications. The alternative is to use a drive cable to connect the rotating elements at the tip of the catheter with an external motor (Fig. 2-1B, C). This simplifies the design of the motor considerably, but at the price of difficulty in designing the cable assembly because this system must rotate with great uniformity, in spite of the long distance (>1.5 m) and possible curves that the catheter takes on its way to the artery being imaged. Any significant rotational nonuniformity will

cause distortion of the image on the screen, since the assumed position of the transducer is based on the motor rotation, while the actual image comes from the direction of the beam. Careful design can reduce this problem to where it seldom affects the image significantly. The other advantage of the cable designs is that further miniaturization, although difficult, is not as difficult as it would be if the entire motor and timing mechanisms have to be miniaturized as well.

Electronic Beam Steering

In contrast to a mechanical catheter, one that uses electronic beam steering has no moving parts, and has many transducers rather than only one (Fig. 2-

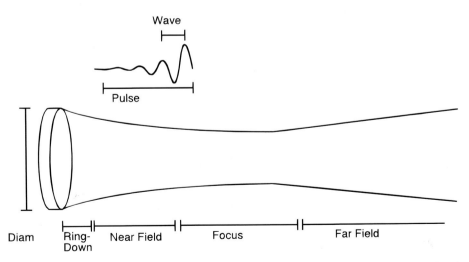

Fig. 2-2. The transducer emits a pulse of sound, which has a fundamental wavelength (*Wave*), and pulse length (*Pulse*). The pulse length determines the longitudinal resolution, while the wavelength and the diameter of the transducer (*Diam*) determine the lateral resolution. The area indicated by *Ring-Down* has marked disturbance due to the vibrations of the transducer caused by pulse transmission. The area marked *Near Field* has wavefront disturbances due to proximity to the transducer face. After the focus, the beam begins to diverge in the far field.

1D). The principle of operation is very similar to that of a phased array, but there are certain differences due to the size constraints. A phased array also consists of a number of transducers used for transmission and reception *almost* in unison. Slight delays are introduced both for transmission and reception to point the beam in different directions. In practice this means that the transducers are excited at slightly different times and the received signals are added together with controlled time delays. This also means that each transducer must be used almost simultaneously for each pulse and therefore must have its own electrical connections. The large number of wires this requires cannot be incorporated into a small catheter, and therefore another solution is necessary.

The solution relies on the fact that the operation of each transducer can be at a completely different time, as long as the structures being imaged have not moved too much. The technique of adding the signals together can work properly, even if the received signals from each transducer occurred at completely different times and were generated by completely different transmitted pulses. Because of the short distances involved for the penetration and return of the pulses, it is possible to send pulses out at a very high rate. By using miniaturized switching circuitry at the tip of the catheter, a limited number of wires can control the switching between the different transducers and the transmission and reception of the ultrasound signals. Because the signals from an array of transducers (aperture) are put together (synthesized) after the fact, this technique is called *synthetic aperture*. The whole process occurs very rapidly, so that the end result is that the images generated appear in real time on the monitor screen, in spite of the sophisticated signal processing that has occurred. Such a system has an advantage in that there are no moving parts, so that the discussion about uniform rotation in the preceding section is irrelevant for this type of catheter. The disadvantage is that there is a limitation of resolution inherent

in the design, so that it will not be able to match a mechanical design of the same size.[17]

Guidewire

The way in which the guidewire is used in conjunction with the catheter is an important part of its design. In general, we can identify four different types of guidewire designs (Fig. 2-3 and Table 2-4).

The simplest is a fixed guide wire, which is attached to the end of the catheter. This results in no additional width to accommodate the guide wire, but it also means that the lesion must be crossed each time that the catheter is exchanged. This type of design was common in the earliest intravascular ultrasound catheters, but has been largely displaced by the designs that are described below.

Next, there is the eccentric design, again analogous to the interventional catheter designs. The guidewire enters the catheter 5–30 cm proximal to the tip, and then is directed to the center by the time it reaches the tip. These allow a shorter exchange wire, but the wire is adjacent to the imaging region of the catheter, in a position where it will interfere with part of the field of view.

Next, in the concentric design, the guidewire is in the center of the tip and is removable. This is completely analogous to interventional catheters and has the same advantages and disadvantages, namely, good pushability, but a long exchange wire is essential.

The last alternative is the *removable core*. This is a variation on the mechanical, rotating cable designs, which has a cable and transducer assembly ("core") that can be withdrawn either fully or partially, leaving the sheath in place. This sheath in turn can accommodate a guidewire in the same channel used for the core. This means that the overall diameter is reduced compared to a similar eccentric design, and that there is no interference due to the guidewire during imaging. An additional advantage of this design is that the transducer assembly can be pulled back within the sheath, so that a pullback is less

Table 2-4. Types of Guidewire Usage

Type	Advantages	Disadvantages
Fixed	Simple, not in imaging field	Crosses lesion every catheter change
Eccentric	Exchangable	In image field
Concentric	Exchangable, not in image field	Long exchange wire
Removable core	Exchangable, no imaging disturbance	Combining with interventions?

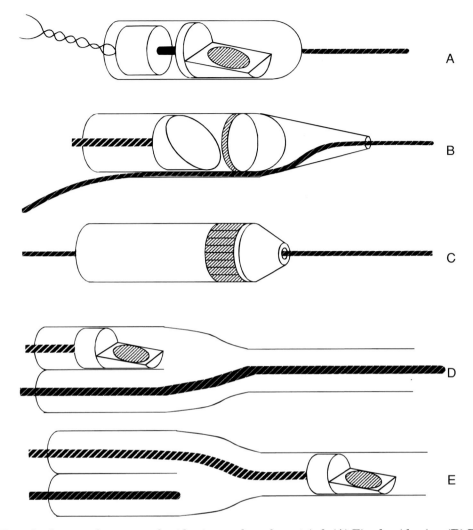

Fig. 2-3. Four fundamental systems of guidewire use have been tried. **(A)** Fixed guidewire. **(B)** Eccentric guidewires or **(C)** concentric guidewires. A recent development is the "removable core": **(D)** with the transducer "parked"; **(E)** with the guidewire "parked". In actual practice, the length of the common segment of catheter is much longer, but it has been shortened here for illustrative purposes.

likely to abrade the endothelium and may be more uniform. This type of design may be at a disadvantage for combined interventional-imaging designs (discussed in the following section) but this can be compensated for if interventional catheters can fit into the "guidewire" lumen.

Combined Devices

Another interesting development is the emergence of combined interventional and imaging catheters. The advantages to this are obvious, since one can image without exchanging catheters, and is more likely to examine the results of an intervention with the imaging system. The disadvantages are the compromises that are necessary in designing a catheter, and these are numerous if the catheter combines several functions. These compromises also add to the cost and may reduce flexibility—for example, if one decides to use a different interventional technique after imaging.

Virtually every interventional catheter has been considered for a combined device. The most common is in combination with a balloon. In spite of this, the techniques that probably have the most to gain are those that are directional in nature, such as atherectomy and lasers. A combined atherectomy and imaging device has been constructed, allowing the operator to see where the tissue will be removed. Similar systems for lasers are more difficult to create, since current lasers "shoot" in a forward direction, and current imaging devices look perpendicular to the catheter. In any case, we can expect that advances in ease of use and combination with interventional procedures will be important in the near future of intravascular ultrasound.

CURRENT INDICATIONS

The following chapters deal in detail with the applications of intravascular ultrasound to particular vascular beds and in combination with interventional procedures. In addition to demonstrating features other techniques do not have, intravascular ultrasound must have a favorable effect on outcome and costs, or both, to be accepted as a routine clinical procedure. Research on these issues is currently under way. For more basic research, however, the criteria are somewhat broader. The ability to observe the atherosclerotic process with a greater sensitivity than existing techniques is of great importance. In particular, in studies of atherosclerotic progression and regression, as well as restenosis, the sensitivity of a technique determines the number of studies necessary to prove a difference. This in turn affects the chances of a false-negative result, and the cost in setting up the study, due to number of patients or experimental animals.

We already know that intravascular ultrasound is much more sensitive to the atherosclerotic process than angiography. Pathologic studies suggested that the early atherosclerotic process involves a "compensatory" *dilation* of the adventitia at the same time as the atheroma develops. The result is that the lumen of the vessel is not affected until there is a very significant atheroma, occluding 45% or more of the area of the lumen.[8] Comparisons of angiography to intravascular ultrasound in vivo have produced similar results.[7] This means that we can have progression from 0% to 45% filling of the lumen with the atherosclerotic process before it will become visible on the angiogram. It also suggests that a treatment that may be effective at *reducing* atheroma load may be judged ineffective by angiography, due to the insensitivity of the technique. Given these results, intravascular ultrasound should be preferred to angiography for the study of regression and progression of lesions. We are able to see much more of the contents of lesions and the details of lesion anatomy with ultrasound imaging. This technique is also preferable for the study of morphology—both before and after interventions—and for obtaining the natural history.

An example of the superior facility of ultrasound imaging can be observed in the placement of stents. Several studies have shown that stents that appear to be adequately placed angiographically are, in fact, correctly apposed to the arterial wall in less than 17% of patients.[18,19] In the remaining patients the stent is not fully expanded, and there is some dead space between the wall of the artery and the stent. It is reasonable to assume that better technical results would lead to better clinical results, and some preliminary studies suggest that ultrasound guidance (1) can increase the percentage of good technical results to more than 70%,[20] (2) can dramatically reduce the need for anticoagulation, and (3) may lead to reduced restenosis. Application of this technique may be limited for some stent designs because they are less visible on the ultrasound image.

OUTLOOK AND POTENTIAL DEVELOPMENT

Intravascular ultrasound provides unique information that is difficult or impossible to obtain with other techniques in vivo. The information on lesion and vessel dimensions, as well as lesion contents, is extremely important to the understanding of the effect of interventions, both intravascular and medical, on the natural history of the atherosclerotic process.

We can expect evolutionary developments in terms of better image quality, smaller catheters, and more convenient handling. In addition, we can expect revolutionary developments with combined catheters changing the way interventions are performed, improvements in tissue identification, and combined use of flow and imaging. It is highly probable that intravascular ultrasound will find a significant clinical and research role in the interventional laboratory.

REFERENCES

1. Cieszynski T. Intracardiac method for investigation of structure of the heart with the aid of ultrasonics. Arch Immunol Ter Dosw 1960;8:551
2. Lancée CT, van Egmond FC. An ultrasonic intracardiac catheter. Ultrasonics 1972;10:72–76
3. Yock PG, Johnsen EL, Linker DT. Intravascular ultrasound: development and clinical potential. Am J Car Imaging 1988;2:185–193
4. Tobis JM, Yock PG. Introduction and synopsis of intravascular ultrasound Imaging. In Tobis JM, Yock PG, Intravascular Ultrasound Imaging. eds. New York: Churchill Livingstone, 1992:1–6
5. Bom N, ten-Hoff H, Lancée CT, et al. Early and recent intraluminal ultrasound devices. Int J Card Imaging 1989;4:79–88
6. Linker DT, Kleven A, Grønningsæther Å, et al. Tissue characterization with intra-arterial ultrasound: spe-

cial promise and problems. Int J Card Imaging 1991; 6:255–263.

7. Escaned J, Haase J, di Mario C, et al. Undetected coronary atheroma during quantitative angiographic analysis demonstrated by intravascular ultrasound and histological morphometry. Eur Heart J 1993;14 (Suppl):426 (abst)

8. Glagov S, Weisenberg E, Zarins CK, et al. Compensatory enlargement of human atherosclerotic coronary arteries. N Engl J Med 1987;316:1371–1375

9. Di Mario C, The SHK, Madretsma S, et al. Detection and characterization of vascular lesions by intravascular ultrasound: an in vitro study correlated with histology. J Am Soc Echocardiog 1992;5:135–146

10. Linker DT, Yock PG, Grønningsæther Å, et al. Analysis of backscattered ultrasound from normal and diseased arterial wall. Int J Card Imaging 1989;4: 177–185

11. Landini L, Sarnelli R, Picano E, Salvadori M. Evaluation of frequency dependence of backscatter coefficient in normal and atherosclerotic aortic walls. Ultrasound Med Biol 1986;12:397–401

12. Picano E, Landini L, Distante A, et al. Angle dependence of ultrasonic backscatter in arterial tissues: a study in vitro. Circulation 1985;72(3):572–576

13. de Kroon MGM, van der Wal LF, Gussenhoven WJ, et al. Backscatter directivity and integrated backscatter power of arterial tissue. Int J Cardiac Imaging 1991; 6:265–275

14. DiMario C, Madretsma S, Linker D, et al. The angle of incidence of the ultrasonic beam: a critical factor for the image quality in intravascular ultrasonography. Am Heart J 1993;125(Pt 1):442–448

15. Fitzgerald PJ, Ports TA, Yock PG. Contribution of localized calcium deposits to dissection after angioplasty: an observational study using intravascular ultrasound. Circulation 1992;86:64–70

16. Honye J, Mahon DJ, Jain A, et al. Morphological effects of coronary balloon angioplasty in vivo assessed by intravascular ultrasound imaging. Circulation 1992;85:1012–1025

17. Angelsen BAJ, Linker DT, Yock P, Brisken A. Comparison between phased array and mechanical scanning for cross sectional intraluminal ultrasound imaging. Adv Laser Med 1990;4:169–174

18. Goldberg SL, Colombo A, Almagor Y, et al. Can intravascular ultrasound improve coronary stent deployment? Circulation 1993;88(Suppl Pt 2):I-597(abst)

19. Kiemeneij F, Laarman GJ, Slagboom T. Suboptimal stent geometry after deployment with the Palmaz-Schatz stent delivery system. Circulation 1993; 88(Suppl Pt 2):I-641(abst)

20. Nakamura S, Colombo A, Gaglioni A, et al. Intravascular ultrasound criteria for successful stent deployment. Circulation 1993;88(Suppl Pt 2):I-598(abst)

3 Ultrasound: Combined Imaging and Therapeutic Approaches

Paul G. Yock
Peter J. Fitzgerald

Intravascular ultrasound is coming of age as a method for high-resolution imaging in the coronary arteries. The latest generation of stand-alone ultrasound catheters provides reliable image quality and can access the majority of lesions that can be reached with angioplasty equipment. Imaging is increasingly being used to understand the pattern of lesion calcification, to assist in device selection, to guide the cutting protocol in directional atherectomy, to help in appropriate sizing of rotational atherectomy burrs, to optimize the deployment of stents, and to assess the results of balloon angioplasty.

In a sense, coronary interventional techniques have lagged behind other less-invasive surgical methods in using high-resolution imaging as an integral part of the procedure. The major advances of arthroscopic, laparoscopic, and thoracoscopic surgery have all been based on on-line, high-resolution imaging guidance. Intracoronary imaging has been slower to develop both because of the technical difficulties involved and the relatively unforgiving environment of the coronary arteries. Recent developments in intravascular ultrasound, however, have led to catheter-based systems that can aquire good quality images rapidly and safely within most coronary segments.

STAND-ALONE IMAGING VERSUS COMBINED DEVICES

Because of the considerable technical challenge in developing intracoronary ultrasound capability, the first platform for coronary ultrasound has been in stand-alone devices (as opposed to combined imaging therapeutic catheters). In fact there are some significant advantages to the stand-alone approach. For the purposes of choosing a therapeutic device and strategy, it is often useful to obtain a preintervention scan of the entire length of the artery to be treated. This is best accomplished by means of an accurate pullback sequence, generally employing a motorized pullback system. This initial scan of the vessel is used to determine the extent and location of calcium deposits, the plaque burden, the degree of remodeling in different segments, and the media-to-media dimensions. These considerations are all used to choose an appropriate device and to determine the proper size of the device. This type of scan is best performed with a stand-alone device for three reasons: (1) from a technical standpoint, the pullback images are more easily and accurately obtained with a stand-alone device; (2) image quality can be optimized in the stand-alone catheters since there is no tradeoff for the therapeutic function; (3) if a device type and size can be more accurately selected based on the ultrasound images, it may be counterproductive to begin with a combined device where the decision about the catheter size must be made before imaging.

Similar considerations apply in assessing the results of an intervention at decision points during the case, for example, whether to "upsize" the device, exchange for a perfusion balloon, place a stent, etc. Again, it is useful to have the most accurate, high-quality images possible, which are obtained from the stand-alone imaging catheters. Of course, there is a

23

significant tradeoff with stand-alone imaging in the form of the time required to exchange catheters. To minimize the barrier to exchanging, all the imaging catheters from the various manufacturers have an option for the "rail" or "rapid exchange" configuration. Other operators prefer the use of exchange devices such as the Trapper or the Magnet (Scimed, Maple Grove, MN).

Another significant consideration in use of the stand-alone imaging catheters is cost. Analysis of the actual costs involved in imaging, however, is not straightforward. On the one hand, the individual catheter costs (currently in the range of $500 to $700) and the system costs (in the range of $50,000 to $80,000) are substantial, particularly in the context of a procedure that is under cost scrutiny. On the other hand, if preprocedure scanning reduces utilization of therapeutic catheters in at least some cases, by picking an appropriate type of device or size of catheter, the savings can offset the cost of imaging. If, in addition, imaging guidance leads to clinically significant differences in outcome, savings will also follow. There are early indications that imaging guidance of stent deployment may substantially reduce hospital stay and perhaps lower rates of recurrence—a level of savings that is considerable compared to the cost of the catheters. To complicate cost analyses further, some of the catheter companies are beginning to include imaging catheters in a "bundled" contract where the laboratories pay for equipment on a per-patient rather than a per-catheter basis so that, from the hospital's point of view, there is no incremental cost to imaging.

The cost/benefit analysis for a stand-alone imaging device therefore depends in a complicated fashion on the characteristics of the lesion, on the procedure performed and—not least—on the type of purchasing contract for the catheters. The clearest evaluation of the utility of combined imaging/therapeutic devices is therefore provided by looking at the technical and clinical benefits obtained from "onboard" imaging guidance with each class of device.

BALLOON ANGIOPLASTY AND STENTING

There is not yet a consensus on the optimal morphologic results of balloon angioplasty as judged from intravascular ultrasound.[1-3] It is clear that in a small proportion of cases—perhaps 10% to 20%—the lumen caliber achieved after percutaneous transluminal coronary angioplasty (post-PTCA) is considerably less favorable when imaged by ultrasound than would be judged from angiography. Typically these

are lesions that are hazy or slightly opaque on the angiogram, but appear to have a reasonable lumen compared to the reference segment. Ultrasound imaging shows that this is not the case and that the lumen is in fact severely compromised. In these cases it seems unquestionable that further dilatation will be of clinical benefit. Beyond this type of case, however, there is no consensus yet available on how to optimize the lumen appearance based on the ultrasound images. For example, whether the presence of dissection—or a particular type of dissection—is favorable or unfavorable is unknown at this point. Some ongoing trials are examining the long-term outcome post-PTCA in lesions with different ultrasound-determined morphologies.

Combined imaging/balloon catheters have been designed in several different configurations. Isner and colleagues[4] tested a balloon ultrasound imaging catheter that incorporated a rotating transducer within the balloon (the balloon material is relatively transparent to ultrasound). This catheter was produced in a prototype for peripheral use and has not been developed in a coronary version. The catheter had the interesting feature of being able to image through the balloon while it was inflated. In favorable cases it was possible to see splits developing in the plaque; following balloon inflation, an immediate assessment of the degree of elastic recoil could be made. Whether or not the ability to visualize plaque during balloon inflation is a significant advantage is unclear. Splitting of plaque is generally an abrupt event, and it seems unlikely that real-time monitoring of the process would lead to a meaningful modification of the inflation protocol in many cases.

J. M. Hodgson and colleagues[5] designed and tested a different configuration of combined imaging/balloon catheter (Fig. 3-1) in which a cylindrical array transducer is mounted immediately behind the balloon on the shaft of an over-the-wire catheter. This catheter has undergone substantial development and is available clinically in Europe as a coronary catheter with a 3.5 F shaft (Endosonics, Inc., Rancho Cordova, CA). FDA approval has recently been granted in the United States. To use this combined device, the operator picks a balloon size based on angiographic criteria and then performs initial inflations in a standard fashion. The catheter is then advanced forward until the imaging element is within the lesion, allowing an immediate assessment of the results of that set of inflations. Further inflations can be performed with the same balloon or, if indicated, a different balloon or device can be substituted. Hodgson and colleagues have documented that the availability of images changed operators' strategies during the angioplasty in over 40% of cases. A

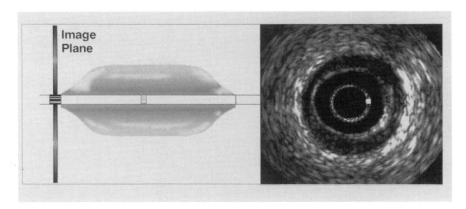

Fig. 3-1. Combined ultrasound imaging/balloon imaging catheter (**A**) and image (**B**) (the Oracle; Endosonics). The transducer is mounted immediately behind the balloon with the imaging plane being the standard two-dimensional cross section. The image on the right shows concentric intimal thickening. The dark circle in the center of the image is the catheter.

multicenter trial with a similar design has recently been initiated.

The application of a combined balloon/imaging catheter may be more straightforward in the case of stenting. Colombo and colleagues[6] have suggested that even after deployment with high-pressure balloons, one-quarter to one-third of stents are not fully expanded over some portion of the stent (typically in the area where the original plaque accumulation was the greatest). If a combined balloon/imaging catheter could be used for initial deployment so that the cases of incomplete expansion were detected immediately using the same catheter, it may be possible to "fine-tune" the deployment using the same balloon or exchange for a high-pressure or larger balloon. Alternatively, the combined imaging catheter could be used as a second, "touchup" balloon. In this case a noncompliant balloon with high-pressure capability would be desirable. The use of an imaging guidewire (see below) would also be useful in this context and, ideally, would also help to position the stent.

DIRECTIONAL PLAQUE REMOVAL

Imaging guidance is particularly well suited for directionally oriented plaque removal techniques, of which directional coronary atherectomy (DCA) is the prototype.[7-9] When DCA was originally introduced into clinical practice in the late 1980s, there was little concern that guidance would be an issue. Operators were encouraged by the excellent angiographic results from the procedure and generally practiced a 360-degree cutting protocol with emphasis on the part of the vessel wall in which the plaque accumula-

tion appeared to be the thickest. Deep cuts—that is, cuts in which portions of media or adventitia were included—were encountered in over 40% of cases but only rarely were associated with significant immediate clinical sequelae such as perforation or aneurysm. A report from the Mayo Clinic raised concerns about the possibility that restenosis may be increased by deep cuts,[10] but subsequent analyses did not appear to support this finding.[11]

In the past two years, several factors have combined to renew interest in the possibility of ultrasound guidance for DCA. First, restenosis data from randomized clinical trials (in particular, the CAVEAT[12] and CCAT[13] studies) have not been highly favorable for DCA. It has become clear from the work of Baim and Kuntz and their colleagues[14] that a key factor in the long-term patency of interventions is the lumen caliber at the end of the procedure. It follows that if more complete plaque removal could be performed safely, restenosis rates should be positively influenced. In parallel with these results from angiographic studies, the use of stand-alone ultrasound imaging in conjunction with DCA emphasized that the device was not accomplishing as much plaque removal as might be expected on the basis of angiography.[7,9] On average, 60% of the cross-sectional area is still occupied by plaque at the end of an angiographically "successful" DCA, despite 10% to 20% stenosis by angiography. These data suggest that more complete plaque removal could double the postprocedure lumen size—a result that would lead to low restenosis rates by the Baim/Kuntz model. Increasing use of intracoronary ultrasound in laboratories performing atherectomy has also provided operators with a day-to-day, practical demonstration of the limitations in using angiography alone to gauge

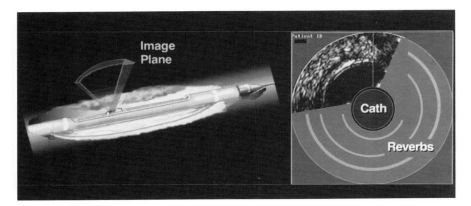

Fig. 3-2. Combined ultrasound imaging/directional atherectomy device. **(A)** The crystal is mounted on the cutter immediately behind the sharp edge. The resulting image is a 120-degree cross section looking out the window of the housing. **(B)** An image generated from a 7 F device in a pig coronary artery (catheter developed by DVI).

the amount or location of plaque within a target segment.

One of the authors (PY) originally suggested a prototype design for a combined imaging/atherectomy catheter (Fig. 3-2), and initial tests were performed with a 9 F, peripheral catheter configuration. In this design, a single ultrasound transducer is incorporated in the body of the cutter, just behind the cutting edge. Because the housing in which the cutter is partially encased is made of metal, the transducer only "looks" out the open window to the portion of the artery that will be subjected to cutting. The image is therefore a 110-degree sector; the round "blank" at the center of the image represents the boundary of the cut. The use of the combined or guided atherectomy device (GDCA) is fairly similar to the standard catheters. The catheter is advanced into the artery with the cutter in the fully forward, safety position. Once the housing is in the general region of the lesion, the motor is activated and the images generated from the rotating transducer used to more precisely position the housing both in the axial and rotational dimensions. The balloon is then inflated while the operator watches the image: the plaque should be seen to move into the area of the blank. The cutter is then retracted, the balloon inflated to the definitive pressure, and the cutting pass is completed.

Recently, we performed in vitro and animal testing with a series of 7 F, fixed-wire coronary prototype catheters (Devices for Vascular Intervention, Inc., Redwood City, CA). The fixed-wire approach was selected initially to help maintain smooth rotation of the drive cable, thereby ensuring good quality images without nonuniform rotational distortion (NURD). A side benefit of the fixed-wire approach has been noted, however, in that the absence of the

central wire increases both the cutting and storage capabilities of the device. This is a particularly favorable feature for the guided device, where the main purpose is to remove larger volumes of plaque more efficiently. The fixed-wire device obviously has the disadvantage of being more difficult to deliver into the artery.

Initial in vivo testing of the GDCA device has been favorable in several respects. Image quality actually exceeded that of the best stand-alone imaging catheters, due to the relatively large aperture (that is, effective transducer area) in the GDCA device (with a diameter of 0.040 in., the GDCA transducer has over three times the area of the transducers in the stand-alone catheters). Torque control of the entire catheter could be directly assessed by means of the images, and was very good using the newest shaft configuration (the GTO design). Another interesting finding with the coronary prototype was the ability of the images to show incomplete contact of the cutter with the vessel wall—providing an early warning of an ineffective cut. This occurred commonly in the animal model, despite the fact that the angiographic clues pointed to good apposition of the device.

The first clinical tests of the GDCA device are under way. Other designs have been considered, including incorporating a multielement transducer in a redesigned nose cone. The excellent image quality of the mechanical design combined with the close physical integration between the imaging plane and the cutting surface have led to the decision to pursue this approach in the initial clinical device.

The same general concepts discussed above for directional atherectomy apply to other directional methods as well, for example, directional excimer laser angioplasty. To date, there are no combined imaging/directional laser catheters that have been reported.

CONCENTRIC PLAQUE REMOVAL

Several studies have addressed the use of intravascular ultrasound in assessing and guiding concentric plaque removal techniques such as rotational atherectomy and laser angioplasty.[15–17] With the Rotablator, ultrasound has documented more effective ablation of plaque in calcified lesions as compared to fibrofatty disease. In our own experience, ultrasound has proven useful in selecting an initial burr size. It is not uncommon that the initial burr selected from angiography is smaller than the preprocedure lumen seen with ultrasound, obviating the need for the small burr. Imaging may also be useful in planning the strategy for upsizing burrs. Most often the images demonstrate that a larger burr than expected can be tolerated from the standpoint of plaque burden (depending on the degree of distal flow in the vessel). On the other hand, we are conservative in upsizing a burr if the plaque is highly eccentric by ultrasound. The same general considerations apply with concentric laser angioplasty. In particular, it may be useful to image bifurcation lesions to determine whether there is a safe margin of plaque on the inner aspect of the branch. With both rotational atherectomy and laser, ultrasound images may help in deciding whether adjunctive angioplasty is desirable.

Because the current concentric ablation devices do not have an option to increase the radius of ablation, the concept of onboard guidance is not particularly compelling. On the other hand, if a concentric device were created with the ability to adjust the size of the abrading/laser tip, it would be extremely useful to have an integrated ultrasound capability.

FORWARD-LOOKING ULTRASOUND

Catheters that project a beam in a forward direction have been discussed since the early development of intravascular ultrasound. One prototype catheter has recently been described that creates a sector-forward beam based on a mechanically oscillated crystal.[18,19] This technology is currently in an early development phase and is limited by the large size required by the transducer aperture and the requirements for side-to-side motion. It is reasonable to expect, however, that the configuration can be miniaturized to the range of 5 F or smaller, which would be usable in the coronary circulation. From the standpoint of a combined device, the most promising application of a forward configuration would be as a guidance strategy for treatment of total occlusions. The ability of the ultrasound to generate an image 5 to 10 mm ahead of the catheter tip, perhaps combined with the ability to steer a guidewire or laser fiber, could provide a safer strategy for penetrating occlusions without perforation. A solid-state approach to forward imaging is a technical possibility, but must solve the same basic problem as the mechanical design: there must be a sufficiently large aperture pointed forward to make a reasonable image, without "growing" the overall size of the catheter beyond the range that would be suitable for coronary use.

IMAGING GUIDEWIRES

In the past several years, there has been increasing discussion in the industry and among interventionalists about the desirability of imaging guidewires. Certainly an imaging guidewire would provide a solution to the issue of onboard guidance while potentially having greater flexibility of use than an integrated imaging/therapeutic catheter. One happy circumstance for guidewire imaging is that most balloon catheter shafts are reasonably transparent to ultrasound. This makes it feasible to image through the catheter with the idea, for example, of facilitating positioning of a balloon.

No doubt part of the enthusiasm for an imaging guidewire has come from the fact that Doppler ultrasound has been successfully miniatured to a 0.014-in. guidewire platform (Cardiometrics, Inc., Mountain View, CA).[20] It is important to understand, however, that the beam characteristics for an imaging transducer are much less forgiving than for a Doppler transducer. With miniaturization of ultrasound transducers the beam tends to diverge quickly, providing a wide, V-shaped pattern. This is actually advantageous in the case of the Doppler transducer, since the broad beam has a better chance of "finding" the peak velocity signal. In the case of imaging, on the other hand, the broad beam causes a substantial loss of resolution. Other important aspects of image quality—particularly penetration and dynamic range or gray scale—are also severely compromised with reduction of transducer aperture.

As stand-alone imaging catheters have been miniaturized, the size of the transducers used has come closer to the range that would be required for guidewire imaging. The smallest transducers currently in

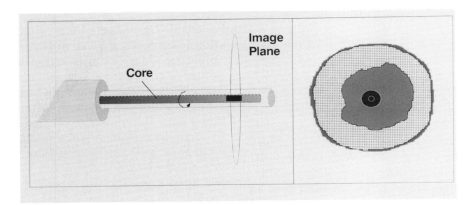

Fig. 3-3. An imaging core. The transducer rotates within a sheath or balloon catheter **(A),** creating a 360-degree cross-sectional image. **(B)** The core can be left in place in the vessel for catheter exchanges.

a production catheter are 0.018 by 0.030 in., with the longer dimension being along the axis of the catheter. In making a guidewire transducer, there would be some portion of the edge of transducer—perhaps the outer 0.002 inches—that would not provide good quality aperture. So to actually create a guidewire transducer for a 0.018-in. wire would require further reduction in the aperture, at least in the thickness dimension. This would decrease resolution and dynamic range (gray scale); however, this worsening of image quality might not be a practical problem in certain clinical circumstances. For example, the struts of stents provide excellent, bright targets for the ultrasound beam, so that measurements of the stent expansion would be possible without a high-quality transducer. A technical approach to improving image quality in guidewire imagers is to use a higher frequency transducer. Current imaging catheters run at a maximum frequency of 30 MHz because at higher frequencies the backscatter from blood becomes so intense that the blood appears to be solid tissue, and the images are confusing. It is

theoretically possible to identify and subtract the blood from the overall image by making use of the unique pattern of ultrasound backscatter created by the flowing blood elements. Even with the blood subtracted from the image, however, penetration of the ultrasound signal at frequencies of 40 MHz or greater may become a limiting issue. Replacing the blood with saline—as is done for angioscopy—is one possible means of overcoming this issue.

Assuming that the capability of small transducers can improve sufficiently to make guidewire imaging feasible, there is still the need to develop a combined system that does not trade off the basic functionality of the guidewire. At present the best quality catheter images come from the mechanical, rotating element systems. It is certainly possible that a solid-state, multilement guidewire can be developed. The key hurdle will be providing enough transducer "real estate" to overcome some of the limitations of the approach—for example, by arranging a linear array of transducers along a short length of wire near the tip. Even this configuration,

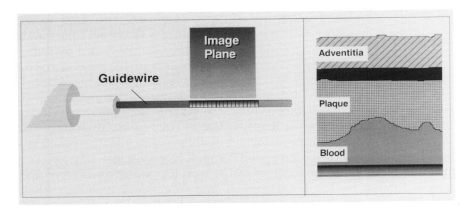

Fig. 3-4. (A & B) Concept for a linear array imaging guidewire. Because the wire does not need to rotate, it can potentially function as a true guidewire. The image plane is along the length of the wire **(B).**

however, would stretch the limits of the solid-state transducer performance.

For the near future, then, it is likely that the first guidewire transducers will be of the rotating, mechanical style (Fig. 3-3). This provides a considerable design challenge, since it is not desirable to have a rotating wire exposed in the coronary artery (certainly not a rotating guidewire tip). One interim solution to this problem is to develop an imaging core of sufficiently small size to fit in the lumen of a catheter and which can be substituted for a conventional guidewire once the catheter is placed across the lesion. This type of imaging core has been developed in prototype form and used in conjunction with peripheral angioplasty and stent deployment balloons in clinical trials.[21] One advantage of this approach is that the core could potentially be reused for purposes of cost reduction. Given an appropriate design, the imaging core could also serve as a place holder for catheter exchange. Developments along these lines are proceeding at several companies, and it is reasonable to expect to see coronary prototype devices within the next year. In the future it may be possible to develop a solid-state configuration for guidewire imaging that combines standard guidewire functionality with imaging. A linear array configuration (Fig. 3-4) would be one reasonable design approach.

SUMMARY

Increasing interest in the information provided by intravascular ultrasound has led to consideration of various combined imaging/therapeutic catheters. Clinical experience is accumulating with the first imaging/balloon catheter and an ultrasound-guided directional atherectomy device is about to begin initial clinical testing. Guidewire imaging is a technically challenging frontier with obvious appeal from a user standpoint. Prototype imaging guidewires for the coronary arteries should enter clinical trials later this year.

REFERENCES

1. Fitzgerald PJ, Yock PG. Mechanisms and outcomes of angioplasty assessed by intravascular ultrasound imaging. J Clin Ultrasound 1993;21:579–588
2. Honye J, Mahon DJ, Jain A, et al. Morphological effects of coronary balloon angioplasty in vivo assessed by intravascular ultrasound imaging. Circulation 1992;85:1012–1025
3. Tenaglia AN, Buller CE, Kisslo KB, et al. Mechanisms of balloon angioplasty and directional coronary atherectomy as assessed by intracoronary ultrasound. J Am Coll Cardiol 1992;20:685–691
4. Isner JM, Rosenfield K, Losordo DW, et al. Combination balloon-ultrasound imaging catheter for percutaneous transluminal angioplasty: validation of imaging, analysis of recoil, and identification of plaque fracture. Circulation 1991;84:739–754
5. Caccione JG, Reddy K, Richards F, et al. Combined intravascular ultrasound/angioplasty balloon catheter: initial use during PTCA. Cathet Cardiovasc Diagn 1991;24:99–101
6. Goldberg SL, Colombo A, Nakamura S, et al. Benefit of intracoronary ultrasound in the deployment of Palmaz-Schatz stents. J Am Coll Cardiol 1994;24:996–1003
7. Yock PG, Fitzgerald PJ, Sudhir K, et al. Intravascular ultrasound imaging for guidance of atherectomy and other plaque removal techniques. Int J Card Imaging 1991;6:179–189
8. Kimura BJ, Fitzgerald PJ, Sudhir K, et al. Guidance of directed coronary atherectomy by intracoronary ultrasound imaging. Am Heart J 1992;124:1365–1369
9. De LJ, Romero M, Medina A, et al. Intracoronary ultrasound assessment of directional coronary atherectomy: immediate and follow-up findings. J Am Coll Cardiol 1993;21:298–307
10. Garratt KN, Edwards WD, Kaufman UP, et al. Differential histopathology of primary atherosclerotic and restenotic lesions in coronary arteries and saphenous vein bypass grafts: analysis of tissue obtained from 73 patients by directional atherectomy. J Am Coll Cardiol 1991;17:422–428
11. Fishman RF, Kuntz RE, Carrozza JP, et al. Long term results of directional atherectomy: predictors of restenosis. J Am Coll Cardiol 1992;20:1101–1110
12. Topol EJ, Leya F, Pinkerton CA, et al. A comparison of directional atherectomy with coronary angioplatsy in patients with coronary artery disease (CAVEAT). N Engl J Med 1993;329:221–227
13. Adelman AG, Cohen EA, Kimball BP, et al. Canadian Coronary Atherectomy Trial (CCAT): a comparison of directional atherectomy with balloon angioplasty for lesions of the left anterior descending coronary artery. N Engl J Med 1993;329:228–233
14. Kuntz RE, Gibson CM, Nobuyoshi M, Baim DS. Generalized model of restenosis after conventional balloon angioplasty, stenting and directional atherectomy. J Am Coll Cardiol 1993;21:15–25
15. Kovach JA, Mintz GS, Pichard AD, et al. Sequential intravascular ultrasound characterization of the mechanisms of rotational atherectomy and adjunct balloon angioplasty. J Am Coll Cardiol 1993;22:1024–1032
16. Mintz GS, Potkin BN, Keren G, et al. Intravascular ultrasound evaluation of the effect of rotational atherectomy in obstructive atherosclerotic coronary artery disease. Circulation 1992;86:1383–1393

4 Intravascular Ultrasound-Guided Revascularization

Kenneth J. Rosenfield
Jeffrey M. Isner

Advances in interventional technology have intensified the need for improved vascular imaging capabilities. Conventional contrast angiography has been the time-honored approach for lesion characterization and assessment. Angiography, however, remains limited by several factors that have been well described previously.[1–11] These limitations relate principally to the fact that contrast angiography depicts the vessel lumen only; plaque and vessel wall are viewed as a "negative imprint" on the contrast-filled lumen. While this allows for characterization of lumen topography, irregularities in the plaque/wall topography may be inferred only from the negative imprint. Thus angiography does not allow visualization or characterization of tissue elements below the intimal surface. This becomes particularly problematic in a vessel with diffuse disease, in which case the vessel may appear angiographically normal due to the ubiquitous distribution of atherosclerotic plaque. Furthermore, contrast angiography is limited to a single planar view per injection; as such, information regarding the circumferential nature of the vessel/lumen interface cannot be directly recorded. Visualization of the vessel from alternative angles is possible, but only at the expense of additional injections of contrast material. As a consequence of uniplanar viewing, direct measurement of luminal cross-sectional area is not feasible; instead, estimates of cross-sectional area must be derived from algorithms based on diameter measurements obtained from a single, potentially nonrepresentative, plane.

Intravascular ultrasound (IVUS) imaging offers a potential solution to many of these limitations inherent in conventional contrast angiography. IVUS imaging is unequivocally superior to contrast angiography in its ability to demonstrate detailed characteristics at the lumen/vessel wall interface, as well as depiction of structures within the plaque and vessel wall. Several investigators[12–16] have demonstrated that IVUS imaging is exquisitely sensitive in detecting plaque and other details that are angiographically "silent." IVUS now provides the opportunity for the first time to accurately assess qualitative and quantitative effects of interventional therapy in vivo.[17–30] As such, the mechanisms by which balloon angioplasty increases luminal patency, as well as the device-specific effects of directional and rotational atherectomy, laser angioplasty, and stent deployment, may be more clearly elucidated.

Recent technological developments, as well as an expanding library of clinical experience with image interpretation, have facilitated the clinical applications of IVUS. In this chapter, we review some of the early studies that laid the foundation for the current and potential future applications of IVUS, describe clinical experience with IVUS, and review the results of both combination (imaging/therapeutic) devices and three-dimensional reconstruction of serial IVUS images.

IN VITRO VALIDATION

Images of vessels derived from IVUS typically demonstrate a layered appearance surrounding the probe. The presentation of distinct layers is a consequence of the differing acoustic reflectivity of different tissues. Dense, hyperreflective tissues are represented by bright echoes, and less dense tissues produce hypoechoic signals. While the acoustic property of each tissue is critical in determining the brightness of the signal produced, it appears that "acoustic discrepancy" or "mismatch" (e.g., change in sonoreflectivity between adjacent structures) is the most important factor in defining the border between structures.[31] Accordingly, even a minor difference between tissue echogenicity can enable delineation of a border.

IVUS enables high-resolution imaging of vessel wall and lumen; because of the intraluminal location of the probe and the ability of ultrasound energy to penetrate tissues, IVUS provides information regarding the arterial wall previously unavailable by in vivo examinations. Indeed, experimental and clinical experience to date indicates that IVUS images correlate remarkably well with histologic examination, qualitatively as well as quantitatively. Numerous in vitro comparison studies have established the relationship between echos seen on IVUS images and structures seen histologically.[10,28,32–37] Each layer of the arterial wall can be recognized by a typical ultrasound "signature": in normal, muscular arteries, intima yields a hyperechoic signal; media, hypoechoic; and adventitia, hyperechoic. Siegel and colleagues[38] further confirmed the pathoanatomic correlates of the three layers by peeling away sequential layers of the vessel using microdissection techniques.[39] IVUS images were obtained at each stage of dissection, and, despite the limitation that vessels were formalin-fixed, the results supported previous assignments of the three layers to intima, media, and adventitia. Pathologic or abnormal elements also have their own characteristic ultrasound appearance: calcium, for example, consistently produces bright echo reflections with acoustic shadowing or dropout of the subjacent ultrasound signal.

In addition to the qualitative similarity between IVUS imaging and histology, quantitative measurements of the thickness of the arterial wall correlate remarkably well; Mallery and coworkers[40] found correlation coefficients for total wall thickness and media alone of 0.85 and 0.83, respectively; Potkin and coworkers[35] found a similar correlation of .92 for linear wall thickness, including plaque and media combined. Despite these results, since the correlation between IVUS and histologic measurements for intima alone is less optimal than when intima and media are combined, some controversy remains regarding the accuracy of IVUS in determining the thickness of the intimal layer. Several investigators[41,42] have demonstrated that the inner echogenic layer shown by IVUS imaging is often thicker than the intimal layer measured histologically. The presumed cause of this is radial spreading or "blooming" of the ultrasound reflections; that is, the signal created by the interface between blood and intima is sufficiently bright relative to the subjacent echolucent media that it "overlaps" into the medial area.

Normal elastic arteries, in contrast to muscular arteries, do not demonstrate a distinct border between intima and media.[17,33,36,43] Consequently, the vessel wall is more homogeneous and lacks the three-layered appearance, which is likely due to the presence of highly sonoreflective elastic and fibrous tissue in the medial layer. The absence of this tissue in muscular arteries renders the media more sonoluscent and, therefore, creates the three-layered appearance.

Nishimura and colleagues[36] observed in vitro that even muscular arteries may not exhibit the typical tripartite appearance if the intima is truly normal (e.g., only a few cell layers thick). This finding was confirmed in vivo by Yeung and colleagues.[44] Although this phenomenon was originally presumed to be due to the relative lack of resolution of the 20 MHz device employed in their study, recent work by Fitzgerald and colleagues[45] confirmed the absence of an intimal signal in histologically normal vessels, even using a higher resolution 30-MHz instrument. Explanted muscular coronary arteries from young patients (mean age: 27) had a homogeneous, nonlayered IVUS appearance; in contrast, older (mean age: 42) vessels demonstrated the typical tripartite layering. Histologic analysis demonstrated that an intimal thickness of 178 μm or more was required to generate sufficient sonoreflectivity to be apparent on IVUS examination; in young, normal patients, intimal thickness was typically less than 178 μm and therefore sonographically silent. The implication of these findings is that intimal thickening advances with advancing age. Previous descriptions[28] of the three-layered appearance as the norm were based on studies from "relatively normal" vessels in patients with high-grade stenoses elsewhere; not unexpectedly, even so-called "normal" sites in these patients had evident intimal thickening. Another factor that may account for the increased echogenicity of the intima with advancing age is a gradual change in the composition of the intima, comprising of more echogenic material; such an age-related change would be consistent with gradual loss in compliance and elasticity. Whether due to subtle intimal thickening or age-related changes in composition of the intimal layer, differences demonstrated between "young" and "old" intima underscore the ability of IVUS imaging to identify subtle abnormalities of the vascular wall.

DETECTION OF "SILENT" PLAQUE

Studies in our own laboratory,[28] as well as those by Tobis and associates,[46] Nissen and colleagues,[46] and Davidson and colleagues[11] have shown that IVUS frequently demonstrates plaque not detected angiographically. Davidson and colleagues[12] observed that, among 46% of patients in whom plaque was identified by IVUS scan, the sites examined were normal by angiography. In a more recent report comparing IVUS examinations to angiography in cardiac transplant recipients, St. Goar and associates[48] demonstrated that among patients studied 1 year after cardiac transplantation, all exhibited intimal thickening by IVUS imaging. Despite this, corresponding angiograms were normal in 42 of the 60 patients studied; in 21 of these 42, the thickening was severe or moderate. The fact that diffuse, uniform intimal thickening would not be detected angiographically has been documented in multiple previous angiographic-histologic correlative studies.[6,9] Interestingly, of the 20 patients studied by St. Goar and coworkers[15] within 1 month after transplant, the intima was visualized in only 7 (35%); this is consistent with the findings described above regarding the "invisible" nature of the intima on IVUS examination in young, normal, muscular arteries and suggests that the thickness of the intimal layer was less than 178 μm in these vessels (i.e., below the resolution of the IVUS instrument).

In our own experience imaging patients during interventional procedures, the finding of angiographically "silent" plaque has been the rule, rather than the exception. Angiographically normal sites that are adjacent to lesions and would typically be identified as "normal reference vessels," are almost always shown to be significantly diseased by IVUS imaging. Again, this highlights one of the major liabilities of angiography: the degree of disease at one site is typically (for lack of any other available standard) evaluated in relationship to a *normal-appearing* adjacent site.[5,28]

TISSUE/PLAQUE CHARACTERIZATION

Previous studies have attemped to use IVUS to discriminate plaque composition.[23,33,35,36,46] Fibrous plaque appears as bright, homogeneous echos. Cal-

cific deposits clearly and consistently generate intensely echogenic bright signals, which create an "acoustic shadow" that shields subjacent structures. In our experience, reproducible characterization of plaque as fibrous versus "fatty" is not as consistently possible by IVUS imaging; this is almost certainly due in part to the fact that few plaques are ever purely "fatty," and the lipid component of most plaques is, in fact, minor.[49] In occasional cases, identification of thrombus by IVUS imaging has been well documented.[21] Although some investigators have suggested that thrombus may be regularly distinguished from low-density plaque,[50] we have not found any reliable characteristics to differentiate these two entities. Indeed, the appearance of thrombus may be variable even in the same patient. Seigel and coworkers[37] likewise found IVUS to be insensitive for the identification of thrombus. Detection of thrombus and associated unstable plaque appears to be one area in which angioscopy is superior to both IVUS imaging and angiography.[51,52]

In occasional cases, IVUS imaging may be uniquely informative with regard to details of plaque/wall pathology. Mecley and collaborators[53] show images recorded from a patient with recent onset of disabling claudication (see their Fig. 4); hypoechoic foci that suggested plaque rupture and hemorrhage were responsible for the patient's accelerated symptoms. Tissue obtained by directional atherectomy documented findings of plaque fissure and hemorrhage confirming plaque rupture as the mechanism for the patient's acute onset of symptoms.

Preliminary investigation using "backscatter" analysis and "ice-pick" imaging may better define the acoustic properties of given tissues and allow more reproducible and accurate tissue characterization in vivo.[54]

QUANTIFICATION OF VESSEL DIMENSIONS

The most critical advantage of IVUS imaging for clinical work derives from its unequivocally superior capability to define luminal dimensions, particularly cross-sectional area. Early in vitro studies by Nishimura and colleagues[36] demonstrated the accuracy (correlation coefficient = .98) of IVUS lumen measurements compared to histology. Nissen and colleagues,[47] using live animals, found a correlation for diameter between quantitative angiography and IVUS of .98 for normal sites, and .89 for experimentally induced concentric stenoses. Subsequent studies in humans found similarly close correlations (.80 to .95) between cross-sectional area in normal or near-normal vessels measured by IVUS imaging versus quantitative angiography.[12,16,55] Diseased, nondilated vessels demonstrated a lesser, but still respectable, correlation (r = .86).[16] While these data demonstrate a good *correlation* between cross-sectional area measured by IVUS and those derived by quantitative angiographic algorithms, the *absolute* values for area may differ substantially. Furthermore, since algorithms developed for quantitative angiography fail to address the problems posed by diffusely diseased vessels,[7] the *relative* degree of compromise of a given site may be better determined by IVUS.

To the extent that IVUS images may directly demonstrate luminal cross-sectional area in cases where angiography is complicated by certain anatomic factors, IVUS may be useful as a *diagnostic* tool. Angiographic assessment of the left main coronary artery, for example, has been a well-documented[5] source of angiographic ambiguity. IVUS imaging has been useful in such cases for elucidating the extent of luminal compromise.[55] IVUS imaging may also resolve lesion severity in instances in which the presence of bends, vessel overlap, or branch points obscures the border of contrast during angiography. IVUS imaging can also be particularly helpful in circumstances where it is necessary to define components of the arterial wall. While difficulty in assessing pathology is not uncommon in the tortuous coronary tree, IVUS images may be specifically useful for defining the severity of aortic ostial lesions in renal and mesenteric vessels[57]; stenoses at these sites are often difficult to visualize angiographically, because of their proximity to the aorta, the brisk flow of contrast, and the abundance of calcium.

After intervention, the discrepancy is significantly greater between vessel dimensions determined by IVUS imaging and the dimensions determined by angiography. This was graphically demonstrated in the assessment of 13 consecutive patients in whom the results of balloon (10 patients) or laser (3 patients) angioplasty were quantified by both quantitative angiographic analysis and IVUS imaging.[24] Minimal luminal diameter and cross-sectional area were calculated for interventional sites and nearby reference sites. Corresponding ultrasound frames from both interventional and reference sites were digitized, and the minimal luminal diameter was measured directly; cross-sectional area was obtained by tracing the perimeter of the lumen. Luminal diameter for reference sites measured 3.9 mm by IVUS imaging versus 3.3 mm by quantitative angiography ($P <$ .05). Regression analysis disclosed a correlation coefficient of .87. For cross-sectional area of *reference sites,* the absolute difference between ultrasound and

angiography—12.6 mm² versus 9.6 mm²—was also statistically significant ($P <$ .05). Regression analysis disclosed a correlation coefficient of .92, similar to that calculated for analysis of luminal diameter. Luminal diameter for *interventional sites* measured 2.8 mm by IVUS versus 1.8 mm by angiography ($P <$ .01). Regression analysis disclosed a poorer correlation—.62—than that calculated for reference sites. Similarly, for cross-sectional area of interventional sites, there was a highly statistically significant difference between absolute measurements made by ultrasound (6.9) versus quantitative angiography (2.8) ($P <$ .01).

There is good reason to believe that cross-sectional area measurements are more accurate by IVUS than by quantitative angiography, especially after intervention.

1. IVUS provides accurate delineation of luminal borders and obviates the need for multiple orthogonal angiographic views.
2. IVUS provides the ability to planimeter the cross-sectional area directly, eliminating the dependence on algorithms which derive area from diameter measurements, algorithms which make potentially incorrect assumptions about luminal geometry.
3. In contrast to quantitative angiography where the catheter used for calibration may be located at a distance from the segment being measured, with IVUS the calibration instrument is, by definition, within the plane of measurement.
4. With IVUS, the area being measured occupies nearly the entire field of view on the screen; in contrast, for angiographic analysis, the vascular region of interest involves only a small fraction of the cine frame from which it is measured.

DEFINING THE MECHANISM OF BALLOON ANGIOPLASTY

The most extensive clinical experience with IVUS to date, and the application in which it appears to offer the greatest practical clinical utility, has been in the assessment of intravascular effects of percutaneous therapy in coronary and peripheral vessels. Contrast angiography, while routinely performed before and after instrumentation, provides only a profile of luminal diameter, rather than depiction of cross-sectional area; this fact, along with other methodological limitations described previously,[1,2,4–6] has compromised its usefulness for the study of angioplasty mechanisms. In vitro studies have demonstrated that IVUS imaging consistently provides exquisite detail regarding morphologic alterations in the arterial wall and subjacent plaque resulting from the barotrauma of balloon inflation.[10,35,58–60]

Experience with in vivo imaging postdilation has confirmed the in vitro data. In the few patients studied at necropsy post-PTA in whom IVUS had also been performed, IVUS images displayed the identical morphologic abnormalities seen by light microscopy.[60,61] The fact that IVUS routinely depicts tomographic full-thickness images of the arterial wall, allows one to gain—in vivo—a perspective similar to that achieved by histologic examination. Furthermore, the ability to perform serial examinations in vivo enables documentation regarding pathologic alterations attributable to specific instrumentation employed. These unique features of IVUS have been used to good advantage to study the mechanisms by which balloon angioplasty improves luminal patency. Observations from IVUS at our own institution[27] and others[62] suggest that plaque fracture and/or dissection is associated with balloon dilation in the overwhelming majority of angiographically and hemodynamically successful procedures. Indeed, recent data[63,64] suggests that at least some degree of plaque fracture must be seen by IVUS in order to achieve a successful long-term result; vessels that display no tearing may be much more prone to recoil or restenosis.

The relative contribution of plaque fractures, as opposed to other factors, to the overall increase in luminal area seen following balloon angioplasty has been elucidated by IVUS imaging. Tobis and associates[10] demonstrated in vitro that diseased vessels subjected to balloon dilation tended to tear longitudinally at the thinnest region of the plaque; they suggested that these tears account for the enlargement of luminal cross-sectional area. Losordo and colleagues[65] evaluated IVUS images obtained before and after percutaneous transluminal angioplasty (PTA) performed in 40 patients, and quantified the relative contributions of plaque fracture, plaque compression, and arterial stretch to the enhanced overall luminal area. Luminal cross-sectional area more than doubled, from 11.5 mm^2 pre-PTA to 25.4 mm^2 post-PTA. The neolumen created by plaque fractures accounted for the majority (72%) of the total increase in luminal area. Compression of plaque was seen in all treated vessels and made an important, but quantitatively less significant, contribution to postangioplasty increase in luminal area. Arterial stretching was demonstrated in only 25% of patients and, even in this group, its contribution to increased area was minimal. These data confirm pre-

vious observations suggesting that plaque fracture constitutes the principal mechanism reponsible for increased luminal patency after balloon angioplasty. These results consequently contradict conclusions based on prior in vitro studies[66,67] and a smaller in vivo study[68] that implicated stretching of the vessel wall as a major factor contributing to increased lumen size.

In an attempt to categorize the degree of plaque fracture observed by IVUS imaging following balloon angioplasty, Honye and coworkers[64] have identified six characteristic morphologic patterns of vessel disruption (Table 4-1). In their proposed scheme, patterns A through D represent increasing degrees of plaque tearing and separation from subjacent structures, while pattern E represents stretching without obvious tearing.

Of 66 coronary lesions subjected to balloon dilation, Honye and coworkers[64] observed fairly equal distribution of the different morphologic subtypes, with a slight predominance in types B, C, and especially E. Interestingly, in their preliminary analysis, Type E1 lesions displayed a greater tendency toward restenosis at 6-month follow-up.

Calcified plaque is detected by IVUS imaging in most vessels undergoing angioplasty, a feature that is underappreciated by angiography and may be important in understanding the mechanism of PTA. Honye and associates,[69] for example, identified calcific deposits in 14% versus 83% of patients studied by angiography and ultrasound, respectively. Our experience has been similar.[23,28] Waller and col-

Table 4-1. Morphologic Patterns of Vessel Disruption Following PTCA

Type A:	Partial-thickness tear in plaque, not extending to subjacent tissue
Type B:	Full-thickness tear in plaque, extending to media, with separation of two edges of torn plaque
Type C:	Full-thickness tear, with separation (dissection) of plaque from underlying media for arc of up to 180 degrees
Type D:	Full-thickness tear, with separation of plaque extending circumferentially >180 degrees. Plaque largely or entirely pulled away from subjacent tissues
Type E:	Stretching of concentric (E1) or eccentric (E2) plaque, without obvious separation or plaque fracture

(Adapted from Honye et al.,[64] with permission.)

leagues[70] have previously suggested that tears and fractures typically occur along the border between calcific plaque and softer tissue; assuming that such is the case, then the increased sensitivity of IVUS in detecting calcific deposits may be clinically relevant. Indeed, recent observations[32,71] lend further support to the notion that the presence of calcium may predict location and extent of plaque fracture. Fitzgerald and colleagues, for example, imaged 41 patients following angioplasty; they found that in 87% of patients with focal deposits of calcium who also demonstrated dissections, the fracture site was located adjacent to the calcified plaque. Furthermore, the extent of dissection was greater in the patients with calcified than in those with noncalcified vessels. To the extent that large dissections may portend a poor angioplasty outcome, including specifically a higher risk of abrupt closure, the detection and localization of calcium may become an important, practical application of IVUS. Further studies are necessary, however, to discriminate the characteristic features or patterns of calcific deposition that might be a harbinger of a poor PTCA result.

Evidence from in vivo IVUS studies has also provided insight regarding the mechanisms by which directional atherectomy, stent deployment, and laser angioplasty enhance luminal area. In contrast to vessels undergoing balloon angioplasty, vessels in which directional atherectomy is performed demonstrate less prominent plaque-arterial wall disruption; instead, the perimeter of the neolumen is typically smooth and uninterrupted. In our initial series of patients,[28] no plaque cracks were observed on postatherectomy IVUS examination. Rather, discrete "bites" corresponding to individual passes of the cutting blade were often observed, consistent with tissue removal. Similar findings have been reported by Yock and colleagues,[72] Smucker and colleagues,[73] and Tenaglia and colleagues,[18] all of whom reported a relatively low incidence of plaque fracture. Controversy persists regarding the extent to which inflation of eccentric balloon of the Simpson Atherocath contributes to increased luminal area; indeed, angiographic studies have suggested that the amount of tissue retrieved is not enough to account for the resultant increase in luminal diameter,[74,75] and in certain cases the Dotter effect of the catheter and the effects of balloon inflation have been documented to produce most of the luminal patency.

Signs of arterial wall trauma are most completely effaced on IVUS images recorded following delivery of an endovascular stent: the fact that extensive trauma is observed at these same sites postballoon (prestent) suggests that stent implantation acutely ameliorates arterial wall pathology.[28,76,77]

GUIDING INTERVENTIONS

Although the ultimate role of IVUS vis-à-vis contrast angiography remains to be determined, we have previously used IVUS as the primary (sole) imaging modality to guide interventional procedures.[78] In a series of 46 patients undergoing iliac or femoro-popliteal revascularization, serial IVUS imaging was performed to assess the results of balloon dilation, directional atherectomy, and/or physiologic low-stress angioplasty. Decisions regarding whether the procedure result was satisfactory and whether to treat further were made on the basis of IVUS examinations alone, without any angiographic information. Repeat intervention was deemed necessary by IVUS in approximately one-third of patients; the specific adjunctive treatment modality, including repeat balloon inflation, adjunctive atherectomy, or stent deployment was determined based upon interpretation of the quantitative and qualitative findings on IVUS examination. Angiograms were performed after completion of the recanalization procedure, both to confirm the adequacy of the result by the traditional standard and to determine if IVUS had failed to define a significant residual narrowing. In only 2 of 46 patients did information obtained on completion angiography indicate the need for repeat intervention.

A number of reports support the findings that IVUS enhances definition of residual luminal narrowing and morphometry postintervention and that this information may influence subsequent therapeutic management.[31,79–81] Several of these recent studies have explored the lesion- and device-specific use of IVUS and, in addition to supporting its use to determine procedural outcome, implicate a potential role for IVUS in identifying the optimal interventional therapy. Examples of this include determination of appropriate device/balloon size based on accurate measurement of vessel dimensions; selection of a directional, rather than a concentric, atherectomy device, based on the finding of eccentric plaque; and choice of a device better suited for debulking of calcium, in the case of a heavily calcified lesion.

IVUS imaging is uniquely suited for guidance in the deployment of endovascular stents. Evaluation of the interface between stent struts and endoluminal surface is difficult by fluoroscopy (where one sees the stent but not the vessel wall) and angiography (where one sees the vessel but the contrast column may obscure the stent), but such evaluation is straightforward by IVUS. IVUS imaging is specifically useful during stent deployment in several respects:

1. IVUS imaging may assist in determining the need to stent a vessel post-PTA, by identifying an inadequate luminal area, severe plaque disruption, or the presence of a flow-limiting flap or dissection not apparent by angiography.
2. The target vessel may be measured by IVUS to ensure appropriate stent sizing. Since balloon/stent undersizing may predispose to abrupt closure and oversizing is associated with a hyperproliferative response leading to increased restenosis, exact sizing may directly affect clinical outcome.
3. IVUS permits identification of the origin, as well as end sites of a dissection, and thus easily identifies the longitudinal extent of vessel that requires stenting.
4. IVUS may identify sites of inadequate stent expansion and, specifically, non-apposition of struts to the underlying arterial wall.
5. For complex deployment, as in the case of stenting the bifurcation of the distal aorta, IVUS may facilitate stent positioning and subsequently can confirm the adequacy of the reconstructed bifurcation.

CURRENT LIMITATIONS

Initial clinical applications of IVUS have also revealed certain limitations of this technology. Perhaps the most decisive limitation concerns the inability of currently available IVUS imaging devices to consistently discriminate boundaries between the three layers of the arterial wall at sites of severe narrowing by atherosclerotic plaque. With advanced degrees of atherosclerosis, the characteristic ultrasound patterns become blurred. This is due principally to two factors: first, emaciation of the media typically accompanies progression of the atherosclerotic process.[82] Second, extensive calcific deposits, because they are often blanketed across the intimal-medial boundary and, because they attenuate or "shadow" the ultrasound reflections from the deeper layers of the wall, further obscure the normal ultrasound depiction of the arterial wall. Ambiguity regarding the boundary between intimal thickening and media reduces the precision with which any given measurement of wall thickness can be determined to represent atherosclerotic plaque versus normal wall.[40]

A second limitation of all currently available IVUS imaging devices is that the design of these devices allows only for side viewing. Because forward viewing is not possible, IVUS cannot be currently employed to determine the composition—for example, thrombus versus plaque—of a total occlusion prior to recanalization. Nor can IVUS direct the advancement of a wire or laser into an occluded segment. For this particular aspect of percutaneous interventional therapy, angioscopy may have superior utility. However, once through the occlusion, the IVUS image may identify whether the neolumen is intravascular or subintimal.[81]

Finally, it should be pointed out that the application of IVUS imaging is not without risk, especially in the coronary circulation. Because of the size of currently available catheters, imaging must be performed more expeditiously than is usually the case in the peripheral circulation. In addition, introduction of the IVUS catheter may occasionally precipitate spasm; accordingly, it is recommended that a final angiogram be recorded following IVUS examination of the coronary circulation.

INSTRUMENTS FOR COMBINED ULTRASOUND IMAGING AND PERCUTANEOUS REVASCULARIZATION

Initial attempts by Mallery and associates[83] to combine intravascular ultrasound imaging with balloon angioplasty and/or mechanical atherectomy employed a 4.5 F balloon dilatation catheter fitted with an array of eight 20-MHz transducers mounted radially around the catheter. The transducers were positioned within and midway between the two ends of a 3.0-cm polyethylene balloon; images were recorded perpendicular to the long axis of the catheter, through the balloon.

Hodgson and coworkers[84] performed in vivo imaging in normal canine coronary arteries using an alternative design in which a ring of modified phased-array transducers were positioned *proximal* to the balloon. The design of this device was intended to permit pre- and postdilation imaging without the requirement for multiple catheter exchanges. Recent in vivo studies using the Oracle in humans during PTCA[79,85] suggest that images obtained immediately pre- and postballoon dilation using this device may influence procedural strategy.

Recent clinical investigation in our laboratory has confirmed that it is feasible to perform on-line IVUS imaging during percutaneous revascularization, monitoring the effects of angioplasty on the arterial wall *during* balloon inflation, as opposed to *post hoc* evaluation described above. The balloon ultrasound imaging catheter (BUIC) (Boston Scientific), which we have employed, is a hybrid device that incorporates both diagnostic and therapeutic functions, imaging through polyethylene balloon material, the thickness of which is standard for peripheral angioplasty balloons.[63] In 8 of 10 patients pre-PTA and 9 of 10 patients post-PTA, images recorded from the BUIC permitted rapid quantitative analysis of minimum luminal diameter and luminal cross-sectional area. The measurements obtained were nearly indistinguishable from those recorded using a nonballoon ultrasound catheter.

Quantitative findings provided by the BUIC were specifically useful in defining the contribution of elastic recoil, long inferred to constitute a mechanical reason for loss of gain achieved during balloon inflation.[61,86,87] Previous investigators employed quantitative angiographic techniques to analyze the extent to which recoil complicates standard PTCA. Nobuyoshi for example, observed that "restenosis" (more than 50% loss of gain in absolute diameter assessed by cinevideodensitometry) was already present in 27 (14.6%) of 185 patients or in 27 (11.4%) of 237 lesions by 1 day post-PTCA, and was therefore interpreted to represent evidence of elastic recoil.

Measurements recorded using the BUIC confirm the observations made using angiographic techniques and establish that the phenomenon of recoil is common to peripheral as well as coronary angioplasty and that such recoil is instantaneous. Interestingly, the single patient in our series in whom clinical evidence of restenosis has thus far been observed was the one in whom recoil was most severe.

Finally, on-line ultrasound monitoring of ballon inflation also facilitates identification of the initiation of plaque fracture. Images recorded from the BUIC disclosed that plaque fractures were initiated by dilatation at low (less than 2 atm) inflation pressures. This is consistent with previous clinical observations. Hjemdahl-Monsen and colleagues[88] for example, found that most improvement in luminal size occurred at inflation pressures less than 2 atm. As suggested by Kleiman and colleagues[89] any technique that permits immediate, on-line recognition of plaque fracture might theoretically be employed to modify the remainder of the dilatation procedure in an attempt to prevent the development of a flow-limiting dissection.

Yock and coworkers[90] have investigated a prototype catheter that combined a 30-MHz transducer with a modified version of the Simpson directional atherectomy catheter. Preliminary experiments performed in vitro and in vivo demonstrated that this device could be used to monitor the depth to which plaque was mechanically excised. Furthermore, the availability of on-line imaging from within the cutting window of the device permits the operator to assign directionality to the subsequent cut(s). The ability to selectively debulk plaque has obvious positive implications: by facilitating more complete and selective plaque remorval and avoidance of normal elements in the arterial wall, the potential beneficial therapeutic effect of the Simpson device may be maximized.

The theoretical advantages of a combined laser/IVUS device are similar to those described above, including the enhanced ability to "aim" and thereby achieve precise tissue ablation and controlled plaque removal. Preliminary attempts to combine IVUS with laser ablation by Aretz and coworkers[91] and Linker and coworkers[92] suggested that the development of microcavitations during laser activation might preclude effective IVUS imaging. More recently we used a combination IVUS/laser catheter in vivo to guide and assess the results of laser-induced ablation of plaque.[93] The catheter consists of a conventional multifiber laser catheter, the wire-lumen of which has been used to accommodate a mechanical ultrasound transducer. Images recorded by IVUS simultaneously with excimer (308 nm) laser irradiation disclosed abrupt formation of cavitations, as previously described, that transiently attenuated the ultrasound image. Upon cessation of laser irradiation, normal blood flow cleared the excimer-generated gas, restoring the ultrasound image, and documenting the extent of reduced plaque volume.

Finally, the combination of IVUS imaging with a catheter for stent deployment would facilitate applications of IVUS to stent deployment described earlier. A prototypical device has been developed.

THREE-DIMENSIONAL RECONSTRUCTION

The introduction of three-dimensional reconstruction[22,57,62,94–106] has solved certain limitations inherent in the spatial display formats of current IVUS imaging systems. Conventional two-dimensional IVUS displays tomographic sections of the lumen and arterial wall in sequential fashion as a video recording. Comparison of individual segments examined by IVUS to adjacent or more distant segments requires repeated review of serially recorded images to reconstruct, in the mind's eye, the spatial relationship of the segments of interest. For example, while one tomographic image obtained during IVUS examination may offer high-resolution definition of a plaque fracture resulting from balloon angioplasty, details regarding the longitudinal distribution of the same plaque fracture at one site relative to proximal and distal sites cannot be displayed in a single image. In contrast, conventional angiography preserves the advantage of displaying each segment in longitudinal relationship to adjacent and more distant segments; once contrast media has opacified the artery of interest, any individual segment may be compared to adjacent and distant segments, limited only by the field of view.

For IVUS imaging to provide the same capability, for example, to compare adjacent segments within the vessel, simultaneous viewing of the data from multiple sequential cross-sectional slices is necessary. The liability of IVUS imaging that provides for only one tomographic view at a time, without a longitudinal perspective, may be resolved by "stacking" sequential IVUS frames recorded during a catheter pullback through a given vascular segment. Computer-based reconstruction of these serially-acquired IVUS frames creates a longitudinal, three-dimensional format for IVUS imaging data. Thus, the benefits of detailed tomographic imaging are preserved, while providing an efficient method to review the cumulative IVUS imaging data.

Original attempts to perform three-dimensional reconstructions in our laboratory involved the use of software (SigmaScan, Jandel Scientific, Corte Madera, CA) that required manual morphometric tracing of each serial tomographic image followed by computer-aided reconstruction.[99] The more detail intended, the more images were required, and consequently the more labor-intensive was the reconstruction. The principal liability of this approach, however, related to the fact that the modeling technique was based exclusively on boundary depiction and therefore allowed three-dimensional reconstruction of the lumen but not the arterial wall. Such an approach would clearly squander one of the chief assets of intravascular ultrasound, namely, the capability to image the vessel wall and thereby evaluate characteristics of the native wall, as well as pathologic alterations resulting from interventional therapies.

Automated three-dimensional reconstruction of intravascular ultrasound images was investigated in a preliminary fashion by Kitney and collaborators[107] using voxel modeling. This approach considers each voxel, or volume element, as an extension to three-dimensional space of the digital image element, or pixel (picture element). Voxel modeling is a particularly attractive option for three-dimensional reconstruction of the vasculature, because it preserves detailed ultrasound data and thereby allows representation of the arterial wall, rather than sim-

ply surface features that would limit the reconstruction to the arterial lumen.

To thereby preserve information regarding the arterial wall and plaque in the reconstructed image, ImageComm Systems (Santa Clara, CA) developed for us a PC-based system using algorithms[108,109] designed specifically for analysis of images recorded during IVUS examination (Omniview, Pura Labs, Brea, CA). This software employs a surface rendering process predicated on segmented boundary formation, but includes interpolative algorithms designed to link boundary elements, and thereby preserve the capability of viewing the arterial wall, as well as lumen. Three distinct display formats are currently available for reconstructed IVUS data: so-called *sagittal, cylindrical,* and *lumen cast* modes. In the sagittal mode, a planar view of the IVUS data is displayed in longitudinal relief and can be revolved around the long axis of the IVUS catheter. Use of the sagittal format, in particular, not only facilitates comparative analysis of adjacent tomographic images, but offers the additional advantage of displaying the ultrasound data in a longitudinal profile-type format more familiar to the angiographer.

While similar in orientation to an angiogram, sagittal reconstruction substantially augments information available from conventional angiography in two important ways. First, limitless orthogonal views can be rendered by incremental rotation of the imaging plane about the reference catheter. Given the documented importance of orthogonal views in the assesment of luminal narrowing[110] on the one hand, and the logistical factors which frequently obviate the possibility of obtaining orthogonal views on the other, this feature may ultimately prove to be the principal advantage of three-dimensional reconstruction. Second, information regarding pathologic alteration of the arterial wall is provided simultaneously with the conventional assessment of luminal diameter narrowing. Experience with patients undergoing percutaneous revascularization indicates that certain features of arterial wall pathology are particularly well defined in such a longitudinal format. For example, three-dimensional reconstruction in the sagittal mode graphically demonstrated that recanalization of a lengthy total occlusion was achieved by tunneling a false lumen through calcified plaque. Such a mechanism of recanalization has been previously described in vitro[111,112] and is frequently inferred to occur in vivo.[113] While the individual tomographic ultrasound images indicated creation of a "double-barrel" lumen, the full extent of pathologic disruption was more immediately apparent from inspection of the sagittal reconstructions. Similarly, sagittal reconstructions of balloon-dilated nonoccluded vessels demonstrates the longitudinal distribution of barotraumatic injury, otherwise evident as only local, isolated plaque fractures on the tomographic two-dimensional IVUS images. Use of the three-dimensional formats facilitates delineation of the extent of a dissection facilitates selection and deployment of endovascular stents.

The cylindrical three-dimensional mode preserves the wall and lumen as an intact cylinder and thus provides true three-dimensional—as opposed to planar—views. Experience with the cylindrical format suggests that this mode of three-dimensional reconstruction—particularly when the reconstructed vascular segment is hemisected—is optimally suited for those cases in which direct inspection of luminal topography is of special interest, such as analysis of implanted endovascular prostheses. Details of the "cobblestoned" neointima lining the stent cannot be appreciated angiographically or even by intravascular ultrasound, when viewed in standard video format;[76] the algorithms developed to accomplish the cylindrical reconstruction serve the dual functions of both joining together the series of adjacent elements representing the neointima, and then rotating the reconstructed image 90 degrees to permit viewing of the endoluminal surface en face. The sagittal reconstruction supplements the cylindrical format by facilitating analysis of arterial contour proximal and distal to the stent; such analysis is otherwise not feasible using the unassembled tomographic images.

While sagittal and cylindrical three-dimensional formats facilitate qualitative assessment of pathologic alterations involving plaque arterial wall, neither format allows quantitative analysis of residual luminal cross-sectional area narrowing. Therefore, in order to take advantage of the unique ability to planimeter cross-sectional area from tomographic IVUS images, the lumen cast format was developed,[94,95,100,103] reconstructing a cast of the lumen by isolating it from the underlying arterial wall. Each sequential stored IVUS frame is analyzed by projecting rays radially outward from the center of the transducer. Based on a preselected threshold valve, these rays automatically detect the luminal border; the borders detected by the rays are integrated to create a disclike cross-sectional area "map" for each IVUS frame. Maps from sequential frames are then stacked to create a three-dimensional cast of the lumen. The area of each map or disc is determined by precalibration with the known size of the IVUS probe, and the resulting series of cross-sectional area determinations is plotted linearly, allowing near-instantaneous quantitative analysis of cross-sectional area along the entire length of the vascular segment examined. Inspection of the plot permits rapid identification of sites of residual cross-sectional narrowing.

Preliminary in vitro[114] and in vivo[100] investigations have provided evidence validating the algorithm employed for quantitative analysis in the lumen cast format. While the lumen cast display forfeits information regarding qualitative alterations in the plaque and underlying wall, this format greatly facilitates on line interpretation of the extent to which satisfactory luminal dimensions have been achieved. The cast graphically depicts residual sites of luminal narrowing, and as a cursor is directed to any suspicious site, provides automated quantitative assessment of luminal cross-sectional area and percentage of narrowing at that site. Moreover, because movement of the cursor to a specific level of the luminal cast simultaneously brings up the corresponding two-dimensional tomographic image on the upper left quadrant of the ImageComm workstation screen, the operator retains the option of inspecting the two-dimensional image to confirm the quantitative readout derived from analysis of the luminal cast. Our experience employing the lumen cast algorithm on line during interventional procedures suggest that it is useful in accurately and rapidly identifying sites of residual narrowing, including sites which might otherwise be overlooked during routine two-dimensional IVUS examination due to their focal nature.

Certain limitations of current attempts to perform three-dimensional reconstruction must be acknowledged. *First,* it is apparent that the quality of the three-dimensional reconstructions can only be as good as the original two-dimensional images. Details which are absent from the original recordings will likewise be absent from the reconstructed images. In those instances when calcific deposits, for example, are observed on the two-dimensional images to attenuate echoes from the subjacent plaque and/or wall, these portions of the plaque and/or wall will not be incorporated into the reconstructed image.

Second, "ring-down artifact," resulting from dead space in the acoustic transmission path and manifested on the two-dimensional image as a white halo immediately peripheral to the transducer, may obscure near-field structure in smaller, particularly stenotic vessels. In our preliminary work such artifact was routinely masked out of the three-dimensional reconstructions; in those cases in which reconstruction is applied to two-dimensional images with little or no lumen peripheral to the transducer, such masking could overestimate three-dimensional depiction of luminal patency. Current attempts by the manufacturers of mechanical transducer systems to eliminate such artifact will it is hoped, resolve this issue.

Third, while major branch points, such as the aortic bifurcation, are accurately depicted in the three-dimensional reconstruction, the two-dimensional images are otherwise reassembled as a straight tube; sharp bends in the artery are not faithfully reconstructed on either the two- or three-dimensional images. While this is typically not a severe liability in evaluation of the peripheral and renal circulations, it may become more significant in the assessment of the more tortuous coronary circulation.

Fourth, three-dimensional reconstruction shares with conventional intravascular ultrasound imaging the difficulty of matching the rotational orientation of the ultrasound transducer to that of the imaged vessel. Furthermore, if the ultrasound probe is inadvertently twisted during the pullback recording, the three-dimensional reconstruction will reflect this rotational event.

Fifth, in most studies performed to date, the two-dimensional images have been acquired during a slow, timed catheter pullback; this strategy is intended to optimize the number of acquired images over a given segment length and provide equal representation for each portion of the artery in the reconstructed image. Such catheter pullback, however, is entirely operator-dependent and small variations in the rate of pullback may ultimately influence the three-dimensional representation. For example, if the catheter withdrawal rate is slowed during pullback through an abnormal segment of vessel, and subsequently accelerated through a more normal segment, the abnormal segment will occupy proportionally more than its true length of the resulting reconstruction. This phenomenon is particularly likely to occur when there is a tendency for the operator to slow catheter movement through abnormal segments to achieve closer inspection of morphologic disruptions. Recent modifications in acquisition technique include automated image registration utilizing motorized pullback devices, rendering the technique less operator-dependent.[27]

Sixth, current software does not gate image acquisition to phases of the cardiac cycle. While this is not a significant liability in three-dimensional reconstruction of peripheral vessels, it remains a major source of artifact in reconstruction of coronary and renal vessels.

Beyond these limitations, many of which are currently being addressed, the extent to which three-dimensional reconstruction will be employed clinically is principally dependent on two factors: the time required for reconstruction and the prognostic implications of the resulting images. With regard to the former, image processing time has been reduced considerably through a combination of modifications in software and memory expansion. While early reconstructions typically required 20 to 40 minutes to assemble, current sagittal reconstructions are performed and visualized real-time, concurrent with catheter pullback.[97] Cylindrical and lumen cast reconstructions are routinely available within 30 seconds of completing the pullback recording[102] Thus, the time required to reconstruct and review the reconstructed images is comparable to that required to review the video playback of a contrast angiogram.

REFERENCES

1. Vlodaver Z, Frech R, Van Tassel RA, Edwards JE. Correlations of the ante-mortem arteriogram and the post-mortem specimen. Circulation 1973;47:162–169
2. Grondin CM, Dyrda I, Pasternac A, et al. Discrepancies between cineangiographic and post-mortem findings in patients with coronary artery disease and recent myocardial revascularization. Circulation 1974; 49:703–708
3. Pepine CJ, Feldman RL, Nichols WW. Coronary arteriography: potentially serious sources of error in interpretation. Cardiovasc Med 1977;2:747–752
4. Arnett EN, Isner JM, Redwood CR, et al. Coronary artery narrowing in coronary heart disease: comparison of cineangiographic and necropsy findings. Ann Intern Med 1979;91:350–356
5. Isner JM, Kishel J, Kent KM, et al. Accuracy of angiographic determination of left main coronary arterial narrowing: angiographic-histologic correlative analysis in 28 patients. Circulation 1981;63:1056–1064
6. Isner JM, Donaldson RF. Coronary angiographic and morphologic correlation. Cardiol Clin 1984;2: 571–592
7. De Feyter PJ, Serruys PW, Davies MJ, et al. Quantitative coronary angiography to measure progression and regression of coronary atherosclerosis. Circulation 1991;84:412–423
8. Marcus ML, Skorton DJ, Johnson MR, et al. Visual estimates of percent diameter coronary stenosis: "a battered gold standard." Am Coll Cardiol 1988;11: 882–885
9. Dietz WA, Tobis JM, Isner JM. Failure of angiography to accurately depict the extent of coronary artery narrowing in three fatal cases of percutaneous transluminal coronary angioplasty. J Am Coll Cardiol 1992;19:1261–1270
10. Tobis JM, Mallery JA, Gessert JM, et al. Intravascular ultrasound cross-sectional arterial imaging before and after balloon angioplasty in vitro. Circulation 1989;80:873–882
11. White CW, Wright CB, Doty DB. Does visual interpretation of the coronary arteriogram predict the physiologic importance of a coronary stenosis? N Engl J Med 1984;310:819–824
12. Davidson CJ, Sheikh KH, Harrison JK, et al. Intravascular ultrasonography versus digital subtraction angiography: a human in vivo comparison of vessel size and morphology. J Am Coll of Cardiol 1990;16: 633–636
13. Gussenhoven WJ, Essed CE, Frietman P, et al. Intra-

vascular echographic assessment of vessel wall characteristics: a correlation with histology. Int J Cardiac Imaging 1989;4:105–116

14. Hodgson JMcB, Graham SP, Savakus AD. Clinical percutaneous imaging of coronary anatomy using an over-the-wire ultrasound catheter system. Int J Cardiac Imaging 1989;4:187–193

15. St. Goar FG, Pinto FJ, Alderman EL, et al. Detection of coronary atherosclerosis in young adult heart using intravascular ultrasound. Circulation 1992;86:756–763

16. Nissen SE, Gurley JC, Grines CL, et al. Intravascular ultrasound assessment of lumen size and wall morphology in normal subjects and patients with coronary artery disease. Circulation 1991;84:1087–1099

17. Pandian NG, Hsu TL. Intravascular ultrasound imaging of the coronary circulation. In: Heart Disease: A Textbook of Cardiovascular Medicine. Philadelphia: Braunwald E, ed. WB Saunders, 1992;65–76

18. Tenaglia AN, Buller CE, Kisslo KB, et al. Mechanisms of balloon angioplasty and directional coronary atherectomy as assessed by intracoronary ultrasound. Am J Cardiol 1992;20:685–691

19. Tenaglia AN, Tcheng JE, Kisslo KB, et al. Intracoronary ultrasound evaluation of excimer laser angioplasty. Circulation 1992;86:I–516(abst)

20. Yock PG, Fitzgerald PJ, Linker DT, Angelsen BA. Intravascular ultrasound giudance for catheter-based coronary interventions. J Am Coll Cardiol 1992;17:39B–45B

21. Comess K, Fitzgerald PJ, Yock PG. Intracoronary ultrasound imaging of graft thrombosis. N Engl J Med 1992;327:1691–1692

22. Rosenfield K, Kaufman J, Pieczek A, Isner JM. On-line three-dimensional reconstruction from 2D IVUS: utility for guiding interventional procedures. J Am Coll Cardiol 1992;19:224A(abst)

23. Rosenfield K, Losordo DW, Ramaswamy K, et al. Qualitative assessment of peripheral vessels by intravascular ultrasound before and after interventions. J Am Coll Cardiol 1990;15:107A(abst)

24. Rosenfield K, Voelker W, Losordo DW, et al. Assessment of coronary arterial stenoses post-intervention by quantitative angiography versus intracoronary ultrasound in 13 patients undergoing balloon and/or laser coronary angioplasty. J Am Coll Cardiol 1991;17:46A(abst)

25. The GUIDE trial investigators. Lumen enlargement following angioplasty is related to plaque characteristics: a report from the GUIDE trial. Circulation 1992;86:I–531(abst)

26. Tobis JM, Mahon DJ, Lehmann KG, et al. Intracoronary ultrasound imaging after balloon angioplasty. Circulation 1990;82:III–676(abst)

27. Mintz GS, Keller MB, Fay KG. Motorized IVUS transducer pullback permits accurate quantitative axial length measurements. Circulation 1992;86:I–323(abst)

28. Isner JM, Rosenfield K, Kelly K, et al. Percutaneous intravascular ultrasound examination as an adjunct to catheter-based interventions: preliminary experience in patients with peripheral vascular disease. Radiology 1990;175:61–70

29. Gussenhoven EJ, The SHK, Serruys PW, et al. Intravascular ultrasound and vascular intervention. J Intervent Cardiol 1991;4:41–48

30. Gurley JC, Nissen SE, Grines CL, et al. Comparison of intravascular ultrasound and angiography following percutaneous transluminal coronary angioplasty. Circulation 1990;82:III–72(abst)

31. Fitzgerald PJ, Muhlberger VA, Moes NY, et al. Calcium location within plaque as a predictor of atherectomy tissue retrieval: an intravascular ultrasound study. Circulation 1992;86:I–516(abst)

32. Fitzgerald PJ, Ports TA, Yock PG. Contribution of localized calcium deposits to dissection after angioplasty: an observational study using intravascular ultrasound. Circulation 1992;86:64–70

33. Gussenhoven WJ, Essed CE, Lancee CT, et al. Arterial wall characteristics determined by intravascular ultrasound imaging: an in vitro study. J Am Coll Cardiol 1989;14:947–952

34. Gussenhoven EJ, Essed CE, Frietman P, et al. Intravascular ultrasonic imaging: Histologic and echographic correlation. Eur J Vasc Surg 1989;3:571–576

35. Potkin BN, Bartorelli AL, Gessert JM, et al. Coronary artery imaging with intravascular high-frequency ultrasound. Circulation 1990;81:1575–1585

36. Nishimura RA, Edwards WD, Warness CA, et al. Intravascular ultrasound imaging: in vitro validation and pathologic correlation. J Am Coll Cardiol 1990;16:145–154

37. Siegel RJ, Ariani M, Fishbein MC, et al. Histopathologic validation of angioscopy and intravascular ultrasound. Circulation 1991;84:109–117

38. Siegel RJ, Fishbein MC, Chae JS, et al. Origin of the three-ringed appearance of human arteries by ultrasound: microdissection with ultrasonic and histologic correlation. J Am Coll Cardiol 1990;15:17A(abst)

39. Coy KM, Maurer G, Siegel RJ. Intravascular ultrasound imaging: a current perspective. J Am Coll Cardiol 1991;18:1811–1823

40. Mallery JA, Tobis JM, Griffith JM, et al. Assessment of normal and atherosclerotic arterial wall thickness with an intravascular ultrasound imaging catheter. Am Heart J 1990;119:1392–1400

41. Yock PG, Linker DT. Intravascular ultrasound: looking below the surface of vascular disease. Circulation 1990;81:1715–1718

42. Webb JG, Yock PG, Slepian MJ. Intravascular ultrasound: significance of the three-layered appearance of normal muscular arteries. J Am Coll Cardiol 1990;15:17A(abst)

43. Lockwood GR, Ryan LK, Gotlieb AI, et al. In vitro high resolution intravascular imaging in muscular and elastic arteries. J Am Coll Cardiol 1992;20:153–160

44. Yeung AC, Ryan TJ, Isner JM. Correlation of intravascular ultrasound characteristics with endothelium-dependent vasodilator function in the coronary arteries of cardiac transplant patients. Circulation 1991;84:II–703

45. Fitzgerald PJ, St. Goar FG, Connolly AJ, et al. Intravascular ultrasound imaging of coronary arteries: is three layers the norm? Circulation 1992;86:154–158

46. Tobis JM, Mallery JA, Mahon DJ, et al. Intravascular ultrasound imaging of human coronary arteries in vivo. Circulation 1991;83:913–926

47. Nissen SE, Grines CL, Gurley JC, et al. Application of a new phased-array ultrasound imaging catheter in the assessment of vascular dimensions: in vivo

comparison to cineangiography. Circulation 1990;81:660–666

48. St. Goar FG, Pinto FJ, Alderman EL, et al. Intracoronary ultrasound in cardiac transplant recipients: in vivo evidence of "angiographically silent" intimal thickening. Circulation 1992;85:979–987

49. Isner JM, Kearney M, Berdan LG, et al. Core pathology lab findings in 425 patients undergoing directional atherectomy for a primary coronary artery stenosis and relationship to subsequent outcome: the CAVEAT Study. J Am Coll Cardiol 1992

50. Pandian NG, Kreis A, Brockway B. Detection of intra-arterial thrombus by intravascular high frequency two-dimensional ultrasound imaging: in vitro and in vivo studies. Am J Cardiol 1990;65:1280–1283

51. Siegel RJ, Chae JS, Forrester JS, Ruiz CE. Angiography, angioscopy, and ultrasound imaging before and after percutaneous balloon angioplasty. Am Heart J 1990;120:1086–1090

52. Johnson C, Hansen DD, Vracko R, Ritchie J. Angioscopy: more sensitive for identifying thrombus, distal emboli, and subintimal dissection. J Am Coll Cardiol 1989;13:146A(abst)

53. Mecley M, Rosenfield K, Kaufman J, et al. Atherosclerotic plaque hemorrhage and rupture associated with crescendo claudication. Ann Intern Med 1992;117:663–666

54. Yock PG, Linker DT. Catheter-based two-dimensional ultrasound imaging. In: Topol EJ, ed. Textbook of Interventional Cardiology. Philadelphia: WB Saunders; 1993:816–827

55. Tabbara M, White RA, Cavaye D, Kopchok G. In vivo human comparison of intravascular ultrasonography and angiography. J Vasc Surg 1991;14:496–502

56. Isner JM, Rosenfield K. Enough with the fantastic voyage: will IVUS pay in Peoria. Cathet Cardiovasc Diagn 1992;26:192–199

57. Rosenfield K, Losordo DW, Harding M, et al. Intravascular ultrasound of renal arteries in patients undergoing percutaneous transluminal angioplasty: feasibility, saftey, and initial findings, including 3-dimensional reconstruction of renal arteries. J Am Coll Cardiol 1992;17:204A(abst)

58. Graham SP, Brands D, Savakus AD, Hodgson JMcB. Utility of an intravascular ultrasound imaging device for arterial wall definition and atherectomy guidance. J Am Coll Cardiol 1989;13:222A(abst)

59. Waller BF, Pinkerton CA, Slack JD. Intravascular ultrasound—a histologic study of vessels during life: the new "gold standard" for vascular imaging. Circulation 1992;85:2305–2310

60. Waller BF, Orr CM, Pinkerton CA, et al. Coronary balloon angioplasty dissections: "The Good, the Bad and the Ugly." J Am Coll Cardiol 1992;20:701–706

61. Waller BF. Pathology of new interventions used in the treatment of coronary heart disease. Curr Prob Cardiol 1986;11:666–760

62. Coy KM, Park JC, Fishbein MC, et al. In vitro validation of three-dimensional intravascular ultrasound for the evaluation of arterial injury after balloon angioplasty. J Am Coll Cardiol 1992;20:692–700

63. Isner JM, Rosenfield K, Losordo DW, et al. Combination balloon-ultrasound imaging catheter for percutaneous transluminal angioplasty. Circulation 1991;84:739–754

64. Honye J, Mahon DJ, Jain A, et al. Morphological effects of coronary balloon angioplasty in vivo assessed by intravascular ultrasound imaging. Circulation 1992;85:1012–1025

65. Losordo DW, Rosenfield K, Pieczek A, et al. How does angioplasty work? serial analysis of human iliac arteries using intravascular ultrasound. Circulation 1992;86:1845–1858

66. Farb A, Virmani R, Atkinson JB, Kolodgie F. Plaque morphology and pathologic changes in arteries from patients dying after coronary balloon angioplasty. J Am Coll Cardiol 1990;16:1421–1429

67. Castaneda-Zuniga WR, Formanek A, Tadavarthy M. The mechanism of balloon angioplasty. Radiology 1980;135:565–571

68. The SHK, Gussenhoven EJ, Zhong Y, et al. Effect of balloon angioplasty on femoral artery evaluated with intravascular ultrasound imaging. Circulation 1992;86:483–493

69. Honye J, Mahon DJ, Nakamura S, et al. Enhanced diagnostic ability of intravascular ultrasound imaging compared with angiography. Circulation 1992;86:I-324(abst)

70. Waller BF, Miller J, Morgan R, Tejada E. Atherosclerotic plaque calcific deposits: an important factor in success or failure of transluminal coronary angioplasty. Circulation 1988;78:II-376.(abst)

71. Mintz GS, Leon MB, Satler LF, et al. Pre-intervention intravascular ultrasound imaging influences transcatheter coronary treatment strategies. Circulation 1992;86:I-323(abst)

72. Yock PG, Fitzgerald PJ, Sykes C, et al. Morphologic features of successful coronary atherectomy determined by intravascular ultrasound imaging. Circulation 1992;82:III-676(abst)

73. Smucker ML, Scherb DE, Howard PF, et al. Intracoronary ultrasound: how much "angioplasty effect" in atherectomy. Circulation 1990;82:III-676(abst)

74. Penny WF, Schmidt DA, Safian RD, et al. Insights into the mechanism of luminal improvement after directional coronary atherectomy. Am Jo Cardiol 1991;67:435–437

75. Safian RD, Gelbfish JS, Erny RE, et al. Coronary atherectomy: clinical, angiographic, and histological findings and observations regarding potential mechanisms. Circulation 1990;82:69–79.

76. Chokshi SK, Hogan J, Desai V, et al. Intravascular ultrasound assessment of implanted stents. J Am Coll Cardiol 1990;15:29A(abst)

77. Rutherford RB, Flanigan DP, Guptka SK, et al. Suggested standards for reports dealing with lower extremity ischemia. J Vasc Surg 1986;4:80–94.

78. Isner JM, Rosenfield K, Mosseri M, et al. How reliable are images obtained by intravascular ultrsound for making decisions during percutaneous interventions? experience with intravascular ultrasound employed in lieu of contrast angiography to guide peripheral balloon angioplasty in 16 patients. Circulation 1990;82:III-440(abst)

79. Hodgson JMcB, Nair R. Efficacy and usefulness of a combined intracoronary ultrasound-angioplasty balloon catheter: results of the multicenter oracle trial. Circulation 1992;86:I-321(abst)

80. Mintz GS, Douek P, Pichard AD, et al. Target lesion calcification in coronary artery disease: an intravascular ultrasound study. J Am Coll of Cardiol 1992;20:1149–1155

detailed preinterventional images of the target ath-

discrepancies between visual assessment of lesion

reconstruct an image. As a result, two very different

blood can prove invaluable in identifying vessel wall

81. Rees MR, Sivananthan MU, Verma SP. The role of intravascular ultrasound and angioscopy in the placement and followup of coronary stents. Circulation 1992;86:I-364(abst)
82. Isner JM, Donaldson RF, Fortin AH, et al. Attenuation of the media in coronary arteries in advanced

lar ultrasound images of iliac arteries. Am J Cardiol 1992;70:412–415
98. Schryver TE, Popma JJ, Kent KM, et al. Use of intracoronary ultrasound to identify the "true" coronary lumen in chronic coronary dissection treated with intracoronary stenting. Am J Cardiol 1992;69:

structures that communicate with the lumen, such as intramural dissection.

Several investigators have characterized normal coronary morphology using intravascular ultrasound.[6,15,16] Such studies report a distinctly laminar appearance to the vessel wall in many, but not all normal subjects. Many normal coronary arteries exhibit an intimal leading edge that poorly reflects ultrasound, resulting in a monolayered appearance (Fig. 5-2). Depending on the studied population, distinct laminations of the vessel wall are inapparent in more than 50% of normal coronary sites, particularly in younger normal subjects. The lack of lamination of the vessel wall in many normal coronaries probably reflects the fact that the endothelium in healthy subjects consists of only a single cell layer—well below the axial resolution of ultrasound devices. For the normal subjects who possess a distinct intimal leading edge, the maximum thickness averages 0.15 ± 0.07 mm; most investigators consider the upper limit of normal intima as less than 0.25 or 0.30 mm.

Virtually all atherosclerotic coronary arteries have sufficient intimal thickening to generate a trilaminar appearance. Typical coronary atherosclerotic plaques appear as textured echogenic intraluminal

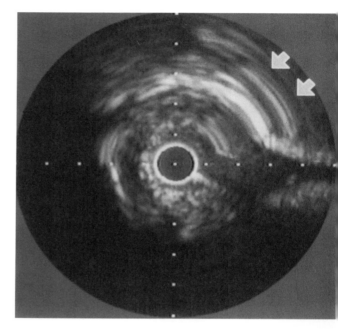

Fig. 5-3. Intravascular ultrasound image showing nonuniform rotational distortion (NURD). Stretching of the image during a portion of the transducer rotation (*arrows*) distorts anatomy.

encroachments. Underlying the atheroma, there usually exists a thin, sonolucent subintimal band, which in vitro studies have demonstrated to represent the media (Figs. 5-3 to 5-12). Coronary atheromas that appear less echogenic than the vessel adventitia are often termed "soft" plaques. In vitro studies have demonstrated a high lipid content in these highly sonolucent lesions. Soft atheromas vary widely in echogenicity, ranging from plaques nearly as sonolucent as blood to more echogenic, highly textured lesions (Fig. 5-4). Differences in the resolution and dynamic range of the differing ultrasound instrumentation may contribute to the variability in appearance.

Atheromata demonstrate markedly increased plaque echogenicity in some vessels (Fig. 5-5). These more echogenic lesions are commonly termed "hard" plaques, because studies indicate the presence of significant fibrosis. Hard coronary plaques behave differently when approached with interventional devices, often requiring higher balloon pressures for effective dilatation. In the most extreme examples of plaque echogenicity, an echodense portion of the lesion attenuates transmission of low-energy, high-frequency ultrasound, thus obscuring the underlying structures of the arterial wall (Fig. 5-6). In lesions that impede the penetration of ultrasound, histologic studies demonstrate the presence of calcium. Calcified lesions exhibit considerable biomechanical

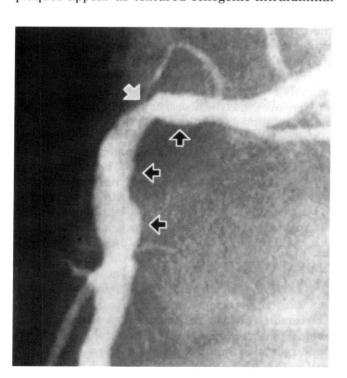

Fig. 5-2. Angiogram showing diffuse coronary disease. Determination of percentage of stenosis for the lesion (*gray arrow*) requires identification of a normal reference segment (*black arrows*). In this case, multiple sites represent possible "normal" reference sites.

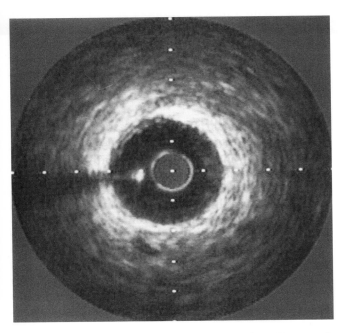

Fig. 5-4. A normal coronary by intravascular ultrasound. The space between each marker of the distance scale in 1.0 mm. The lumen is round with intimal thickness never exceeding 0.25 mm.

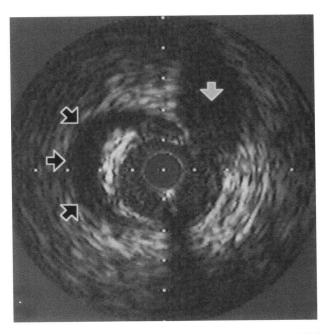

Fig. 5-6. A complex coronary atheroma with a "hard" fibrous cap overlying a lipid core, showing a large sonolucent zone with an echogenic fibrous cap (*black arrows*) and a sidebranch (*gray arrow*).

rigidity and often require higher balloon pressures to achieve adequate luminal gain during angioplasty. Dense calcified atheromata also resist plaque removal by directional atherectomy.

DIAGNOSTIC APPLICATIONS

Angiographically Unrecognized Disease

Coronary ultrasound commonly detects atherosclerotic abnormalities at sites containing no apparent lesion by angiography (Fig. 5-7).[6,17-19] In patients with minimal to moderate coronary disease, virtually the entirety of the coronary arterial tree exhibits abnormal intimal thickness by intravascular ultrasound. Several phenomena explain the greater sensitivity of ultrasound in the detection of coronary atherosclerosis. To classify sites as diseased, angiography relies on identification of a coronary segment with apparent luminal encroachment. However, not all atherosclerotic segments are narrowed in comparison to adjacent disease-free sites. This conundrum reflects a phenomenon first described by Glagov and colleagues[20] in which compensatory remodeling of the vessel wall preserves angiographic lumen size in atherosclerotic arteries (Fig. 5-8). In such segments, adventitial enlargement opposes luminal encroach-

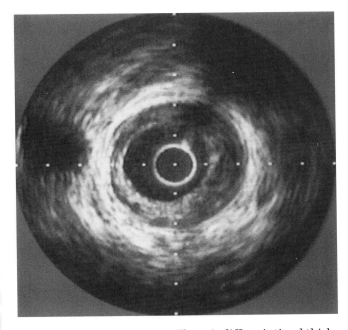

Fig. 5-5. A "soft" atheroma. There is diffuse intimal thickening with an average echogenicity much less than the adventitia. Maximum atheroma thickness exceeds 1 mm (3 o'clock).

Fig. 5-9. Coronary remodeling. **(A)** The midcircumflex is free of disease. **(B)** The proximal circumflex contains a large crescentic atheroma; however, the adventitia has remodeled outward, thereby concealing the atherosclerosis from the angiographer.

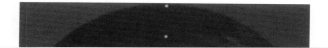

angiography arises from lesion eccentricity. In the absence of an unlimited number of angiographic projections, the operator cannot identify small eccentric

relatively large standard error, exceeding 0.50 mm. This phenomenon presents a complex problem for the interventionist who must select a specific device for the revascularization procedure. A device that is too small may compromise results, while a device that is too large will risk complications.

Preliminary data from our laboratory indicates that differences between ultrasound and angiographic "reference" diameters represent an important factor, affecting both initial results and long-term clinical outcome.[22] These data demonstrate that diffuse atherosclerosis reduces luminal diameter by more than 50% in approximately one-third of angiographically normal reference segments. In this subgroup of patients, the operator selects a smaller interventional device than that employed for patients without reference segment disease. Intuitively, the systematic undersizing of interventional devices could significantly impair the success of percutaneous revascularization procedures.

No prospective randomized data exist that document a clear advantage for device-sizing by intravascular ultrasound. Potentially, improved device-sizing by intravascular ultrasound may impact upon both the acute complication and recurrence rates for coronary lesions. However, this approach must contend with a critical confounding variable, coronary remodeling, in which the vessel adventitia expands outward during the early stages of atherosclerosis.

Balloon Angioplasty Results

Measurement of percent stenosis, typically expressed either as diameter or cross-sectional area reduction, represents the standard approach to assessment of procedural success. Several studies have revealed a strikingly poor correlation between ultrasound and angiographic measurement of percentage of stenosis following coronary angioplasty, typically approximately $r = .30$.[5] Analysis of comparative studies have shown that disparities in percentage of stenosis determination arise from differences in both lesional and reference vessel measurements.

Lumen shape represents the most important phenomenon responsible for disagreement between angiography and ultrasound. Intravascular ultrasound demonstrates a diverse spectrum of morphologic findings following balloon angioplasty that often include complex fractures or dissections in the vessel wall (Fig. 5-9). The extreme distortion of lumen shape produced by balloon dilatation represents the most adverse environment for angiographic quantitation of lesion severity. Theoretically, extravasation of contrast through narrow dissection channels within the intima, media, or adventitia of the vessel

can enhance the apparent angiographic diameter of the vessel. In this setting, the angiographic appearance consists of a large, but "hazy" lumen, in which intravascular ultrasound reveals minimal balloon augmentation of lumen size.

The ability of ultrasound to provide images before, as well as after, angioplasty, has enabled routine evaluation of the mechanism and extent of luminal enlargement. In some patients, intimal fracture constitutes the sole or principal mechanism responsible for luminal enlargement. In these cases, ultrasound can readily determine the depth of the dissection, which may range from superficial intimal disruption to extensive periadventitial tears. Plaque dissections typically consist of single fracture but can occasionally comprise multiple tears. The typical site for dissection consists of a junction between hard and soft plaque elements.

Although dissection represents the most common mechanism of luminal enlargement, intravascular imaging in some patients identifies an alternative mechanism responsible for balloon enlargement of the lumen, most often stretching of the vessel wall. Analysis of the intravascular images can confirm this dilation effect whenever ultrasound measurements of media-adventitia diameter at the lesion site increase substantially after the procedure. In a few patients, luminal enlargement results primarily from an apparent reduction in the cross-sectional area of the atheromatous plaque. Whether this phenomenon represents true plaque compression or simply axial redistribution of atheroma remains controversial.

However, the acute and long-term implications of each of the various mechanisms of luminal enlargement remain uncertain. Preliminary data suggest that vessels exclusively enlarged by media-adventitia stretching are more susceptible to restenosis secondary to acute or chronic recoil. However, there exist no prospective data describing the relationship between these morphologic patterns and long-term prognosis. The relatively poor correlation between angiographic and ultrasonic dimensions following angioplasty raises provocative clinical and scientific issues. In certain patients, it remains possible that "restenosis" represents a failure to adequately augment the luminal area, rather than subsequent cellular proliferation. Several multicenter clinical trials will examine whether ultrasound imaging can predict or favorably affect long-term outcome.

Directional Atherectomy

Intravascular ultrasound has proven particularly valuable in the guidance of directional coronary atherectomy (DCA).[23,24] Most clinicians consider the location and distribution of the atheroma as important

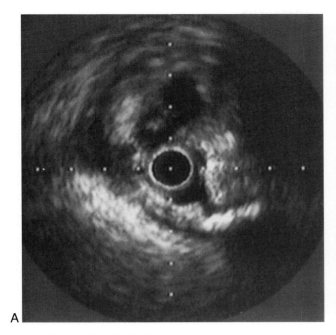
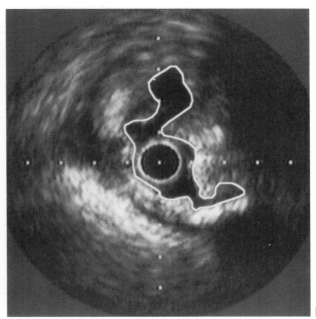

Fig. 5-10. (A & B) A complex coronary dissection following balloon angioplasty. The manual tracing of the lumen borders is shown **(B)**.

factors in the selection of patients for directional atherectomy (Fig. 5-10). Angiographic studies have suggested that eccentric plaque would represent the optimal target for atherectomy. However, recent comparative studies have shown that the apparent distribution of the atheroma by angiography correlates poorly with plaque location determined by intravascular ultrasound. Thus, lesions that appear concentric by angiography are often highly eccentric when examined by ultrasound and conversely, angiographically eccentric lesions are frequently concentric by ultrasound. The poor correlation for plaque distribution reflects the disadvantages of a silhouette imaging method such as angiography in comparison to a tomographic technique such as ultrasound.

The presence and extent of vessel wall calcification constitute important determinants of the efficacy of directional atherectomy. Traditionally, significant fluoroscopic calcification has constituted a contraindication to atherectomy. However, studies have confirmed that intravascular ultrasound reveals vessel calcification more frequently than fluoroscopy. Unlike radiographic methods, ultrasound can readily determine the circumferential location and depth of calcification. Vessels with extensive superficial calcification resist plaque removal by directional atherectomy, but arteries with extensive deep calcification can undergo successful atherectomy if ultrasound demonstrates only deep calcium. Conversely, vessels with little or no calcium on fluoroscopy may actually contain extensive superficial calcification thus precluding successful atherectomy.

In ultrasound-guided atherectomy, the extent, location, and distribution of the atheroma determine the device size and orientation of atherectomy cuts. However, successful application of this approach requires experience, patience, and careful planning. Although ultrasound provides an excellent view of the circumferential distribution of plaque, precise orientation of the intravascular image remains difficult. Experienced practitioners will carefully examine the target segment before atherectomy to locate anatomic landmarks, particularly side branches, which are subsequently used to orient the ultrasound image. For example, a plaque in the left anterior descending can be described as contralateral or ipsilateral to the septal perforators. The operator can subsequently direct atherectomy cuts toward the appropriate side of the vessel.

Rotational Ablation

Although experience remains limited, coronary intravascular ultrasound can significantly benefit clinical application of the Rotablator, a high-speed diamond-coated burr for percutaneous coronary revascularization. This device is particularly effective at removing calcium from lesions—precisely the type of lesion least suitable for directional atherectomy (Fig. 5-11). Intravascular ultrasound evidence

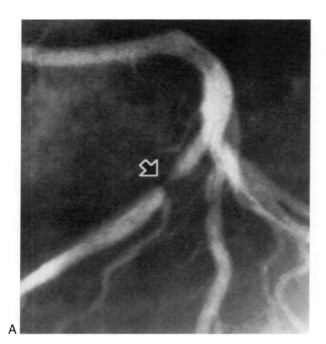 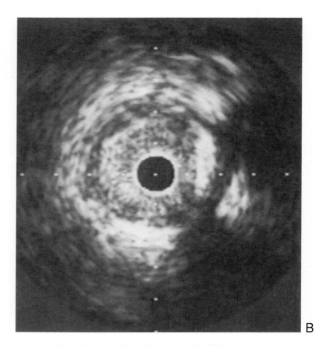

Fig. 5-11. Coronary lesion preatherectomy in which plaque distribution by ultrasound differs greatly from angiography. **(A)** The angiogram shows a highly eccentric atheroma, while **(B)** the ultrasound demonstrates that plaque is actually distributed concentrically.

of the location and extent of calcification enables differentiation of lesions most suitable for rotablation from vessels more appropriate for directional atherectomy.[25,26] Furthermore, the precise vessel-sizing provided by ultrasound facilitates selection of the appropriately sized burr for rotational ablation. Intravascular ultrasound following each pass of the device can readily quantitate the size of the neolumen and characterize the morphology of the remaining atherosclerotic plaque. The operator can subsequently select the optimal technique and size of device used for further luminal enlargement. If little or no calcium remains following rotablation, directional atherectomy may be feasible. Conversely, the presence of extensive calcification will require the use of a larger Rotablator burr or adjunctive balloon angioplasty.

Ultrasound Guidance of Stent Placement

The importance of coronary stenting has increased following publication of data demonstrating a reduction in the risk of restenosis with this therapy. However, studies have shown an increased risk of hemorrhagic complications following coronary stenting secondary to the aggressive anticoagulation and large sheath sizes required by most devices. Recent

intravascular ultrasound studies have demonstrated failure to fully deploy coronary stents in a significant subset of patients in which the procedure was guided solely by angiography (Fig. 5-12). Presumably, the porous nature of these stents results in the angio-

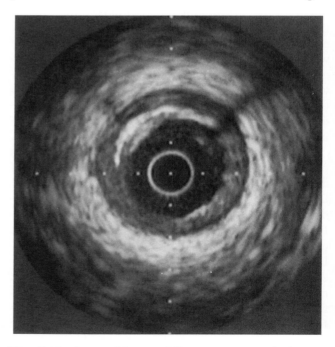

Fig. 5-12. A round lumen following rotational ablation (Rotablator).

graphic appearance of an enlarged lumen, even when some stent struts are not fully apposed to the vessel wall. Some investigators have proposed that routine application of intravascular ultrasound to determine the adequacy of stent deployment could improve clinical outcome and reduce anticoagulation requirements. Employing ultrasound to assist stent deployment, a preliminary report from a single European center has reported a low stent thrombosis rate without vigorous anticoagulation. However, widespread application of this approach will require careful testing through prospective randomized trials.

New Coronary Ultrasound Devices

Important technical advances in intravascular imaging technology will emerge during the next few years. Industry engineers anticipate further reductions in the size of imaging catheters and a guidewire-sized device (less than 0.025 in.) has already begun animal testing. This guidewire-sized ultrasound probe would enable simultaneous imaging during many revascularization procedures, regardless of the device. Very small devices would also enable imaging of virtually any coronary stenosis prior to treatment. Several investigators have demonstrated three-dimensional reconstruction of cross-sectional ultrasound images, but artifacts and other limitations have pre-

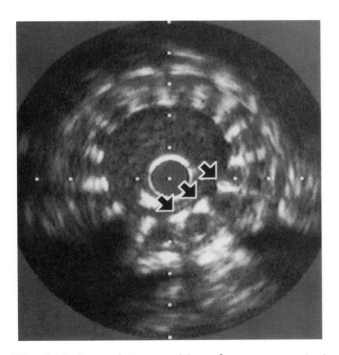

Fig. 5-13. Incomplete apposition of a coronary stent; showing three struts that are not completely expanded, (*arrows*).

cluded any practical application of this technique. Several industry and academic centers are jointly developing combination devices incorporating both diagnostic ultrasound imaging and therapeutic capability.

SUMMARY

Recent advances in microelectronic and piezoelectric technology have permitted development of miniaturized ultrasound devices capable of real-time tomographic intravascular imaging. Initial studies have successfully employed intravascular ultrasound to augment angiography in both diagnostic and therapeutic catheterization. The cross-sectional perspective of intravascular ultrasound appears ideally suited for precision measurements of luminal diameter and cross-sectional area. In addition, ultrasound improves assessment of problem lesions such as ostial stenoses or disease at bifurcations. Intravascular imaging provides unique, detailed cross-sectional images of the arterial wall not previously obtainable in vivo by any other technique and is more sensitive than angiography in the detection of atherosclerosis. Intravascular ultrasound images of atherosclerotic wall abnormalities have the potential to greatly augment the understanding of the anatomy and pathophysiology of coronary disease.

For interventional applications, ultrasound analysis of lesion characteristics offers many potential advantages. Evaluation of the "normal" reference segment used for device-sizing constitutes an important emerging application for intravascular imaging. After the procedure, intravascular ultrasound imaging often yields smaller luminal size measurements than angiography and greater stenosis severity. These differences likely reflect augmentation of the "apparent" angiographic diameter by extraluminal contrast within cracks, fissures, or dissection planes. New ultrasound instruments under development combine an imaging transducer with an interventional device, permitting on-line guidance during the procedure. Although the clinical value of routine ultrasound imaging following mechanical revascularization has not been tested by randomized trials., it seems likely that this new imaging modality will provide valuable insights into diverse phenomena such as abrupt occlusion and restenosis.

REFERENCES

1. Bom N, Lancee CT, Van Egmond FC. An ultrasonic intracardiac scanner. Ultrasonics 1972;10:72–76
2. Yock PG, Johnson EL, Linker DT. Intravascular ultra-

sound: development and clinical potential. Am J Card Imag 1988;2:185–193

3. Nissen SE, Grines CL, Gurley JC et al. Application of a new phased-array ultrasound imaging catheter in the assessment of vascular dimensions: in vivo comparison to cineangiography. Circulation 1990;81:660–666

4. Hodgson J, Graham SP, Savakus AD et al. Clinical percutaneous imaging of coronary anatomy using an over-the-wire ultrasound catheter system. Int J Card Imaging 1989;4:187–193

5. Tobis JM, Mallery J, Mahon D et al. Intravascular ultrasound imaging of human coronary arteries in vivo: analysis of tissue characterizations with comparison to in vitro histological specimens. Circulation 1991;83:913–926

6. Nissen SE, Gurley JC, Grines CL et al. Intravascular ultrasound assessment of lumen size and wall morphology in normal subjects and coronary artery disease patients. Circulation 1991;84:1087–1099

7. Pandian NG, Kreis A, Brockway B et al. Ultrasound angioscopy: real-time, two-dimensional, intraluminal ultrasound imaging of blood vessels. Am J Cardiol 1988;62:113–116

8. Zir LM, Miller SW, Dinsmore RE et al. Interobserver variability in coronary angiography. Circulation 1976;53:627–632

9. Roberts WC, Jones AA. Quantitation of coronary arterial narrowing at necropsy in sudden coronary death. Am J Cardiol 1979;44:39–44

10. Vlodaver Z, Frech R, van Tassel RA, Edwards JE. Correlation of the antemortem coronary angiogram and the postmortem specimen. Circulation 1973;47:162–168

11. White CW, Wright CB, Doty DB et al. Does visual interpretation of the coronary arteriogram predict the physiologic importance of a coronary stenosis? N Engl J Med 1984;310:819–824

12. Waller BF. "Crackers, breakers, stretchers, drillers, scrapers, shavers, burners, welders, and melters": the future treatment of atherosclerotic coronary artery disease? a clinical-morphologic assessment. J Am Coll Cardiol 1989;13:969–987

13. Cacchione JG, Reddy K, Richards F et al. Combined intravascular ultrasound/angioplasty balloon catheter: initial use during PTCA. Cathet Cardiovasc Diagn 1991;24:99–101

14. Pinto FJ, St. Goar FG, Gao SZ et al. Immediate and one-year safety of intracoronary ultrasonic imaging: evaluation with serial quantitative angiography. Circulation 1993;88:1709–1714

15. St. Goar FG, Pinto FJ, Alderman EL et al. Detection of coronary atherosclerosis in young adult hearts using intravascular ultrasound, Circulation 1992;86:756–763

16. Fitzgerald PJ, St. Goar FG, Connolly AJ et al. Intravascular ultrasound imaging of coronary arteries: is three layers the norm? Circulation 1992;86:154–158

17. Hermiller JB, Buller CE, Tenaglia AN et al. Unrecognized left main coronary artery disease in patients undergoing interventional procedures. Am J Cardiol 1993;71:173–176

18. White CJ, Ramee SR, Collin TJ et al. Ambiguous coronary angiography: clinical utility of intravascular ultrasound. Cathet Cardiovasc Diagn 1992;26:200–203

19. Tuzcu EM, Hobbs RE, Rincon G et al. Occult and frequent transmission of atherosclerotic coronary disease with cardiac transplantation. Insights from intravascular ultrasound. Circulation 1995;91:1706–1713

20. Glagov S, Weisenberg E, Zarins CK et al: Compensatory enlargement of human coronary arteries. N Engl J Med 1987;316:1371–1375

21. Nissen SE, De Franco AC, Raymond RE et al. Angiographically unrecognized disease at "normal" reference sites: a risk factor for sub-optimal results after coronary interventions. Circulation 1993;88I:412A

22. Nissen SE, Tuzcu EM, De Dranco AC et al. Intravascular ultrasound evidence of atherosclerosis at normal reference sites predicts adverse clinical outcomes following mechanical coronary interventions. J Am Coll Cardiol 1995

23. Suarez de Lezo J, Romero M, Medina A et al: Intracoronary ultrasound assessment of directional coronary atherectomy: immediate and follow-up findings. J Am Coll Cardiol 1993;21:298–307

24. Tenaglia AN, Buller CE, Kisslo KB et al. Mechanisms of balloon angioplasty and directional coronary atherectomy as assessed by intracoronary ultrasound. J Am Coll Cardiol 1992;20:685–691

25. Kovach JA, Mintz GS, Pichard AD et al. Sequential intravascular ultrasound characterization of the mechanism of rotational atherectomy and adjunct balloon angioplasty. J Am Coll Cardiol 1993;22:1024–1032

26. Mintz GS, Potkin BN, Keren G et al. Intravascular ultrasound evaluation of the effect of rotational atherectomy in obstructive atherosclerotic coronary artery disease. Circulation 1992;86:1383–1393

6 Angioscopy: Introduction

James S. Forrester
Neal Eigler
Frank Litvack

Angioscopy, the use of flexible small-diameter fiberoptics to visualize the surface and lumen of blood vessels, began in the mid-1980s when Spears and colleagues[1] and Litvack and colleagues[2] reported the use of 3.3- to 1.8-mm diameter endoscopes in blood vessels. All early angioscopic studies were performed during surgery.

In the last five years, major improvements in technology have made it possible to perform percutaneous coronary and peripheral angioscopy. The unique value of angioscopy is that we can examine the vascular surface directly during surgery or angioplasty. The vascular surgeon can inspect anastomoses or determine the completeness of thrombectomy. The interventional cardiologist can determine the etiology of unstable coronary chest pain syndromes, the trauma created by angioplasty, the appropriateness of stent placement and the completeness of thrombolysis. Despite the unique information provided by coronary angioscopy, the method probably will not evolve into routine use during coronary angiography or angioplasty because patient care decisions are only infrequently contingent on such information. On the other hand, angioscopy is, and will remain, a superb tool for clinical vascular research and for specific clinical applications in peripheral vascular surgery.

RECENT ADVANCES IN FIBEROPTIC TECHNOLOGY

The central challenges in fiberoptic technology have been flexibility, miniaturization, and guidance (Table 6-1).[3-5] The first two problems are intrinsic to the structure of angioscopes. Each fiber in a fiberoptic bundle is composed of two glass materials: an inner core that conveys light, and a surrounding cladding that traps the light within the inner core. When the ratio between the refractive indices of the core and cladding material is appropriately chosen, light is completely reflected within the core, resulting in transmission of light around bends with minimal loss of intensity. Individual fibers are assembled into a bundle, such that each fiber forms one pixel of the intravascular image. A lens attached to the distal end of the bundle focuses the output, which is transmitted to a television monitor and videotape recorder.

In one form of fiberoptic technology, all the fibers are fused throughout the length of the angioscope, resulting in a device that is relatively stiff, and less practical for cardiovascular application. One way to increase flexibility is to decrease the total diameter (Table 6-2). A fused imaging bundle becomes flexible when angioscope diameter is less than 0.5 mm. This

In principle, angioscopy can be used to assess the magnitude of diameter stenosis.[12-14] Spears and coworkers[12] used a transverse circle of light emitted from a guideline passed a known distance beyond the

angiography , and frequency of angioscopically detected dissection (77%) greatly exceeded that of angiography (29%). In the largest series yet reported, Mizuno and associates[18] compared coronary angioscopy

Table 6-1. Synopsis of the Major Technical Problems of Commercially

in some devices by use of a wide-angle 90-degree lens with a focal length as short as 0.5 mm.

Guidance refers to steering the angioscope through tortuous vessels, and to central alignment of the lens

siderations when choosing a recorder: quality, durability, and frame accuracy. Quality can be measured by the number of horizontal lines recorded. Durability is a function of the tape width; wider tapes are more durable. Frame accuracy requires the presence of *time code*. If at all possible a video recorder that accepts a Y/C video signal should be used.

Image Quality

When evaluating an angioscopic imaging system it is important to remember that the quality of the video imaging is determined by signal loss. The best possible image a video system can deliver is directly related to the worst individual component within the system. With catheter size constraints that limit a fiberoptic bundle's imaging capabilities, angioscopic imaging magnifies the total image loss. It is regrettable that the digital recording revolution that has transformed the catheterization laboratory is currently too expensive for angioscopic use.

By its very nature video is an imaging system based on motion; electronically capturing a series of moments on magnetic tape. When these moments are shown sequentially at high speed, the human eye sees a motion picture. What goes unnoticed is that each single frame is of relatively low resolution. For example, photographic film recording exposes thousands of silver grains per inch whereas a video signal records only 72 dots per inch. These resolution limitations of video play an important part in the selection of computer imaging equipment.

Digital technology provides a set of tools for image manipulation that improve image content. As the personal computer has become increasingly powerful, imaging software that was only available on expensive workstations is now available for the desktop computer. It is important to choose a software package designed specifically for image *retouching* rather than software designed for graphic artists.

Acquiring the desired image from video tape requires the use of a video capture card. Our experience has been that the capability of a video card to capture a sequence of frames is an important feature. A single frame of a video image passes by in 1/30 second. Capturing a sequence of frames, bracketing the desired frame, reduces the amount of time spent attempting to capture a specific frame. Computer capture cards rely upon a synchronization signal that is recorded on the control track of the videotape. Unfortunately, a video deck in the "pause" mode does not provide the necessary synchronization signal, so images must be captured "on the fly."

Video capture yields a low-resolution picture measuring 640 by 480 pixels on the computer screen. Even worse, the angioscopic image takes up only a small portion of this space. The expensive video capture cards offer little to improve resolution; however they do provide increased control over the color information.

Hard Copy Output

Composing pre- and postangiographic and angioscopic images into one image yields an image suitable for publication. Color printing technology for computers is an ever-hanging world. To optimize the quality of the print, a continuous tone color printer that prints images on glossy photographic stock paper should be used. Kodak has been one of the leaders in the field of digital imaging, and their printers are some of the best. There are a number of impressive technologies employed in color printers, including ink jet, dye sublimation, and thermal wax transfer.

The latest imaging equipment for personal computers are the desktop video cards. They support either Microsoft's Audio Video Interface (AVI) or Apple's QuickTime systems. Desktop video cards record both video and audio information directly onto the hard disk of the computer. Although it remains to be seen which of these competing systems will ultimately prevail, it is a virtual certainty that desktop video will grow in acceptance and may replace the video recording device currently used in angioscopy. The reasons for this are clear, easy, transmission, random access, digital clarity, and multiuser access. Multimedia software is now the forefront in the software battles taking place in the computer community.

Given the pace of change in personal computers, traditional video editing suites will be replaced by the personal computer in a very short while. Although a frame accurate recording deck is not imperative today, future imaging computers will require frame accuracy. The gold standard is SMPTE time code, which uses videotapes that have a prerecorded frame number that occupy either an audio channel or are part of the video control track.

ANGIOSCOPE DELIVERY CATHETER

The development of the percutaneous coronary angioscope required solving several major obstacles not encountered by the initial investigators who performed intraoperative angioscopy. The ideal coronary angioscope must be thin, and flexible with high-resolution optics for reliable imaging. Unlike the early intraoperative devices, percutaneous angioscopes must also be able to maintain a blood-free field, be steerable, and give the operator control over his field of view.

Blood-Free Field

Coronary angioscopy was first performed in surgical patients in whom a blood-free field could be easily maintained in the arrested heart during cardiopulmonary bypass.[1] Maintaining a blood-free field in the beating heart requires occlusion of antegrade arterial flow and perfusion of the viewing field with a crystalloid solution without causing trauma, arrhythmias, or persistent ischemia.

There are two basic methods of creating a blood-free field of view within the coronary artery for the angioscope. The first involves "wedging" the guiding catheter in the coronary ostium to occlude native blood flow and flushing an optically clear solution through the guiding catheter to clear the artery of blood. This method is effective but has the disadvantage of potentially causing dangerous trauma to the coronary artery and also renders the entire distribution of that coronary artery ischemic during viewing.

The second method employs a soft, atraumatic, balloon on the distal tip of the angioscope that can be inflated when imaging is desired and deflated to allow coronary blood flow to resume. When the occlusion balloon is inflated small amounts of optically clear flush solution can be delivered through the distal tip of the angioscope to displace a small amount of blood. The advantages of this system are that it restricts the ischemic territory to that portion of the myocardium distal to the occlusion balloon, smaller volumes of flush solution are necessary to clear the imaging field of blood, and the balloon may also help to center the angioscope within the coronary lumen. The disadvantages of the distal occlusion balloon, include the requirement for a lumen within the angioscope to inflate and deflate the balloon, which adds to the total diameter of the catheter, and there is the potential for local arterial trauma as a result of the balloon inflation.

Steerability

The ability to navigate the angioscope through the coronary vasculature to the target area without damaging the delicate intimal surface has been a more difficult task. The development of thinner, more flexible fiberoptic bundles incorporated into catheters that track over steerable guidewires (analogous to PTCA systems) has enabled operators to select any major coronary vessel for viewing.

Once the angioscope is in position for viewing it is desirable to have a mechanism of deflecting or centering the tip of the scope to allow circumferential viewing of the lumen of the artery. A distal balloon may be attached to the angioscope, which, when inflated, helps to bring the imaging element of the angioscope away from the wall of the artery, but this alone is not sufficient to allow the operator to control the alignment to circumferentially image the lumen of the artery.

More precise control over the orientation of the distal tip of the angioscope can be achieved in two ways. The first is by embedding two wires along the length of the angioscope catheter and attaching them to the distal end of the scope. By shortening one of the

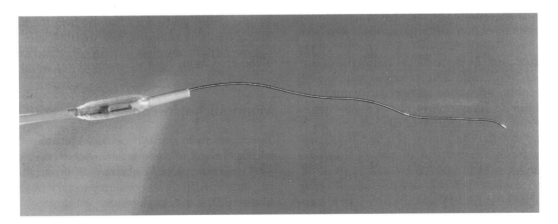

Fig. 7-2. Angioscope guidewire (Microvision System, Advanced Cardiovascular Systems, Santa Clara, CA). The sinusoidal curves of the wire passively deflect the tip of angioscope. By advancing the scope over the curves and rotating the tip of the wire, the scope can be directed in a multitude of directions.

ous coronary angioscopy in patients with restenosis after coronary angioplasty. J Am Coll Cardiol 1991; 17:46B–49B(abst)

13. White CJ, Ramee SR, Collins TJ, et al. Percutaneous angioscopy of saphenous vein coronary bypass grafts. J Am Coll Cardiol 1993;21:1181–1185

14. Hoeher M, Hombach V, Hoepp H, et al. Percutaneous coronary angioscopy during cardiac catheterization. J Am Coll Cardiol 1988;2(Suppl A):65A(abst)

15. Mizuno K, Arakawa K, Shibuya T, et al. A serial observation of coronary thrombosis in vivo by a new angioscope. J Am Coll Cardiol 1988;2(Suppl A):30A(abst)

8 Angioscopy: Comparison With Intravascular Ultrasound

Berthold Höfling
Tanya Y. Huehns

Angiography can define coronary artery anatomy when the lumina of arteries are injected with contrast medium; lesion presence is ascertained by the irregularities on the wall surface. In a crude manner, angiographic fluoroscopy can also show if there is calcification in the wall. It is well recognized that this form of imaging has several limitations. First, angiography images the coronary arteries one plane at a time, although pictures can be taken at several angles to extend its usefulness. However, these multiple views give a variable representation of what is happening in any arterial segment because of foreshortening and overlapping of branches. Second, pathologic studies of arteries have shown that coronary angiography may be misleading because the lumen picture gives no indication of disease in the wall. Arterial segments that appear to be normal at angiography can actually have extensive atherosclerosis, which is often seen at postmortem examination. Compensatory enlargement by the vessel with increasing deposition of atheroma allows the lumen to appear unobstructed until it is more than 40% narrowed.[1] Third, in some instances angiographic imaging is not able to distinguish plaque from thrombus or dissection. After intracoronary intervention, despite the use of multiple views, the vessel is often hazy, which makes it difficult to establish whether a flap or thrombus is present.

Certain of the limitations of angiography can now be resolved to some extent with angioscopy, which increases information about the lumen, and intravascular ultrasound imaging, which gives an additional picture of the wall layers. These imaging modalities provide data on the pathogenesis of coronary artery disease and aid operators in decision-making at intervention. Experience with both these methods is accumulating.

EQUIPMENT

Angioscopy allows an operator to visualize the inside of a vessel. The first studies in humans with coronary artery disease were reported ten years ago.[2] The technique involves the cannulation of arteries with a fine, flexible, steerable catheter containing bundled optic fibers that illuminate the lumen (Fig. 8-1). The proximal end of the catheter has a radiopaque marker so that it can be visualized in the artery at fluoroscopy. Systems are designed to be compatible with standard guiding catheters and wires. To obtain a detailed picture, a compliant balloon that temporarily interrupts blood flow when inflated is incorporated in the system (Fig. 8-2). Concurrent with inflation at this point in the procedure, perfusion through a standard power injector with saline or other transparent solution clears the view, and three-dimensional color images of the surface characteristics of the interior of a vessel can be viewed through an eyepiece or on a monitor. The operator can simultaneously record a commentary at the same time that the images are preserved on videotape. Once the balloon is inflated, the angioscope can pass forward through the artery to view the 5-cm segment distal to the balloon. A pass such as this takes 30 to 40 seconds.

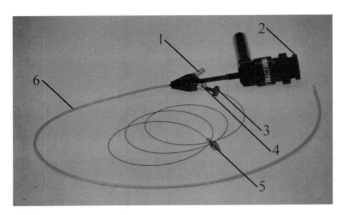

Fig. 8-1. Equipment for angioscopy: *1,* flush port; *2,* viewing lens; *3,* valve for introduction of wire; *4,* light source port; *5,* external connection to light source; *6,* angioscope.

Another imaging technique, intracoronary ultrasound, incorporates a high-frequency (30 to 40 Hz) miniature ultrasound transducer in the tip of an intracoronary catheter, which is introduced into a vessel over the guidewire. The vessel is viewed perpendicular to the catheter axis, creating a cross-sectional image with the potential to accurately define both arterial wall and plaque morphology. Rather than simply exhibiting a shadowgram of the vascular lumen or a picture of the inner arterial surface, intravascular ultrasound provides an insight into various components of the vessel wall. The three arterial wall layers of intima, media, and adventitia are acoustically distinctive, and detailed analysis of plaque, including extent, composition, and morphology, is also possible as a result of varying backscatter power.[3,4]

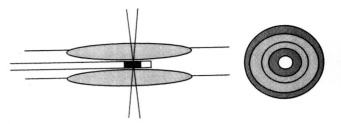

Fig. 8-3. Proximal end of ultrasound catheter in plaque-filled artery, with concentric layers as would be visualized (*right*).

Characteristic ultrasound images of arteries show a central echo-free lumen surrounded by concentric rings of variable density representing the arterial wall layers (Fig. 8-3). With both angioscopy and intravascular ultrasound imaging pictures are displayed on an external monitor and can be recorded.

CLINICAL USES

Angioscopic and Ultrasonic Assessment of Wall and Plaque Components

Although contrast angiography provides a standard imaging method for the entire coronary artery tree, it only outlines the lumen and any irregularities. Both angioscopy and intravascular ultrasound imaging have several advantages in that they are able to distinguish normal arterial wall from stable atheroma, disrupted atheroma, or thrombus.[5]

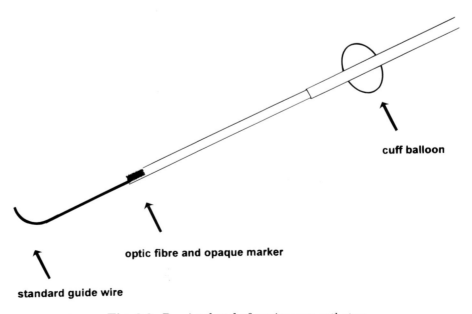

cuff balloon

optic fibre and opaque marker

standard guide wire

Fig. 8-2. Proximal end of angioscopy catheter.

Histologic validation demonstrates that both modalities are relatively accurate in distinguishing atheroma from normal vessel segments. The color and surface characteristics of a plaque seen angioscopically correlate with clinical presentation.[6] Plaques seen in patients with stable angina tend to look white or yellow while those related to unstable angina are usually yellow and ulcerated, with thrombus (Plate 8-1).[7] This agrees with previous angiographic work in which complex irregular lesion morphology was

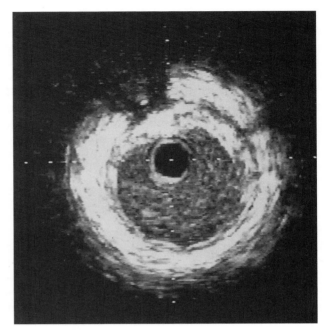

Fig. 8-5. Concentric plaque with calcium seen as a shadow (*top left*) at intravascular ultrasound.

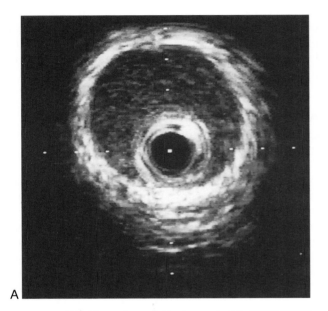

A

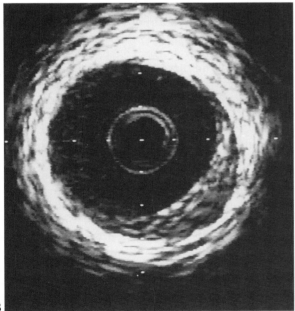

B

Fig. 8-4. (A) Normal artery as seen at intravascular ultrasound. **(B)** Eccentric plaque (*bottom right*) in an artery as seen at intravascular ultrasound.

more commonly found in patients with unstable symptoms.[8] Intravascular ultrasound imaging identifies the amount of atheroma by the increased wall thickness measured (Fig. 8-4). Predominantly lipid-filled plaques, which are dangerous and prone to rupture, but may respond to lifestyle change (for example, cholesterol modification), look echolucent; those that are fibrous result in denser reflections, and calcium deposition within the plaque can be identified by the bright echoes that shadow the image (Fig. 8-5).[9] Extensive calcified plaques are less easily treated with angioplasty or atherectomy. The sensitivity of ultrasound in detecting calcium deposits in plaques may be clinically relevant in predicting tears at angioplasty; in addition, a larger amount of calcified plaque leads to more extensive dissection at intervention, with the possibility of acute closure. Tears themselves can be imaged and usually are seen as separation of plaque from the medial layer.

All intraluminal filling defects suggesting the presence of thrombus by the relatively crude method of angiography can be confirmed by angioscopy to be thrombus. However, much thrombus occurs in angiographically unremarkable vessels[10]; as well as confirming the existence of thrombus, angioscopy also enables the clinician to estimate its components and age. Angioscopically, thrombus can appear red or white: Red indicates that it contains an abundance of fibrin, with coagulated red blood cells and platelets; by contrast, white or grayish thrombus appears to be made up mainly of platelet aggregations.[11] Knowledge of these appearances may be used to decide appropriate further management, including selection of the most relevant device for intervention. A large amount of thrombus suggests that intracoronary thrombolysis will be the most useful course of action.[12] In comparison with angioscopy, ultrasound imaging is poorer at detecting thrombus,[5] as both thrombus and soft atheroma have similar acoustic characteristics, and it is therefore difficult to discriminate plaque from plaque with superimposed thrombus.[3]

Angioscopy and Intravascular Ultrasound Imaging at Angiography

Both angioscopy and ultrasound imaging can add essential information when coronary angiography appears relatively normal. This may be important in the subgroup of patients who are investigated after an acute event, suggesting either coronary thrombosis that has been thrombolyzed or a resolved episode of unstable angina, and yet the coronary arteries appear undiseased at angiography. In such patients, establishing a probable coronary cause for their symptoms will direct further management, especially concerning lifestyle and secondary prevention. Angioscopy is more sensitive than angiography and intravascular ultrasound imaging at detecting thrombi and small frondlike dissections,[3] which may aid in diagnosis if the primary problem was thrombotic; however, intravascular ultrasound can demonstrate diffuse disease in arteries that have a smooth outline at angiography because of compensatory enlargement.[1]

Although quantitative computerized angiography is the current gold standard in measuring arteries and their stenoses,[13] this method relies on catheter size to calibrate subsequent arterial measurements and thus is subject to certain errors. The catheter may be some distance from the vessel segment being analyzed and perhaps also at an angle relative to the plane in which the vessel is traveling. With intravascular ultrasound imaging, calibration takes place where the segment is, making on-line arterial diameter measurement more accurate, which is important in selecting an appropriately sized intervention device. Left main stem disease is notoriously difficult to assess accurately at angiography, and the use of quantitative algorithms is not possible because of difficulty in ascertaining reference diameter; intravascular ultrasound imaging may be able to provide more detailed information.

Total occlusions can be visualized with angioscopy because it permits the clinician to look ahead along the vessel, but this cannot be done with conventional intravascular ultrasound. In occluded peripheral arteries, the angioscopy catheter can also be used to push aside occluding plaque.[14] In one study, advancement of the angioscope further through several long occlusions revealed multiple segmental stenoses separated by relatively normal arterial wall.[15] In the presence of tortuous vessels with bends, branching, or overlap, the accuracy of angiography, even with multiple views, is compromised, and intravascular ultrasound imaging has particular value in visualizing lesions. In a similar fashion, angioscopy and ultrasound imaging are able to distinguish particularly eccentric plaques and thus enable the operator to select an appropriate device for intervention.

Angioscopy and Intravascular Ultrasound Imaging During Angioplasty

Preprocedural vessel wall and plaque characteristics identified by angioscopy or intravascular ultrasound imaging will help in the decision as to which intervention is the most appropriate. After a recent acute myocardial infarction, angioscopy may play a particular role in the assessment of whether a severe residual culprit lesion is atherosclerotic or whether it is minimal underlying plaque with superimposed thrombus. Knowledge of the thrombus may enable the operator to decide on the best subsequent intervention. In addition, if any thrombus is initially present, the operator should be especially alert to acute closure after intervention.[10]

Angioscopy and intravascular ultrasound imaging complement angiography in the assessment after angioplasty—in understanding the mechanism of action, and in directing further intervention. After angioplasty, mere assessment of the lumen created with angiography is relatively limited information; more useful would be an awareness of the morphologic changes occurring, for example, the amount of damage created or where dissections and wall stretching are taking place. From angioscopy studies, it appears that thrombus is not removed or dislodged during an angioplasty procedure, especially when the thrombus looks old and is white.[16] Angioplasty appears to distend the segment both transaxially and longitudinally,[17] and small flaps are commonly present after the procedure.[16] The hazy appearance common after dilatation is now attributed to dissection, rather than to thrombus as previously thought. Angioscopy can, however, miss obvious flaps seen at angiography; thus the two techniques are complementary in this situation.[10] Subintimal hemorrhage, as well as dissection, can be seen by angioscopy after angioplasty, although the clinical significance of this is not yet clear.

Both angioscopy and intravascular ultrasound imaging help to optimize the acute end result after intervention with the ultimate aim of improving long-term outcome. When acute occlusion occurs after angioplasty, it is vital to be able to distinguish thrombus from dissection, and here angioscopy is especially helpful.[10] By contrast, intravascular ultrasound produces full-thickness pictures of the wall that add a different complementary perspective to angioplasty and allow the selection of further intervention to be based on objective evidence of events occurring in the wall. Most hemodynamically and angiographically successful angioplasty procedures are associated with plaque fracture and dissection[18]; intimal flaps appear as discrete reflective protrusions into the echolucent lumen.[19] Ultrasound imaging is better than angioscopy at delineating the extent and depth of dissection.[3] It has been demonstrated that tears tend to occur longitudinally at the thinnest part of a plaque,[20] at the junction between calcific and softer tissue.[21] These tears explain most of the increase in lumen gained at angioplasty, in contrast to previously held beliefs that stretching of the artery accounts for this enlargement. In addition, there is plaque compression, with some reduction in plaque area although this makes a smaller contribution to lumen area increase.[22] From studies of ultrasound

imaging, restenosis has been shown to be particularly associated with a concentric result immediately after angioplasty.[23] Combined imaging and balloon catheters are undergoing clinical trials: the ultrasound transducer is mounted behind the balloon to preserve lesion-crossing profile. On-line monitoring of balloon angioplasty identifies the start of plaque fracture, further studies are needed to assess the significance of acquiring this knowledge. Intravascular ultrasound imaging has also been used instead of angiography to guide angioplasty; this could be useful, for example, where contrast medium carries a risk of renal failure.[24]

Thus, after angioplasty, angioscopy or intravascular ultrasound imaging can identify a poor lumen increase or delineate dissections or flaps not seen at angiography. Identification of the extent of a larger dissection directs therapeutic intervention appropriately. If further angioplasty or stenting is to be carried out, these imaging techniques are beneficial in ensuring that the flap is fully plastered to the wall.

Angioscopy and Intravascular Ultrasound Imaging During Other Interventions

Angioscopy and intravascular ultrasound imaging can both be used to compare the ways in which newer interventions create a larger lumen after the procedure. Adjunctive angioscopy has been evaluated in

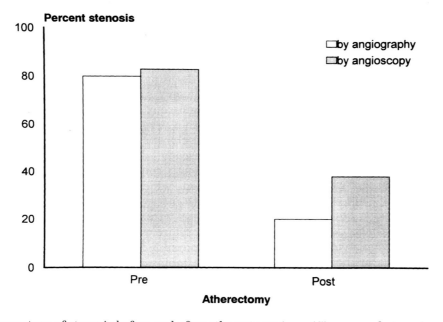

Fig. 8-6. Percentage of stenosis before and after atherectomy ($n = 15$), assessed at angiography and at angioscopy.

THE DOPPLER PRINCIPLE OF FLOW VELOCITY

A sound source moving toward a stationary point will be transmitted with higher frequency than at rest and similarly with lower frequency when moving

nearly parallel to blood flow, with φ near zero (cosine φ) to measure maximum velocity. With continuous sinusoidal ultrasound waves (continuous-wave Doppler), all the flow velocities encountered by the exploring ultrasound beam will be reflected and measured. In contrast, a pulsed-wave emitter permits determination of both magnitude and direction of the

procedure is prolonged or for certain patients; this is more of a potential problem in endoscopy of large peripheral vessels.[33] Ultrasound has the practical

CONCLUSION

Angioscopy and intravascular ultrasound imaging

Table 9-1. Clinical Applications of Intracoronary Doppler Guidewire Flow Velocity

Applications	Reference
Angioplasty	
Endpoint	Ofili et al.,[2,4] Segal,[3] Kern et al.[5]
Monitoring complications	Kern et al.,[6] Eichhorn et al.,[7] Anderson et al.,[8]
Assessing additional lesions	Donohue et al.,[9] Kern et al.[10]
Collateral flow	
Stent	Ofili et al.[11] Donohue et al.,[12] Kern et al.[13]
Atherectomy	Younis et al.,[14] Bach et al.,[15] Kern et al.[16]
Laser	Segal,[3] Deychak et al.[17]
Intermediate coronary lesion assessment	Segal[3]
Coronary vasodilatory reserve	Donohue et al.,[9,18] Kern et al.,[19] DiMario et al.[20]
Syndrome X	Wilson,[21] Wilson et al.,[22] McGinn et al.[23]
Transplant coronary arteriopathy	Treasure et al.[24]
Coronary physiology research	
Pharmacologic studies	
Intraaortic balloon pumping	Kern et al.[16]
Perfusion imaging correlation	Donohue et al.[9]
Saphenous vein graft, internal mammary artery flow characteristics	Bach et al.[25]
Endothelial function	Treasure et al.[24]

flow velocity at a predetermined distance (range) from the transducer. Doppler flow velocity measures the velocity of red blood cells, allowing a continuous assessment of flow without requiring flow marker substances to be introduced. There is a direct relationship between velocity and volumetric flow, where volumetric blood flow (cm³/s) = vessel cross-sectional area (cm²) × mean flow velocity (cm/s). Changes in coronary flow velocities can be used to represent changes in absolute coronary flow when the vessel cross-sectional area remains constant.

Intracoronary Doppler velocity measurements have limitations. Flow velocity data may be affected by coronary stenosis geometry, intracoronary veloc-

ity profile,[26] the angle between the piezoelectric crystal and the main stream of the blood,[27] and a limited sample volume.[28] These limitations have been partially overcome by spectral signal analysis of the Doppler guidewire instrumentation.

CHARACTERISTICS OF THE DOPPLER ANGIOPLASTY GUIDEWIRE AND VELOCITY SYSTEM

Subselective 3 F Doppler catheters have been proposed for assessing the hemodynamic significance of coronary lesions and interventions, but have not been incorporated into routine practice because of the large catheter size, measurements limited to velocity proximal to a lesion, the necessity to exchange the catheter for the interventional device, and difficulty in ascertaining optimal signals with the zero cross technique.[21,29–31]

The Doppler angioplasty guidewire (FloWire, Cardiometrics, Inc., Mountain View, CA) is a 175-cm long, 0.014- to 0.018-in. diameter flexible steerable angioplasty-style guidewire with a 12-MHz piezoelectric ultrasound transducer integrated into the tip, which sends and receives the emitted ultrasound waves (Fig. 9-2). As described and validated by Doucette and colleagues,[32] the forward-directed ultrasound beam diverges in a 27-degree arc from the long axis (measured to the 6-dB roundtrip points of the ultrasound beam pattern) (Fig. 9-3). The pulse

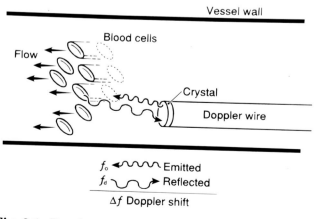

Fig. 9-1. Doppler principle measures velocity of moving red cells by the change between the emitted ultrasound frequency (f_o) and the reflected frequency (f_d).

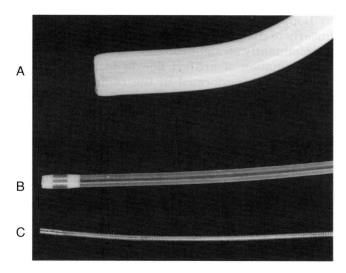

Fig. 9-2. **(A)** 8 F angiographic catheter. **(B)** 2.2 F tracking (Tracker, Target Therapeutics) pressure catheter; **(C)** 0.01-in. FloWire (Cardiometrics, Inc., Mountain View, CA).

repetition frequency of more than, 40 kHz, pulse duration of + 0.83 ms, and sampling delay of 6.5 ms is standard for clinical usage. The system is coupled to a real-time spectrum analyzer, videocassette recorder, and video page printer. The quadrature/ Doppler audio signals are processed by the spectrum analyzer using on-line fast Fourier transformation. The frequency response of the system calculates approximately 90 spectra per second. Blood flow velocities up to 6 m/s can be quantitated without aliasing a sample volume 5 mm (×2 mm) from the tip of the wire. The small diameter of the wire ensures that

the blood velocity is not affected by the turbulent wake of flow across the wire. Flow velocity is observed in real time by a gray scale spectral scrolling display. An automatic peak velocity tracking algorithm is provided, which yields accurate key parameters that remain relatively positionally insensitive and reliable. Simultaneous electrocardiographic and arterial pressure are also put into the video display.

Flow velocity spectra are printed on an integrated video page printer. Automatic variables of intracoronary flow velocity are peak and mean diastolic and systolic velocities, diastolic and systolic velocity integrals (total area under the peak instantaneous velocity profile). Mean velocities and the velocity integral are obtained from averaged data over two cardiac cycles (Fig. 9-3). The velocity parameters have been validated using a custom software program and manual tracing of the spectral peak Doppler velocity signal on a digital computer bit pad.[4,32,33]

Technique of Translesional Velocity Measurements

To assess a coronary lesion, the Doppler guidewire is passed through a Standard angioplasty Y-connector attached to either a diagnostic or guiding catheter. Heparin (5,000 to 10,000 units intravenously) is always administered before inserting the guidewire. The guidewire is then advanced into the artery. Baseline flow velocity data are acquired at least 1 cm proximal to the lesion in question. The wire is then advanced at least 5 to 10 artery-diameter lengths (≈ 2 cm) beyond the stenosis, avoiding placement in any side branches. At this distance, laminar flow has been reconstituted, and accurate distal velocity values can then be obtained. Diffuse disease and serial or tandem lesions will elevate distal velocity. Coronary hyperemia is induced with intracoronary adenosine (6 to 18 μg) as previously described.[22] The translesional velocity assessment requires approximately 10 minutes. In over 700 patients studied in our laboratory, no complication of this methodology has occurred.

On traversing a lesion, an intralesional high jet velocity may be observed. The jet velocity is not routinely sought because of the difficulty in obtaining a stable signal and potential for excessive lesion manipulation and activation in a critical area.

Limitations and Assumptions of Doppler Velocity for Lesion Assessment

Despite the ease of application for clinical practice, the Doppler guidewire has several limitations. Signal acquisition may be at times difficult and depen-

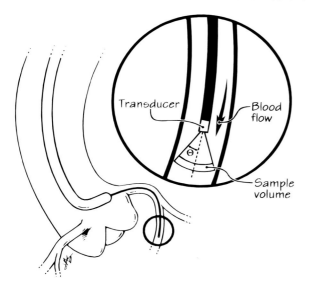

Fig. 9-3. FloWire in an angiographic diagnostic catheter. Transducer has a 27-degree beam spread from the midaxis. Sample volume is 5 mm from the tip. See text for description. (From Ofili et al.[2] with permission.)

Table 9-2. Baseline and Hyperemia Velocity Parameters in Individual Coronary Arteries

	Baseline			Hyperemia[a]		
	LAD (n = 24)	LCX (n = 19)	RCA (n = 12)	LAD	LCX	RCA
Proximal						
Peak D Vel	49 ± 20	40 ± 15	37 ± 12	104 ± 28[c]	79 ± 20	72 ± 13
Mean Vel	31 ± 15	25 ± 8	26 ± 7	66 ± 18[c]	50 ± 14	48 ± 13
D Vel Int	18 ± 11[b]	13 ± 5	11 ± 4	37 ± 55[c]	27 ± ?	22 ± 9
⅓ FF (%)	45 ± 4[b]	44 ± 5	40 ± 5	44 ± 5	43 ± 6	41 ± 4
D/S	2.0 ± 0.5[b]	1.8 ± 0.7	1.5 ± 0.5	2.0 ± 0.5	1.9 ± 0.6	1.9 ± 0.8
Distal						
Peak D Vel	35 ± 16	35 ± 8	28 ± 8	70 ± 17	71 ± 22	67 ± 16
Mean Vel	23 ± 11	21 ± 6	21 ± 9	45 ± 12	45 ± 12	42 ± 9
D Vel Int	13 ± 9	10 ± 3	8 ± 5	9 ± 6	11 ± 8	9 ± 2
⅓ FF (%)	46 ± 2	45 ± 9	39 ± 6	45 ± 3	42 ± 7	40 ± 9
D/S	2.4 ± 0.8[b]	2.1 ± 0.8	1.4 ± 0.3	2.2 ± 1.0	1.9 ± 0.8	1.6 ± 0.3

Abbreviations: LAD, left anterior descending coronary artery; LCX, left circumflex artery; RCA, right coronary artery, D, diastolic; D/S, peak diastolic/systolic velocity; D Vel Int, diastolic flow velocity integral (units); Vel, velocity (cm/s); ⅓ FF, one-third flow fraction.
ANOVA: Scheffe F test $P < .05$.
[a] All 3 coronary arteries had significantly higher absolute velocity parameters during hyperemia ($P < .001$).
[b] LAD vs RCA.
[c] LAD vs LCX and RCA.
(Modified from Ofili et al.,[4] with permission.)

at baseline or at peak hyperemia (Fig. 9-7). There were differences among the three major coronary arteries, with the diastolic velocity integral at baseline significantly higher for the proximal left anterior descending compared to the proximal right coronary artery. Furthermore, hyperemic mean velocity, peak diastolic velocity, and diastolic velocity integral were significantly higher in the proximal left anterior descending coronary artery compared to proximal left circumflex and right coronary arteries.[4] The average proximal left anterior descending and circumflex flow velocity values are approximately 30 cm/s (mean diastolic velocity). Peak diastolic velocity ranges from 40 to 80 cm/s and peak systolic velocity from 10 to 20 cm/s. Right coronary artery and distal locations may be slightly reduced (≤15%).[2]

The maintenance of proximal to distal flow velocity results from 2 anatomic features of the coronary circulation. Coronary volumetric flow is normally distributed from the proximal to distal regions of the myocardium through branches of each major artery. Coronary arteries gradually taper in diameter from the proximal to distal regions on average about 0.5 to 1 mm in diameter. Absolute volumetric flow is necessarily lower in the distal compared to proximal vessel regions. Since volumetric flow is calculated as the product of vessel cross-sectional area and velocity (mean velocity or velocity integral), flow velocity, but not volume, is maintained along the epicardial con-

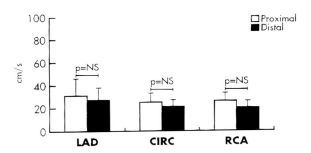

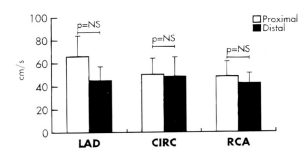

Fig. 9-7. Normal and hyperemic flows in the left anterior descending, right coronary and circumflex arteries. (From Ofili et al.,[2] with permission.)

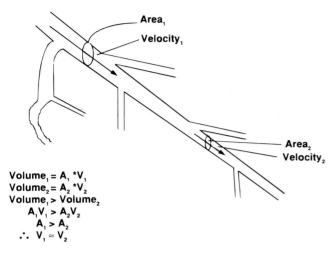

Fig. 9-8. Branching coronary artery: Volumetric flow and cross-sectional vessel area gradually diminish from proximal to distal regions resulting in normalization of flow velocity.

duit from the proximal to distal part of the large epicardial arteries (larger than 2.0 mm diameter) (Fig. 9-8). The ratio of proximal to distal flow velocity is approximately 1, while the ratio of proximal/distal flow volume is often higher than 2.

APPLICATION OF FLOW VELOCITY MEASUREMENTS IN CORONARY DISEASE

The flow velocity findings distal to severe coronary stenoses demonstrate four common findings (Fig. 9-9).[2,5,18,33]

1. Decrease in mean velocity, usually less than 20 cm/s
2. A mean proximal/distal flow velocity ratio higher than 1.7
3. An impaired diastolic/systolic phasic pattern of coronary flow
4. Impaired distal coronary hyperemia (less than 2.0 × basal values)

Normally, the diastolic component of phasic flow velocity is nearly two times the systolic component. A normal DSVR is 1.8 or more for the left coronary artery.[33] This value may vary normally among vessels, but in severe lesions, DSVR is usually less than 1.4.

Coronary Vasodilatory Reserve

Coronary vasodilatory reserve is calculated as the ratio of hyperemic/basal mean flow velocity and can be normalized for arterial pressure by dividing each flow value by the corresponding mean arterial pressure producing the reserve ratio.[27,36]

Hyperemic blood flow velocity can be induced with a variety of vasodilatory agents, such as nitroglycerin,[37] papaverine,[38] adenosine,[22,39] and contrast media.[46] Only adenosine and papaverine produce maximal hyperemia. Coronary flow reserve measurements in our laboratory are obtained by comparing baseline flow with peak flow following administration of intracoronary adenosine (6 to 8 μg in the right coronary artery and 12 to 18 μg in the left coronary artery).[22]

Proximally measured coronary flow reserve has not been accepted as a determinant of lesion significance in human because of the wide range of normal values and lack of angiographic correlations. Factors such as infarcted myocardium, hypertension, and microvascular disease impair normal hyperemia. Basal flow may be increased with tachycardia or hypertension, also reducing the coronary vasodilatory reserve ratio.[23] Coronary reserve measurements obtained only in proximal vessel locations reflect the vasodilatory capacity of the vessel in question, as well as all proximal branches. This weighted average cannot give a true reflection of stenosis severity.

Using the Doppler guidewire allows direct assessment of the coronary flow reserve distal to a stenosis. This is the most accurate assessment of any particular perfusion bed microvascular reactivity. In our laboratory, we have found that a distal coronary flow reserve of 2.0 or less has a high correlation with abnormal stress perfusion imaging.

Using the distal velocity data after angioplasty, coronary vasodilatory reserve ratios obtained with the FloWire, as in other similar studies,[36,41] were not significantly increased after angioplasty, averaging 2.3 ± 0.8 both before and after the procedure.[33]

Flow Velocity During Coronary Interventions

Balloon Angioplasty

A satisfactory angioplasty flow velocity result is demonstrated by improvement or normalization of the distal mean velocity, diastolic/systolic velocity ratio, proximal/distal flow velocity ratio, and coronary vasodilatory reserve (Fig. 9-10). After successful angioplasty, the distal mean velocity is increased (usually >20 to 30 cm/s), or at least equal to the proximal preprocedural basal flow velocity. The distal coronary flow velocity appeared to be more predictive of successful angiographic outcome of balloon angioplasty than did measurements performed proximal

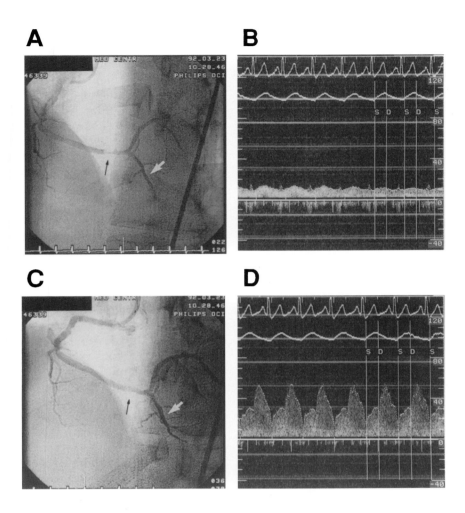

Fig. 9-9. Coronary flow velocity beyond significant stenoses. **(A)** The right coronary artery (left anterior oblique projection) shows severe narrowing (*small black arrow*) with distal velocity measured in the posterior descending branch (*white arrow*) showing **(B)** abnormal distal flow with blunted diastolic/systolic velocity ratio and low mean velocity (10 cm/s). **(C)** Post-PTCA angiogram with minimal right coronary artery (RCA) lesion (black arrow). **(D)** Normal distal RCA velocity measured at *white arrow* in (C). Phasic diastolic/systolic velocity ratio is now normal and mean velocity is increased to 30 cm/s.

to the stenosis.[33] Average peak velocity increased significantly from 19 ± 12 to 35 ± 16 cm/s ($P <$ .01) in the distal vessel following angioplasty, while changes in proximal average peak velocity were increased but to a lesser degree (preangioplasty 34 ± 18 cm/s vs postangioplasty 41 ± 14 cm/s, $P =$ .04) (Fig. 9-11).[2] Coronary flow reserve was unchanged after angioplasty whether measured in either the distal or proximal coronary artery.

In 38 patients undergoing balloon angioplasty and 12 patients without significant coronary artery disease serving as controls, velocity and diastolic/systolic velocity patterns were measured.[33] Luminal stenosis diameter was reduced from 80 ± 17% to 33 ±

23%. Flow velocity signals demonstrated a marked improvement in the diastolic/systolic average velocity ratio from 1.9 ± 0.6 to 2.8 ± 1.1, a 46% increase from preangioplasty values (normal ratios; >2.0) (Fig. 9-12). Phasic velocity patterns were noted to normalize with significant increases in diastolic/systolic flow ratios within 10 to 15 minutes following successful balloon angioplasty. When measurements were performed in the proximal vessel, phasic diastolic/systolic flow patterns were not significantly different than normal vessel (diastolic/systolic flow ratios = 1.8 ± 0.8 vs 1.8 ± 0.5, $P =$ NS), and diastolic/systolic flow ratios did not increase significantly after angioplasty was performed.

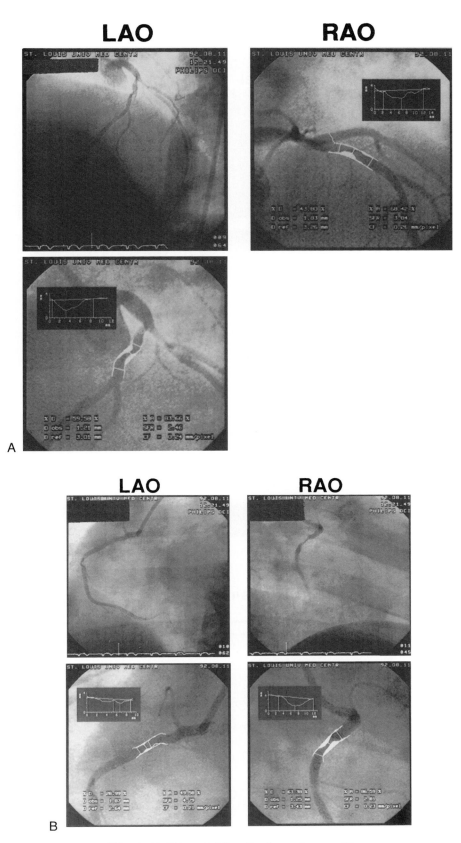

Fig. 9-10 (A) and **(B).** See legend on p. 95.

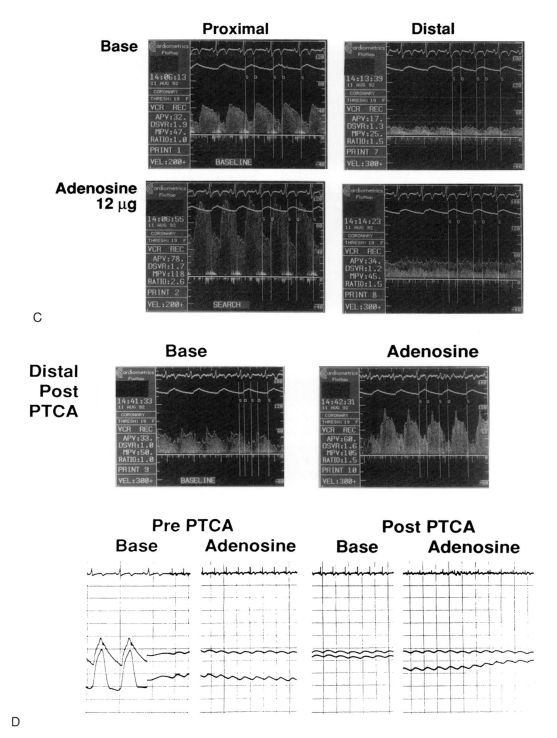

Fig. 9-10 (C) and (D).

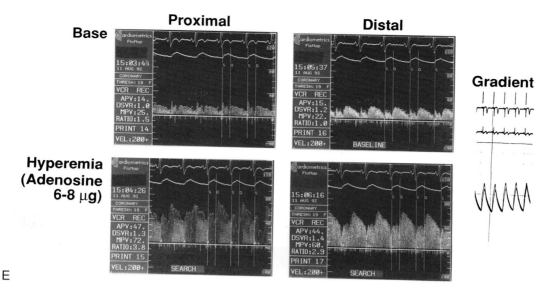

Fig. 9-10. Forty-three year old man at one week postanterior myocardial infarctions. **(A)** Coronary cineangiogram in the left anterior oblique projection (LAO) and right anterior oblique projection (RAO) of the left anterior descending artery demonstrating a 60% diameter narrowing of the proximal segment by QCA in the "worst" projections. **(B)** Coronary cineangiogram in the left anterior oblique projection (LAO) and right anterior oblique projection (RAO) of the right coronary artery also demonstrating a 60% diameter narrowing of the proximal segment by, QCA in the "worst" projections. **(C)** Left anterior descending coronary blood flow velocity proximal and distal to the stenosis at baseline and during maximal hyperemia with 12 μg of intracoronary adenosine (flow velocity scale = 0–200 cm/s) before angioplasty. The distal flow velocity is abnormal. The phasic DSVR pattern is 1.1 (normal: >1.7). The ratio of proximal to distal flow velocity is 1.9 (normal: <1.7). Distal hyperemia was impaired with a flow reserve ratio of approximately 1.42 (normal: >2.0). Note the normal proximal hyperemia, which does not reflect flow limitation beyond the stenosis. **(D)** (*Top*) Translesional pressure gradient before and after left anterior descending angioplasty at baseline and during maximal hyperemia with adenosine. Hemodynamic tracings show electrocardiogram, aortic pressure, and distal coronary pressure (from the top down, 0–200 mmHg scale). Resting gradient is 40 mmHg, which widens to approximately 50 mmHg at maximal hyperemia. Following angioplasty, baseline gradient is 8 mmHg, which widens to approximately 20 mmHg during maximal hyperemia. (*Bottom*) There is an increase of the distal velocity equivalent to proximal velocity before angioplasty with restoration of the phasic DSVR. Distal hyperemia is 2.1 times basal flow velocity in association with the reduction in the translesional gradient and angiographic stenosis. **(E)** Flow velocity data for the right coronary artery, proximal and distal to the eccentric stenosis. The DSVR is normal for a proximal right coronary artery. Proximal/distal flow velocity ratio was 0.9. Distal hyperemia was 2.9 times baseline flow. There was no translesional gradient at rest or during hyperemia in this artery. Angioplasty was not performed. (From Kern et al.,[5] with permission.)

Failure to observe post-PTCA balloon (ischemic) hyperemia likely indicates continued obstruction to flow at or below the level of the angioplasty site.

Atherectomy and Stents

Studies are under way to provide comparisons of atherectomy, laser, and Rotoblator influences on postprocedural flow characteristics.[14] Preliminary studies by Deychak and colleagues[17] and Segal[3] suggest suboptimal improvement in flow after atherectomy and laser angioplasty compared to standard balloon angioplasty.[34] Other studies have indicated normalization of flow velocity after stent and atherectomy comparable to that found in angiographically normal vessels (Fig. 9-13).[14]

Monitoring Flow Velocity Trends During and After Coronary Interventions

Immediate postintervention coronary flow velocity alterations may occur due to slowly progressive dissection, thrombus accumulation, or vasospasm. Flow velocity monitoring is easily incorporated into the postinterventional observation periods using the mean velocity trend plot. Cyclical flow variations have been associated with early thrombus formation

p=NS

p 0.0001

In a preliminary study in our laboratory,[19] the use of continuous measurement of blood flow velocity

10 Fiberoptic Pressure Recording

Håkan Emanuelsson

Intracoronary pressure measurement has been employed ever since the introduction of diagnostic coronary angiography. Recording of the pressure level through the catheter offers improved safety since a drop in blood pressure may be avoided by monitoring. When the percutaneous transluminal coronary angioplasty (PTCA) era began in the late 1970s, it was realized early on that simultaneous pressure measurement via the guiding and balloon catheters offered important information on the stenosis characteristics in addition to the angiographic picture. However, the pressure gradients obtained were not optimal from a technical point of view. The pressure from the balloon catheter was measured through a thin, liquid-filled lumen, producing a signal with a low-frequency response that gave a damped pressure waveform. A mean pressure was acquired, precluding analysis of the phasic changes of the pressure gradient and positioning the balloon catheter in the stenotic segment exaggerated the pressure gradient through additional obstruction to coronary flow.[1] Nevertheless, since many investigators considered the pressure measurement to be of significant clinical value, this technique became a common practice for several years. Further miniaturization of balloon catheters and the introduction of the monorail technique led to abandonment of pressure gradient recording during PTCA by most operators.

In recent years, tip-manometer pressure transducers have circumvented the drawbacks of previous techniques.[2,3] The fiberoptic principle allows further miniaturization and avoids introduction of electricity into the heart, with its potential hazards. Thus, a 0.35-mm-diameter fiberoptic device has been developed that can be incorporated into a 0.014″ PTCA guidewire; it offers the possibility of high-fidelity recordings without significantly affecting blood flow through the artery.

This chapter reports on experiences with pressure gradient recording during PTCA gives recommendations, and discusses the future of the technique.

INDICATIONS FOR PRESSURE GRADIENT RECORDINGS

Decision Making for Coronary Interventions

Angiographic coronary artery stenosis (70% stenosis or more) in combination with unequivocal signs of myocardial ischemia as detected by exercise electrocardiography (ECG) or myocardial scintigraphy constitutes an accepted basis for recommending a myocardial revascularization procedure. Conversely, in lesions of borderline significance (i.e., 40 to 60% stenosis and equivocal findings form provocation studies), further physiological assessment is required before a decision regarding an intervention can be made. A pressure gradient measurement is of great value in this situation. Ideally this could be performed during the initial angiographic procedure. However, since it implies an invasive component that would potentially increase the risk of the catheterization, this practice cannot be recommended as routine at the present time. Instead, measurements are usually performed during the angioplasty session, and their results are important for deciding on which lesions, if any, to treat.

is most pronounced in patients with a baseline gradient in the range of 10 to 30 mmHg.

The ideal agent to produce maximal hyperemia should have rapid onset, short duration, and be free of side effects. In practice, papaverine and adenosine are the two most widely used substances. Papaverine is usually administered as an intracoronary bolus of 6 to 8 mg in the right and 12 mg in the left coronary artery. Some QT prolongation is usually seen on the ECG, and serious ventricular arrhythmia has been reported. The maximal effect of papaverine is usually observed after about 30 seconds, with return to baseline values within 2 to 3 minutes. Adenosine is administered in a dose of 12 to 18 μg i.c.; the maximal effect as well as return to baseline occurs earlier than for papaverine. Although anginal chest pain and hyperventilation may be observed with high doses of adenosine, these signs are virtually never seen with low doses. This also holds true for asystole caused by atrioventricular (AV)-block III, which usually requires doses of 1 mg or more i.c.

It is important recognize that obstruction of flow caused by the position of the guiding catheter in the coronary ostium must be avoided. If this occurs, the catheter should be temporarily dislodged from the artery to prevent distortion of the pressure gradient.

LIMITATIONS OF THE TECHNIQUE

In spite of eliminating several of the drawbacks of conventional intracoronary pressure measurements, the fiberoptic method still carries some limitations. The transducer has been miniaturized down to 0.35 mm in diameter, yet it must be realized that even this size of guidewire placed across a narrow lesion will to some extent affect the true pressure gradient. It has been shown during in vitro studies that an overestimation of the pressure gradient can be expected in small coronary arteries with a tight stenosis (more than 85% area reduction)[4] or if the diameter of the sensing catheter or wire is more than 40% of the stenosis diameter.[5] This implies that accurate measurements will be acquired in lesions more than 0.9 mm in diameter. For practical purposes, this is sufficient, since in most cases recordings are performed in lesions of moderate degree to assess their clinical significance, or in the post-PTCA situation when the obstruction diameter usually considerably exceeds 1.0 mm.

Another question relates to the tip manometer principle and the problem of pressure calibration. In some instances, it has been observed that a sudden shift of the zero line occurs. It has been demonstrated

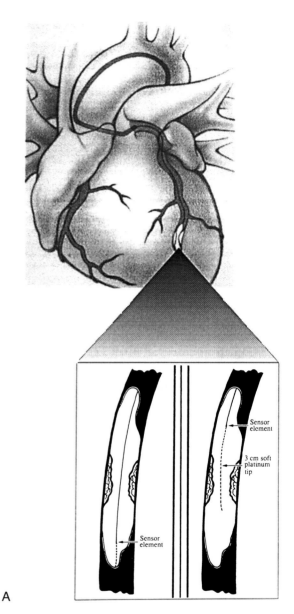

A

Fig. 10-3. Pressure measurements by the pull-back method (**A**) and by simultaneous recording from the wire and guiding catheter (**B**). (*Figure continues.*)

in vitro that this phenomenon may be induced if the transducer is positioned in curvatures of sufficient degree.[6] This zero line shift was seen in a former generation of the wire (0.018″) and should theoretically be less pronounced with the 0.014″ version. Other factors may influence the tendency toward offset of the zero line; hopefully, optimization of production control of the wire will reduce this unwanted phenomenon in the future. If a shift of the baseline is observed, the wire should be withdrawn from the

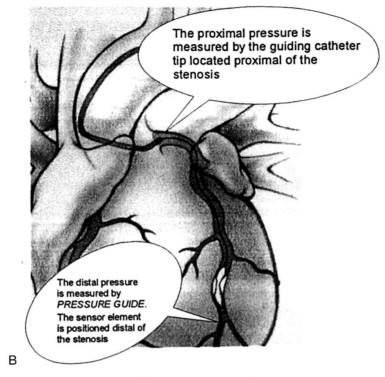

Fig. 10-3 (*continued*).

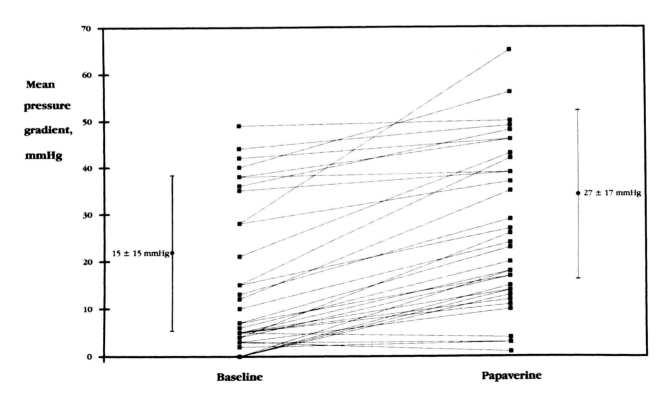

Fig. 10-4. Pressure gradients in individual patients at baseline and during papaverine-induced hyperemia.

catheter to be recalibrated before the procedure is continued.

CORRELATION WITH ANGIOGRAPHIC PARAMETERS

A curvilinear relation has been found between pressure gradients and stenosis diameter and area (Fig. 10-5). A mean gradient of more than 15 mmHg

was highly predictive of a less than 2 mm^2 obstructed area.[3] However, this concordance should be viewed against the fact that only lesions suitable for quantitative coronary angiography were included in that study. It is probable that the correlation is considerably poorer if no specific selection of stenoses is performed, thus emphasizing the independent information acquired from pressure measurement.

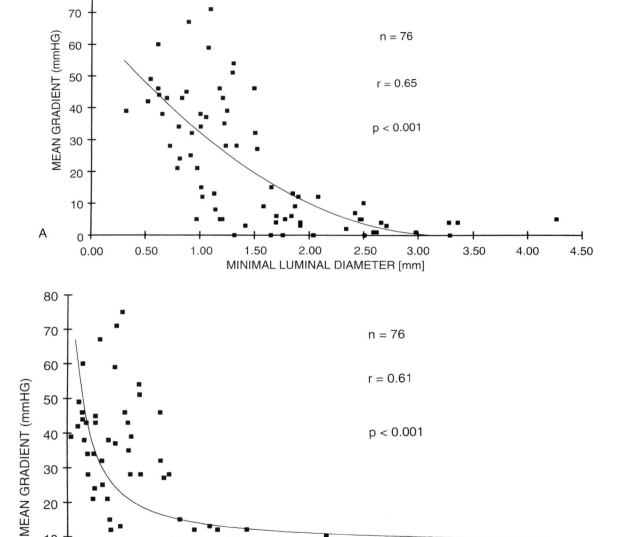

Fig. 10-5. Relationship between minimal luminal diameter **(A),** minimal luminal cross-sectional area **(B),** and the mean pressure gradient. Regression lines are shown.

CALCULATION OF CORONARY FLOW RESERVE

The concept that the absolute coronary flow reserve (CFR) could provide an accurate and clinically useful measure of the physiologic severity of a coronary stenosis was first suggested by Gould et al.[7] However, attractive as this hypothesis may be, several important limitations have been recognized. Since the traditional way of calculating CFR is by determining the ratio of hyperemic and baseline flow, all factors that influence baseline or maximal perfusion, or both, will also affect CFR.

This problem is clinically highly relevant, not least of all in the setting of coronary angioplasty. Therefore, several attempts have been made to find a denominator of flow reserve that is not dependent on the resting condition or a changing hemodynamic situation. One such parameter is the stenotic flow reserve (SFR), which may be calculated from angiographic parameters assuming standardized values for aortic pressure and coronary flow velocity.[8]

The fractional flow reserve (FFR) is an alternative parameter to describe functional stenosis severity independent of physiologic conditions that may affect absolute CFR. FFR is defined as the ratio of maximal flow in a stenotic artery and the maximal flow in the absence of stenosis. It has been demonstrated theoretically and in animal experiments that this quotient can be calculated from intracoronary pressure measurements alone and can be expressed as

$$FFR = 1 - \frac{\Delta P_{max}}{P_a}$$

where ΔP_{max} is the maximal pressure gradient and P_a aortic pressure.[9,10] By measuring the coronary wedge pressure, the contribution of collateral circulation may be calculated. However, in moderately severe stenoses, where collaterals have little impact, the original formula above can be used.

Figure 10-6 shows the correlation between FFR and the percent diameter and area of stenosis. As can be seen, the correlation coefficient is high and the tolerance levels are relatively low, implying that this calculation is also of value in the individual case. Interestingly, the correlation between SFR and FFR was also good (r = 0.87; P <0.001), even though these two denominators of CFR were derived in two completely different ways (Fig. 10-7), FFR from pressure values and SFR from angiographic data. Again, the reason for this result was probably that only lesions optimal for angiographic analysis were included for comparison. The consequence would be that in angiographically complex lesions, particularly those post-PTCA, SFR would tend to yield less reliable information, whereas calculation of FFR should be independent of morphologic features.

ASSESSMENT OF THE RESULTS

Since coronary flow in normal vessels, as well as across mild-to-moderate stenoses, is higher in diastole than in systole, it is not unexpected that the pressure gradient generally reaches maximum in diastole. However, with increasing severity of the lesion, the systolic gradient may reach the same level as the diastolic. It may be difficult to choose a single level that is representative of the pressure gradient as a whole. Should we use the maximal gradient, the mean gradient, the end-diastolic gradient, or some other variable? Obviously, no single parameter will adequately describe the dynamic situation. On the other hand, the pressure gradient curve during the entire cardiac cycle contains considerably more information. Therefore, continuous display of the pressure gradient curve online during the catheterization could be helpful for guidance of the procedure. However, even this curve may be difficult to interpret, and an index derived from the pressure curve would be helpful in this situation.

One way of taking advantage of all the pressure gradient curve information would be to combine the phasic pressure gradient levels with corresponding values for coronary flow or flow velocity into a pressure gradient/flow velocity relation loop. In the animal model, the relationship between the transstenotic pressure gradient and the coronary flow velocity has been extensively studied by Gould and associates.[11] As can be expected from equations of flow dynamics, it has been demonstrated that this relationship in diastole during maximal hyperemia characterizes stenosis severity, with steeper curves for tighter lesions.

The recent miniaturization of pressure as well as flow velocity transducers has resulted in initial studies in humans using this technique with promising results (Fig. 10-8). However, further studies will be needed before it can be determined whether this method of describing the characteristics of coronary lesions is clinically useful.[12] The feasibility of the procedure would be greatly enhanced if the pressure and flow sensors were incorporated into one guidewire and not separated into two wires, as they are today.

CASE STUDY

Figure 10-9 shows pressure curves and angiographic pictures for a patient with an initially moderate stenosis but with resting mean gradient of 19 mmHg.

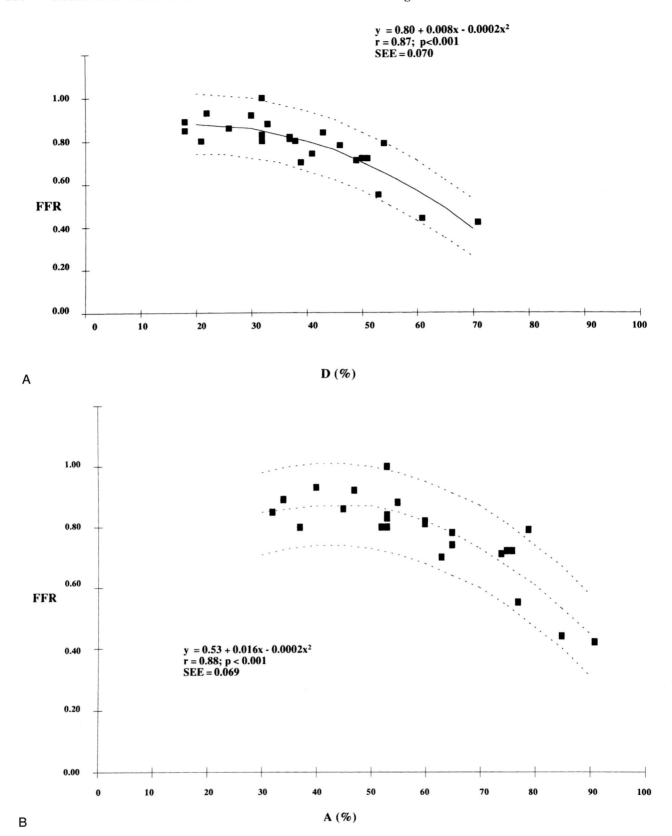

Fig. 10-6. Relationships including 95% tolerance levels are shown between FFR and the percent diameter (**A**) and area stenosis (**B**).

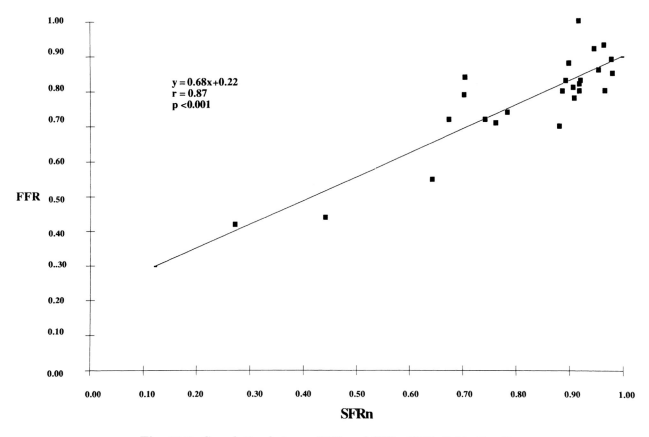

Fig. 10-7. Correlation between FFR and SFRn (SFR divided by 5).

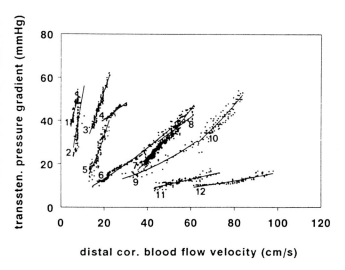

Fig. 10-8. Instantaneous hyperemic diastolic pressure gradient/flow velocity relationship for 12 stenoses of increasing hemodynamic severity (from left to right and from bottom to top).

After 2 balloon dilations, the angiographic appearance was acceptable, whereas the gradient was still not significantly reduced. After two additional dilations with high pressure, the gradient was virtually abolished. Interestingly, the angiographic picture was not further improved. In fact, there was a discordance between the effect on the gradient and angiography. Realizing the shortcomings of angiography in the post-PTCA situation, guidance from the pressure gradient data could be recommended in this situation.

FUTURE DIRECTIONS

In the face of continuing evolution of the angioplasty technique, little doubt exists that angiographic evaluation alone of the results of the procedure will be insufficient in many clinical situations. A physiologic assessment with pressure gradient measurements may be attractive for many investigators. However, for a more widespread use of this technique, feasibility should be improved in several ways. The properties of the guidewire on which the fiberoptic transducer is mounted must be improved with regard to

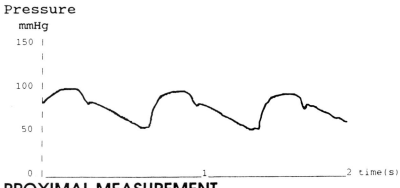

PROXIMAL MEASUREMENT

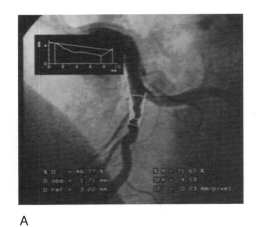

A

DISTAL MEASUREMENT

B

PROXIMAL MEASUREMENT

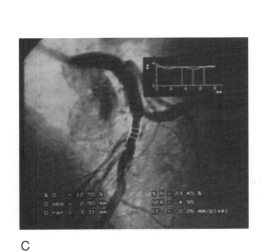

C

DISTAL MEASUREMENT

D

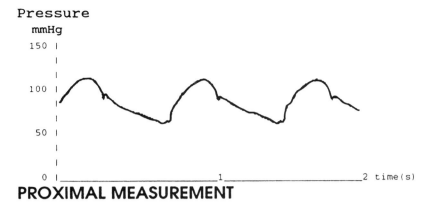

PROXIMAL MEASUREMENT

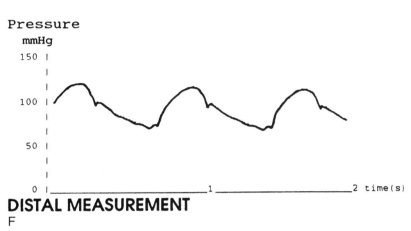

DISTAL MEASUREMENT

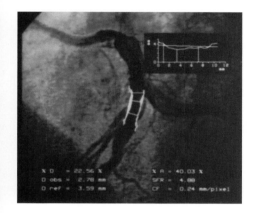

E

F

Fig. 10-9. **(A)** Angiograph and **(B)** pressure curves in a patient before coronary angioplasty (proximal measurement: systolic pressure, 105; mean pressure, 82; diastolic pressure, 54; distal measurement: 98, 63, and 36 respectively; gradient: 7, 19, and 18 respectively). **(C)** Angiography and **(D)** pressure curves in the same patient after second coronary angioplasty (proximal measurement: systolic pressure, 120; mean pressure, 92, and diastolic pressure, 48; distal measurement: 111, 77, and 48 respectively; gradient: 9, 15, and 14, respectively). **(E)** Angiograph and **(F)** pressure curves in the patient after fourth coronary angioplasty (proximal measurement: 129, 99, and 74, respectively; distal measurement: 124, 94, and 70 respectively; gradient: 5, 5, and 4, respectively).

torque and steerability, and it should be extendable like regular guidewires. Furthermore, the pressure gradient should be presented as an online curve on the monitor in order for the operator to have direct information from the measurement. Ideally, additional biosensors should be incorporated into the pressure wire. Of particular value would be a flow velocity probe, since this would greatly facilitate the acquisition of pressure gradient/flow velocity loops, which could be an optimal way of describing the severity of a coronary lesion.

REFERENCES

1. Sigwart U, Grbic M, Gray JJ, Essinger A. High fidelity pressure gradients across coronary artery stenoses before and after transluminal angioplasty (PTCA). J Am Coll Cardiol 1985;5:520

2. Emanuelsson H, Dohnal M, Lamm C, Tenerz L. Initial experiences with a miniaturized pressure transducer during coronary angioplasty. Cathet Cardiovasc Diagn 1991;24:137

3. Lamm C, Dohnal M, Serruys PW, Emanuelsson H. High-fidelity translesional pressure gradients during percutaneous transluminal coronary angioplasty: correlation with quantitative coronary angiography. Am Heart J 1993;126:66

4. De Bruyne B, Pijls N, Paulus W et al. Transstenotic coronary pressure gradient measurement in man: in vitro and in vivo evaluation of a new pressure monitoring PTCA guide-wire. Circulation 1993;85:(in press)

5. Leiboff R, Bren G, Katz R et al. Determinants of transstenotic gradients observed during angioplasty: an experimental model. Am J Cardiol 1983;52:1331

6. Görge G, Erbel R, Niessing S, Schön F. Evaluation of a PTCA guidewire-mounted pressure sensor, abstracted. Circulation 1992;86:1

7. Gould KL, Lipscomb K, Hamilton G. Physiological basis for assessing critical coronary stenosis. Am J Cardiol 1974;33:87

8. Kirkeeide RL, Gould KL, Parsel L. Assessment of coronary stenoses by myocardial perfusion imaging during pharmacologic coronary vasodilation. VII. Validation of coronary flow reserve as a single integrated functional measure of stenosis severity reflecting all its geometric dimensions. J Am Coll Cardiol 1986;7:103

9. Gould KL, Kirkeeide RL, Buchi M. Coronary flow reserve as a physiologic measure of stenosis severity. J Am Coll Cardiol 1990;15:459

10. Pijls N, Kirkeeide RL, Gould KL et al. Quantitation of relative coronary flow reserve and collateral flow by pressure measurements during maximal hyperemia: a rapid accurate method for assessing funtional stenosis severity at PTCA. Circulation 1993;86:1354

11. Gould KL, Kelley K, Bolson E. Experimental validation of quantitative coronary arteriography for determining pressure-flow characteristics of coronary stenosis. Circulation 1982;66:930–937

12. Serruys PW, Di Mario C, Meneveau N et al. Intracoronary pressure and flow velocity with sensor-tip guidewires. A new methodologic approach for assessment of coronary hemodynamics before and after coronary interventions. Am J Cardiol 1993;71:41D–53D

Fluid-Filled Catheters for Intracoronary Pressure Measurements

11

Bernard De Bruyne
Jozef Bartunek
Guy R. Heyndrickx
Nico H. J. Pijls

The transstenotic coronary pressure gradient reflects the total amount of energy lost when blood traverses a stenosis.[1] Since this pressure drop incorporates all dimensional features of the narrowing for a given coronary blood flow, translesional pressure gradient is a straightforward index of functional severity of an epicardial coronary narrowing. The usefulness of coronary pressure monitoring to assess stenosis severity and postangioplasty results was recognized by the pioneers in balloon angioplasty, as testified by the presence of a fluid-filled lumen in the first generation of balloon catheters. In addition, coronary wedge pressure (or coronary pressure during balloon coronary occlusion) has been shown to reflect collateral circulation during occlusion[2] and has proved useful in cases of acute vessel closure as well as for predicting restenosis[3] and the occurrence of ischemic events after percutaneous transluminal coronary angioplasty (PTCA).[4,5] However, the interest in measuring coronary pressure has oscillated between enthusiasm for a simple index of coronary hemodynamics[6–9] and disillusion caused by the inconsistency of the results.[10] The latter may be related to at least two reasons.

First, the translesional pressure gradient is highly dependent on coronary flow. When measured under baseline conditions, the transstenotic pressure gradient will be determined by autoregulated coronary flow. Since, in practice, the absolute coronary blood flow is unknown, the interpretation of a given value of a resting transstenotic pressure gradient remains difficult for clinical decision making in individual patients. The transstenotic pressure gradient would be more related to stenosis severity during maximal coronary vasodilation. From the clinical point of view the hyperemic rather than the resting transstenotic pressure gradient is more warranted as an index of stenosis severity since functional capacity and the patient's symptomatology in the presence of coronary artery disease are more determined by maximal achievable flow than by resting myocardial perfusion.

Second, the device used for pressure measurements (in most cases the balloon catheter itself) is unsuitable because its size is too large compared with the size of the stenotic coronary segment (Fig. 11-1). Clinical practice showed that a marked reduction in coronary flow often accompanies the placement of the deflated balloon catheter across the lesion. Accordingly, it was admitted that, even with the presently available ultra-low-profile balloon angioplasty catheters, a marked overestimation in gradient could occur. The development of monorail angioplasty catheters, precluding pressure measurements, further prompted the trend away from measuring distal pressures during PTCA. Nevertheless,

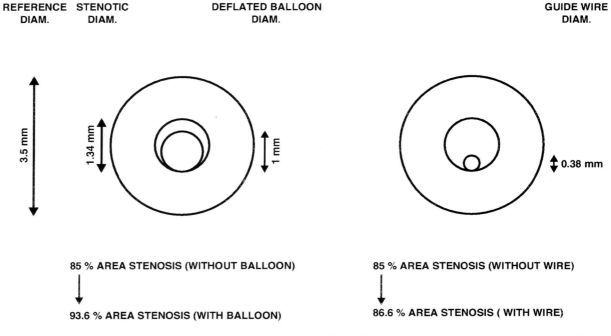

Fig. 11-1. Schematic representation of the room occupied in an 85% area stenosis (72% diameter stenosis) in a 3.5-mm vessel by a balloon catheter and by a 0.015″ guidewire, respectively. The additional resistance to coronary blood flow induced by the wire is expected to be minimal.

knowledge of the transstenotic pressure gradient can still be of aid in the setting of PTCA. Moreover, the recent introduction of the concept of coronary and myocardial fractional flow reserve, which makes the interpretation of pressure gradients easier and independent of hemodynamic changes, could revive interest in coronary pressure measurements.[11] Accordingly, a fluid-filled pressure-monitoring guidewire was developed.

TECHNICAL CHARACTERISTICS OF THE GUIDEWIRE

The pressure-monitoring guidewire is a steerable angioplasty wire (Premo wire, Advanced Cardiovascular Systems, Santa Clara, CA; Although Premo wire is no longer being produced, another fluid-filled pressure-monitoring guidewire is currently being developed). The pressure is transmitted through a fluid column. The proximal 129-cm section consists of a Teflon-coated hypotube with an external diameter of 0.015″. The next 45 cm are made of a second hypotube, which is coaxial to a core wire. These two hypotubes communicate via 10 0.002″ diameter ports. A second series of 10 0.002″ diameter pressure-monitoring ports is located 3 cm from the tip, at the junction of the nonradiopaque portion and the radiopaque tip of the wire. The 3-cm tip is radiopaque and flexible, and may be shaped (Fig. 11-2). The wire is to be connected to a conventional pressure transducer for pressure monitoring. The inner lumen is flushed with heparinized saline and attached via a small screwable valve and a three-way high-pressure

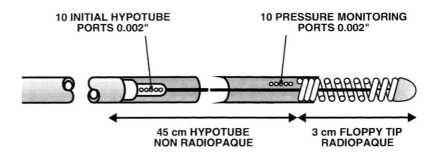

Fig. 11-2. Scheme of the fluid-filled pressure-monitoring guidewire (Premo wire; see text for details).

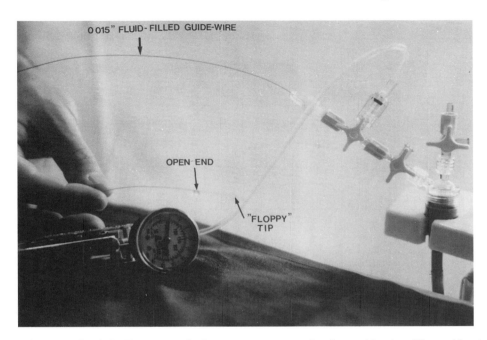

Fig. 11-3. Photograph of the Premo angioplasty pressure-monitoring guidewire. The guidewire is connected to a pressure transducer via two three-way stopcocks. This allows the operator to flush the wire with an inflation device during the procedure without disconnecting the wire from the pressure transducer.

stopcock to the pressure transducer. The side arm of the distal stopcock can be connected to a high-pressure syringe filled with heparinized saline to flush the wire (Fig. 11-3).

IN VITRO VALIDATION STUDIES

To investigate the accuracy of pressure measurements as well as the frequency-response characteristics of the guidewires, five pressure-monitoring guidewires were tested in a hydrostatic model consisting of a water-filled barrel, connected to a Silastic tube with a Y-shaped distal end. A tip micromanometer (Millar SP-780C) was introduced in one leg of the Y, and the pressure-monitoring guidewire to be tested as well as a 5-F right Judkins coronary catheter were introduced in the other leg. By adjusting the height of the barrel, measurements at different pressures were performed. The five pressure-monitoring wires were tested consecutively in eight steps, as follows: from 0 to 50, from 50 to 100, from 100 to 150, from 150 to 0, from 0 to 150, from 150 to 100, from 100 to 50, and from 50 to 0 cmH$_2$O. At each level, pressures measured with the Millar manometer and the pressure-monitoring guidewire were simultaneously recorded until the wire pressure reached a plateau. The absolute pressures measured

with both the microtip manometer and the fluid-filled guidewire were compared and the percent differences calculated. The time constant of the pressure-monitoring wire, defined as the time required for the signal to reach 63.2% of its final value, was calculated for every step. The actual hydrostatic pressure and the pressure recorded by the tip manometer were identical, and therefore the latter was used as an equivalent of the true pressure.

An excellent correlation ($r = 0.98$) was found between the pressure measurements performed with the tip manometer and the fluid-filled pressure-monitoring guidewire. However, the pressure recorded by the Premo wire slightly underestimated the true pressure in all cases. The percent difference between both measurements was $-3 \pm 5\%$ ($n = 15$). The time constant for all steps was almost identical in a single pressure-monitoring guidewire. However, wide variations in time constant (from 9 to 27 seconds; mean, 16 ± 5 seconds) (Fig. 11-4) were found among the five pressure-monitoring guidewires tested.

IN VIVO VALIDATION STUDIES

To investigate in humans the accuracy and feasibility of coronary pressure measurements with a Premo wire, 37 patients undergoing PTCA for single-vessel

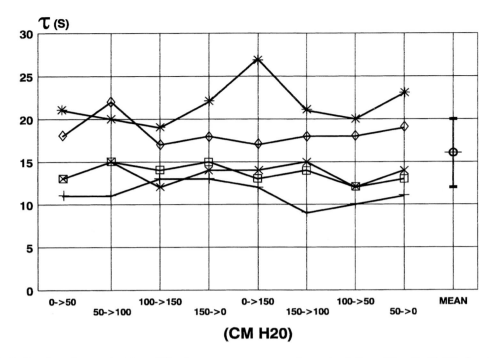

Fig. 11-4. In vitro determination of the frequency-response characteristics of five fluid-filled guidewires. The time constant τ of each wire was calculated for each pressure step.

disease (14 left anterior descending, 15 right, and 8 left circumflex coronary arteries) were studied. Before catheterization patients were given Molsidomine 4 mg tid. Total coronary occlusions were excluded from this study. The ability to perform quantitative coronary angiography in at least two projections was a prerequisite. An 8-F introduction sheath was inserted in the right femoral artery and a 7- or 8-F Judkins guiding catheter was used to cannulate the coronary ostium. Both the side arm of the sheath and the guiding catheter were connected to a pressure transducer (Spectranetics P 23 Statham). The three pressure transducers were zeroed at the midchest level. The pressure-monitoring guidewire was placed at the tip of the guiding catheter, where mean and phasic guiding pressure and guidewire pressure were simultaneously recorded. The wire was advanced through the stenosis while the operator continuously recorded the phasic pressures of the femoral sheath, of the guiding catheter, and of the pressure-monitoring guidewire. Pressure recordings were performed at least 3 minutes after the last contrast medium injection. In most cases the pressure-monitoring wire could cross the lesion while remaining connected to the pressure transducer. When this was not possible, the wire was disconnected from the transducer for better torque control. Only the radiopaque tip was placed distally to the narrowing so that the side holes remained proximally to the stenosis. The proximal end of the wire was again connected to the pressure transducer. Under continuous pressure monitoring the guidewire was then advanced so that the side holes were positioned across the stenosis. After equilibration of the pressures, the mean pressure gradient was recorded between the guiding catheter and the pressure-monitoring guidewire (ΔP_w). These recordings were repeated after completion of balloon angioplasty.

The use of monorail angioplasty catheter systems facilitated the manipulation of the wire and the pressure recordings. Clotting of the lumen of the wire occurred in two patients and precluded further measurements of distal pressures. This emphasizes the need for frequent flushing of the wire.

The correlation between the mean pressures recorded by the guiding catheter and by the Premo wire advanced up to the tip of the guiding catheter was close to unity both before and after PTCA. Only three patients showed a difference in mean pressure larger than 5%. The target vessel could be reached in all cases. All lesions except one were crossed (97%) with the pressure-monitoring guidewire without any particular difficulty, and angioplasty could be successfully performed without the need for another guidewire. There were no complications. The only lesion that could not be crossed with the Premo wire was an eccentric 88% area stenosis in the mid-left anterior descending artery followed by a bend of ap-

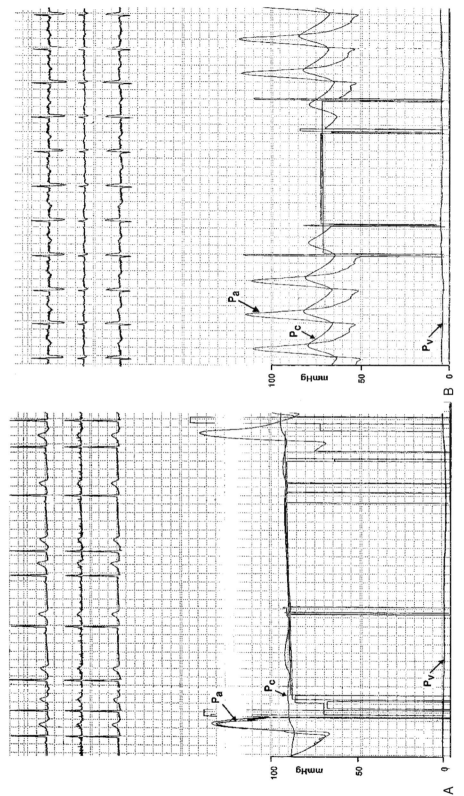

Fig. 11-5. Examples of pressure recordings performed with the pressure-monitoring guidewire advanced at the tip of the guiding catheter. The large differences in time constant between different pressure-monitoring guidewires are reflected by the different damping of the pressure recorded through the wire. **(A)** pressure tracing with oscillation of less than 4 mmHg. **(B)** Pressure tracing shows differences between systolic and diastolic pressure of more than 20 mmHg. However, the mean pressures recorded by the guidewire and by the guiding catheter are identical in both cases. P_a, mean aortic pressure; P_c, distal coronary pressure; P_v, mean right atrial pressure.

were found in severe lesions, when the catheter is totally occlusive since even without a catheter these lesions induced a large pressure drop. In mild or intermediate lesions the overestimation caused by the presence of the catheter was spread over a very large value range, precluding any predictive value of the measurement.

In contrast to the theoretical model of Leiboff et al.,[15] who found that overestimation of the "true" transstenotic pressure gradient was predictable, our results suggest that the overestimation is poorly predictable in vivo. Hence, the pressure gradient measured by means of the balloon catheter is relatively accurate when this information is not needed (i.e., in critical lesions, in which angiography most often suffices) but is inaccurate when this information is most desirable (i.e., in intermediate lesions and in post-PTCA segments, where functional information can be clinically helpful).

ADVANTAGES AND LIMITATIONS OF THE FLUID-FILLED COMPARED WITH MICROMANOMETER-TIPPED GUIDEWIRES

The main advantages of a fluid-filled guidewire is its simplicity of use and its low cost. Since it has essentially the same technical characteristics of most of the currently available PTCA guidewires, it could be routinely used to cross the majority of the lesions scheduled for angioplasty and could even be proposed to measure gradients across dubious lesions during diagnostic catheterization. Moreover, since the fluid-filled pressure wire simply needs to be connected to a conventional pressure transducer, it is immediately usable in every catheterization laboratory without additional cost or material. Thanks to the small cross-sectional area of the wire, only very limited hindrance to coronary hemodynamics is to be expected. The main limitation of the fluid-filled pressure-monitoring guidewire consists in the inability to measure phasic pressure tracings. In contrast to micromanometer-tipped wires, systolic and diastolic components of the gradients cannot be distinguished with the fluid-filled pressure-monitoring guidewire.[16] Since coronary blood flow occurs predominantly during diastole, a gradient may occur exclusively during diastole in mild stenoses and in post-PTCA segments. However, for assessing the impact of a stenosis on the underlying myocardium, only mean transstenotic pressure gradient should be measured. Hence, this disadvantage (not allowing phasic pressure recordings) is counterbalanced by several practical advantages.

CLINICAL APPLICATIONS OF FLUID-FILLED CORONARY PRESSURE RECORDINGS

The relationship between distal coronary pressure and myocardial perfusion during maximal coronary hyperemia has been synthesized in the concept of myocardial fractional flow reserve (FFR_{myo}).[11] The theoretical bases are summarized in Chapter 12. The accuracy of the FFR_{myo} measurements in humans has been demonstrated.[17] Pressure-derived indices were compared with relative myocardial perfusion reserve assessed by positron emission tomography in 22 patients with an isolated proximal stenosis in the left anterior descending artery. This study showed a close correlation between FFR_{myo} and relative flow reserve ($r = 0.87$).

To explore the use of coronary pressure measurements in clinical practice we studied 60 patients with an isolated epicardial coronary stenosis to define the values of pressure-derived indexes associated with exercise-induced myocardial ischemia detected by exercise electrocardiography.[18] In the whole population, the magnitude of ST segment depression during maximal exercise correlated well with FFR_{myo} ($r = -0.75$). The correlation between resting transstenotic pressure gradient and ST segment depression was weaker than with a maximal hyperemic pressure gradient ($r = 0.71$ versus $r = 0.53$, $P < 0.001$). More importantly from a clinical point of view, an FFR_{myo} value greater than 0.72 and a hyperemic transstenotic pressure gradient less than 21 mmHg were uniformly associated with the absence of inducible ischemia during exercise electrocardiography. In the settings of both interventional cardiology and diagnostic coronary angiography, these cutoff values of pressure-derived indexes should help in clinical decision making in cases with questionable angiographic findings.

REFERENCES

1. Young DF, Cholvin NR, Roth AC. Pressure drop across artificially induced stenosis in the femoral arteries of dogs. Circ Res 1975;36:735–743
2. Meier B, Luethy P, Finci L et al. Coronary wedge pressure in relation to spontaneously visible and recruitable collaterals. Circulation 1987;75:566–572
3. Urban P, Meier B, Finci L et al. Coronary wedge pressure: a predictor of restenosis after coronary balloon angioplasty. J Am Coll Cardiol 1987;10:504–509
4. Redd DC, Roubin GS, Leimgruber PP et al. The transstenotic pressure gradient trend as a predictor of acute

complications after percutaneous transluminal coronary angioplasty. Circulation 1987;76:792–801

5. Pijls NHJ, Bech JW, De Bruyne et al. Quantitative assessment of recruitable collateral blood flow by intracoronary pressure measurements at PTCA. Circulation 1993;88:I–650

6. Rothman MT, Baim DS, Simpson JB, Harrison DC. Coronary hemodynamics during percutaneous transluminal coronary angioplasty. Am J Cardiol 1982;49:1615–1622

7. Haraphongse M, Tymchak W, Burton JR, Rossal RE. Implication of transstenotic pressure gradient measurement during coronary artery angioplasty. Cathet Cardiovasc Diagn 1986;12:80–84

8. Leimgruber PP, Roubin GS, Hollman J et al. Restenosis after successful coronary angioplasty in patients with single-vessel disease. Circulation 1986;73:710–717

9. Anderson HV, Roubin GS, Leimgruber PP et al. Measurement of transstenotic pressure gradients during percutaneous transluminal coronary angioplasty. Circulation 1986;73:1223–1230

10. Serruys PW, Wijns W, Reiber JHC et al. Values and limitations of transstenotic pressure gradients measured during percutaneous coronary angioplasty. Herz 1985;10:337–342

11. Pijls NHJ, Van Son JAM, Kirkeeide RL et al. Experimental bassis of determining maximum coronary, myocardial, and collateral blood flow by pressure measurements for assessing functional stenosis severity before and after percutaneous transluminal coronary angioplasty. Circulation 1993;87:1354–1367

12. Reiber JHC, Serruys PW, Kooijman CJ et al. Assessment of short-, medium and longterm variations in arterial dimensions from computer-assisted quantification of coronary cineangiograms. Circulation 1985;71:280–288

13. Sigwart U, Grbic M, Goy JJ, Essinger A. High fidelity pressure gradients across coronary artery stenoses before and after transluminal angioplasty (PTCA), abstracted. J Am Coll Cardiol 1985;5:521

14. Gould KL, Lipscomb K. Effects of coronary stenosis on coronary flow reserve and resistance. Am J Cardiol 1974;34:48–55

15. Leiboff R, Bren G, Katz R. Determinants of transstenotic gradients observed during angioplasty: an experimental model. Am J Cardiol 1983;52:1311–1317

16. Emanuelsson H, Dohnal M, Lamm C, Tenerz L. Initial experiences with a miniaturized pressure transducer during coronary angioplasty. Cathet Cardiovascular Diagn 1991;24:137–143

17. De Bruyne B, Baudhuin T, Melin JA et al. Coronary flow reserve calculated from pressure measurements in humans. Validation with positron emission tomography. Circulation 1994;89:1013–1022

18. De Bruyne B, Bartunek J, Sys SY, Heyndrickx GR. Relation between myocardial fractional flow reserve calculated from coronary pressure measurements and exercise-induced myocardial ischemia. Circulation 1995;92:39–46

method for assessment of flow reserve in the coronary circulation by pressure measurements. This method is easy to apply, accurate, inexpensive, and hardly prolongs the procedure. It is independent of changes in driving pressure and permits separate assessment of coronary arterial and collateral blood flow to total myocardial perfusion.

coronary pressure recordings are interpreted in combination with aortic and right atrial pressure, FFR of the coronary artery, the myocardium, and the collateral flow can be reliably assessed, thereby providing a complete description of the effect of the stenosis on the coronary circulation.

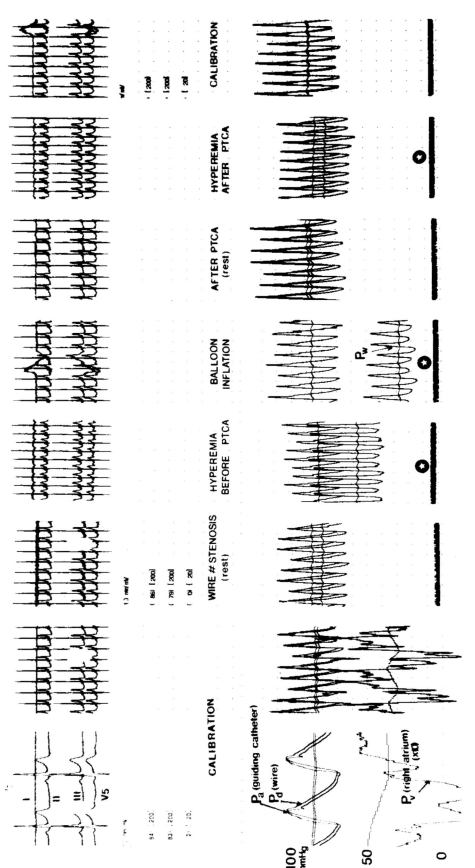

Fig. 12-4. Simultaneous recording of the three relevant pressures (P_a, P_d, and P_v) during the different steps of a PTCA of the LAD artery in a 64-year-old man. For clarity, P_v is only displayed in Fig. A. **(A)** Calibration before the wire enters the coronary artery. Arterial pressure (P_a), measured by the guiding catheter, equals the pressure measured by the wire. **(B)** The wire has passed the stenosis. Resting P_a and P_d are obtained. **(C)** Maximum hyperemia, obtained by intravenous adenosine. Simultaneously recorded P_a, P_d, and P_v at steady-state hyperemia are used to calculate FFR_{myo} before PTCA. **(D)** Balloon occlusion. P_a, P_w, and P_v are obtained. **(E)** Resting P_a and P_d after PTCA. **(F)** Hyperemic pressures after PTCA, obtained by intravenous adenosine. **(G)** Calibration at the end of the procedure and control for drift or other mistakes. The values of all pressures in this patient are discussed further in Case Study 4. The angiogram of this patient is shown in Figure 11-6.

Because P_w at balloon occlusion is also known, FFR_{cor} and the contribution of collateral blood flow to myocardial blood flow are also available, both before and after the PTCA. Moreover, recruitable collateral flow at balloon occlusion is easily calculated by $(P_w - P_v)/(P_a - P_v)$ or by P_w/P_a in case P_v is undetermined. The matrix describing the complete distribution of flow throughout the coronary circulation is already known, as illustrated in the examples.

In our laboratory, the three pressures P_a, P_d, and P_v are always displayed by different colors on the monitor (i.e., orange, blue, and yellow, respectively) together with their digital values (Fig. 12-3). Because of the simplicity of the equations. This display permits direct evaluation of all steps by the operator. For example FFR_{myo} equals blue minus yellow, divided by orange minus yellow, and so forth. The pressure recordings are also displayed on paper at a speed of 5 mm/sec, as shown in Figure 12-4.

After a satisfactory result has been obtained, the procedure is finished and calibrations are performed as described above (Fig. 12-4G). All these steps prolong the total length of the PTCA in our laboratory by approximately 15 minutes. In diagnostic catheterization, P_w is unknown and therefore only FFR_{myo} can be determined. As already explained, however, this is the most important parameter from the point of view of the patient because it tells immediately to what degree maximum achievable myocardial blood flow is affected.

Maximum Vasodilatory Stimuli

Maximum vasodilation of the coronary circulation can be obtained in a number of ways.

- Papaverine i.c. (12 mg left coronary artery; 8 mg right coronary artery)
- Adenosine i.c. (18 μg left coronary artery; 10 μg right coronary artery)
- Adenosine i.v. (140 μg/kg/min)
- Dipyridamole i.v. (0.56 mg/kg over 4 minutes)

Papaverine, Intracoronary

Intracoronary papaverine is considered the standard for induction of maximum coronary and myocardial hyperemia. In our lab, 1 ampulla (= 1 ml = 50 mg) is diluted with 9 ml of saline. After administration of 2.5 ml of that dilution (= 12.5 mg) in the left coronary artery or 1.5 to 2 ml (= 7.5 to 10 mg) in the right coronary artery through the guiding catheter, followed by 3 ml of saline, steady-state hyperemia is obtained from approximately 30 to 60 seconds after the administration. In the United States, some concern exists about intracoronary papaverine with regard to QT prolongation and polymorphous ventricular tachycardia. In our experience of over 600 cases, only twice has ventricular fibrillation occurred, which is no different from the incidence after regular contrast injection. Intracoronary papaverine should not be used in connection with hexabrix.

Adenosine, Intracoronary

In most patients, 18 μg of adenosine into the left coronary artery and 12 μg into the right is a maximum hyperemic stimulus. However, the peak hyperemia occurs early and lasts for only 5 to 10 seconds, which is too short for reliable steady-state pressure recording. Another disadvantage of intracoronary administration of the hyperemic stimulus is that the pressure signal by the guiding catheter has to be interrupted.

Adenosine, Intravenous

If adenosine is infused intravenously at a rate of 140 μg/kg/min, maximum hyperemia is reached within 2 minutes without significant influence on arteriovenous conduction. Thus stable hyperemic pressure recordings are possible. A side effect of intravenous adenosine infusion is a burning sensation in the chest, which is harmless but mimics angina pectoris. After stopping the infusion, the effect disappears within 2 minutes. The advantage of intravenous administration of an hyperemic stimulus is that the signal by the guiding catheter does not have to be interrupted. Intravenous administration of this dosage of adenosine is accompanied by a decrease in mean arterial pressure of approximately 10 to 15%. All effects vanish within 2 minutes after stopping the infusion.

Dypiridamole, Intravenous

Administration of dypiridamole i.v. 0.56 mg/kg over 4 minutes results in long-lasting maximum hyperemia. However, this is associated with significant decrease in blood pressure in some patients. The hyperemic effect lasts for at least 20 minutes (and sometimes much longer) but can be directly counteracted by 250 mg of aminophylline intravenously.

P_w Before and After PTCA

For PTCA, one further remark should be made. Because P_a and P_v are not necessarily constant during the procedure, and because P_w can only be determined at balloon occlusion, Equation 4 must be used to assess the value of P_w as it would be at that particular P_a and P_v as observed before and after PTCA. This is illustrated in Examples 2, 3, and 4.

Example 1

First, two imaginary examples are given to demonstrate how the calculation of flow reserve by pressure data should be performed. Later, a number of "real" examples are given.

The first example refers to a PTCA and is based on the simple hemodynamic case in which systemic pressures (P_a and P_v) are unchanged during the procedure. Therefore, according to Equation 4, wedge pressure P_w is also constant. The superscript $^{(1)}$ indicates values before PTCA and the superscript $^{(2)}$ values after. Before and after a PTCA of one of the coronary arteries, pressure measurements are performed by the pressure-monitoring guidewire at maximum coronary hyperemia, induced by administration of intracoronary papaverine or intravenous adenosine. Mean arterial pressure P_a is 90 mmHg both before and after the procedure, distal coronary pressure equals 40 mmHg before and 80 mmHg after the procedure, and venous pressure P_v is 0 both before and after the procedure. Coronary wedge pressure, measured during balloon inflation, is 20 mmHg. Therefore:

$$P_a^{(1)} = P_a^{(2)} = 90 \text{ mmHg}$$

$$P_d^{(1)} = 40 \text{ mmHg}$$

$$P_d^{(2)} = 80 \text{ mmHg,}$$

$$P_v^{(1)} = P_v^{(2)} = 0 \text{ mmHg}$$

$$P_w^{(1)} = P_w^{(2)} = 20 \text{ mmHg}$$

By using Equations 1, 2, and 3 (both before and after PTCA), one obtains the values of all flow parameters, expressed as a fraction of normal maximum myocardial blood flow Q^N expected in the absence of a stenosis, normalized for pressure changes:

$$FFR_{myo}^{(1)} = (40 - 0)/(90 - 0) = 0.44$$

$$FFR_{myo}^{(2)} = (80 - 0)/(90 - 0) = 0.89$$

$$FFR_{cor}^{(1)} = (40 - 20)/(90 - 20) = 0.29$$

$$FFR_{cor}^{(2)} = (80 - 20)/(90 - 20) = 0.86$$

$$Q_c^{(1)} = 0.44 - 0.29 = 0.15$$

$$Q_c^{(2)} = 0.89 - 0.86 = 0.03$$

Moreover, it can be noted that maximally achievable blood flow through the myocardium increased by a factor 2, maximally achievable blood flow through the dilated artery increased by a factor of 3, and collateral blood flow decreased by a factor of 5. Finally

Table 12-2. Flow Distribution Before and After PTCA When Systemic Pressures Are Unchanged[a]

	Before PTCA	At Balloon Inflation	After PTCA
FFR_{myo}	0.44	0.22	0.89
FFR_{cor}	0.29	0	0.86
Q_c/Q^N	0.15	0.22	0.03

[a] Such a matrix completely describes the distribution of flow in the coronary circulation both before and after PTCA. It is independent of changes in driving pressure or other hemodynamic parameters. Moreover, it indicates maximum recruitable collateral blood flow during coronary artery occlusion.

maximum recruitable collateral flow during coronary artery occlusion, expressed as a fraction of normal maximum myocardial perfusion, can be calculated by the equation $Q_c/Q^N = (P_w - P_v)/(P_a - P_v) = 20/90 = 0.22$.

This information is summarized in Table 12-2.

Example 2

The second example demonstrates the calculations when mean arterial and venous pressures change during PTCA. A PTCA of one of the coronary arteries is performed. At maximum coronary hyperemia, mean arterial pressure is 96 mmHg before and 80 mmHg after the procedure. Distal coronary pressure equals 51 mmHg before and 65 mmHg, after, and venous pressure is 6 mmHg before and 5 mmHg after. Coronary wedge pressure is 23 mmHg during balloon inflation. Mean arterial pressure during balloon inflation is 92 mmHg, and mean venous pressure during balloon inflation is 6 mmHg.

In this case, with changing P_a and P_v, first the values of $P_w^{(1)}$ and $P_w^{(2)}$ must be calculated as they would be at the arterial pressure encountered before and after PTCA, using the fact that $(P_a - P_v)/(P_w - P_v)$ is constant according to Equation 4. Therefore, $P_w^{(1)} = 24 \text{ mmHg}$ and $P_w^{(2)} = 20 \text{ mmHg}$. Thereafter, in an identical way as in Example 1, Equations 1, 2, and 3 are used to calculate that:

$$FFR_{myo}^{(1)} = (51 - 6)/(96 - 6) = 0.50$$

$$FFR_{myo}^{(2)} = (65 - 5)/(80 - 5) = 0.80$$

$$FFR_{cor}^{(1)} = (51 - 24)/(96 - 24) = 0.38$$

$$FFR_{cor}^{(2)} = (65 - 20)/(80 - 20) = 0.75$$

$$Q_c^{(1)} = 0.50 - 0.375 = 0.12$$

$$Q_c^{(2)} = 0.80 - 0.75 = 0.05$$

Table 12-3. Flow Distribution Before and After PTCA When Systemic Pressures Change[a]

	Before PTCA	At Balloon Inflation	After PTCA
FFR_{myo}	0.50	0.20	0.80
FFR_{cor}	0.38	0	0.75
Q^c/Q^N	0.12	0.20	0.05

[a] This matrix completely describes the distribution of flow in the coronary circulation both before and after PTCA and at balloon inflation and is independent of pressure changes.

Therefore, it can be noted that maximally achievable blood flow through the myocardium increased by a factor of 1.6, maximally achievable blood flow through the dilated artery increased by a factor of 2, whereas collateral flow decreased by a factor of 2.5. In this way, by using Equations 1, 2, and 3 (both before and after PTCA), one obtains the values of all flow parameters, expressed as a fraction of normal maximum myocardial blood flow expected in the absence of a stenosis, normalized for pressure changes, whereas maximum recruitable collateral flow at coronary artery occlusion is calculated by $Q_c/Q^N = (P_w - P_v)/(P_a - P_v) = (23 - 6)/(92 - 6) = 17/86 = 0.20$. This is shown in Table 12-3.

INTERPRETATION OF PRESSURE DATA AND FRACTIONAL FLOW RESERVE

As sufficiently explained, the transstenotic pressure gradient ΔP alone does not hold much significance for evaluation of coronary blood flow and it is virtually impossible to define a range of ΔP indicating inducible ischemia. Only simultaneous use of hyperemic P_a, P_d, and preferably P_v will allow calculation of FFR and permit a correct assessment of the functional significance of the coronary artery stenosis (Fig. 2-1).

Fractional Myocardial Flow Reserve

Although the interventional cardiologist is prone to focus on the *coronary* artery, it should be realized that from the point of view of the patient, maximum achievable *myocardial* blood flow is the most relevant parameter because this index determines the functional capacitance and the threshold of exercise at which angina occurs.

Therefore, in both diagnostic and interventional procedures FFR_{myo} is the most important and can be easily obtained by simply calculating $(P_d - P_v)/(P_a - P_v)$ after administration of a hyperemic stimulus. If right atrial pressure is not elevated, P_v might be ignored and FFR_{myo} equals P_d/P_a. In our experience we were unable to demonstrate ischemia if FFR_{myo} exceeded 0.77 (by regular exercise testing, by thallium, or by Dobutrex stress echoing). On the other hand, so far in all patients in whom FFR_{myo} was less than 0.73, we were able to demonstrate ischemia by at least one of those testing modalities. Therefore we believe that in diagnostic studies a FFR_{myo} value of over 0.75 is a reason to consider the stenosis as functionally nonsignificant, whereas a post-PTCA value of FFR_{myo} exceeding 0.75 indicates functionally successful PTCA even if the angiogram is suboptimal. One of the unique features of FFR_{myo} is that it represents both the blood flow through the coronary artery and the collateral blood flow.

Fractional Coronary Flow Reserve

FFR_{cor} cannot be calculated separately during diagnostic procedures but only during PTCA. If there is no stenosis at all, FFR_{cor} equals FFR_{myo} and is equal to 1. As the stenosis increases, FFR_{cor} and FFR_{myo} both decrease, but FFR_{cor} will be progressivily lower than FFR_{myo}, due to an increasing contribution of collateral blood flow. At total occlusion, $FFR_{cor} = 0$, whereas FFR_{myo} equals recruitable collateral blood flow. As is clear by the examples, increase of FFR_{myo} and FFR_{cor} by PTCA are not equal. Whereas the increase in FFR_{myo} describes the improvement of the *patient*, an increase in FFR_{cor} describes the improvement of the dilated *artery*.

Because, in contrast to FFR_{myo}, FFR_{cor} does not incorporate the extent of collateral flow, no threshold value of FFR_{cor} exists below which ischemia is absent or present. This is an important fact that elucidates why methods that only assess coronary blood flow are fundamentally limited to understanding the influence of the stenosis on the myocardium and thereby for the patient.

In one patient coronary flow may be less than in another, but, due to a larger collateral contribution, inducible ischemia may be absent in the first but present in the second. Therefore, even theoretically, no sharp border between "normal" and "abnormal" is possible if only the coronary artery flow is studied.

This also explains the large overlap between normal and pathologic values for other methods such as Doppler velocimetry and videodensitometry. By using FFR_{myo}, this overlap is avoided. Because FFR_{cor} is always less than or equal to FFR_{myo}, a value of FFR_{cor} of more than 0.77 excludes ischemia.

Collateral Blood Flow

Collateral blood flow (Q_c) expressed as a fraction of normal maximum myocardial blood flow (Q^N), is calculated by Equation 3 and provides insight into the distribution of flow through the coronary circulation. In fact this method is the first approach that permits real quantification of collateral flow in a conscious human and also allows assessment of the separate contributions of coronary artery and collateral blood flow to total myocardial perfusion.

An especially valuable index is the maximum recruitable collateral blood flow at coronary artery occlusion, expressed as:

$$Q_c/Q^N = (P_w - P_v)/(P_a - P_v)$$

because this index determines whether ischemia at rest will occur in case of occlusion of the coronary artery. Recently we demonstrated that if Q_c/Q^N at occlusion exceeds approximately 25% (or 30% if venous pressure is not incorporated), no ischemia at rest could be demonstrated in 36 of 41 patients, whereas in 79 of 79 patients with Q_c/Q^N less than 23%, ischemia at rest was present.[12] During a follow-up of 24 months, seven patients experienced a myocardial infarction and all of them belonged to the "poor collaterals" group. Therefore, recruitable collateral flow at balloon occlusion is a reliable index of sufficient collateral protection and can be used for future risk stratification.

Example 3

Figure 12-5 shows the left coronary artery of a 55-year-old man who was referred because of stable angina class III and a positive exercise test. A moderate stenosis is seen in the proximal left anterior descending artery, a more severe stenosis in the proximal left circumflex artery, and another moderate stenosis in the distal left circumflex artery artery. How to proceed and what artery to dilate? At first, the left anterior descending artery stenosis was crossed by a fiberoptic pressure-monitoring guidewire. Intracoronary papaverine (12 mg) was administered, and simultaneous values of P_a, P_d, and P_v at steady-state maximum hyperemia were recorded of 75, 66, and 3 mmHg, respectively. Therefore, FFR_{myo} artery supplied by the left anterior descending equals $(66 - 3)/(75 - 3) = 0.87$, indicating that maximum blood flow in this artery equals 87% of its normal value (i.e., its value in case no stenosis would be present). This means that no ischemia can be caused by that stenosis. Consequently no PTCA was performed in this artery. Thereafter the wire was placed across the proximal left circumflex artery stenosis and after ad-

ministration of another 12 mg of papaverine i.c., FFR_{myo} of the left circumflex artery myocardium proved to be 54%, which is considerably less than the marginal value (cut-off point) of 0.75 (75%). Therefore, this lesion was dilated by a 3.0 balloon and FFR_{myo}, determined after PTCA was 0.81, indicated a successful procedure.

However, another interesting observation may be made in this patient: as can be seen in Figure 12-5, the left circumflex artery has three distal branches, two of which are filled by collaterals from the left anterior descending and right coronary arteries, respectively. When the balloon was inflated in the proximal left circumflex artery stenosis, P_a, P_w, and P_v equaled 71, 22, and 2 mmHg, respectively. No ECG changes occurred at occlusion (the pre-existing abnormalities remained unchanged), and the patient, resting on the table, experienced no angina. Recruitable collateral blood flow to the left circumflex artery myocardium was calculated by: $Q_c/Q^N = (22 - 2)/(71 - 2) = 0.27$, which is sufficient to protect the myocardium at rest, according to our studies.[12] The balloon was then inflated in the distal left circumflex artery, thereby occluding the atrioventricular sulcus branch, which is not visibly filled by collaterals. Severe ECG abnormalities occurred, the patient experienced angina at rest, and P_a, P_w, and P_v equaled 69, 11, and 2 mmHg, respectively, resulting in a recruitable collateral flow that was 13% of normal maximum myocardial flow and therefore insufficient. The exercise test was normal 7 days later. This example demonstrates the ease and power of this approach for a complete understanding of the influence of multiple stenoses on the coronary circulation.

Example 4

The next example is a 64-year-old man who had experienced an aborted anterior wall infarction 3 weeks earlier and was refered because of postinfarct angina. The pressure recordings obtained in this patient are displayed in Figure 12-4 and the angiogram in Figure 12-6.

As can be observed, P_a, P_d, and P_v are 81, 56, and 5 mmHg at steady-state hyperemia before PTCA; 85, 21, and 5 mmHg during balloon occlusion; and 83, 76, and 6 mmHg at steady-state hyperemia after PTCA. Maximum hyperemia was obtained in this patient by intravenous adenosine. By Equation 4 it is calculated that P_w, if measured at P_a and P_v as these are before and after PTCA, would be 19 mmHg before and 21 mmHg after. Using Equations 1, 2, and 3, this results in the next matrix as shown in Table 12-4.

The matrix shows that the functional result of the

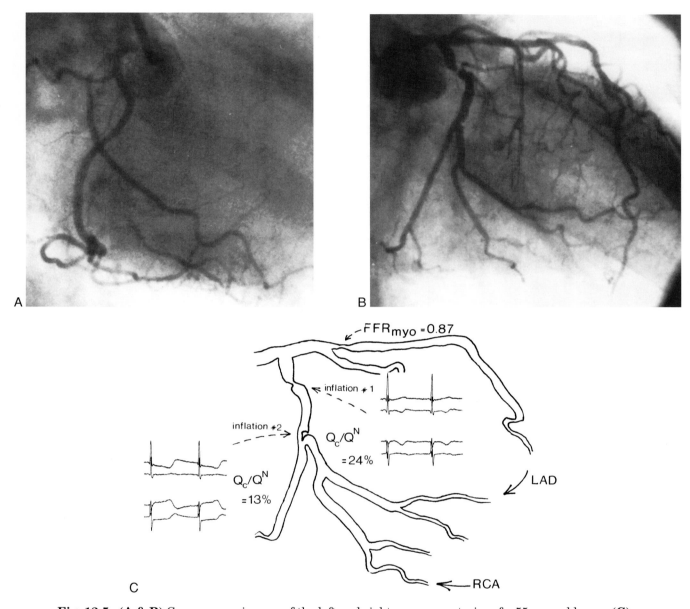

Fig. 12-5. (A & B) Coronary angiogram of the left and right coronary arteries of a 55-year-old man. **(C)** A schematic representation of the data obtained by the pressure-flow equations. See Example 3.

PTCA is excellent, despite a residual stenosis of about 30%. As can be seen, recruitable collateral flow in this patient is 0.20 at balloon occlusion, which is below the clinical cut-off point of 25%, and therefore it is not surprising that ischemia was present on ECG at balloon inflation.

Example 5

A 53-year-old man was admitted because of chest pain at rest with typical biphasic T-wave abnormalities in the anterior wall leads, indicating proximal or mid-left anterior descending artery stenosis. After this single episode, the ECG normalized within a few days; at angiography, a moderate 50 to 70% left anterior descending artery stenosis was found. The patient was referred to our center for PTCA. At maximum exercise testing 1 day before PTCA, however, no ischemia was inducible and at the planned PTCA, a fiberoptic pressure monitoring guidewire was placed across the stenosis and intravenous adenosine was administered. P_a, P_d, and P_v were 89, 78, and 1, respectively, resulting in $FFR_{myo} = (78 - 1)/(89 - 1) = 0.88$, indicating *almost normal maximum blood flow in the left anterior descending artery*. No PTCA was performed, but instead ergonovine testing

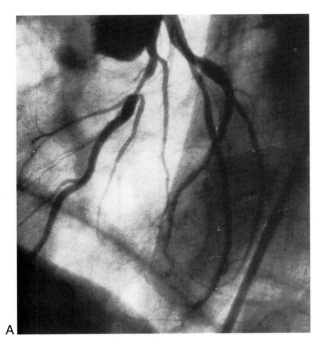 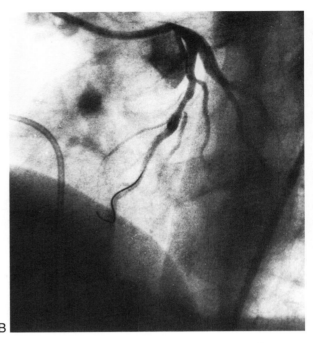

Fig. 12-6. Angiogram of the patient discussed in Example 4 before **(A)** and after PTCA **(B)**. FFR_{myo} of the LAD-supplied myocardium is 0.67 and FFR_{cor} 0.60. After PTCA both values almost normalized. The pressure recordings of this patient are displayed in Figure 12-4 and described in the text.

was performed resulting in severe spasm and occlusion superimposed on the left anterior descending artery lesion and revealing the true nature of the coronary disease of this patient. *Standard PTCA would not only have been senseless in this patient but could have been accompanied by severe complications.*

Example 6

A 51-year-old man was admitted because of typical anginal complaints at exercise and an abnormal resting ECG 2 weeks before admission (Fig. 12-7). Standard bicycle testing and thallium scintigraphy were normal. At cardiac catheterization, the only suspicious view was the left anterior oblique (LAO) 45/20 view of the left coronary artery, showing a trifunction

where the origin of the first and second diagonal branches and the left anterior descending artery itself were difficult to analyze (Fig. 12-8). Using a fiberoptic guidewire, FFR_{myo} was determimined in all three branches, and turned out to be 1.0 and 0.88 in the respective diagonal branches. In the left anterior descending artery, however, FFR_{myo} was seriously decreased to 0.42 (Fig. 12-9). Based on this observation, the patient had cardiac surgery with a LIMA on the left anterior descending artery and has been free of complaints.

COMPARISON WITH OTHER TECHNIQUES FOR INVASIVE CORONARY FLOW ASSESSMENT

At present, only three techniques have emerged from the purely experimental stage and are available for flow assessment in the catheterization laboratory. These are ECG-triggered digital subtraction angiography, Doppler velocimetry, and FFR assessment by pressure-flow equations. ECG-triggered digital subtraction angiography is time consuming, expensive, and only feasible in a minority of patients.[17] Moreover, its less complex variant, using appearance-time contrast-density ratios, is unreliable and lacks a scientific basis.[19,27] Finally, only information about the

Table 12-4. Flow Distribution Before and After PTCA in a Patient with Postinfarct Angina

	Before PTCA	At Balloon Inflation	After PTCA
FFR_{myo}	0.67	0.20	0.91
FFR_{cor}	0.60	—	0.89
Q_c/Q^N	0.07	0.20	0.02

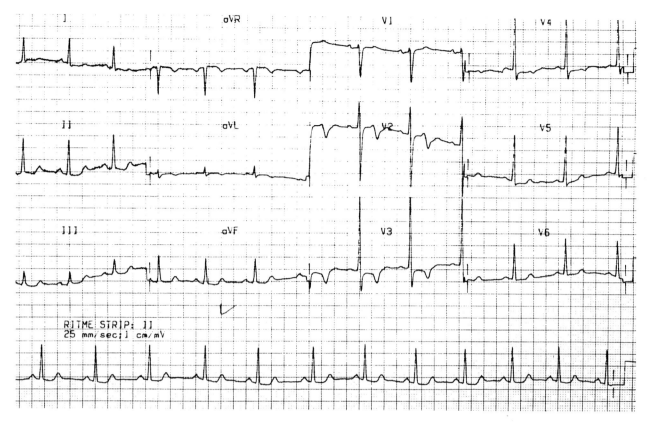

Fig. 12-7. ECG of a 51-year-old man in whom thallium scintigraphy was normal and whose angiogram showed only minor abnormalities (Fig. 11-8).

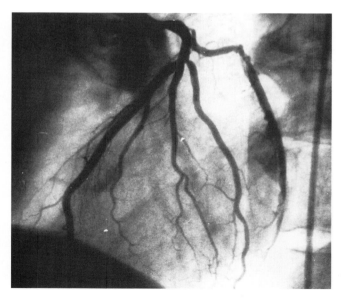

Fig. 12-8. Angiogram of the left coronary artery of the patient from Figure 12-7. This LAO 45/20 was the only one that raised concern as to the left anterior descending artery and both diagonal branches. See text.

coronary artery is obtained, and collateral flow is neglected.

Doppler velocimetry is easily and safely to performed at present, as repeatedly demonstrated by Kern and co-workers[5,28] and by Serruys and Di Mario and their colleagues,[29] using crystal-mounted guidewires. It shares, however, the disadvantages of videodensitometry in that it provides an index of coronary flow alone without taking into account the collateral contribution. Moreover, data must be interpreted on an empirical basis, and a sound scientific explanation for why, for example, the proximal-to-distal flow ratios should be useful is still disputable. In addition, videodensitometry and Doppler velocimetry are strongly dependent on changes in blood pressure, and normal values are not circumscript.

Pressure-derived assessment of FFR is easy, safe, and rapidly performed. It is supported by a sound theoretical scientific basis and, of all the current methods, it has been best validated in both animal and human studies.[7-12] Unlike the other methods, it is not dependent on pressure and heart rate changes, and a clear range of normal and pathologic values is known. In a diagnostic procedure, it provides infor-

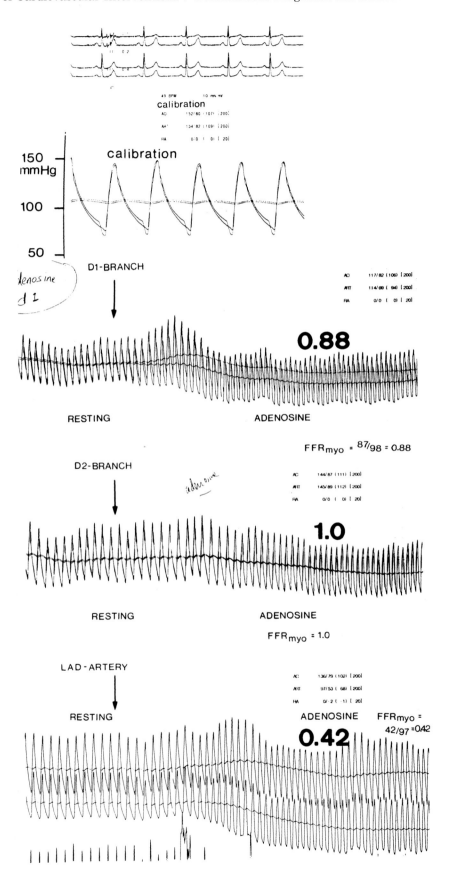

mation on myocardial perfusion, including the collaterals. Therefore, in the diagnostic situation Doppler velocimetry and pressure measurements are complementary by assessing coronary flow and myocardial flow, respectively. In the interventional situation, the pressure-flow equations are superior to both other methods in giving a complete insight into coronary, myocardial, and collateral flow both before and after PTCA. The advantages of FFR_{myo} may be summarized as follows:

- Based upon firm scientific background
- Well-validated in animals and humans
- Independent of changes in pressure and heart rate
- Normal value (1.0) identical in every coronary artery, in every patient, and at every hemodynamic state
- Clear cut-off point between normal and pathologic values (0.70 to 0.75)
- Includes contribution of collateral circulation
- Applicable in multivessel disease
- Applicable in both diagnostic and interventional procedures
- Easily and rapidly obtained by pressure recordings at maximum hyperemia
- If right atrial pressure is not elevated, then

$$FFR_{myo} = P_d/P_a$$

which gives a *superior index of functional stenosis severity*.

For the time being, the fiberoptic wire has some technical disadvantages and limitations that need further improvement. The most important points are that its steerability and torquability should be improved and made comparable to regular PTCA guidewires. The present wire is sometimes hard to manipulate in tortuous vessels and bifurcations. For an interventional cardiologist this will not be a large problem and if necessary the wire can be used in connection with a balloon catheter with an exchangeable guidewire to ensure proper placement within the coronary artery. However, to make it safely available for diagnostic use outside an interventional laboratory, these characteristics need further improvement. Moreover, the diameter should be decreased to 0.014″ to make it suitable for simultaneous use

with all present balloon catheters. These improvements are expected to be accomplished at the end of 1994.

CLINICAL IMPLICATIONS, CONCLUDING REMARKS, AND FUTURE DEVELOPMENTS

Patients with ischemic heart disease are limited in their activity as soon as the maximum amount of blood flowing to their myocardium is no longer sufficient to provide an adequate amount of oxygen and a substrate to maintain cardiac function. Therefore the best parameter for reflecting the functional status of a coronary artery is the maximum achievable amount of blood that can flow through that artery or to its depending myocardium. In our studies, maximum flow in the presence of a stenosis is related to normal maximal flow, resulting in the FFR concept, which has considerable advantages compared with CFR and RFR (Table 12-1).

From the theory and studies described in this chapter, we see that maximum coronary and myocardial blood flow can be determined by the pressure-flow equations during PTCA just by performing the correct pressure measurements under vasodilated circumstances, using a tiny pressure-monitoring guidewire for distal coronary pressure recording. The measurements can be performed safely, easily, and rapidly in a conscious human in the catheterization laboratory. The calculations are highly accurate and superior to anatomic data if compared with positron emission tomography as a standard for myocardial flow assessment in humans.[9,30] To calculate flow reserve from pressure measurements, no expensive equipment is needed, and the complete procedure is prolonged by only a few minutes. Moreover, the separate contributions of coronary and collateral blood flow to total myocardial flow can be assessed. Because this method only uses pressures as an end point without concern for how these pressures are generated, most physiologic phenomenon affecting other methods for flow assessment are already accounted for because these phenomena are reflected by their influence on pressure.

The definitive value of this method must be investigated further, but studies being performed in our laboratories indicate that the threshold value of

Fig. 12-9. Pressure recordings during intravenous adenosine-induced hyperemia in the ascending aorta and the three different branches of the patient seen in Figures 11-7 and 11-8. It is easy to see that the FFR_{myo} supplied by both diagonal branches is (almost) normal, whereas the FFR_{myo} of the LAD distribution is severely decreased.

FFR_{myo} for indicating or excluding inducible ischemia is approximately 0.75. Additional confirmation studies in humans are warranted. As far as collateral flow is involved, methodology is limited because no standard exists for collateral flow assessment in a conscious human. Our initial results, however, provide strong indirect evidence for the correctness and applicability of our equation for collateral flow calculation. For diagnostic catheterization, FFR_{cor} and collateral blood flow cannot be separately calculated because knowledge of P_w is necessary for calculation of those two parameters. However, FFR_{myo} can be easily determined, also in diagnostic studies, by simply crossing a stenosis with the pressure-monitoring guidewire and a single administration of a maximum hyperemic stimulus (Example 3, 5, and 6). Pressure-derived functional stenosis assessment can be especially useful in intermediate stenosis and in the post-PTCA setting, where the limitations of the coronary arteriogram are most pronounced. It can also help in a better understanding of data obtained by newer techniques such as angioscopy and intravascular ultrasound imaging. Finally it has been hypothesized that some patients with early restenosis (notwithstanding an apparently satisfactory anatomic result) never had adequate functional improvement. Using pressure recordings, further functional improvement at the initial PTCA could be possible in those patients and the restenosis rate accordingly decreased.

REFERENCES

1. Gould KL, Kirkeeide RL, Buchi M. Coronary flow reserve as a physiologic measure of stenosis severity. J Am Coll Cardiol 1990;15:459–474
2. Pijls NHJ. pp. 27–37. Maximal Myocardial Perfusion as a Measure of the Functional Significance of Coronary Artery Disease. Kluwer Academic Publishers, Dordrecht, 1991
3. Gould KL. Identifying and measuring severity of coronary artery stenosis. Quantitative coronary arteriography and positron emission tomography. Circulation 1988;78:237–245
4. Kirkeeide RL, Gould KL, Parsel L. Assessment of coronary stenoses by myocardial perfusion during pharmacologic coronary vasodilation. VIII. Validation of coronary flow reserve as a single integrated functional measure of stenosis severity reflecting all its geometric dimensions. J Am Coll Cardiol 1986;7:103–113
5. Ofili EO, Labovitz J, Kern MJ. Coronary flow velocity dynamics in normal and diseased arteries. Am J Cardiol 1993;71:3D–9D
6. Pijls NHJ. pp. 109–139. Maximal myocardial perfusion as a measure of the functional significance of coronary artery disease. Kluwer Academic Publishers, Dordrecht, 1991
7. Pijls NHJ, Van Son JAM, Kirkeeide RL, De Bruyne B, Gould KL. Experimental basis of determining maximum coronary, myocardial, and collateral blood flow by pressure measurements for assessing functional stenosis severity before and after percutaneous transluminal coronary angioplasty. Circulation 1993;87:1354–1367
8. De Bruyne B, Pijls NHJ, Paulus WJ et al. Transstenotic coronary pressure gradient measurement in humans: in vitro and in vivo evaluation of a new pressure monitoring angioplasty guide wire. J Am Coll Cardiol 1993;22:119–126
9. De Bruyne B, Baudhuin T, Melin JA et al. Coronary flow reserve calculated from pressure measurements in man. Validation with positron emission tomography. Circulation 1994;89:1013–1022
10. Pijls NHJ, De Bruyne B, El Gamal MIH. Revival of pressure measurements. pp. 15.1–15.20. In Topol EJ, Serruys PW (eds): Current Review of Interventional Cardiology 1994. Current Medicine, Philadelphia, 1994
11. Pijls NHJ, De Bruyne B, El Gamal M et al. Fractional flow reserve: the ideal parameter for evaluation of coronary, myocardial and collateral blood flow by pressure measurements at PTCA. J Interv Cardiol 1993;6:331–344
12. Pijls NHJ, Bech GJW, De Bruyne B et al. Quantitative assessment of recruitable collateral blood flow by intracoronary pressure measurements at PTCA. Circulation 1993;88:I–650
13. Anderson HV, Roubin GS, Leimgruber PP et al. Measurement of transstenotic pressure gradient during percutaneous transluminal coronary angioplasty. Circulation 1986;73:1223–1230
14. Rothman MT, Baim DS, Simpson JB, Harrison DC. Coronary hemodynamics during percutaneous transluminal coronary angioplasty. Am J Cardiol 1982;49:1615–1622
15. Chokshi SK, Meyers S, Abi-Mansour P. Percutaneous transluminal coronary angioplasty: ten years' experience. Prog Cardiovasc Dis 1987;30:147–210
16. MacIsaac HC, Knudtson ML, Robinson VJ, Manyari DE. Is the residual translesional pressure gradient useful to predict regional myocardial perfusion after percutaneous transluminal coronary angioplasty? Am Heart J 1989;117:783–790
17. Pijls NHJ, Aengevaeren WRM, Uijen GJH et al. Concept of maximal flow ratio for immediate evaluation of percutaneous transluminal coronary angioplasty result by videodensitometry. Circulation 1991;83:854–865
18. Nissen SE, Gurley JC. Assessment of the functional significance of coronary stenoses. Is digital angiography the answer? Circulation 1990;81:1431–1435
19. Pijls NHJ, Uijen GJH, Hoevelaken A et al. Mean transit time for the assessment of myocardial perfusion by videodensitometry. Circulation 1990;81:1331–1340
20. Meier B, Luethy P, Finci L et al. Coronary wedge pressure in relation to spontaneously visible and recruitable collaterals. Circulation 1987;75:906–913
21. Gould KL, Lipscomb K, Hamilton GW. Physiologic basis for assessing critical coronary stenosis. Instantaneous flow response and regional distribution during coronary hyperemia as measures of coronary flow reserve. Am J Cardiol 1974;33:87–94

22. Gould KL. Functional measures of coronary stenosis severity at cardiac catheterization. J Am Coll Cardiol 1990;16:198–199
23. Hoffman JIE. Maximal coronary flow and the concept of coronary vascular reserve. Circulation 1984;70: 153–159
24. Klocke FJ. Measurements of coronary flow reserve: defining pathophysiology versus making decisions about patient care. Circulation 1987;76:1183–1189
25. Serruys PW, Wijns W, Reiber JHC et al. Values and limitations of transstenotic pressure gradients measured during percutaneous transluminal coronary angioplasty. Herz 1985;10:337–342
26. Gould KL. Pressure-flow characteristics of coronary stenoses in unsedated dogs at rest and during coronary vasodilation. Circ Res 1978;43:242–253
27. Hess OM, McGillem MJ, De Boe SF et al. Determination of coronary flow reserve by parametric imaging. Circulation 1990;82:1438–1448
28. Kern MJ, Donohue TJ, Aguirre FV et al. Assessment of angiographically intermediate coronary artery stenosis using the Doppler Flowire. Am J Cardiol 1993; 71:26D–33D
29. Di Mario C, Menevaeu N, Gil R et al. Maximal blood flow velocity in severe coronary stenoses measured with a Doppler guidewire. Am J Cardiol 1993;71: 54D–61D
30. Bol A, Melin JA, Vanoverschelde JL et al. Direct comparison of N^{13}-ammonia and O^{15}-water estimates of perfusion with quantification of regional myocardial blood flow by microspheres. Circulation 1993;87: 512–525

lems of acute occlusion and late coronary stenosis. Four to 6% of all angioplasty procedures are complicated by acute coronary occlusion or threatened acute occlusion. Half of these patients require repeat angioplasty or emergency bypass surgery, suffer myocardial infarction, or (less commonly) die. Late coronary restenosis at the site of angioplasty was re-

is a factor in determining intra-arterial pressure, transmission of the pressure pulse, and rheologic characteristics of the vessel. The mechanical characteristics of blood vessels depend on both passive and active tissue components present in the arterial wall.[2] The passive components comprise the fibrous connective tissues, including elastin, collagen, glycosoaminoglycan ground substance, and the water content of the tissues. The smooth muscle cells represent the active tissues present in the blood vessel wall determining the mechanical characteristics. Smooth muscle cell tone is affected by the sympathetic nervous system and by various pharmacologic agents. This in turn imparts variability in vessel diameter and tone under physiologic stimuli.

In the coronary arteries, as in all arterial structures, the principal elastic property is imparted by the elastin present in the internal and external elastic laminae. Elastin is a unique protein containing proline- and glycine-rich helical regions that stretch easily. Furthermore, the elastic fibers are arranged in such a fashion that they are displaced longitudinally relative to each other at very low stresses and allow an increase in linear length of up to 300% without rupture. Elastin has a tensile modulus of about 750 mmHg and mechanically behaves in a similar fashion to a linear elastic material like rubber. The other important determinants of the elastic properties are collagen fibers, which, in contrast to elastin, are stiffer and have a tensile modulus of 3.7×10^6 mmHg, which is several thousand times higher than elastin.[3] Thus, collagen imparts rigidity to the arterial structure. With age, the elastin content decreases, whereas collagen increases in human arteries, partially explaining the increased vascular stiffness with age.

The presence of atherosclerosis decreases the elasticity and compliance of the artery by contributing relatively rigid fibrous tissue and a varying amount of calcium. Similarly, restenotic lesions, because of their higher smooth muscle cell content, are relatively rigid.

MECHANICAL PROPERTIES OF LARGE CORONARY ARTERIES

Mechanically, the arteries behave as orthotropic, cylindrical bodies in which all net strains are oriented along the three different axes, namely, the longitudinal axis (along the length of the artery), the radial axis (the outward distentional forces), and the circumferential axis (Fig. 13-1). The forces acting in the arterial wall are represented by *stress*, which is the force acting on the surface per unit area.

$$\text{stress} = \text{force/area}$$

Circumferential wall stress is defined by the equation

$$\text{wall stress} = P \times R/Th$$

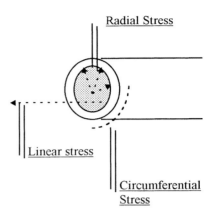

Fig. 13-1. Directions of stress on the arterial wall. Linear stress, tending to elongate the artery; radial stress, due to a force directed from center to circumference of the artery; and circumferential stress, tending to stretch the arterial wall.

where P is the distending pressure, R is the lumen radius, and Th is the wall thickness. This force may be external or compressive, may be applied intraluminally in a radial direction as distention force, or may be applied parallel to the internal surface (called *shear stress*). Radial distention force as applied by the mean arterial blood pressure or intracoronary angioplasty balloon is balanced by the circumferential tensile stress in the vessel wall. Any stress applied to the vessel wall may be counterbalanced by the circumferential tensile stress generated in the walls. When the applied force exceeds the tensile stress, in deformation or distention of the vessel wall results, producing *strain*. Strain is defined as the change in the length of a material upon application of force and is usually expressed as a percent or fraction of the initial length. The relationship between stress and strain is described by the elastic modulus (E), or DeYoung's modulus, as:

$$E = \text{stress/strain}$$

The elastic modulus may be constant and is called linear elastic behavior, or the relationship between stress and strain may become nonlinear with increasing application of force and is then described as nonlinear mechanical behavior.[3] Most biologic materials, including arterial wall, exhibit nonlinear mechanical behavior such that, with application of increasing stress forces, there is a decreasing amount of strain. In other words, the material becomes stiffer as larger forces are applied.

Compliance is defined as change in volume per unit change in the pressure. When dealing with arteries, the volume may be replaced by the cross-sec-

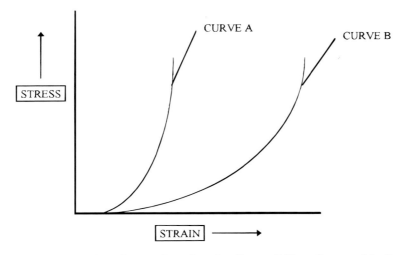

Fig. 13-2. Compliance curves. Compliance describes the distensibility of a vessel in the circumferential direction. It is obtained by measuring the degree of strain or stretch produced over a range of stress or pressure. Curve A reflects a relatively noncompliant vessel, and curve B represents a more compliant vessel.

tional area and compliance, defined as the fractional increase in the diameter per unit increase in the intraluminal pressure.[2] Thus compliance describes the distensibility of a vessel in the circumferential direction. It is an easily derived parameter and is independent of wall thickness. Due to the nonlinear elastic properties of arterial wall, arterial compliance varies with intraluminal pressure. When arterial compliance is measured over a range of pressures, a curve of compliance versus pressure can be obtained (Fig. 13-2). Compliance expressed as a fraction of baseline volume corrects for the vessel size. This characterization can enable more meaningful comparison of different vessels.

$$C = \Delta V/\Delta P$$

or compliance can be expressed as diameter change or percent diameter change per unit of pressure, which is a measure of arterial distensibility.

$$C = [\Delta D/(Ddia \times \Delta P)] \times 100$$

where C is compliance, ΔV change in volume, ΔP change in pressure, ΔD change in diameter, and Ddia diastolic diameter. Dynamic compliance is measured when oscillating pressure changes are superimposed on a baseline distention pressure, as is seen in systemic arterial circulation or coronary arteries.

Upon application of a force or stress, a material may or may not revert to its original dimension on removal of the applied force. If it does, the material is considered *elastic,* and the deformation is considered elastic deformation; if it doesn't, the material is said

to exhibit plastic deformation. Most elastic materials, when subjected to a high level of stress, distend or deform with elastic properties until they reach the point when a further increase in applied force results in permanent change and they do not return to their normal state. This is known as *yield stress.*

Most biologic tissues exhibit a form of elasticity whereby application of a constant tensile force or stress results in a gradually progressive increase in deformity over a period of time until a new mechanical balance is achieved. This is described as *viscoelasticity* of the material. Two other physical properties pertaining to the vessel wall and its mechanics are important for interventional cardiologists, namely, recoil and creep. *Recoil,* sometimes referred to as elastic recoil, is a property of elastic tissues when they return to their original shape or form after removing the deforming stress. By definition, the recoil is instantaneous, or elastic. However, in most biologic tissues, including the arterial wall, the process of recoil is gradual and time dependent and is then referred to as *creep*[2,3] (Fig. 13-3).

EXPERIMENTAL BACKGROUND

The compliance of epicardial coronary arteries was first measured in isolation by Gregg et al.[4] in 1935 using an isolated canine coronary artery segment. These investigators injected lycopodium spores into the coronary arteries of dogs to plug the small arteries; they then studied the static pressure volume characteristics of the anterior descending coronary artery by infusing mercury at different pressures.

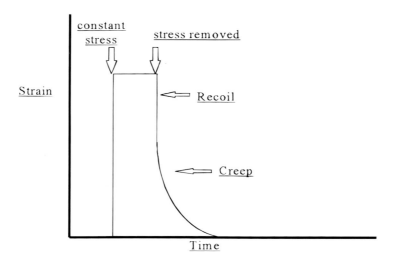

Fig. 13-3. Recoil and creep. Once a force tending to stretch a vessel is removed, the elastic components of the wall attempt to restore the original dimension. Recoil refers to the more rapid return of the vessel to its original configuration. Most biologic tissues, however, recoil more gradually, a phenomenon referred to as creep.

They estimated compliance to be 1×10^{-3} ml/mmHg^{-1}. Patel et al.[5] reported the static elastic properties of the left coronary circumflex artery and the common carotid artery in dogs in 1970. Stepwise increased perfusion pressure in the isolated arterial segments resulted in increased external vascular diameter, which was measured on the microscopic scale, and elasticity and compliance were thereby calculated. They measured compliance at 0.5×10^{-3} ml/mmHg^{-1}. In 1961, Bergel[6,7] reported on the static and dynamic elastic properties of the arterial wall. For static arterial elasticity segments of the aorta, femoral artery, and carotid artery taken from dogs within 2 hours of death were used. The segments were subjected to stepwise incremental pressures from 0 to 240 mmHg at 20-mm steps and the diameter measured with a collimated light beam and a photomultiplier tube. It was demonstrated that the vessel wall became progressively less extensible with increasing pressures. The dynamic elastic properties were also studied by using a similar preparation in which a constant pressure of 100 mmHg was maintained, on which superimposed oscillations of 5 to 10 mmHg of pressure were made.

In 1970 Douglas and Greenfield[8] reported on epicardial coronary artery compliance in an in situ canine model. Intramyocardial portions of the circulation were occluded by injecting a mixture of 200 μm glass beads in liquid silicone. Saline infusion was perfused to provide a stepwise incremental pressure with superimposed injections of 1.0 ml of saline at a rate of 30 pulses/min. Pressure in the system was monitored continuously, and static radiographs with

dye injections were taken. The results indicated that dynamic compliance decreases as the distending pressure rises. Calculated dynamic compliance was 0.7×10^{-3} ml/mmHg^{-1}. In 1981 Klassen and Wong[9] reported on the arterial compliance for canine coronary arteries. They invasively measured the coronary arterial pressure and flow (radioactive microspheres) in an anesthetized open chest dog model using controlled conditions, left stellate ganglion stimulation, dipyridamole intracoronary injection, and glutaraldehyde perivascular injection. The reported average values were 0.21×10^{-3} ml/mmHg^{-1} in the control group.

Several other investigators have attempted to measure compliance in animal coronary arteries. Noninvasive assessment of compliance has also been described using externally applied strain gauges and ultrasonic crystals. All these experiments were complicated because measurement of compliance required either ex vivo experimentation or, at least, dissection, isolation, and exposure of the artery. These changes per se affect arterial compliance. The differing values reported reflect the different preparations used. These were nonatherosclerotic vessels, and compliance measurements were done at physiologic pressures only.

IN VIVO COMPLIANCE ESTIMATION

All the above animal studies suffer from the basic lack of reproducibility and practical application in the human in vivo models. Despite extensive experience with intracoronary manipulation of various devices, data are scarce on invasive evaluation of intracoronary compliance in humans. Some potential and established methods for in vivo measurement of compliance in human coronary arteries are described below.

Absolute Induction Angiometer

A device used to evaluate intravascular elasticity and compliance, the angiometer consists of two loops (primary and secondary) of a resilient beryllium copper wire pair insulated with barium sulfate-impregnated polyurethane varnish.[10] The loops are connected to wires that run through a probe. One of the loops carries an alternating current and acts as a primary transformer, while the second loop acts as a secondary transformer in which the primary current induces an alternating electromotive force that constitutes the angiometer signal. Upon introduction into the target vessel, the loops expand until the sides contact the inner vessel wall and the vascular movements are followed as the vessel contracts and expands. Measurements of the secondary loop voltage permit determination of the absolute value of the vascular diameter and its changes. The loop's signal is amplified by a phase amplifier connected to a recorder. The sensitivity is high enough to detect variations of a few microns in a vessel comparable to canine aorta. This system has been used to estimate compliance and elasticity in peripheral vessels and vascular grafts. No human coronary studies have thus far been performed with the system.

Angioplasty Balloons for Compliance Evaluation

In 1987 Jain et al.[11] reported on a series of elegant experiments using a percutaneous transluminal coronary angioplasty (PTCA) balloon to characterize the process of vascular dilation in vivo and to plot the pressure volume changes in the angioplasty balloon during inflation within a stenosis. They utilized an inflation syringe attached to the balloon port through a three-way connector. The plunger of the syringe was connected to a linear displacement transducer, providing a high-resolution indication of the plunger position and thus the fluid volume transmitted to the balloon. An electronic pressure transducer was attached to the system through the three-way connector for continuous pressure monitoring of the balloon catheter system, and a rotary crank was used to obtain smooth inflation pressures. The pressure

volume signals were displayed on an X-Y storage oscilloscope (Fig. 13-4). The authors initially performed several in vitro studies utilizing a 1:1 solution of normal saline solution with the coronary dye used to inflate the balloon. A polyethylene coronary angioplasty balloon (ACS) was used for in vitro tests and patient studies. The in vitro experiments included expansion of the balloon in Silastic tubing, Styrofoam, and dry, hollow macaroni, representing three forms of mechanical behavior (i.e., stretching, compaction, and cracking, respectively). A series of balloon inflations were performed in 3- to 10-mm segments of these materials, and pressure volume curves were obtained. In vivo studies were done in 46 patients undergoing PTCA. Control curves were obtained by inflating the balloons in open air before and after the angioplasty. The control curves for individual balloons were reproducible over multiple inflations, indicating that the behavior of the balloon and the recording system were stable. The results of the in vitro experiments showed three distinct patterns of inflation characteristic of the compliance and elasticity of the three materials used for in vitro testing. Silastic tubing showed a leftward displacement of the curve at the lower pressures, but at the higher pressures it was nearly superimposed over the control curve. This represented the elastic behavior. The inflation of the balloon embedded in a piece of Styrofoam showed an initial deviation of the curve to the left caused by the constraint of the balloon by Styrofoam. Increasing pressures and compaction of the surrounding Styrofoam resulted in an abrupt shift of the curve to the right and superimposition on the control curve for the remainder of the inflation. Inflation of the balloon in hollow, dry macaroni resulted in a distinct pattern: at low pressures the curve was shifted to the left of the control curve, as seen with rigid tubing. When cracking occurred the pressure fell abruptly, creating a notch and a rightward shift in the curve, which was then superimposed on the control curve (Fig. 13-5).

In vivo conduction of these experiments in humans during PTCA showed that 56% of the lesions exhibited a pressure-volume relationship compatible with stretching, 27% showed the compaction pattern, and only 17% showed cracking. Lesions manifesting a stretching pattern tended to be longer and had calcific deposits, as seen on the cineangiogram. Lesions exhibiting predominantly a compaction pattern tended to be shorter, and only 17% had visible calcium deposits. The compaction pattern was most evident during the first inflation, and subsequent inflations tended to superimpose on the control curve. Of the eight lesions that showed a pattern consistent with cracking, six had angiographic evidence of dis-

balloon pressure. Pressure volume coordinates at each 0.1-ml increment in volume were used to plot pressure-volume curves for each inflation. Before dilation, each balloon catheter was inflated up to 10 atm at least seven times, with and without radiofrequency heating, to obtain superimposable curves. This pressure-volume curve measured the intrinsic compliance of the balloon material and served as a control. The results showed that heating caused an immediate increase in arterial compliance in the dilated segment, and the pressure-volume curves obtained at 60°C were shifted rightward in comparison to curves obtained from nonheated inflations of the contralateral vessel. The radiofrequency-heated inflations increased luminal cross-sectional area by 80 to 146% more than nonheated inflations. They performed histologic examinations that revealed increased thinning and compression of the arterial wall, with some variable medial smooth muscle necrosis and straightening of elastic tissue fibers in comparison with nonheated controls. Although these were nonatherosclerotic and nonstenosed vessels, the increase in compliance obtained translated into an improved dilation by the experimental device. This may have clinical relevance and shows how evaluation of the mechanical properties may help to improve the results of the procedure.

Ultrasound Methods

With the advent of ultrasound and echocardiography it became possible to measure the arterial dimensions and thickness of arteries noninvasively. Measurement of compliance for large peripheral arteries, including femoral and carotid arteries, as well as aortic compliance, has been done by various investigators using ultrasound to measure vessel diameters and dimensions with simultaneous invasive measurement of the arterial filling pressure.[14–17]

In 1986 Megerman et al.[18] used a pulsed ultrasound echo tracking device to measure the arterial dimensions noninvasively over a wide range of pressures. Nonlinear compliance curves were obtained from the femoral arteries of dogs. They used controlled hemorrhage, nitroprusside, halothane anesthesia, and norepinephrine to vary the systemic pressures. They also studied the arterial segment in vivo before and after surgical exposure and demonstrated its effect on the calculated compliance. The compliance curves obtained with bleeding induced hypotension, halothane, nitroprusside, or norepinephrine were similar regardless of the method utilized to alter the perfusion pressure. The pressure compliance curves showed nonlinear progression, as previously described for other models.

High-frequency intravascular ultrasound (IVUS) provides high-quality tomographic images of the coronary artery lumen, atherosclerotic plaque, vessel wall, and total vessel area.[19] Several studies have documented its validity for measurement of lumen area, plaque area and morphology, and external elastic lamina area. Changes in arterial diameter with pulse pressure can be measured and compliance estimated. Botas et al.[20] used quantitative coronary angiography and IVUS before and after angioplasty to measure segmental coronary distensibility. IVUS-acquired images were used to calculate the largest (systolic) and smallest (diastolic) lumen areas during cardiac cycle. A distensibility index was calculated as follows:

$$\text{distensibility index} = (\Delta \text{ lumen/diastolic lumen}) \times 100$$

They showed that distensibility index improved with angioplasty. Reddy et al.[20a] reported a lumen change during the cardiac cycle of 14% in normal and 4% in diseased coronary segments. Hansen et al.[21] recently reported the use of IVUS to estimate in vivo compliance of common and external iliac arteries. They measured diameter changes with systolic and diastolic blood pressure and expressed compliance as diameter change/100 mmHg, as follows:

$$C = (\Delta D/D \text{dia} \times \Delta P) \times 10^4$$

where ΔD is change in diameter, Ddia is diastolic diameter, and ΔP is the change in blood pressure. These reports are exciting because standardization and validation of IVUS for compliance assessment may lead to further insight and understanding of the mechanism and effects of various interventional devices in the future.

PRACTICAL CONSIDERATIONS

Most invasive cardiologists encounter many of the physical and mechanical properties of coronary vessels during procedures in the catheterization laboratory. It is a common fact that arterial diameter changes with the systolic and diastolic pressures, with a physiologic pulse pressure of only 40 to 80 mmHg. However, further distention of arterial lumen size during angioplasty requires several atmospheres of pressure, which are much greater than mean or peak arterial pressures. This is a manifestation of the nonlinear compliance in which arterial stiffness increases at increasing diameters. Presence of yield stress is often noted when progressive increase in the angioplasty balloon diameter results in a sudden increase in the arterial diameter that does not revert to its original narrowing once the balloon is deflated. Viscoelasticity is seen when prolonged inflation at a fixed pressure is utilized for resistant arterial stenosis and a delayed, time-dependent improvement of stenosis severity is seen over a period of several minutes. The prolonged stress allows vessel wall strains to increase gradually until the critical fracture point or yield stress is reached. Similarly, several studies on angioplasty subjects show that the immediate postangioplasty vessel diameter is often less than the maximal diameter obtained by the angioplasty balloon during the final inflation, the difference representing the elastic recoil. The presence of gradual recoil over the next 24 hours to several days has variably been shown in some studies and is a manifestation of the creep phenomenon.

In diseased, atherosclerotic arteries, compliance varies not only in different parts of the vessel but may also differ at different points along the circumference of the stenotic segment. Lesion compliance depends on geometry as well as the composition of the atherosclerotic plaque. Thus a long-standing fibrocalcific lesion is rigid, noncompliant, and noncompressible. It is more likely to fracture or dissect rather than stretch or compress, when subjected to high inflation pressures. The relatively acute lesions seen in unstable angina or acute myocardial infarction are usually soft, bulky, and easy to compress with stretching of underlying media.

Differential compliance is often encountered in eccentric lesions when balloon dilation results in distention of the more compliant, relatively disease-free arc of the circumference, with little impact on the plaque itself. Upon balloon deflation, the greater recoil of the relatively compliant segment results in rapid loss of the lumen gained. The difference in compliance within the lesion is reflected in the pathologic studies showing that plaque rupture and dissections frequently occur at the junction of the plaque with the normal vessel wall. Because of nonhomogeneous compliance, large, eccentric bulky lesions appear to be best treated with directional atherectomy, which allows debulking of the lesion. Similarly, in tight, heavily calcified lesions, due to very poor compliance, balloon dilation alone often leads to unsatisfactory results. Rotational atherectomy in these lesions selectively pulverizes the hard noncompliant components of the plaque into particles less than 30 μm in size.[22] Both directional and rotational atherectomy debulk the lesion, releasing the media from the cicatrizing effects of the plaque. Adjunctive balloon dilation can then be performed on a relatively more compliant residual lesion to obtain an optimal result.

The operative compliance during the angioplasty procedure is the net effect of the balloon and the lesion compliance together. Angioplasty balloons are available in different materials with differing properties. Polyterphthelate (PTP) and polyethelene (PE) balloons are noncompliant, polyvinylchloride (PVC) balloons have intermediate compliance, and polyolefincopolymer (POC) balloons are compliant.[23,24] Although two retrospective studies showed no difference in outcome using different balloon types, lesion-dependent choice of balloon and operator bias cannot be fully excluded.[23,25] Jain et al.[24] demonstrated a linear $\Delta D/\Delta P$ relationship in PVC and PE balloons over 1 to 10 atm pressures. However, PE balloons reached the specified diameter at 5 atm, and PVC balloons reached specified diameter at 10 atm. At any given pressure, the diameter for PVC balloons was higher than for PE balloons.

The differing balloon compliances can be exploited to interact optimally with the anticipated lesion compliance. A compliant balloon at low pressures may be sufficient for a soft lesion. On the other hand, an old calcific lesion may require much higher pressures (10 to 18 atm). If a compliant balloon is used, plaque fracture and sudden yield with uncontrolled balloon expansion may lead to an adverse outcome. A noncompliant balloon in this situation would allow the operator to use high pressures with more controlled expansion. Similarly, after intracoronary stent deployment, noncompliant balloons at high pressures may be used to obtain maximum stent expansion.

Coronary stents, when deployed, change the segmental compliance. The decrease in compliance would vary depending on the type of stent used. The compliance mismatch between the stented and the adjacent segments can potentially alter the rheology of the vessel and create abnormal shear forces. The additional rigidity provided by the stents makes the dilation of a diseased segment much more predictable and controllable.

SUMMARY

Mechanical properties of the coronary arteries generally and the target lesion specifically are of paramount importance to the invasive cardiologist. Compliance can be determined invasively, but its accurate measurement is tedious and cumbersome. Understanding of vascular mechanics, knowledge of disease pathology, and careful, meticulous attention to detail during the review of coronary angiograms can enable the discerning cardiologist to make reasonable estimates. Such an understanding will lead to a better planned revascularization strategy, a rational choice of the devices used, and anticipation of possible complications. Further experience with IVUS and use of novel devices combined with or incorporated in the interventional devices may make it possible to assess compliance during the procedure.

REFERENCES

1. Hoffman JI, Spaan JA. Pressure-flow relations in coronary circulation. Physiol Rev 1990;70:331–390
2. Dobrin PB. Mechanical properties of arteries. Physiol Rev 1978;58:397–459
3. Lee RT, Kamm RD. Vascular mechanics for the cardiologist. J Am Coll Cardiol 1994;23:1289–1295
4. Gregg DE, Green HD, Wiggers CJ. Phasic variations in peripheral coronary resistance and their determinants. Am J Physiol 1935;115:362–373
5. Patel DJ, Janicki J. Static elastic properties of the left coronary circumflex artery and the common carotid artery in dogs. Circ Res 1970;27:149–158
6. Bergel DH. The static elastic properties of the arterial wall. J Physiol 1961;156:445–457
7. Bergel DH. The dynamic elastic properties of the arterial wall. J Physiol 1961;156:458–469
8. Douglas JE, Greenfield JC, Jr. Epicardial coronary artery compliance in the dog. Circ Res 1970;27:921–929
9. Klassen GA, Wong AY. Coronary artery compliance in the dog. Can J Physiol Pharmacol 1982;60:942–951
10. Kaolin A. Absolute induction angiometer. Blood Vessels 1980;17:61–77
11. Jain A, Demer LL, Raizner AE et al. In vivo assessment of vascular dilatation during percutaneous transluminal coronary angioplasty. Am J Cardiol 1987;60:988–992
12. Hjemdahl-Monsen CE, Ambrose JA, Borrico S et al. Angiographic patterns of balloon inflation during percutaneous transluminal coronary angioplasty: role of pressure-diameter curves in studying distensibilty and elasticity of the stenotic lesion and the mechanism of dilatation. J Am Coll Cardiol 1990;16:569–575
13. Mitchel JF, Fram DB, Aretz TA et al. Effect of low-grade conductive heating on vascular compliance during in vitro balloon angioplasty. Am Heart J 1994;128: 21–27
14. Buntin CM, Silver FH. Noninvasive assessment of mechanical properties of peripheral arteries. Ann Biomed Eng 1990;18:549–566
15. Gamble G, Zorn J, Sanders G et al. Estimation of arterial stiffness, compliance, and distensibility from M-mode ultrasound measurements of the common carotid artery. Stroke 1994;25:11–16
16. Marcus RH, Korcarz C, McCray G et al. Noninvasive method for determination of arterial compliance using Doppler echocardiography and subclavian pulse tracings. Validation and clinical application of a physiological model of the circulation. Circulation 1994;89: 2688–2699
17. Shankar R, Bond MG. Correlation of noninvasive arterial compliance with anatomic pathology of atherosclerotic nonhuman primates. Atherosclerosis 1990;85: 37–46
18. Megerman J, Hasson JE, Warnock DF et al. Noninvasive measurements of nonlinear arterial elasticity. Am J Physiol 1986;250:H181–H186
19. Potkin BN, Bartorelli AL, Gessert JM et al. Coronary artery imaging with intravascular high frequency ultrasound. Circulation 1990;81:1575–1585
20. Botas J, Clark DA, Pinto F et al. Balloon angioplasty results in increased segmental coronary distensibility: a likely mechanism of percutaneous transluminal coronary angioplasty. J Am Coll Cardiol 1994;23: 1043–1052
20a. Reddy KG, Suneja R, Nail RN et al. Measurement by intracoronary ultrasound of in vivo arterial distensibility within atherosclerotic lesions. Am J Cardiol 1993;72:1232–1237
21. Hansen ME, Yucel EK, Megerman J et al. In vivo determination of human arterial compliance: preliminary investigation of a new technique. Cardiovasc Intervent Radiol 1994;17:22–26
22. Mintz GS, Pichard AD, Popma JJ et al. Preliminary experience with adjunctive directional coronary atherectomy after high-speed rotational atherectomy in the calcific coronary artery disease. Am J Cardiol 1993; 71:799–804
23. Bach RG, Kern MJ, Aguirre FV et al. Effects of percutaneous transluminal coronary angioplasty balloon compliance on angiographic and clinical outcomes. Am J Cardiol 1993;72:904–907
24. Jain A, Demer LL, Raizner AE, Roberts R. Effect of inflation pressures on coronary angioplasty balloons. Am J Cardiol 1986;57:26–28
25. Moony FR, Moony JF, Longe TF, Brandenburg RO. Effect of balloon material on coronary angioplasty. Am J Cardiol 1992;69:1481–1482

14 Cardiopulmonary Bypass Support

Robert A. Vogel

Coronary angioplasty has been increasingly utilized in patients with extensive coronary disease, severe and acute chest pain syndromes, and poor ventricular function.[1-5] This process was facilitated by technical advances, increased operator experience, improved imaging equipment, and use of circulatory support. Although it was unexpected by early investigators, patients with limited coronary disease and good ventricular function rarely experience circulatory collapse during balloon inflation. The same is not true for the increasing numbers of high-risk patients undergoing angioplasty. Perfusion balloons and the intra-aortic balloon pumps were the first techniques employed to support the coronary and systemic circulations, respectively. A closed circuit cardiopulmonary bypass system utilizing femoral cannulation was reported for emergency management of shock, trauma, and hypothermia in 1983.[6] In 1988, our group reported the first elective use of this system for circulatory support of high-risk angioplasty and valvuloplasty patients.[7] The introduction of percutaneous cannulation and standby techniques subsequently led to the increased applicability of this approach.

In comparison with other techniques for circulatory support, such as the intra-aortic balloon pump[8-11] and autoperfusion catheters,[12-14] cardiopulmonary bypass provides the greatest degree of systemic circulatory augmentation, but it is also the most complex and invasive.[15-20] The intra-aortic balloon pump and cardiopulmonary bypass support are compared in Table 14-1. This chapter summarizes the technique of cardiopulmonary bypass in patients undergoing high-risk angioplasty and identifies those circumstances in which prophylactic, standby, and emergency support have been found helpful.

INSTRUMENTATION AND MECHANISM OF ACTION

The cardiopulmonary bypass systems employed (Fig. 14-1). utilize a closed circuit system consisting of, in series, a centrifugal pump, heat exchanger, and membrane oxygenator. It provides 4 to 6 L/min nonpulsatile flow through 17- to 20-F cannulas inserted in the femoral artery and vein.[7,18,20] Unlike the intra-aortic balloon pump, full systemic circulatory support is provided irrespective of intrinsic cardiac output or rhythm.[21,22] Although left ventricular volume and systolic pressure are decreased on bypass, myocardial ischemia distal to balloon occlusion is not reduced, and myocardial lactate production occurs upon placing a patient on bypass even before balloon inflation. The system only minimally unloads the left ventricle, necessitating restoration of sinus rhythm for operation more than a few minutes. In some instances, left ventricular venting via an 8- to 10-F pigtail catheter has been employed during cardiopulmonary bypass.

Techniques

Procedures are performed in the catheterization laboratory by an interventional cardiologist, perfusionist, and technical team using mild sedation and local anesthesia.[7,18,20] Coagulation, blood gases, and

Table 14-1. Comparison of Circulatory Support Devices

	IABP	CPS
Arterial access	10 F	17–20 F
Venous access	No	18–20 F
Augments CO	1 L/min	4–6 L/min
Unloads LV	Min-Mod	Min
Augments CBF	Min-Mod	Min
Rhythm dependent	Yes	No (chart-term)
		Yes (long-term)
Support duration	Days	Hours

Abbreviations: Min, minimal; Mod, moderate; IABP, intra-aortic balloon pump; CPS, cardiopulmonary support; LV, left ventricle; CBF, coronary blood flow.

electrolytes are routinely monitored. Although femoral cannulation was initially performed using surgical cutdown, the more recently developed percutaneous technique[17,18] is associated with lesser morbidity and allows for standby support.[19,20] Iliofemoral angiography is routinely performed prior to cannulation to ensure vessel adequacy. The percutaneous technique utilizes placement of flexible, followed by stiff, guidewires over which progressive vessel dilation

(10, 14 F) is accomplished. Under fluoroscopic guidance, the 18- to 20-F venous cannula is positioned at the right atrial-inferior vena caval junction and the 17- to 19-F arterial cannula in the distal aorta. Activated clotting times are maintained at greater than 400 and 300 seconds for standard and heparin-bonded oxygenators, respectively.

Coronary angioplasty is performed after the initiation of circulatory support. Pump flow is adjusted to reduce pulmonary artery wedge pressure to less than 5 mmHg and maintain mean blood pressure above 70 mmHg (usually 2 to 3 L/min). Fluid administration is frequently found necessary to maintain adequate venous return. Ventricular tachycardia or fibrillation is promptly cardioverted to prevent ventricular dilation. Following successful angioplasty, pump flow is gradually decreased over a few minutes. Cannula removal is accomplished either immediately using surgical closure or percutaneously 4 to 6 hours later following decrease in the activated clotting time to about 240 seconds. In the latter instance, a mechanical groin clamp is used to achieve hemostasis after cannula removal. Progressively lesser clamp pressure is employed over a period of 2 to 6 hours. In approximately 10% of cases, hemostasis cannot be maintained and surgical closure is performed. Other

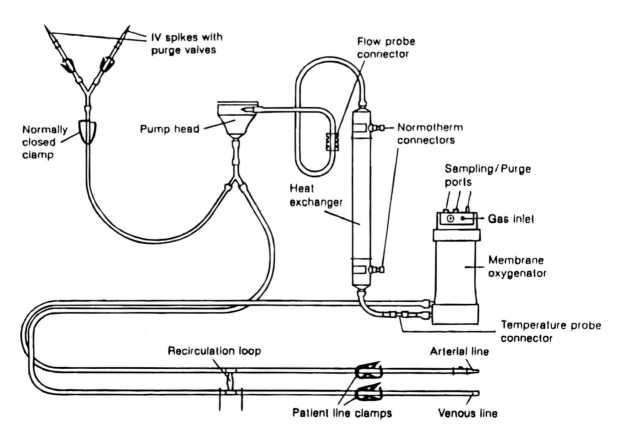

Fig. 14-1. Schematic flow diagram of cardiopulmonary bypass system used with coronary angioplasty.

centers prefer to perform direct surgical closure immediately following the procedure, even if cannulas were placed percutaneously. This allows continued use of heparin. Packed red cells are retrieved from the bypass circuit and returned to the patient.

Standby support has been increasingly employed for high-risk, but not critical, individuals.[19,20] Standby support requires the same teamwork, perfusion expertise, and bypass system availability as does prophylactic support. Iliac angiography is performed, followed by placement of 5-F sheaths in the artery and vein contralateral to the guiding catheter. Pump priming is performed in about half of standby cases. If hemodynamic instability or vessel closure occurs, cannulation and initiation of cardiopulmonary bypass can be initiated in less than 5 minutes in at least 90% of instances. Laboratories performing standby supported angioplasty have found that only 5 to 10% of patients require circulatory support, although it is very difficult to select those who will require it in advance. Emergency initiation of cardiopulmonary support following unexpected protracted circulating collapse or cardiac arrest has also been employed in centers with technical expertise.[15-17]

Most patients sustaining vessel closure during supported angioplasty have not required emergency bypass surgery due to the circulatory stability, which allows time for correction of the coronary occlusion. Those patients requiring surgical bypass can be taken to the operating room on support. Autoperfusion catheters have been found additionally helpful following sustained vessel closure since cardiopulmonary bypass does not augment myocardial perfusion distal to the occluded vessel. As left ventricular venting is used only occasionally, it is important to maintain sinus rhythm to prevent ventricular dilation.

PATIENT POPULATION AND RESULTS

The multicenter experience of 25 centers performing elective supported angioplasty has been collected in a National Registry since March 1988.[19,20,23,24]

Through March 1992, the data on 801 elective procedures have been collated. Patients were considered candidates for prophylactic or standby support if they had severe or unstable angina, a dilatable lesion, and a target vessel supplying more than one-half the residue of viable myocardium or a left ventricular ejection fraction less than 25%. Of the 801 patients, 76% were male, their mean age was 65 years, and 85% had either class III or IV angina. Multivessel disease was present in 90%, left main coronary disease was present in 15%, and dilation of the only patent coronary vessel including bypass grafts was undertaken in 21%.[25-27] Using local criteria, 20% of patients were deemed bypass surgery inoperable. The mean left ventricular ejection fraction was 30%, with 28% of patients having an ejection fraction of 20% or less.

Prophylactic and standby support were undertaken in 73% and 27% of patients, respectively. The characteristics of these two groups of patients were the same except for a higher ejection fraction in the patients undergoing standby support (32.8% versus 28.4%, $P < 0.01$). Angioplasty was undertaken at 1.9 vessel sites/patient, with a primary success rate of 93% (final diameter stenosis less than 50%). Acute myocardial infarction occurred in 0.87%, emergency bypass surgery was required in 2.6% and the hospital mortality rate for the entire group was 6.9%. Only the presence of age more than 70 years and left main coronary disease were associated with increased mortality (12% each). Unexpectedly, patients with ejection fraction of 20% or less, surgical inoperability, and those undergoing dilation of their only patent vessel did not experience significantly higher mortality than the group mean. Table 14-2 lists morbidity and mortality according to the use of percutaneous or cutdown prophylactic support or standby support. In general, the fewest vascular complications and need for transfusions occurred in the standby support group and the most in the cutdown cannulation-prophylactic support. These data raise the question of whether any specific subgroup benefited from prophylactic support. As seen in Table 14-

Table 14-2. National Registry of Elective Supported Angioplasty: Morbidity and Mortality by Technique (%)

	Prophylactic Support (Cutdown) (n = 100)	Prophylactic Support (Percutaneous) (n = 476)	Standby Support (n = 217)
Transfused	69	31	14
Vascular complications	19	15	6.1
Acute myocardial infarction	1.9	0.6	0.9
Emergency bypass surgery	1.9	2.5	3.2
Death	11	6.3	6.0

Table 14-3. National Registry of
Elective Supported Angioplasty:
Mortality by Ejection
Fraction (EF)[a]

	EF ≤20%	EF >20%
Standby support	7/39 (18)	7/178 (3.9)
Prophylactic support	13/187 (7)	28/397 (7.1)
P value	<0.05	NS

[a] Data are number/total, with percent in parentheses.

Table 14-4. Summary of Follow-Up
Data (%)

	Anginal Status NYHA Class III/IV	Mean LVEF	Survival (2-Year)
Pre-PTCA	85	27	
Follow-up	11	36	80

Abbreviations: LVEF, left ventricular, ejection fraction; NYHA, New York Heart Association; PTCA, percutaneous transluminal coronary angioplasty.

3, those with a left ventricular ejection fraction of 20% or less had significantly less hospital mortality when prophylactic support was employed compared with standby support. An opposite trend was observed for those with an ejection fraction of more than 20%. No other subgroup clearly benefited from prophylactic support.

Ninety-one percent of the 217 patients undergoing standby support underwent successful coronary dilation without protracted hypotension or cardiopulmonary arrest (Fig. 14-2). This finding underscores the lack of need for circulatory support in most high-risk patients undergoing coronary angioplasty. Three patients (1.4%) underwent emergency bypass surgery following unsuccessful dilations unassociated with circulatory collapse. Sixteen patients (7.4%) on standby required emergency initiation of bypass support. Of these, support was initiated successfully in 15 cases in less than 5 minutes. Most (75%) of the patients requiring circulatory support underwent successful angioplasty without the need for bypass surgery, of whom seven survived in the long term. Four patients required emergency bypass surgery

following initiation of circulatory support, of whom 2 survived in the long term. These findings suggest that standby support reduces the need for emergency bypass surgery by about two-thirds and reduces the mortality of high-risk angioplasty by about one-half. Although five standby support patients underwent angioplasty on intra-aortic balloon support, the Registry did not attempt to compare or randomize these therapies. Good experience in high-risk patients using intra-aortic balloon support has been reported, but these studies also have not directly compared support therapies.[9,28,29] Moreover, only patients with very poor ventricular function appear to benefit from prophylactic support.

FOLLOW-UP

Follow-up of 527 prophylactic and standby support patients was reported, although this was not an initial goal of the registry. At follow-up, 90% had class I or II angina, and the mean ejection fraction had risen from 27.3 to 35.7% (P <0.05) (Table 14-4). Addi-

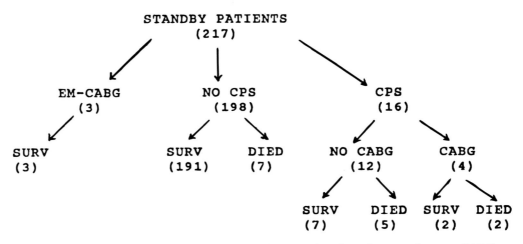

Fig. 14-2. Outcome of 217 patients undergoing standby use of cardiopulmonary bypass. CABG, coronary artery bypass; graft; CPS, cardiopulmonary bypass support, EM, emergency; SURV, survived. Five of the CPS patients received IABP.

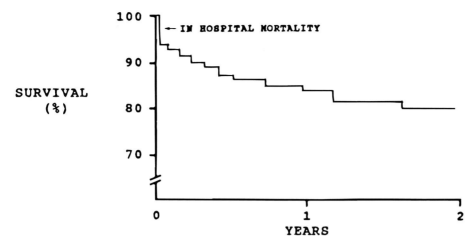

Fig. 14-3. Overall survival following elective use of cardiopulmonary bypass during high-risk angioplasty.

tional procedures were required as follows: unsupported angioplasty, 36; supported angioplasty, 22; bypass surgery, 34; automatic implantable cardioverter defibrillator placement, 5; and cardiac transplantation, 4. Survival rates including hospital mortality at 1, 2, and 3 years were 82, 80, and 77%, respectively. (Fig. 14-3)

EMERGENCY TECHNIQUE AND FOLLOW-UP

Percutaneous cardiopulmonary bypass was originally envisioned as an emergency technique to support patients with hemodynamic collapse or profound hypothermia.[6] It has continued to be employed in this fashion, initiation generally occurring in the catheterization laboratory, coronary care unit, or emergency room. Overlie[15] has collated the National Registry experience of the last 4 years, now totaling 210 patients. The most frequent clinical situations requiring emergency support have been angioplasty complicated by vessel occlusion, acute myocardial infarction associated with shock, and post-cardiac surgery hemodynamic collapse. The Registry's experience underscores the need for prompt initiation of support. Of 140 patients, in whom cardiopulmonary bypass was initiated in less than 20 minutes, 49% survived in the long term. In the comparison, only 19% of 70 patients in whom support was initiated more than 20 minutes from hemodynamic collapse survived in the long term.

CURRENT INDICATIONS

Percutaneous cardiopulmonary bypass support, initiated in either a prophylactic or a standby fashion, has been successfully employed in conjunction with high-risk angioplasty. Multicenter experience suggests that only patients with an ejection fraction of 20% or less clearly benefit from prophylactic support. Lesser morbidity and equally good outcomes are experienced in patients with an ejection fraction greater than 20% using standby support. Only 5 to 10% of the standby patients appear to require any form of circulatory support. Patients requiring support are difficult to predict in advance, however. With experience, cardiopulmonary bypass can be initiated in the standby situation promptly in almost all cases. Emergency use of bypass support is most successful when initiated in less than 20 minutes. The indications may be summarize as follows:

- Prophylactic support: left ventricular ejection fraction 20% or less
- Standby support: other high-risk patients
- Emergency support: initiated within 20 minutes

COSTS

The cardiopulmonary bypass system costs about $25,000 and cannula sets and disposable oxygenators and tubing about $1,100. Many centers also employ cardiopulmonary bypass technicians, which adds an additional $500 a case. By nature, these high-risk cases tend to require more prolonged hospitalizations than routine cases. An important financial consideration is whether to "prime" the bypass system during standby use, which is currently the most frequently employed technique. This decision is difficult to reach, as circulatory collapse is often unpredictable. The clinician must integrate the patient's clinical status with the likelihood of untoward outcome to decide whether or not to "prime" the system. In a positive sense, the ability to initiate bypass support in the standby circumstance reduces the need for emergency bypass surgery by about two-thirds and procedural mortality by about one-half.

CURRENT OUTLOOK

The experience to date suggests that high-risk patients are appropriate candidates for coronary angioplasty since they undergo intervention with acceptable morbidity and mortality, improvement in anginal status and ventricular function, and good long-term survival. In evaluating the use of circulatory support, it has become clear that the vast majority of high-risk patients do not need any form of circulatory support, although the availability of stents, intra-aortic balloon pumps, perfusion balloons, and circulatory support may be required to allow successful completion of the interventional procedure. Unfortunately, the need for any of these "bail-out" devices is difficult to predict in advance. The use of prophylactic circulatory support has clearly decreased in the past few years as operators have grown in confidence in undertaking high-risk cases. This presents a problem for laboratories utilizing cardiopulmonary bypass that wish to maintain current skills. Although used only occasionally, circulatory support remains an important prophylactic interventional tool for the very high-risk patient and a life-saving emergency technique for the occasional patient with circulatory collapse.

REFERENCES

1. Bentivoglio LG, Van Raden MJ, Kelsey SF et al. Percutaneous transluminal coronary angioplasty (PTCA) in patients with relative contraindications: results of the National Heart, Lung and Blood Institute PTCA Registry. Am J Cardiol 1984;53:82C–88C
2. Ellis SG, Topol EJ. Results of percutaneous transluminal angioplasty of high-risk angulated stenosis. Am J Cardiol 1990;66:932–937
3. Hartzler GO, Rutherford BD, McConahay DR et al. "High-risk" percutaneous transluminal coronary angioplasty. Am J Cardiol 1988;61:33G–37G
4. Kohli RS, DiSciascio G, Cowley MJ et al. Coronary angioplasty in patients with severe ventricular dysfunction. J Am Coll Cardiol 1990;16:807–811
5. Tommaso CL. Management of high-risk coronary angioplasty. Am J Cardiol 1989;64:33E–37E
6. Phillips SJ, Ballentine B, Slonine D et al. Percutaneous initiation of cardiopulmonary bypass. Ann Thorac Surg 1983;36:223–225
7. Vogel R, Tommaso CL, Gundry S. Initial experience with angioplasty and aortic valvuloplasty using elective semipercutaneous cardiopulmonary support. Am J Cardiol 1988;62:811–813
8. Alcan KE, Stertzer SH, Walsh JE et al. The role of intra-aortic balloon counterpulsation in patients undergoing percutaneous transluminal coronary angioplasty. Am Heart J 1983;105:527–530
9. Kahn JK, Rutherford BD, McConahay DR et al. Supported "high-risk" coronary angioplasty using intraaortic balloon pump counterpulsation. J Am Coll Cardiol 1990;15:1151–1155
10. Margolis JR. The role of percutaneous intra-aortic balloon in emergency situations following percutaneous transluminal coronary angioplasty. pp. 145–150. In Kaltenbach M, Gruentzig, Rentrop P, Bassman W-D (eds): Transluminal Coronary Angioplasty and Intracoronary Thrombolysis. Springer-Verlag, Berlin, 1982
11. Morrison DA, Barbierre C, Cohan A et al. Percutaneous transluminal coronary angioplasty for rest angina pectoris requiring intravenous nitroglycerin and intra-aortic balloon counterpulsation. Am J Cardiol 1990;66:168–171
12. Anderson HV, Leimgruber PP, Roubin GS et al. Distal coronary artery perfusion during percutaneous transluminal coronary angioplasty. Am Heart J 1985;110:720–726
13. Stack RS, Quigley PJ, Collins G et al. Perfusion balloon catheter. Am J Cardiol 1988;61:77G–80G
14. Turi ZG, Campbell CA, Gottimukkala MV et al. Preservation of distal coronary perfusion during prolonged balloon inflation with an autoperfusion angioplasty catheter. Circulation 1987;75:1273–1280
15. Overlie PA. Emergency use of portable cardiopulmonary bypass. Cathet Cardiovasc Diagn 1990;20:27–31
16. Reichman RT, Joyo CL, Dembitsky WP et al. Improved patient survival after cardiac arrest using a cardiopulmonary support system. Ann Thorac Surg 1990;49:101–105
17. Shawl FA, Domanski MJ, Hernandez SP. Emergency percutaneous cardiopulmonary support in cardiogenic shock from acute myocardial infarction. Am J Cardiol 1989;64:967–970
18. Shawl FA, Domanski MJ, Wish MH et al. Percutaneous cardiopulmonary bypass support in the catheterization laboratory. Technique and complications. Am Heart J 1990;120:195–203
19. Teirstein PS, Vogel RA, Dorros G et al. Prophylactic versus standby cardiopulmonary support for high-risk percutaneous transluminal coronary angioplasty. J Am Coll Cardiol 1993;21:590–6
20. Tommaso CL, Johnson RA, Stafford JL et al. Supported coronary angioplasty and standby supported coronary angioplasty for high-risk coronary artery disease. Am J Cardiol 1990;66:1255–1257
21. Pavlides GS, Hauser AM, Stack RK et al. Effect of peripheral cardiopulmonary bypass on left ventricular size, afterload and myocardial function during elective supported coronary angioplasty. J Am Coll Cardiol 1991;18:499–505
22. Stack RK, Pavlides GS, Miller R et al. Hemodynamic and metabolic effects of venoarterial cardiopulmonary support in coronary artery disease. Am J Cardiol 1991;67:1344–1348
23. Vogel RA, Shawl F, Tommaso C et al. Initial report of the national registry of elective cardiopulmonary

bypass supported coronary angioplasty. J Am Coll Cardiol 1990;20:22–26

24. Vogel RA, Tommaso CL. Elective supported angioplasty: initial report of the National Registry. Cathet Cardiovasc Diagn 1990;20:22–26

25. Freedman RJ, Wrenn RC, Gudley ML et al. Complex multiple percutaneous transluminal coronary angioplasty with vortex oxygenator cardiopulmonary support in the community hospital setting. Cathet Cardiovasc Diagn 1989;17:237–242

26. Muller DWM, Ellis SG, Topol EJ. Atherectomy of the left main coronary artery with percutaneous cardio-pulmonary bypass support. Am J Cardiol 1989;64:114–116

27. Vogel JHK, Ruiz CE, Jahnke EJ et al. Percutaneous (nonsurgical) supported angioplasty in unprotected left main disease and severe ventricular dysfunction. Clin Cardiol 1989;12:297–300

28. Lincoff AM, Popma JJ, Ellis SE et al. Percutaneous support devices for high-risk or complicated coronary angioplasty. J Am Coll Cardiol 1991;17:770–780

29. Topol EJ. Emerging strategies for foiled percutaneous transluminal coronary angioplasty. Am J Cardiol 1989;63:249–250

15 Anterograde Perfusion

Jean-Christian Farcot
Charles N.S. Chan
Jacques Berland

Percutaneous transluminal coronary angioplasty (PTCA) is now an established technique for the treatment of angina in patients with single or multivessel disease.[1-3] During early use of the technique, Andreas Grüentzig,[4] proposed the idea of distal perfusion of the coronary artery during balloon inflation to prevent myocardial ischemia. However, experience has shown that brief coronary occlusions were usually well tolerated with an acceptable primary angioplasty success rate and therefore more prolonged balloon inflation was not attempted routinely.[5,6] Despite increased operator experience and improved PTCA hardware, acute vessel closure still occurs in 3 to 6% of elective PTCA cases. Acute vessel closure is mainly responsible for most of the early morbidity (myocardial infarction and emergency bypass surgery) and mortality associated with PTCA.[7-9] Ellis et al.[10] have determined that several independent factors, including long lesions, lesions associated with thrombus, lesion at a bend, postangioplasty residual stenosis greater than 50%, and presence of significant dissection, are independent predictors of acute closure.[10]

Transient coronary occlusion during PTCA results in acute hemodynamic, electrophysiologic, biochemical, and functional changes in the myocardium.[11-13] These changes are particularly important in high-risk cases such as patients with severe triple-vessel disease, patients with depressed left ventricular function, and patients with no collaterals to the vessel dilated. The risks may be summarized as follows:

- Proximal large vessel with large myocardial distribution
- Left ventricular ejection fraction less than 35%
- Severe triple-vessel disease
- Complex lesion morphology (i.e., types B2 or C lesions)
- Prolonged inflation required for reparative angioplasty in abrupt closure or threatened closure
- Bridge to surgical revascularization after failed PTCA
- Dilating the only remaining coronary artery supplying a large viable myocardium

Perfusing the myocardium distal to the occlusion allows more prolonged balloon inflation without jeopardizing myocardial viability or producing necrosis or patient discomfort.[14-17] Recent data have suggested that a more prolonged and gradual balloon inflation may influence the acute angiographic results and primary success rate of PTCA.[18-20] Chan et al.[21] have demonstrated a significant reduction in elastic recoil in 123 consecutive patients undergoing elective PTCA if the inflation time is longer than 200 seconds, resulting in greater acute gain. In a prospective randomized study of prolonged inflation (longer than than 12 minutes) versus standard inflation (less than 3 minutes), prolonged inflation was associated with a decreased incidence of severe dissection, presumably due to improvement in plaque molding and treatment of any dissection caused by PTCA.[22]

CORONARY BLOOD FLOW PHYSIOLOGY

The coronary perfusion that takes place under a mean aortic pressure is characterized by the difference between the distribution of perfusion between the epicardium and myocardium.[23] Chilian and Marcus[24] have demonstrated that the coronary flow occurs mainly in diastole in the epicardial arteries and that only 20% of the total blood flow is distributed during the systolic phase. In fact, the coronary flow in the intramyocardial arteries virtually ceases in systole because of the increase in the intramyocardial pressure. This phenomenon becomes more pronounced in the deeper layers of the myocardium.[25,26] Spaan et al.[27] have observed that although the coronary flow is markedly reduced in systole, the diameter of the epicardial coronary vessels measured by ultrasound in fact increases slightly. This phenomenon is caused by the development of retrograde flow from endocardium to epicardium during compression of intramyocardial vessels by the ventricular contraction.[28,29] The endothelial cells lining the coronary arteries play an important physiologic role in the antithrombotic property and smooth muscle tone of the artery through their secretory vasoactive substances such as prostaglandins, histamine, and endothelium-derived relaxing factor.[30,31] In addition, the endothelial function is dependent on the phasic coronary flow, a nonpulsatile flow results in a significant decrease in the secretory activity of the endothelial cells, and therefore may result in thrombus formation, vasospasm, and arterial occlusion.[31]

CHOICE OF ANTEGRADE PERFUSION SYSTEM

Passive Hemoperfusion

Passive perfusion of autologous blood (autoperfusion) during coronary occlusion has been achieved with a perfusion balloon catheter (High-Flow CPC Mainz, Schneider/Pfizer Europe AG, ACS Stack, or ACS RX Flow Track perfusion catheter, Mountain View, CA), which has side ports proximal and distal to the balloon allowing simultaneous dilation of the coronary artery with antegrade flow.[32–34] This method has several advantages with respect to its wide availability and simplicity of use; it also does not require a complex pumping mechanism and

therefore avoids the possibility of air embolism, red cell hemolysis, and distal endothelial trauma. The amount of blood flow is significantly influenced by the pressure gradient among the proximal and distal side ports, the internal diameter of the catheter and blood viscosity.[32,35,36] In clinical studies coronary perfusion catheters have permitted balloon inflations of 10 minutes or more without significant electrocardiographic (ECG) or echocardiographic evidence of ischemia.[32–36] Nevertheless, a significant number of patients do not tolerate prolonged inflation periods, because of either obstruction to a major side branch or inadequate flow relative to the demands of the myocardium at risk. Coghlan et al.[37] found that production of free radical and sinus lactate content were consistent with significant ischemia after only 3 minutes of inflation with a perfusion balloon catheter. Recently, observational data have suggested that a very long inflation (average, 23 minutes) with an autoperfusion catheter may in fact salvage an initially unsuccessful PTCA (i.e., abrupt closure, occlusive type dissection, and suboptimal angiographic results in about 50 to 70% of cases).[21,38–40] Jackman et al.[41] reported that in 40 patients treated with a Stack catheter for major dissection or acute closure, a mean inflation time of 30 minutes resulted in angiographic success in 32 (80%) patients, without death, myocardial infarction, or coronary artery surgery during hospitalization. The mechanism by which prolonged inflation achieves salvage is not completely understood but could be explained by better remodeling of the atherosclerotic plaque, less elastic recoil, and a sealing effect on intimal flaps.[21,22] Limitations of the autoperfusion catheter include its dependence on the systemic blood pressure for passive flow, its relative stiffness and large profile, and its susceptibility to thrombosis. Finally, the actual flow rate achieved in vitro (compared with the 40 to 60 ml/min in vivo) is more likely to be around 35 to 45 ml/min and is usually not sufficient to provide full myocardial protection especially in patients with multivessel disease and poor left ventricular function.

Active Perfusion With Oxygenated Perfluorocarbons (Fluosol)

Fluosol consists of perfluorochemicals—perfluorodecolin and perfluoro tri-n-propylamine in a 7:3 ratio; it is chemically inert and is not metabolized by the body. It is slowly excreted through gaseous exchange in the lungs and by the reticuloendothelial system. Because of its high oxygen transport capability, some workers have perfused perfluorocarbons enriched with oxygen distally through a standard balloon catheter and found a reduction in myocardial ischemia.[42-44] Kent et al.[45] found that intracoronary infusion of Fluosol distal to the occlusion was associated with a reduction in severity of anginal, ST segment changes and regional wall abnormality during balloon occlusion when compared with routine coronary angioplasty. In the same report, adverse reactions were rare (2%) including ventricular fibrillation, chest pain, dypsnea, and bradycardia. However, Fluosol has certain limitations. First, it may take up to 30 minutes to oxygenate the solution and it may not be useful in an emergency situation. Second, the amount of Fluosol infused is limited because of slow removal from the lungs and reticuloendothelial system. Third, the extra volume of the solution may be just enough to precipitate left ventricular failure in patients with low ejection fraction.

Active Distal Coronary Hemoperfusion

Active antegrade perfusion is a form of autologous blood perfusion during balloon angioplasty in which arterial blood is mechanically injected through the angioplasty catheter either manually or by a mechanical pump such as the Angiomat, Leocor, or roller pump, thus allowing more prolonged inflation times and a lesser degree of ischemia without relying on the physiologic pressure gradient of the patient.[46-51] In a multicenter prospective series of 110 patients undergoing elective PTCA, distal hemoperfusion with the Leocor pump achieved at least a 50% increase in tolerated inflation times (from 1.3 ± 0.9 to 7 ± 4 minutes, P <0.001), resulting in less ST depression and chest pain during balloon inflation.[49] The Leocor system consists of a battery-operated portable pump with a large lumen over the wire balloon

catheter (0.032[11]) designed to infuse the patient's own oxygenated blood. The blood is driven by a piston pump in a semicontinuous flow pattern at a rate of up to 80 ml/min. However, this usually requires very high pressure of up to 200 psi, may induce distal endothelial trauma or spasm, and might explain the occurrence of a paradoxical shorter inflation period in some patients and transient complete heart block in the right coronary artery perfusion. In this series, three patients developed echocardiographic evidence of persistent left ventricular dysfunction despite full balloon deflation after hemoperfusion. This system has several advantages: first, it does not depend on the mean systemic aortic pressure, and the flow rate is adjustable; and second, it is portable and can be easily transported with the patient to the operating theatre. The disadvantages are that the flow rate is semicontinous, resulting in filling and distension of the artery in systole and may cause endothelial trauma. This system requires a specially designed balloon catheter for blood delivery.

We have developed a physiologic anteroperfusion system (PAS) that allows flow mainly in diastole in concordance with the phasic physiology of the coronary blood flow through a standard angioplasty catheter.[49,51-53] In contrast to the continuous pump system, in which a high perfusion is required due to the competitive action of intramyocardial contraction in systole, the physiologic pump requires less driving force thus, avoiding coronary spasm, thrombus formation, or hemolysis (Fig. 15-1).

PHYSIOLOGIC ANTEROPERFUSION SYSTEM

The system is shown in Figure 15-2 and consists of the following elements:

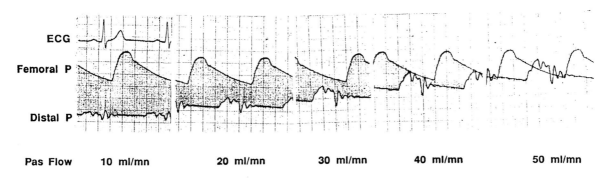

Fig. 15-1. Pressure distal to the balloon (Distal P) given by different perfusion flows from 10 ml/min to 50 ml/min. Note the excellent phasism of the flow. Between 40 and 50 ml/min, the diastolic perfusion pressure equals the diastolic aortic pressure.

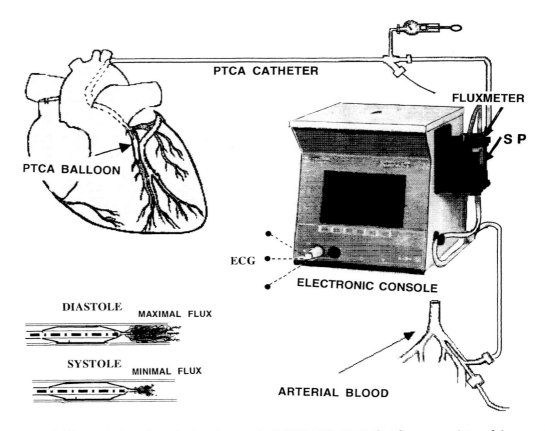

Fig. 15-2. PAS, consisting of an electronic console (PERFANT 1000) that houses a piston-driven motor, a disposable unit (SP), a fluxmeter, and ECG connections.

1. An electronic console that is battery operated and that drives a piston synchronized on the patient's ECG so that the maximum flow is achieved in diastole and minimal flow in systole. The flow rate is adjustable, with a mean of 44 ± 12 ml/min, is driven under a physiologic pressure equal to the mean arterial pressure of the patient, and is automically cut off if the driving pressure is too high by an intrinsic flow-sensing mechanism built into the console. The blood flow at the distal end of the catheter is phasic rather than continuous, like the normal physiologic flow of the coronary artery.

2. A disposable pulsatile unit consisting of a piston and a reservoir of 10 ml.

3. Autologous blood is obtained, either from a 6 F sheath introduced in the contralateral femoral artery or from a special 6.5 F PTCA introducer sheath (INTROLAT), and is connected to the pulsatile unit. After removing the guiding wire from the balloon catheter, the proximal end of the catheter is connected to the outflow port of the pulsatile unit.

CLINICAL FEASIBILITY AND VALIDATION

From 1990 to 1992, the PAS system was utilized during angioplasty of a proximal left anterior descending artery stenosis in 30 patients with stable angina. All patients had only single-vessel disease, normal left ventricular function, and absence of significant collateral circulation at baseline coronary angiogram.

At that time the PTCA procedure was performed in a standard manner using a standard 8 F guiding catheter introduced via the right femoral artery. [Today, clinical procedures are performed through a 6 F guiding catheter, and the blood may be obtained by the lateral arm of this slightly modified sheath (Fig. 15-2)]. A 6 F sheath (USCI, Bard) was then introduced into the contralateral femoral artery, so that autologous blood could be obtained via its side arm. Patients were given 10,000 IU heparin, at the start of the procedure. The target lesion was then crossed with a 0.014 floppy wire (ACS), and a standard over-the-wire balloon catheter (UCSI Profile

Plus) was placed across the lesion. Several balloon angioplasty catheters were tested in vivo and in animal studies, and the USCI Profile Plus provided the optimal distal perfusion. A control balloon inflation without perfusion was performed routinely for 60 seconds. If there was marked ST-segment elevation with or without chest pain, the patients were enrolled in the study. The protocol consisted of three balloon inflations; the first (OC 1) was performed without antegrade perfusion for 90 seconds. Subsequent inflation (OC 2) with hemoperfusion was performed for a total duration of 15 minutes with progressive pressure ramping (1 atm/min), and the last inflation (OC 3) was repeated without hemoperfusion for 90 seconds. During each balloon inflation, myocardial ischemia was assessed by severity of angina, continuous ECG, and two-dimensional echocardiography (apical four-chamber view).

During the same period we operated on 60 patients with proximal left anterior descending artery stenosis who had similar baseline characteristics; this group constitutes our control. The clinical features and PTCA procedural data are shown in Table 15-1. All 30 patients with PAS could tolerate the 15 min-

utes of balloon inflation without significant chest discomfort or ST-segment elevation (Fig. 15-3). Simultaneous two-dimensional echocardiography shows that the segmental wall motion was completely preserved for the whole 15 minutes of inflation with PAS; when compared with the control group, all the patients had regional wall motion abnormality within 90 seconds of coronary artery occlusion (Fig. 15-4). Quantitative coronary analyses were performed using online edge detection for all the patients, and angioplasty with PAS was shown to yield a greater gain in percent luminal diameter and less elastic recoil compared with the control group (Table 15-2). Acute PTCA complications (defined as significant coronary artery dissection and acute closure) were also significantly higher in the conventional angioplasty group. Three patients required emergency coronary bypass surgery in the conventional PTCA group and none in the PAS group (Table 15-3). Following the procedure, blood was taken for cardiac enzymes, complete blood count, serum myoglobin, and bilirubin. No significant hemolysis or cardiac enzymes increase were seen in the patients undergoing 15 minutes of balloon inflation with PAS.

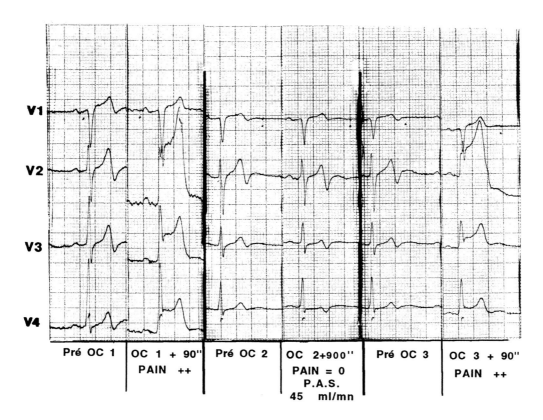

Fig. 15-3. ECG of a patient in our study protocol: Coronary occlusion (OC) in phases I and III without PAS and phase II during PAS support.

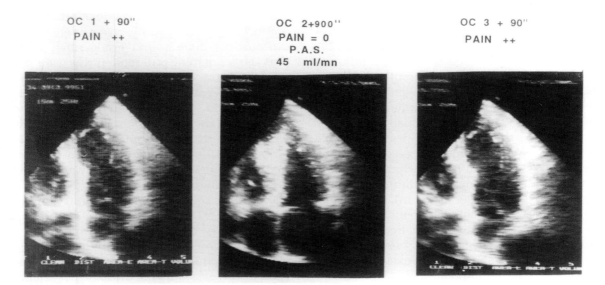

Fig. 15-4. Example of continuous two-dimensional echocardiography (apical view) in the study protocol. Note that in coronary occlusions (OC 1 and OC 2) without PAS, the left ventricular end-systolic still frame chamber is dilated and the left free wall is akinetic, in contrast to angioplasty with PAS (OC 3), in which the left ventricular chamber is normal and contracts normally.

We therefore conclude that the PAS (1) allows prolonged and gradual pressure ramping (1 atm/min) dilation of proximal left anterior descending artery lesions without myocardial ischemia, (2) results in greater acute gain in luminal diameter because of better plaque remodeling and less elastic recoil, and (3) shows a reduction in the incidence of coronary intimal tear and acute closure.

POTENTIAL CLINICAL APPLICATIONS IN HIGH-RISK PTCA

PAS would be a valuable tool in the angioplasty of high-risk patients such as those with proximal stenosis of large dominant coronary arteries and severe triple-vessel disease with impaired left ventricular function (ejection fraction less than 35%). In such patients, transient ischemia caused by balloon inflation is poorly tolerated because of chest pain and he-

Table 15-1. Effects of PAS versus Conventional Angioplasty in Severe Proximal Left Anterior Descending Coronary Artery Stenosis

	Conventional PTCA (n = 60)	PAS (n = 30)
Male/female	40/20	27/3
Age (years)	58 ± 8	53 ± 10
Lesion type		
A	39	13
B	21	17
Balloon size (mm)	2.88 ± 0.53	3.02 ± 0.28
Total inflation time (sec)	274 ± 164	637 ± 10[a]
No. of inflations	3.2 ± 1.9	1[a]
Inflation pressure (atm)	7.9 ± 2.9	5.1 ± 0.8[a]

[a] P <0.01.

Table 15-2. Quantitative Coronary Analysis of Dilated Coronary Arteries

	Conventional PTCA (n = 60)	PAS (n = 30)
% Diameter stenosis		
Pre-PTCA	81.0 ± 8.1	85 ± 7.6
Post-PTCA	34.4 ± 26.0	14.5 ± 8.1[a]
% Luminal gain	57.5 ± 17	82.0 ± 9.7[a]
Balloon area (mm²)	6.73 ± 2.3	7.15 ± 1.3
Post-PTCA area (mm²)	3.45 ± 1.4	5.93 ± 0.9[a]
Recoil (%)	48.7 ± 13.4	17.0 ± 8.7[a]

[a] P <0.01.

Table 15-3. Angioplasty Success and Acute Complications

	Conventional PTCA (%)	PAS (%)
Angioplasty success	95	100
Intimal tear	31	3[a]
Reocclusion (3 days)	18	0[b]
Emergency coronary artery bypass graft	5	0

[a] $P < 0.01$.
[b] $P < 0.05$.

modynamic and electrical instability. PAS allows gradual and prolonged inflation with full myocardial protection and therefore provides greater safety in performing PTCA for high-risk patients.[52]

BRIDGE TO SURGERY

The occurrence of myocardial infarction and mortality during emergency bypass surgery after failed PTCA is dependent on the duration of ischemia before revascularization. In cases in which coronary patency could not be maintained after coronary angioplasty, the PAS system could be set up very quickly in the catheterization laboratory. This simple system will reduce ischemic time by hemodynamic support in maintaining physiologic anterograde autologous blood flow in the jeopardized territories while the patient is awaiting surgical intervention. This system can be transported easily with the patient, it has its own battery power source, and it differs from the Leocor anteroperfusion system, which requires specific catheters.

PREVENTION AND TREATMENT OF CORONARY ARTERY DISSECTION COMPLICATING PTCA

The aim of PAS is to achieve prolonged and gradual inflation without regional ischemia, thus avoiding angina, cardiac arrhythmia, and regional wall abnormality. This technique of inflation may lead to a decrease in the incidence of dissection, better plaque remodeling, reduction of elastic recoil (as demonstrated by our clinical study), and normal secretory activity of the endothelial cells of the dilated segment of the artery. Several data have shown that extremely prolonged balloon inflation (more than 20

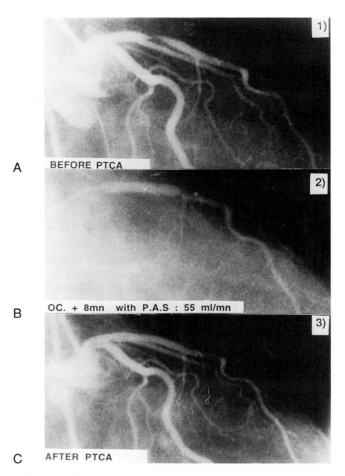

Fig. 15-5. (A) Preangiogram of a patient undergoing angioplasty for a severe proximal left anterior descending artery stenosis. **(B)** At 8 minutes of inflation with PAS, autologous blood mixed with contrast medium was perfused distally. **(C)** The post-PTCA angiogram revealed an excellent result with no visible tear and minimal elastic recoil.

minutes) is useful in about 70% of cases in salvaging an initially failed PTCA due to occlusive dissection. The PAS is an ideal flow support device in this situation, allowing prolonged balloon inflation (up to 6 hours) independent of the patient's blood pressure and free from the thrombotic or hemolytic complications encountered in other perfusion devices.

STAGED REPERFUSION DURING THE ACUTE PHASE OF MYOCARDIAL INFARCTION

Sudden distal reperfusion of an infarct-related artery may result in acute reperfusion injury, which may manifest in cardiac arrhythmias and myocardial stunning. Since the distal flow rate of the PAS is adjustable, a gradual reperfusion of the distal artery during coronary dilation is possible; furthermore, drugs such as nitrates, thrombolytic agents, cardioplegic solution, and free radicals scavengers could be infused distally.

POTENTIAL INVESTIGATIONAL RESEARCH AREAS

Local Drug Delivery System

PAS has been tested in animals and has proved to eradicate ischemia in the dependent myocardium in over an hour[52]; it may thus offer a simple, safe, and less costly device (through a balloon or a recently developed catheter design) for long-term drug delivery at the angioplasty site.

Physiologic Perfusion Support During Coronary Angioscopy

During imaging, warmed physiologic saline solution is usually infused through the distal angioscopic irrigation port, at a rate of 30 to 45 ml/min by means of a power injector. PAS is proposed to achieved the goal of salin or Fluosol perfusion in a physiologic manner to ease and assist the dependent myocardium during the prolonged angioscopic perfusion time.

Physiologic Perfusion Support During Coronary Artery Surgery

Recently interest has been devoted to a reappraisal of open-heart surgery without external extracorporeal circulation assistance. PAS is proposed for open heart surgery through a PTCA balloon catheter, on the beating heart, to ensure regional protection for the dependent myocardium during the grafting period, providing more ease and sewing time for the surgeon.

REFERENCES

1. Gruentzig AR, Senning A, Siegenthaler WE. Non-operative dilatation of coronary artery stenosis: percutaneous transluminal coronary angioplasty. N Engl J Med 1979;301:61
2. Detre K, Holubkov R, Kelsey S et al. Percutaneous transluminal coronary angioplasty in 1985–86 and 1977–81. The National Heart, Lung and Blood Institute Registry. N Engl J Med 1988;318:265
3. Weintraub WS, Jones EL, King SB III et al. Changing use of coronary angioplasty and coronary bypass surgery in the treatment of chronic coronary artery disease. Am J Cardiol 1990;65:183
4. Meier B, Gruentzig AR, Brown JE. Percutaneous arterial perfusion of acutely occluded coronary arteries in dogs, abstracted. J Am Coll Cardiol, 505, 1984; suppl. A.:3
5. Cohen M, Rentrop KP. Limitation of myocardial ischemia by collateral circulation during sudden controlled artery occlusion in human subjects: a prospective study. Circulation 1986;74:1124
6. DiSciascio G, Vetrovec GW, Lewis SA et al. Clinical and angiographic recurrence following PTCA for nonacute total occlusions: comparison of one versus five minute inflations. Am Heart J 1990;120:529
7. Simpfendorfer C, Belardi J, Bellamy G et al. Frequency, management and follow-up of patients with acute coronary occlusions after percutaneous transluminal coronary angioplasty. Am J Cardiol 1987;59:267
8. de Feyter PJ, van den Brand M, Jaarman G et al. Acute coronary artery occlusion during and after percutaneous transluminal coronary angioplasty. Frequency, prediction, clinical course, management and follow-up. Circulation 1991;83:927
9. Sinclair IN, McCabe CH, Sipperley ME, Baim DS. Predictors, therapeutic options and long-term outcome of abrupt closure. Am J Cardiol 1988;61:619
10. Ellis SG, Roubin GS, King SB et al. Angiographic and clinical predictors of acute closure after native vessel coronary angioplasty. Circulation 1988;77:372
11. Serruys PW, Wijns W, van den Brand M et al. Left ventricular performance, regional blood flow, wall motion and lactate metabolism during transluminal angioplasty. Circulation 1984;70:25
12. Hauser AM, Gangadharan V, Ramus RG et al. Sequence of mechanical, electrocardiographic and clinical effects of repeated coronary arterial occlusion of human beings. Echocardiographic observations during coronary angioplasty. J Am Coll Cardiol 1985;5:193
13. Wohlgelertner D, Cleman M, Highman et al. Regional myocardial dysfunction during coronary angioplasty: evaluation by two-dimensional echocardiography and 12-lead electrocardiography. J Am Coll Cardiol 1986;7:1245
14. Lehman KG, Atwood JE, Snyder EL, Ellison RL. Autologous blood perfusion for myocardial protection during coronary angioplasty: a feasibility study. Circulation 1987;76:312
15. Azpiri JR, Chisholm RT, Watson KR, Amstrong PW. Effects of hemoperfusion during percutaneous transluminal coronary angioplasty on left ventricular function. Am J Cardiol 1991;67:1324
16. Turi ZG, Campbell CA, Gottimukkala MV, Kloner RA. Preservation of distal coronary perfusion during prolonged balloon inflation with an autoperfusion angioplasty catheter. Circulation 1987;75:1273
17. Angelini P, Heibig J, Leachman DR. Distal hemoperfusion during percutaneous coronary angioplasty. Am J Cardiol 1986;58:252
18. Kaltenbach M, Koberg G. Can prolonged application of pressure improve the results of percutaneous trans-

luminal coronary angioplasty (PTCA)? Circulation II-123 1982;suppl. II.:66

19. Remetz MS, Cabin HS, Mc Connel S, Cleman M. Gradual balloon inflation protocol reduces arterial damage following pércutaneous transluminal coronary angioplasty, abstracted. J Am Coll Cardiol, 131A 1988; suppl. A.:11

20. Berland J, Farcot J-C, Stix G et al. Gradual, low-pressure and sustained inflations with the physiologic antero-perfusion system improve the immediate results of LAD angioplasty, abstracted. J Am Coll Cardiol, 350A 1992;suppl. A.:19

21. Chan C, Berland J, Stix G et al. Effects of prolonged balloon inflation on elastic recoil immediately after PTCA. Circulation, I-332 1992;suppl. I.:86

22. Cribier A, Eltchaninoff H, Chan C et al. Comparative effects of long (> 12 min) versus standard (3 min) sequential balloon inflations in PTCA, abstracted. J Am Coll Cardiol, 713–58A 1994;suppl. A.:23

23. Klocke FJ. Coronary blood flow in man. Prog Cardiovasc Dis 1976;19:117

24. Chilian WM, Marcus ML. Phasic coronary blood flow velocity in intramural and epicardial coronary arteries. Circ Res 1982;50:775

25. Cutarelli R, Levy MN. Intraventricular pressure and the distribution of coronary flow. Circ Res 1963;12:322

26. Sullivan JM, Taylor WJ, Elliot WC, Gorlin R. Regional myocardial blood flow. J Clin Invest 1967;46:1402

27. Spaan JAE, Brenls NPW, Laird JD. Diastolic-systolic coronary flow differences are caused by intramyocardial pump action in the anaesthetized dog. Circ Res 1981;49:584

28. Baird RJ, Manktelow RT, Shah VA, Ameli FM. Intramyocardial pressure: a study of its regional variation and its relationship to intraventricular pressure. J Thorac Cardiovasc Surg 1970;59:810

29. Hoffman JIE. The effects of intramyocardial forces on the distribution of intramyocardial flow. J Biomed Eng 1979;1:33

30. Palmer RM, Ashton DS, Mucada S. Vascular endothelial cells synthesize nitric oxide from L-arginine. Nature 1988;333:664

31. Yao SK, Ober JC, Wilterson JT et al. Endogenous nitric oxide protects against platelet aggregation and cyclic flow variation in stenosed and endothelial injured arteries. Circulation 1992;86:1302

32. Stack RS, Quigley PJ, Collins G, Phillips HR. Perfusion balloon catheter. Am J Cardiol 1988;61:77G

33. Erbel R, Clas W, Busch U et al. New balloon catheter for prolonged percutaneous transluminal coronary angioplasty and bypass flow in occluded vessels. Cathet Cardiovasc Diagn 1986;12:116

34. Turi ZG, Campbell CA, Gottimukkala M, Kloner R. Preservation of distal coronary perfusion during prolonged balloon inflation with an autoperfusion angioplasty catheter. Circulation 1987;75:1273

35. Christensen CW, Lassar TA, Dailey LC et al. Regional myocardial flow with a reperfusion catheter and an autoperfusion catheter during total coronary occlusion. Am Heart J 1990;119:242

36. Zalewski A, Berry C, Kosman ZK et al. Myocardial protection with autoperfusion during prolonged coronary artery occlusion. Am Heart J 1990;119:41

37. Coghlan J, Fitter W, Paul V et al. Myocardial protection with ACS Rx perfusion balloon catheterischemic or nonischemic?, abstracted. J Am Coll Cardiol, 293A 1992;suppl. A.:19

38. Palazzo AM, Gustafson GM, Santilli E, Kemp HG. Unusually long inflation times during percutaneous transluminal coronary angioplasty. Cathet Cardiovasc Diagn 1988;14:154

39. Quigley PJ, Hinohara T, Phillips HR et al. Myocardial protection during coronary angioplasty with an autoperfusion balloon catheter in humans. Circulation 1988; 78:1128

40. Arie S, Checchi H, Coelho W et al. Coronary angioplasty: unstable lesions and prolonged balloon inflation time. Cathet Cardiovasc Diagn 1990;19:77

41. Jackman JD, Zidar JP, Tcheng JE et al. Outcome after prolonged balloon inflations > 20 minutes for initially unsuccessful percutaneous transluminal coronary angioplasty. Am J Cardiol 1992;69:1417

42. Anderson HV, Leimgruber PP, Roubin GS et al. Distal artery perfusion during percutaneous transluminal coronary angioplasty. Am Heart J 1985;110:720

43. Cleman M, Jaffe CC, Wohlgelernter D. Prevention of ischemia during percutaneous transluminal coronary angioplasty by transcatheter infusion of oxygenated Fluosol DA 20%. Circulation 1986;74:355

44. Cowley MJ, Snow FR, DiSciasccio G et al. Perfluorochemical perfusion during coronary angioplasty in unstable and high-risk patients. Circulation, III-27 1990; suppl. III.:81

45. Kent K, Cleman M, Cowley M et al. Reduction of ischemia during percutaneous transluminal coronary angioplasty with oxygenated Fluosol. Am J Cardiol 1990;60:261

46. Lehmann KC, Atwood JE, Snyder EL. Autologous blood perfusion for myocardial protection during coronary angioplasty. Circulation 1987;76:312

47. Heibig J, Angelini P, Leachman R et al. Use of mechanical devices for distal hemoperfusion during balloon catheter coronary angioplasty. Cathet Cardiovasc Diagn 1988;15:143

48. Banka VS, Trivedi A, Patel R et al. Prevention of myocardial ischemia during coronary angioplasty. A simple new method for distal antegrade arterial blood perfusion. Am Heart J 1989;118:830

49. Farcot J-C, Berland J, Derumeaux G et al. Results of physiologic anteroperfusion system to support prolonged PTCA inflations in 40 patients, abstracted. J Am Coll Cardiol 1992;19:34

50. DiSciascio G, Angelini P, Vandormael MG et al. Reduction of ischemia with a new flow-adjustable hemoperfusion pump during coronary angioplasty. J Am Coll Cardiol 1992;19:657

51. Berland J, Farcot J-C, Barrier A et al. Clinical evaluation of a phasic coronary anteroperfusion system during PTCA, abstracted. Circulation, 272 1989;suppl. II.: 80

52. Farcot J-C, Berland J, Derumeaux G et al. Perfusion antérograde synchronisée pendant l'angioplastie coronaire: Etude clinique préliminaire. Arch Mal Coeur 1995;88:371

53. Martinot S, Farcot J-C, Franck M et al. Etude des effets de la perfusion active pulsatile synchronisée longue durée chez l'animal. Arch Mal Coeur 1996 (in press)

16 Aortic Counterpulsation During Percutaneous Intervention

Jean-François Tanguay
Ian Shearer
E. Magnus Ohman

Applications of coronary angioplasty in the treatment of cardiovascular disease have expanded tremendously since 1977, when the technique was introduced by Gruentzig. Patients who had unstable ischemic syndromes (unstable angina and acute myocardial infarction), multivessel disease, markedly impaired left ventricular function, and target vessels that supply large areas of myocardium were typically considered to have prohibitively higher risks of morbidity and mortality from angioplasty. However, these patients are now undergoing percutaneous transluminal coronary angioplasty (PTCA) as part of the daily workload in most high-volume centers.

Concomitant with increasing technical expertise and equipment improvements, developments in left ventricular support have provided interventional cardiologists with an array of mechanical strategies to achieve revascularization in high-risk patients. The clinical challenges are to recognize the need for a support device and to determine which device will provide maximum benefit with minimum complications. In this era of economic constraint, the cost effectiveness of a particular device is also relevant.

In this chapter we discuss the use of intra-aortic balloon pumping (IABP) in the context of circulatory support during PTCA. The mechanisms of action, indications, operative techniques, results, and role of IABP with respect to other devices are discussed. The intent is to be as practical as possible and to reflect our experience at Duke University Medical Center.

HISTORICAL BACKGROUND

Over the last four decades, technologic advances have permitted development of devices that employ principles of counterpulsation: augmenting diastolic pressure and reducing impedance to ventricular ejection, thus reducing the work of the heart. In 1953 Kantrowitz and Kantrowitz[1] first reported that retarding systolic pulse pressure can augment the arterial diastolic or coronary pressure and lead to an estimated increase in coronary blood flow of 22 to 53%. In 1962 Moulopoulos et al.[2] were the first to construct an inflatable latex balloon, which they inserted into the descending aorta of dogs through the femoral artery. With pulsed, electrocardiographically (ECG) synchronized inflation, the balloon displaced blood during diastole, augmenting arterial diastolic blood flow and pressure, with rapid deflation in systole, it effectively emptied the left ventricle. The first human use of aortic counterpulsation was reported in 1968 by Kantrowitz et al.,[3] who supported two patients with infarction and refractory cardiogenic shock. Both had reversal of hemodynamic shock with IABP, although one died of irreversible ventricular fibrillation after discontinuation of IABP. This experience was followed by reports on larger cohorts. In 1969 Summers et al.[4] further noted that emergency coronary angiography and left ventriculography can be performed during IABP support.

Since then, IABP has become one of the easiest

and most commonly used systemic support devices. Patients have undergone IABP support for indications that include: *refractory unstable angina* while awaiting coronary angiography and PTCA or coronary artery bypass graft (CABG); *acute myocardial infarction* while awaiting PTCA or with cardiogenic shock or mechanical complications (acute ventricular septal defect or mitral regurgitation); *severe left ventricular dysfunction* with refractory heart failure or while awaiting transplantation; and *prophylactic placement* before high-risk PTCA or for incipient complications, as a bridge to cardiac surgery.

MECHANISMS OF ACTION

Support systems can be divided into regional myocardial and systemic support techniques. Intra-aortic balloon counterpulsation, femoral-femoral percutaneous cardiopulmonary bypass (CPS), and the Hemopump are *systemic* support techniques. These can be combined with perfusion balloon catheters, passive hemoperfusion, coronary sinus retroperfusion techniques, and oxygenated perfluorocarbons to achieve *regional* myocardial support during PTCA.

The IABP is the simplest left ventricular support device and employs the principles of counterpulsation mentioned previously.[5] By inflating during diastole, the IABP displaces blood from the aorta and increases the diastolic pressure. Then rapid deflation triggered by the QRS complex (before aortic valve opening) creates a vacuum during early systole. This reduces aortic volume, thus decreasing the afterload and the work required from the left ventricle to eject blood (Fig. 16-1).

The net *hemodynamic effects* of IABP are dependent on many physical and biologic variables (Table 16-1). By affecting global IABP performance, they explain the wide range of hemodynamic and clinical effects observed in different patients. The augmentation of mean aortic diastolic pressure (MADP) is a function of *IABP volume:* with increasing balloon volume, MADP is augmented at all levels of mean arterial pressure, but more so at the lowest levels (Fig. 16-2). MADP of patients in cardiogenic shock could thus be expected to increase by 30 to 40%. The *timing and duration of IABP cycles* also influence augmentation of MADP. Optimal balloon inflation should begin at the end of ejection, coincident with aortic valve closure. The onset of inflation has been synchronized best with either the dicrotic notch of the arterial pressure or the second half of the T wave on ECG. The duration of inflation should be individualized by heart rate and mean aortic pressure to ensure

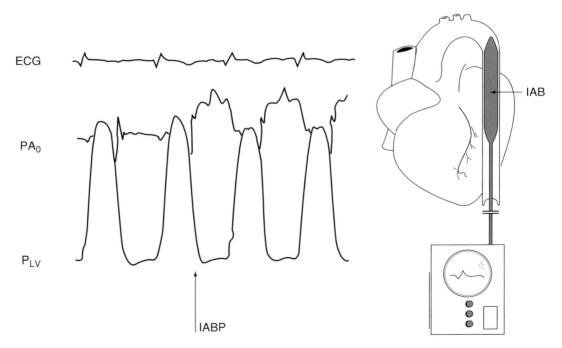

Fig. 16-1. Principles of intra-aortic balloon counterpulsation. The intra-aortic balloon (IAB) is positioned in the thoracic aorta and driven synchronous to the ECG by an external console. Shown are the effects of IABP on aortic root (P_{AO}) and left ventricular (P_{LV}) pressures (i.e., augmentation of aortic diastolic pressure and reduction in ventricular systolic pressure, respectively). (From Weber and Janicki,[5] with permission.)

Table 16-1. Variables That Influence IABP

Goal	Physical Variables	Biologic Variables
Diastolic pressure augmentation	Position Volume Diameter Occlusivity Configuration Driving gas Timing	Arterial pressure Heart rate Aortic pressure/volume ratio
Impedance and work reduction	Volume Occlusivity Inflation duration	Arterial pressure Heart rate Aortic pressure/volume ratio Afterload reduction Preload reduction Augmented shortening

(From Weber and Janicki,[5] with permission.)

optimal reduction of afterload. Deflation should occur before aortic valve opening and isovolumetric contraction. The *duration of balloon cycles* will also influence aortic flow velocity and thus coronary perfusion. Other important variables are the position of the balloon in the aorta, size ratio of balloon to aorta, heart rate and rhythm, compliance of the aorta, and resistance of the arterial bed. The net effects of IABP on *coronary perfusion* have been a subject of controversy. Recently, Kern et al.,[6] using a 0.018″ Doppler guidewire, noted a lack of significant flow improve-

ment beyond most critical stenoses, but showed an unequivocal, IABP-mediated augmentation of both proximal and distal coronary blood flow velocities after successful PTCA (Fig. 16-3).

INSTRUMENTATION

Percutaneous placement of IABP requires less resources compared with other systemic support devices. Insertion must be performed under sterile conditions, and fluoroscopy should be used to ensure proper placement. With PTCA, these issues are easily resolved, and the IABP device can be inserted efficiently before the procedure. The smaller diameters of the catheters and sheaths have made percutaneous insertion easier overall and possible for smaller patients. Typically, the primary operator is assisted with insertion and fluoroscopy, while a third person is responsible for the balloon pump console. While a typical insertion takes 15 to 20 minutes, IABP can be done within 5 minutes in an emergency.

OPERATIVE TECHNIQUE

After standard preparation for percutaneous catheterization and appropriate local anesthesia, a small incision is made to facilitate insertion of the dilators. In a nonemergency case, the equipment and balloon catheter are prepared while the anesthetic takes effect. Then arterial puncture can begin with the necessary equipment within reach. The intra-aortic balloon is carefully removed from the tray, and a 60-ml syringe with a one-way valve is used to aspirate

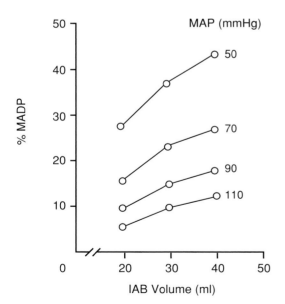

Fig. 16-2. Percent augmentation in aortic root mean diastolic pressure (MADP), as a function of IAB volume for four mean arterial pressures (MAP). (From Weber and Janicki,[5] with permission.)

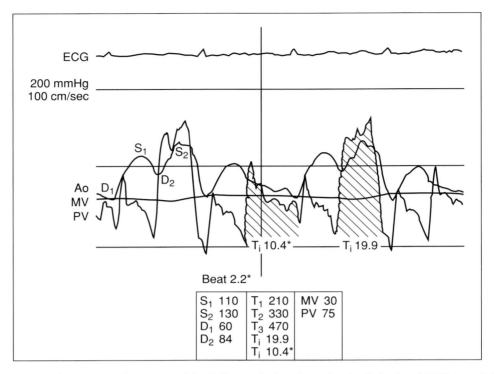

Fig. 16-3. Hemodynamic and coronary blood flow velocity data obtained during IABP in a 2:1 mode. Aortic pressure (A_o) demonstrates augmentation of diastolic pressure (S_2) with augmentation of the peak phasic velocity (PV) and diastolic flow velocity integral (T_i). Hemodynamic effects of balloon pumping are indicated by points S_1, S_2, D_1, and D_2. Augmentation of diastolic pressure to 130 mmHg corresponded to an increase in diastolic flow velocity integral from 10.4 to 19.9 U. Although the mean velocity (MV) is unchanged, peak flow velocity is nearly doubled, from 40 to about 80 cm/sec. Intra-aortic balloon pumping increases proximal coronary flow velocity measured directly within the coronary artery. (From Kern et al.,[6] with permission.)

slowly at least 30 ml, creating a vacuum that is maintained throughout the insertion (Fig. 16-4). After removal of the inner stylet, the distance from the angle of Louis to the umbilicus and obliquely to the femoral insertion site is measured with the balloon catheter. This distance is noted relative to catheter markings. The angiographic needle is inserted into the common femoral artery (Fig. 16-5). Since the IABP is usually kept in place for several hours post-PTCA, only the

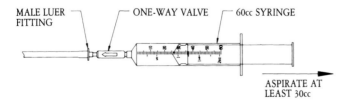

Fig. 16-4. Preparation of the IABP catheter. Connect the 60 ml-syringe to the one-way valve and slowly aspirate at least 30 ml. Remove the syringe, leaving the one-way valve in place until the IABP is inserted and ready to be connected to the console. (From Datascope Corp,[20] with permission.)

anterior wall is punctured. This minimizes posterior wall bleeding in high-risk patients. The guidewire is inserted through the needle and advanced carefully, avoiding dissection of the arterial wall. The needle is then removed, leaving the guidewire in place.

The tapered end of the vessel dilator is placed over the guidewire, and the artery is dilated by gently pushing and rotating the dilator into the artery. The dilator is then removed (keeping the wire in place), and pressure is applied to the wound site to prevent bleeding. Blood is wiped from the wire with a wet, lint-free sponge. The secured introducer sheath and dilator are placed over the wire and then advanced gently with a rotary motion into the lumen. Newer IABP catheters have allowed insertions without sheaths. This has generally reduced the access site diameter from 10.5 to 9.5 F.

The IABP is inserted and advanced while securing the guidewire and avoiding excessive force and kinking. Under fluoroscopy, the IABP is positioned in the descending thoracic aorta, approximately 2 cm distal to the left subclavian artery (Fig. 16-6). The guidewire is removed and blood is aspirated. The pressure

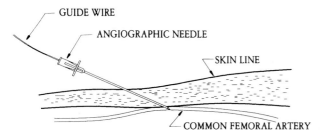

Fig. 16-5. Insertion of the angiographic needle. After local anesthesia and preparation for percutaneous catheterization, the needle is inserted into the common femoral artery, keeping the angle of the insertion as shallow as possible. The guidewire is then inserted through the needle into the artery, and the needle is removed, leaving only the guidewire in place. (From Datascope Corp,[20] with permission.)

line is connected and the vacuum released, by removing the one-way valve from the IABP and coupling its lumen to an actuator device that synchronizes balloon cycles with the patient's ECG. Most control consoles will automatically purge the system and fill it with helium before balloon inflation. To allow proper inflation and deflation of the balloon, the sheaths are pulled back to expose them above the skin line: 1″ for a 6″ sheath, 6″ for an 11″ sheath. The IABP and sheath can then be secured by suturing. Balloon expansion is confirmed by fluoroscopy. Radiographs are also obtained to confirm proper positioning of the IABP in the descending aorta.

The insertion site must be checked for unusual bleeding or hematoma, and peripheral pulses are evaluated bilaterally. Intravenous heparin must be administered to prevent thrombosis in the peripheral vasculature and clot formation on the balloon.

INDICATIONS AND SELECTION OF PATIENTS

IABP in High-Risk PTCA

IABP is increasingly used in high-risk PTCA, due to its ease of use and reliability in reducing myocardial

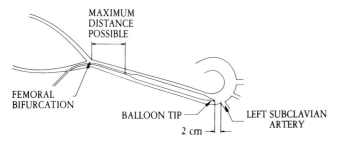

Fig. 16-6. Proper position of the IABP. Under fluoroscopy, advance the IABP to the proper position in the descending aorta, just distal (about 2 cm) to the left subclavian artery. Place the IABP as high above the femoral bifurcation as possible. (From Datascope Corp,[20] with permission.)

ischemia. This is done by decreasing left ventricular filling pressure, augmenting diastolic pressure, and increasing blood flow velocity. In patients with stable ventricular rhythms and intrinsic cardiac output, IABP can increase the cardiac index by 0.2 to 0.8 L/min/m^2 while reducing myocardial oxygen demand through afterload reduction.[5] While anatomic and technical risks influence early PTCA success, clinical parameters have a much stronger impact on the risk of procedural and long-term outcomes after PTCA. Furthermore, experienced operators with increasingly better skills and advanced technologies have reduced the relative importance of anatomic risk (American College of Cardiology/American Heart Association lesion classifications that predict the likelihood of successful dilation). Low-risk PTCA is associated with a procedural mortality of about 0.25%. Clinical variables related to higher mortality include patient age over 70 years (1.3% mortality), multivessel angioplasty (1.4%), left ventricular ejection fraction below 40% (2.9%), and left main coronary artery disease (3.4%).[7] Other clinical features can also increase procedural risk: unstable angina, acute myocardial infarction, hemodynamic instability, or dilation of vessels that supply large areas of myocardium. The patient may also have a higher risk of subsequent mortality due to abrupt reocclusion.

Although few prospective randomized trials have compared prophylactic IABP with other systemic support devices or with standby support in patients with high-risk PTCA, several reports suggest that patients do well when IABP is initiated before angioplasty.[8–12] The results of five small retrospective studies are summarized in Table 16-2. Patients who had ejection fractions below 30%, those undergoing multivessel PTCA, those who had dilation of a vessel supplying more than 50% of the viable myocardium, those who presented with or developed systemic hypotension, and those presenting with moderate-to-severe mitral insufficiency appeared to be best suited for prophylactic IABP. For borderline or high-risk patients, IABP could be used on a standby basis, and for those in whom rapid insertion may be necessary, a 5-F sheath could be inserted in the contralateral femoral artery before the procedure.

Since the goals of any support strategy are to provide oxygenated blood to the ischemic myocardium and to support systemic circulation, simultaneous IABP and perfusion balloon catheters (PBCs) could be used synergistically when augmented diastolic pressure is adequate. By allowing longer inflations and reducing major dissections, PBCs increased acute angiographic success with PTCA in a recent randomized trial of "average" patients. Although we cannot extrapolate these results to a high-risk popu-

Table 16-2. IABP Before High-Risk PTCA: Early Angiographic Success

Study	No. of Patients	High-Risk Features	PTCA Success[a]	IABP Complications[b]
Alcan et al.[8]	9	Unstable angina (n = 7) Cardiogenic shock (n = 2)	9/9 (100)	3 (33)
Szatmary et al.[11]	16	Unstable angina (n = 16) Ejection fraction <40% (n = 10) Sustained hypotension (n = 6)	27/30 (90)	0 (0)
Voudris et al.[12]	27	Ejection fraction <40% (n = 24) Multivessel disease (n = 3)	39/39 (100)	1 (4)
Kahn et al.[9]	28	Ejection fraction <30% (n = 25) Left main disease (n = 7) Single remaining circulation (n = 11)	90/94 (96)	3 (11)
Kreidieh et al.[10]	21	Ejection fraction <30% (n = 16) Multivessel disease (n = 14) Unstable angina (n = 12)	38/42 (90)	2 (10)

[a] Numerator is the number of successes, and denominator is the total number of stenosed arteries. Percentages are indicated within parentheses.
[b] Values are numbers (percentage) of patients who had complications.
(Adapted from Wilson and Ohman,[19] with permission.)

lation, this strategy certainly merits further evaluation.

IABP in PTCA During Myocardial Infarction

Primary and salvage PTCA successfully restore patency during acute myocardial infarction. Unfortunately, they carry a reocclusion rate as high as 20%. By increasing coronary blood flow velocity, IABP would be expected to maintain patency of the infarct artery. Recent reports have shed light on the optimal use of IABP with PTCA during acute myocardial infarction. Several small, nonrandomized trials suggest that IABP may also reduce reocclusion rates of infarct-related arteries.

We conducted a multicenter, prospective, randomized trial to evaluate the optimal strategy for using IABP after emergency PTCA for acute myocardial infarction.[13] Patients who underwent emergency catheterization and in whom patency was restored to the infarct artery by angioplasty or intracoronary thrombolytics were randomized to 48 hours of IABP or conventional post-PTCA care. Patients were excluded if they had spontaneous or thrombolytic-induced reperfusion and fewer than three epicardial arteries with 75% or more stenosis, if they presented in cardiogenic shock, unresponsive hypotension, or pulmonary edema, or if they had histories of severe peripheral vascular disease or aortic aneurysm or insufficiency.

Patients who received IABP had significantly lower reocclusion rates. They also showed significant reductions in recurrent ischemia and emergency repeat PTCA. Moreover, there was no significant difference in the rates of peripheral vascular complications between the groups. These findings suggest that careful use of IABP can improve clinical outcomes in patients who undergo emergency PTCA for acute infarction.

IABP in PTCA with Cardiogenic Shock

Without aggressive management, cardiogenic shock is associated with a mortality rate of 70 to 90%. Balloon pumping alone can produce temporary clinical stabilization, but improved survival is achieved only with rapid, complete revascularization. Thrombolytic therapy results in reperfusion in less than 50% of patients. Bolooki,[14] reviewing the literature of 20 years' experience, reported a 66% survival rate after emergency revascularization for acute myocardial infarction with cardiogenic shock. When reperfusion was achieved in nonrandomized studies, inpatient survival rates of 56 to 71% were reported, compared with only 7 to 29% survival for incomplete or failed revascularization.[15–18] Bengtson et al.,[15] reporting a series of 200 consecutive patients admitted with acute myocardial infarction and cardiogenic shock, found that these survival benefits continued for at least 1 year. The best predictors of postdischarge mortality were age, peak creatine kinase level, ejection fraction, and infarct artery patency. Furthermore, the use of IABP and mechanical revascularization appeared to be superior to IABP alone.

In patients who develop cardiogenic shock after failed PTCA or abrupt closure after PTCA, IABP with PBC has also been useful in stabilizing blood pressure and limiting the final size of the infarct before bypass is attempted.[14] Despite the lack of adequate clinical trials, IABP and PTCA have become standard therapies in the management of cardiogenic shock.

POSTPROCEDURE MANAGEMENT

Patients on IABP should be anticoagulated such that an activated partial thromboplastin time of 50 to 80 seconds is maintained. They should be screened for any active bleeding and placed on prophylactic H_2 blockers to prevent gastrointestinal stress ulcers. The insertion site must be kept clean using standard sterile precautions. Complete bed rest is required, but the patient can be carefully turned toward one side or sedated for comfort while the leg is held straight.

Peripheral pulses as well as distal perfusion must be monitored, and rapidly restored if any deterioration is noted. If ischemia progresses, the IABP often must be removed. It may be placed in the other limb if required for hemodynamic support. Any active bleeding or major hematoma formation at the insertion site must be evaluated and properly treated. Rarely, thrombocytopenia will develop. Removal of the IABP should be considered if the platelet count falls below 80,000/ml, depending on the clinical situation.

Pressure monitoring through the central lumen is necessary when the pump is functioning, to detect malfunctions or changes in clinical status. Augmentation not within the normal range may be related to several problems. The balloon could be expanding incorrectly, which can be corrected by pulling back the sheath until it clears the balloon membrane. If the balloon is adhering to itself, it should be flushed with 60 ml of helium, preferably by means of a stopcock. The IABP could be malpositioned in the aortic arch or even in a false lumen. The synchronization could be suboptimal, or the augmentation/volume control could be set inappropriately. The patient's physiologic state may change: blood pressure or vascular resistance can become reduced, volume can be depleted, and the heart beat can become so rapid or irregular that it compromises ventricular filling and ejection. All these situations require thorough evaluation and efficient correction.

Anticoagulation is discontinued 4 to 6 hours before IABP removal, with weaning if clinically indicated. After administration of local anesthesia, the sutures are removed, the balloon is disconnected from the pump, and the deflated balloon is slowly withdrawn. If a sheath was used, the IABP is not withdrawn through it, but both are removed as a unit. Any undue resistance is a warning that a thrombus may have formed within the balloon, and removal by arteriotomy may be necessary. Once the balloon is removed, free bleeding is allowed for a few seconds, and then hemostasis is achieved by applying pressure to the puncture site for at least 30 minutes. The distal limb should be examined for adequate perfusion. If any ischemic indications are present, a vascular surgical consultation should be obtained without delay.

OUTCOMES WITH AORTIC COUNTERPULSATION

Several small, nonrandomized trials have reported beneficial short-term effects of prophylactic IABP in high-risk PTCA patients.[8-12] These are summarized in Tables 16-2 and 16-3. Nonemergency IABP was effective in the short term, with minimum complications. A definitive benefit was not shown, however, due to the lack of a control group. The long-term prognoses of these patients were much less favorable, with high cardiac and overall mortality that most likely reflected the poor general condition of this population. Unfortunately, none of the studies was designed or had the power to detect significant differences in long-term event-free survival or reocclusion rates.

In a series of 200 patients treated at Duke University who had acute myocardial infarction complicated by cardiogenic shock, IABP use coupled with angioplasty to restore patency was associated with an improved in-hospital survival. In one randomized trial of 182 patients, prophylactic IABP for 48 hours reduced the rate of reocclusion (8 vs. 21%, $P < 0.03$) of the infarct-related artery compared with control treated patients. In addition, in-hospital morbidity was reduced with IABP. Patients assigned to IABP had less recurrent ischemia (4 vs. 21%, $P < 0.001$), need for emergency PTCA (2 vs. 11%, $P < 0.02$), and reinfarction (3 vs. 8%). These clinical benefits were not offset by an increased incidence of vascular or hemorrhagic complications.

However, IABP can be associated with several complications. The absolute incidence of events is difficult to determine because of changes in techniques, use of smaller catheters, and better patient selection. Consequently, a lower complication rate is now reported compared with early results. Nonetheless,

Table 16-3. IABP Before High-Risk PTCA: Short-Term and Long-Term Follow-Up[a]

	No. of Patients	Mean Follow-up (months)	In-Hospital Events				Follow-Up Events			
			MI	Death	CABG	Repeat PTCA	MI	Death	CABG	Repeat PTCA
Alcan et al.[8]	9	—	—	1 (11)	1 (11)	—	—	0	—	—
Szatmary et al.[11]	16	22	0	1 (6)	0	0	0	2 (13)	1 (6)	1 (6)
Voudris et al.[12]	27	13.1	0	0	0	0	0	2 (7)	1 (4)	6 (22)
Kahn et al.[9]	28	—	0	2 (7)	0	—	—	—	—	—
Kreidieh et al.[10]	21	14	0	0	1 (5)	0	—	2 (10)	3 (14)	5 (24)

Abbreviation: MI, myocardial infarction.

[a] Values are given as the number (percentage) of patients having each event.

(Adapted from Wilson and Ohman,[19] with permission.)

vascular complications remain the primary adverse events associated with IABP. In a recent randomized trial, rates of vascular and hemorrhagic complications were low: severe hemorrhage in 1% of the IABP patients and vascular repair or thrombectomy in 5%. Both of these rates were similar to the standard PTCA (control) group. In the literature, rates of limb ischemia range from 5 to 28%, vascular repair from 0 to 6%, and bleeding requiring transfusion from 6 to 24%. Of several predictors of vascular complications, the most important is a history of vascular disease, followed by diabetes and female sex.

Comparison With Cardiopulmonary Support

Without controlled data comparing IABP with percutaneous CPS, no definitive guidelines can be given, but clearly the approach must be individualized to the patient, hospital expertise, and operator experience and judgment. IABP can be applied in a larger number of hospital settings, while CPS usually requires high-volume centers with pools of high-risk patients adequate to maintain peak skills while minimizing complications.

Patients with reduced ejection fractions (20 to 30%) or target arteries that supply more than 50% of the myocardium, or both, can probably benefit from either IABP or stand-by CPS. In those with severely depressed systolic function (ejection fraction <15%) or current or prior hemodynamic collapse, however, prophylactic CPS is probably the strategy of choice. Since IABP increases patency in patients undergoing emergency PTCA for acute infarction, CPS may not be necessary unless hemodynamic collapse occurs.

Since CPS requires much greater resources, an international trial in several high-volume centers is needed to determine the best systemic support strategies for various types of patients.

CONCLUSIONS

The role of IABP in coronary interventions has evolved over the last two decades. Aortic counterpulsation represents one of the simplest and easiest support devices to use in conjunction with angioplasty. Over the last decade the placement of IABP catheters by well-trained interventional cardiologists has made the procedure more accessible to cardiology. Coupled with advances in catheter designs, clinical observations and randomized trials have suggested an acceptable benefit-to-risk ratio in patients with acute myocardial infarction, in particular in patients with hemodynamic compromise. Aortic counterpulsation in patients undergoing high-risk angioplasty remains unproven, but several observational series have suggested that this approach may be useful. In the future, with further refinements in catheters and IABP techniques, this support device may be applied to a broader spectrum of patients.

REFERENCES

1. Kantrowitz A, Kantrowitz A. Experimental augmentation of coronary flow by retardation of arterial pressure pulse. Surgery 1953;34:678
2. Moulopoulos SD, Topaz S, Kolff WJ. Diastolic balloon pumping (with carbon dioxide) in the aorta—a mechanical assistance to the failing circulation. Am Heart J 1962;63:669

3. Kantrowitz A, Tjønneland S, Freed P et al. Initial clinical experience with intraaortic balloon pumping in cardiogenic shock. JAMA 1968;203:135
4. Summers DN, Kaplitt M, Norris J et al. Intraaortic balloon pumping: hemodynamic and metabolic effects during cardiogenic shock in patients with triple coronary artery obstructive disease. Arch Surg 1969;99:733
5. Weber KT, Janicki JS. Intraaortic balloon counterpulsation: a review of physiological principles, clinical results, and device safety. Ann Thorac Surg 1974;17:602
6. Kern MJ, Aguirre F, Back R et al. Augmentation of coronary blood flow by intra-aortic balloon pumping in patients after coronary angioplasty. Circulation 1993;87:500
7. Hartzler GO, Rutherford BD, McConahay DR et al. "High-risk" percutaneous transluminal coronary angioplasty. Am J Cardiol 1988;61:33G
8. Alcan KE, Stertzer SH, Walls E et al. The role of intraaortic balloon counterpulsation in patients undergoing percutaneous transluminal coronary angioplasty. Am Heart J 1983;105:527
9. Kahn JK, Rutherford BD, McConahay DR et al. Supported "high risk" coronary angioplasty using intraaortic balloon pump counterpulsation. J Am Coll Cardiol 1990;15:1151
10. Kreidieh I, Davies DW, Lim R et al. High-risk coronary angioplasty with elective intra-aortic balloon pump support. Int J Cardiol 1992;35:147
11. Szatmary LJ, Marco J, Fajadet F et al. The combined use of diastolic counterpulsation and coronary dilation in unstable angina due to multivessel disease under unstable hemodynamic conditions. Int J Cardiol 1988;19:59
12. Voudris V, Marco J, Morice MC et al. "High-risk" percutaneous transluminal coronary angioplasty with preventive intra-aortic balloon counterpulsation. Cathet Cardiovasc Diagn 1990;19:160
13. Ohman EM, George BS, White CS et al. The use of aortic counterpulsation to improve sustained coronary artery patency during acute myocardial infarction: results of a randomized trial. Circulation 1994;90:792
14. Bolooki H. Emergency cardiac procedures in the patients in cardiogenic shock due to complications of coronary artery disease. Circulation, suppl. I, 1989;79:I137
15. Bengtson JR, Kaplan AJ et al. Prognosis in cardiogenic shock after acute myocardial infarction in the interventional era. J Am Coll Cardiol 1992;20:1482
16. Gacioch GM, Ellis SG, Lee L et al. Cardiogenic shock complicating acute myocardial infarction: the use of coronary angioplasty and the integration of the new support devices into patient management. J Am Coll Cardiol 1992;19:647
17. Hibbard MD, Holmes DR, Bailey KR et al. Percutaneous transluminal coronary angioplasty in patients with cardiogenic shock. J Am Coll Cardiol 1992;19:639
18. Moosvi AR, Khaja F, Villanueva L et al. Early revascularization improves survival in cardiogenic shock complicating acute myocardial infarction. J Am Coll Cardiol 1992;19:907
19. Wilson JS, Ohman EM. Supported coronary angioplasty. p. 243. In White CJ, Ramee S (eds): Advances in Interventional Cardiology: New Technologies and Strategies for Diagnosis and Treatment. Marcel Dekker, New York, 1995
20. Datascope Corp. Abbreviated Guide for Optional Sheathless Insertion. Datascope Corp, Fairfield, New Jersey, 1992

17 Hypertrophic Obstructive Cardiomyopathy

Ulrich Sigwart

Hypertrophic obstructive cardiomyopathy (HOCM) is dominated by a dynamic left ventricular outflow tract obstruction due to asymmetrical septal hypertrophy.[1–4] Surgical resection of the septal myocardial bulge often remains the only acceptable therapeutic option. The results of surgery are palliative, but in nonrandomized series they seem to compare favorably with conservative treatment.[5] This chapter describes a new technique based on nonsurgical ablation of the septal bulge in advanced hypertrophic cardiomyopathy.

PROCEDURE

Patients with symptomatic HOCM are studied invasively by transeptal and retrograde cardiac catheterization. Pressures are measured by fluid-filled catheters in the ascending aorta and simultaneously in different locations in the left ventricle. A transeptally introduced Brockenbrough catheter is placed in the left ventricular inflow tract. Left ventricular outflow tract pressure gradients are recorded at rest, during the Valsalva maneuver, following induction of premature ventricular contraction, after administration of amyl nitrate and pacing, and during isoproterenol infusion. The left coronary artery ostium is then intubated using an 8-F coronary angioplasty guiding catheter and, with the help of a 0.014″ steerable guidewire, a small-diameter over-the-wire angioplasty balloon is advanced into the first large septal branch of the left anterior descending coronary artery. Contrast injections through the balloon cathe-

ter are used to delineate the area of the interventricular septum supplied by this artery and to correlate it with the location of the myocardial bulge. The artery is then occluded by balloon inflation with pressures ranging from 2 to 5 bar, and intracavity and aortic pressures are recorded simultaneously during the same provocations as before.

If the intraventricular pressure gradients react typically with increase during preload reduction as well as during the Valsalva, maneuver, pacing, and isoproterenol infusion, and if the post-extrasystolic beats show a large gradient, all findings are normalized during balloon occlusion of the first major septal branch. The salutary effects of balloon occlusion are reversed immediately after balloon deflation. Following intravenous administration of 5 mg diamorphine, 5 ml of absolute alcohol are then slowly injected through the inflated balloon into the vessel and left in situ for 5 minutes before the balloon is deflated. Seconds after the alcohol injection, the pressure gradient is again abolished and fails to reappear after balloon deflation. Patients report moderate chest discomfort but only at the initiation of the alcohol injection. Often a transient complete AV block is seen in patients with a permanent pacemaker. The postprocedure gradients remain absent or very low on provocation.[6] The systolic anterior movement of the mitral valve remains visible on echocardiography despite the absence of a significantly accelerated flow. Postprocedure creatinine phosphokinase normally rises to about 2,500 IU within hours and falls rapidly thereafter. After uneventful recovery the patient is discharged 2 days after the intervention on low-dose aspirin and β-blockers.

DISCUSSION

β-Adrenoreceptor blockers remain the first-line treatment in symptomatic patients with HCOM.[3,7] β-Blockers reduce overall myocardial contractility, which includes systolic thickening of the septal bulge. As the intracavity gradient largely depends on the instantaneous catecholamine level, this effect is more pronounced during exercise than at rest.[7] Other negative inotropic substances like verapamil[8] and disopyramide[9–12] have been given with satisfactory acute results, but none of them has clearly changed the natural history of the disease.

Atrioventricular sequential pacing has been shown to reduce intracavity pressure gradients in HCOM[13,14] by a more favorable left ventricular excitation pattern and through optimal timing of atrial contraction.[15] DDD pacing is therefore often recommended as a first-line treatment before surgery.[16,17] Several surgical techniques aiming at resection of the offending myocardial bulge have been evaluated in symptomatic patients with severe outflow tract obstruction.[18–20] All require extracorporeal circulation and are associated with a moderate surgical risk on the order of 5%.[18,21] Most patients derive long-term benefit from surgery in respect to symptoms and exercise capacity without significant impairment of left ventricular function.[22–25] As a last resort, cardiac transplantation has been advocated.[26]

The idea of producing a septal infarction by catheter techniques was born out of the observation that systolic and diastolic myocardial function of selected areas of the left ventricle can be selectively suppressed by balloon occlusion of the supplying artery during coronary angioplasty[27,28] and that intracavity pressure gradients in hypertrophic cardiomyopathy diminish markedly when the major first septal artery is temporarily occluded by an angioplasty balloon.[28] The feasibility of diagnostic temporary interruption of blood flow to the first major septal coronary vessel has recently been confirmed by others.[29] The attraction of the procedure resides in its simplicity, minimal morbidity, and the fact that the outcome of the definite ablation can be estimated by temporary occlusion of the target vessel.

REFERENCES

1. Morrow AG, Braunwald E. Functional aortic stenosis: a malformation characterized by resistance to left ventricular outflow without anatomic obstruction. Circulation 1959;20:181

2. Braunwald E. Hypertrophic cardiomyopathy—continued progress. N Engl J Med 1989;320:800

3. Maron BJ, Bonow RO, Cannon RO et al. Hypertrophic cardiomyopathy: interrelations of clinical manifestations, pathophysiology, and therapy. N Engl J Med 1987;316:780

4. Jarcho JA, McKenna W, Pare JAP et al. Mapping a gene for familial hypertrophic cardiomyopathy to chromosome 14ql. N Engl J Med 1989;321:1372

5. Bonow RO, Maron BJ, Leon MB. Medical and surgical therapy of hypertrophic cardiomyopathy. Cardiovasc Clin 1988;19:221

6. Grbic M, Sigwart U. Relationship between preload and afterload and gradient in hypertrophic obstructive cardiomyopathy, abstracted. Circulation 1982;66:268

7. Bonow RO, Dilsizian V, Rosing DR et al. Verapamil-induced improvement in left ventricular diastolic filling and increased exercise tolerance in patients with hypertrophic cardiomyopathy. Short and long-term effects. Circulation 1985;72:853

8. Chatterjee K. Calcium antagonist agents in hypertrophic cardiomyopathy. Am J Cardiol 1987;59:146B

9. Sherrid M, Delia E, Dwyer E. Oral disopyramide therapy for obstructive hypertrophic cardiomyopathy. Am J Cardiol 1988;62:1085

10. Cokkinos DV, Salpeas D, Ioannou NE, Christoulas S. Combination of disopyramide and propranolol in hypertrophic cardiomyopathy. Can J Cardiol 1989;5:33

11. Pollick C, Kimball B, Henderson M, Wigle ED. Disopyramide in hypertrophic cardiomyopathy. I. Hemodynamic assessment after intravenous administration. Am J Cardiol 1988;62:1248

12. Duncan WJ, Tyrrell MJ, Bharadwaj BB. Disopyramide as a negative inotrope in obstructive cardiomyopathy in children. Can J Cardiol 1991;7:81

13. Hassenstein P, Storch H, Schmitz W. Erfahrungen mit der Schrittmacher Dauerbehandlung bei Patienten mit obstruktiver Kardiomyopathie. Thoraxchirurgie 1975;23:496

14. McDonald K, McWilliams E, O'Keefee B, Maurer B. Functional assessment of patients treated with permanent dual chamber pacing as a primary treatment for hypertrophic cardiomyopathy. Eur Heart J 1988;9:893

15. Jeanrenaud X, Goy J-J, Kappenberger L. Effects of dual-chamber pacing in hypertrophic obstructive cardiomyopathy. Lancet 1992;339:1318

16. Fananapazir L, Cannon RO, Tripodi D, Panza JA. Impact of dual-chamber permanent pacing in patients with obstructive hypertrophic cardiomyopathy with symptoms refractory to verapamil and β-adrenergic blocker therapy. Circulation 1992;85:2149

17. Kappenberger L. Pacing for obstructive hypertrophic cardiomyopathy, editorial. Br Heart J 1995;73:107

18. McIntosh CL, Maron BJ. Current operative treatment of obstructive hypertrophic cardiomyopathy. Circulation 1988;78:487

19. Seiler C, Hess OM, Schoenbeck M et al. Long term follow-up of medical versus surgical therapy for hypertrophic cardiomyopathy: a retrospective study. J Am Coll Cardiol 1991;17:643

20. Chahine RA. Surgical versus medical therapy of hypertrophic cardiomyopathy: is the perspective changing? J Am Coll Cardiol 1991;17:643

21. Mohr R, Schaff HV, Danielson GK et al. The outcome of surgical treatment of hypertrophic obstructive cardiomyopathy: Experience over 15 years. J Thorac Cardiovasc Surg 1989;97:666

22. Leachman RD, Krajcer Z, Azic R, Cooley DA. Mitral valve replacement in hypertrophic cardiomyopathy: ten year follow-up in 54 patients. Am J Cardiol 1987; 60:1416

23. Walker WS, Reid KG, Cameron EWJ et al. Comparison of ventricular septal surgery and mitral valve replacement for hypertrophic obstructive cardiomyopathy. Ann Thorac Surg 1989;38:528

24. Krajcer Z, Leachman RD, Cooley DA et al. Mitral valve replacement and septal myomectomy in hypertrophic cardiomyopathy: ten year follow-up in 80 patients. Circulation 1988;78:35

25. McIntosh CL, Greenberg GJ, Maron BJ et al. Clinical and hemodynamic results after mitral valve replacement in patients with obstructive hypertrophic cardiomyopathy. Ann Thorac Surg 1989;47:236

26. Warren SE, Cohn LH, Schoen FJ et al. Advanced diastolic heart failure in familial hypertrophic cardiomyopathy managed with cardiac transplantation. J Appl Cardiol 1988;3:415

27. Sigwart U, Grbic M, Essinger A, Rivier JL. L'effet aigu d'une occlusion coronarienne par ballonet de la dilatation transluminale, abstracted. Schweiz Med Wschr 1982;45:1631

28. Sigwart U, Grbic M, Payot M, Essinger A, Sadeghi H. Wall motion during balloon occlusion. In Sigwart U, Heintzen PH (eds.): Ventricular Wall Motion. George Thieme, New York, 1983

29. Gietzen F, Leuner C, Gerenkamp T, Kuhn H. Relief of obstruction in hypertrophic cardiomyopathy by transient occlusion of the first septal branch of the left coronary artery, abstracted. Eur Heart J 1994;15: 125

30. Sigwart U. Nonsurgical myocardial reduction: a new treatment for hypertrophic obstructive cardiomyopathy. Lancet 1995;346:221

31. Sigwart U. Non-surgical myocardial reduction for hypertrophic obstructive cardiomyopathy, letter. Lancet 1996;346:1624

18 Catheter-Based Techniques of Local Drug Delivery

Raymond G. McKay

Percutaneous coronary angioplasty continues to be plagued by abrupt vessel closure and late vascular restenosis. In part, these limitations are related to mechanical factors such as coronary dissection and elastic recoil. Equally important, however, are biologic factors such as intracoronary thrombus formation and smooth muscle cell hyperplasia as major causes of suboptimal angioplasty results. Newer adjunctive angioplasty techniques, including intracoronary stents, coronary atherectomy, and laser angioplasty, have provided some benefit in ameliorating the mechanical deficiencies of balloon dilation. All these devices, however, have either worsened the biologic consequences of arterial injury or had no effect on limiting them.

Given the limitations of mechanical approaches to vascular dilation, there has been renewed interest in pharmacologic measures to combat the problems of intracoronary thrombus formation and smooth muscle cell hyperplasia. Some degree of success in treating intracoronary thrombus has been achieved with systemic administration of antiplatelet, antithrombin, and thrombolytic agents, as well as with the intracoronary and subselective administration of thrombolytic agents directly to the thrombus site. In spite of these advances, however, percutaneous intervention of thrombus-containing stenoses is still associated with an unacceptably high incidence of myocardial infarction, emergency coronary bypass, and death.

Systemic pharmacologic therapy for preventing smooth muscle hyperplasia has likewise been largely unsuccesful. Animal studies have provided a large number of therapeutic agents that appear to inhibit neointimal thickening following balloon injury, but no agent has been shown to reduce the incidence of restenosis consistently in patients undergoing angioplasty.

One theory why systemic pharmacologic therapy has been unsuccessful in limiting the biologic consequences of balloon injury is that patients are unable to tolerate the high systemic drug concentrations needed for prolonged periods to impact on suboptimal angioplasty results. As a result, there has been recent interest in the development of strategies designed to achieve a local therapeutic drug effect at the angioplasty site without the risk of systemic side effects. These strategies have included the development of a number of local drug delivery catheters for intraluminal drug administration, as well as various other experimental techniques including drug-coated metallic stents, endovascular and extravascular drug-eluting polymers, periadventitial drug pumps, and cell-targeting techniques designed to activate intravenously administered agents locally.

OVERVIEW OF CATHETER-BASED DRUG DELIVERY

The field of catheter-based local drug delivery is currently in its infancy. Based on in vitro and animal studies, the list of possible agents that might have a therapeutic effect is enormous and includes antiplatelet agents, antithrombin agents, thrombolytic agents, steroids, antiproliferative agents, specific growth factor inhibitors, antisense oligonucleotides, calcium blocking agents, and many others. Apart from not knowing which agent should be used, the specific drug dose, the optimal time of administration, and the necessary intramural residence time have not been established for any given agent. Moreover, the individual pharmacokinetics of each drug, in terms of the efficiency of intramural delivery, depth of penetration, and wash-out from the arterial wall, are presumably different for each agent, depending on its molecular weight, charge, lipophilicity, ability to bind to specific receptors, and affinity for macrophage ingestion.

A catheter-based, locally administered drug would have to exert its therapeutic effect by either acting intraluminally during the time of catheter administration, or by persisting at the angioplasty site by being deposited into the arterial wall. At least three mechanisms of intramural delivery are possible: passive diffusion, active bulk transfer, or facilitated diffusion. In passive diffusion techniques, drugs are infused via catheters into a closed intraluminal space and allowed to bathe the arterial wall, with intramural deposition by simple diffusion down a concentration or electrochemical gradient. With active bulk transfer, agents are introduced directly into the wall by physical means. With facilitated diffusion, agents are intramurally distributed by means of a substrate-carrier complex that may undergo translational or rotational diffusion. Some or all of these mechanisms are operant in the catheter-based delivery systems that have been developed, depending on the individual drug being used.

At least sixteen different types of catheter-based delivery systems are currently in development. At the present time, two of these catheters are approved by the United States Food and Drug Administration for intramural drug delivery. All these systems differ with respect to efficiency of drug delivery, homogeneity of drug deposition, degree of vascular disruption, ability to deliver drug and dilate vascular stenoses simultaneously, and ability to maintain perfusion during drug delivery. Very little comparative information is available on the relatively efficacy of these systems.

In addition to the ongoing refinement of catheter-based drug delivery systems, current research is aimed at maintaining drugs within the arterial wall following initial intramural deposition. Some locally administered agents may exert a therapeutic effect on abrupt closure and late restenosis with only a short intramural residence time. Alternatively, given the time course of thrombus formation, smooth muscle cell division, smooth muscle cell migration, and extracellular matrix production following balloon injury, other agents may require an intramural residence time of days to weeks to achieve a beneficial impact. Possible techniques of increasing drug persistence at the angioplasty site that are under active investigation include the delivery of drug-containing liposomes and biodegradable microspheres.

SPECIFIC DRUG-DELIVERY SYSTEMS

Double-Balloon Catheter

The earliest approach to local drug delivery, the double-balloon catheter (Boston Scientific, Watertown, MA) consists of a standard angioplasty shaft with two latex balloons separated by 2 cm mounted on its distal end[1] (Fig. 18-1). The catheter has four lumens, two for inflating/deflating the balloons, one for a central guidewire, and a fourth for drug infusion. When the catheter is placed in an artery over a guidewire and the two balloons are inflated, drug may be infused into the closed space between the inflated balloons. The arterial wall is thus bathed in a local intraluminal reservoir of drug, and intramural penetration occurs by passive diffusion.

The double-balloon catheter has been used in several experimental models for the delivery of horseradish peroxidase and therapeutically active

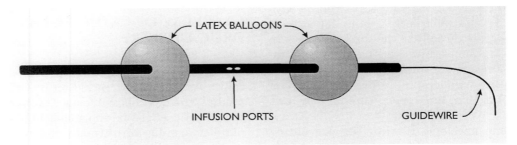

Fig. 18-1. The double-balloon catheter. Drug is infused into the closed intraluminal space between the two latex balloons and bathes the arterial wall. Intramural deposition occurs by passive diffusion.

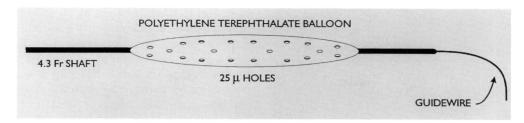

Fig. 18-2. The perforated (Wolinsky) balloon. Drug is infused intramurally through 28 25-μm holes arranged in longitudinal rows.

compounds including gene transfer. Intramural penetration of agents has been documented with low infusion pressures. In one study, the depth of penetration of horseradish peroxidase was shown to be related to infusion pressure, with complete penetration of the arterial media at 300 mmHg. At least three groups have reported successful in vivo gene transfer with the double-balloon catheter.

The specific advantages of the double-balloon catheter include its ability to deliver agents at low pressure atraumatically and homogeneously, and its ability to limit the site of drug therapy while minimizing systemic exposure. Disadvantages of the catheter, however, include the need for total arterial occlusion during drug infusion, loss of drug from side branches that originate from the site of drug administration, and inability to dilate vascular stenoses.

Perforated Balloon Catheter

The perforated balloon catheter (Wolinsky Infusion Catheter, USCI, Billerica, MA) consists of a triple-lumen shaft with a distal balloon made of polyethylene terephthalate[2] (Fig. 18-2). The balloon has 28 holes 25 μm in diameter arranged in longitudinal rows. During balloon inflation, drug is infused into the balloon and is intramurally deposited by bulk transfer through the balloon's pores.

The perforated balloon catheter has been utilized to deliver horseradish peroxidase, heparin, tissue plasminogen activator (t-PA), methotrexate, doxorubicin, colchicine, thiol protease inhibitor, and angiopeptin. In all cases, successful intramural delivery of the agent has been reported. In an initial series of reports studying horseradish peroxidase and fluoresceinated heparin, the depth of penetration of infused fluid was shown to correlate with both the infusion pressure and the duration of infusion. Following local delivery of agents, intramural persistence of agents has been reported for up to 48 hours for heparin and up to 2 weeks for methotrexate.

In spite of successful intramural delivery, there has been no beneficial effect of perforated balloon delivery. Studies with heparin, methotrexate, doxo-

rubicin, colchicine, thiol protease inhibitor, and angiopeptin have all failed to demonstrate any reduction in neointimal thickening in animal models. Similarly, studies with heparin, t-PA, and aurin tricarboxylic acid have failed to show any local inhibition of thrombus formation.

The disappointing results from the perforated balloon catheter may be related to the fact that the catheter traumatizes the angioplasty site from high-pressure fluid jets that emanate from the balloon pores. Histologic examination after local delivery of heparin at 5 atm has shown a moderate degree of medial necrosis. The disruption of the arterial wall caused by the system may therefore result in more platelet deposition, thrombus formation, and late restenosis.

Attempts to limit vascular trauma from the perforated balloon catheter have involved increasing the number of holes in the balloon surface. In vitro studies have demonstrated that the "jet streaming" effect of a drug infusion at any infusion pressure is significantly diminished with larger number of pores for delivery.

Microporous Balloon Catheter

The microporous balloon catheter (Cordis Corporation, Miami Lakes, FL) is a variant of the perforated balloon catheter in which an outer membrane contains thousands of pores less than 1 μm in diameter.[3] This catheter theoretically allows for the delivery of drug at low pressure without significant jet effects. A recent study with horseradish peroxidase has demonstrated successful drug delivery to the inner layers of the arterial wall with catheter-induced injury confined to the endothelium.

Channel Balloon

The channel balloon (Boston Scientific, Watertown, MA) consists of a standard polyethylene balloon that has intramural channels in the balloon surface (Fig. 18-3). Located in the channels are multiple external pores 75 μm in diameter that connect to a proximal

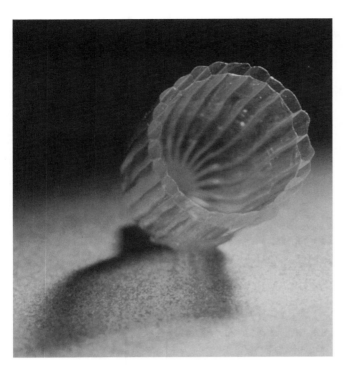

Fig. 18-3. The channel balloon. Cross section of balloon demonstrating intramural channels. Drug is infused via 75-μm pores located within the channels.

catheter port independent of the balloon inflation port. When the balloon is inflated at normal pressure through the inflation port, drug can be infused at lower pressures through the proximal port. The infused drug exits the balloon through the pores in the channel and bathes the arterial wall at low pressures, thus avoiding the "jet streaming" effect of the perforated balloon catheter.

Successful in vivo delivery of both horseradish peroxidase and fluoresceinated heparin has been accomplished with the channel balloon in rabbits. Drug infusion at 2 atm for 1 minute has resulted in full-thickness penetration of the drug. Histologic studies have demonstrated no evidence of medial dissection or intimal disruption.

The major advantage of the channel balloon is that successful drug delivery can be achieved with low pressure, atraumatic drug infusions during simultaneous angioplasty of an arterial stenosis. The disadvantages of the catheter include a nonhomogenous distribution of drug related to the location of the channels on the balloon surface and the need for arterial occlusion during drug administration.

Hydrogel-Coated Balloon

The hydrogel-coated balloon (Boston Scientific, Watertown, MA) consists of a standard polyethylene balloon coated with a hydrogel polymer[5] (Fig. 18-4). The hydrogel coating consists of an interlacing network of polyacrylic acid chains that adhere to the balloon surface. When the hydrogel comes in contact with an aqueous environment, it absorbs water and the lattice begins to swell, forming a stable matrix of polymer and water. Any agents that are dissolved in the water will also be incorporated into this matrix. The thickness of the coating ranges from 5 μm when dry to 25 μm when fully saturated with water.

Intramural drug delivery is achieved with the hydrogel system during balloon inflation when the hydrogel polymer comes in contact with the arterial intimal surface. Hydrogel compression during pressurized inflation results in accelerated diffusion of a given agent from the polymer directly into the vessel wall.

Drugs may be loaded onto the hydrogel balloon surface either by immersion of the inflated balloon into a concentrated drug solution or by "painting" the balloon surface with known aliquots of the drug. Using the immersion technique, in vitro studies have demonstrated maximum drug loading onto the hydrogel with immersion times as short as 30 to 60 seconds. The amount of fluid (and drug) absorbed by the hydrogel coating is proportional to the balloon surface area and amount of hydrogel available for binding. Relatively larger quantities of drug on the balloon surface can be achieved by "painting" the balloon surface with small aliquots of a drug solution, allowing for drying of the surface in between drug applications.

The hydrogel balloon has been used for in vivo delivery of horseradish peroxidase, heparin, antisense oligonucleotides, urokinase, and PPACK. In all cases, homogeneous intramural penetration of drug has been demonstrated without disruption of the vessel architecture. Studies with heparin, antisense oligonucleotides, and urokinase have demonstrated that between 2 and 33% of the drug on the balloon surface is intramurally deposited during balloon inflation. Studies with horseradish peroxidase have also demonstrated that the depth of drug delivery into the arterial wall is proportional to the balloon inflation pressure and inflation time. Following local delivery, heparin has been noted to persist in the arterial wall for as long as 48 hours, and antisense oligomers have been detected for at least 24 hours.

All hydrogel studies have demonstrated significant wash-off of drug from the balloon surface when the drug-coated balloon is exposed to the intact circulation. For this reason, use of a protective sheath to cover the balloon surface is recommended.

At the present time, the hydrogel balloon is one of the few drug delivery systems that has been shown to produce beneficial physiologic effects at the angio-

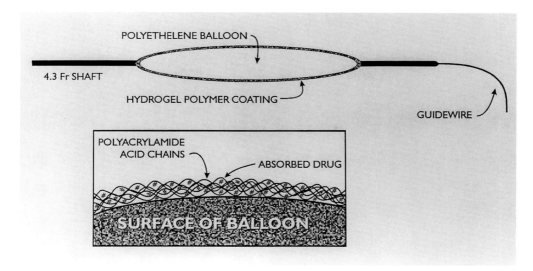

Fig. 18-4. The hydrogel-coated balloon. An interlacing network of polyacrylic acid chains absorbs aqueous drug solutions on the balloon surface.

plasty site. The in vivo delivery of heparin and urokinase in the porcine model has been shown to decrease platelet deposition significantly following balloon injury. Studies with heparin and antisense oligomers to c-*myb* have also demonstrated a significant decrease in smooth muscle cell proliferation 1 week after local delivery.

Preliminary studies with urokinase-coated hydrogel balloons have also demonstrated efficacy of this system in patients. In one recent study involving 20 patients, locally delivered urokinase reversed abrupt thrombotic closure and lysed intracoronary thrombus without evidence of distal embolization.

The major advantage of the hydrogel system is that it results in homogenous, atraumatic drug delivery at the same time that an arterial lesion is being dilated. Deficiencies of the hydrogel system, however, include the wash-off of drug from the balloon surface, the relatively small amount of drug that can be loaded onto the balloon surface, and the need for vessel occlusion during drug delivery.

D^3 Infusion Catheter

The D^3 Infusion Catheter (Dispatch Catheter, Scimed Life Systems, Maple Grove, MN) consists of an over-the-wire, nondilation catheter with a POC-6 helical, inflation coil on its distal tip[6] (Fig. 18-5). When the helical coil is inflated, the coil supports an inner urethane sheath that allows for distal blood flow. Drug is infused through a separate infusion port and is delivered locally through slits in the shaft of the device, allowing the arterial wall to be bathed in protected spaces in between the coils of the device.

Successful in vivo delivery of methylene blue, heparin, hirudin, and horseradish peroxidase has been accomplished with the D^3 catheter in several animal models. In the case of heparin, the amount of intramurally deposited drug has been shown to be proportional to the drug infusion time and the concentration of infused drug. Preliminary studies have also been performed in patients and have demonstrated successful intracoronary use of the catheter for periods as long as 30 minutes, without significant alteration of coronary blood flow or ventricular function.

Unlike other local drug delivery systems, the specific advantages of the D^3 catheter are that it allows for prolonged localized drug delivery at an angioplasty site with simultaneous perfusion of the artery. Although loss of drug from side branches and ischemia from side branch occlusion by the catheter's coils have been noted, newer generation D^3 catheters are currently being designed to avoid these problems. One additional limitation of the catheter is that it does not provide sufficient inflation pressure for stenosis dilation.

Iontophoresis Catheter

Local drug delivery by iontophoresis is based on the concept that an electrical field can be used as a driving force to intramurally deliver charged agents at an angioplasty site[7] (Fig. 18-6). The iontophoresis system (CorTrak Medical, Roseville, MN) consists of a standard angioplasty catheter shaft with a microporous balloon membrane mounted on its distal end. The middle portion of the balloon membrane, which

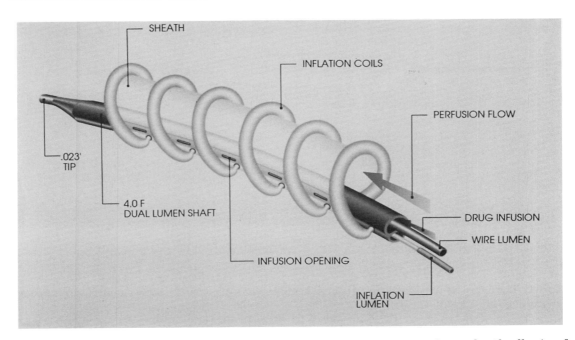

Fig. 18-5. The D³ catheter. The inflated POC-6 coil supports an inner urethane sheath allowing for distal perfusion. Drug is infused via slits in the catheter shaft in between the balloon coils.

is in contact with the arterial wall during balloon inflation, contains millions of submicron pores for drug delivery. These submicron pores as well as impermeable proximal and distal ends of the balloon membrane minimize drug loss into the blood stream during balloon inflation/deflation and during drug delivery. Located under the microporous balloon membrane is an electrode (e.g., Ag/AgCl) that wraps around the catheter shaft. This electrode is connected to a power source, with a return electrode placed within or on the body. When the balloon membrane is inflated with drug solution at low pressure (e.g., 1 atm) and an electric current is applied by the power source, charged drug molecules are preferen-

tially transported through the balloon pores into the arterial wall in response to the voltage differential between the catheter electrode and return electrode.

Successful in vivo delivery of hirudin has been accomplished with the iontophoresis catheter in both pigs and rabbits. Iontophoretic delivery in the porcine model resulted in tissue concentrations as much as 80 times greater than passive delivery. The subsequent retention of hirudin in the intact vessel was time dependent. Minimal systemic drug levels could be detected after iontophoretic delivery in the rabbit. In both animal models, iontophoretic delivery was atraumatic and homogenous and resulted in drug distribution throughout the three layers of the vessel wall.

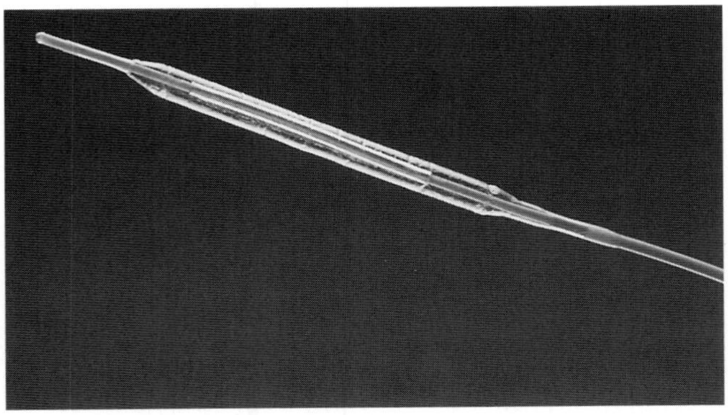

CONCLUSIONS

The field of catheter-based drug delivery is currently in its infancy. Multiple catheter designs are being developed and will probably be available for clinical research in the next several years. Comparative studies are needed to assess the relative merits of the different systems under investigation with respect to efficiency of drug delivery, effect on vessel architecture, homogeneity of drug deposition, ability to dilate vascular stenoses simultaneously, and ability to limit ischemia from vessel and side branch occlusion. Beneficial therapeutic effects on platelet deposition

Fig. 18-6. The iontophoresis catheter. The iontophoresis electrode is coiled around the catheter shaft below the balloon membrane.

and smooth muscle cell physiology have been documented in several instances, but very little information on the pharmacokinetics of individual drugs is available. Although the technique is promising, the ultimate impact of local drug delivery on thrombotic closure and restenosis remains uncertain at the present time.

REFERENCES

1. Goldman B, Blanke H, Wolinsky H. Influence of pressure on permeability of normal and diseased muscular arteries to horseradish peroxidase: a new catheter approach. Atherosclerosis 1987;65:215
2. Wolinsky H, Thung SN. Use of a perforated balloon catheter to deliver concentrated heparin into the wall of the normal canine artery. J Am Coll Cardiol 1990; 15:475
3. Lambert CR, Leone J, Rowland S. The microporous balloon: a minimal trauma local drug delivery catheter, abstracted. Circulation 1992;86:1–381
4. Hong MK, Farb A, Unger EF et al. A new PTCA balloon catheter with intramural channels for local delivery of drugs at low pressure, abstracted. Circulation 1992;86: 1–380
5. Fram DB, Aretz TA, Mitchel JF et al. Localized intramural delivery of a marker agent during balloon angioplasty: a new technique using hydrogel-coated balloons and active diffusion, abstracted. Circulation 1992;86: 1–380
6. Fram DB, Mitchel JF, Eldin AM et al. Intramural delivery of heparin with a new site-specific drug delivery system: the D^3 catheter, abstracted. J Am Coll Cardiol 1994;23:186A
7. Fernandez-Ortiz A, Meyer BJ, Mailhac A et al. Intravascular local delivery: an iontophoretic approach, abstracted. Circulation 1993;88:1–309

19 Iontophoretic Transmyocardial Drug Delivery

Boaz Avitall

The poor efficacy of antiarrhythmic agents administered at clinically tolerable doses may be partly related to an inadequate concentration of the drug in the target tissue. Delivery of a drug such as procainamide (PA) directly into an arrhythmogenic substrate using the technique of iontophoresis could lead to high tissue concentrations and avoidance of systemic toxicity.

Iontophoresis uses electrical current to transport charged molecules into tissue or the blood stream. Presently, this process is used to deliver drugs through the skin. Although the myocardium should provide a much lower resistance to iontophoretic drug transport than the skin, this idea has never been explored in cardiovascular pharmacology. In recent years, implantable devices utilizing direct myocardial electrode patches have increasingly been used to treat ventricular tachycardia (VT) and ventricular fibrillation. These electrode patches could be a convenient way to deliver an antiarrhythmic drug directly into the myocardium using iontophoresis.

In a study carried out in dogs, iontophoretic transport was used to deliver PA into infarcted myocardium and was shown to be effective in suppressing VT. The results obtained with iontophoretic transport of PA were superior to intravenous administration and passive diffusion of this drug.

METHODS

Drug-Delivery System

To develop and test a direct epicardial drug-delivery system, a Cardiac Pacemaker Incorporated automatic implantable cardioverter-defibrillator platinum mesh patch electrode was trimmed to 9 cm^2 and modified to contain a 4-mm-deep chamber that was sealed with dialysis membrane (chamber volume, 3.6 ml). The pore size of the permeable membrane is 400 A, which allowed the PA molecule to pass through the membrane and onto the epicardial surface. The chamber was equipped with ports to allow infusion of the drug (Fig. 19-1). PA hydrochloride at a concentration of 100 mg/ml was the initial prototype drug used to test the efficacy of iontophoretic versus passive and intravenous delivery into a 7-day infarct canine model. PA, supplied at pH 5, is a charged molecule with a molecular weight of 271.79, and is suitable for iontophoretic delivery.[1]

Surgical Preparation

The left anterior descending coronary artery (LAD) was ligated just proximal to the second diagonal branch. In addition, other small arteries from the apex and lateral wall that feed into the LAD area were also ligated. The chest was repaired, and the animal was allowed to recover for 7 days. The heart was exposed through a median sternotomy and suspended in the pericardial cradle. The coronary sinus was cannulated with a 6-F catheter, which was placed in the great cardiac vein. The femoral vein was cannulated for venous blood sampling. A 3-mm stainless steel wire electrode was threaded to approximately 4 mm below the epicardial surface in the center of the infarcted zone. Wide margins allowed for entrance and exit of the wire to prevent overlap between the drug-delivery patch (described below) and the myocardial puncture sites. A second wire

197

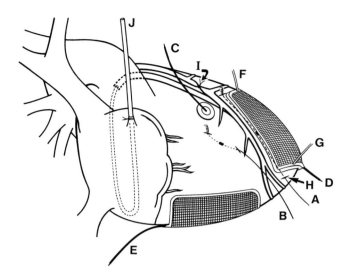

Fig. 19-1. Schematic diagram of the instrumented heart. **(A)** Infarcted tissue stimulation electrode embedded 4 mm into the myocardium. **(B)** Normal tissue stimulation electrode. **(C)** Bipolar-ring recording electrode. **(D)** Iontophoresis patch electrode and chamber with inlet and outlet tubing **(F & G)** for antiarrhythmic drugs. **(E)** Reference-patch electrode. **(H)** Infarcted tissue stimulation electrode insertion site outside the margins of the iontophoretic chamber. **(I)** Site of left anterior descending coronary artery ligation. **(J)** Great cardiac vein cannulated with a 6-F catheter for blood sampling.

was placed in the right ventricle away from the infarcted zone. These electrodes were used for the evaluation of the effective refractory period (ERP), end-diastolic threshold (EDT), and the initiation of VT. A bipolar ring electrode was sutured to the border of the infarcted zone between the two stimulating electrodes (Fig. 19-1). This electrode permitted recording of discrete signals free of far-field artifact. The recording electrode was connected to a Bloom recording system for monitoring the electrical activity of the heart. A 14-cm^2 reference electrode for stimulation was imbedded subcutaneously in the hind leg, and a 14-cm^2 platinum mesh patch electrode was secured to the posterior surface of the heart and used as a reference electrode for the iontophoretic current. The sinus node was crushed, and the heart was paced at 150 bpm using a 2-msec cathodal pulse with an amplitude of twice diastolic threshold. The pacing pulse was delivered to the wire electrodes implanted in either the infarcted or normal tissue (Fig. 19-1, sites A and B), as were the test stimuli for the determination of the ERP and EDT. The open chest cavity was covered with thick pads to prevent cooling. The delivery patch, lined with platinum mesh and equipped with two ports to allow the infusion of either the drug or normal saline, was connected to a

constant-current pulse generator. The output of the constant-current unit was electrically isolated to prevent any current loops other than the current between the patches (Fig. 19-1).

The efficacy of iontophoretic PA transport into infarcted myocardial tissue was compared with passive drug diffusion and intravenous administration. For 10 minutes, PA at a concentration of 100 mg/ml was passively exposed to the myocardial surface or was delivered iontophoretically for 10 minutes with 1 mA/cm^2-80 ms pulsed current, synchronized with ventricular pacing at 150 pulses/min. During VT, the iontophoretic pulses were limited to 150 pulses/min synchronized with the R wave recorded from the ring electrode. The iontophoretic current pulse pathway was between the modified anterior patch containing the drug and the posterior patch, as shown in Figure 19-1. After each of these interventions, the patch containing PA was removed from the heart, and any moisture was blotted from the epicardial surface that had been exposed to the PA. Intravenous PA was infused slowly at a 15-mg/kg loading dose followed by a 0.6-mg/kg/min constant infusion.

Study Groups

Measurements were determined in three groups of dogs as follows: (1) sixteen dogs that received 15 mg/kg PA IV followed by 0.6 mg/kg/min PA infusion—15 were followed for 3 hours, and 1 was followed for 30 minutes; (2) five dogs in which infarcted epicardial tissue was exposed to PA administered by passive diffusion from the drug-delivery patch for 10 minutes—the drug-delivery patch was then removed from the heart, and the epicardium blotted dry; these dogs were followed for 3 hours; and (3) sixteen dogs in which infarcted epicardium was exposed to pulsed-current PA iontophoresis for 10 minutes—the drug-delivery patch was then removed from the heart and the epicardium was blotted dry; these dogs were followed for 3 hours.

Electrophysiologic and Sampling Methods

Coronary sinus and venous blood samples were taken at 1, 5, 15, 30, 60, 120, and 180 minutes, timed from the beginning of PA exposure. ERP, EDT, and inducibility for arrhythmia were measured before and after PA exposure at the same intervals as blood sampling using the Bloom Associates stimulation system. Ventricular stimulation was performed with cathodal impulses 2 msec in duration at two times

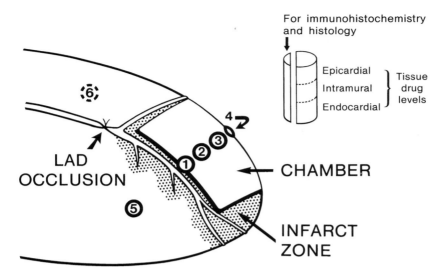

Fig. 19-2. Schematic diagram shows locations of the transmural biopsies traversing the drug-exposed infarcted zone and two remote biopsies. Biopsies were sectioned as shown. LAD, left anterior descending coronary artery.

diastolic threshold. Two different basic cycle lengths were used: 600 and 400 ms. Up to four premature beats were delivered to the infarcted and noninfarcted zones via electrodes A and B (shown in Fig. 19-1). The initial coupling interval of an extrastimulus was 300 ms, which was decremented by 10-ms intervals until VT was induced or ventricular effective refractory period was achieved. This extrastimulus was then fixed at 10 ms above refractoriness, and an additional premature beat was inserted that was similarly decremented.

By using this stimulation protocol, the inducibility of VT was tested every 30 minutes over a 2-hour period before PA exposure to ensure reproducibility of VT induction in 12 dogs before PA exposure and after PA exposure for 3 hours. Electrical current and saline may cause electrophysiologic changes comparable to those seen after PA exposure, and VT induction and stability may change over time. Electrophysiologic evaluations were performed in 12 dogs with inducible VT before drug exposure by measuring the ERP, EDT, VT suppression, and changes in VT cycle length. The infarcted epicardium was exposed to a saline-filled drug-delivery patch with pH similar to that of the PA (pH 5) for 10 minutes with pulsed iontophoretic current. Drug-delivery patch temperature was maintained at the dog core temperature. Intramyocardial pH was evaluated with a Corning pH/C 107 meter and Microelectrodes Inc. MI-407 miniature needle electrode in four of the dogs. The intramyocardial pH needle electrode was inserted into the myocardium immediately after iontophoretic PA delivery. No measurable pH changes were

recorded intramyocardially under the iontophoretic patch. Although the iontophoretic current could pace the heart, it was synchronized with ventricular systole with a total pulse duration of 80 ms. When appropriately triggered, no arrhythmias were recorded during or after iontophoretic current application.

At the end of the 3-hour observation period, the patches and all other electrodes were removed from the heart, and the heart was removed. The hearts were rinsed in saline, and four transmural punch biopsies traversing the drug-exposed infarcted zone were taken (Fig. 19-2). Two additional biopsies were taken from the site of right ventricular stimulation and the left ventricular free wall. Both of these sites were remote from the drug-exposed zone. Core biopsies were sectioned longitudinally. These sections were used for histology and immunohistochemistry, whereas the remaining core biopsies were divided into three equal segments containing the endocardial, intramural, and epicardial tissues (Fig. 19-2). The right ventricular biopsy was divided into only two segments. From these samples, drug concentrations were measured using high-performance liquid chromatography (HPLC). In addition, myocardial biopsies were taken for immunohistochemical analysis to define the distribution of PA within the myocardial wall.

Statistical Analysis

One-way analysis of variance technique was used to define the statistical significance of the ERP and EDT changes, as well as myocardial and blood drug

Table 19-1. Changes in Ventricular Tachycardia After Iontophoresis and Intravenous Procainamide Administration

	Before PA VTCL	15 Min After PA		3 Hours After PA		3 Hours After PA			Venous PA	
		VTCL	ΔERP	VTCL	ΔERP	Endo	Intra	Epi	15 Min	3 Hrs
Iontophoresis										
1	250	NI	10	NI	40	9	81	1065	4.1	5.3
2	165	NI	0	NI	20	4	5	28	4.7	3.3
3	260	NI	NC	NI	NC	40	187	814	2.2	3.5
4	310	NI	30	NI	30	29	394	1432	1.0	1.4
5	210	NI	70	210	90	14	69	2360	2.0	3.6
6	190	NI	40	230	0	2	2	22	0.8	1.5
7	150	NI	0	NI	10	2	7	42	1.0	0.5
8	210	NI	NC	240	NC	19	27	1336	2.8	1.3
9	150	NI	0	NI	10	15	8	125	0.4	0.5
10	220	NI	20	NI	40	17	54	344	7.3	4.7
Intravenous administration										
1	140	NI	40	NI	10	11	13	10	16.0	5.7
2[a]	NI	380	0	320	10	2	4	5	24.0	17.2
3[a,b]	NI	150	30			27	26	46	47.7	
4	200	290	40	180	10	9	12	16	48.2	16.1
5	160	140	30	NI	0	9	14	17	16.4	7.7
6	140	170	50	NI	10	3	3	5	14.6	7.9
7[a]	NSVT	NSVT	10	140	0	4	3	6	13.9	9.0
8	170	170	30	190	0	15	20	24	22.5	9.5
9	170	190	20	230	20	19	22	32	25.4	22.3
10	210	280	50	260	30	13	5	28	44.3	27.6

Abbreviations: PA, procainamide; VTCL, ventricular tachycardia cycle length (msec); ΔERP, change in effective refractory period from before PA (msec); Endo, PA tissue level in the endocardium (μg/g of tissue); Intra, intramyocardium; Epi, epicardium; NI, noninducible; NC, noncapture (infarcted tissue end-diastolic threshold of >10 mA); NSVT, nonsustained ventricular tachycardia.

[a] Dogs that developed ventricular tachycardia after intravenous PA.

[b] This dog was followed for 30 minutes.

concentrations at the different time intervals. Data are presented as mean ± SD; results with a value of $P < 0.05$ were considered statistically significant.

RESULTS

The results reported here are based on data collected in the 37 canine experiments. In 12 dogs in which sustained monomorphic VT could be induced with programmed stimulation, the reproducibility of VT induction was followed after 10 minutes of saline iontophoresis every 30 minutes for 2 hours. In 11 dogs the ERP and EDT were evaluated throughout the 2-hour follow-up period (in dog 8, Table 19-1, the EDT was above 10 mA). In these dogs, VT morphology, mode of induction, and termination were the same. No statistically significant changes in ERP, EDT, or VT cycle length were observed. In one dog, the VT could not be reinduced after saline iontophoresis; however, the same tachycardia was induced 15 minutes later.

Tissue Concentration and Distribution of Procainamide After Passive, Iontophoretic, and Intravenous Delivery Into Infarcted Myocardium

Three hours after iontophoretic PA delivery into the infarcted tissue, the concentration of PA was considerably higher than the concentration of PA delivered with passive diffusion from the drug-delivery patch or intravenous administration (Fig. 19-3). The greatest amount of drug was retained in the epicardial layer at the center of the infarcted zone (840 ± 853 μg/g of tissue versus 93 ± 90 μg/g with passive diffusion and 15 ± 8 μg/g with intravenous administration), whereas the lowest concentrations were found in the endocardial layer. However, in the center of the infarcted zone, the endocardial layer PA concentrations with iontophoresis were still higher (38 ± 57 μg/g) than those achieved with either passive diffusion (4 ± 2 μg/g), or with intravenous delivery (11 ± 6 μg/g, $P < 0.05$). Passive diffusion showed no sig-

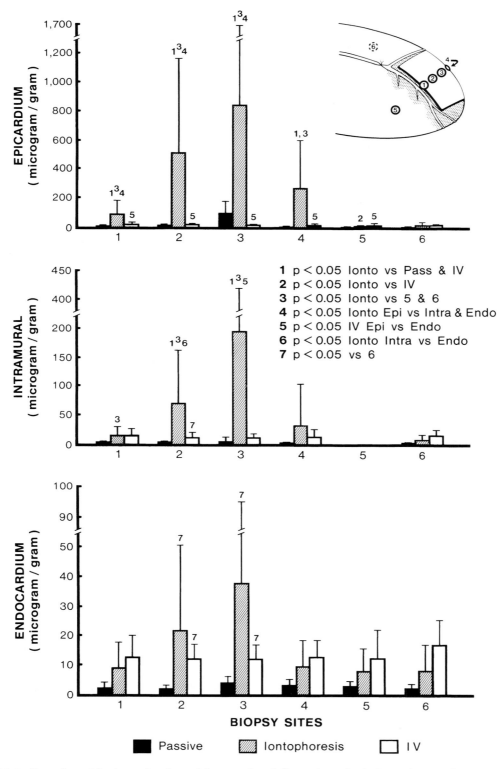

Fig. 19-3. Procainamide tissue levels at 3 hours after delivery into the infarcted tissue by passive diffusion (Pass), iontophoretic delivery (Ionto), and intravenous (IV) administration. Note scale differences for the three tissue layers. Epi, epicardium; Intra, intramural; Endo, endocardium.

nificant differences between the normal and infarcted zones in all three layers 3 hours later. However, 3 hours after intravenous PA, the concentration of the PA in the normal tissue was higher than in the center of the infarcted zone intramural and endocardial samples. Only iontophoretic PA delivery produced very high concentrations of the drug in the epicardial and intramural layers, which were distributed across the infarcted zone (P <0.05). HPLC determination of PA tissue and serum concentrations showed no shifts in PA retention time, which indicates that by using the HPLC method, no changes in the PA structure occurred after iontophoresis or passive and intravenous PA delivery.

Coronary Sinus and Venous Procainamide Blood Concentrations

High concentrations of PA were recorded in the coronary sinus (49 ± 33 μg/ml) and venous blood (58 ± 16 μg/ml) immediately after intravenous PA administration. By contrast, iontophoretic delivery resulted in initial high concentrations of PA in the coronary sinus (11 ± 8 μg/ml), but very low concentrations in the venous circulation (0.3 ± 0.3 μg/ml, P <0.0001). Whereas coronary sinus PA concentration slowly decreased after the completion of PA delivery by passive or iontophoretic diffusion, venous PA concentration slowly increased over 30 minutes and remained stable thereafter. After 3 hours, passive diffusion of PA resulted in venous levels of 0.85 ± 0.67 μg/ml (range, 0.3 to 2 μg/ml); 3 hours after iontophoresis, the venous level was 2.4 ± 3.35 μg/ml (range, 0.52 to 13.3 μg/ml). In only one of the 16 dogs was the venous blood level at a high theraputic level, whereas in all other dogs, the maximum level did not exceed 5.3 μg/ml. These levels were recorded with very high infarcted tissue PA concentrations and are significantly lower (P <0.05) than the PA levels in the circulation after intravenous infusion. In contrast to passive and iontophoretic delivery, intravenous administration resulted in a venous blood level of 11.4 ± 6.7 μg/ml (range, 5.1 to 27.6 μg/ml) (Fig. 19-4).

Electrophysiologic Changes

In the infarcted tissue, iontophoresis and intravenous PA administration resulted in similar ERP prolongation of 20 ms, and there was no statistical difference between these two groups. Iontophoretic PA delivery to the infarcted zone caused no ERP prolongation in the normal tissue. Intravenous PA resulted in a significant prolongation of the ERP in the normal tissue, which is, however, smaller than the prolongation recorded in the infarcted tissue. The EDT rose transiently following iontophoresis, and no other significant changes were noted for either iontophoresis or intravenous delivery. The ERP prolongation following iontophoretic PA delivery was recorded with venous PA levels that were markedly lower than the PA levels recorded with intravenous PA infusion.

Suppression of Ventricular Tachycardia

Sixteen dogs received PA iontophoretically. Ten of these dogs had sustained monomorphic VT. Sixteen dogs received PA intravenously, and 10 of these dogs had VT. As shown in Table 19-1, iontophoretic PA delivery was effective in terminating and preventing the reinduction of VT for up to 3 hours in 7 of 10 dogs. In three dogs in which the VT was reinduced, the time of reinduction was 60 to 120 minutes. The ERP evaluated in the intramural tissue in the center of the infarcted zone did not show consistent ERP prolongation immediately after PA iontophoresis (21 ± 23 ms; range, 0 to 70 ms, with a circulating blood level of 2.6 ± 2 μg/ml). The ERP prolongation was more pronounced 3 hours later, with the exception of one dog (30 ± 26 ms; range, 0 to 90 ms, with circulating PA levels of 2.6 ± 1.7 μg/ml). Measurements of the ERP in the intramural tissue changed little initially and increased as the PA passively diffused deeper into myocardial tissues. Tissue PA levels show wide variations from one dog to another. Low tissue PA levels in the center of the infarct do not translate to ineffective VT suppression. PA venous blood levels were below the therapeutic range. In 10 dogs with VT that received intravenous PA, 9 could be reinduced with programmed stimulation after PA infusion. Two dogs with no inducible VT (dogs 2 and 3) and one with nonsustained VT (dog 7) became inducible for sustained VT after intravenous PA. ERP prolongation was noted in all except one dog immediately after intravenous PA (30 ± 15 ms; range, 0 to 50 ms, with PA venous levels of 27.3 ± 13 μg/ml). These changes in ERP were associated with high circulating drug levels as a result of the bolus effect. ERP prolongation decreased in all the dogs (10 ± 9 ms; range, 0 to 30 ms as circulating blood PA levels decreased to 13.7 μg/ml) 3 hours later with therapetic drug levels. In the center of the infarcted zone, epicardial PA tissue levels (20 ± 12 μg/g) were greater than intramural and endocardial levels (12 ± 8 and 11.5 ± 7 μg/g of tissue, respectively; P <0.05).

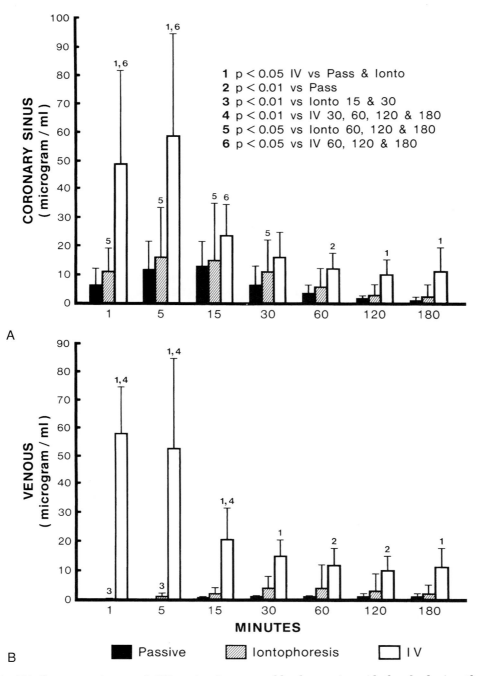

Fig. 19-4. (A) Coronary sinus and **(B)** systemic venous blood procainamide levels during the 3-hour follow-up period for passive (Pass), iontophoretic (Ionto), and intravenous (IV) delivery.

None of the dogs in which PA was delivered iontophoretically into the infarcted myocardium developed VT that was otherwise not induced before delivery of the drug. In an additional animal, a hemodynamically stable, sustained monomorphic VT was induced with a cycle length of 200 msec. PA delivered iontophoretically into the infarcted zone successfully terminated the tachycardia after 2 minutes. VT was noninducible with only a trace level of systemic PA (1.3 μg/ml). After 90 minutes, VT could be reinduced. Intravenous PA was then administered, increasing the venous PA level to 26 μg/ml. Despite this high blood level, VT (cycle length, 340 ms) was easily induced throughout the 1-hour follow-up period. However, after reinitiation of iontophoretically delivered PA, VT was again rapidly suppressed.

Procainamide Tissue Distribution by Immunohistochemical Analysis

An example of the PA distribution in the 7-day infarcted tissue 3 hours after 10 minutes of PA iontophoresis is shown in Plate 5-1C. This section demonstrates intense granular cytoplasmic staining and appears similar to the staining seen in normal myocardial cells that were soaked in 100 mg/ml of PA for 24 hours, shown in Plate 5-1B. The control section taken from a normal canine heart that was not exposed to PA shows no such staining (Plate 5-1A). In contrast to the iontophoretic zone, the staining intensity in the remote section (Plate 5-1D) is considerably less intense. PA staining was noted transmurally within viable cells and included the endocardial surface. Upon histologic examination of the hematoxylin and eosin-stained sections, neither passive diffusion nor iontophoresis caused any epicardial tissue injury beyond that which one would expect from a chronically infarcted myocardium.

DISCUSSION

Less than 40% of patients with life-threatening VT are treated successfully with antiarrhythmic agents.[2,3] In 18%, these drugs may be proarrhythmic, and side effects are encountered in 52%.[4] This necessitates the discontinuation of the drugs in 23% of the patients treated with drug therapy.[2] In only 18% of patients with sustained monomorphic VT was the arrhythmia suppressed by intravenous PA or quinidine administered during electrophysiologic study.[5] In the same report, ERP prolongation, determined in the right ventricle, was not predictive of the effect of PA on VT. It has been shown that high systemic doses of PA significantly increase the effectiveness of the drug but often cause intolerable side effects.[6] These sobering data suggest that transportation of the drug by the systemic circulation is not an effective route to suppress VT without the use of toxic drug levels. Furthermore, surgical therapy for VT has been shown to be effective in only 60 to 70% of patients in whom surgery was attempted.[7,8] Poor ventricular function and multiple VT morphologies with diffuse, nondescript infarcts eliminate many patients from surgical therapy. Implantable defibrillators do not prevent initiation of the VT, and, as a result, many patients receive frequent multiple shocks, which in turn may lead to further damage to the myocardium.[9] At this time, there is no other effective therapy for these patients. It has been shown that retroperfusion of the infarcted myocardium was considerably more effective in suppressing ventricular arrhythmias in the dog than intravenous PA infusion.[10] However, a chronically implanted, indwelling coronary sinus catheter may cause severe complications.

An alternative approach to this problem would be to deliver locally high concentrations of the effective antiarrhythmic agents, independent of blood flow, to the areas of injured myocardium containing the arrhythmogenic foci. Drug effectiveness would therefore be increased where it is needed most, and systemic drug exposure and its side effects would be minimized. Direct iontophoretic delivery of antiarrhythmic drugs will not result in toxic levels of the drug in the normal myocardium, because the drug will be rapidly removed and diluted by the circulating blood. Furthermore, this method of drug delivery may provide a new insight to the mechanism of proarrhythmia by contrasting the electrophysiologic side effects of intravenous drug delivery (causing global changes) and iontophoretic delivery (causing local changes). Our data demonstrate that high drug concentrations occur in the infarcted regions of the myocardium where the slow-conducting reentrant circuits are likely to be present.[11]

In this study, the iontophoretic current was set at 1 mA/cm^2. This current density will cause ventricular depolarization if it is not delivered during the ventricular refractory period. Because iontophoretic drug delivery is a linear function of the intensity of the current and the duration of application, reduction in current density to levels below the ventricular capture threshold will not only decrease the possibility of arrhythmia, but also will decrease the amount of drug delivered into the myocardium. However, a proportional increase in the epicardial exposure time to the iontophoretic drug delivery will increase the amount of drug transported and will compensate for the reduction of current. In this study we did not record any significant local pH changes nor did we observe any increase in ventricular irritability as a result of local ionic shifts. Furthermore, despite high local PA concentrations recorded in this study, no spontaneous arrhythmia occurred.

The results of PA concentrations recorded in this study show that the epicardial tissue contains the highest concentration of drug and serves as a reservoir of PA, which diffuses down the concentration gradient into the endocardium, and from there into the ventricular cavity. In addition, the drug diffuses into peripheral tissues where it may be cleared by the coronary circulation. The rate of diffusion determines the elimination rate of the drug from the myocardium. The data presented here suggest that the rate of PA elimination from the 7-day infarcted myocardium is much slower than that of normal tissue.

This conclusion is supported by the fact that the myocardial PA concentration remained high after the 3-hour follow-up period and that PA concentration in the blood was low throughout this period. For the antiarrhythmic agent to be effective in suppressing VT, it has to be delivered to the arrhythmogenic substrate in therapeutic concentrations. In this study, no specific attempt was made to map the site of early activation and adjust the site of PA exposure. Furthermore, the drug-delivery patch covered only a portion of the infarcted zone. Despite these limitations, in the dogs that developed inducible VT, the VT was suppressed shortly after the initiation of PA iontophoresis. In 7 of 10 dogs, the VT was suppressed for the duration of the 3-hour monitoring period after 10 minutes of iontophoretic drug delivery without adverse effects and with subtherapeutic PA levels in the systemic circulation. In three dogs with VT, iontophoretic delivery of PA resulted in long-term suppression of the VT despite low tissue PA levels in the center of the infarcted zone. In the same dogs, iontophoretic current applied to the saline-filled chamber did not suppress the VT, and the VT was reproducible for 2 hours before the iontophoretic delivery of PA. These observations may suggest that VT suppression after PA iontophoresis may depend on the concentration of PA at the site of slow conduction that was possibly located at the epicardial surface.

In the human heart, the activation sequence during ventricular tachycardia was mapped and correlated with histologic studies of the infarcted tissue in the Langendorff-perfused human hearts of transplant recipients.[11] It was concluded that "the location of the tracts is not confined to the subendocardial surface, but many run intramurally or even subepicardially." In the canine VT model, it has been shown that the inducibility of VT peaks after 1 week of infarction after single-stage permanent coronary occlusion.[12,13] Electrophysiologic mapping of these tachycardias revealed intramural and endocardial slow activity in 9 of 13 VTs. In the remaining VTs, epicardial reentry was identified, and only two were suppressed by epicardial cooling and cryoablation.[14] Histologic evaluation of the dogs with sustained VT revealed surviving myocardial cells interlaced with acellular tissues. These observations suggest that VT induced in the 7-day infarct in canine heart may originate from different myocardial layers. This is similar to what was observed in the human heart.

One would expect that with high concentrations of PA in the epicardial tissues and to a lesser extent in the intramural and endocardial tissues, the electrophysiologic changes should correspond to the PA tissue concentrations; however, that is not the case. At this time, we can only speculate why, and further studies are required to elucidate these findings. Because the PA concentration in the circulation is low, a large tissue-to-circulation gradient is present. The drug diffuses passively from the necrotic tissue in the infarcted zone, which is not well perfused, to islands of myocytes within the infarcted tissue that are capable of responding to the electrical stimulation. These myocytes are alive as a result of blood supply or passive diffusion of oxygen. Any blood supply to these tissues results in removal of the PA. The PA concentration and perhaps the drug electrophysiologic effects on the surviving cells within the infarcted zone are influenced by several factors: the concentration gradient between the tissues, the blood flow in the infarcted tissue, and the mobility of the drug. Because the effect of the PA is a function of its concentration, it is conceivable that the electrophysiologic effects recorded in this study represent the amount of drug present within surviving cells in the infarcted zone. These cells are exposed to much greater levels of PA than is present in the circulation because of their proximity to necrotic tissues that serve as a reservoir of PA, as documented by the HPLC drug tissue levels in the infarcted tissue. However, the PA level in the islands of viable cells is probably not the same level present in the necrotic tissues. In addition, it is possible that the electrophysiologic effects of PA delivered directly into the infarcted tissue, bypassing the circulation, result in electrophysiologic effects that are unlike those recorded with intravenous drug application and yet are effective in suppressing VT. Iontophoretic current may result in PA structure changes, leading to diminution of the drug's electrophysiologic effects. However, using HPLC analysis, no changes in the elution profile were observed.

Potential Limitations and Future Studies

Large myocardial infarctions that involve the septum may cause VT that is sustained by a deep septal reentrant circuit distant from the iontophoretic site. Such a VT may be resistant to this mode of drug delivery as well as to systemic antiarrhythmic drugs. It is possible that combined systemic and iontophoretic drug application may enhance the suppression of VT that is otherwise resistant to either method alone. However, in all the dogs in which VT was induced, the VT was successfully suppressed by iontophoretic PA delivery for at least 60 minutes, and in 7 of 10 dogs, the VT was suppressed for over 3 hours with iontophoretic PA delivery. Furthermore, the center of the drug-delivery patch should be placed as close as possible to the area of the reentrant circuit. For this reason, electrophysiologic mapping may provide valuable information for proper patch placement. In addition, it may be necessary to modify several other experimental parameters to achieve optimum therapeutic effect. These additional parameters include drug concentration, duration of drug exposure, patch size and configuration, and type of drug being delivered. Another potential limitation is the possibility that other ionic species with a charge similar to that of PA that are used in the preparation of the drug may act as antiarrhythmics when delivered in high concentrations into the infarcted tissues. High PA concentration may cause depression of contractility. In preliminary canine model studies using echocardiographic techniques, iontophoretic PA delivery caused only transient, mild depression of nontransmural 4-week infarcts, and did not affect the mechanical function of the normal myocardium.

Significance

This work documents for the first time that sustained monomorphic VT caused by myocardial infarction can be suppressed for a significant period of time by epicardial iontophoretic drug delivery. Rapid high concentrations of PA were achieved within the infarcted tissue and sustained even after 3 hours fol-

lowing the removal of the drug-delivery patch from the heart. This new approach to drug delivery may be further developed into an implantable drug-delivery system capable of recognizing ventricular arrhythmias and containing a subcutaneous pump and chamber that can be replenished through a subcutaneous port. The system may deliver electrical current to a specially designed patch affixed to the surface of the heart directly over the arrhythmogenic site. When spontaneous runs of VT are detected, the antiarrhythmic drug will be pumped into the patch and transported into the myocardium iontophoretically by pulsed electrical current. This system may also be incorporated into the automatic implantable defibrillator, which already has the capability of recognizing ventricular arrhythmias. A system such as this is shown in Figure 19-5. The design of an implantable system capable of delivering drugs to the arrhythmogenic site may pose a significant challenge. However, given the current technology of implantable pumps and the implantable defibrillator, it is believed that such a system can be successfully developed. This method of drug delivery will minimize the systemic effect of the drug and maximize the effect within the affected myocardium. It will provide a new modality for the treatment of life-threatening arrhythmias that are otherwise refractory to conventional forms of medical and surgical therapy. The potential use of such a drug-delivery system extends beyond antiarrhythmic drugs, because its uses

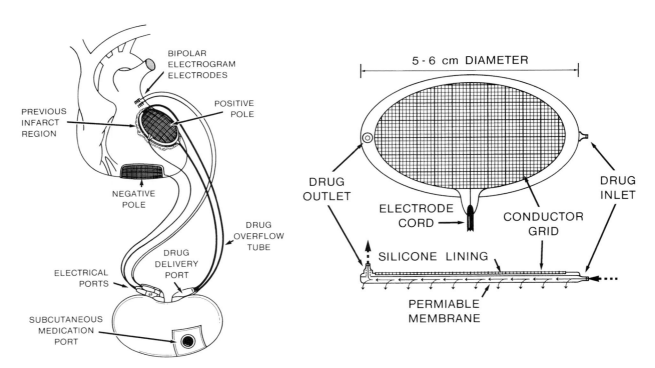

Fig. 19-5. Diagrammatic representation of the drug-delivery system.

can be expanded to deliver inotropic agents such as dobutamine, vasodilators, β-blockers, or any cardioactive agents that can be transported directly into the myocardium passively or iontophoretically. Furthermore, because most of the drug effect is limited to the infarcted tissue, it has the potential of increasing the efficacy of the drugs and may provide valuable insights into the antiarrhythmic and proarrhythmic action of antiarrhythmic drugs

CONCLUSIONS

The delivery of high concentrations of PA directly into infarcted myocardium is both feasible and effective, PA concentrations in the infarcted tissues were significantly above therapeutic levels for over 3 hours after 10 minutes of iontophoretic drug exposure, with only minimal levels detected in the circulation, and PA was distributed transmurally within the infarcted tissue. PA delivery into the infarcted myocardium using iontophoresis is much more effective than either passive diffusion or intravenous administration and in this model, VT is suppressed by the iontophoretic delivery of PA into the infarcted area.

REFERENCES

1. Gangarosa LP, Park NH, Fong BC, Scott DF, Hill JM. Conductivity of drugs used for iontophoresis. J Pharm Sci 1978;67:1439–1443
2. Cain ME. The role of newer antiarrhythmic drugs in the management of patients with ventricular arrhythmias. Presented at the 29th Annual Meeting of the International College of Angiology, Montreux, Switzerland, International Symposium, July 25, 1987
3. DiMarco JP, Garan H, Ruskin JN. Quinidine for ventricular arrhythmias: value of electrophysiologic testing. Am J Cardiol 1983;51:90–95
4. Podrid PJ, Lampert S, Graboys TB, Blatt CM, Lown B. Aggravation of arrhythmia by antiarrhythmic drugs—incidence and predictors. Am J Cardiol 1987; 59:38E–44E
5. Gold RL, Haffajee CI, Alpert JS. Electrophysiologic and clinical factors influencing response to class IA antiarrhythmic agents in patients with inducible sustained monomorphic ventricular tachycardia. Am Heart J 1986;112:9–13
6. Greenspan AM, Horowitz LN, Spielman ST, Josephson MK. Large dose procainamide therapy for ventricular tachyarrhythmia. Am J Cardiol 1980;46:453–462
7. Josephson ME, Harken AH, Horowitz LN. Long-term results of endocardial resection of sustained ventricular tachycardia in coronary disease patients. Am Heart J 1982;104:51–57
8. Miller JM, Kienzle MG, Harken AH, Josephson ME. Subendocardial resection for ventricular tachycardia: predictors for surgical success. Circulation 1984;70: 624–631
9. Avitall B, Port S, Gal R et al. Automatic implantable cardioverter/defibrillator discharges and acute myocardial injury. Circulation 1990;81:1482–1487
10. Karagueuzian HS, Ohta M, Drury JK et al. Coronary venous retroinfusion of procainamide: a new approach for the management of spontaneous and inducible sustained ventricular tachycardia during myocardial infarction. J Am Coll Cardiol 1986;7:551–563
11. de Bakker JMT, Coronel R, Tasseron S et al. Ventricular tachycardia in the infarcted, Langendorff-perfused human heart: role of the arrangement of surviving cardiac fibers. J Am Coll Cardiol 1990;15:1594–1607
12. Hunt GB, Ross DL. Influence of infarct age on reproducibility of ventricular tachycardia induction in a canine model. J Am Coll Cardiol 1989;14:765–773
13. Garan H, Ruskin JN, McGovern B, Grant G. Serial analysis of electrically induced ventricular arrhythmias in a canine model of myocardial infarction. J Am Coll Cardiol 1985;5:1095–1106
14. Garan H, Fallon JT, Rosenthal S, Ruskin JN. Endocardial, intramural, and epicardial activation patterns during sustained monomorphic ventricular tachycardia in late canine myocardial infarction. Circ Res 1987; 60:879–896

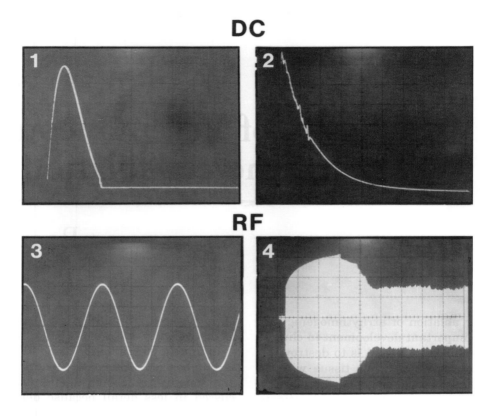

Fig. 20-1. (*1*) The output waveform from a Zoll external defibrillator used in DC ablation (each vertical division represents 200 V, and each horizontal division represents 2 ms). The charge was recorded across a 50-Ω resistor. (*2*) The same power using a 7-F, 2-mm tip electrode placed within the left ventricle of a dog heart. (*3*) Sinusoidal waveform of RF power (each horizontal division represents 30 V, and each vertical division represents 0.5 μsec). (*4*) A 20-second sweep of RF current delivered to the left ventricle of a dog heart using a 7-F, 4-mm tip ablation electrode. Initially the current increases as the tissue impedance decreases. Once the tissue is overheated and gas bubbles are formed under the catheter tip, the RF current drops and fluctuates for the duration of the ablation.

R2-type skin patch is 70 to 200 Ω. The catheter's internal resistance is only 3 to 4 Ω, while the large remaining resistance is due to the electrode-tissue interface. Much energy is dissipated across the electrode-tissue interface (the largest impedance in the series resistor network). The maximum current density (defined as the current per area [amperes/meter^2]) is at the electrode-tissue interface, which is the location of maximum power dissipation and, therefore, heat production. Despite the high power used in DC ablation, it is believed that only minimal intramural tissue heating takes place, primarily because of the short duration of the power application. Because the electrode and the tissue are immersed in flowing blood and the time of resistive heating is short, tissue heating is probably limited to the direct vicinity of the electrode-tissue interface.

Electrical Arcing and Incandescent Globe Formation

During DC ablation it is likely that the blood in contact with the catheter tip reaches the boiling state within the first few milliseconds of current application. To reduce gas formation and arcing, it was determined that connecting the catheter tip electrode to the cathodal pole of the defibrillator, as opposed to the anodal pole, is preferable because it produces a smaller shock wave and less hemolysis.[6,7] In addition, reducing the duration of the electrical pulse to 10 μs with a current of up to 30 A and voltage of 3,000 V results in decreased gas formation and arcing. The total energy delivered by such an electrical pulse is less than 0.65 J.[8] This produces complete heart block with no complications. Much of the therapeutic incentive for the use of transcatheter DC shock for cardiac tissue ablation stems from its ability to produce a large area of tissue damage, as noted with high-energy multiple shocks.[9] Since VT is often a result of diffusely scarred tissue, one advantage of this technique is the generation of lesions larger in area than those produced by other forms of ablation energy.

Catheters, Monitoring, and Safety Considerations

During high-energy DC ablation, the catheter insulation has to withstand high voltages without breakdown. The insulation on the catheters should be reinforced and braided. By monitoring the voltage and current output during ablation, one can detect sharp fluctuations that are most commonly caused by arc formation, breakdown of the catheter insulation, or both. The loss of recording or pacing capabilities is sometimes noted and results from conductor meltdown. With lower energy levels, the possibility of catheter breakdown and extensive tissue injury is less likely. However, decreasing the energy will result in a decrease in the efficacy of the procedure.

Clinical Use and Experience

Atrioventricular Nodal Reentry Tachycardia

Since AV nodal re-entry is a common cause of paroxysmal supraventricular tachycardia, percutaneous transcatheter ablation for this indication has wide applications in the field of cardiac electrophysiology. Ablation or modification of the AV node is critically important in managing drug-refractory supraventricular tachycardia and is being done successfully at many institutions.[10,11] Initial experience involved high-voltage DC shock as the source of ablative energy, and this method is still in use at some centers. Transcatheter DC high-energy pulses have been used clinically to treat supraventricular and ventricular tachycardias since 1982.[5,12]

A standard multipolar catheter is inserted percutaneously across the tricuspid valve to record the His bundle potential. An R2-type patch electrode serves as the indifferent electrode and is connected to the positive pole of the defibrillator. A standard cardioverter/defibrillator is used to deliver the DC shock, usually in the range of 50 to 360 J. The procedure is done under general anesthesia or heavy sedation because of the discomfort associated with a high-energy shock. The average time required to complete the procedure has been reported to be 131 ± 48 minutes.[13]

The percutaneous cardiac mapping and ablation registry includes data on 552 patients who were followed for 23 ± 18 months after AV node ablation by DC energy.[14] Ablation was successful in 354 patients (75%), all of whom were asymptomatic during the follow-up period and did not require any antiarrhythmic medication. Forty patients (8%) had resumption of AV conduction after the procedure but remained asymptomatic and did not need antiarrhythmic medication. In sixty-four patients (12%), AV conduction recurred, and antiarrhythmic medications were needed to control arrhythmias. The procedure failed to ablate the AV node in 88 patients (16%). In comparison, the success rate of AV nodal ablation/modification using RF power varies from 80 to 100%.[1]

A major disadvantage of AV node ablation with high-energy DC shock is the frequent subsequent need for permanent pacemaker placement. Rosenqvist et al.[15] reported late development of complete heart block in 2 of 47 patients after high-energy DC shock delivered to the AV junction.

Using DC energy, a high rate of success has been reported when ablating the His bundle[14] and accessory pathways.[16,17] A more than 96% success rate was reported in 284 patients with accessory pathways.[18] Ventricular fibrillation occurred in two patients, resulting in the death of one. Complete AV block occurred in four patients. A high-energy DC pulse from 160 to 240 J was used and multiple shocks were delivered. Bardy et al.[19] have used energies of 150 to 500 J. In their report, the posterior septal accessory pathway was eliminated in 13 of 19 patients with the shock delivered within the coronary sinus. Three patients required a sternotomy for control of cardiac tamponade from coronary sinus rupture, and one patient had a small posterior infarction due to a spasm of a branch of the right coronary artery. An 85% success rate was reported in 47 patients undergoing ablation of the AV junction. AV conduction resumed in two patients, and a new onset of congestive heart failure occurred in four. After an average follow-up of 31 months, a 17% mortality rate was recorded in this patient group.[15]

Accessory Pathways

With high-energy DC ablation of accessory pathways, the reported success rate has ranged from 68 to 96%[18,19] (Table 20-1). The Percutaneous Cardiac Mapping and Ablation Registry provides important data on a small number of patients treated for this indication.[14] Among the 26 reported patients who underwent DC catheter ablation of an accessory

Table 20-1 High-energy Direct Current and Radiofrequency Ablation: Summary of Clinical Studies

Study	No.	Energy Source	Diagnosis	Age Range (yr.)	Initial Success	Complications	Postablation Antiarrhythmic Therapy
Bardy et al.[19]	19	DC	Posterior accessory pathways	9–56	68% a 10/13	AV block: 5/9 patients Myocardial infarction: 1 patient Pericardial tamponade: 3 patients	
Warin et al.[18]	248	DC	Refractory anteroseptal AP: 24 patients Right parietal: 16 patients Posteroseptal AP: 86 patients Left parietal: 120 patients Mohaim AP: 4 patients	6–65	96% Follow-up 3–64 mo	Ventricular fibrillation: 2 patients Sudden cardiac death: 1 patient AV block: 5 patients	All patients received this prophylactically
Rosenqvist et al.[15]	47	DC	Refractory SVC	20–77	86% Follow-up 41 ± 23 mo	Hypotension: 1 patient Pericarditis: 1 patient Nonsustained VT: 1 patient Sudden cardiac death: 1 patient	7 patients
Tchou et al.[23]	7	DC	Bundle branch reentrant VT	62–81		AV block: 1 patient Postablation bradycardia: 3 patients All received permanent pacemakers	0
Langberg et al.[44]	16	RF followed by DC in 6 patients (failed RF)	Refractory SVT AV nodal ablation	26–73	10/16 Follow-up 4.2 mo	None	2 patients
Jackman et al.[41]	166	RF	AP Left free wall: 106 patients Anteroseptal: 13 patients Posteroseptal: 43 patients Right free wall: 15 patients	6–78	99% Follow-up 8 mo	AV block: 1 patient Pericarditis: 1 patient Pericardial tamponande: 1 patient (no thoracotomy) Vascular injury: 2 patients	6 patients
Leather et al.[11]	75	RF	AP	8–67	71% (1st 3 months) 90% (last 3 months)		
Van Hare et al.[35]	17	RF	Refractory SVT: 12 patients Junctional ectopic tachycardia: 1 patient AV nodal reentrant tachycardia: 4 patients	1–17	89% 82%	None	
Calkins et al.[40]	106	RF	SVT: 66 patients AP: 40 patients	15–79	92% 93%	Myocardial infarction: 1 patient AV block: 1 patient	2 patients
Lee et al.[37]	39	RF	Refractory AV nodal tachycardia	14–86	82%a Follow-up 8 ± 3 months	AV block: 3 patients Deep venous thrombosis: 2 patients	1 patient
Jazayeri et al[37]	35	RF	AV nodal reentrant tachycardia	9–82	100% 92%	None	

Abbreviations: AP, accessory pathway; AV, atrioventricular; DC, direct current; RF, radiofrequency; SVT, supraventricular tachycardia; VT, ventricular tachycardia; WPW, Wolff-Parkinson-White syndrome; SVC, superior vena cava.
a Cure.

pathway, the targeted tissue was located in the posteroseptal region in 14. The greatest success was achieved with the pathways located in the right posteroseptal region, close to the coronary sinus. There were four cases of cardiac tamponade and one death related to the procedure, however. The incidence of complications has since decreased with improved understanding of the procedure. Electrophysiologists have become aware that the application of any form of energy inside the coronary sinus is not a benign process and can cause coronary sinus rupture leading to pericardial tamponade, as reported in several patients.[14] Since high-energy DC ablation produces a far greater complication rate, RF power is now more commonly used to ablate accessory pathway tissues,

Ventricular Tachycardias

Ablation of AV nodal tissues and the His bundle requires a well-defined injury to a small tissue mass of only a few cubic millimeters. However, unlike the specific anatomic locations of both AV nodal pathways and the His bundle, the anatomic origin of VT is often poorly defined and is usually within a large volume of previously injured myocardium. The energy for ablation may have to reach tissues remote from the electrode contact area, which greatly reduces the probability of successful ablation. For these reasons, the success rate with high-energy DC ablation of VT substrates, as reported by the Percutaneous Mapping and Ablation Registry, has been only 18% among 164 patients, with a total mortality of 24% (40 patients, including 5 who died from noncardiac causes and 11 whose deaths were procedure related).[14] Patients considered for percutaneous transcatheter ablation should have inducible and hemodynamically stable monomorphic VT.[20]

Accurate mapping of the VT is an important determinant of the success of ablation. Currently, this is done by multiple electrode endocavitary mapping catheters positioned inside the ventricular chambers. VT is induced using standard electrophysiologic techniques. During the mapping procedure, the earliest endocavitary pre-segment of electrocardiogram (QRS) activity (relative to the surface recording) defines the area for ablation. To verify whether the early activation location during VT is close to the area of slow conduction causing the reentrant circuit, the VT is terminated, and pacing is initiated at the same location in which early activation is detected. The 12-lead electrocardiograms obtained during VT and during ventricular pacing should be very similar in axis and form. This finding enhances the probability of VT ablation.[21]

The difficulty in identifying the exact location for

ablation is a major factor in the failure of catheter ablation for the treatment of VT. Theoretically, DC shock should be effective in eradicating the arrhythmogenic substrate for VT because it produces large lesions. However, this would be accompanied by a higher risk of myocardial perforation through barotrauma, especially in the right ventricular region.

Catheter ablation therapy for the treatment of VT is still far from rewarding, except in the case of bundle branch reentry VT.[22,23] Tchou et al.[23] reported very good outcomes with DC catheter ablation of this arrhythmia substrate (Table 20-1). In this study, seven patients each received two electrical shocks of 170 to 310 J via catheter to the right bundle branch. The macroreentry circuit was ablated, and right bundle branch block developed. During electrophysiologic studies conducted 2 to 3 days following the procedure, the VT was no longer inducible.

Complications of High-Energy Direct Current Ablation

Although the long-term mortality following high-energy DC ablation of VT has been reported to be 24%, many of these deaths were not a result of the ablation procedure.[14] The complication and mortality rates after high-energy DC shock are significant but can be reduced with increased operator experience. There is a theoretical possibility that VT may be worsened with the injury of more myocardium by catheter ablation; however, this has not been substantiated in the literature. The occurrence of ventricular fibrillation and sudden cardiac death after DC catheter ablation is another complication.[10,15,18] In one study, sudden cardiac death was reported in 1 of 47 patients 2 weeks after DC ablation of the AV node.[15] Total mortality was 17% in this study, and the rate was significantly higher among the patients with structural heart disease. In a group of 10 patients treated by DC ablation, 2 patients developed asymptomatic pericardial effusion, 1 patient had nonsustained VT, 1 patient became hypotensive, and 1 experienced chest pain believed to be due to shock-induced perforation of the right ventricle.[13]

Other complications of DC ablation include arrhythmias, cardiac tamponade, coronary sinus rupture, thrombosis,[24] circumflex artery lesions, and ventricular dysfunction.[25]

RADIOFREQUENCY ENERGY AND CARDIAC TISSUE ABLATION

For DC ablation, the diffuse nature of its tissue injury, its high rate of serious complications, and the limited operator control of the energy delivered have been the major catalysts for the development of an alternative ablation energy source such as RF energy. RF energy has been used since the turn of the century for cutting and coagulation in the surgical disciplines of clinical medicine.[26] Electrosurgery is used in every surgical discipline and most recently has been introduced into internal medicine through the endoscope (gastroenterology) and transcatheter ablation procedures (cardiac electrophysiology).

Physics and Engineering

RF energy is an alternating current with a frequency between 10 kHz and 900 MHz. Frequencies above this are in the microwave spectra. The frequency range used in electrosurgery ranges from 200 to 1,200 kHz. At these frequencies, the electrical current does not directly depolarize excitable tissues, and the heat generated by this energy is dissipated into the area that is close to the electrode-tissue interface.[27] Frequencies significantly greater than these (in the microwave range) are transmitted to tissues more distant from the electrode, and, unless the energy is focused, the heat dissipation can occur over a much larger tissue mass. In contrast to the instantaneous energy output associated with high-energy DC shock, the relatively low RF energy is applied for a variable time period and intensity, giving the operator the ability to control the size of the lesion. In addition, the ease of delivery makes RF energy the current choice for cardiac tissue ablation. Unlike the DC ablation technique, which requires considerable patient sedation or general anesthesia, RF energy causes minimal discomfort to the patient during ablation, does not directly depolarize cardiac tissue, and rarely triggers arrhythmias. However, arrhythmia induction does sometimes occur during RF ablation. This is probably a result of increased tissue temperature leading to increased excitability.

Technical Aspects of Radiofrequency Ablation

The RF generator currently in use for electrosurgery is often a sufficient source of energy. These generators are capable of producing three forms of RF current: sinusoidal alternating current (continuous at a frequency of several hundred kilohertz) used for tissue cutting, modulated current (burst-like forms of energy) used for coagulation, and a combination of the two called a blend. Since the goal of cardiac tissue ablation is tissue destruction with preservation of tissue mechanical integrity, lower power levels are applied to a large electrode-tissue contact area with unmodulated sinusoidal current. Using unmodulated current at power levels lower than those used for tissue cutting allows better control of the power delivered without arcing (Fig. 20-1, 3 and 4). To avoid arcing, the electrode-tissue impedance should be closely monitored, and the power should be terminated at the first indication of impedance rise. When using electrosurgery cutting/coagulation equipment, the bipolar output is used at power levels of 10 to 60 W.

Many factors play important roles in determining the characteristics of lesion formation. Among them are the intensity of the power, the total energy delivered, the area of the electrode-tissue contact, the electrode-tissue impedance, the tissue heat dissipation characteristics, and the type of electrodes used (i.e., electrode to reference patch or between two electrodes on a catheter).

To control the total energy delivered better, dedicated lesion generators have been developed (Fig. 20-2) in which the power source is controlled by a timer that contains a display of the elapsed time, impedance, current output, and voltage of the delivered power. This control unit is connected to a steerable catheter from which the power is emitted between the catheter tip electrode and a reference electrode. The reference electrode is a large electrosurgery patch placed on the patient's upper back. Ablation may also be achieved between the tip electrodes of two ablation catheters positioned across the tissue to be ablated (sandwich approach) or between the tip and a more proximal electrode.

Gas and Coagulum Formation

Because the heat causes tissue dehydration, dynamic decreases in tissue thermal conductance occur, which in turn result in an increase in temperature at the electrode-tissue interface. We have noted that at the initial application of RF energy, the tissue surrounding the electrode retracts to form a crater-like depression around the catheter tip electrode from which the RF energy is emitted, and the tissue also forms a bond with the electrode. These changes may increase the electrode-tissue contact area and decrease the impedance. Moreover, if the electrode-tissue interface temperature increases rapidly above the boiling point, any liquids under the electrode will be vaporized. If RF energy continues to form vapor, high pressure develops under the electrode and eventually overcomes the electrode's opposing mechanical pressure. This leads to sudden dislodgment of the electrode and an explosive burst that can cause a

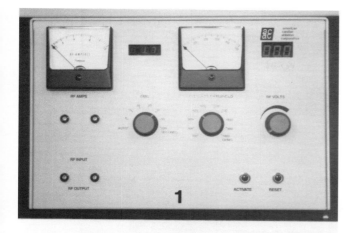

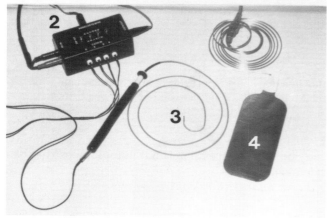

Fig. 20-2. Basic equipment used in transcatheter ablation. The RF generator (*1*) provides output voltage, current, impedance, and power, which are displayed in digital or analogus form, or both. The knobs control ablation time, impedance level cutoff, and voltage or power output. The device allows for automatic cutoff when the impedance increases above a predetermined level. Other generators provide temperature sensing and automatic temperature control, which require a thermistor to be placed within the ablation electrode. The generator's positive and negative outputs are connected to a switching box (*2*). This box switches the ablation/mapping catheter (*3*) tip electrode from a recording mode to an ablation mode. The RF ablation circuit is completed by way of the large electrosurgery patch electrode, which is covered with highly conductive adhesive gel (*4*).

significant amount of tissue damage.[28] As evaporation may also occur intramurally, a gas bubble may develop within the tissue under the electrode. Continued application of RF energy will cause the bubble to expand and its pressure to increase. This may lead to eruption of the gas bubble through the weakest path, leaving behind a gaping hole. The release of the gas pressure is associated with a popping sound similar to the popping of a kernel of corn. When such

a sound is heard during the application of RF power, it is likely that tissue tearing has occurred.[29] An example of such a tear is shown in Figure 20-3. Furthermore, if blood is trapped between the electrode and tissue during the delivery of RF energy, a rapid increase in temperature results, causing a coagulum to be formed on the metallic surface of the electrode. Coagulum formation causes a rapid increase in voltage across the rising impedance, which may result in arcing and tissue charring.

Electrode-Tissue Contact and Impedance

The most commonly used RF ablation catheter is a 7-F steerable catheter with a 4-mm-long platinum tip electrode. If the ablation electrode is firmly embedded in tissue, the impedance is greater (130 to 180 Ω, rarely more) than the impedance of a catheter with its tip electrode floating in blood. With the 7-F catheter, the average impedance is 116 $\pm$ 17 Ω (range, 80 to 140 Ω).[29] During the first few seconds of energy delivery, the impedance tends to decrease. The reason for this decrease is not totally clear. However, as mentioned before, the retraction of the endocardial surface around the electrode tip enlarges the area of electrode-tissue contact. Electrode-tissue bonding and tissue heating will also reduce the impedance. Many electrode configurations were devised to improve electrode-tissue contact and stability, decrease impedance, direct the current into the tissue, and minimize the amount of current diverted to blood. Such electrodes include needle and screw-in electrodes[30] and suction electrodes,[31] which increase the efficacy of lesion formation but may cause a significant amount of trauma.

Practical Considerations for the Application of Radiofrequency Power

Electrode-tissue contact is an important parameter in the creation of effective myocardial lesions during RF ablation. Since the electrode-tissue contact may not be adequately assessed prior to the initiation of RF power, monitoring the temperature rise (if available) or the decrease in impedance can provide important information regarding electrode-tissue contact.

In a recent electrode-tissue contact evaluation study, it was found that as the electrode-tissue contact increases, so does the rate and level of temperature.[32] With the electrode floating in blood, the maxi-

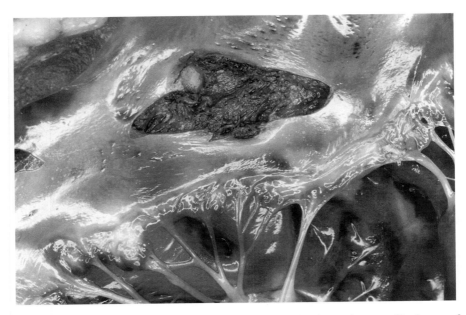

Fig. 20-3. Left atrial tear above the mitral valve annulus in a dog heart is a result of an explosion using 40 W of RF power. The tear, measuring 17 mm long and 7.5 mm wide, is not associated with atrial wall perforation.

mum temperature increase with 20 and 30 W was only $7° \pm 1°C$ and $11° \pm 2°C$, respectively, and plateaued after a few seconds of power application. With the electrode in good contact with the tissue, the temperature increase with 20 and 30 W reached $31° \pm 11°C$ and $60° \pm 1°C$, respectively, after 60 seconds of power application.

As the electrode-tissue contact increases, so does the rate and level of impedance decrease. However, the rate of the decrease is slower compared with the rate of temperature rise. With the electrode floating in blood, the maximum impedance decrease with 20 and 30 W was 6 ± 6 and $9 \pm 5 \, \Omega$, respectively, and plateaued after a few seconds of power application. With the electrode in good contact with the tissue, the maximum impedance decrease with 20 and 30 W was 23 ± 3 and $20 \pm 7 \, \Omega$, respectively. The impedance plateaued after 40 seconds of power application.

During RF ablations, the increase in lesion diameter and depth correlates well with decreasing impedance and increasing temperature. However, lesion depth appears to correlate better with impedance than temperature. The lesion maturation rate is not uniform for diameter and depth. The diameter of the lesion is established within 10 to 20 seconds, especially with power levels of 40 to 50 W. However, using power levels of greater than 20 W may lead to impedance rise, frequent explosions, and tissue shredding. Since the electrode-tissue contact is not known prior to the initiation of power, the following approaches

may be useful once an optimal mapping position has been established.

For a temperature-controlled system:

1. Set the temperature to 85°C and turn the power on.
2. Good contact is indicated if the temperature rises to the desired level within the first 10 to 20 seconds and is accompanied by a greater than 15 Ω impedance decrease after 20 seconds of power application. Full lesion maturation may evolve over 90 seconds.
3. If no therapeutic results are noted, then remap and reposition.

For an impedance-monitoring system:

1. Start at 5 W and gradually increase the power every 10 seconds up to 20 W.
2. A greater than 15-Ω impedance decrease after 20 to 40 seconds indicates good contact. Lesion depth can be maximized by maintaining the power for 90 seconds.
3. If no therapeutic results are noted, then remap and reposition.
4. If the impedance decrease is less than 10 Ω, the power may be increased, but *it would be best to reposition the catheter for better contact.*

It is important that the initial RF power be limited to 10 to 20 W or less and then increased slowly in 5-

W increments to levels of no more than 40 W. This approach may decrease the incidence of sudden impedance rise and explosions, which can cause severe tissue shredding.[20] An impedance rise to several hundred ohms with a concomitant decrease in current is an indication that coagulum has formed on the electrode. Continued application of energy in the presence of high impedance leads to high voltages and may result in arcing, charring, and increasing the size of coagulum formation on the tip electrode. This coagulum may become detached and may embolize. In addition, once impedance has increased, it is unlikely that repeated power application will deliver any significant amount of energy to the tissue. Therefore, removing the catheter and scraping and coagulum from the tip is necessary in this situation. Unfortunately, removing the catheter from what may be the optimal location for ablation can result in many hours of effort to reposition the catheter and, therefore, prolonged radiation exposure.

Several published reports have evaluated catheters with a temperature sensor (thermistor) mounted on the tip electrode.[28,33] It is important to note that the tip of the RF delivery electrode is not the source of heat. The tissue under the electrode is heated, and then this heat is conducted into the catheter tip containing the temperature sensor. RF generators with a feedback loop feature that adjusts the current flow to maintain the tip electrode at a fixed, preselected temperature below the boiling point would be desirable because this would provide the capability of generating a lesion without the fear of coagulum formation and increasing impedance.

During RF application, it is desirable to observe both the limb lead electrocardiograms and several intracardiac electrograms for arrhythmias, interruption of tachycardia, changes in pre-excitation, and changes in the AV and His-ventricular intervals. Because the highest frequencies that compose the limb leads and intracardiac recordings do not exceed 3,000 Hz, digital or linear notch filters can be applied to filter the RF interference without compromising the quality of the recordings.

Clinical Use and Experience

Sinus Node Tachycardias

No large studies have been published concerning the treatment of sinus node re-entry and automatic tachycardias. However, several abstracts suggest that RF ablation is effective for these arrhythmias. This technique may involve the insertion of the ablation catheter into the superior vena cava and retracting the catheter to the sinus node region while mapping for the earliest electrogram activity during the tachycardia. Possible complications include right phrenic injury and sinus node dysfunction.

Atrial Tachycardias

Common atrial flutter has been successfully treated with RF power applied to the posterior septal region of the tricuspid valve. Mapping of the tricuspid ring during atrial flutter defined the reentry circuit where the AV node slow pathway and the flutter share a common path.[22,34] Currently, atrial fibrillation has no treatment using a percutaneous catheter approach other than ablation of the AV node (to slow the ventricular response) or total ablation of the AV junction or His bundle in combination with the placement of a permanent pacemaker to control ventricular rate. It has been shown that ablation of supraventricular reentrant tachycardias improves ventricular function.[35]

Atrioventricular Nodal Reentry Tachycardia

In sharp contrast to ablation with high-energy DC shocks, RF ablation lesions are small and localized, and the ablation process can be interrupted. This makes it possible to produce lesions that modify AV nodal conduction by disrupting the re-entrant circuit while maintaining normal pathways, thus obviating the need for permanent pacing.[35] Such modification was successful in four of five pediatric patients who underwent the procedure for AV nodal reentrant tachycardia and junctional ectopic tachycardia. It failed in one case, for an overall success rate of 80%.[36]

Lee et al. reported a success rate of 82% at 8 ± 3 months following RF perinodal ablation for AV nodal reentrant tachycardia.[37] Only 3 of the 39 patients developed complete AV block and required permanent pacemaker placement. AV nodal modification is the treatment of choice for AV nodal reentrant tachycardia due to its high success and low complication rates. In a more recent paper, selective AV nodal slow pathway ablation was performed using the stepwise anatomic approach (the most commonly used approach).[39] AV nodal re-entry tachycardia was eliminated in 91% of the patients with none of the 35 patients requiring a pacemaker due to complete AV block. The RF lesion placements were started at the most posterior septal region of the tricuspid valve. Power levels of 40 to 50 W were used for 40 to 60 seconds. An accelerated junctional rhythm was often an indication of a successful outcome. Slow pathway electrograms can be mapped in most pa-

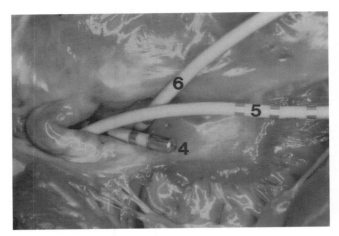 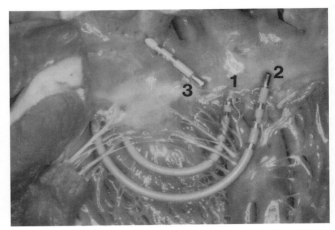

Fig. 20-4. Because of the limited lesion size, the deflectable ablation catheter has to be placed close (within 3 to 4 mm) to the arrhythmogenic tissue. Ablation of bypass tracks in this dog heart can be approached retrogradely through the aortic valve with the ablation catheter tip placed either under the mitral valve in the left ventricle (*1*) or just above the valve in the atrium (*2*). Ablation in the left atrium can also be achieved through a transseptal approach with the catheter introduced by way of the venous system and through the atrial septum (*3*). AV node modification for patients with AV node reentrant pathways or ablation of accessory pathways that insert into the right atrium most commonly require placing the ablation catheter at the posterior septal region of the right atrium in close proximity to the tricuspid valve (*4*). Additional catheters are placed across the tricuspid ring superiorly for atrial, His, and ventricular electrogram recordings (*5*) and a catheter positioned in the coronary sinus (*6*).

tients with AV nodal reentry tachycardia. The application of 30 W of RF power for 40 to 60 seconds results in a success rate as high as 97%. This high success rate can be attributed to the superficial location of the specific tissue to be ablated, the ability to place the catheters in accessible, well-defined locations (Fig. 20-4), and the small amount of tissue that needs to be ablated (Fig. 20-5). Patients with persistent AV nodal echoes are at a much higher risk for recurrence of the tachycardia.[39] Since there are few complications with RF power, it is the first line of therapy for AV nodal reentry tachycardias.[40,41]

Accessory Pathways

Following the first successful catheter ablation of an accessory pathway by Borggrefe and co-workers in 1987,[42] experience with this technique has grown at a rapid pace. The procedure involves electrophysiologic mapping for the precise location of the accessory pathway, followed by its ablation. A single deflectable catheter can be used both for mapping (of the electrical activity around the mitral ring for the earliest AV coupling interval) and for ablation.[40]

At most centers, electrophysiologic mapping involves placing a catheter with multiple, closely spaced, bipolar electrodes in the coronary sinus. Additional catheters are placed in the right ventricular apex for stimulation, His bundle electrogram recording, and high right atrium stimulation and recording. The electrograms recorded from each bipolar

electrode in the coronary sinus catheter show atrial and ventricular deflections that allow evaluation of the location of the shortest AV conduction during the orthodromic tachycardia and the location of the shortest ventriculoatrial conduction time during ventricular pacing.

Right-sided posterior septal pathways are mapped and ablated using a deflectable catheter that is introduced through the femoral vein so the tip can be positioned on the atrial side of the tricuspid ring posterior wall. Anterior and lateral right-sided pathways are more readily approached from the internal jugular vein. The deflectable catheter is inserted into the right ventricle and curved to position the tip over the tricuspid ring. The major complication encountered with anterior septal pathway ablation is inadvertent damage to the His bundle or to the right bundle branch.

Techniques used to ablate left-sided accessory pathways are somewhat different. One of these involves a retrograde approach in which the catheter is passed through the femoral artery, aorta, and aortic valve into the left ventricle. The tip is then positioned either under the mitral valve (as close as possible to the AV ring) or above the valve in the left atrial chamber on the AV ring (Fig. 20-4, 1 and 2). The catheter tip is guided into position by coronary sinus mapping as well as the recording from the catheter tip bipolar electrode demonstrating the shortest AV coupling interval (Fig. 20-6).

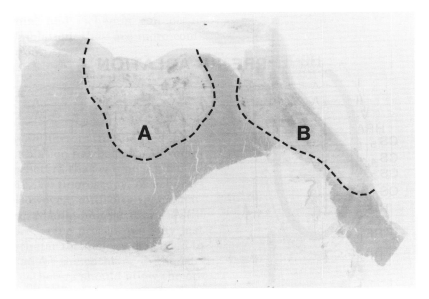

Fig. 20-5. Micrograph showing a cross section of the junction between the left atrium (thinner wall segment) and the left ventricle (the thicker wall segment). A segment of the mitral valve is shown in the center. Supra- and infravalvular lesions were generated in a dog heart with 40 W power applied for 40 seconds. After healing for 4 weeks, the two lesions are dense, well-demarcated, and consist of necrotic tissues and regions of hemorrhage within the lesions. The ventricular lesion (*A*) measured 9.5 mm in diameter and 6.5 mm in depth. The atrial lesion (*B*) measured 8 mm in diameter and 3 mm in depth. The indentation seen on the endocardial surface of the left ventricular lesion is a result of tissue retraction under and around the catheter during the application of energy.

Another method of left-sided accessory pathway ablation involves a transeptal approach in which the interatrial septum is punctured from the right side using a Brockenbrough needle, and a Mullen sheath is placed across the septum (Fig. 20-4, 3). The catheter is inserted from the right atrium into the left atrium via the sheath. The tip is then positioned at the ablation site just over the AV ring where the accessory pathway may be located. The anatomic position of the coronary sinus, which is in close proximity to the atrial tissues along the AV groove, provides the mapping information used to define the site of the left-sided accessory pathway. The deflectable catheter tip is guided to the most appropriate location using the electrodes of the coronary sinus catheter showing the shortest AV conduction interval during ventricular pacing or during reciprocating tachycardia. The operator is aided by fluoroscopy and, at some centers, by transesophageal echocardiography. Ablation is carried out between the tip electrode (connected to the RF generator) and a large conductive electrode placed on the patient's upper back.

In one study, the average procedure time was 114 ± 55 minutes, a mean of 35 ± 12 minutes was required for the insertion and positioning of the catheters, and patients were discharged on the third day after the procedure.[40] Overall, the success rate using RF power for accessory pathway ablation has ranged from 83 to 99%.[1,9,43] Among a total patient population of 378, those with procedural complications have included two patients with complete AV block, one with pericarditis, one with cardiac tamponade, one with femoral hematoma, and one who developed a myocardial infarction as a result of inadvertent delivery of RF power inside the left coronary artery.

Because of its safety and success, it appears that percutaneous transcatheter ablation of accessory pathways may totally obviate the need for surgical resection in the future.

Ventricular Tachycardias

Currently, RF ablation of VT is only 10 to 30% successful. The reason for the high failure rate may be that the regional response to the RF current is affected by structural changes (scarring) in the diseased myocardium.[43] Transcatheter RF ablation has also been shown to be feasible for postinfarction and bundle branch reentry VT management.[44] In one study, the procedure-related in-hospital mortality for VT management was 3.3% among 92 patients, 65 of whom were treated with high-energy DC ablation and 27 of whom received RF ablation.[45]

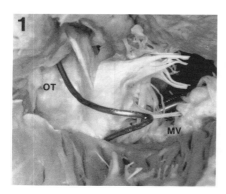
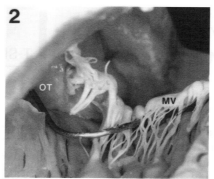
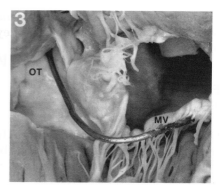

Fig. 20-8. Retrograde approach with the wire tip positioned under the mitral leaflets. OT, left ventricular outflow tract; MV, mitral valve posterior leaflet.

short-tip (5-cm) catheter when approached retrogradely (Fig. 20-11A) or transseptally (Fig. 20-11B), whereas the longer tip (7-cm) catheter is better for the lateral position.

Pigtail-Type Mapping and Ablation Electrode

Figure 20-12 shows a 7-F deflectable catheter placed just above the mitral valve in a patient with a lateral accessory pathway.[47] Although the catheter tip is stable above the mitral ring during ventricular systole, during diastole the anterior leaflet of the mitral valve exerts a downward force on the catheter, causing the catheter tip to dislodge from its position above the mitral ring.

The anatomic junction of the mitral ring, the atrium, and the ventricle create a depression in the atrium just above the mitral ring. A catheter with a pigtail-type end equipped with six 4-mm-long electrodes (used for both recording and ablation) has been constructed to fit the left atrium just above the mitral ring.[48] To assess mobility around the mitral ring and stability of recording and ablation, this catheter was inserted into the left ventricle of an intact dog heart under fluoroscopic guidance with the

pigtail end positioned retrogradely across the mitral valve on the atrial side of the AV ring (Fig. 20-13). The pigtail and a secondary curve allow the catheter to cross the mitral valve apparatus and adapt to the curvature of the atrial mitral ring structure. The secondary curve stabilizes the deflectable tip across the valve so that the opening and closing of the leaflets only minimally affects the catheter's position. The catheter is secured in the mitral ring and is less prone to drop back into the ventricle. As shown in Figure 20-14, the electrograms from the electrodes on the pigtail portion of the catheter show the transition from the atrium to the ventricle across the mitral ring. Torquing the catheter shaft results in rotation of the pigtail and the ability to map and apply lesions around the mitral ring. This catheter can be used with a standard 8-F introducer.

Variable Deflection Length, Lateral Deflection, and Bidirectional Deflection

The optimal catheter deflection length cannot always be established prior to catheter insertion. Therefore, a variable deflection length catheter is currently under

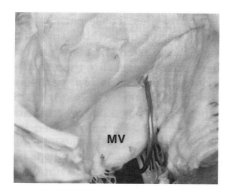
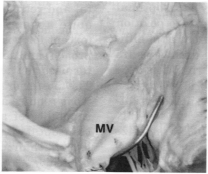
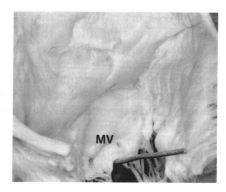

Fig. 20-9. Retrograde supravalvular approach. MV, mitral valve posterior leaflet.

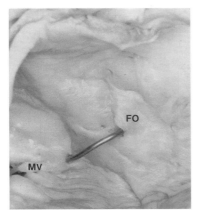

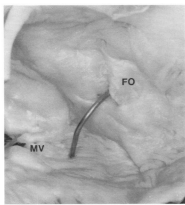

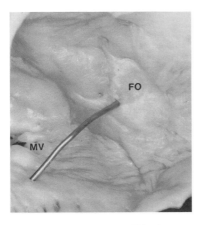

Fig. 20-10. Transeptal approach. FO, foramen ovale; MV, mitral valve posterior leaflet.

development. Another catheter system under testing at this time has lateral deflection and bidirectional deflection capabilities. These catheters may decrease procedure time and increase ablation success rates.

Deflectable Loop Catheter

Ablation of right-sided accessory pathways, modification of AV nodal reentry tachycardia, and His bundle ablation all require mapping and ablation along the perivalvular atrial tissues of the tricuspid ring. Since the tricuspid valve ring is directly accessible to catheters introduced from the major veins, it provides the setting for a loop-type structure that adapts to the valve ring. The most effective approach for ablation around the tricuspid ring would be to map and then apply RF power through the recording electrode that identified the desired area for ablation. A deflectable loop catheter equipped with 16 electrodes (4 mm long, spaced 4 mm apart) can be used for both recording and ablation (Fig. 20-15A & B). The distal portion of the catheter is equipped with a small secondary loop. The catheter, introduced into the right atrium from the femoral vein, is capable of adapting to the shape of the tricuspid ring when opened and is also capable of rotation across the valve plane by a separate deflection control.[47] The smaller secondary loop is anchored in the right ventricular outflow, and the proximal end is anchored by the inferior vena cava, as shown in Figure 20-16. Simultaneous recordings from the electrodes can show both atrial and ventricular electrograms (Fig. 20-17). Adjustments can be made by moving the catheter vertically, by rotating it, or by changing the deflection angle of the loop. As shown in Figure 20-18, the mapping/ablation electrodes on the loop catheter adapt well to the tricuspid ring orifice. Discrete, sequential, perivalvular, atrial lesions were produced around the tricuspid valve without the need to readjust the catheter (Fig. 20-18B).

Right Atrial Mapping and Ablating Multielectrode Array Designed for the Ablation of Atrial Fibrillation

The highly invasive maze operation has been shown to be effective in the treatment of atrial fibrillation. We tested a catheter approach using RF power to ablate atrial fibrillation in a sterile pericarditis dog model. A 7-F monorail sliding catheter system was constructed that allows the catheter to curve and adapt to the endocardial surface of the right atrium. The catheter is equipped with 20 closely spaced 4-mm electrodes that are used for both mapping and ablation. The catheter was tested in seven dogs. It was initially positioned at the posterolateral right atrium with the electrodes in contact with the superior vena cava, right atrium, and inferior vena cava tissues. Following the ablation, the catheter was positioned over the anterior wall of the right atrium, and the ablations were repeated. Six of the seven dogs had sustained atrial fibrillation (more than 3 minutes). Following this ablation, atrial fibrillation could not be sustained and lasted only 20 ± 48 seconds. Examina-

Table 20-2. Measurements (mm) of Different Parameters of Deflectable Catheters for Different Approaches to the Left Atrium

	TL	T-SH	R	L-DEF
PS RETRO	45 ± 7	12 ± 3	8 ± 1	10 ± 4
PS TRANS	38 ± 6	18 ± 5[a]	8 ± 1	8 ± 4
P RETRO	48 ± 6	19 ± 6	10 ± 1	15 ± 6
P TRANS	36 ± 8[a]	26 ± 7	10 ± 3	4 ± 3[a]
PL RETRO	52 ± 9[b]	36 ± 5[b]	18 ± 4[b]	7 ± 10
PL TRANS	39 ± 11[a]	29 ± 7[a]	19 ± 6[b]	1 ± 2[b]
L RETRO	59 ± 8[b]	42 ± 5[b]	24 ± 7[b]	0.5 ± 2[b]
L TRANS	52 ± 13[b]	40 ± 9[b]	27 ± 6[b]	3 ± 8[b]

Abbreviations: PS, posterior septal; P, posterior; PL, posterior lateral; L, lateral; RETRO, retrograde; TRANS, transeptal; TL, tip length; T-SH, tip to shaft distance; R, vertical curvature; L-DEF, lateral curvature.

[a] P <0.01 TRANS vs. RETRO.
[b] P <0.01 vs. RETRO, TRANS PS, and P.

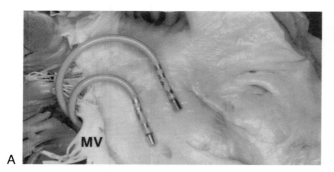
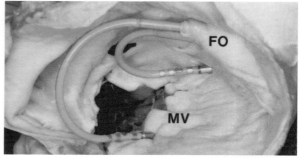

Fig. 20-11. Posterior septal position of the mitral valve AV ring approached retrogradely **(A)** or transseptally **(B)**. MV, mitral valve; FO, foramen ovale.

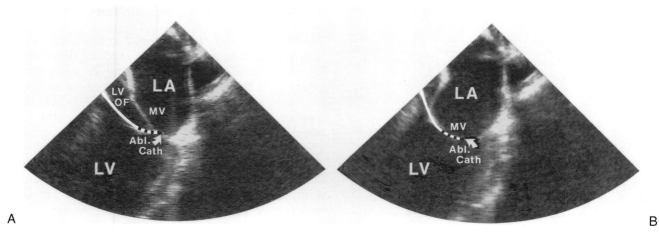

Fig. 20-12. Transesophageal echocardiography with the ablation catheter positioned at the lateral wall of the LA/AV junction during ventricular systole **(A)** and diastole **(B)** showing the anterior leaflet forcing the catheter tip off the AV junction. LVOF, left ventricular outflow tract; LA, left atrium; MV, mitral valve; ABL. cath, ablation catheter.

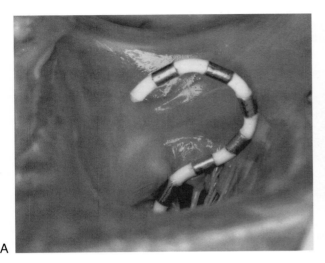
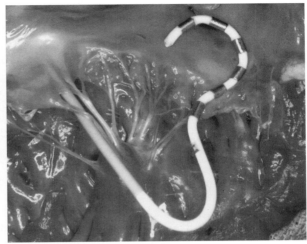

A   B

Fig. 20-13. A pigtail-type catheter equipped with 4-mm ablation ring electrodes. **(A)** The pigtail positioned in the left atria on the AV ring of a dog heart. **(B)** The same heart was opened to expose the mitral apparatus.

tion of each heart revealed continuous, transmural lesions bisecting the right atrium posterolaterally and anteriorly. This catheter system holds promise for the treatment of atrial fibrillation and other arrhythmias originating from the right atrium.

Segmented Ablation Electrode: Flexible Lesion Size and Discrete Localized Mapping

Enlarging the ablation electrode size will result in a larger lesion by increasing electrode-tissue contact if the amount of RF power is increased proportionally.

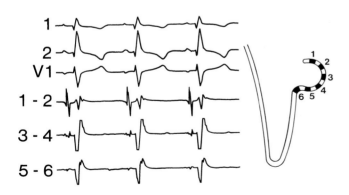

Fig. 20-14. The electrograms recorded from the pigtail portion of the catheter show the transition of the atrial and ventricular electrograms across the mitral ring. The upper three tracings show the scalar leads 1, 2, and V1 and the bottom four tracings show the bipolar recordings from the 4-mm ring electrodes shown on the right.

However, this commits the operator to a large lesion and may significantly decrease the ability to map localized electrical activity discretely. To allow the operator more control of lesion size and to provide high-quality electrograms, a 2-mm tip electrode followed by three 2-mm ring electrodes (spaced 0.5-mm apart) were mounted on a 7-F deflectable catheter. These electrodes yield sharp and discrete high-frequency content intracardiac electrograms. RF lesions were created by applying 60 W of power through the following electrode combinations: the 2-mm tip electrode plus the first ring electrode (2 + 2), the tip plus the first and second ring electrodes (2 + 2 + 2), and the tip plus all three ring electrodes (2 + 2 + 2 + 2). These combinations were compared with lesions created with a standard 4-mm electrode (Table 20-3). It was concluded that segmented ablation electrode configurations 2 + 2 and 2 + 2 + 2 result in a significantly greater lesion depth than the standard 4-mm electrode. These electrode configurations provide the operator with the flexibility to increase lesion size without compromising mapping ability.

Basket-Type Mapping Catheters

A collapsible basket-type catheter for intra-right-atrial mapping was recently introduced and is currently undergoing testing. It contains multiple spines with 5 pairs of small rings on each spine, for a total of 25 pairs.[48] A similar catheter designed for ventricular mapping was recently introduced. It is constructed from spiral-like spines equipped with small recording electrodes. These catheters do not

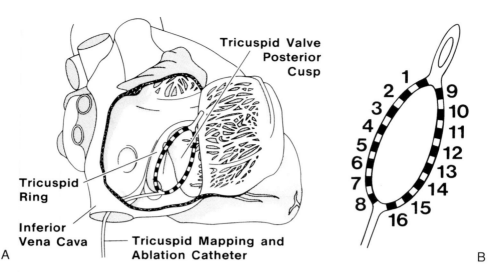

Fig. 20-15. (A) The loop catheter is introduced from the femoral vein into the inferior vena cava and across the tricuspid valve. The loop is equipped with 16 4-mm-long electrodes spaced 4 mm apart. (B) The most distal portion of the catheter is equipped with a small secondary loop.

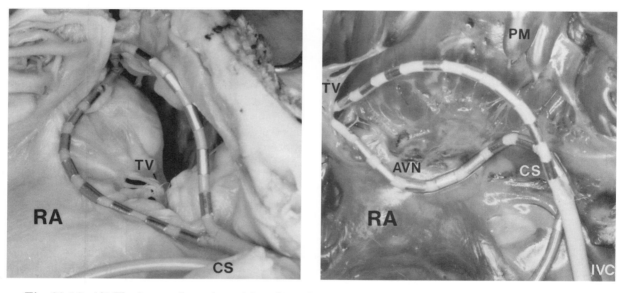

Fig. 20-16. (A) The loop catheter is positioned in a human cadaver heart with an intact tricuspid orifice. (B) A dog heart with the orifice open showing the septal leaflet of the tricuspid ring. RA, right atrium; TV, tricuspid valve; CS, coronary sinus; AVN, atrial ventricular node; IVC, inferior vena cava; PM, papillary muscle.

allow for the transmission of RF power for ablation. They require the introduction of ablation catheters once the ablation site is identified.

Rotating Tip Electrode for Mapping and Ablation

A deflectable catheter was constructed with a rotating tip electrode, which allows the catheter's de-flectable section to move over the endocardium (Fig. 20-19). Since the electrode-tissue contact surface area is large, application of RF power to this electrode results in a large, dense lesion, as shown in Figure 20-20. Because controlled movements can be achieved with this catheter, mapping and RF ablation can be performed on ventricular or atrial tissue in small incremental steps to create a continuous lesion.

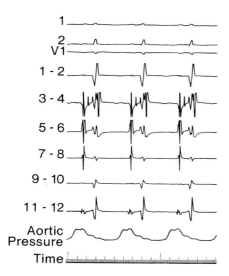

Fig. 20-17. Scalar electrocardiogram leads I, II, and VI are the top three tracings, and aortic pressure is shown on the bottom tracing. Simultaneous recordings from the ring electrodes: 1–2, 3–4, 5–6, 7–8 are from the posterior septum, and 9–10, 11–12 are from the anterior wall.

Actively Cooled Tip Electrode

Temperature control of RF power level has greatly enhanced the ability to generate lesions while minimizing the incidence of impedance rise, intramyocardial boiling, pressure rise, and tissue shredding. Since the maximal temperature is generated at the electrode-tissue interface, the lesion size and, more importantly, lesion depth is limited to 7 to 9 mm. Ventricular tachycardias originating from intramyocardial or near-epicardial circuits require deeper lesions for successful ablation. Recently an ablation catheter with a saline-irrigated tip was introduced. Saline infusion cools the tip electrode and allows much greater power to be applied.[50] The ablation electrode has six circumferential holes (0.4 mm in diameter) connected to a central infusion tubing that irrigates the electrode at 20 ml/min. Although the tissue-electrode interface is actively cooled, the increased power results in greater intramyocardial current density, increased tissue heating, and, therefore, a significantly larger lesion size than a standard RF ablation catheter (depth, 6.1 ± 0.5 versus 9.9 ± 1.1 mm; width, 11.3 ± 0.9 versus 14.3 ± 1.5 mm).

Discussion

Electrophysiology mapping/ablation catheter specifications should be based on anatomic and electrical requirements, clinical need, and safety. The design characteristics of mapping ablation catheters are important factors in the efficient, successful completion of ablation procedures. To maximize power transfer to the tissue, catheter design characteristics should be based on the ability of a catheter to adapt to the anatomic location of the arrhythmogenic tissue, maneuverability of the catheter's mapping/ablation electrodes, and optimal electrode-tissue contact.

As demonstrated in the cadaver heart, left-sided

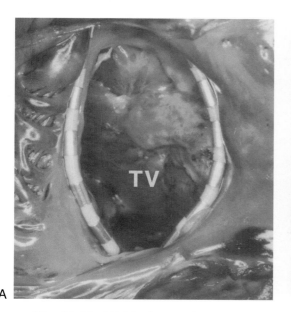

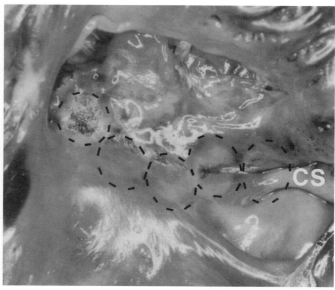

Fig. 20-18. (A) The loop catheter is seen from the open right atrium at the tricuspid valve (TV) orifice of a dog heart. **(B)** Discrete perivalvular atrial sequential lesions were produced around the tricuspid valve.

Table 20-3. Lesion Measurements (mm) Using Various Electrode Configurations

	2 + 2	2 + 2 + 2	2 + 2 + 2 + 2	4 mm
Length	11.4 ± 1.6	11.9 ± 0.9[a]	12.3 ± 0.7[a]	9.1 ± 0.4
Width	7.8 ± 1.1[b]	6.5 ± 1.1	5.4 ± 0.2	6.9 ± 1.2
Depth	7.1 ± 1.4[a]	7.1 ± 1.2[a]	6.8 ± 1.3	5.3 ± 0.6

[a] $P < 0.05$ vs. 4 mm.
[b] $P < 0.95$ vs. 2 + 2 + 2 + 2.

accessory pathways located in the posterior half of the mitral ring are much more accessible using specifically designed catheters that adapt to the desired anatomic location.[51]

A pigtail-shaped catheter tip improves the positioning capabilities and stability of the catheter when directed at the atrial side of the mitral ring. This design can be optimized by varying the length of deflection segment as well as the lateral movement capability.

The accessibility of the tricuspid ring allows for the introduction and anchoring of a loop-type catheter. The lesions generated by RF power applied to the 4-mm ring electrodes were similar to those generated with a 4-mm tip ablation electrode. To produce adequate lesions with RF power, good electrode-tissue contact must be maintained. Since all the ablation electrodes are placed on deflectable ring shafts, it is possible that the electrode-tissue contact may vary

from one location to another. However, because of the deflection, expansion, and rotational capabilities of the catheter, electrode-tissue contact can be optimized prior to the application of maximal RF power.

The more radical designs are the variable deflection catheter, the large multielectrode array catheters for mapping/ablation, and the rotating tip catheter.

ENERGY SOURCES

Laser Ablation

Laser energy can be delivered via a catheter into the cardiac chambers for tissue ablation. The laser energy wavelengths used range from infrared to ultraviolet and are characterized by their monochromatic and coherent form. Several forms of laser energy can

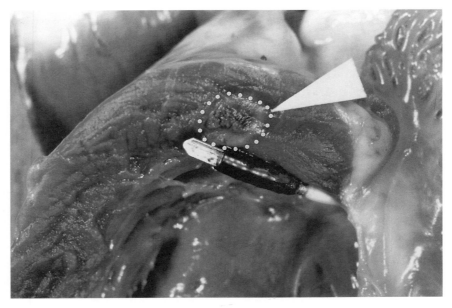

Fig. 20-19. A rotating tip electrode with three elongated teeth were curved 120 degrees apart into the electrode surfaces shown against left ventricular free wall intramural lesion (dotted line) created with 40 W for 40 seconds.

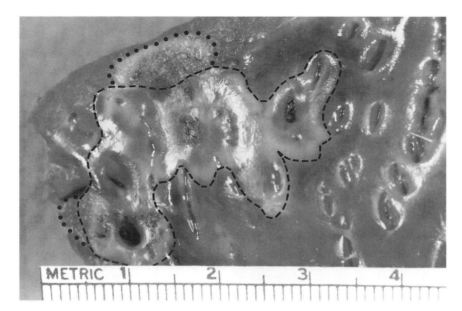

Fig. 20-20. Application of 40 W of RF power for 40 seconds to this electrode at each location after a movement of 0.5 to 1 cm results in a large dense lesion (note metric scale at the bottom) that is deep within the left ventricular free wall. Dotted line outlines the depth of the lesion and the broken line outlines the surface area of the lesion.

be used including argon, carbon dioxide (CO_2), and neodymium:yttrium-aluminum-garnet (Nd:YAG). Each of these sources requires a unique delivery system. The CO_2 laser utilizes optical prisms and mirrors to direct its beam, whereas the argon and Nd:YAG lasers use fiber optic tubes to transmit light energy. These laser beams can be used in either a continuous or a pulsed manner. The lesion produced by myocardial irradiation with a laser beam is a direct result of tissue heating, which is a function of the laser beam power density on the tissue. The laser beam power decreases within the tissue in an exponential decay manner. The rate of this decay is related to the laser beam scatter, absorption, and distance from the laser source. With a CO_2 laser beam, the tissue scatter compared with absorption is minimal. As a result, maximal heating occurs at the interface between the laser beam and the tissue, causing tissue evaporation. This energy is ideal for tissue cutting. The Nd:YAG laser beam yields high tissue scatter and low absorption. It causes heating of deeper tissues and creates larger lesions.[51] Because of the characteristics of this laser, many of the experimental and clinical attempts at arrhythmogenic tissue ablation by photocoagulation have been made with the Nd:YAG laser.

Thus far, experience with laser ablation has been limited to intraoperative endocardial laser ablation for VT.[52] It has also been used in conjunction with surgical endocardial resection.[53] Successful arrhyth-mia suppression was achieved in 60% of patients with VT and in a high percentage of patients with supraventricular tachycardia.[53] With advancement of fiberoptic technology, it is possible to deliver laser energy through a catheter.[12] The complications associated with transcatheter laser application in myocardial tissue range from tachyarrhythmias to perforation.[54] However, arrhythmias were not noted in patients who underwent intraoperative laser application for arrhythmia control.[52]

The development of a pulsed delivery system, which allows cooling to occur between pulses, has reduced the incidence of myocardial perforation and optical fiber tip degradation. Saksena et al.[53] demonstrated that the diseased myocardium has a higher safety margin for perforation from laser energy than normal myocardium. The lesion dimensions, including depth and diameter, were greater in the normal myocardial tissue than in the diseased fibrotic myocardium, with other variables being constant. Atrial tissue has the lowest safety margin for perforation with laser energy because of the thinness of the atrial wall. In other studies, application of 300 J of argon laser energy to a single site in the normal ventricular myocardium was not associated with perforation.[55,56]

Initial experience with laser ablation did not show a significant risk of embolization because the laser ablative process generates gaseous, soluble byproducts about 3 μm in size.[57] The lack of sufficient safety data, the complex nature of fiberoptic technology, and poor flexibility of the energy delivery systems (catheters) have been the major limiting factors in the use of widespread laser transcatheter ablation. Currently, fiberoptic technology is expensive to install and maintain. It has yet to be shown that this technology provides clear advantages over other types of ablation treatment.

Cryoablation

The ideal approach to arrhythmogenic tissue ablation is by freezing rather than by heating. By cooling excitable tissues, refractory periods and conduction times are prolonged, and excitability is reduced. Localized cooling of arrhythmogenic tissue slows or interrupts tachycardia. Cooling is easily reversible and no tissue damage occurs as long as freezing does not take place. Freezing the tissue disrupts the cell membrane and causes coagulation injury, leading to a dense, homogeneous, well-demarcated scar tissue.[58,59] Cold mapping has been applied in the operating room for AV node cryosurgical ablation of reciprocating tachycardias and VT. Recently, a method has been developed to introduce it through a transvenous approach.[60,61]

The standard cryoablation system consists of a high-pressure nitrous oxide or nitrogen storage tank that pumps pressurized gas into a probe. Within the probe, the gas expands, resulting in a rapid temperature decrease at the tip to as low as $-60°C$. The gas flow is maintained through a return conduit. The temperature can be controlled by adjusting the flow rate of gas into the tip. A cryoprobe placed in water will produce an expanding ice ball that is limited in size by the temperature gradient between the ice and the surrounding water. When the probe is immersed in 37°C blood and placed against the perfused myocardium, the cooling capabilities of the probe largely depend on the rate of nitrous oxide gas expansion within the cooling chamber. Recently an experimental 11-F cryoprobe for transvenous application has been developed and tested.[60] This catheter can be inserted to create lesions around the tricuspid ring; however, manipulation of the catheter to ablate left-sided arrhythmogenic tissues may not be possible.[60] The use of pressurized gas systems represent both safety and delivery problems.

Attempts are being made to produce controlled cooling using deflectable catheters and pulsed direct current electrical energy into a thermocoupled semiconductor junction, a concept called the Peltier effect. When electrical energy is delivered into the junction, one element is rapidly cooled while the second element is heated. Using this technology, the cooling element can be directed to contact the tissues whereas the heat can be vented by the blood. Whether such a system can cool a useful amount of tissue remains to be determined.

Chemical Ablation

Transcatheter injectable necrotizing agents such as formalin, alcohol, radiopaque solutions, and other mixtures have been used to cause local sclerosis and necrosis in cardiac tissue. This method was initially used to cause total AV block in experimental animals by injection into the perinodal area.[62,63] Local injection for ablative purposes had variable success in the experimental animal protocols. The nonsurgical approach of perinodal sclerosis with formalin in a dog model was introduced in the 1960s. Fisher et al.[64] reported a 50% success rate in producing heart block in 38 dogs by injecting 40% formaldehyde in the vicinity of the His bundle.

Intracoronary injection of alcohol and drugs have been explored in several studies.[65,66] Brugada et al.[67] studied three patients with incessant ventricular tachycardia who had coronary artery disease and who failed several antiarrhythmic drug trials. Ethanol was injected into the coronary artery branches that supplied the arrhythmogenic areas. VT suppression was successful in two patients. All patients experienced chest pain, although technetium pyrophosphate scans did not reveal an area of myocardial infarction. Kay et al.[65] reported similar work with ethanol injection into the AV node artery in 12 patients. Six patients had medically refractory arrhythmias that could not be ablated in previous DC or RF attempts. In this study, immediate heart block associated with mild transient chest discomfort was noted in 10 patients. Similar selective administration of antiarrhythmic agents into the AV node artery has been performed, demonstrating its feasibility in human subjects.[66] This procedure involves occlusion of the coronary blood supply to a poorly defined territory, which may cause a significant amount of tissue infarction and possible additional arrhythmias.

Microwave Ablation

The dominant factor in heat production using RF power at frequencies of 200 to 750 kHz is electrical resistance. A rapid decrease in current density is noted only a few millimeters away from the ablation electrode and, as a result, lesions are produced with limited depth of penetration. This may be one of the primary factors limiting the successful ablation of ventricular tachycardia using RF power.

Recently, we have seen a growing interest in microwave technology as a means of transmitting energy into cardiac tissues and causing tissue destruction by heat.[62,68] Microwaves are electromagnetic waves with frequencies in the range of 30 to 3000 MHz. These high-frequency waves can propagate in free space or in a conductive medium. The waves, however, are reflected and scattered at the interfaces of media with different impedance levels.[69] As the impedance increases, the energy scatter and reflection increases. As the electric field is oscillating, so do ions within the exposed media. This oscillation is the primary mechanism of heat generation within physiologic tissues. The oscillation of charges and changes in electric dipoles (causing loss of dielectric properties) generates an increase in the kinetic energy of these molecules and thus an increase in tissue temperature. The increase in kinetic energy is a function of the frequency of the electromagnetic field and the tissue's dielectric constant and electrical conductivity. The high water content of cardiac tissue provides for a high tissue dielectric constant and conductivity and, therefore, high power absorption. However, as the frequency of the electromagnetic field increases, the conductivity increases and the dielectric property decreases. Consequently, at higher frequencies the power absorption of deeper tissues decreases. A rapid decrease of power density (to 10%) has been noted at 3.5 cm. with a frequency of 918 MHz, whereas at a frequency of 27 MHz, 60% of the power density is noted at the same distance.[69] Although at higher frequencies the electromagnetic transmission allows better focusing of energy to affect limited regions of tissue, the power dissipation at distant tissues is decreased, and thus distant tissue destruction is decreased. The transmission of microwave energy into the cardiac chambers through the arterial or venous system requires a specially designed cable (called a coaxial transmission line) to be incorporated into a catheter. The catheter tip can be a helical antenna designed to radiate a prespecified frequency and to match the transmission line impedance.[68] Different shapes of a needle-like protrusion from the coaxial cable can be formed to improve the uniformity of the transmitted electromagnetic field.[62] Temperature maps of microwave radiation revealed nonuniform heating around the antenna, where the maximum heat production is generated laterally to the shaft of the catheter. These transmission characteristics can be improved with an inverted coil design of the catheter tip antenna.[62] Successful modification of the AV node has recently been reported in dogs.[68] However, it has yet to be proved that this form of energy is superior to RF for the ablation of cardiac tissues, especially for tissues causing VT, where deeper lesions are needed to eradicate the reentrant circuits.

Ultrasound Ablation

Ultrasound is the latest addition to the cardiac tissue ablation energy group. Ultrasound has been used for many years to heat joints and deep tissues. However, the delivery of this form of energy via a small-caliber catheter into a resonating crystal at the catheter tip presents significant challenges.[70] The advantages of this energy include tissue heating without the need for good electrical contact and potentially deeper lesions if enough energy can be delivered into the tissue.

CONCLUSIONS

Table 20-4 summarizes the physical and engineering aspects of each of the seven transcatheter cardiac tissue ablation techniques discussed.

Table 20-4. Summary of Seven Transcatheter Cardiac Tissue Ablation Techniques

	Success Rate			Complication Rate	Ease of Delivery	Lesion Size: Width, Penetration	Potential Arrhythmogenesis
Technique	AVNRT	AP	VT				
1. DC[a]	Very high	Very high	Low[b]	High	Easy	Large, shallow	High
2. RF[a]	Very high	Very high	Low[b]	Low	Easy	Small, shallow	Low
3. Microwave	Unknown	Unknown	Unknown	Unknown	Complex	Large, deep	Unknown
4. Cryothermia	High	High	Unknown	Low	Complex	Small, shallow	Low
5. Laser	High	High	High	High	Complex	Large, deep	Low
6. Chemical	High	Low	Unknown	High	Complex	Large, deep	Unknown
7. Ultrasound	Unknown	Unknown	Unknown	Unknown	Unknown	Unknown	Unknown

Abbreviations: AVNRT, atrioventricular node reentry tachycardia; AP, accessory pathway dependent reentry tachycardia; VT, ventricular tachycardia; DC, direct current high-energy shock; RF, radiofrequency power.
[a] Methods currently in clinical use.
[b] Other than bundle branch reentrant VT.

Similar to the field of angioplasty 15 years ago, the technology of ablative catheters and energy sources is still in its infancy. As the newer generation of catheters (designed to perform specific tasks) is introduced and new energy sources are applied, ablative procedures may become easier and more successful. There is a need for more easily steerable catheters, which will allow for better mapping and ablation results. Such catheters will also reduce radiation exposure time. Electrophysiologic testing and therapeutic ablation in a single session is already being done, resulting in decreases in morbidity and length of hospital stay.[40]

Because of the encouraging results with supraventricular tachycardia, AV nodal reentry, and accessory pathways, transcatheter ablation should be considered the procedure of choice in many patients with these indications. It has been proved to be safe and economical.[1] It has been shown that the number of hospital admissions per year after percutaneous catheter ablation of the AV node decreased from 2.4 ± 2 to 0.3 ± 0.5 ($P < 0.001$) in patients with refractory supraventricular tachycardia.[15]

Although the success rate for surgical management of these tachyarrhythmias is close to 100%, it involves prolonged morbidity that cannot be ignored. Potential complications of anesthesia, the need for thoracotomy and cardiopulmonary bypass, and the possibility of postpericardiotomy syndromes, constrictive pericarditis, and valvular insufficiency postoperatively are all significant considerations. In addition, life-long antiarrhythmic therapy, especially for child-bearing women and younger individuals, carries its own risks. Percutaneous transcatheter ablation is indispensable in this select group of patients.

Percutaneous catheter ablation procedures currently used for VT are not very effective (except those originating from bundle branch reentry). The surgical approach may be appropriate in these patients, especially when there is need for cardiac surgery for other reasons (e.g., revascularization, valve replacement, or aneurysm resection).[20]

It is expected that the rapid technologic and methodologic advancement that has taken place since the introduction of coronary and peripheral angioplasty will also be seen with the treatment of cardiac arrhythmias. Innovative investigators in both industry and medicine will provide practitioners with an assortment of catheters and techniques that will enhance the currently available modalities and provide insight as to the safest and most effective approach for cardiac arrhythmia ablation.

REFERENCES

1. Buitleir M, Sousa J, Bolling SF et al. Reduction in medical care cost associated with radiofrequency catheter ablation of accessory pathways. Am J Cardiol 1991;68:1656
2. Vedel J, Frank R, Fontaine G et al. Bloc auriculo-ventriculaire intra-Hisien définitif induit au cours d'une exploration endoventriculaire droite. Arch Mal Coeur 1979;72:107
3. Gonzalez R, Scheinman RR, Margaretten W, Rubinstien M. Closed-chest electrode catheter technique for His bundle ablation in dogs. Am J Physiol 1981; 241:H283
4. Gallagher JJ, Svenson H, Kasell JH et al. Catheter technique for closed chest ablation of the atrioventricular conduction system: a therapeutic alternative for the treatment of refractory supraventricular tachycardia. N Engl J Med 1982;306:194
5. Fontaine G, Volmer W, Nienaltowska E et al. Approach to the physics of fulguration, In Fontaine G, Scheinman MM (eds): Ablation in Cardiac Arrhythmias. Futura, Mt. Kisco, NY, 1987;101:381
6. Bardy GH, Coltorti F, Ivey TD et al. Some factors affecting bubble formation with catheter-mediated defibrillator pulses. Circulation 1986;73:525
7. Holt P, Boyd E. Haematologic effects of high energy endocardial ablation technique. Circulation 1986;73: 1029
8. Holt PM, Boyd E. His bundle ablation using impulses below one joule, abstracted. J Am Coll Cardiol 1988; 11:16A
9. Scheinman MM, Bharati S, Wang Y, Shapiro W, Lev M. Electrophysiologic and anatomic changes in the atrioventricular junction of dogs after direct-current shocks through tissue fixation catheters. Am J Cardiol 1985;55:194
10. Davies DW, Nathan AW, Camm AJ. Three sudden deaths after attempted high-energy catheter ablation of ventricular tachycardia. Br Heart J 1986;55:506
11. Leather RA, Leitch JW, Klein GJ et al. Radiofrequency catheter ablation of accessory pathways: a learning experience. Am J Cardiol 1991;68:1651
12. Saksena S, Lime F, Prasher S, An HL. Feasibility of transcatheter argon laser ablation for ventricular tachyarrhythmias, abstracted. Circulation 1987;76: 278
13. Langberg JJ, Chin MC, Rosenqvist M et al. Catheter ablation of the atrioventricular junction with radiofrequency energy. Circulation 1989;80:1527
14. Evans GT, Scheinman MM et al. The percutaneous cardiac mapping and ablation registry: final summary of results. PACE 1988;11:1621
15. Rosenqvist M, Lee MA, Moulinier L et al. Long term follow-up of patients after transcatheter direct current ablation of the atrioventricular junction. J Am Coll Cardiol 1990;16:1467
16. Morady F, Scheinman MM. Transvenous catheter ablation of a posteroseptal accessory pathway in a patient with the Wolff-Parkinson-White syndrome. N Engl J Med 1984;310:705
17. Morady F, Scheinman MM, Winston SA et al. Efficacy and safety of transcatheter ablation of posteroseptal accessory pathways. Circulation 1985;72:170
18. Warin JF, Haissaguerre M, D'Ivernois C, Metayer PL,

Montserrat P. Catheter ablation of accessory pathways: technique and results in 284 patients. PACE 1990;1609

19. Bardy GH, Ivey T, Coltórti F et al. Developments, complications, and limitations of catheter-mediated electrical ablation of posterior accessory atrioventricular pathways. Am J Cardiol 1988;61:309
20. Morady F. A perspective on the role of catheter ablation in the management of tachyarrhythmias. PACE 1988;11:98
21. Morady F, Scheinman M, Di Carlo L. Catheter ablation of ventricular tachycardia with intracardiac shocks: results in 33 patients. Circulation 1987;75:1037
22. Kirkorian G, Canu G, Atallah G et al. Radiofrequency ablation: a promising approach to the treatment of atrial flutter, abstracted. Am Coll Cardiol, suppl. A. 1993;21;2:374A
23. Tchou P, Jazayeri M, Denker S et al. Transcatheter electrical ablation of right bundle branch. A method of treating macroreentrant ventricular tachycardia attributed to bundle branch reentry. Circulation 1988;78:246
24. Fisher JD, Brodman R, Kim SG et al. Attempted nonsurgical electrical ablation of accessory pathway via the coronary sinus in the Wolff-Parkinson-White syndrome. J Am Coll Cardiol 1984;4:685
25. Abbot JA, Eldar M, Segar JJ et al. Noninvasive assessment of myocardial function following attempted catheter ablation of ventricular tachycardia foci. Circulation 1985;72:III-388
26. Clark W. Oscillatory desiccation in the treatment of accessible malignant growth and minor surgical conditions. J Adv Ther 1911;29:169
27. Borggrefe M, Haverkamp W, Budde T, Breithardt G. Radio frequency ablation. p. 997. In Zipes DP, Jalife J, (eds.): Cardiac Electrophysiology. WB Saunders, Philadelphia, 1990
28. Haines D, Verow A. Observations on electrode-tissue interface temperature and effect on electrical impedance during radiofrequency ablation of ventricular myocardium. Circulation 1990;82;82:1034
29. Avitall B, Morgan M, Hare J, Khan M, Lessila C. Intracardiac explosions during radio frequency ablation: histopathology in the acute and chronic dog model, abstracted. Circulation, suppl. I. 1992;86:I-191
30. Bloiuin LT, Marcus FI. The effect of electrode design on the efficacy of delivery of radiofrequency energy to cardiac tissue in vitro. Pace 1989;12:136
31. Lavergne T, Plumer L et al. Transcatheter radiofrequency ablation of atrial tissue using a suction catheter. PACE 1989;12:177
32. Mughal K, Krum D, Hare J et al. Time course of lesion maturation as a function of radiofrequency power and time: correlation with changes in impedance. J Am Col Cardiol 1993;21:375A
33. Haines D. The biophysics of radiofrequency catheter ablation in the heart: the importance of temperature monitoring. PACE 1993;16:586
34. Lesh M, Van Hare G, Kwasman M et al. Curative radiofrequency (RF) catheter ablation of atrial tachycardia and flutter, abstracted. J Am Coll Cardiol suppl. A. 1993;21;2:374A
35. Chen S, Yang C, Chiang C et al. Reversibility of left ventricular dysfunction after successful catheter ablation of supraventricular reentrant tachycardia. Am Heart J 1992;124:1512
36. Van Hare GF, Lesh MD, Scheinman M, Langberg JJ. Percutaneous radiofrequency catheter ablation for supraventricular arrhythmias in children. J Am Coll Cardiol 1991;17:1613
37. Lee MA, Morady F, Kadish A et al. Catheter modification of atrioventricular junction with radiofrequency energy for control of atrioventricular nodal reentry tachycardia. Circulation 1991;83:827
38. Jazayeri M, Hempe S, Sra S et al. Selective transcatheter ablation of the fast and slow pathways using radiofrequency energy in patients with atrioventricular nodal reentrant tachycardia. Circulation 1992;85:1318
39. Thibault B, Talajic M, Roy D. Prognostic importance of single AV nodal echoes after slow pathway ablation, abstracted. Circulation, suppl. 1993;88;4;2:I-61
40. Calkins H, Sousa J, El-Atassi R et al. Diagnosis and cure of the Wolf-Parkinson-White syndrome or paroxysmal supraventricular tachycardia during a single electrophysiologic test. N Engl J Med 1991;324:1612
41. Jackman WM, Wang X, Friday KJ et al. Catheter ablation of accessory atrioventricular pathways (Wolf-Parkinson-White syndrome) by radiofrequency current. N Engl J Med 1991;324:1605
42. Borggrefe M, Budde T, Podczeck A, Breithardt G. High frequency current ablation of an accessory pathway in humans. J Am Coll Cardiol 1987;10:576
43. Hunalin A, Saksena S. Comparative effects of radiofrequency and laser ablation in normal and diseased ventricular myocardium, abstracted. J Am Coll Cardiol 1989;13:175A
44. Langberg JJ, Desai J, Dallet N. Treatment of macroreentrant ventricular tachycardia with radiofrequency ablation of a tight bundle branch. Am J Cardiol 1989;63:1010
45. Breithardt G, Borggrefe M, Wichter T. Catheter ablation of idiopathic right ventricular tachycardia. Circulation 1990;82:2273
46. Avitall B, Hare J, Lessila C et al. New generation of catheters for mapping and ablation: a rotating tip and lateral deflectable catheters, abstracted. Circulation, suppl. II. 1991;84:I-96
47. Avitall B, Hare J, Khan M et al. A new catheter for mapping and radiofrequency ablation of the AV node and right-sided accessory pathways, abstracted. J Am Coll Cardiol suppl. A. 1993;21;2:418A
48. Avitall B, Hare J, Krum D, Silverstein E, Blanck Z. A new pigtail type catheter for retrograde atrial left-sided accessory pathway mapping and ablation, abstracted. Circulation, suppl. 1993;88;4;2:I-63
49. Jenkins KJ, Walsh EP, Colan SD et al. Multipolar endocardial mapping of the right atrium during cardiac catheterization: description of a new technique. J Am Coll Cardiol 1993;22:1105
50. Nakagawa H, Yamanashi W, Pitha J et al. Comparison of in vivo tissue temperature profile and lesion geometry for radiofrequency ablation with a saline-irrigated electrode versus temperature control in a canine thigh muscle preparation. Circulation 1995;8:2264
51. Avitall B, Hare J, Krum D et al. The anatomical determinants for the design of intracardiac mapping and ablation catheters. PACE 1994;17:908
52. Saksena S. Catheter ablation of tachycardias with laser energy: Issues and answers. PACE 1989;12:196

53. Saksena S, Ciccone J, Chandran P et al. Laser ablation of normal and diseased human ventricle. Am Heart J 1986;112:52
54. Lee BI, Gottdiener JS, Fletcher RD, Rodriguez ER, Ferrans VJ. Transcatheter ablation: comparison between laser photoablation and electrode shock ablation in the dog. Circulation 1985;71:579
55. Saksena S, Gadhoke A. Laser therapy for tachyarrhythmias: a new frontier. PACE 1986;9:531
56. Saksena S, Ciccone J, Chandran P et al. Laser ablation of normal and diseased human ventricle. Am Heart J 1986;112:52
57. Presosti LG, Cook JA, Bonner RF. Comparison of particulate debris size from excimer and argon laser ablation, abstracted. Circulation 1987;76:410
58. Gallagher LA, Sealy WC, Anderson W et al. Cryo-surgical ablation of accessory atrioventricular connections: a method for correction of the pre-excitation syndrome. Circulation 1977;55:471
59. Hollman WL, Ikeshita M, Douglas JM et al. Cardiac cryosurgery: effects of myocardial temperature on cryolesion size. Surgery 1983;92:268
60. Gillette PC, Swindle MM, Thompson RP, Case CL. Transvenous cryoablation of the His. PACE 1991;14:504–510
61. Hollman WL, Hakel DB, Lease JG, Ikeshita M, Cox JL. Cryosurgical ablation of atrioventricular nodal reentry: histologic localization of the proximal common pathway. Circulation 1988;77:1356
62. Williams JP, Lambert EH. Production of heart block in dogs without thoracotomy. Fed Proc 1964;23:413
63. Williams JP, Lambert EH, Titus JL. Use of intracardiac A-V nodal potentials in producing complete heart block in dogs. J Appl Physiol 1969;27:740
64. Fisher VJ, Lee RJ, Christianson LC, Kavaler F. Production of chronic atrioventricular block in dogs without thoracotomy. J Appl Physiol 1966;21:1119
65. Kay GN, Bubien RS, Daily SM, Epstein AE, Plumb VJ. A prospective evaluation of intracoronary ethanol ablation of the atrioventricular conduction system. J Am Coll Cardiol 1991;17:1634
66. Wang PJ, Guillerimo SS, Friedman PL. Modification of human atrioventricular nodal function by selective atrioventricular nodal artery catheterization. Circulation 1990;82:817
67. Brugada P, Swart H, Smeet JL, Wellens HJ. Transcoronary chemical ablation of ventricular tachycardia. Circulation 1989;79:475
68. Langberg JJ, Diel K, Gallagher M, Harvey M. Catheter modification of the AV junction using a microwave antenna, abstracted. J Am Coll Cardiol 1992;19:3:26A
69. Whayne JG, Haines DE. Comparison of thermal profile produced by new antenna designs for microwave catheter ablation, abstracted. PACE 1992;5:II:580
70. Paliwal BR, Shrivastava PN. Microwave hyperthermia principles and quality assurance. Radiol Clin North Am 1989;27:3:489
71. He D, Zimmer J, Hynynen K, Marcus F, Lampe L. The effect of acoustic power, sonication time and transducer temperature of myocardial lesion size, abstracted. Circulation, suppl. 1993;88:4:2:I-399

21 Radiofrequency Catheter Ablation of Arrhythmias

Hans Kottkamp
Gerhard Hindricks
Martin Borggrefe
Günter Breithardt

In 1979, Vedel and coworkers[1] reported the accidental application of a direct-current cardioversion shock through an electrode catheter that induced complete atrioventricular (AV) block. Gonzales et al.[2] described in 1981 their experience with closed-chest catheter application of high-energy direct-current discharges ("fulguration") in dogs. Subsequently, Scheinman et al.[3] and Gallagher et al.[4] reported in 1982 on the intentional creation of complete AV block using endocardial catheter fulguration. These first series started the era of catheter ablation since it was soon recognized that selectively applied fulguration shocks could also provide successful treatment for other types of supraventricular and ventricular tachyarrhythmias. In the following years, accessory atrioventricular pathways, ventricular tachycardias, and ectopic atrial tachycardias were targeted for endocardial catheter fulguration. However, Fisher et al.[5] were the first to report on the significant risk of delivering direct-current shocks to the coronary sinus since they had observed coronary sinus rupture with subsequent cardiac tamponade.

The most important factors during endocardial fulguration that cause tissue injury are barotrauma due to shock waves, high-voltage electrical field, and, to a lesser degree, tissue heating in the direct vicinity of the catheter-tissue interface. The complications after high-energy direct-current discharges in clinical studies included ventricular tachyarrhythmias, sudden death, ventricular dysfunction and pump failure, coronary artery lesions, cardiac tamponade, and others.[6] Additionally, in a striking portion of direct-current ablations, tissue effects and therefore ablation success were only of a transient nature. Thus, because of this unfavorable efficacy-risk profile, there was a definite need for other energy sources. Laser techniques had been recognized as an alternative to induce tissue effects for the treatment of arrhythmias.[7] However, the limited flexibility of the energy-delivering catheters, the complexity and costs of the laser technology, and the insufficiently known efficacy-safety profile of laser catheter ablation have prevented a widespread use in humans so far.

In 1987, our group introduced radiofrequency alternating current in the setting of supraventricular tachyarrhythmias for ablation of accessory AV pathways and His bundle ablation.[8,9] It was soon recognized that radiofrequency catheter ablation offers significant advantages compared with high-energy direct-current discharges with respect to the safety, efficacy, and controllability and reproducibility of the extent of induced tissue injury. Additionally, radiofrequency ablation, in contrast to direct-current discharges, does not require general anesthesia since little pain or discomfort are caused during its application. Therefore, radiofrequency alternating current has definitely replaced high-energy direct current as the primary energy source for catheter ablation techniques. In recent years, this technique has been widely used for the curative treatment of patients with accessory pathway, AV node reentrant tachycardia, and for ablation of the AV conduction system. For these indications, radiofrequency catheter ablation has been established as a first-line therapy. The feasibility of radiofrequency ablation for curing patients with atrial tachycardia and atrial flutter as well as ventricular tachycardia is presently under extensive clinical investigation.

BIOPHYSICAL CHARACTERISTICS

Radiofrequency generator systems used for catheter ablation procedures deliver a continuous sinusoidal unmodulated waveform with a frequency of 350 to 1,000 kHz. Radiofrequency current is usually applied with a power output of 10 to 50 W for 30 to 90 seconds. In most cases, radiofrequency energy is delivered between the 4-mm tip electrode of a 7-F deflectable ablation catheter and an external backplate electrode placed at the back of the patient (so-called unipolar configuration). Alternatively, the energy may be applied between the distal and proximal electrodes of the ablation catheter (bipolar configuration) or, in very rare instances, between the distal electrodes of two ablation catheters that might be placed at both sides of the interventricular septum (e.g., ablation of septal accessory pathways).

Biophysical Aspects

Tissue effects due to radiofrequency energy application are mainly induced by conversion of electrical energy into heat dissipating into the areas in the vicinity of the catheter tip electrode-tissue interface where current density is high and electrical conductivity is low. A permanent myocardial tissue injury results from temperatures exceeding 50°C by cell dehydration and denaturation of membrane proteins.[10] The extent of tissue coagulation induced by radiofrequency current is governed by multiple variables that influence each other dynamically. The size and shape of the catheter electrode, the impedance of the electrical circuit, the power output, and the duration of the energy application are parameters that have been shown in in vitro studies to correlate with the magnitude of the induced tissue effects.[11,12] However, the electrode-tissue contact pressure and the extent of heat generated at the electrode-tissue interface are the most important variables determining the extent of tissue coagulation in vivo. Therefore,

current, voltage, and impedance, which are usually continuously monitored during energy application in the clinical setting, failed to predict lesion size when radiofrequency energy was delivered in the beating heart since they were not indicative of the quality and the stability of the electrode-tissue contact.[13] Nevertheless, impedance measurements during energy application are mandatory since a regular flow of current within the electrical circuit can be ensured, and sudden rises in impedance are indicative of disturbances of current flow that may result in dramatic overheating of the catheter electrode. Thus, energy application must be stopped immediately after impedance rise.

Role of Catheter Tip Temperature

In several in vitro and in vivo studies, it has been shown that catheter tip temperature, measured via built-in thermistors in the active electrode, indicates whether the catheter tip electrode is in sufficiently good contact to the tissue to be ablated.[13] Additionally, the incidence of impedance rise caused by overheating of the catheter electrode and subsequent clot formation can be reduced by limiting the electrode-tissue interface temperature.[14] Therefore, radiofrequency energy applications with power output guided by actual catheter tip temperature instead of constant power output are currently under clinical investigation. In this setting, power output is adjusted automatically via a feedback mechanism to reach and maintain a preselected catheter tip temperature of 60° to 80°C (Fig. 21-1). Sudden rises in impedance, however, cannot be completely prevented by temperature-guided energy applications, especially during current applications with a poor electrode tissue contact. Additionally, other determinants including convective heat loss, the heat transfer properties of the tissue (e.g., fibrotic scar tissue in coronary artery disease), and the extent of phase displacement between current and voltage cannot be controlled during radiofrequency energy application in vivo. It thus becomes clear that it is presently impossible to predict accurately the individual tissue effect of a radiofrequency pulse in the beating heart. In summary, the most important and instructive parameters to be continuously monitored during radiofrequency energy application at this time are impedance and catheter tip temperature.

ABLATION OF ACCESSORY ATRIOVENTRICULAR PATHWAYS

Patients with Wolff-Parkinson-White syndrome or only retrogradely conducting (concealed) accessory AV pathways often present with drug-refractory AV

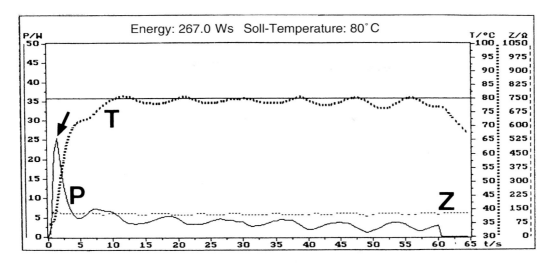

Fig. 21-1. Simultaneous recordings of catheter tip-tissue interface temperature (T), power output (P), and impedance (Z) during radiofrequency current application in a patient who underwent successful radiofrequency catheter ablation of an accessory AV pathway. Current application was guided by a constant preselected temperature of 80°C. Note that an initial peak of applied power (25 W) resulted in a temperature rise to the preselected level. Thereafter, power output was automatically downregulated and only 4 to 5 W was sufficient for maintenance of the preselected temperature, resulting in a cumulative applied energy of only 267 J during the application time of 60 seconds.

reentrant tachycardias or atrial fibrillation with rapid anterograde conduction via the accessory pathway. Since its first application in humans, radiofrequency catheter ablation has become an established first-line treatment modality for definite cure of patients with accessory AV connections and has almost completely replaced surgical interruption of accessory pathways.[8] In experienced centers, the overall success rate for ablation of left- and right-sided accessory pathways exceeds 90%.[15–17]

General Approach

For electrophysiologic study, standard multipolar electrode catheters are introduced percutaneously from femoral veins and positioned in the high right atrium, and right ventricular apex and across the tricuspid valve to record the His bundle potential. Another multipolar catheter may be positioned in the coronary sinus via the right internal jugular or subclavian vein (Fig. 21-2). All antiarrhythmic agents should be discontinued at least 5 half-lives before the procedure. The stimulation protocol includes introduction of single and (rarely) double extrastimuli from the high right atrium and right ventricular apex during different basic cycle lengths.[18] Antegrade and retrograde conduction properties of the accessory pathway are assessed by incremental atrial and ventricular pacing, beginning at a rate just exceeding the sinus rate until accessory pathway conduction block occurs, respectively. A concealed accessory pathway is diagnosed when there is no preexcitation during sinus rhythm or atrial pacing from the high right atrium and coronary sinus.

During the mapping procedure, electrograms are recorded from the tip electrode (unipolar configuration) and from the distal pair of electrodes (bipolar configuration) of the mapping catheter. Distinct patterns of the morphology of the unipolar "unfiltered" electrogram indicate different distances to the accessory pathway.[19] By definition, a *positive* deflection in an unipolar electrogram reflects an activation *toward* the electrode, whereas a negative deflection represents electrical forces away from the electrode location (Fig. 21-3). Therefore, a so-called PrS morphology suggests a substantial distance to the accessory pathway whereas the PQS morphology indicates a close proximity to the AV accessory pathway (Fig. 21-3). Additionally, the timing of the intrinsic deflection of the unipolar electrogram, indicating the onset of local ventricular activation, can be related to the onset of the δ-wave in the surface electrocardiogram (ECG) and to the onset of the local ventricular activation in the bipolar electrogram recorded by the mapping catheter. Bipolar electrogram characteristics obtained from target sites for ablation of accessory AV pathways (filter setting, 40 to 500 Hz) include recording of discrete atrial and ventricular potentials, early ventricular activation relative to

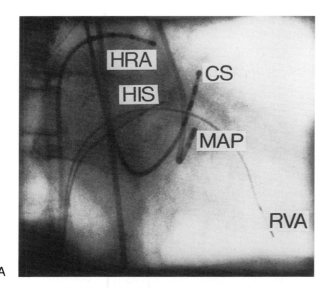

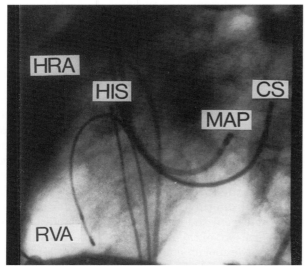

Fig. 21-2. Radiograph in (**A**) right anterior oblique 30° and (**B**) left anterior oblique 60° projections obtained from a patient with a left-sided accessory pathway. Multipolar catheters for electrophysiologic study were placed in the high right atrium (HRA), right ventricular apex (RVA), His bundle region (HBE), and coronary sinus (CS). The ablation catheter (MAP) is positioned underneath the mitral valve annulus at the ventricular insertion of the accessory AV pathway directly opposite the proximal pair of electrodes of the coronary sinus catheter recording the earliest anterograde ventricular activation.

the onset of the δ-wave in the surface ECG, continuous AV activation, and recording of accessory pathway potentials (Fig. 21-4). Accessory pathway potentials are considered to be present if a discrete sharp potential exists between local atrial and ventricular activation during pre-excited sinus rhythm or atrial pacing that precedes the onset of the δ-wave and the

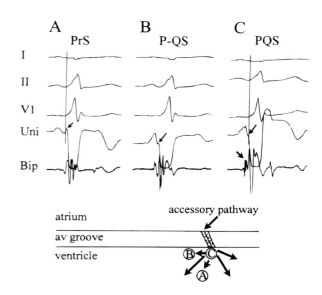

Fig. 21-3. The principles of the unipolar recording mode for localization of accessory pathways. (**Top**) Surface ECG leads I, II, and V1 and unipolar (Uni) and bipolar (Bip) intracardiac recordings of the mapping catheter during sinus rhythm mapping in a patient with a left-sided accessory pathway. (**Bottom**) Schematic drawing illustrating representative locations of the mapping catheter with different distances to the AV groove and accessory pathway. (**A**) The P wave in the unipolar electrogram is followed by a clear R wave (*arrow*), and the intrinsic deflection indicating the start of the unipolar ventricular downstroke inscribes later than the onset of the δ-wave in the surface ECG (*vertical line*) (PrS-morphology). The R wave represents the electrical forces of the pre-excited ventricular myocardium (via the accessory pathway) toward the mapping electrode. The distance of the mapping electrode to the insertion of the accessory pathway is also evident from the bipolar electrogram, where no local atrial potential is recorded, indicating a substantial distance to the AV groove. (**B**) No R wave is recorded in the unipolar electrogram; however, the QS-like ventricular deflection is separated from the atrial potential by a short "shoulder" (P-QS morphology). The location of the mapping catheter at the mitral malve annulus is evident by the local atrial potential in the bipolar electrogram, which is, however, separated from the local ventricular electrogram by a short isoelectric line. (**C**) The QS-like ventricular deflection of the unipolar electrogram is superimposed on the the P wave (PQS morphology). The pure negative QS morphology of the ventricular deflection in the unipolar electrogram indicates that all electrical ventricular forces are moving away from the mapping electrode site reflecting the vicinity of the electrode to the ventricular insertion of the accessory pathway. The close proximity of the mapping electrode to the accessory pathway can also be appreciated by the bipolar electrogram where the local atrial potential is connected to the local ventricular potential by a distinct sharp deflection representing the activation of the accessory pathway (accessory pathway potential, *thick arrow*). Additionally, the intrinsic deflection is synchronous with the onset of the δ-wave in the surface ECG (*vertical line*) and is preceded by the inscription of the accessory pathway potential.

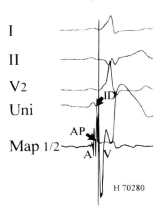

Fig. 21-4. Surface ECG leads I, II, and V2 and unipolar (Uni) and bipolar (Map 1/2) intracardiac recordings from the mapping/ablation catheter during sinus rhythm in a patient with a right posteroseptally located accessory atrioventricular pathway. The local bipolar atrial potential (A) is followed by a sharp deflection presumed to be an accessory pathway potential (AP, *arrow*) that occurred immediately before the local bipolar ventricular potential (V). The accessory pathway potential inscribed shortly before the intrinsic deflection (ID) in the unipolar electrogram (*arrow*). Both accessory pathway potential and local ventricular activation preceded the onset of the δ-wave in the surface ECG leads (*vertical line*). At this site, the accessory pathway was successfully ablated.

intrinsic deflection in the unipolar electrogram and disappears after effective energy application or atrial extrastimulation inducing accessory pathway conduction block.

Left-Sided Accessory Pathways

For localization of left-sided accessory pathways, a multipolar catheter is positioned in the coronary sinus and advanced anteriorly in the great cardiac vein. Bipolar electrograms obtained from a catheter within the coronary sinus record local atrial and ventricular potentials from adjacent sites of the AV groove. During sinus rhythm or atrial pacing, the catheter is slowly withdrawn in search of the site of earliest antegrade ventricular activation and continuous AV activation, indicative of a site adjacent to the accessory pathway. Additionally, earliest retrograde atrial activation may be sought during orthodromic AV reentrant tachycardia or ventricular pacing. After localization of the AV accessory pathway with the catheter placed within the coronary sinus, the ablation/mapping catheter (7-F deflectable catheter, 4-mm tip electrode) is usually retrogradely advanced via the femoral artery to the aortic root. The catheter tip is then deflected and the catheter ad-

vanced across the aortic valve into the left ventricle. After positioning the ablation catheter at the mitral valve annulus, careful mapping is performed at the *ventricular* insertion of the AV connection directly opposite the electrodes of the coronary sinus catheter recording the earliest antegrade ventricular activation by rotating the catheter in steps of a few millimeters anteriorly and posteriorly at the mitral annulus. However, the accessory pathway may take an oblique course through the AV groove, and the ventricular insertion of the accessory pathway may thus be some millimeters away from the atrial insertion localized via the coronary sinus catheter. In a retrospective and prospective analysis of local electrograms recorded at successful and unsuccessful sites of ablation, we could demonstrate that recording of an accessory pathway potential, ventricular activation preceding the onset of the δ-wave during sinus rhythm, presence of a distinct atrial electrogram, and stability of the local electrograms were the most powerful predictors of success when mapping was performed during pre-excited sinus rhythm at the ventricular insertion side.[18] When mapping was performed during orthodromic tachycardia, recording of the earliest atrial activation during orthodromic tachycardia and a presumed accessory pathway activation potential were the best predictors of success[18] (Fig. 21-5).

In about 10% of left-sided accessory pathways, attempted ablation may be unsuccessful at the ventricular insertion, suggesting an intramural or even epicardial course of the ventricular insertion of accessory AV connections. In these cases, different approaches for ablation can be used. First, the accessory pathways can be ablated at the *atrial* insertion using the *retrograde* approach via the mitral valve.[20] With this approach, the ablation catheter is positioned toward the inflow tract of the left ventricle, and the tip of the catheter is deflected and advanced to reach the left atrium via the mitral valve. The catheter is then slowly withdrawn and straightened until an atrial and relatively small ventricular potential (A/V ratio 1 or more) is recorded indicating a position of the ablation catheter at the atrial aspect of the mitral valve annulus. Anterior and posterior annular regions of the left atrium can then be mapped by careful clockwise and counterclockwise rotation of the ablation catheter, respectively. Second, the *transseptal* approach via the interatrial septum can be used for ablation.[20,21] Using right and left anterior oblique fluoroscopic projections, transseptal puncture is performed using a Brockenbrough needle. An 8-F sheath is then advanced over the needle into the left atrium. The transseptal approach can be guided fluoroscopically using a 5-F pigtail

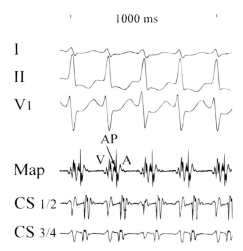

Fig. 21-5. Surface ECG leads I, II, and VI and bipolar intracardiac recordings from the mapping/ablation catheter (Map) and distal (CS 1/2) and proximal (CS 3/4) pair of electrodes of a coronary sinus catheter during orthodromic tachycardia in a patient with a concealed left lateral accessory pathway. Continuous activity between local ventricular (V) and atrial (A) activation with a sharp stable deflection in between which was presumed to be an accessory pathway potential (AP) was recorded from the ablation catheter, whereas a clear isoelectric line was seen between the local ventricular and atrial deflection recorded from the coronary sinus catheter. Delivery of a radiofrequency pulse at this site terminated orthodromic tachycardia and achieved complete block of the accessory pathway.

catheter inserted in the femoral artery and advanced to the aortic root as a landmark or echocardiographically (transesophageal technique). The ablation catheter is advanced via the sheath into the left atrium, and mapping is performed by positioning the catheter at the atrial aspect of the mital valve annulus. Third, radiofrequency catheter ablation may be performed within the *coronary sinus*. Effective target site electrograms recorded within the coronary sinus have been described to be characterized by larger accessory pathway potentials than the corresponding atrial or ventricular electrograms.[22]

Right-Sided Accessory Pathways

For right-sided accessory pathways, the ablation catheter is advanced through a femoral vein to the tricuspid annulus, and ablation is performed at the *atrial* insertion of the AV pathways. During sinus rhythm or atrial pacing, the catheter is rotated in steps of a few millimeters along the atrial aspect of the tricuspid annulus in search of the site of earliest antegrade ventricular activation and continuous AV activation, indicative of a site adjacent to the acces-

sory pathway. Additionally, earliest retrograde atrial activation may be sought during orthodromic AV reentrant tachycardia or ventricular pacing. In rare cases, mid- to posteroseptal accessory pathways cannot be ablated using the conventional unipolar approach from the tricuspid or mitral valve annulus. For successful ablation of these pathways, a *bipolar* electrode configuration with application of radiofrequency current between the distal electrodes of two catheters placed against both the tricuspid septal and mitral septal annulus may be used.[23] In very rare instances, posteroseptal accessory AV connections are associated with coronary sinus diverticula.

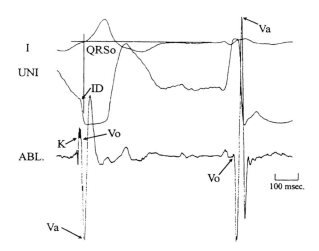

Fig. 21-6. Surface ECG lead I, unipolar electrogram (UNI) recorded from the tip electrode of the ablation catheter, and bipolar electrogram (ABL) from the distal pair of electrodes of the ablation catheter in a patient with a left posteroseptal accessory pathway obtained directly before successful ablation of the pathway during sustained atrial fibrillation. The onset of pre-excitation (QRSo) is indicated by the vertical line. Marked by arrows are the intrinsic deflection (ID) from the unipolar electrogram, the activation potential of the accessory pathway [K (Kent)], and components of the ventricular electrogram (Vo, onset of ventricular electrogram; Va, ventricular activation time). Irregular atrial activation recorded in a bipolar fashion from the ablation catheter is clearly present and indicative of the position of the ablation catheter close to the mitral annulus. The tracings show an example of two successive beats during atrial fibrillation with anterograde conduction over the accessory pathway (first beat) and with predominant conduction over the AV node (second beat). Note the marked difference of the configuration of the unipolar electrogram during pre-excitation (QS morphology) compared with the non-pre-excited beat. A rapid sharp potential (K) preceding local ventricular activation and the intrinsic deflection in the unipolar electrogram is clearly present during pre-excitation but not during the non-pre-excited beat. (From Hindricks et al.,[25] with permission.)

Biplane coronary sinus venograms usually reveal diverticula attached to the coronary sinus near the ostium by a relatively narrow neck. These pathways can be ablated when radiofrequency energy is applied in the neck of the diverticula.[24]

Atrial Fibrillation in Wolff-Parkinson-White Syndrome

The onset of paroxysmal or sustained atrial fibrillation in patients with Wolff-Parkinson-White syndrome may complicate and prolong the ablation procedure. Usually, antiarrhythmic drugs are administered or direct-current cardioversion is performed for termination of atrial fibrillation. However, antiarrhythmic drugs may fail to convert atrial fibrillation into sinus rhythm or may induce accessory pathway conduction block, making localization of the accessory pathway impossible. Recently, we therefore assessed the feasibility and electrophysiologic criteria for ablation of left-sided accessory pathways during atrial fibrillation.[25] Mapping and ablation were performed at the *ventricular* insertion during atrial fibrillation using the conventional retrograde approach (see above). The recording of an accessory pathway potential, the earliest activation time of the local ventricular electrogram relative to the δ-wave in the surface ECG, and the recording of atrial activation from the ablation catheter indicated successful target sites (Figs. 21-6 and 21-7). Recently, this experience was extended to ablation of right-sided accessory pathways during sustained atrial fibrillation with rapid anterograde conduction over the accessory pathway.[26] Appropriate target sites could be identified by recording an accessory

pathway activation potential, early onset and activation time of the local ventricular electrogram, and a QS morphology of the unipolar electrogram.

Complications and Future Developments

Although radiofrequency catheter ablation has been shown in specialized centers to be highly effective and relatively safe for ablation of AV accessory pathways, future developments should aim at reducing radiation exposure and procedure-related complications. Additionally, no standardized anticoagulation regimen during and after the ablation session so far exist. In our clinic, a heparin bolus of 5,000 IE is given intravenously after insertion of the catheters with an additional 1,000 IE/hr thereafter. Systemic anticoagulation is maintained for 24 hours, and aspirin 100 mg/d is administered for 3 months. The Multicenter European Radiofrequency Survey investigators recently reported a 4.4% incidence of complications in 2,222 patients who underwent ablation of accessory pathways.[27] It is noteworthy that a 0.63% incidence of complete AV block was reported. This risk is highest when ablation of anteroseptal accessory pathways is attempted because of the proximity of the ablation site to the bundle of His.

ABLATION OF ATRIOFASCICULAR PATHWAYS (MAHAIM PATHWAYS)

So-called Mahaim pathways represent a distinct subset of accessory pathways and pre-excitation syndromes with unique electrophysiologic properties.

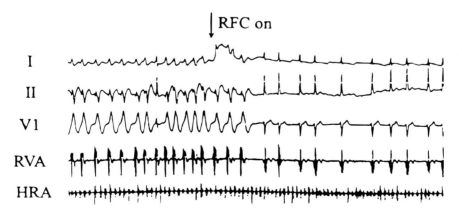

Fig. 21-7. Successful radiofrequency ablation of a left posterior accessory pathway during atrial fibrillation. Approximately 1 second after the onset of radiofrequency application (RFC on) pre-excitation disappeared. Note that the tachyarrhythmic pattern during rapid anterograde conduction via the accessory pathway during atrial fibrillation is followed by normofrequent conduction via the atrioventricular node. HRA, high right atrium; RVA, right ventricular apex. (From Hindricks et al.,[25] with permission.)

The original concept of Mahaim fibers consisted of accessory pathways originating in the AV node and inserting into the distal right bundle branch (nodo-fascicular pathways) or the right ventricle (nodoven-tricular pathways). This understanding has been challenged by surgical interventions identifying the atrial insertion of Mahaim pathways at the *parietal* tricuspid annulus. Electrophysiologic and surgical studies have confirmed the antero- to posterolateral atrial origin of these accessory pathways remote from the AV node. Therefore, the concept of nodoven-tricular pathways has been replaced by the concept of *atriofascicular* pathways. Overall, the current knowledge about atriofascicular pathways is indicative of a proximal AV node-like component and a distal bundle branch-like component, therefore suggesting an accessory AV conduction system.

General Approach

During sinus rhythm, pre-excitation is minimal or absent, whereas incremental atrial stimulation reveals pre-excitation with a left bundle branch block-like morphology. Mahaim fibers exhibit long conduction times, decremental conduction properties by atrial extrastimuli or incremental atrial pacing, and conduction only in the anterograde direction. The typical AV reentrant tachycardia incorporating a Mahaim pathway is a pre-excited antidromic tachycardia with anterograde conduction over the accessory pathway and retrograde conduction over the AV node. Mahaim fibers may be associated with dual AV node physiology or common AV accessory pathways (Fig. 21-8). The initial mapping approach is similar to that described for right-sided accessory AV pathways (i.e., the ablation catheter is advanced through a femoral vein to the tricuspid annulus and ablation is performed at the atrial insertion of the atriofascicular pathways). However, catheter mapping along the atrial aspect of the tricuspid annulus does not reveal the site of earliest antegrade ventricular activation, because the earliest ventricular activation during anterograde conduction over the atriofascicular pathway is close to the right ventricular apical region in the area of the distal right bundle branch and, therefore, no continuous AV activation can be recorded at the tricuspid annulus. Additionally, earliest retrograde atrial activation cannot be mapped since atriofascicular accessory pathways do not conduct retrogradely.

Mapping and Ablation

The atrial insertion of atriofascicular pathways can be localized to sites where the shortest interval between atrial activation during constant pacing from

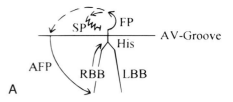

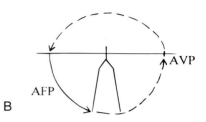

Fig. 21-8. Schematic presentation of AV reentrant tachy-cardias incorporating atriofascicular accessory pathways (Mahaim pathways). **(A)** Pre-excited antidromic AV reentrant tachycardia with anterograde conduction over the atriofascicular pathway (AFP) and retrograde conduction over the right bundle branch (RBB), His bundle, and fast pathway (FP) of the AV node. In rare cases, the left bundle branch (LBB) and the slow pathway (SP) of the AV node may serve as parts of the retrograde limb. **(B)** Pre-excited AV reentrant tachycardia with anterograde conduction over the atriofascicular pathway (AFP) and retrograde conduction over an accessory AV pathway (AVP). *Dashed lines,* conduction through normal atrial or ventricular myocardium. (From Kottkamp et al.,[31] with permission.)

the atrial side of the tricuspid annulus and the onset of pre-excitation (δ-wave) in the surface ECG can be recorded.[28] However, it may be difficult to obtain a stable catheter position at the lateral tricuspid annulus during atrial pacing and, additionally, the conduction times over the atriofascicular pathways may change according to the state of the autonomic nervous system. Distinct, high-frequency activation potentials of atriofascicular accessory pathways can be recorded at the atrial insertion at the antero- to posterolateral tricuspid annulus and along the entire ventricular course up to the ventricular insertion in the right ventricular apical region near or at the distal right bundle branch. Radiofrequency current application for ablation of atriofascicular pathways can be accomplished at their atrial insertion and along their entire ventricular course where target sites for ablation are identified by recording activation potentials of the atriofascicular pathways[29–32] (Fig. 21-9). However, the ventricular insertion site should not be the initial target site for ablation since presumed activation potentials of the atriofascicular pathways at their ventricular insertion may instead be part of the distal right bundle branch. Ablation at these

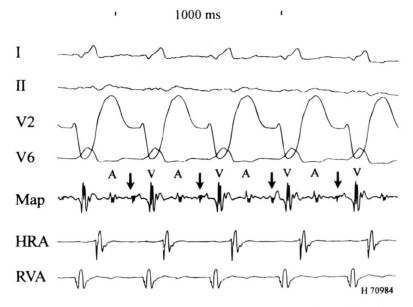

Fig. 21-9. Surface ECG leads I, II, V2, and V6 and intracardiac recordings from the mapping/ablation catheter (Map), high right atrium (HRA), and right ventricular apex (RVA) during antidromic AV reentrant tachycardia (cycle length, 410 ms) in a patient with a right lateral atriofascicular accessory pathway (Mahaim pathway). At the subannular level of the tricuspid annulus, an activation potential of the atriofascicular pathway could be recorded (*arrow*). The interval from the local atrial potential to the atriofascicular pathway activation potential measured 150 ms, and the interval from the atriofascicular pathway activation potential to the onset of the QRS in the surface ECG measured 40 ms. Note that, in contrast to common AV accessory pathways, the *basal* ventricle at the atrial insertion site is activated late (35 ms after the onset of the QRS), indicating the distal insertion of this type of accessory pathway.

sites may result in prolongation of the retrograde conduction over the septal muscle or the left bundle branch and may even provoke incessant AV reentrant tachycardia. Transient mechanical conduction block by catheter manipulation at the subannuluar level of the atrial insertion has also been introduced as a marker for successful ablation of these unusual accessory pathways.[29] Using this technique, radiofrequency application is performed after resumption of pre-excitation at the site of mechanical block.

ABLATION OF ATRIOVENTRICULAR NODE REENTRANT TACHYCARDIA

In 1985, the introduction of curative surgery for AV node reentrant tachycardia (AVNRT) revealed successful elimination of AVNRT by disconnection of the *perinodal atrium* from the AV node.[33] Thus the conventional theory of a purely *intra*nodal reentry circuit was challenged. The advent of catheter ablation techniques for elimination of AVNRT has further stimulated interest in detailed delineation of the morphology of the AV node since the components for maintenance of AVNRT and the location of critical parts of circus movement pathways remain a matter of speculation. The current concept of the anatomic arrangement of the reentrant pathways is depicted in Figure 21-10. The reentry circuit in AVNRT consists of two different pathways with distinct electrophysiologic properties. In the common type (about 90% of cases), the wavefront propagates anterogradely through the slow pathway and retrogradely through the fast pathway (slow-fast) and vice versa (fast-slow) in the uncommon type of AVNRT. The so-called fast pathway is usually located in the anterior-superior area of the interatrial septum whereas the so-called slow pathway is situated posterior at the septal annulus of the tricuspid valve. Selective ablation of either pathway has been demonstrated to cure patients with AVNRT.

General Approach

For electrophysiologic study, multipolar electrode catheters are introduced percutaneously from femoral veins and positioned in the high right atrium and right ventricular apex, across the tricuspid valve to record the His bundle potential, and within the coro-

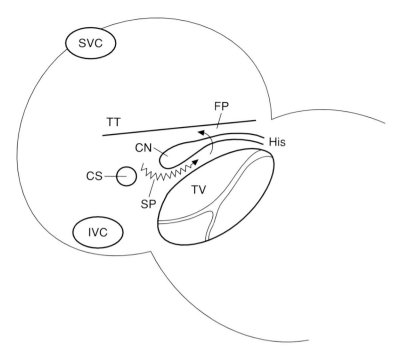

Fig. 21-10. Diagrammatic representation of the AV junctional area with delineation of the components and location of distinct parts of the circus movement pathways in AVNRT. The AV node is located within the triangle of Koch, which is formed by a collagen bundle inserting into the central fibrous body (tendon of Todaro), the ostium of the coronary sinus, and the septal annulus of the tricuspid valve. In the common type of AVNRT (about 90% of cases), the wavefront propagates anterogradely through the slow pathway and retrogradely through the fast pathway (slow-fast), and vice versa (fast-slow) in the uncommon type of AVNRT. The so-called fast pathway (*curved arrow*, FP) is usually located in the anterior-superior area of the interatrial septum, whereas the so-called slow pathway (*zigzag arrow*, SP) is situated posterior at the septal annulus of the tricuspid valve. CN, compact AV node; CS, coronary sinus ostium; IVC, inferior vena cava; SVC, superior vena cava; TT, tendon of Todaro; TV, tricuspid valve.

nary sinus. During programmed atrial stimulation, the anterograde fast pathway usually exhibits a longer effective refractory period than the anterograde slow pathway. The switch from anterograde fast pathway conduction to anterograde slow pathway conduction results in the typical manifestation of dual-pathway physiology [increase in the A_2H_2 intervals of more than 50 ms in response to a 10-ms decrement in the A_1A_2 interval during application of premature atrial extrastimuli (AH jump)]. The common type of AVNRT is usually induced by atrial extrastimuli that block anterogradely in the fast pathway, slowly conduct anterogradely via the slow pathway, and reexcite the fast pathway retrogradely, which has already recovered from anterograde conduction block.

Fast Pathway Ablation

In most institutions, catheter-induced modifications of the AV node in patients with AVNRT were initially performed by ablation of the fast pathway. The "exit"

of retrograde fast pathway conduction during AVNRT or ventricular pacing has been demonstrated in mapping studies to be located near the apex of the triangle of Koch adjacent to the central fibrous body (Fig. 21-10). The fast pathway exit was usually located adjacent to the bundle of His and anterosuperior to the compact AV node. Therefore, the simplicity of positioning the ablation catheter in the area of the maximal His bundle recording site and performing catheter ablation merely after slight withdrawing of the catheter seemed to be promising. Target site criteria usually only included a His bundle recording amplitude of less than 0.1 mV and an atrial/ventricular potential amplitude ratio of more than 1. However, application of several radiofrequency pulses using this approach resulted in inadvertent complete AV block in about 10% of the patients.[15,34]

We recently introduced a new anatomically and elctrographically guided stepwise approach for effective and safe ablation of the fast pathway for elimination of AVNRT.[35] Thereby, a 7-F quadripolar catheter with a 4-mm tip electrode is introduced in the right vena femoralis and advanced to the septal area of the tricuspid annulus. Bipolar endocardial electrograms obtained by the ablation catheter are recorded with a filter bandwidth of 40 to 500 Hz. Surface ECG leads and endocardial electrograms are displayed and recorded simultaneously with a paper speed of 100 or 200 mm/sec. Biplane fluoroscopy with

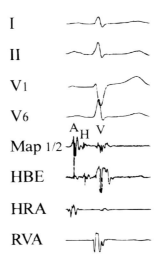

Fig. 21-12. Simultaneous recordings of surface leads I, II, V1, and V6 and intracardiac recordings of the distal pair of electrodes of the ablation catheter (Map 1/2), His bundle region (HBE), high right atrium (HRA), and right ventricular apex (RVA) in a patient with recurrent AVNRT. Recordings during sinus rhythm are depicted for a representative target site electrogram for fast pathway ablation. The ablation catheter was positioned posterior to the site of maximal His bundle recording. A small proximal His bundle potential and an atrial/ventricular potential amplitude ratio of 3.6 was obtained in this position. Application of radiofrequency current at this site resulted in an increase of the atrial-His bundle interval and complete retrograde block, indicating successful ablation of the fast pathway.

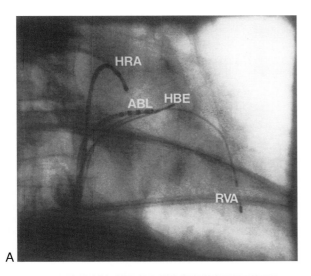

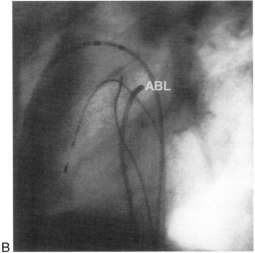

Fig. 21-11. Radiograph in (**A**) right anterior oblique 30° and (**B**) left anterior oblique 60° projection are shown presenting a typical location of the mapping/ablation catheter (ABL) for ablation of the fast pathway for elimination of AVNRT. Additionally, catheters were placed in the high right atrium (HRA), right ventricular apex (RVA), and His bundle region (HBE). The ablation catheter was positioned *posterior* to the site of typical His bundle recording by clockwise rotation of the catheter. A more stable position of the ablation catheter at the interatrial septum rather then across the tricuspid annulus may thus be achieved. (Modified from Kottkamp et al.,[35] with permission.)

right anterior oblique 30° and left anterior oblique 60° projections is used to determine the position of the catheters. The ablation catheter is initially positioned posterior and slightly superior to the site of the maximal His bundle recording area by advancing the catheter to the region of the maximal His bundle recording and then rotating the catheter in a clockwise fashion posteriorly (Fig. 21-11). Slightly superior sites are reached by gently pushing the ablation catheter forward or by a slight straightening of the deflection of the catheter tip. At these sites, the amplitude of the local atrial potential is usually at least twice as high as the local ventricular potential, and a small proximal His bundle potential can be recorded (Fig. 21-12). When the amplitude of the His bundle potential exceeds that obtained in the typical His bundle region, the ablation catheter is slightly rotated clockwise and positioned more posterior. When the first pulse in this area is ineffective or no adequate potentials can be recorded, the ablation catheter tip is further deflected and moved slightly inferior toward more midseptal sites stepwise. The end points of the ablation session are an increase of the atrial-His bundle interval of more than 50% or elimination or marked slowing of ventriculoatrial conduction (or both), and the noninducibility of AVNRT before and during isoproterenol infusion. By contrast, the AV node Wenckebach block cycle length or the AV node anterograde effective refractory period do not change after fast pathway ablation. After a median of 2 pulses, AVNRT was noninducible in 51 of 53 patients (96%) in our series, and no inadvertent complete AV block occurred.[35]

Slow Pathway Ablation

Recently, several groups targeted the slow pathway for radiofrequency catheter ablation and reported success rates between 90 and 100% with less or even no incidence of complete AV block.[36,37] The anterograde slow pathway is located posteroinferior to the compact AV node in proximity to the coronary sinus orificium (Fig. 21-10). In most centers, an anatomically guided approach for slow pathway elimination is used, and ablation is attempted at the posterior-inferior aspect of the interatrial septum near the coronary sinus ostium. Therefore, a 7-F quadripolar catheter with a 4-mm tip electrode is introduced in the right vena femoralis and advanced to the septal area of the tricuspid annulus close to the coronary sinus ostium. If the ablation attempt at this site fails, the catheter is positioned stepwise toward more midseptal areas by slightly straightening the catheter tip deflection. Local bipolar electrograms recorded from the ablation catheter at these sites should reveal an AV amplitude ratio of less than 1 and no His bundle potential. Another technique for slow pathway ablation consists of attempted ablation at sites where so-called slow pathway potentials are recorded.[36,37] However, different characteristics of these potentials have been described. In the study from Haissaguerre et al.[36] low-amplitude/low-frequency "humps" were recorded in the mid- to posterior septum anterior to the coronary sinus ostium and posteroinferior to the compact AV node. On the other hand, in the study from Jackman et al.,[37] high-amplitude/high-frequency potentials were recorded close to or within the coronary sinus ostium. The sensitivity and specificity of these potentials is presently unknown since the low-amplitude/low-frequency slow pathway potentials were also found in 80% of control patients without AVNRT.[36] Therefore, so-called slow pathway potentials may be epiphenomena instead of recordings of the depolarization of the slow pathway. In our institution, we follow a combined anatomically and electrographically guided approach for slow pathway ablation. Mapping and ablation using our approach is started at the posterior portion of the septal leaflet of the tricuspid valve

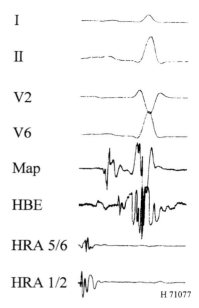

Fig. 21-13. Simultaneous recordings of surface leads I, II, V2, and V6 and intracardiac recordings from the ablation catheter (Map), His bundle region (HBE), and high right atrium (HRA 5/6 and 1/2) in a patient with recurrent AVNRT. Recordings during sinus rhythm are depicted for a representative target site electrogram for slow pathway ablation. The ablation catheter was positioned at the posterior part of the septal leaflet of the tricuspid valve close to the annulus. The local electrogram obtained by the ablation catheter showed a typical broad and fragmented atrial potential without a visible His bundle potential.

close to the annulus, where a broad and fragmented atrial potential can be recorded (Fig. 21-13). However, no attempts are made in our institution to validate so-called slow pathway potentials. Overall, the only randomized study comparing the anatomically and electrographically guided mapping approaches for ablation of the slow pathway in AVNRT revealed comparable results with respect to efficacy and duration of the procedure.[38] The end points of slow pathway ablation are noninducibility of AVNRT before and during isoproterenol infusion. Induction of single AV nodal reentrant beats has been reported after successful slow pathway ablation.[39] However, debate continues on whether residual slow pathway conduction is associated with a higher incidence of recurrence compared with complete slow pathway ablation with elimination of even single AV nodal reentrant beats.[39,40]

Junctional Tachycardia During Energy Application

The occurrence of junctional ectopic rhythms during energy application for ablation of either fast or slow pathway ablation should be analyzed for each radiofrequency pulse by continuously monitoring and recording the ECG during current delivery. Recently, it has been suggested that junctional tachycardia heralding complete AV block can be recognized by a faster junctional rate and ventriculoatrial block.[41] However, during junctional ectopic activity, the integrity of anterograde AV conduction and the persistence of ventriculoatrial conduction in some instances cannot be assessed with certainty. Therefore, at least when fast pathway ablation is attempted, atrial pacing should be performed at sufficiently short cycle lengths until one-to-one AV conduction is achieved. Otherwise, radiofrequency application should be immediately interrupted.

Summary and Complications

Radiofrequency catheter ablation has been established as a first-line curative treatment modality in patients with recurrent symptomatic AVNRT. As clearly indicated by the Multicenter European Radiofrequency Survey,[42] slow pathway ablation carries a significantly lower risk of complete AV block (2.0%) compared with fast pathway ablation (6.2%, $P < 0.05$) and therefore should be the initial target site for ablation to cure patients with AVNRT. However, some groups experienced in the selective ablation of the fast pathway showed that this approach can also be performed with an acceptable incidence of unintended complete atrioventricular block. The data reported by the Multicenter European Radiofrequency Survey[42] include the early experience with modification of the AV node and therefore also include the learning curve. In experienced centers, slow and fast pathway ablation can be performed with a risk of complete AV block of about 1 to 2% or even less.

ABLATION OR MODIFICATION OF THE ATRIOVENTRICULAR JUNCTION

General Approach

Control of the ventricular response constitutes a challenge in patients with chronic or paroxysmal atrial fibrillation resistant to antiarrhythmic drugs since symptomatic palpitations, tachycardia-induced left ventricular dysfunction, and other sequels may result. Permanent interruption of AV conduction followed by pacemaker implantation may be the only method of ameliorating palpitations, which re-

sult from the rapid ventricular response in atrial fibrillation. Ablation of the AV junction is usually performed from the right atrium. Energy is applied to target sites showing a large atrial potential and a proximal His bundle potential by positioning the ablation catheter slightly inferiorly and proximally to the reference catheter placed near the central fibrous body using the right and left anterior oblique fluoroscopy view. A permanent pacemaker is usually inserted within 48 hours after the ablation procedure. In our institution, however, a permanent pacemaker is implanted prior to ablation of the AV junction. If a patient has received a pacemaker before the ablation session, careful control of the pacemaker function is necessary after ablation because pacemaker dysfunction following radiofrequency ablation has been reported.

Ablation From the Left Side

In patients in whom the above-described approach fails, ablation can be performed from the left ventricular septum. Souza et al.[43] reported unsuccessful radiofrequency energy applications from the conventional right-sided approach in 6 of 30 patients. However, complete AV block was achieved in all these patients through a retrograde arterial approach. A 7-F deflectable catheter was introduced via the femoral artery, advanced across the aortic valve into the left ventricle, and placed at the AV septum where the largest His bundle potential could be recorded. Overall, success rates exceeding 90% have been reported.[44,45]

Modification of Atrioventricular Conduction

Slowing of the ventricular response in atrial fibrillation by modulation of AV conduction may be an alternative to complete ablation of the AV junction since no pacemaker dependency would result. First attempts at applying radiofrequency energy to the *anteroseptal* area have yielded only modest success rates.[46] By contrast, radiofrequency modification of AV conduction for control of rapid ventricular response could be achieved recently in patients with medically refractory atrial fibrillation, possibly by ablation of the *posterior* AV nodal input.[47–49] Radiofrequency current was initially applied to the posteroseptal right atrium close to the coronary sinus orificium. When no change in the ventricular rate resulted, the catheter was repositioned more anterior to midseptal sites. However, a rather large number of radiofrequency energy applications was necessary in these studies, and complete AV block resulted in 4 of 19 patients in the series of Williamson et al.[49] and in 2 of 14 patients in the series of Della Bella et al.,[47] indicating that damage to the central body of the AV node rather than selective ablation of the so-called slow pathway might have been accomplished. It is noteworthy that in three of the four patients in the study of Williamson et al.[49] who developed third-degree AV block, complete block occurred 36 to 72 hours after the procedure. Therefore, patients should be monitored after modification of AV conduction to control the ventricular rate during atrial fibrillation for at least 3 days following the procedure. However, because of the relatively high risk of complete AV block, this procedure should presently be reserved for patients in whom otherwise intended complete AV block would have been induced.

ABLATION OF ATRIAL FLUTTER

Atrial flutter is a common and often highly symptomatic supraventricular arrhythmia. Termination of atrial flutter with antiarrhythmic drugs and prevention of recurrences is often difficult. Irrespective of the underlying structural heart disease there is a remarkable consistency in the common type of atrial flutter (type I) with respect to atrial rate and the so-called sawtooth morphology of the flutter waves in the inferior ECG leads II, III, and aVF. Recent studies in humans using intraoperative mapping as well as endocardial catheter mapping have demonstrated that type I atrial flutter is due to a "counterclockwise" macroreentrant circuit with upward (caudocranial) activation of the interatrial septum and downward (craniocaudal) activation of the right atrial free wall, whereas the left atrium is activated secondarily[50,51] (Fig. 21-14).

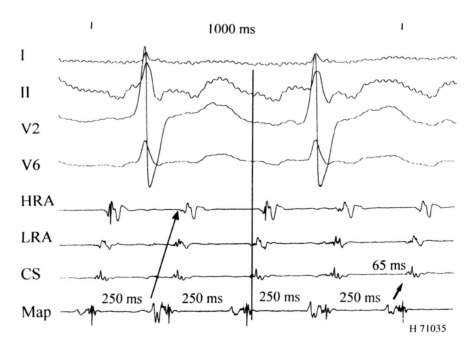

Fig. 21-14. Simultaneous recordings of surface leads I, II, V2, and V6 and intracardiac recordings from the high right atrium (HRA), low right atrium close to the His bundle area (LRA), coronary sinus ostium (CS), and mapping and ablation catheter (Map), which was placed slightly inferior to the coronary sinus ostium. The tracings show the typical activation sequence during the *common type* of atrial flutter (type I) with activation of the interatrial septum in an *upward* (caudocranial) direction (*long arrow*). Note the typical polyphasic, fragmented potential that can be recorded in the area of slow conduction inferior to the coronary sinus ostium (Map). The activation time from the local potential recorded with the mapping catheter to that recorded at the coronary sinus ostium measured 65 ms (*short arrow*) [i.e., approximately 25% of the whole atrial flutter cycle length (250 ms)], although the recording electrodes were only a few millimeters apart. The vertical line indicates the beginning of the downstroke of the negative flutter waves in the inferior leads. Note that the polyphasic fragmented potential recorded from the mapping catheter (Map) slightly inferior to the coronary sinus ostium precedes the onset of the flutter wave.

General Approach

For electrophysiologic study, standard multipolar electrode catheters are introduced percutaneously from femoral veins and positioned in the high right atrium, right ventricular apex, across the tricuspid valve to record the His bundle potential, and in the coronary sinus via the right internal jugular vein. Alternatively, a so-called halocatheter with 10 bipoles might be advanced for right atrial activation mapping covering the posteroseptal and anterolateral areas or a multipolar ellipsoidal basket catheter incorporating four to six spokes.

Two different strategies for radiofrequency catheter ablation of atrial flutter currently exist, one anatomically guided and one guided by endocardial activation and entrainment mapping. However, even when the anatomically guided strategy is used for

ablation, a detailed electrophysiologic preablation study is mandatory for the exact localization of the reentrant circuit (Fig. 21-15).

Ablation Using Anatomic Landmarks

Perioperative mapping studies indicated that early potentials relative to the negative deflection of the so-called sawtooth flutter waves could be recorded in the vicinity of the coronary sinus ostium.[50] A clustering of isochronal lines during multielectrode epicardial mapping in the posteroseptal region indicative of an area of slow conduction suggested that this anatomically well-defined area might be critical for the maintenance of the reentrant circuit.[50] Cosio and coworkers[52] introduced successful radiofrequency in-

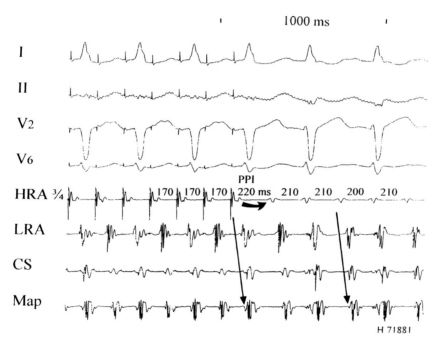

Fig. 21-15. Simultaneous recordings of surface leads I, II, V2, and V6 and intracardiac recordings from the proximal pair of electrodes of the high right atrium catheter (HRA 3/4), low right atrium close to the His bundle area (LRA), coronary sinus ostium (CS), and mapping and ablation catheter (Map), which was placed slightly inferior to the coronary sinus ostium. The tracings show the activation sequence during the *uncommon type* of atrial flutter (type II). Note that in this case the interatrial septum was activated in a *downward* (craniocaudal) direction (*long arrows*). Pacing from the distal pair of electrodes of the HRA catheter with a cycle length of 170 ms resulted in acceleration of atrial flutter to the pacing cycle length without a change in the activation sequence at the interatrial septum and toward the area of the coronary sinus ostium (i.e., entrainment with orthodromic activation at the interatrial septum). After termination of pacing, atrial flutter continued with the same activation sequence at the interatrial septum and toward the area of the coronary sinus ostium. The postpacing interval (220 ms) closely matched the atrial flutter cycle length (200 To 210 ms), indicating that pacing was performed within or close to the reentrant circuit pathway. In this case, *uncommon* atrial flutter was successfully ablated by repetitive radiofrequency energy applications, creating a contiguous line of ablation from the coronary sinus ostium to the inferior vena cava.

terruption using anatomic landmarks. With this technique, the ablation catheter is advanced from the inferior vena cava to the right ventricle and then slowly withdrawn until bipolar recordings from the distal pair of electrodes of the ablation catheter reveal atrial electrograms. Along the withdrawal line from the tricuspid annulus to the inferior vena cava, radiofrequency energy is applied at multiple sites every 3 to 4 mm until atrial flutter is interrupted or until no atrial electrograms are recorded, indicating the orifice of the inferior vena cava. If the approach was ineffective, this procedure may be repeated along the same line at points where sharp atrial electrograms can still be recorded, indicating that the line of ablation is not contiguous at these sites. Alternatively, the ablation catheter might be introduced from the superior vena cava via the right internal jugular vein or a subclavian vein in an attempt to obtain a better catheter tip electrode-tissue contact. Fischer and coworkers[53,54] recently reported on radiofrequency energy application for ablation of common atrial flutter in three different anatomic zones of the right atrium: between the posterior tricuspid annulus and the orifice of the inferior vena cava (zone 1), between the septal leaflet of the tricuspid valve and the ostium of the coronary sinus (zone 2), and between the orifice of the inferior vena cava and the ostium of the coronary sinus (zone 3). Ablation of atrial flutter in their series was most successful in zone 1. In patients in whom a single line in one of the three zones is not effective, three lines of conduction block may be sequentially created by ablation in all three zones described.[55] Recently, Kirkorian et al.[56] reported that catheter ablation at the atrial isthmus between the inferior vena cava and the tricuspid ring might also be effective for termination of *atypical* atrial flutter.

Electrophysiologically Guided Ablation

Feld et al.[57] reported the results of attempted electrophysiologically guided radiofrequency catheter ablation of type I atrial flutter. These authors found that successful ablation sites were located inferior or posterior to the ostium of the coronary sinus. The successful sites in this area were characterized by discrete electrograms with activation times of -20 to -50 ms before the onset of the P wave. Additionally, entrainment mapping resulting in concealed fusion and stimulus-to-P-wave intervals of 20 to 40 ms consistent with the exit site from the area of slow conduction was indicative of ablation success.[57] Another approach using electrophysiologic criteria for selection of target sites for ablation of atrial flutter was

reported by Calkins et al.[58] These authors, in agreement with the results of other groups, found that fractionated potentials or so-called double potentials were not associated with successful ablation. However, the combination of electrophysiologic and anatomic criteria might help to reduce the number of radiofrequency energy applications for successful ablation of atrial flutter when compared with ablation guided merely by anatomic landmarks.

Summary and Limitations

A discrete area in the low posteroseptal right atrium is critical for the maintenance of the macroreentrant circuit in atrial flutter and is amenable to radiofrequency catheter ablation. Ablation strategies using anatomic landmarks or a combination of anatomic and electrophysiologic criteria may result in high initial success rates for ablation. However, the number of patients with atrial flutter treated with radiofrequency energy so far is limited and the duration of the follow-up period is relatively short. Therefore, more experience and a longer follow-up is needed to define clearly the role of radiofrequency catheter ablation for definite treatment of atrial flutter. Late recurrences of the same or different kinds of atrial flutter as well as the late development of atrial fibrillation might limit the role of catheter ablation as a long-term therapy for patients with atrial flutter.

ABLATION OF ATRIAL TACHYCARDIAS

Atrial tachycardia, a relatively rare arrhythmia that may occur in all age groups, may be defined as a regular arrhythmia originating within the right or left atrium outside the sinus or AV node. Atrial tachycardias may be clinically relevant as a paroxysmal type of tachycardia or as a permanent type of so-called incessant tachycardia. The latter frequently occurs in pediatric patients and may lead to tachycardia-related cardiomyopathy. Especially in this situation, antiarrhythmic drugs often fail to control the atrial tachycardias. Most important, left ventricular dysfunction has been shown to be reversible after curative therapy of atrial tachycardia including surgery or radiofrequency catheter ablation.[59]

General Approach

Different electrophysiologic mechanisms have been proposed to underlie atrial tachycardia, including abnormal automaticity, triggered activity due to afterdepolarizations, and reentrant activation. Atrial tachycardias due to abnormal automaticity usually cannot be initiated or terminated with programmed electrical stimulation; however, the arrhythmia may often be provoked during continuous intravenous infusion of isoproterenol. Reentrant activation is the presumed mechanism if the tachycardia can be reproducibly initiated and terminated with programmed electrical stimulation and the demonstration of manifest or concealed entrainment. Criteria for atrial tachycardias related to triggered activity, however, are less well defined, although recording of monophasic action potentials might add important information in the future.[60]

For mapping and ablation of atrial tachycardias arising from the right atrium, a deflectable mapping catheter is usually introduced from the right or left femoral vein and advanced to the right atrium. The *transseptal* approach via the interatrial septum may be used for mapping and ablation of atrial tachycardias originating within the left atrium (Figs. 21-16 and 21-17). Using right and left anterior oblique fluoroscopic projections, transseptal puncture is performed using a Brockenbrough needle. An 8-F sheath is then advanced over the needle into the left atrium. Alternatively, the *retrograde* approach may be used

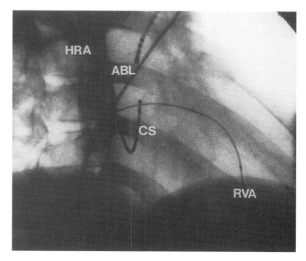

A

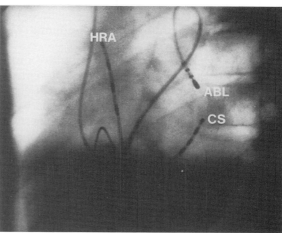

B

Fig. 21-17. Radiographs in (A) right anterior oblique 30° and (B) left anterior oblique 60° projection obtained from a patient with an incessant form of left atrial tachycardia (same patient as in Fig. 21-16). Multipolar catheters for electrophysiologic study were placed in the high right atrium (HRA), right ventricular apex (RVA), His bundle region (HBE), and coronary sinus (CS). Using right and left anterior oblique fluoroscopic projections, transseptal puncture was performed to gain access to the left atrium. The position of the mapping and ablation catheter (MAP) indicates the area where the earliest endocardial atrial activity during ongoing atrial tachycardia was recorded close to the orifice of a pulmonary vein (see also Fig. 21-18).

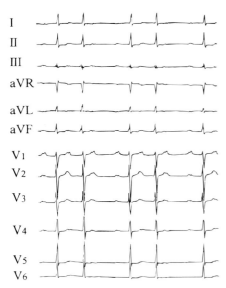

Fig. 21-16. Twelve-lead surface ECG leads in a 23-year-old man with an incessant form of ectopic atrial tachycardia. The cycle length of the tachycardia measured 470 ms and the Wenckebach periodicity allows analysis of the P-wave morphology. Note that the isoelectric P wave in lead I and the negative P wave in aVL is indicative of a left atrial origin of the tachycardia. Seven different antiarrhythmic drug regimens had previously failed to control this incessant form of atrial tachycardia, and there was progressive left ventricular enlargement and dysfunction (see also Figs. 21-17 and 21-18).

to gain access to the left atrium by advancing the mapping catheter from the femoral artery across the aortic valve into the left atrium and retrograde across the mitral valve. Catheter positions are identified using biplane fluoroscopy. During the mapping procedure, atrial angiograms may be performed to clarify the atrial anatomy and to identify anatomic landmarks.

Ectopic (Automatic) Atrial Tachycardia

Ectopic atrial tachycardia is characterized by a rapid atrial rate that is inappropriate for sinus rhythm, by a P-wave axis and configuration differing from that during sinus rhythm, and by a different atrial activation sequence compared with sinus rhythm. Additionally, ectopic atrial tachycardias may exhibit a relatively wide variation in cycle length that is often related to the state of the autonomic nervous system and a so-called warm-up and cool-down phenomenon at the initiation and termination of the tachycardia, respectively. Mapping studies have identified a clustering of the sites of origin of ectopic atrial tachycardias in the atrial appendages, along the crista terminalis, and around the orifices of the pulmonary veins. Occasionally, ectopic atrial tachycardias may arise from atrial myocardium *within* a pulmonary vein (K. H. Kuck, personal communication).

For electrophysiologic study, standard multipolar electrode catheters are introduced percutaneously from femoral veins and positioned in the high right atrium and right ventricular apex and across the tricuspid valve to record the His bundle potential. Another multipolar catheter may be positioned in the coronary sinus via the right internal jugular or subclavian vein. The local atrial activation time obtained by the distal pair of electrodes of the mapping catheter during ongoing ectopic atrial tachycardia is related to the onset of the P wave in the surface ECG. However, the onset of the P wave during tachycardia is often obscured by the QRS complex or the T wave, especially in cases with 1:1 or 2:1 conduction via the AV node (Fig. 21-18). In these cases, a stable intracardiac electrogram (e.g., the electrogram obtained by the catheter positioned in the right atrial appendage or within the coronary sinus) may serve as a more reliable reference (Fig. 21-18). Precise mapping is performed to search for the earliest detectable atrial activity. When the atrial tachycardia originates within the right atrium, a second deflectable catheter may be advanced for mapping. Using two mapping catheters, an alternating movement of the catheters is possible (i.e., the first is left in place serving as a reference until the second has recorded an earlier atrial activation). The second catheter is then left in place as the new reference, and the first serves as the new mapping catheter. Target sites for ablation are identified by local atrial activation preceding the onset of the P wave in the surface ECG by more then 20 ms.[61–63] In many cases, the origin of the atrial tachycardia is characterized by fragmentation of the atrial potential (Fig. 21-18). Additionally, "pace mapping" may be performed. The P-wave mor-

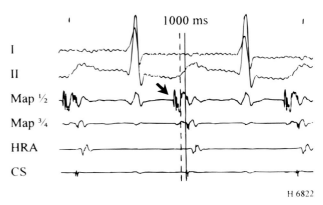

Fig. 21-18. Simultaneous recordings of surface leads I and II, and intracardiac recordings from the distal (1/2) and proximal (3/4) pair of electrodes of the mapping and ablation catheter (Map), high right atrium (HRA), and coronary sinus (CS) during ongoing ectopic atrial tachycardia originating in the left atrium (same patient as in Figs. 21-16 and 21-17). The local atrial activation time obtained by the distal pair of electrodes of the mapping catheter during ongoing ectopic atrial tachycardia was related to the onset of the P wave in the surface ECG. However, the onset of the P wave during tachycardia was obscured by the T wave (*dashed line,* presumed onset of the P wave). Therefore, a stable intracardiac electrogram (i.e., the electrogram obtained by the catheter positioned in the lateral coronary sinus) served as a more reliable reference (*solid line*). Precise mapping indicated the earliest detectable atrial activity 30 ms prior to the presumed onset of the P wave and 55 ms prior to the reference potential from the coronary sinus. Note that the atrial potential at this site revealed a fragmented morphology (*arrow*). At this site, the previously incessant atrial tachycardia was successfully ablated. It is noteworthy that left ventricular dysfunction and enlargement due to tachycardia-related cardiomyopathy normalized within the next 6 months.

phology during endocardial stimulation at the presumed "site of origin" is compared with the P-wave morphology of the atrial tachycardia. A very similar or identical P-wave morphology during pacing and during atrial tachycardia in at least 11 or 12 ECG leads is used to select appropriate target sites for ablation. However, the morphology of the P wave may be indistinct by the T wave and, therefore, the usefulness of this mapping criterium is limited.

Intra-atrial and Sinoatrial Reentrant Tachycardia

Sinoatrial reentrant tachycardia is electrophysiologically characterized by a similar P-wave morphology and atrial activation sequence compared with normal sinus rhythm, reproducible inducibility, and termination using programmed electrical stimulation with critically timed extrastimuli, as well as termination of the tachycardia with vagal maneuvers and adenosine.[64,65] For ablation of intra-atrial or sinoatrial reentrant tachycardias, a combination of endocardial atrial activation mapping and entrainment mapping is used to identify target sites for energy application.[65-67] Earliest atrial activation times more than 35 ms relative to the onset of the P wave, significantly prolonged and fractionated electrograms, and a concealed entrainment mapping with a stimulus-P-wave interval of about 20 ms have been reported to be associated with ablation success.[65,66] In the series reported by Lesh and coworkers,[67] all patients with intra-atrial reentrant tachycardia had previous surgery for congenital heart disease and reentry around a surgical scar, anatomic defect, or atriotomy incision. The mechanism by which ablation was successful in their series of patients was similar to that previously described for ablation of atrial flutter (i.e., ablation was performed at a critical narrow isthmus bounded by anatomic or structural obstacles).[67]

ABLATION OF VENTRICULAR TACHYCARDIA IN PATIENTS WITH CORONARY ARTERY DISEASE

Sustained monomorphic ventricular tachycardia in the setting of chronic myocardial infarction has been suggested to be due to reentrant activation as indicated by its response to programmed electrical stimulation and other electrophysiologic characteristics. The reentry circuit is localized in many cases in the border zone of normal myocardium and myocardial scar tissue or aneurysm. One of the key problems for radiofrequency catheter ablation of ventricular tachycardia in patients with remote myocardial infarction is the identification of the optimal site for ablation. This site should be an essential part of the reentry circuit and should consist of a circumscribed isthmus since the lesions generated by radiofrequency energy are relatively small. The situation is further complicated by the fact that in a significant portion of patients with ventricular tachycardia and a history of myocardial infarction, the substrate of the reentrant circuit consists of a three-dimensional structure involving not only the subendocardium but also intramural and subepicardial myocardium.[68] Additional features in patients with coronary artery disease and ventricular tachycardia may limit the applicability of catheter ablation. These include endocardial thrombus formation, hemodynamic or elec-

trically unstable ventricular tachycardia, multiple reentrant circuits, and others. To reduce the risk of thromboembolic complications, intracavitary thrombus formation should be excluded prior to the ablation session with transthoracic echocardiography and, if necessary, with transesophageal echocardiography.

General Considerations

Antitachycardia surgery using mapping guided subendocardial resection, encircling endocardial ventriculotomy, and other techniques have been proved effective in treating selected patients with chronic recurrent ventricular tachycardia in the setting of chronic myocardial infarction.[69] However, operative mortality has averaged 12% and postoperative reinducibility rate 24%, indicating the need for additional treatment modalities. The introduction of catheter ablation has stimulated the search for more precise localization techniques for identifying areas critical for the perpetuation of ventricular tachycardia since the lesion size produced by catheter ablation, in contrast to antitachycardia surgery, is limited. Selection criteria for patients with remote myocardial infarction and chronic recurrent ventricular tachycardia for radiofrequency catheter ablation usually include the following: documentation of the ventricular tachycardia on a 12-lead ECG; inability to control the ventricular tachycardia by at least one antiarrhythmic drug; reproducible inducibility of the clinically documented ventricular tachycardia and termination in the electrophysiology laboratory using programmed ventricular stimulation; and the presence of monomorphic and hemodynamically stable ventricular tachycardia to allow catheter mapping during ongoing ventricular tachycardia.

Mapping and Ablation

For endocardial mapping and ablation, a 7-F deflectable catheter with a 4-mm distal electrode and a 2-mm interelectrode spacing is used. The ablation catheter is introduced via a femoral artery and advanced retrogradely into the left ventricle. Rarely, target sites for catheter ablation of ventricular tachycardia in the setting of remote myocardial infarction must be approached from the right ventricle. In these instances, the ablation catheter is inserted into a femoral vein and advanced through the right atrium into the right ventricle. After catheter insertion, a heparin bolus of 5,000 IE is given intravenously with an additional 1,000 IE/hr thereafter. Systemic anticoagulation is maintained for at least 24 hours. In our clinic, aspirin 100 mg/d is administered for 3 months.

Bipolar electrograms are recorded from the distal and proximal pair of electrodes throughout the ablation session (filter setting, 40 to 500 Hz). For endocardial pacing, bipolar or unipolar stimulation is performed from the distal pair of electrodes or the distal electrode of the mapping/ablation catheter, respectively. The endocardial mapping procedure for selection of appropriate target sites for delivery of radiofrequency energy in our clinic is guided by the following protocol.[95]

Initially, catheter mapping during sinus rhythm is performed. According to a given scheme, the left and, if necessary, the right ventricle are mapped during sinus rhythm.[70] Endocardial signals are analyzed with respect to their timing in relation to the surface ECG and their morphology. Low-amplitude fragmented potentials occurring after the QRS complex in the surface ECG may be considered areas of impaired and/or slow conduction ("late potentials") (Fig. 21-19A). The next step includes the induction of the ventricular tachycardia and "activation mapping" during ongoing tachycardia. Again, endocardial signals are analyzed with respect to their timing in relation to the surface ECG and their morphology. The activation sequence of the "late potentials" during sinus rhythm is different during ventricular tachycardia. Low-amplitude fragmented potentials participating in the so-called area of slow conduction of the reentrant circuit may be inscribed in early diastole, mid-diastole, or presystole. In the case of a "micro-reentrant" circuit, the whole activation of the area of slow conduction may be shown by recording to exhibit *continuous* diastolic activity (Fig. 21-19B). Recordings of areas participating in critical regions for the perpetuation of the reentrant circuits are usually characterized by low-amplitude fragmented potentials generated by surviving myocardial fiber strands interspersed within the scar tissue or located at the border zone of necrotic tissue. Additionally, more sophisticated mapping criteria such as entrainment mapping are necessary to determine target sites for radiofrequency ablation.[71] Thus, pacing maneuvers are performed during ongoing ventricular tachycardia at cycle lengths 20 to 100 ms shorter than the ventricular tachycardia cycle length, resulting in constant ventricular fusion beats on the surface ECG except for the last captured beat, which is entrained but not fused.

Another entrainment criteria includes progressive fusion (i.e., different degrees of fusion beats at different pacing cycle lengths). During entrainment with so-called concealed fusion, pacing *within* the reen-

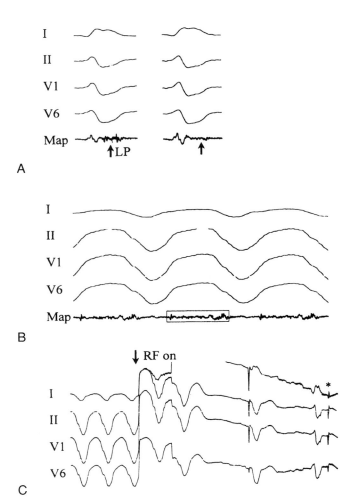

Fig. 21-19. Surface ECG leads I, II, V1, V6 and local bipolar electrograms from the distal pair of electrodes of the mapping/ablation catheter (Map) in a patient with remote anterior wall myocardial infarction and chronic recurrent ventricular tachycardia. **(A)** Left, a fragmented low-amplitude potential inscribing at the end of the QRS complex in the surface ECG could be recorded at the left ventricular septum during sinus rhythm mapping (LP, "late potential," *arrow*). **(B)** After induction of ventricular tachycardia with programmed ventricular stimulation, "activation mapping" during ongoing ventricular tachycardia revealed continuous diastolic activity (framed potential) at the recording site of a late potential during sinus rhythm. **(C)** Radiofrequency current was applied at the site where fragmented late potentials during sinus rhythm and continuous diastolic activity during ventricular tachycardia had been recorded. Ventricular tachycardia terminated about 1 second after institution of energy application. Termination of ventricular tachycardia was followed by ventricular stimulation by a pacemaker system that had been implanted several years previously because of sick sinus syndrome. At the end of the registration, malfunction of the pacemaker system was recorded (*asterisk*). Sensing defects are frequently seen during application of radiofrequency energy. Note that after successful radiofrequency application, no fragmented late potential could be recorded at the site of ablation (**A,** right panel, *arrow*). (From Hindricks et al.,[95] with permission.)

trant circuit results in an orthodromic wavefront along a pathway similar to that seen during ventricular tachycardia and in an antidromic wavefront that collides near the "entrance" of the area of slow conduction and does not activate the surrounding normal myocardium. Therefore, during concealed entrainment, the paced QRS complex identically matches the QRS morphology of the ventricular tachycardia (Fig. 21-20). Thus the pacing maneuvers mentioned above may indicate sites that are critically involved in the perpetuation of the ventricular tachycardia. However, the characteristics described may also be observed in so-called bystander areas not participating in the reentrant circuit itself. Additional criteria for the differentiation between sites within the reentrant circuit and bystander areas include the stimulus-QRS interval and the postpacing interval (Fig. 21-20). The stimulus-QRS interval of trains of stimuli is the interval from the last stimulus to the last entrained QRS complex, and the postpacing interval is the interval from the last stimulus to the local activation following at the site of stimulation.[72]

Radiofrequency catheter ablation is performed when the mapping criteria described above indicate that the target site is probably critically involved in the reentrant circuit. When endocardial mapping does not reveal presystolic or mid-diastolic poten-

tials, the ventricular tachycardia is terminated and "pace mapping" may be performed. The QRS morphology during endocardial stimulation at the presumed "site of origin" is compared with the QRS morphology of the clinical ventricular tachycardia. A very similar or identical QRS morphology during pacing and during ventricular tachycardia in at least 11 or 12 ECG leads is used to select appropriate target sites for ablation. However, the value of pace mapping to identify critical sites within the reentrant circuit is limited because, although the paced QRS complex may mimic the QRS complex of the ventricular tachycardia, this does not imply that the site of pacing represents an adequate site for radiofrequency application. Instead, the critical isthmus of the "common pathway" that might be the best target site for ablation may be relatively far away from the so-called exit point of the common pathway where pacing would result in an identical QRS complex compared with the QRS complex of the ventricular tachycardia.

Radiofrequency energy is usually applied during ongoing ventricular tachycardia for immediate assessment of the efficacy of current delivery (Fig. 21-19C). The ablation procedure may be considered acutely successful when the target ventricular tachycardia is no longer inducible by standard programmed ventricular stimulation 15 to 30 minutes

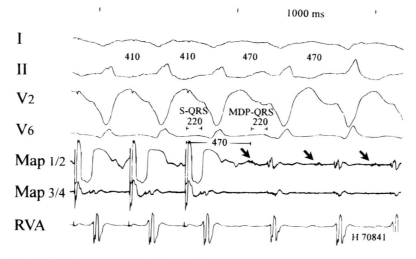

Fig. 21-20. Surface ECG leads I, II, V2, V6, and local bipolar electrograms from the distal (Map 1/2) and proximal (Map 3/4) pair of electrodes of the mapping/ablation catheter in a patient with remote anterolateral wall myocardial infarction and chronic recurrent ventricular tachycardia. Entrainment mapping with concealed fusion is performed with a cycle length of 60 ms less than the ventricular tachycardia cycle length (i.e., pacing resulted in acceleration of the ventricular tachycardia to the pacing cycle length without a change in the morphology of the surface ECG). During pacing a stimulus-QRS interval (S-QRS) of 220 ms resulted that exactly matched the interval of the isolated mid-diastolic potential to the onset of the QRS complex (MDP-QRS) recorded during ventricular tachycardia. Additionally, the postpacing interval (i.e., the interval from the last stimulus to the following local activation at the site of stimulation) measured 470 ms and thus exactly matched the cycle length of the ventricular tachycardia, indicating that pacing was performed within the reentrant circuit and not from a bystander area.

after radiofrequency application. In our clinic, repeat programmed stimulation is performed 4 to 6 days and 3 to 6 months after the ablation session for assessment of long-term ablation success.

Recently, Stevenson and coworkers[72] developed criteria for identifying target sites for ablation using computer simulations that were then applied to patients with ventricular tachycardia late after myocardial infarction. In this study, entrainment with concealed fusion, a postpacing interval approximating the tachycardia cycle length, a stimulus-QRS interval of more than 60 ms but less than 70% of the tachycardia cycle length, and recording of isolated diastolic potentials or continuous electrical activity during ventricular tachycardia were helpful in identifying target sites for successful radiofrequency catheter ablation. However, 4 of the 10 successfully treated patients in the series of Stevenson et al.[72] and all 11 successfully treated patients from Morady et al.[73] continued to take the previously ineffective antiarrhythmic medication. Our group recently analyzed the results of 53 consecutive patients undergoing radiofrequency catheter ablation of ventricular tachycardia related to coronary artery disease and remote myocardial infarction. In 39 of 53 patients (73%), the clinical ventricular tachycardia was rendered noninducible at the end of the ablation session. Seventeen of 39 patients (44%) with an early success were free from recurrences during a mean follow-up of 15 ± 9 months, indicating that long-term success can presently only achieved be in a limited number of patients.

Incessant Ventricular Tachycardia

Incessant ventricular tachycardia usually occurs in patients suffering from severe organic heart disease. In these patients, ventricular tachycardia covers more than 50% of all cardiac beats, and recurrent episodes of ventricular tachycardia are only occasionally interrupted by a few sinus beats. In most cases, incessant ventricular tachycardia is difficult to control by antiarrhythmic drugs or even results from excessive antiarrhythmic drug therapy. The patients are often significantly hemodynamically compromised by the ongoing arrhythmia, and an intervention to stop the arrhythmia is badly needed. In this emergency situation, we performed radiofrequency catheter ablation in a total of 22 patients. The incessant tachycardia could be successfully terminated in 20 patients (91%) by radiofrequency ablation (unpublished data). The recurrence rate of the same tachycardia or ventricular tachycardia of other morphologies is high in these patients, and most of them require additional types of antiarrhythmic therapy (antiarrhythmic drugs, antitachycardia surgery, implantable cardioverter/defibrillators). However, the results show that the patients can be effectively treated in the dangerous situation of incessant ventricular tachycardia and stabilized until additional forms of therapy are applied.

Catheter Ablation as an Adjunctive Treatment

The role of radiofrequency catheter ablation for ventricular tachycardia as a complementary therapy is further highlighted by a recent report from our group illustrating the results of catheter ablation in patients following implantation of an automatic cardioverter/defibrillator.[74] Six of 180 patients with an implanted cardioverter/defibrillator developed frequent or incessant episodes of monomorphic ventricular tachycardia. Despite recurrences of ventricular tachycardia in four patients, all episodes could be controlled after catheter ablation by the implantable cardioverter/defibrillator. In addition, the incidence of cardioverter/defibrillator therapies (antitachycardia pacing or shock delivery) was markedly reduced after the ablation procedure.

Summary and Complications

Overall, radiofrequency catheter ablation is presently only feasible in a highly selected patient group with ventricular tachycardia and remote myocardial infarction. Prerequisites for this indication include the reproducible inducibility of the clinical ventricular tachycardia as well as a monomorphic appearance and hemodynamic stability during ventricular tachycardia. Additionally, the substrate of the reentrant circuit should be circumscribed and should be accessible by catheter techniques. In 7.5% of 320 patients who were reported to the Multicenter European Radiofrequency Survey,[27] complications occurred in relation to the ablation of ventricular tachycardia. By taking into consideration the severe organic heart disease of this patient population, the low morbidity and mortality is indicative of the relative safety of radiofrequency catheter ablation for this indication.

ABLATION OF VENTRICULAR TACHYCARDIA IN PATIENTS WITH IDIOPATHIC DILATED CARDIOMYOPATHY

The histopathologic and electrophysiologic characteristics of sustained ventricular tachycardia in idiopathic dilated cardiomyopathy are even less well defined when compared with ventricular tachycardia related to coronary artery disease. A variety of factors may contribute to the genesis of ventricular tachyarrhythmias in nonischemic dilated cardiomyopathy. Histopathologic investigations revealed hypertrophy of the ventricular myocytes in all patients with idiopathic dilated cardiomyopathy.[75] The degree of cardiomyopathic changes detected by electron microscopy was found to be different in patients with inducible and noninducible ventricular tachycardia.[75] Additionally, a tendency was seen toward more interstitial fibrosis and myocyte hypertrophy in the cases with more severe cardiomyopathic changes. Presently, therapeutic options for ventricular tachycardia in patients with idiopathic dilated cardiomyopathy include antiarrhythmic drugs, implantable cardioverter/defibrillators, and, as a last resort, heart transplantation. However, some of these patients suffer from incessant ventricular tachycardia refractory to antiarrhythmic drugs or provoked by antiarrhythmic agents. Furthermore, patients with incessant or frequent, recurrent ventricular tachycardia may not be adequately treated by the implantable cardioverter/defibrillator, and emergency heart transplantation is only exceptionally available.

Mapping and Ablation

We recently investigated the feasibility of radiofrequency catheter ablation as a treatment option for ventricular tachycardia in patients with idiopathic dilated cardiomyopathy who could not be adequately treated by conventional treatment modalities.[76] We adopted the endocardial mapping techniques developed for mapping of ventricular tachycardia in the setting of chronic myocardial infarction (see above), since the electrophysiologic criteria of the ventricular tachycardias in our group of patients with dilated cardiomyopathy also seemed to be compatible with a reentrant mechanism (Fig. 21-21). The results of our study indicated that radiofrequency current application for ablation of ventricular tachycardia in a highly selected group of patients with idiopathic dilated cardiomyopathy is feasible. Potential target sites for radiofrequency current application were identified by concealed entrainment and activation mapping during ongoing ventricular tachycardia as well as by pace mapping in those patients in whom no fragmented potentials could be recorded during sinus rhythm or ventricular tachycardia.[76] The efficacy of radiofrequency ablation was high in patients

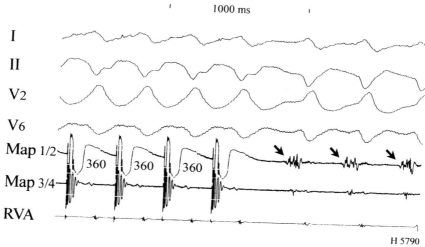

Fig. 21-21. Surface ECG leads I, II, V2, V6 and local electrograms from the distal (1/2) and proximal (3/4) pair of electrodes of the mapping/ablation catheter (Map) and right ventricular apex (RVA). Electrophysiologic recordings during entrainment mapping for ablation of ventricular tachycardia in a patient with idiopathic dilated cardiomyopathy at a site of successful radiofrequency current application are depicted. The patient presented with an incessant ventricular tachycardia with right bundle branch block pattern and left axis deviation with a cycle length of 420 ms. Pacing from the distal pair of electrodes of the mapping/ablation catheter with a cycle length of 360 ms at the left anteroseptal region resulted in acceleration of the incessant ventricular tachycardia to the pacing cycle length without a change in the morphology of the surface ECG ("concealed entrainment"). The stimulus-QRS interval during entrainment mapping measured 95 ms. At the pacing site, a presystolic fragmented potential inscribing 70 ms before the onset of the QRS complex in the surface ECG was recorded during ventricular tachycardia (*arrows*). (From Kottkamp et al.,[76] with permission.)

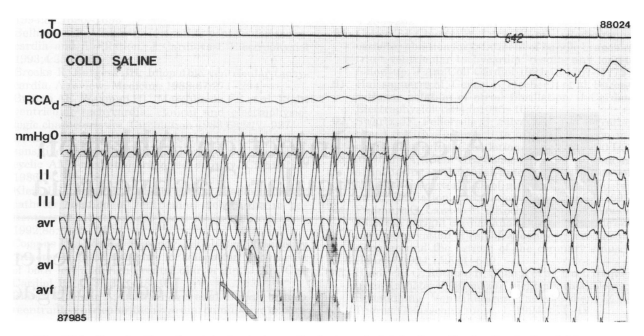

Fig. 22-1. Termination of ventricular tachycardia during administration of iced saline in the right coronary artery. Six electrocardiographic leads and the arterial pressure in the right coronary are shown.

The mechanism of action seems therefore to be a destruction of surviving cells by the production of a new infarct, with all the possible complications associated with this condition.[8] At the atrial level, it is clear that when the atrioventricular node is necessary to perpetuate a tachycardia, ablation or destruction of the node stops the tachycardia circuit.

INSTRUMENTATION

Coronary angiographic findings, along with information from programmed electrical stimulation of the heart, endocardial mapping techniques, and the techniques and materials used during percutaneous coronary angioplasty, can be used to identify and catheterize very small branches of the coronary arterial circulation, which is the blood supply to the site of origin or pathway of a tachycardia. The instrumentation needed for these procedures is the routine equipment for electrophysiologic investigations, coronary angiography, and percutaneous coronary angioplasty.

PATIENT POPULATION

Table 22-1 summarizes the clinical characteristics of the study patients. Fourteen patients with incessant ventricular tachycardia unresponsive to medical therapy, and with a suitable coronary anatomy, were selected for transcoronary chemical ablation. The incessant character of the ventricular tachycardia precluded the use of antitachycardia pacing or a cardioverter defibrillator. In three patients an attempt to ablate with radiofrequency energy had failed. All patients except one had coronary artery disease, and the arrhythmia originated in an infarcted area.

PRETREATMENT

The chemical ablation procedure requires an intensive electrophysiologic study of the coronary anatomy and arrhythmia substrate. For the comfort of the patient, we routinely perform the procedures of coronary angiography and electrophysiologic investigation separately before the ablation procedure and it is helpful to us to be able to discuss all the therapeutic possibilities in advance.

Coronary Angiography

A routine diagnostic left ventriculogram and coronary angiogram was performed on each patient using routine 6 or 7 F Judkins catheters. Supplementary injections in steep cranial and caudal inclinations helped guide our search for the origin of all diagonal and obtuse marginal and septal branches.

Table 22-1. Clinical Characteristics of 14 Patients with Incessant Ventricular Tachycardia

N	Age	Sex	Clinical Diagnosis	Proc.	FU (months)	Death
1	61	M	Anteroinferior MI IVT	OK	56	—
2	62	M	Anterior MI IVT	OK	52	—
3	44	M	Anteroinferior MI IVT	OK	47	+(TX)
4	58	M	Anterior MI IVT	OK	2 weeks	+(PROC)
5	59	M	Anterior MI IVT	OK	11	+HF
6	62	M	Anterior MI IVT	OK	36	—
7	64	M	Inferoposterior MI IVT	OK	30	—
8	67	M	Idiopathic cardiomyopathy IVT	OK	21	—
9	68	M	Anteroinferior MI IVT	—	1	+
10	63	M	Inferoposterior MI IVT	OK (BYP)	3	+(SUD)
11	70	M	Posterior MI IVT	OK (PTCA)	15	—
12	64	M	Inferior MI IVT	—	14	—
13	61	F	Anterior MI IVT	OK (EPIC)	2	—
14	67	M	Anteroinferior MI IVT	OK	1	+HF

Abbreviations: M, male; F, female; MI, myocardial infarction; +, death; IVT, incessant ventricular tachycardia; PROC, procainamide; HF, heart failure, Tx, transplantation; EPIC, epicardial; PTCA, percutaneous transcoronary coronary angioplasty; SUD, sudden death; BYP, bypass surgery.

Electrophysiologic Study

In all patients ventricular tachycardia was induced by programmed electrical stimulation of the atria and ventricles according to a standard protocol, which consisted of delivery of progressively earlier single, double, and then triple premature stimuli to the point of ventricular refractoriness. Stimulation was applied first during sinus rhythm, and thereafter an eight-beat ventricular paced train at two or more basic cycle lengths (600 ms or 500 ms and 400 ms) was introduced. Sustained monomorphic ventricular tachycardia corresponding to the patient's clinical arrhythmia was induced; at this time endocardial mapping was performed with unipolar and bipolar recordings to localize the earliest activity during the arrhythmia.[9]

The site of origin of the tachycardia was localized by using the results of endocardial mapping, pace mapping, the morphology and axis of the QRS complex during clinical ventricular tachycardia, and the electrocardiographic location of myocardial infarction during sinus rhythm.[10,11]

ABLATION TECHNIQUE

Combining the information obtained from the routine coronary and left ventricular angiograms and the electrophysiologic study, we were able to identify the coronary artery supplying blood to the site of origin of the tachycardia. Only coronary arteries seen with standard angiographic techniques could be considered for possible selective catheterization. After we introduced a venous 7-F sheath into the femoral vein, a 6-F electrode catheter was advanced to the right ventricular apex. Then we introduced an 8-F

sheath into the femoral artery, and administered 10,000 U of heparin to the patient. An 8-F left or right Judkins coronary angioplasty guiding catheter was positioned in the ostium of the appropriate coronary artery.

The coronary branch supplying blood to the site of origin of the tachycardia was selectively catheterized with a 0.014″ diameter guidewire. After the guidewire was positioned, an infusion catheter (2.2 F with a radiopaque tip marker) (Cook Inc., Bloomington, IN, USA), or, when possible, an angioplasty catheter (Cordis Corp., Miami, FL, USA) was advanced over the guidewire and positioned in the artery. Proper positioning of the catheter was confirmed by injection of radiographic contrast material through the guiding catheter. When the infusion catheter was properly positioned, the guidewire was removed, and arrhythmia was induced by programmed ventricular stimulation. After iced saline or lidocaine was administered to reproduce the tachycardia, 96% ethanol was given at a dose of 1.5 to 6 ml until the tachycardia stopped. Thereafter, programmed electrical stimulation was repeated to assess whether the arrhythmia substrate had been destroyed; if not, a supplementary dose of ethanol was given. After the infusion catheter was withdrawn, repeat coronary arteriography was performed to assess continued patency or closure of the vessel as well as other branches of the coronary artery.

POSTOPERATIVE MANAGEMENT

Patients received continuous electrocardiographic monitoring during the remainder of their hospital stay. Serum creatine kinase isoenzymes were measured every 6 hours during the first postprocedure day. All patients also had repeat noninvasive assessment of left ventricular ejection fraction and regional wall motion after the procedure.

FOLLOW-UP AND RESULTS

All 14 patients in this study were treated with transcoronary chemical ablation for incessant ventricular tachycardia. The tachycardia-related coronary artery was identified in 12 of them. One patient collapsed during tachycardia, probably due to ischemia, when the artery (septal branch) was selectively catheterized with the guidewire, and the procedure was stopped. In another patient the tachycardia-related artery could not be catheterized for anatomic reasons; a subselective injection was not possible because there was too much myocardium in jeopardy. Ethanol was injected epicardially after thoracotomy. In summary, in our series catheter ablation was successfully performed in 12 of 14 patients.

On a short-term basis, incessant ventricular tachycardia recurred after 4 weeks in one patient due to the development of collateral circulation from a right ventricular and a conus branch to the ventricular septum. Chemical ablation through these two branches cured the tachycardia. On a long-term basis, three patients died of heart failure. In one of them, heart failure was provoked by procainamide, which his physician had prescribed to treat ventricular premature beats. Another patient died as a result of heart transplant rejection. The third patient died suddenly, probably of recurrent arrhythmia.

COMPLICATIONS

Selective catheterization of the coronary arteries and the administration of iced saline are not devoid of theoretical and practical complications. Minor complications, such as coronary spasm, caused by manipulation of catheters and guidewires and the injection of cold saline are frequent, especially in the right coronary artery. These complications can be prevented by administering nitrates and reducing the amount of iced saline. During the administration of ethanol all patients complained of chest pain, which was, however, short-lived, and was probably caused by the immediate destruction of nerve terminals. Since chemical ablation is aimed at destroying an anatomic arrhythmia substrate, a myocardial infarction can occur as a consequence of the rise in cardiac enzymes. The rise in enzyme levels we observed, however, was only moderate.

In another patient group, we performed an ablation of the atrioventricular node to control atrial fibrillation or flutter with fast ventricular rates; in one patient an inferior wall infarction developed due to occlusion of the right coronary artery, backflow of alcohol while the perfusion catheter was wedged. Patients with incessant ventricular tachycardia received enormous benefits from the destruction of a small myocardial area in terms of control of the arrhythmia and improvement in their functional capacity. Complete atrioventricular block occurred in two patients treated for incessant ventricular tachycardia; we anticipated this complication regarding the arrhythmia-related artery (first septal branch). Neal Kay and colleagues[12] describe myocardial rupture and tamponade in a patient whose operation was complicated by rupture and plication in the same region. The occurrence of Dressler syndrome has also been reported in a patient who received a relatively high dose of alcohol (8 ml) and required three ablation procedures.

COSTS

In Belgium the cost of the ablation procedure itself is 32,000BF (US$900). The average total cost of a chemical ablation is very reasonable, and 250,000BF, includes coronary angiography, pre- and postelectrophysiologic investigations, ablation procedure, catheter material, pre- and postechocardiography gated radionuclide ventriculogram, laboratory, hospital stay, and drugs.

CURRENT INDICATIONS

Most laboratories have attempted to perform transcoronary chemical ablation, but all of them, including our own, have reserved the technique (Fig. 22-2) to be used for those forms of incessant ventricular tachycardia that do not respond to medical therapy, including amiodarone, and for those patients in whom radiofrequency ablation was unsuccessful, but whose coronary anatomy is suitable for chemical ablation. Although we first reserved the technique for ventricular tachycardia after myocardial infarction, the procedure was successful in a patient with idiopathic cardiomyopathy and also in patients with ventricular tachycardia caused by Chagas' disease.[13]

DISCUSSION

Transcoronary chemical ablation of ventricular tachycardia is clearly feasible, and, although the technique is still experimental, it represents an im-

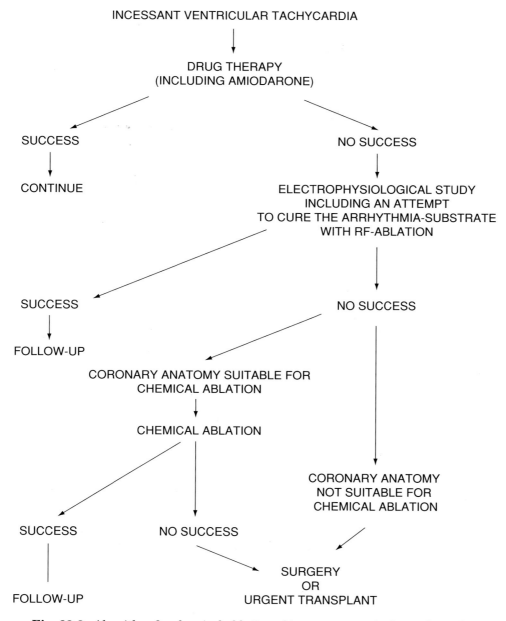

Fig. 22-2. Algorithm for chemical ablation of incessant ventricular tachycardia.

portant development in arrhythmia control and is of enormous value for patients with an incessant form of ventricular tachycardia that does not respond to any medical therapy. Indeed, these patients often have severely depressed left ventricular function, and a surgical procedure would put them at high risk for myocardium destruction, thoracotomy, cardiopulmonary bypass, and cardioplegia.[14] On the other hand, pacing or an implantable defibrillator cannot be offered to these patients because of the incessant character of the arrhythmia.[15]

Radiofrequency ablation is still experimental, be-

cause lesions created by this technique are small, an exact localization of the site of origin or pathway of the tachycardia is required. Also, many of these patients have a thickened and fibrotic endocardial surface that probably prevents radiofrequency energy from creating a sufficiently large lesion to destroy the arrhythmogenic substrate. These two factors may account for the relatively poor results achieved with radiofrequency ablation in patients with ventricular tachycardia after myocardial infarction.

The risks and benefits of chemical ablation have to be compared with the risks of surgery or radiofrequency ablation. We must keep in mind that incessant ventricular tachycardia is often a complication of severe left ventricular dysfunction, and the ablation procedure can be considered as a bridge to transplant.[16–19]

For nonincessant recurrent forms of ventricular tachycardia occurring late after myocardial infarction, chemical ablation has never been given a fair chance to prove its potential. An exception was the study by Neal Kay and colleagues,[12] which documented a 60% success rate, using a very conservative approach. Since most laboratories reserve the technique as a last resort, its use is obviously influenced by a negative bias. The a priori probability of success in these "last resort" cases would necessarily be lower than if the technique had been used at an earlier stage or even as first choice. In spite of this very conservative approach, the results remain good, and

actually very good, when one considers the type of patients who have undergone the procedure.

While transcoronary chemical ablation of ventricular tachycardia has the same electrophysiologic background as is used for other ablation techniques, the anatomic background is very peculiar and offers many more possibilities than radiofrequency, direct current shock, or surgical resection techniques. First, transcoronary administration of iced saline allows the clinician to test whether the site chosen (the so-called "tachycardia-related coronary artery") is the correct one, thereby avoiding unnecessary damage by administering the ethanol directly. Second, because of the transcoronary administration of the chemical, a transmural lesion is created that avoids the problems related to intramurally or epicardially located reentry circuits. Third, even when exact data are missing, transcoronary ethanol ablation appears

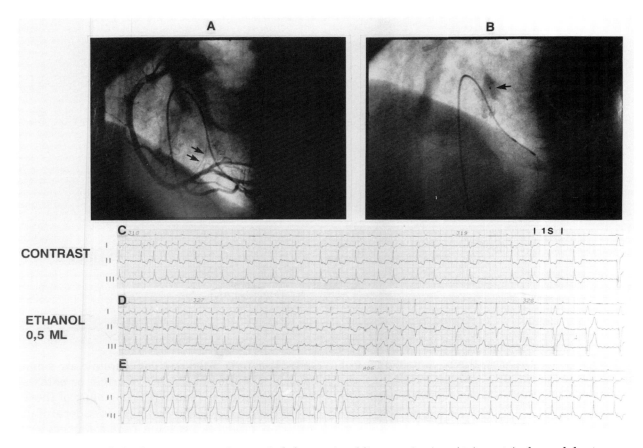

Fig. 22-3. (A) Right coronary angiogram in left anterior oblique projection. Atrioventricular nodal artery is indicated by *arrow*. **(B)** Selective catheterization of atrioventricular nodal artery with a 2.2 F catheter (*arrow*). Contrast material is given showing myocardial staining and no backflow. **(C)** Effects of contrast material on ventricular rate during atrial fibrillation. Transient complete atrioventricular block and pacemaker rhythm is observed in the right part of the electrographic strip. Leads I, II, and III are shown. **(D)** Effects of administration of 0.5 ml 96% ethanol. After series of premature ventricular beats, complete atrioventricular block and pacemaker rhythm occur. **(E)** Escape rhythm after interruption of pacing.

to cause a lesion that is sufficient in size—larger than the lesions created by radiofrequency energy—but does not reach the dimensions of an endocardial resection. In this sense, transcoronary chemical ablation, when correctly executed, may be the only technique to produce sufficient, but not excessive, myocardial damage. Because of the effects of iced saline, it is also the only technique that allows the ablation site to be targeted before the definitive destruction of the area is undertaken. This technique deserves a fair chance to prove (or disprove) its value in the setting of sustained ventricular tachycardia that occurs late after myocardial infarction.

Important questions still to be answered are (1) how often will the new collateral blood supply lead to recurrence of the arrhythmia and (2) whether the lesion created by ethyl alcohol is homogeneous and will not result in new arrhythmic strands or pathways. Improvement in catheter and radiologic techniques holds promise that yet smaller vessels can be cannulated, resulting in a greater selectivity for damage and enabling us to reach an infarct-related vessel in retrograde fashion from collaterals. This will help to reduce the amount of myocardial damage while still obtaining the desired effect.

Finally, it must be realized that transcoronary chemical ablation requires specialized teamwork where the most refined electrophysiology and angioplasty techniques are used. This procedure should not be performed in centers that do not have all these resources.

TRANSCORONARY ABLATION OF THE ATRIOVENTRICULAR NODE

Before the era of radiofrequency ablation, alcohol ablation was also performed on the atrioventricular node by injection, using the same technique—96% ethanol—in the atrioventricular-nodal artery (Fig. 22-3). We studied 19 patients in this setting and were able to ablate 12 of the 14 patients in whom the atrioventricular nodal artery originated from the right coronary artery, but in only 1 of the 5 patients in whom the artery was a branch of the circumflex coronary artery. Technical problems, especially catheter design, were the major shortcomings. Since the clinical success rate of radiofrequency ablation is much higher than that of chemical ablation, we abandoned the technique.

REFERENCES

1. Ellman Ba, Parkhill BJ, Marcus PB: Renal ablation with absolute ethanol: mechanism of action. Invest Radiol 1984;19:416–23

2. Chilson DA, Peigh PS, Molomed Y et al: Chemical ablation of ventricular tachycardia in the dos. Am Heart J 1986;111:1113–8

3. Inoue H, Waller BF, Zipes DP: Intracoronary ethyl alcohol or phenol injection ablates aconitine-induced ventricular tachycardia in dogs. J Am Coll Cardiol 1987;10:1342

4. Brugada P, Lemery R, Taljic M et al: Treatment of patients with ventricular tachycardia or fibrillation: first lessons from the "parallel study." In: Brugada P, Wellens HJJ, eds.: Cardiac Arrhythmias: Where to Go From Here? Mt. Kisco, NY: Futura Publishing, 1987:457–70

5. Brugada P, de Swart H, Smeets J: Transcoronary chemical ablation of ventricular tachycardia. Circulation 1989;29:475–82

6. Brugada P, de Swart H, Smeets J, Wellens HJJ: Transcoronary chemical ablation of atrioventricular conduction. Circulation 1990;81:757–61

7. Friedman PL, Steward JR, Fenoglio JJ Jr: Survival of subendocardial Purkinje fibers after extensive myocardial infarction in dogs. Circ Res 1973;33:597–611

8. Nicolosi A, Weng ZC, Detwiler PW: Transcatheter coronary artery injection of ethanol in swine. Circulation 1989;80:II40

9. Miller J, Harken AH, Hargrove C: Pattern of endocardial activation during sustained ventricular tachycardia. J Am Coll Cardiol 1985;6:1280–7

10. Coumel P: Diagnostic significance of the QRS form in patients with ventricular tachycardia. In Barold SJ, ed. Lead Electrocardiography. Philadelphia: WB Saunders; 1987:527–40

11. Josephson ME, Horowitz LN, Farshidi A: Recurrent sustained ventricular tachycardia: II. Endocardial mapping. Circulation 1978;57:440–7

12. Neal Kay G, Epstein AE, Bubien RS: Intracoronary ethanol ablation for the treatment of recurrent sustained ventricular tachycardia. J Am Coll Cardiol 1992;19:159–68

13. De Paola AA, Gomes JA, Miyamoto MH: Transcoronary chemical ablation of ventricular tachycardia in chronic chagasic myocarditis. J Am Coll Cardiol 1992;20:480–2

14. Harken AH, Josephson ME: Surgical Management of ventricular tachycardia. In Josephson ME, Wellens HJJ, eds. Tachycardias: Mechanisms, Diagnosis and Treatment. Philadelphia: Lea & Febiger; 1984:475–87

15. Mirowski M, Reid PR, Watkins L: Clinical treatment of life-threatening ventricular tachyarrhythmias with the automatic implantable defrillator. Am Heart J 1981;102:265–70

16. Hartzler GO: Electrode catheter ablation of refractory focal ventricular tachycardia. J Am Coll Cardiol 1983;21:1107–13

17. Verna E, Repetto S, Saveri C: Myocardial dissection following successful chemical ablation of ventricular tachycardia. Eur Heart J 1992;13:844–6

18. Wit AL, Dillon S, Ursell PC: Influences of anisotropic tissue structure on reentrant ventricular tachycardia. In: Brugada P, Wellens HJJ, eds. Cardiac Arrhythmias: Where To Go From Here? Mount Kisco, NY: Futura Publishing, 1987:27–50

19. Zipes DP, Heger JJ, Miles WM: Early experience with an implantable cardioverter. N Engl J Med 1984:485–90

23 | Pulmonary Valve in Children

P. Syamasundar Rao

Pulmonary valve stenosis may occur as an isolated congenital cardiac anomaly or may be seen in association with other congenital cardiac anomalies. The treatment approach has been surgical relief of the stenosis by direct enlargement (valvotomy) of the constricted site, especially in isolated obstructions, or to bypass the obstruction by systemic-to-pulmonary artery anastomosis if total surgical correction is not feasible. Since the description by Kan and associates[1] of the application of balloon dilatation techniques in children, we and others have used this technique to relieve congenital and acquired obstructive lesions in infants and children. The role of balloon dilatation in the management of right ventricular outflow tract obstructions is examined in this chapter in two sections: isolated valvar pulmonary stenosis and pulmonary stenosis with ventricular right-to-left shunts.

ISOLATED PULMONARY VALVE STENOSIS

Valvular pulmonary stenosis constitutes 7.5 to 9.0% of all congenital heart defects. The pathologic features of pulmonary stenosis vary, but the most commonly found pathology is what is described as the "dome-shaped" pulmonary valve. The "fused" pulmonary valve leaflets protrude from their attachment into the pulmonary artery as a conical or dome-shaped structure. The size of the orifice of the pulmonary valve may vary from a pinhole to several millimeters, most commonly central in location, but can be eccentric. Raphae, presumably representing fused

valve leaflet commissures, extend from the stenotic valve orifice to a varying extent down into the base of the dome-shaped valve. The number of raphae varies from none to seven. Other, less common pathologic variants include unicommissural, bicuspid, and tricuspid pulmonary valves. Hypoplastic pulmonary annulus and valve leaflets and dysplastic pulmonary valve leaflets are also present in a small but definite number of cases of pulmonic stenosis.

Children with pulmonic stenosis usually present with asymptomatic murmurs, although they can present with signs of systemic venous congestion (usually interpreted as congestive heart failure) due to severe right ventricular dysfunction or cyanosis because of right-to-shunt across the atrial septum. Clinical findings of ejection systolic click and ejection systolic murmur at the left upper sternal border, right ventricular hypertrophy on an electrocardiogram, prominent main pulmonary artery segment on a chest radiograph, and increased Doppler flow velocity in the main pulmonary artery are characteristic for this anomaly. Until recently, surgical valvotomy was the only treatment available, but, at the present time, relief of pulmonary valve obstruction can be accomplished by balloon valvuloplasty.

In the early 1950s Rubio-Alvarez and Limon-Lason described a technique by which pulmonic valve stenosis could be relieved via a catheter; they used a ureteral catheter with a wire. More recently, Kan and her associates[1] used a static dilatation technique (similar to that used by Dotter and Judkins and Gruntzig and their colleagues for dilating femoral, renal, and coronary arteries) in which they introduced a deflated balloon across the pulmonic valve and inflated the balloon; the radial forces of balloon inflation produced relief of pulmonary valve obstruction.

Technique

The diagnosis and assessment of the pulmonary valve obstruction are made by the usual clinical, radiographic, electrocardiographic, and echo-Doppler data. Once a moderate-to-severe obstruction is diagnosed, cardiac catheterization and cineangiography are performed percutaneously to confirm the clinical impression and to consider for balloon dilatation of the pulmonary valve. The indications for catheter intervention (described below) and for surgical intervention are usually the same.[2]

Informed Consent

Despite a decade of use, the balloon dilatation procedures are relatively new and sometimes are considered experimental. It is important that a full explanation of the balloon dilatation procedure be given to the parents and to the patients old enough to understand. Potential complications associated with the procedure should also be explained. The advantages and disadvantages of both surgical and balloon therapy should be mentioned. Such informed consent is essential, especially in view of the fact that acute complications can occur, and long-term effects of the balloon procedure are not yet available.

Patient Preparation

In neonates and infants, a neutral thermal environment, a normal acid-base state, normoglycemia, and normocalcemia should be maintained by appropriate monitoring and correction, if needed. In the neonate with ductal-dependent pulmonary blood flow (e.g., critical pulmonary stenosis), the ductus arteriosus should be kept patent by an infusion of prostaglandin E_1 (PGE$_1$): 0.05 to 0.1 μg kg min. PGE$_1$ may be quite helpful in stabilizing the infant and restoring normal metabolic status. In addition, complete occlusion of circulation during balloon inflation may be better tolerated in the presence of an open ductus.

All infants and children should have blood available before initiating the balloon dilatation procedure so that blood transfusion may be given for significant blood loss or for use during surgery, if required. An intravenous line should be established before the procedure so as to serve as access for infusion of fluids and medications, should they be re-

quired during and after the procedure. Surgical standby is no longer recommended.

Sedation and Anesthesia

We usually perform balloon dilatation with the patient sedated with a mixture of meperidine (1.0 mg/kg, maximum 50 mg), promethazine (0.6 mg/kg, maximum 15 mg), and chlorpromazine (0.6 mg/kg, maximum 15 mg), given intramuscularly. If necessary, this can be supplemented with intermittent doses of midazolam (0.1 mg/kg, given intravenously). Other workers use ketamine or general anesthesia. Although there is no consensus with regard to the type of analgesia/anesthesia, we have not encountered significant problems with the use of sedative mixture for angioplasty/valvuloplasty procedures in children. We have performed more than 500 such procedures, and only three of these children required additional sedation with ketamine. However, institutional practices should be respected with regard to the type of sedation used and whether general anesthesia is employed.

Procedure

A complete hemodynamic and angiographic study should be performed first. Once balloon dilatation is decided upon, the following is undertaken:

1. A 4- to 7-F multi-A-2 (Cordis) catheter is introduced percutaneously into the femoral vein and advanced across the pulmonic valve, and then into the left pulmonary artery. Alternatively a 5- or 6-F right coronary catheter may be used.
2. A 0.014″–0.035″ J-shaped or straight extrastiff guidewire is passed through the catheter into the distal left pulmonary artery.
3. A 4- to 9-F balloon dilatation catheter is advanced over the guidewire, and the balloon is positioned across the pulmonary valve.
4. The balloon is inflated with diluted contrast material (Fig. 23-1) to approximately 3 to 5 atm of pressure. I recommend monitoring pressure of inflation with the help of any of the commercially available pressure gauges. The recommended duration of inflation is 5 seconds. Usually a total of three to four balloon inflations are performed, 5 minutes apart. We use a double-balloon technique (two balloons simultaneously inflated across the stenotic region) when the valve annulus is too large to dilate with a commercially available single balloon.
5. An arterial line (3 F) is inserted into the femoral artery to monitor blood pressure during the proce-

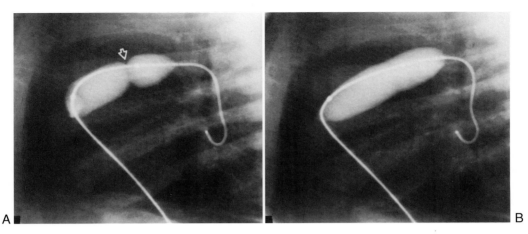

Fig. 23-1. Selected cineradiographic frames of a balloon dilatation catheter placed across the pulmonic valve. **(A)** Note waisting of the balloon (*arrows*) during the initial phases of balloon inflation, which is **(B)** almost completely abolished during the later phases of balloon inflation.

dure. Oxygen saturation by pulse oximetry and heart rate by electrocardiogram are also monitored. (See the section on "Monitoring" for further details.)

6. We do not routinely heparinize right heart balloon dilatations. However, heparinization is advisable if there is evidence for intracardiac right-to-left shunting. If we chose heparinization, a single intravenous dose of heparin, 100 U/kg (maximum 2,500 U), is used. This is administered immediately before introduction of balloon dilatation catheter. If the procedure is prolonged (>1 hour following the introduction of the balloon dilatation catheter), an additional amount of heparin (one-half the above dose) is administered. The heparin is not continued, nor its effect reversed, after the procedure. The major reason for heparin administration is to prevent clot formation on the balloon. Thrombus formation on the deflated balloon is a potential hazard in all balloon dilatation procedures; such a thrombus could dislodge, paradoxically embolize, and produce cerebrovascular accident. Therefore, it is prudent to anticoagulate adequately if there is intracardiac right-to-left (usually a patent foramen ovale or an atrial septal defect) shunt.

7. Measurement of gradient across the pulmonic valve and angiographic demonstration of relief of obstruction are performed. Recordings of heart rate, systemic pressure, and cardiac index before and after balloon dilatation are made to ensure that change in pressure gradient is not related to change in cardiac index but is indeed related to the procedure.

Other aspects of importance for successfully accomplishing balloon angioplasty are as follows:

1. *Difficult femoral venous access.* Sometimes, it may be difficult to cannulate the femoral vein percutaneously either because of technical problems or because of femoral vein thrombosis secondary to previous catheterization or surgery. Cutdown and isolation of saphenous vein-femoral vein junction may be performed, and catheterization and balloon valvuloplasty can be accomplished via saphenous venous bulb. When femoral venous access is not possible, balloon pulmonary valvuloplasty may be performed by the axillary venous or internal jugular venous approach. The latter two approaches are also useful in the presence of infrahepatic interruption of the inferior vena cava with azygos or hemiazygos continuation.

2. *Passing an end-hole catheter across the pulmonic valve.* This may be difficult in some patients, particularly young children and neonates. In such occasions, we employ several maneuvers:

   a. Use end-hole catheter (usually a multi-A-2), position it just underneath the pulmonary valve, and advance the floppy end of a straight guidewire through the tip of the catheter into the main pulmonary artery.

   b. Use a balloon-wedge catheter, position it just beneath the pulmonic valve, and quickly deflate the balloon and advance the catheter into the main pulmonary artery. Failing this, use a guidewire, as described earlier.

   c. Use flexible, steerable coronary guidewires or Nitinol wires through an end-hole catheter.

   d. We have encountered one child in whom we could not advance any catheter across the right ventricular infundibulum because of severe infundibular constriction. In this child, administration of propranolol (0.1 mg/kg IV slowly) made it possible to pass a catheter across the pulmonary valve and eventually perform balloon pulmonary valvuloplasty.

3. *Choice of size of balloon dilatation catheter.* The current recommendations are to use a balloon that is 1.2 to 1.4 times the size of the pulmonary valve annulus. These recommendations are formulated on the basis of immediate[3] and follow-up results.[4,5] Balloons larger than 1.5 times the size of the pulmonary valve annulus are not recommended because of potential damage to the right ventricular outflow tract caused by use of large balloons. However, it may be advisable to use a large balloon to produce a balloon/annulus ratio of 1.5 when pulmonary valve dysplasia is present. When the pulmonary valve annulus is too large to dilate with a single balloon, valvuloplasty with simultaneous inflation of two balloons across the pulmonary valve annulus (Fig. 23-2) should be performed. When two balloons are used, the following formula is used to calculate the effective balloon size:[4]

$$\frac{D_1 + D_2 + \pi\,(D_1/2 + D_2/2)}{\pi}$$

where D_1 and D_2 are diameters of the balloons used. Although we do not believe that double-balloon technique is superior to single-balloon technique, it reduces injury to the femoral veins because smaller catheters can be used.

Some workers have advocated bifoil and trefoil balloons with the idea that there will be forward flow around the balloon during balloon inflation. While such attempts to allow forward flow during balloon inflation are laudable, I do not believe that there will be any significant forward flow in view of the fact that the balloons used for pulmonary valve dilatation are larger than the valve annulus.

4. *Guidewire* On occasion, it may be difficult to advance the balloon angioplasty catheter across the pulmonic valve. It is important to avoid kinking or looping of the guidewire to prevent such a problem. Replacement of the guidewire with an extrastiff wire, if such was not used initially, may be helpful.

5. *Predilation with smaller balloon catheter.* Sometimes it may not be feasible to advance an appropriate-sized balloon dilatation catheter across the pulmonic valve even after having a guidewire across it. In such situations, we use smaller 4 to 6 mm balloons on a 3.5, 4- or 5-F catheter initially to predilate and then use larger, more appropriate-sized balloons (Fig. 23-3). This technique is also helpful when dilating very severely stenotic pulmonary valves and in small infants.

6. *Advancing the guidewire in the neonate.* In the neonate, the technique is much more difficult than in an older child. Advancing the guidewire from the main pulmonary artery into the descending aorta through the patent ductus arteriosus (Fig. 23-4) may give more torque and stability to the guidewire for the balloon catheter to be positioned across the stenotic pulmonary valve (Fig. 23-3D).

Monitoring

During the balloon dilatation procedure, there is complete or almost complete obstruction to blood flow. This causes a fall in systemic pressure. Reflex

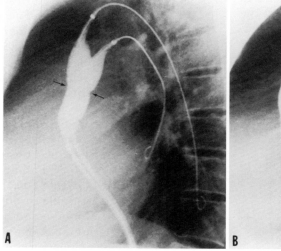
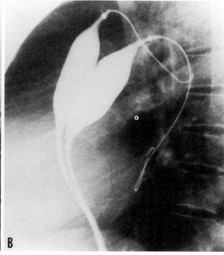

Fig. 23-2. Selected cine frames of two balloon catheters placed across the pulmonary valve showing **(A)** waisting of the balloons (*arrows*) during the initial phases of balloon inflation, which is **(B)** completely abolished after incomplete inflation of the balloons. (From Rao,[2] with permission.)

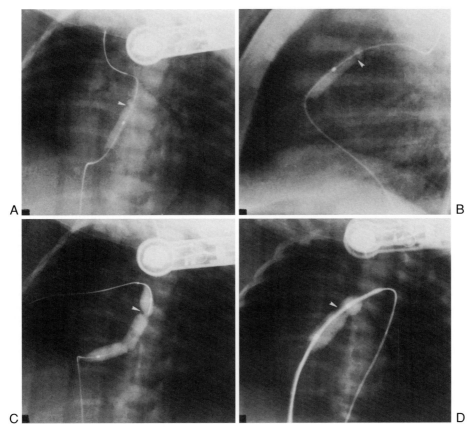

Fig. 23-3. Selected cineradiographic frames demonstrating use of progressively larger balloons in a 1-day-old infant with critical pulmonary stenosis. Initially, a 0.014″ coronary guidewire (*GW*) was advanced into the pulmonary artery via a 5-F multi-A2 catheter positioned in the right ventricular outflow tract. A 3.5-F catheter carrying a 4-mm balloon was positioned across the pulmonary valve. **(A)** Posteroanterior and **(B)** lateral view cine frames showing waisting (*arrows*) of the balloon during the initial phases of balloon inflation. After two additional inflations, this balloon was replaced with **(C)** a 5-F catheter carrying a 6-mm balloon and finally **(D)** a 5-F catheter carrying an 8-mm balloon.

bradycardia during balloon inflation is also common. Premature beats are also commonly seen, presumably related to ventricular stimulation. In patients with intracardiac right-to-left shunting, hypoxemia may result from right heart dilatation procedures. Most of the effects described above are transient and revert back to normal following balloon deflation. However, monitoring the patients is generally recommended to document transient nature of the side effects and to intervene if the abnormalities are severe or do not return to normal. Monitoring of (1) heart rate by electrocardiogram, (2) systemic pressure via an arterial line, and (3) arterial oxygen saturation by pulse oximetry is generally performed. If there is persistence of these abnormalities, the balloon should be withdrawn from the site of balloon dilatation. Short duration of balloon inflation (5 seconds) is likely to result in transient effects and prompt recovery. In our total experience with balloon

dilatation—more than 500 patients—we had only two patients requiring brief cardiac massage. One was a child with severe pulmonary stenosis, in whom, because of technical difficulties, the balloon could not be rapidly deflated, and extreme bradycardia ensued. Brief cardiac massage and withdrawal of balloon into the inferior vena cava resulted in prompt restoration to normal. The second patient was an infant with aortic stenosis who sustained ventricular fibrillation. Removal of the balloon from across the aortic valve, brief cardiac massage, and administration of lidocaine (Xylocaine) were rapidly undertaken. The rhythm reverted to normal before countershock was considered. Meticulous attention to the details of the technique is necessary during the procedure to minimize the complication rate. Limited monitoring, as described above, is adequate to successfully carry out the balloon dilatation procedure.

After balloon valvuloplasty, we monitor the pa-

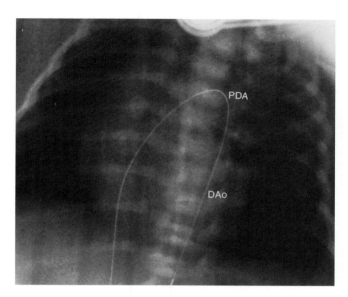

Fig. 23-4. The guidewire was advanced from the main pulmonary across the patent ductus arteriosus (*PDA*) into the descending aorta (DAO). This gave greater stability while positioning a balloon catheter across the stenotic pulmonary valve (Fig. 23-3D).

tient in an intermediate care setting; the electrocardiogram is continuously monitored; vital signs (temperature, pulses, respiration, and blood pressure) are measured intermittently, and perfusion of the extremity is checked. The intravenous line that was started before the procedure is maintained. An echo-Doppler study is performed several hours after the procedure to assess the adequacy of the dilatation procedure. The patient is gradually allowed to re-

cover from sedation and feeding initiated, starting with clear liquids. The patients are monitored overnight and discharged home on the morning following the balloon dilatation procedure.

Other Issues Related to the Technique

Balloon Size

Radtke's group[3] and our group[4,5] evaluated the influence of balloon size on the results of pulmonary valvuloplasty and recommended a balloon/pulmonary valve annulus ratio of 1.2 to 1.4. Such recommendations are arbitrary and were based on (1) small number of patients;[3,4] (2) no follow-up results;[3] or (3) follow-up results on a few patients.[4] Our experience with 64 consecutive balloon dilatation procedures performed in 56 patients with isolated valvar pulmonic stenosis and 39 follow-up catheterizations in 36 patients was reviewed to examine this issue.[5–7] Five repeat valvuloplasty procedures were performed at follow-up catheterization, and three patients had valvuloplasty sequentially with balloons, resulting in increasingly larger balloon/annulus ratios.

First, the 56 patients who received 64 valvuloplasty procedures were divided into two groups: in Group I, the balloon/annulus ratio was 1.0 or less, 12 dilatations; and in Group II, the balloon/annulus ratio was more than 1.0, 52 dilatations. The two groups had similar ($P > .1$) prevalvuloplasty valvar

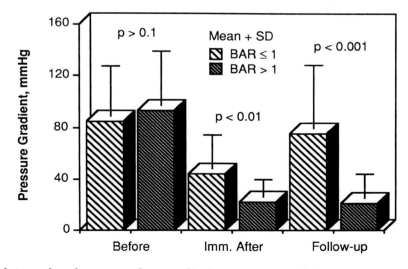

Fig. 23-5. Peak-to-peak pulmonary valvar gradients were compared between two groups of patients. Both the groups with balloon/annulus ratios ≤1.0 and >1.0 had similar prevalvuloplasty gradients, while higher gradients were found in the smaller balloon group both immediately following balloon valvuloplasty ($P < .01$) and at follow-up ($P < .001$). (From Rao,[2] with permission.)

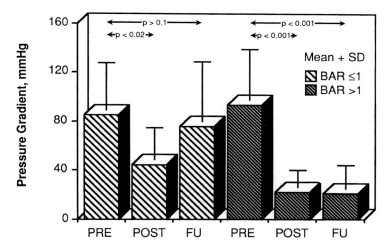

Fig. 23-6. Results of balloon pulmonary valvuloplasty in patient groups with balloon/annulus ratios ≤1.0 and >1.0. Note statistically significant ($P < .02$ and $< .01$) fall in peak-to-peak gradients immediately after valvuloplasty in both groups. In the groups with balloon/annulus ratios ≤1.0, the gradient returned toward prevalvuloplasty values ($P > .1$). (From Rao,[2] with permission.)

gradients (84.3 ± 39.2 vs 92.8 ± 42.1 mmHg) (Fig. 23-5). Immediately after valvuloplasty, there was a significant reduction in pulmonary valve gradient (Fig. 23-6) in both Group I (84.3 ± 29.2 vs 43.6 ± 26.8 mmHg; $P < .02$) and Group II (92.8 ± 42.1 vs 22.4 ± 13.6 mmHg; $P < .001$), although there was a greater fall in the gradient in Group II with larger balloons (Fig. 23-5). On intermediate-term follow-up (which ranged between 6 and 34 months), residual pulmonary valve gradients were significantly lower ($P < .001$) in Group II (20.8 ± 18.5 mmHg) than in Group I (75.0 ± 49.4 mmHg), suggesting restenosis in Group I with small balloons (Fig. 23-5). At follow-up, repeat balloon valvuloplasty was required in four of Group I patients and only one from Group II ($P < .005$) (Table 23-1). Similarly, a higher ($P < .005$)

number of patients with residual pulmonary valve gradient in excess of 30 mmHg were present in Group I than in Group II (Table 23-1). These data suggest that, although good immediate results are seen with either small or large balloons, balloons larger than the pulmonary valve annulus produce more sustained relief of pulmonary stenosis.

Second, the balloon/annulus ratio cutoff point was increased to 1.2, and balloon valvuloplasties were divided into another two groups: in Group III, the ratio was 1.2 or less, 32 balloon dilatations (mean ratio: 1.03 ± 0.13); and in Group IV, the ratio was more than 1.2, also 32 balloon dilatations (mean ratio: 1.43 ± 0.13). Both groups had similar ($P > .1$) prevalvuloplasty gradients (Fig. 23-7), and significant ($P < .001$) reduction in pulmonary valve gradients both

Table 23-1. Prevalence of Repeat Valvuloplasty and Significant Residual Gradients in Various Groups

Groups	No. of Patients Needing Repeat Valvuloplasty	P*	No. of Patients With Pulmonary Valve Gradient >30 mmHg	P*
Group wit B/A ratio of ≤1.0 N = 7	4	.002	5	.001
Group with B/A ratio >1.0 N = 32	1		2	
Group with B/A ratio of ≤1.2 N = 32	5	.05	7	.001
Group with B/A ratio >1.2 N = 32	0		0	

Abbreviations: B/A ratio, balloon/annulus ratio; *N*, number of patients with intermediate-term follow-up catheterization.
* Fisher's exact test.
(Modified from Rao PS,[6] with permission.)

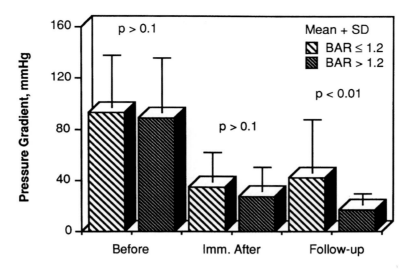

Fig. 23-7. Comparison of gradients similar to Figure 23-5, but the balloon/annulus ratios were ≤ 1.2 and > 1.2. Note similar gradients ($P > .1$) prior to and immediately after valvuloplasty. However, at follow-up, the gradients were higher ($P < .01$) in the group with balloon/annulus ratios of ≤1.2 than the group balloon/annulus ratios <1.2. (From Rao,[2] with permission.)

immediately after valvuloplasty and on follow-up (Fig. 23-8). However, the follow-up gradients in Group IV, with larger balloons, were lower ($P < .01$) than those in Group III, with small balloons (Fig. 23-7). Five patients from Group III required repeat balloon dilatation at follow-up, while none from Group IV required repeat valvuloplasty ($P < .001$) (Table 23-1). Also, seven patients from Group III had gradients above 30 mmHg, while none in Group IV had a gradient that high on follow-up ($P < .001$) (Table 23-1). Based on these data patients who have valvuloplasty with balloons smaller than 1.2 times

the pulmonary valve annulus are at significant risk for residual pulmonary stenosis on follow-up; therefore, balloons of this size are not recommended.

Third, the results of balloon valvuloplasty with a balloon/annulus ratio of 1.21 to 1.5 (Group V) were compared with those in which the ratio was greater than 1.5 (Group VI) because balloons larger than 1.5 times the size of the valve annulus are reported to produce damage to the right ventricular outflow tract. The 23 patients in Group V had a mean balloon/annulus ratio of 1.36 ± 0.08, and the 9 patients in Group VI had a mean ratio of 1.6 ± 0.09. The

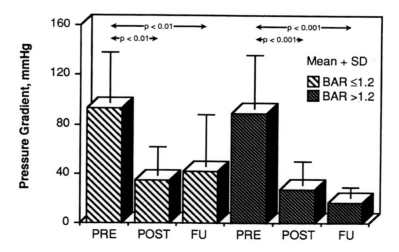

Fig. 23-8. Results of valvuloplasty depicted in a manner similar to that shown in Figure 23-6 but with balloon/annulus ratio groups were ≤1.2 and >1.2. Note significant ($P < .01$) fall in the gradients in both groups immediately following valvuloplasty and at follow-up. The residual gradients were higher in the smaller balloon/annulus ratio group. (From Rao,[2] with permission.)

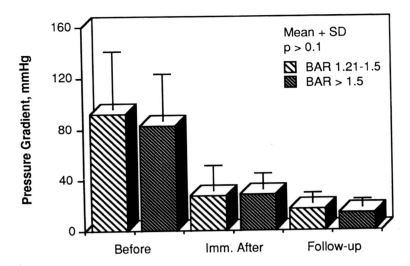

Fig. 23-9. Comparison of peak-to-peak systolic pressure gradients across the pulmonic valve in a manner similar to that done in Figures 23-5 and 23-7 but for balloon/annulus ratio groups of 1.21 to 1.5 vs >1.5. Note that the gradients are similar ($P > .1$) prior to and immediately after valvuloplasty and at follow-up, signifying that the group with >1.5 is not better off than the group with balloon/annulus ratios of 1.21 to 1.5 with regard to residual gradients. (From Rao,[2] with permission.)

pulmonary valve gradients were similar ($P > .1$) (Fig. 23-9) before valvuloplasty in both groups. Significant ($P < .001$) reduction of gradient occurred in both groups immediately after valvuloplasty as well as at follow-up catheterization (Fig. 23-10). Residual pulmonary valvar gradients immediately after balloon dilatation and on follow-up (Fig. 23-9) were similar ($P > .1$). None of the patients in either group required repeat balloon dilatation, nor was there any patient with residual pulmonary valvar gradient in excess of 30 mmHg. These data signify that balloons larger than 1.5 times the size of the pulmonary valve annu-

lus do not offer any advantage over the balloons with a ratio of 1.21 to 1.5.

The data presented in this section indicate that balloons larger than 1.2 times the diameter of the pulmonary valve annulus should be used for pulmonary valvuloplasty if restenosis is to be prevented and that there is no advantage to the use of balloons larger than 1.5 times the size of the pulmonary valve annulus. Therefore, balloons that are 1.2 to 1.5 times the diameter of the pulmonary valve annulus are most ideal for relief of pulmonary stenosis and are recommended.

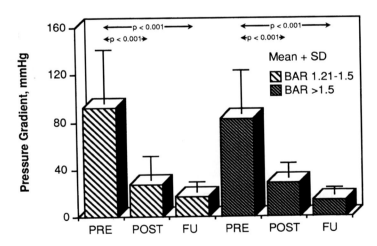

Fig. 23-10. Results of balloon valvuloplasty in the groups with balloon/annulus ratios of 1.21 to 1.5 and > 1.5. Note excellent fall in gradients ($P < .001$) both immediately after and at follow-up in both groups. (From Rao PS,[2] with permission.)

ticularly the use of balloon/annulus ratio of 1.2 to 1.5, should result in better results than previously documented. Further refinement of the catheters and technique may further reduce the complication rate and prevalence of restenosis.

The major mechanism by which pulmonary valve

Pulmonary Valve Dilatation

Indications

The indications for balloon pulmonary valvuloplasty that we have used[24,25] were cardiac defects not amenable to surgical correction at the age and size at the

of such gradients appears to be more frequent with increasing age and severity of valve stenosis. Some of these children may develop systemic or suprasystemic pressures in the right ventricle because of hyperreactivity of the right ventricular infundibulum and may need β-blockade. The infundibular stenosis regresses to a great degree at follow-up. The poten-

sure at follow-up was 75% of prevalvuloplasty measurements. The question to be asked is whether this modest reduction in the right ventricular pressure is worth the risk, morbidity, and expense associated with cardiac catheterization and balloon pulmonary valvuloplasty. The answer (my answer) is "no," especially in view of a benign natural course of the disease

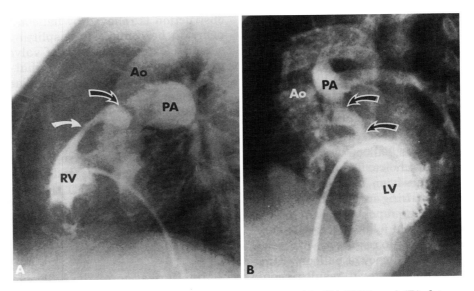

Fig. 23-28. Selected cineangiographic frames from patients with **(A)** TOF, and **(B)** d transposition of the great arteries, demonstrating two sites of pulmonary outflow obstruction (*two arrows*). When the pulmonary valve obstruction is relieved by balloon valvuloplasty, the subvalvar obstruction remains and prevents flooding of the lungs. *Ao,* aorta; *LV,* left ventricle; *PA,* pulmonary artery; *RV,* right ventricle. (From Rao et al.,[25] with permission.)

time of presentation but, at the same time, requiring palliation for pulmonary oligemia. Symptoms related to hypoxemia and polycythemia are indications for intervention. Hypoplasia of the pulmonary valve ring, main or branch pulmonary arteries, is another indication even if symptoms are not present. The presence of two or more sites of obstruction to pulmonary blood flow (Fig. 23-28) was considered a prerequisite when employing balloon valvuloplasty because if valvar stenosis is the sole obstruction, relief of such

an obstruction may result in a marked increase in pulmonary blood flow and elevation of pulmonary artery pressure and resistance.

Technique

The technique of balloon pulmonary valvuloplasty in this group of patients is similar to that used in isolated valvar pulmonic stenosis described earlier in this chapter, although, at times, it may be more diffi-

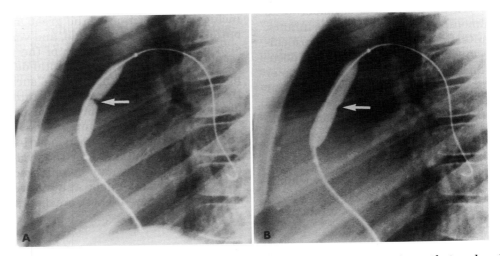

Fig. 23-29. Selected cineradiographic (lateral view) frames of a balloon dilatation catheter placed across the pulmonic valve in an infant with TOF. **(A)** Note waisting of the balloon during the initial phases of balloon inflation, which is **(B)** almost completely abolished during the later phases of balloon inflation. (From Rao et al.,[25] with permission.)

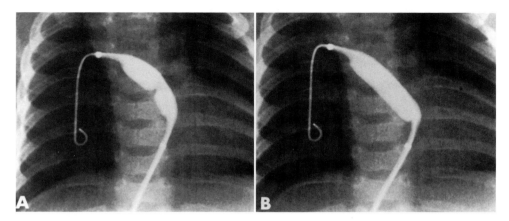

Fig. 23-30. Selected cineradiographic (posteroanterior view) frames demonstrating the position of a balloon dilatation catheter across the pulmonic valve in a patient with TOF. **(A)** Note the indentation (waist) of the balloon, which **(B)** disappeared after full inflation. Although we prefer to place the guidewire in the left pulmonary artery, balloon valvuloplasty can also be successfully performed with the guidewire positioned in the right pulmonary artery, as in the illustrated case. (From Rao,[2] with permission.)

cult to accomplish balloon valvuloplasty in this group than in simple pulmonary valve stenosis group. Examples of balloon catheters across the pulmonary valve is shown in Figures 23-29 to 23-31. A balloon size that is 1.2 to 1.4 times the size of the pulmonary valve annulus is recommended.

Immediate Results

Balloon pulmonary valvuloplasty for infants with cyanotic congenital heart defects with pulmonary oligemia was used by us and others to augment pulmonary blood flow, and the results have been reviewed in detail elsewhere.[14] Our experience with this procedure, including that previously reported,[24,25] was in 11 infants with cyanotic congenital heart defects, aged 3 months to 3 years (median: 10 months), weighing 5.4 to 16 kg (median: 8.0 kg), who underwent balloon pulmonary valvuloplasty as a palliative procedure to improve pulmonary oligemia. The diagnoses were as follows: seven cases of TOF; three cases of transposition of the great arteries, with ventricular septal defect and valvar and subvalvar pulmonary stenosis; and one case of dextrocardia, ventricular inversion with ventricular septal defect, and valvar and subvalvar pulmonary stenosis. Following balloon pulmonary valvuloplasty, the arterial oxygen saturation increased from $67 \pm 13\%$ to $83 \pm 13\%$ ($P < .01$). The pulmonary blood flow index (2.1 ± 0.8 L/min/m² vs 3.2 ± 1.2 L/min/m²; $P < .05$), Qp:Qs (0.7 ± 0.4 vs 1.2 ± 0.5; $P < .02$), and pulmonary artery pressure (16 ± 5 vs 21 ± 11 mmHg; ($P < .02$)) increased after balloon dilatation (Table 23-8). The pulmonary valve gradients (52 ± 16 vs. 32 ± 22 mmHg) fell ($P < .05$), while infundibular gradients

(33 ± 12 vs. 42 ± 16 mmHg) and total pulmonary ventricular outflow tract (valvar plus subvalvar) gradients (77 ± 14 vs. 66 ± 12 mmHg) remained unchanged ($P > .1$) after valvuloplasty. An example is shown in Figure 23-32. None required immediate surgical intervention. No complications were encountered during the procedure. All children were discharged home within 24 hours of the procedure.

From our group all 11 children have been followed for 6 to 36 months (13 ± 10 months) with pulse oximetry and hemoglobin determinations. Cardiac catheterization was also performed in all 11 children 4 to 12 months (median: 11 months) after valvuloplasty. Arterial oxygen saturation ($82 \pm 9\%$), pulmonary blood flow (4.0 ± 1.7 L/min/m²), and Qp:Qs (1.3 ± 0.7) remain unchanged ($P > .1$) from the immediate postvalvuloplasty values, but remain improved ($P < .05$ to .001) when compared to prevalvuloplasty values (Table 23-8). The hemoglobin level (15.8 ± 2.7 g%) did not change ($P > .1$) when compared to prevalvuloplasty value of 16.5 ± 2.9 g%. The pulmonary valve gradient (18 ± 7 mmHg) remains improved when compared to that recorded before ($P < .001$) and immediately after ($P < .05$) valvuloplasty (Table 23-8). The subvalvar (53 ± 18 mmHg) and total pulmonary ventricular outflow tract (69 ± 13 mmHg) gradients remain unchanged ($P > .1$). An example is shown in Figure 23-32. None of the patients had significant elevation of peak systolic pulmonary artery pressure: 22 ± 6 mmHg; range: 12 to 30 mmHg.

Five children with TOF underwent successful total surgical correction 4 to 24 months (12 ± 9 months) following valvuloplasty. These children had very

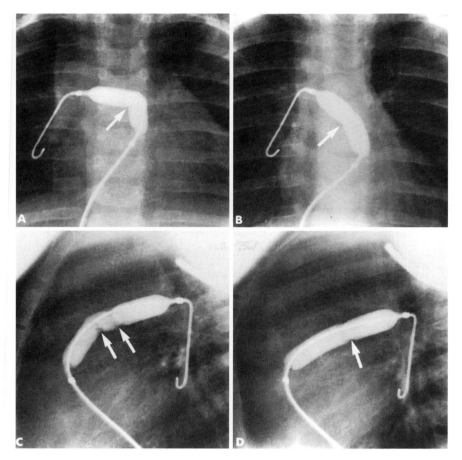

Fig. 23-31. Selected cineradiographic views in **(A,B)** posteroanterior and **(C,D)** lateral projections showing a balloon catheter during the initial (**A** and **C**) and final (**B** and **D**) phases of inflation. Note the waisting is prominent initially which subsequently was almost completely abolished (*arrows*). In this patient with TOF, a lower waist (*lower arrow,* Figure **C**) produced by infundibular constriction is also seen, which completely disappeared after balloon inflation **(D)**. (From Rao,[2] with permission.)

Table 23-8. Results of Balloon Pulmonary Valvuloplasty—Ventricular Right-to-Left Shunt

	Before BPV	Immediately After BPV	P^a	4–36 Months After BPV	P^a
Arterial O_2 sat, %	67 ± 13	83 ± 13	<.01	82 ± 9	<.01
Qp:Qs	0.7 ± 0.4	1.2 ± 0.5	<.02	1.3 ± 0.7	<.05
Qp, L/min/m²	2.1 ± 0.8	3.2 ± 1.3	<.05	4.0 ± 1.7	<.01
PA pressure, mmHg	16 ± 5	26 ± 11	<.02	22 ± 6	>.05
Pulmonary valve gradient, mmHg	52 ± 16	32 ± 22	<.05	18 ± 7	<.001
Infundibular gradient, mmHg	33 ± 12	42 ± 16[b]	>.1	53 ± 18[b]	<.02
Total gradient across, PV outflow, mmHg	77 ± 14	66 ± 12	>.05	69 ± 13	>.1
Hemoglobin, g%	16.5 ± 2.9	—	—	15.8 ± 2.7	>.1

Abbreviations: BPV, balloon pulmonary valvuloplasty; PA, pulmonary artery; PV, pulmonary ventricle; Qp, pulmonary flow; Qp:Qs, pulmonary-to-systemic flow ratio.

[a] Compares with value obtained prior to BPV.

[b] $P > .1$.

(From Rao et al.,[25] with permission.)

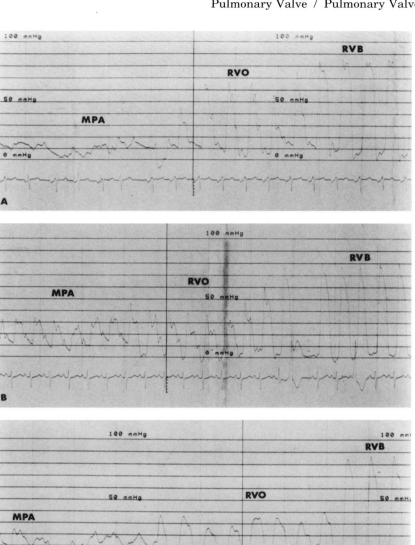

Fig. 23-32. Pressure pullback tracings across the pulmonic valve and right ventricular outflow tract **(A)** before, **(B)** 15 minutes after, and **(C)** 12 months after balloon pulmonary valvuloplasty in a patient with TOF. Note both valvar and infundibular gradients were present prior to valvuloplasty **(A)**, whereas the valvar gradient almost completely disappeared and infundibular gradient persisted immediately after **(B)** and 12 months **(C)** after valvuloplasty. *MPA*, main pulmonary artery; *RVB*, right ventricular body; *RVO*, right ventricular outflow tract. (From Rao et al.,[25] with permission.)

small pulmonary arteries before valvuloplasty and were initially considered unsuitable for total surgical correction. Approximately 12 months later, the pulmonary artery anatomy improved (Fig. 23-33), and total surgical correction was performed without incident. The remaining two children were operated on 4 and 5 months after balloon valvuloplasty because they experienced cyanotic spells.

Two children in the transposition group showed

evidence of significant hypoxemia on follow-up, and Blalock-Taussig (BT) shunts were performed 6 and 18 months after initial balloon valvuloplasty. Increase in the size of the pulmonary artery (Fig. 23-34), as previously reported,[24] was observed. The remaining transposition patients and the single patient with corrected transposition (ventricular inversion) are clinically well and no further intervention is planned.

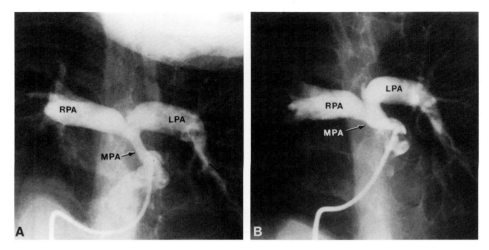

Fig. 23-33. Selected frames from pulmonary artery cineangiograms in a "sitting-up" view in a patient with TOF **(A)** before and **(B)** 12 months after balloon pulmonary valvuloplasty. Note significant improvement in the size of the valve annulus and main and branch pulmonary arteries, following valvuloplasty. *LPA,* left pulmonary artery; *MPA,* main pulmonary artery; *RPA,* right pulmonary artery. (From Rao et al.,[25] with permission.)

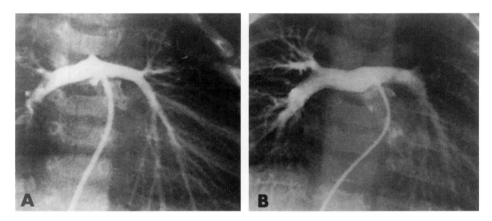

Fig. 23-34. Pulmonary arteriogram immediately **(A)** before and **(B)** 6 months after balloon pulmonary valvuloplasty in an infant with transposition of the great arteries, ventricular septal defect, and valvar and subvalvar pulmonic stenosis. Note increase in the size of the pulmonary arteries after pulmonary valvuloplasty. There were differences in the magnification between both cineangiographic frames; catheters in both frames were 5 F. After correcting for magnification, the right pulmonary artery size increased from 5.0 mm to 9.4 mm, while the left pulmonary artery increased from 3.3 mm to 7.8 mm. Part of the growth was attributed to increase in forward flow following balloon valvuloplasty. (From Rao and Brais,[24] with permission.)

Two additional patients aged 15 years and 27 years could not undergo total surgical correction because of anatomic difficulties and refusal of surgery by the legal guardian, respectively. The 15-year-old patient had very small pulmonary arteries and multiple collateral vessels to the lungs and was considered unoperable. Balloon dilatation of an extremely stenotic pulmonary valve (though the valve ring is markedly hypoplastic) resulted in improvement of arterial oxygen saturation from the low 70s to the high 80s and has improved symptomatically. The 27-

year-old patient with deLange syndrome (and mental retardation) increased his saturations from the low 60s to the low 90s after balloon pulmonary valvuloplasty and has done extremely well during a 4-year follow-up.

Complications

Complications have been remarkably minimal. Transient decrease in systemic arterial saturation occurs while the balloon is inflated, but rapidly improves following balloon deflation. Surprisingly, cyanotic spells following balloon valvuloplasty have not been a problem, presumably because of improvement of pulmonary blood flow following the procedure. However, increasing cyanosis has been observed by some workers. Hypotension during balloon inflation, which is so common in balloon dilatation of pulmonic stenosis with intact ventricular septum, is usually not seen in this group of patients, presumably the flow through the ventricular septal defect provides adequate systemic flow. Pulmonary arterial tear has been reported in a 3-year-old child by other workers, which was noted at the time of total surgical correction 15 months after valvuloplasty.

Comments

The immediate results of balloon pulmonary valvuloplasty in this group of patients appear good and attained the objective of improving pulmonary oligemia and systemic arterial hypoxemia. Immediate surgical intervention was avoided in most cases. Intermediate-term results are also good, the augmentation of pulmonary blood flow continuing to be present at follow-up in most children. The size of the pulmonary arteries improved in most patients, making them more suitable for further palliative or total surgical corrective procedure.

Battistessa and coworkers[26] reported their observations at surgery for TOF patients who had previously undergone balloon pulmonary valvuloplasty. Results in 27 patients (which included 15 patients previously reported by Qureshi and probably form a subgroup of their larger experience[27]) were scrutinized. They found anatomic alterations in the right ventricular outflow tract in 20 (74%) patients, while no change was seen in 7 (26%). They also noted that there was no evidence for significant growth of the pulmonary valve annulus and that the need for a transannular patch was not abolished at the time of intracardiac repair. In view of the damage to pulmonary valve mechanism and no evidence for enough growth of the pulmonary valve to obviate the need for a transannular patch at a later corrective surgery, they were not very supportive of balloon valvuloplasty as a palliative procedure. While these observations are important, we[24,25] and others[27,28] have documented an increase in the size of the pulmonary artery or annulus following balloon pulmonary valvuloplasty. The increase in the pulmonary artery/annulus size is demonstrated in a larger group of patients,[27] which included Battistessa's patients. The increase ($P < .001$) in pulmonary valve annulus size was demonstrated in 24 patients who also increased their systemic arterial oxygen saturations following balloon valvuloplasty, and this increase in pulmonary annulus size was greater ($P < .005$) than expected from normal growth. This improvement in the size of the pulmonary arteries is similar to that observed after the Brock procedure and systemic-to-pulmonary arterial shunts.

In view of the varied observations, it would seem prudent that balloon pulmonary valvuloplasty in TOF (or any other cyanotic defects) should be performed only in selected patients. The following criteria are proposed:

1. The infant/child requires palliation of pulmonary oligemia but is not a candidate for total surgical correction either because of the size of the patient, the type of the defect, or because of anatomic aberrations.
2. Valvar obstruction is a significant component of the right ventricular outflow tract obstruction.
3. Multiple obstructions in series (Fig. 23-28) are present so that there is residual subvalvar obstruction after relief of pulmonary valvar obstruction and flooding of lungs is prevented.

Once balloon valvuloplasty is decided upon, balloons large enough to give a balloon/annulus ratio of 1.2 to 1.4 are recommended.

New Developments

Obstruction to pulmonary outflow tract is usually at multiple levels in TOF; the sites of obstruction are pulmonary arteries, pulmonary valve leaflets, pulmonary valve ring, and infundibulum. Relief of valvar obstruction can, in some patients, increase forward flow and encourage growth of the pulmonary valve ring and pulmonary arteries, as discussed above. If severe infundibular stenosis is present, relief of pulmonary valve stenosis alone may not accomplish the objectives of relieving systemic hypoxemia and encouraging growth of the pulmonary arteries. Qureshi and associates[29] used a Simpson coronary atherectomy catheter to perform infundibular myectomy in a 14-month-old child with TOF. The systemic arterial saturation improved from 78% before the procedure to 85% a month later, and the right ventricular outflow tract became wider. They suggested that this type of transcatheter resection of the infundibulum may be important in the palliation of TOF. Further clinical trials of this method in selected patients are warranted, and this method may serve as a useful adjunct to balloon pulmonary valvuloplasty in the management of TOF.

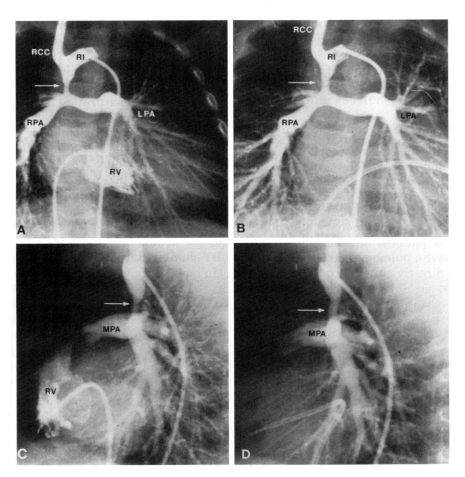

Fig. 23-37. Selected cineangiographic frames of BT shunt **(A,C)** before and immediately **(B,D)** after balloon angioplasty. Anteroposterior (**A** and **B**) and lateral views (**C** and **D**) are shown; the *arrows* point to the narrow BT shunt. Note angiographic improvement in both views. (From Rao et al.,[30] with permission.)

BT shunt, a balloon-on-a-wire* (2 or 3 mm) should be advanced across the narrowed BT shunt (Fig. 23-36). Three successive inflations at 3 to 10 atm pressure, depending on the catheter manufacturer's recommendations, of 5 to 10 seconds duration each, is performed with a 5-minute interval between each dilatation. The procedure of dilatation with the balloon-on-a-wire and with 4-F coronary dilation catheter can be performed through a 5-F sheath placed into the femoral artery at the beginning of the procedure. Larger balloon catheters may either be advanced via a 6-F sheath or dilatation could be performed without the use of a sheath. At 15 minutes following the last balloon dilatation, pulmonary artery to aorta pressure pullback across the BT shunt

and aortic saturation are obtained and innominate or subclavian artery cineangiogram repeated.

Acute Results

Balloon angioplasty of a narrowed BT shunt was initially reported by Fischer and colleagues[31] and subsequently by others. Fischer and colleagues[31] dilated a narrowed classical BT shunt in a 4-year-old child and increased systemic arterial saturation from 68% to 80%.

Our experience with this procedure, including that previously reported,[2,30] is in eight children: four boys and four girls, with a weight range of 6.2 to 19.6 kg (mean: 11.0 kg). The diagnoses in these children were as follows: four cases of pulmonary atresia (one with intact ventricular septum; two with large ventricular septal defects; and one with mitral atresia, hypoplastic left ventricle, and double-outlet right ventricle); three cases of tricuspid atresia; and one

* The balloon-on-a-wire that we used is USCI Probe balloon-on-a-wire.[30] Other available alternatives are ACS Hartzler MicroXR and Sci Med Dilating Guidewire.

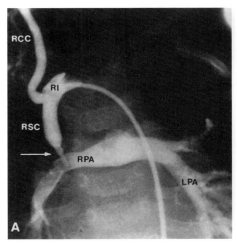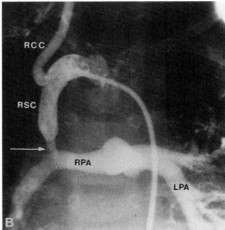

Fig. 23-38. Right innominate artery (*RI*) cineangiographic frames (**A**) before and (**B**) immediately after balloon angioplasty. Note slight, but significant, improvement in the narrowed segment of the right subclavian artery (*RSC*) and the anastomotic site (*arrow*). *LPA,* left pulmonary artery; *RCC,* right common carotid artery; *RPA,* right pulmonary artery. (From Rao,[2] with permission.)

case of single ventricle, single atrium, and severe valvar and subvalvar pulmonic stenosis. Each of these children underwent a BT shunt either in the neonatal period (five patients) or in early infancy (three patients). All children were cyanotic with increased hemoglobin values, 19.0 ± 2.7 g% (mean ± SD), with a range of 14.8 to 22.1 g%. Three children were severely symptomatic and were unable to attend school. Three toddlers were severely cyanotic with hyperpnea. The remaining two children were cyanotic and tolerated normal activity. There was moderate to severe hypoxemia with a mean oxygen saturation of 71% (SD = 7%), with a range of 62 to 82%. The pulmonary artery pressure was low normal in four children in whom the pulmonary artery pressure could be measured before angioplasty. In one child with long segmental narrowing of the left subclavian artery (in a patient with right aortic arch) proximal to its entry into the left pulmonary artery, there was no significant improvement in the oxygen saturation or in the angiographic appearance of the BT shunt. The angioplasty was considered to be a failure, and the child underwent a right BT shunt within several weeks after balloon angioplasty. The remaining children showed significant improvement. The arterial oxygen saturation increased from 71 ± 7 to 81 ± 4% following balloon angioplasty. Pulmonary artery pressure was measured in each case following angioplasty, and the peak systolic pressure was 14 ± 5 mmHg, with a range of 9 to 23 mmHg; none had elevated pulmonary artery pressures. Angiographic improvement of the BT shunt with greater degree of opacification of the pulmonary circuit was observed in each of the seven children. Examples are shown in Figures 23-37 to 23-39. No

complications were encountered during the procedure.

Follow-up Results

Follow-up data after balloon angioplasty of narrowed BT shunts is scanty. From our series, the single child with failed balloon angioplasty (of left BT shunt) underwent successful right BT shunt and improved arterial oxygen saturation. The remaining seven children were followed for 3 to 24 months (mean: 12 months). The children with symptoms of exercise intolerance improved markedly, although all of them remained cyanotic. Hemoglobin level decreased from 19.0 ± 2.7 g% to 17.1 ± 1.9 g%. Arterial oxygen saturation by pulse oximeter remains improved as a group (78 ± 10%). Auscultation revealed continuous murmur of the shunt in five patients, but on echo-Doppler study, the shunt was patent in six children.

Repeat catheterization was undertaken in two children because of progressive hypoxemia. The O₂ saturations decreased. Although the shunts were patent, because of continued hypoxemia BT shunts were successfully performed on the contralateral side 8 and 10 months after the balloon angioplasty. The remaining children were doing well clinically with continued palliation of pulmonary oligema.

Complications

No complications were detected either in our series or in the patients reported by other workers. It is somewhat surprising that there was no significant hypoxemia during balloon inflation (and consequent

---

Table 24-3. Anatomic Classification of the Mitral Valve: Echocardiographic Examination

Leaflet Mobility
1. Highly mobile valve with restriction of only the leaflet tips
2. Midportion and base of leaflets have reduced mobility
3. Valve leaflets move forward in diastole mainly at the base
4. No or minimal forward movement of the leaflets in diastole

Valvular Thickening
1. Leaflets near normal (4–5 mm)
2. Midleaflet thickening, marked thickening of the margins.
3. Thickening extends through the entire leaflets (5–8 mm)
4. Marked thickening of all leaflet tissue (>8–10 mm)

Subvalvular Thickening
1. Minimal thickening of chordal structures just below the valve
2. Thickening of chordae extending up to one third of chordal length
3. Thickening extending to the distal third of the chordae.
4. Extensive thickening and shortening of all chordae extending down to the papillary muscle

Valvular Calcification
1. A single area of increased echo brightness
2. Scattered areas of brightness confined to leaflet margins
3. Brightness extending into the midportion of leaflets
4. Extensive brightness through most of the leaflet tissue

(From the Massachussetts General Hospital,[1] with permission.)
The final score is found by adding each of the components.

---

pends on the results previously obtained by surgery and PMC in any given institution.

TECHNICAL ASPECTS

The two approaches are the retrograde transarterial approach without transseptal catheterization, and the transvenous approach with transseptal catheterization.

Retrograde Transarterial Approach

In the retrograde technique, the balloons are introduced through the femoral artery. The passage from the left ventricle to the left atrium is effected by using preshaped externally steerable catheters. The specific advantage in this approach is that it avoids transseptal catheterization, which makes it potentially more widely usable. However, retrograde left atrial catheterization is not always easy, and it carries the risk of inserting the guidewire between the chordae tendinae, thus damaging the subvalvular apparatus on balloon inflation and causing severe mitral regurgitation. It has been used with good results, but the number of patients treated in this way has been limited, and further studies are needed to evaluate its place.

Transvenous Approach

The transvenous approach is the most widely used. Transseptal catheterization is the first step and one of the most crucial. Its proper performance avoids cardiac perforation and also allows subsequent easy positioning of the balloon in the mitral orifice. Transseptal puncture is carried out conventionally by using several fluoroscopic views under continuous pressure monitoring. Transesophageal echocardiographic guidance may be a useful adjunct to fluoroscopy on the rare occasions when difficulties are encountered in performing the transseptal puncture.

Balloon Techniques

Where the balloons themselves are concerned, there are currently two main techniques: the double-balloon technique and the Inoue technique.

Double Balloon Technique

In the double-balloon technique: after catheterization of the left ventricle by a floating balloon catheter, two long exchange guidewires are positioned in the apex of the left ventricle. The interatrial septum is dilated, using a peripheral angioplasty balloon 8 mm or, more recently, 6 mm in diameter. The balloons then used are two round conventional balloons or a combination of a trefoil balloon and a conventional balloon.

Inoue Technique

The Inoue technique, which was the first described, is detailed elsewhere in this book. Briefly, it appears today that a stepwise dilatation with Inoue's balloon under echocardiographic guidance allows the best use of the mechanical properties of the balloon, and thereby optimizes the results.[4]

Single and Bifoil Balloons

Short preliminary series have reported the results of the use of single low-profile balloons of large diameter up to 30 mm, or bifoil balloons, which have two separate compartments with a common shaft. They provide a rather simple and inexpensive technique, which does, however, require the use of a stiff guidewire with its inherent risk of left ventricular perforation.

Comparison of Balloon Techniques

A small number of studies, mainly retrospective, with the inherent bias this implies, have compared the efficacy of the Inoue technique and the double-balloon technique, or other single-balloon techniques. These data suggest that the Inoue technique eases the procedure and is safer, particularly as regards the risk of perforation or of severe mitral regurgitation when the stepwise technique is used, although it gives slightly less improvement in valve area. Any definite conclusion as to the relative merits of the different balloon techniques must await data from larger randomized series with follow-up.

Balloon Size

The following guidelines are currently used in selecting balloon size, usually chosen according to the patient's characteristics:

Height: when using Inoue's technique, the recommended maximum balloon diameter is 24 mm if height is under 1.47 m, 26 mm between 1.47 and 1.60 m, 28 mm between 1.60 and 1.80 m, and 30 mm if over 1.80 m

Body surface area: a ratio of effective balloon area/body surface area greater than 3.9 is a predictor of an increase in the degree of mitral regurgitation more than 2 grades
Diameter of the mitral annulus assessed by echocardiography: an increase in mitral regurgitation occurs if the ratio of the diameter from the balloon to annular size is greater than 1.1

Pregnancy

In the specific circumstances of pregnancy, PMC should be performed by experienced practicioners, keeping the length of the procedure to a minimum. Protection against radiation should include the use of a shield to surround the patient's abdomen, and fluoroscopy time should be limited. Finally, injection of contrast material should be avoided.

MONITORING THE PROCEDURE AND ASSESSING THE IMMEDIATE RESULTS

During the Procedure

The following criteria have been suggested for the guidance of the procedure:

1. *Mean left atrial pressure and mean valve gradient.* These can be criticized because of variations that may occur because of changes in heart rate or cardiac output.

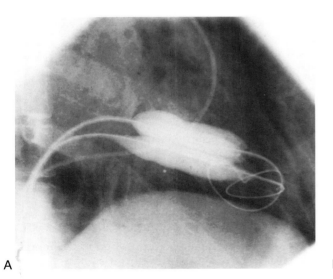
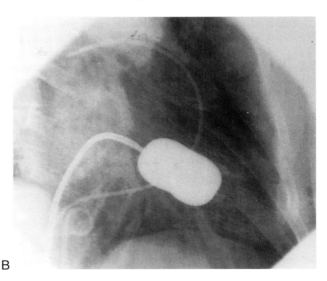

A B

Fig. 24-1. Technique. **(A)** Double-balloon technique: trefoil + conventional balloon. **(B)** Inoue balloon.

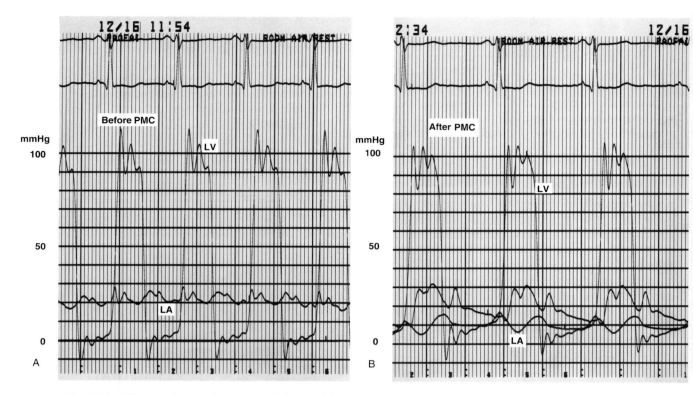

Fig. 24-2. Mitral valve gradient. **(A)** Before PMC. **(B)** After PMC. *L.A.,* left atrium; *L.V.,* left ventricle.

2. *Valve area.* Its repeated evaluation during the procedure by hemodynamic measurements lacks practicality and may be subject to error because of the instability of the patient's condition and the inaccuracy of Gorlin's formula in the presence of atrial shunts, or in cases of mitral regurgitation. The accuracy of Doppler measurements during PMC is low, so that planimetry from two-dimensional echocardiography appears to be the method of choice when it is technically feasible.
3. *Changes in the degree of regurgitation.* Color Doppler assessment is the method of choice.
4. *Commissural morphology.* This can be assessed by two-dimensional echocardiography using the short axis view.

Although, for logistic reasons, echocardiography may be difficult to perform in the catheterization laboratory, it provides essential information and is of utmost importance when using the stepwise Inoue technique.

Ending the Procedure

The following criteria have been proposed for ending the procedure: (1) mitral valve area greater than 1 cm^2/m^2 body surface area, (2) complete opening of at least one commissure, or (3) appearance or increment of regurgitation greater than one-fourth. The strategy must be tailored to the individual circumstances taking into account clinical factors together with anatomic factors and the cumulative data of periprocedural monitoring. For example, balloon size, increments of size, and expected final valve area will be smaller in elderly patients, in cases of very tight mitral stenosis, extensive valve and subvalvular disease, and nodular commissural calcification.

After the Procedure

After the procedure, the most accurate evaluation of valve area is given by echocardiography. To allow for the slight loss occurring during the first 24 hours, this should be performed 1 to 2 days after PMC, when calculation of the valve area may be done by planimetry, and also from the half-pressure time method, or the continuity equation method.

The assessment of the degree of regurgitation may be made by angiography or also by color Doppler flow. Transesophageal examination is recommended in cases of severe mitral regurgitation to determine the mechanisms involved.

The most sensitive method for the assessment of

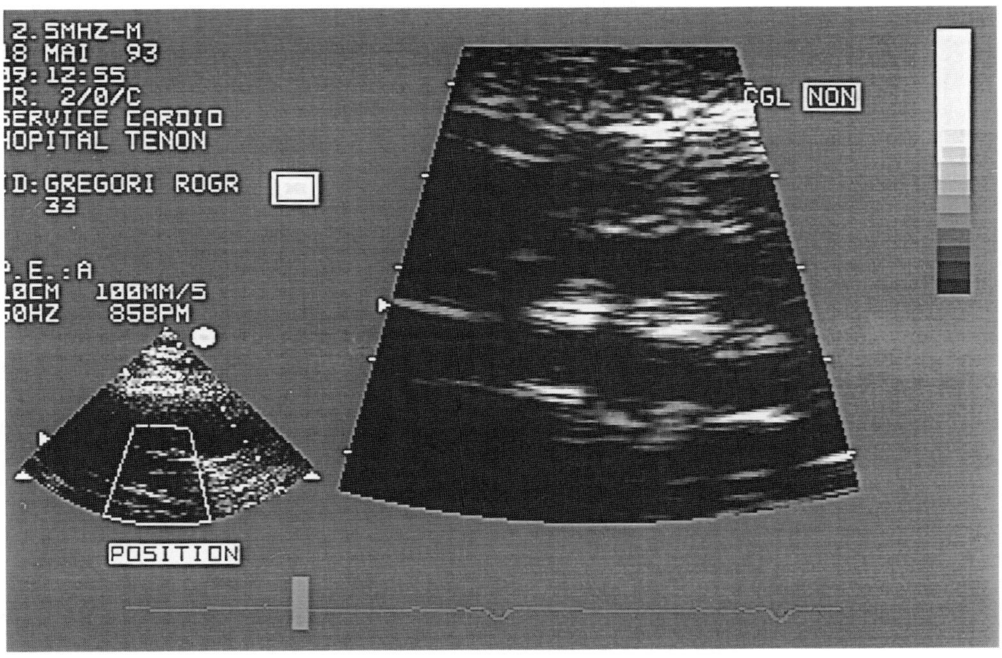

Fig. 24-3. Echocardiography after PMC. Short axis view: transthoracic approach. Bicommissural opening.

shunting is color Doppler flow, especially when using transesophageal examination, which shows the importance of the defect and detects shunting in a more sensitive way than hemodynamics.

Finally, the persistence of spontaneous echocardiographic contrast can be detected by transesophageal echocardiography.

CONCOMITANT MEDICAL TREATMENT

Anticoagulant Treatment

Oral anticoagulant therapy is necessary for at least 2 months before PMC in case of atrial fibrillation, a history of thromboembolic events, or the presence of spontaneous echocardiographic contrast on transesophageal echocardiography. After transseptal catheterization, heparin must be administered intravenously (5,000 U or 100 U/kg). After PMC, low doses of heparin should be given for 24 hours. Oral anticoagulation must be continued in the case of atrial fibrillation or persistence of spontaneous echocardiographic contrast on transesophageal echocardiography.

Antibiotherapy

No prophylactic antibiotherapy is recommended before or during the procedure.

FINANCIAL ASPECTS

The advantages of the Inoue technique may be outweighed by the price of the balloon, which is somewhat higher than that of the various devices needed in the other techniques (balloons + guidewires + floating balloon catheters). Such calculations are of course only indicative and depend on regional variations in the sales price, and, more important, in the number of reuses, which is frequently high in developing countries.

The most important comparison of cost is not between different techniques of PMC but between PMC and surgery. The results of this latter comparison vary from one country to another. In industrialized countries, surgery is more expensive than PMC, whereas in developing countries, this situation is reversed. The large-scale use of PMC in the developing countries is fundamentally dependent on solving logistic and therefore economic problems.

SELECTION OF CANDIDATES

Absolute Contraindications

1. Recent thromboembolism (<2 months) or left atrial thrombosis. If the left atrial thrombus is large, mobile, or if the clinical condition of the pa-

symptomatic and hemodynamic improvement after this procedure has been reported.[2,3] Although its clinical application has been widely adopted, its indications and potential complications have not been thoroughly defined, and only a few follow-up studies have been reported.

The study reported in this chapter was designed to review the immediate and midterm follow-up results after successful balloon commissurotomy at Kokura Memorial Hospital, Japan and to identify the predictive factors for successful commissurotomy.

METHOD

Patients

From February 1987 to May 1992, PTMC was attempted in 357 patients with symptomatic mitral stenosis; 75 were men and 282 were women. The mean age was 54 ± 11 years (24 to 78). Two hundred and twenty patients were in atrial fibrillation, and the remainder were in normal sinus rhythm. Thirty-one patients had undergone open or closed mitral commissurotomy previously.

1. Fresh left atrial thrombus
2. Atrial septal thrombus
3. Severe mitral regurgitation defined as 3 or more by contrast cineventriculography.[4]

Inoue Balloon Catheter

The Inoue balloon catheter (Toray, Tokyo, Japan) is a 12 F polyvinylchloride tube with coaxial lumina. The balloon section is stiffened and slenderized when stretched by the insertion of a metal tube (Fig. 25-1). This allows a smooth entry of the balloon cathter into the femoral vein and left atrium. The Inoue balloon catheter is made of a double atrium. The balloon is made of a nylon micromesh between a double layer of latex rubber. The proximal half of the nylon mesh is wound with thin rubber bands, more tightly in the central region and more loosely at the two ends, so that the shape of the balloon changes in three stages, depending on the extent of inflation. Inflation occurs first at the distal half, then the proximal half, and constriction remains in the middle section until full

tient requires urgent treatment, surgery must be carried out. On the other hand, if the patient is clinically stable, anticoagulant therapy can be given for 2 months and if a new transesophageal examination shows the disappearance of the thrombus, PMC can be attempted.

2. Mitral regurgitation greater than 2/4.
3. Patients with mitral stenosis and severe coronary artery disease, who require coronary bypass surgery.

Relative Contraindications

1. Massive valve calcification or echocardiographic score greater than 12.
2. Severe aortic valve disease associated with mitral stenosis.

In these conditions, PMC is usually excluded, except in cases of contraindications for surgery.

Indications

1. Well-accepted indications
   • Patients with favorable anatomy (pliable valves

suitable anatomy when the major mechanism of restenosis is commissural fusion and not only valve thickening.
   • Pregnant women. PMC can be performed on pregnant patients with refractory symptoms despite medical treatment, preferably in the last trimester.

CONCLUSIONS

The good results that have been obtained with PMC enable us to say that, currently, this technique has an important place in the treatment of mitral stenosis alongside surgery or most often to postpone a need for surgery.

REFERENCES

1. The National Heart, Lung, and Blood Institute Balloon Valvuloplasty Registry Participants. Multicenter experience with balloon mitral commissurotomy: NHLBI balloon valvuloplasty registry report on immediate and 30-day follow-up results. Circulation 1992;85:448–61
2. Vahanian A, Michel PL, Cormier B et al. Immediate and mid-term results of percutaneous mitral commissurotomy. Eur Heart J 1991;12(Suppl B):84–9

---

an 8 F Mullins transseptal dilator (USCI, Billerica, Massachusetts). After entry in the left atrium, 10,000 U heparin were administered. A 5-F pigtail catheter was positioned in the left ventricle from the left femoral artery, and simultaneous pressure tracings of the left atrium and the ventricle were recorded. The previously inserted 7-F Swan-Ganz catheter that had been temporarily removed was reinserted through the right jugular vein, and cardiac output was measured just before the balloon commissurotomy. A 0.28″ stainless steel guidewire was advanced into the left atrium and was used to place the Inoue balloon catheter in the left atrium. Once the balloon catheter tip traversed the interatrial septum, the stiffening cannula for the central lumen was used to facilitate passage of the balloon portion into the left atrium. Once in the left atrium, the tip of the balloon was inflated with 1 to 2 ml of contrast material, allowing blood flow to direct the balloon tip into the left ventricle. The contrast material was removed, and the balloon was inflated with diluted contrast material until the waist of the balloon disappeared.

Immediately after the procedure, all hemodynamic measurements were repeated, including the determination of transvalvular gradient and cardiac output. To evaluate the severity of the resultant mitral regurgitation, if any, cine left ventriculography in the left anterior oblique view was performed. The severity of mitral regurgitation was graded 0 to 4+. One day after PTMC, right heart oximetric study and supine ergometer exercise test were performed to evaluate the interatrial septal perforation and its resultant left-to-right shunt as well as the exercise response. Most patients were discharged 2 days after PTMC.

Serial Echocardiographic Studies

Two-dimensional and Doppler echocardiography were performed the day before and after balloon commissurotomy. The Toshiba SSH 65A and 160A were used for this study. Mitral ejection fraction slope, mitral valve excursion, left atrial diameter, and mitral valve area by the pressure half-time method and tracing method were determined. The presence and severity of mitral regurgitation was assessed by pulsed Doppler and real-time two-dimensional flow imaging system before and after balloon commissurotomy. The severity of mitral regurgitation was graded as none, mild, moderate, or severe based on the extension of the regurgitant jet in the left atrium. In addition, Doppler echocardiography was used to assess the atrial septal defect after balloon commis-

surotomy. Based on the echocardiographic characteristics of the anatomic structures of the mitral valve, primarily the leaflets; second, the commissural disease; and third, the subvalvular apparatus, echo score was determined as follows:

Pliability

Score 1: Pliable leaflets with minimal restriction of the leaflet tip mobility.
Score 2: Semipliable valves with restriction of the leaflets' body mobility.
Score 3: Minimal forward movement of the leaflets.

Commissural Disease

Score 1: No commissural disease.
Score 2: One commissural disease.
Score 3: Both commissural disease.
Score 4: Diffuse disease.

Subvalvular Disease

Score 1: Minimal thickening of the subvalvular chordae.
Score 2: Thickening and shortening of the chordae.
Score 3: Fused subvalvular apparatus.

Clinical Follow-up

With the exception of a few patients living far from the hospital who were followed up by telephone interview, most patients were followed up in our department with two-dimensional and Doppler echocardiographic assessment.

Data and Statistical Analysis

Two-dimensional and Doppler echocardiographic recordings were analyzed by experienced echocardiographers who were unaware of the hemodynamic results.

Mean and standard deviations were determined for all hemodynamic variables and for calculated mitral valve areas. Student's t-test and chi-square test were used for comparing hemodynamic parameters and clinical results.

Multiple regression analysis was used to identify the predictive factors for mitral valve area immediately after and during the follow-up period and for production of mitral regurgitation. The examined

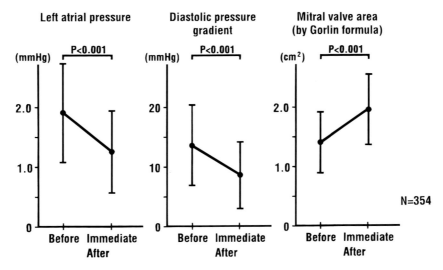

Fig. 25-6. Resting hemodynamic variables before and after PTMC.

factors were age, sex, cardiac rhythm, history of previous commissurotomy, echocardiographic subgrouping, mitral valve area before and after procedure, and balloon diameter-normalized mitral annular diameter. A probability value less than 0.05 was considered significant.

RESULTS

Immediate Clinical and Hemodynamic Improvement

The balloon could be dilated as planned in 354 of 357 patients (99%). Significant symptomatic improvement defined as reclassification by one or more New York Heart Association (NYHA) functional classes was achieved in 325 of 357 patients (91%). The resting hemodynamic variables are shown in Figure 25-6. The mean left atrial pressure decreased from 19 ± 8 to 13 ± 7 mmHg ($P < 0.001$), and the mean diastolic mitral valve pressure gradient measured from simultaneous left atrial and left ventricular pressure tracing fell from 14 ± 7 to 9 ± 6 mmHg ($P < 0.001$). The mitral valve area by Gorlin's formula increased significantly from 1.41 ± 0.51 to 1.96 ± 0.61 cm^2. The echocardiographically estimated mitral valve area also increased significantly (pressure half-time method: 1.28 ± 0.42 to 1.81 ± 0.52 cm^2; tracing method; 1.24 ± 0.34 to 1.71 ± 0.42 cm^2, $P < 0.001$, Fig. 25-7). More than 25% gain in mitral valve area was obtained in 67% patients. Distribu-

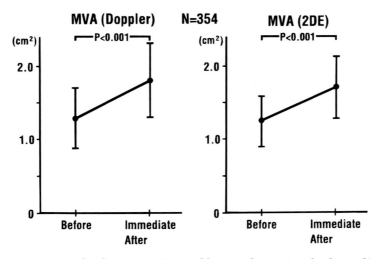

Fig. 25-7. The changes in mitral valve area estimated by two-dimensional echocardiography before and after the procedure. MVA, mitral valve area; 2DE, two-dimensional.

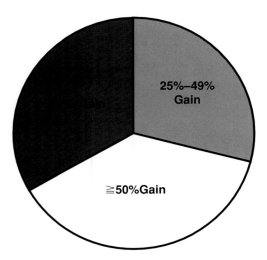

Fig. 25-8. Distribution of the initial gain in mitral valve area.

Table 25-1. Complications After Percutaneous Transvenous Mitral Commissurotomy	
Complication	No.
Mitral regurgitation (≥1°)	57/354 (16%)
Mitral regurgitation (≥3°)	15/354 (4%)
Mitral valve replacement	11/354 (3%)
Atrial septal defect	43/354 (12%)
Cardiac tamponade	9/354 (3%)
Bleeding (requiring BTF)	6/354 (2%)
Thromboembolism	3/354 (0.8%)
Death	1/354 (0.3%)

tions of the valve area gain were less than 25% gain in 29% of the patients, 25 to 49% gain in 32% of the patients, and more than 50% gain in 39% of the patients (Fig. 25-8).

Hemodynamic Response to Exercise

Supine ergometer exercise test revealed a significant decrease in peak pulmonary artery wedge pressure (35 ± 12 to 26 ± 11 mmHg, $P < 0.001$) and a significant increase in cardiac index (from 4.63 ± 1.68 to 5.67 ± 2.16 l/min/m², $P < 0.001$) before and after balloon commissurotomy (Fig. 25-9).

Complications

Complications of balloon commissurotomy are shown in Table 25-1. Three thromboembolic episodes occurred after a successful procedure. One of them resulted in transient cerebral ischemic syndrome, and one patient died as a result of massive pulmonary embolism immediately after the procedure. Renal embolism occurred in another patient. The severity of mitral regurgitation increased in 57 of 354 patients (16%) as evaluated by cine left ventriculography or Doppler echocardiography. Severe mitral regurgitation (greater than 3) occurred in 15 patients, and 11 of them required subsequent mitral valve replacement (emergency, three; elective, eight). Mitral valve replacement was uneventful in all patients. Bleeding from the right femoral vein associated with balloon catheter insertion requiring blood transfusion occurred in six patients (2%). Doppler echocardi-

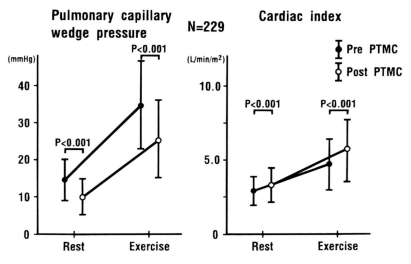

Fig. 25-9. Hemodynamic response to exercise. PTMC, percutaneous transvenous mitral commissurotomy.

Table 25-2. Comparison of Clinical and Hemodynamic Results Among
the Three Patient Groups

	No. of Patients	Age	Previous Mitral Commissurotomy	Atrial Fibrillation	MVA (Post)	Left Atrial Pressure (Post)	Balloon/Mitral Annular Diameter
Group 1	136	52 ± 11	8 (6%)	72 (53%)	2.01 ± 0.42	11 ± 5	0.96 ± 0.07
Group 2	183	56 ± 10	16 (9%)	125 (68%)	1.78 ± 0.29	13 ± 6	0.93 ± 0.14
Group 3	35	60 ± 11	7 (20%)	25 (71%)	1.48 ± 0.68	18 ± 12	0.97 ± 0.08

Abbreviation: MVA, Mitral valve area.
*$P < 0.05$.
**$P < 0.01$.

ography showed the presence of a hemodynamically insignificant interatrial shunt in 43 patients (12%). In nine patients (3%), transseptal puncture resulted in cardiac tamponade requiring emergency subxyphoid drainage.

Valvular Morphology and Immediate Results

To evaluate the relationship between valvular morphology and acute clinical outcome, we divided patients into three groups according to their echocardiographic score:

Group 1: patients with a total echo score of less than 3.
Group 2: patients with a total echo score of 4 to 7.
Group 3: patients with a total echo score of more than 8.

Clinical and hemodynamic results among the three patient groups are shown in Table 25-2. Group 2 and 3 patients were significantly older and had a higher incidence of history of previous commissurotomy than group 1 patients. After balloon commissurotomy, significant severe residual stenosis was prominent in group 2 and 3 patients. Similarly, hemodynamic improvement correlated well with echocardiographic subgrouping, and group 3 patients were least benefited hemodynamically. In group 1 and 3 patients, the balloon diameters normalized to the mitral annular diameters were significantly larger than in group 2 patients. Significant improvement in mitral valve area defined as more than 25% initial gain by pressure half-time method was obtained in 72% of group 1 patients, and in 68% of

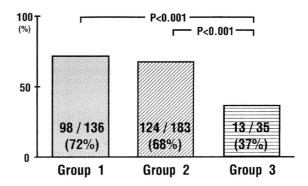

Fig. 25-10. Comparison of initial gain in mitral valve area between the three patient groups.

group 2 patients, as compared to 37% of group 3 ($P < 0.001$, Fig. 25-10). The incidence of production of severe mitral regurgitation defined as 3 or more by cine ventriculography was 0% in group 1, 4% in group 2, and 23% in group 3, which was significantly higher than the other two groups (Fig. 25-11).

Multiple linear regression analysis identified (1)

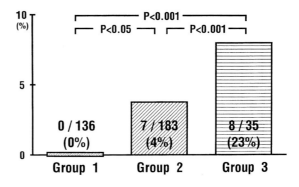

Fig. 25-11. Comparison of production of mitral regurgitation between the three patient groups.

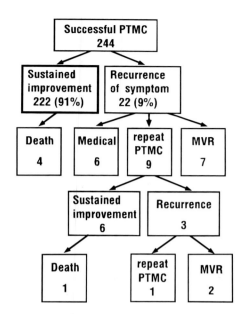

Fig. 25-12. Chart of follow-up data. PTMC, percutaneous transvenous mitral commissurotomy; MVR, mitral valve replacement.

the mitral valve area before the procedure, (2) the echocardiographic subgrouping, and (3) the history of previous commissurotomy as significant predictors for postprocedural mitral valve area. Significant predictors for production of mitral regurgitation were the echocardiographic subgrouping and age.

Follow-up Study

After the initial procedure, 263 patients had a follow-up of more than 2 years. Follow-up study was completed in 244 of 266 patients (92%). The mean follow-up interval was 23 ± 16 months; the end point of follow-up study was death, mitral valve replacement, or repeat balloon commissurotomy. Twenty-two pa-

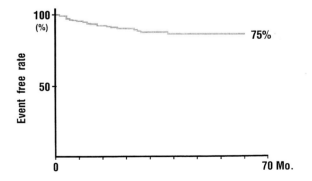

Fig. 25-13. Actuarial event-free curve by Kaplan-Meier method. MO, month.

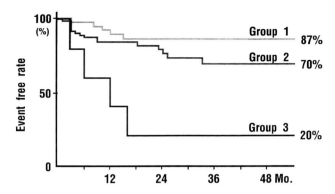

Fig. 25-14. Actuarial event-free curve by proportional hazard model comparing the three patient groups. MO, month.

tients had recurrence of symptoms (Fig. 25-12); 6 patients were observed medically, 9 patients underwent repeat balloon commissurotomy, and 7 patients underwent mitral valve replacement. The reasons for mitral valve replacement were restenosis in 2, symptomatic deterioration that was due to subsequent mitral regurgitation in 3, infective endocarditis in 1, and fresh left atrial thrombus in 1 (Fig. 25-12). Of the 9 patients with repeat balloon commissurotomy, 3 patients had recurrence of symptoms requiring subsequent mitral valve replacement and repeat PTMC. Two patients died from cerebral infarction and three patients died from unknown causes. The actuarial event-free rate by Kaplan-Meier method at 63 months after successful balloon commissurotomy was 75% (Fig. 25-13). *Event* was defined as death, mitral valve replacement, or repeat balloon commissurotomy. The correlating echocardiographic subgrouping and event-free curve, event-free rate in group 3 patients was only 20%, which

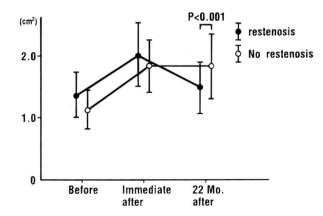

Fig. 25-15. Plot of calculated mitral valve area before, immediately after, and 22 months after percutaneous transvenous mitral commissurotomy (PTMC). MO, month.

Table 25-3. Comparison of Clinical Characteristics Between Two Groups

Clinical Characteristics	With Recurrence	Without Recurrence	P
No. of patients	22	222	
Age	53 ± 10	54 ± 11	
History of previous commissurotomy	18%	7%	
Total echo score	5.8 ± 1.6	4.7 ± 1.9	0.01
MVA (immediately after)	1.80 ± 0.42	1.87 ± 0.51	
Initial gain (MVA)	0.45 ± 0.26	0.53 ± 0.54	
MVA (follow-up)	1.46 ± 0.34	1.88 ± 0.43	0.001
Loss of initial gain (%)	−74.8 ± 74.3	−17.0 ± 35.2	0.001

Abbreviation: MVA, mitral valve area.

Table 25-4. Comparison of Clinical Characteristics Between Two Patient Groups

Clinical Characteristics	With Restenosis	Without Restenosis	P
No. of patients	19	124	
Age	57 ± 11	52 ± 11	0.001
History of previous commissurotomy	11%	5%	
Initial gain (MVA)	0.68 ± 0.34	0.70 ± 0.34	
Total echo score	5.21 ± 1.43	4.81 ± 1.82	

Abbreviation: MVA, mitral valve area.

was significantly lower than that of the other two groups (group 1, 87%; group 2, 70%; Fig. 25-14).

The total echo score in patients with reccurrence was significantly higher than those without reccurrence (Table 25-3). Their mitral valve area at follow-up was significantly smaller, and the loss of initial gain in mitral valve area was also higher (Table 25-3). Echocardiographic follow-up was achieved in 87% of 244 patients. Suboptimal cases defined as less than 25% initial gain in mitral valve area were excluded, and the remaining 143 patients were enrolled in this study. Restenosis defined as a loss greater than 50% of the initial gain in mitral valve area occurred in 13% of 143 patients. The changes in mitral valve area, before, immediately after, and 22 months after the first procedure in patients with restenosis were 1.34 ± 0.34, 2.08 ± 0.61, and 1.44 ± 0.44 cm², respectively (Fig. 25-15). In patients without restenosis, the mitral valve area changed from 1.16 ± 0.32 to 1.86 ± 0.43 immediately after the procedure and to 1.84 ± 0.51 cm² at follow-up (Fig. 25-15). In comparing clinical characteristics between patients with and without restenosis, the only statistically significant difference was age (Table 25-4). Multiple linear regression analysis identified (1) echocardiographic subgrouping and (2) age as the significant predictors for mitral valve area at follow-up.

CONCLUSIONS

The present study demonstrates that percutaneous transvenous mitral commissurotomy could induce excellent immediate and midterm follow-up results only in patients with favorable anatomy.

The most important factors determining the hemodynamic and clinical outcome after PTMC are the anatomic and pathologic features of the mitral apparatus. Patients with rigid valves should be scrutinized very carefully. Further follow-up study is needed to assess the long-term efficacy of the procedure.

REFERENCES

1. Inoue K, Owani T, Nakamura T et al: Clinical application of transvenous mitral commissurotomy by a new balloon catheter. J Thorac Cardiovasc Surg 1984; 394–402
2. Lock LE, Khalilnllah M, Shrivdsta S et al: Percutane-

Catheterization of the Left Atrium

The hemostatic valve that stabilizes the steering arm of the steerable left atrial catheter is released, and the catheter tip is straightened. Then, using the right femoral artery route, the catheter is advanced to the

Valvuloplasty Procedure

After recording of left atrial pressures, a stiffer guidewire (0.038″, 260 cm, J-tip, heavy duty) is inserted into the left atrium and stabilized as above.

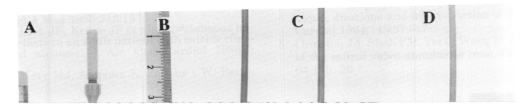

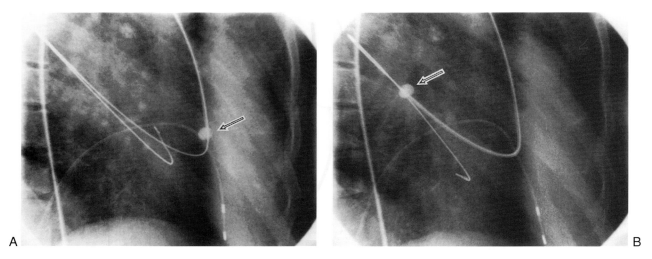

Fig. 26-4. Ventriculographic projection shows test for correct insertion of guidewire (right anterior oblique projection). Free movement of an inflated Swan-Ganz balloon shows that there is no involvement with the chordae tendineae. **(A)** The balloon (*arrow*) is inflated in the outflow region of the left ventricle. **(B)** The balloon (*arrow*) moves freely through the mitral valve into the left atrium.

The pigtail catheter is then removed (Fig. 26-2). As a final check on the route of the guidewire, a flow-directed catheter is introduced over this wire into the left ventricle. The balloon is inflated in the outflow tract of the left ventricle, with carbon dioxide or with a dilute dye solution, and advanced toward the mitral valve. If this movement is unobstructed, it proves that the guidewire passes correctly through the inflow tract of the left ventricle and has not become involved with the chordae tendineae (Fig. 26-4).

Thereafter, the right femoral arterial sheath is replaced with either a 14 F sheath or an adjustable introducer (Medina, Schneider, Europe) and the balloon catheter is advanced over the guidewire under fluoroscopy and positioned across the mitral valve. The balloon is then inflated by hand until the waist of the balloon at the level of the mitral valve disappears (Fig. 26-5). Although the same technique can be employed with two different balloon catheters using both femoral arteries,[15] this bifemoral technique is not presently preferred because current balloon technology meets every demand.

After the removal of the balloon catheter, the hemodynamic measurements are repeated. Thereafter cine left ventriculography is repeated in all patients to assess any change in mitral regurgitation severity.

POSTOPERATIVE MANAGEMENT

On completion of the hemodynamic and ventriculographic measurements, protamine sulfate is administered; the patients are kept in the intensive care unit and the sheaths are removed. Hemostasis is performed by compression applied initially by hand for about 10 minutes and then by a controlled pressure device, so that the arterial pulse can be felt in the lower leg, until complete hemostasis is achieved. Most of the patients are discharged 24 hours after the procedure. If there are any arterial or other complications, the patient remains under observation; most are discharged 1 day later.

RESULTS

Evaluation of Patients

Patients undergoing RNBMV are evaluated before and after valvuloplasty, as well as in routine follow-up examinations performed on the 3rd, 6th, and 12th month after valvuloplasty, and annually thereafter. Right and left heart pressures, transmitral valve gradient, cardiac output, and hemodynamic mitral valve area are measured before and after RNBMV. M-mode, two-dimensional, and Doppler echocardiography studies are performed before, immediately after, and 1 to 2 days after valvuloplasty in all patients, and they are repeated during the follow-up period. Transesophageal echocardiography also is used before the procedure routinely. Evaluation of functional capacity of the patients before valvuloplasty and over the follow-up period is based on clinical criteria according to the New York Heart Association (NYHA) functional classification and on exercise duration and maximal oxygen consumption obtained during cardiopulmonary stress testing according to the Weber protocol.

Immediate Results

See the flow chart in Figure 26-6. The immediate invasive hemodynamic results and the Doppler echocardiographic measurements performed 24 to 48 hours after the procedure are shown in Table 26-2. A significant increase in mitral valve area was shown with both invasive and noninvasive measurements. A successful procedure was achieved in 183 of the 205 attempts (89.3%).

Multiple stepwise linear regression analysis on demographic and hemodynamic variables before valvuloplasty revealed that the degree of increase in mitral valve area was directly related to balloon size and inversely related to the quality of the mitral valve (especially valvular thickening and calcification, and subvalvular fibrosis) and to older age.

Complications

Major complications, such as cardiac perforation, cardiac tamponade, or embolic events, were not encountered in our study population (Table 26-3).

Death

One patient (0.5%) was operated on urgently because she developed severe mitral regurgitation (grade 4 +), and died shortly after mitral valve replacement.

Mitral Regurgitation

Evolution of mitral valve regurgitation as a result of RNBMV is shown in Figure 26-7, and treatment of patients who developed severe mitral regurgitation is shown in the flow chart of patients in Figure 26-6. In all patients who were treated surgically, surgery revealed that mitral regurgitation was associated exclusively with torn mitral valve leaflets. Multiple stepwise linear regression analysis identified effective balloon area normalized to body surface area, mitral valve leaflet rigidity, and mitral valve regurgitation before the procedure as the most significant predictors for an increase in mitral valve regurgitation after the procedure.

Bleeding and Vascular Complications

Bleeding requiring blood transfusion occurred in 1.5% of the patients, and 2% of the patients showed hematoma in the region of the right femoral artery,

which disappeared without affecting the vessel's blood flow. In three patients (1.5%) there was reduced blood flow in the femoral artery. No patient required surgery, and all were treated either with balloon angioplasty or medically.

Long-term Results

The 202 patients treated by valvuloplasty were followed for a mean period of 24 ± 14 months (range: 1 to 66 months) after the procedure (Figs. 26-6 and 26-8). There were no deaths. Of these 202 patients, 183 (91%) had sustained improvement, while 12 patients (6%) had valve restenosis at a mean time of 12 ± 1.4 months after valvuloplasty.

Of the 186 patients who were treated by valvuloplasty alone, 166 have been followed for a period of more than 6 months (mean: 28 ± 12 months). Of these 166 patients, 162 were in NYHA classes I and II, and only 4 were in class III during follow-up. The mitral valve area (Doppler) was 1.02 ± 0.24 cm^2 before valvuloplasty, 2.17 ± 0.47 cm^2 immediately after valvuloplasty, and 2.08 ± 0.45 cm^2 at follow-up.

Two-Year Follow-Up

Up to the time of this writing, 106 of the first 116 consecutive patients of our series have been followed for at least a 2-year period. Mean mitral valve area evolution during follow-up is shown in Figure 26-8. Of these 106 patients, 72 underwent cardiopulmonary exercise stress testing. Before valvuloplasty, and at the 3-, 6-, 12-, and 24-month follow-ups, the durations of the stress tests were 6.7 ± 2.1, 10.1 ± 2.2, 11.6 ± 2.1, 12.5 ± 2.5, 12.8 ± 2.7 minutes, respectively, $(P < .001)$, while the trend of the maximal oxygen consumption was similar (10.5 ± 2.8, 14.4 ± 2.7, 16.1 ± 2.5, 17 ± 2.7, 17.3 ± 3.2 ml kg^{-1} min^{-1}, respectively, $P < .001$). The main improvement in these test scores occurred during the first and, to a lesser degree, the second trimesters.

CURRENT OUTLOOK AND DEVELOPMENTS

Retrograde Catheterization of the Left Atrium

Although percutaneous balloon mitral valvuloplasty employing the transseptal route is considered to be a safe technique when performed by experienced operators in large volume centers, serious complications do occur in a low percentage of patients. Hemo-

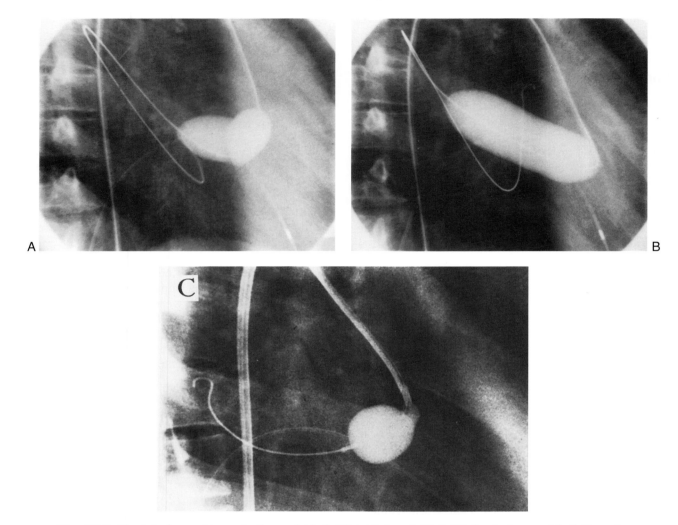

Fig. 26-5. Ventriculographic projections of **(A & C)** initial and **(B & D)** final stages of inflation of a single valvuloplasty balloon **(A & B)** and a modified Inoue balloon **(C & D)** in the mitral valve (right anterior oblique projection). (*Figure continues*)

dynamically significant iatrogenic atrial septal defect[8–10] is a consequence of transseptal catheterization itself, while other complications, such as cardiac perforation and tamponade,[6,7] may be also associated with this procedure. A purely retrograde method of balloon mitral valvuloplasty not requiring transseptal catheterization would thus be desirable. However, retrograde catheterization of the left atrium poses considerable technical difficulties. Moreover, improper positioning of catheter and the guidewire through the mitral chordae would subsequently lead to improper positioning of the valvuloplasty balloon that could result in chordal rupture.

The first clinical attempt of retrograde catheterization of the left atrium was made for diagnostic purposes by Shirey and Sones.[22] In order to perform balloon mitral valvuloplasty employing the purely retrograde route, other investigators used conventional[11] or preshaped[12] catheters. However, these attempts have had limited use, probably due to the aforementioned limitations. A simple, effective, and safe technique for the retrograde catheterization of the left atrium was developed in the Department of Cardiology, Athens Medical School.[13] This technique is based on the use of a specially designed steerable cardiac catheter of which the tip may be configured into the desired form by external manipulations. The effectiveness and safety of this technique have been demonstrated by extensive clinical studies.[15,19,20]

Retrograde Nontransseptal Balloon Mitral Valvuloplasty

Based on the steerable left atrial catheter, RNBMV is a method for balloon mitral valvuloplasty that avoids transseptal catheterization and its inherent

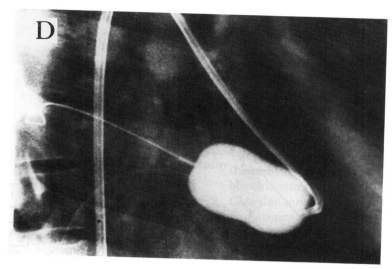

Fig. 26-5. (*Continued*).

complications. The immediate and long-term results are comparable with those of surgical commissurotomy[23] and percutaneous balloon mitral valvuloplasty using the transseptal route,[24,25] while the complication rate is low.

Mechanism

The mechanism of mitral valvuloplasty with the retrograde technique appears to be the same with the transseptal techniques, that is, the splitting of fused calcific or noncalcific commissures and possibly of subvalvular matting. However, the observation that balloons of smaller diameter than those used in the transseptal techniques appear to be effective may be related to a different distribution of the dilating forces when the balloon has been advanced and positioned on the stenotic valve retrogradely.

Effectiveness

Both the immediate and long-term results of RNBMV may be considered very satisfactory. A significant immediate hemodynamic and clinical improvement is accomplished in the majority of the patients, and this initial effect is maintained during long-term follow-up. The restenosis rate during follow-up is approximately 6%, similar to that of the

Table 26-2. Initial Results[a] of Retrograde Nontransseptal Balloon Mitral Valvuloplasty in 203 Completed Procedures

	Before Valvuloplasty	After Valvuloplasty	P
Heart rate (bpm)	82 ± 12	83 ± 16	NS
Mean left atrial pressure (mmHg)	25 ± 6	15 ± 4	<.001
Mean transmitral gradient (mmHg)	15 ± 5	6 ± 2	<.001
Mitral valve area (cm²)			
Gorlin formula[b]	0.96 ± 0.24	2.18 ± 0.55	<.001
Doppler echocardiography	1.03 ± 0.25	2.19 ± 0.49	<.001
Cardiac output (L/min)	3.8 ± 0.5	4.5 ± 0.7	<.001
Mean pulmonary artery pressure (mmHg)	38 ± 10	29 ± 8	<.001

Abbreviations: bpm, beats per minute; NS, not significant.
[a] Values are mean ± SD
[b] Estimated in 197 patients; patients with severe mitral regurgitation were excluded.

└───── **FOLLOW-UP** ─────┘

Fig. 26-8. Mean mitral valve area assessment before and after valvuloplasty by the Gorlin method and Doppler echocardiography and during 24-month (mo) follow-up by Doppler echocardiography.

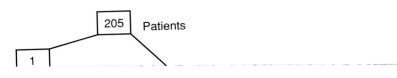

Balloon Aortic Valvuloplasty in Children With Aortic Stenosis

Alain Cribier

Milan Kothari

Brice Letac

Transluminal balloon angioplasty is presently accepted as an alternative to surgical techniques for dilating stenotic arteries in the peripheral and coronary circulation.[1,2] Recently, balloon dilation techniques have been extended to infants and children to relieve congenital, acquired, and postoperative stenotic lesions.[3-8] The initial description of balloon dilation of valve stenosis, given by Rubio and Limon Lason[9] in 1954, and later by Semb et al.[10] in 1979, was that of a pullback technique. However, a static technique as initially described by Kan et al[7] for dilation of the pulmonary valve, is now followed universally. Lababidi[11] was the first to dilate the aortic valve successfully in children. Several other authors have reported since that valvuloplasty can successfully treat valvar aortic stenosis in the pediatric age group.

Congenital valvar aortic stenosis is a relatively common anomaly, occurring in 5 to 7% of all patients with congenital heart disease.[12] The congenitally malformed aortic valve may be unicuspid, bicuspid, or tricuspid, or at times there may be a dome-shaped diaphragm.[13] The congenital bicuspid valve is not inherently stenotic at birth. It may become progressively stenotic, primarily because of fibrosis, and at times calcification, both of which occur secondary to turbulent flow.[14-16] Not uncommonly it may become regurgitant or remain totally normal.[14] Isolated aortic stenosis is more likely to be congenital, while aortic stenosis with associated mitral valve disease is usually caused by a rheumatic pathology. Patients with aortic stenosis may be asymptomatic for many years, despite the presence of severe obstruction.[17] However, the onset of symptoms (i.e., angina, syncope, and exertional dyspnea) heralds the beginning of a rapid downhill course, with mean survival periods after symptom onset being 5, 3, and 2 years, respectively.[18,19] The incidence of sudden death varies between 3 and 15%[20-22] but is usually seen only in previously symptomatic patients.[23,24] Aortic stenosis is a progressive disorder,[17,25] with 40% of patients progressing from mild to severe stenosis over a period of 5 to 7 years.[26] The Natural History Study on aortic stenosis compared the long-term results (more than 15 years) of medical versus surgical management.[27,28] Broad conclusions from this study are that patients with gradients less than 50 mmHg have a 41% chance of requiring valvotomy over a period of 25 years and hence should be followed up medically. Those with gradients more than 50 mmHg have a high risk of sudden death and a 71% chance that intervention will be eventually required and hence should be treated immediately.

Surgical valvotomy, initially regarded as the treatment of choice in patients with aortic valve stenosis, has an average operative mortality of less than 2%.[29-40] However, aortic valvotomy is palliative, since reoperation is indicated in approximately 25 to 40% of patients within 15 to 20 years, the main indications being restenosis and aortic regurgitation.[32,38,40] Hence, the need for an alternative to surgery; balloon valvuloplasty has emerged as a viable option for treatment of congenital valvar aortic stenosis.

MECHANISM OF ACTION

The mechanism of aortic balloon valvuloplasty was assessed by Walls et al.[41] by direct inspection of the valve at surgery. They found that tearing and avulsion of the valve leaflets are the possible mechanisms for relief of aortic valve obstruction. Stretching of valve tissue, splitting of the commissural fusion, and annular dilation all contribute to the relief. Some of the immediate improvement seen after valvuloplasty may be due to leaflet stretching, which may not confer long-term benefit.[42] The splitting of the fused commissures is the most important mechanism. The circumferential dilating force exerted by the balloon during inflation is likely to rupture the weakest part of the valve mechanism (i.e., the fused commissures).[43] However, when the fused commissures are strong, and cannot be torn, tears in the valve cusps or avulsion of the valve leaflets can occur with resultant aortic regurgitation.[41]

TECHNIQUE

The most commonly used method is the retrograde technique by the femoral approach. A brachial approach using the retrograde technique can be used, if the femoral artery is obstructed or the iliac arteries are tortuous. A transvenous approach with a transeptal puncture using a Brockenbrough needle can be used, if there is no arterial access.[44] However, the procedure is longer and carries the added risk of the transeptal puncture.

The most commonly followed technique is described below,[45,47,51] followed by the modified technique used at our Institute.[50] Balloon valvuloplasty is performed in the catheterization laboratory, with the patient lightly sedated. Baseline hemodynamic measurements are obtained by performing a right heart catheterization with a thermodilution balloon flotation catheter using the femoral vein approach. A 5- to 7-F pigtail catheter is positioned in the ascending aorta through the sheath in the femoral artery. Simultaneously another 5- to 7-F pigtail catheter is introduced into the contralateral femoral artery. Through the pigtail catheter, central aortic pressure is measured and biplane aortograms are performed. The patient is then heparinized with 100 U/kg of heparin (maximum dose, 2,500 U). The aortic root angiograms are carefully viewed to determine the degree of regurgitation, the number of leaflets, the size and location of the orifice, and the diameter of the aortic annulus. The aortic valve is generally crossed using a 0.035″ straight-tipped guidewire over an end-hole catheter, like the multipurpose, Gensini, or Schoonmaker catheter. After entering the left ventricle, it is exchanged for a pigtail catheter over a 0.035″ J-tipped exchange wire. Before the exchange, it is important to form an exaggerated curve in the distal part of the wire to protect the myocardium from perforation. Through the pigtail catheters in the left ventricle and aorta, simultaneous aortic and left ventricular pressures are obtained. The transvalvular aortic pressure gradient is measured and the cardiac output is obtained by the thermodilution technique. The valve area is then calculated using Gorlin's formula.[46] After the baseline hemodynamic measurements have been obtained, a left ventricular angiogram is performed in the right anterior oblique projection to determine the left ventricular function, the aortic root diameter, and the presence of mitral regurgitation.

Additional lidocaine is infiltrated at the puncture site and 0.01 mg/kg atropine is given intravenously to avert any vagal reaction, which might otherwise occur during manipulation of the catheters and sheaths at the femoral entry site. Then the diagnostic catheter is removed over a regular 0.035″ or a 0.038″ exchange guidewire, or an extrastiff wire. An extrastiff wire helps in stabilizing and anchoring the balloon across the aortic valve and also prevents the recoil of the inflated balloon into the aorta during systole.[47] Careful fluoroscopic monitoring during all catheter exchanges is very important both to keep the guidewire from being pulled out the left ventricle, as well as to prevent myocardial injury.

The balloon catheters (Meditech, Surgimed & Cook) generally used are 3 to 4 cm long. At times, longer (5.5 cm) balloons are used. The balloon sizes used vary from 4 to 20 mm in diameter. The initial balloon catheter is selected to yield a balloon-to-annulus diameter ratio of 90 to 100%, or whose diameter is 1 to 3 mm smaller than the diameter of the aortic annulus. The chosen balloon is purged with saline, and the air is removed by deflating the balloon and applying strong negative pressure. The central lumen of the balloon catheter is flushed with heparinized saline. The balloon catheter is then introduced over the exchange guidewire. Under fluoroscopic visualization of the tip of the guidewire, the balloon catheter is rapidly advanced until the distal end reaches the left ventricle. The two radiopaque markers at either end of the balloon are used as guide to optimize the position of the balloon across the stenotic valve.

Balloon inflation is performed with a hand-held syringe filled with dilute contrast medium, until the hourglass shape of the balloon disappears. During balloon inflation, three surface electrocardiographic (ECG) leads and the aortic pressure via the catheter in the contralateral femoral artery are monitored. The balloon is kept inflated for 5 to 10 seconds. The balloon is deflated immediately, if significant hypotension occurs, or if marked ST segment shifts or arrhythmias are noted. Before the next inflation, time should be allowed for the aortic pressure and the ECG changes to return to baseline. Two to three inflations are usually performed. However, unlike calcific aortic stenosis in adults, multiple inflations are usually not necessary in congenital aortic stenosis.[48]

The balloon catheter is then replaced by the previous pigtail catheter. The transvalvular gradient, cardiac output, and valve area are obtained, once the heart rate and the aortic pressure return to their prevalvuloplasty levels. If the measurements are considered suboptimal, a larger balloon is used. When a sufficiently large balloon is not available, a double-balloon technique can be used, with simultaneous inflation of both balloons across the stenotic valve.[49] An aortic root angiogram is then done to quantify any dilation-induced aortic regurgitation. Immediately after the procedure is completed, the catheters are removed. Manual pressure is applied to the entry site until complete hemostasis is obtained. Patients remain supine in bed for 24 hours. Most of them are discharged from the hospital 48 hours following valvuloplasty.

At Rouen, our experience in this field is limited to adolescents and young adults with valvar aortic stenosis of either congenital or rheumatic etiology. Following the success of our technique in adults with calcific aortic stenosis, we applied the same technique in adolescents.[50] The major differences between our and the outlined above are as follows:

1. The aortic valve is crossed using a 7-F type B Sones catheter, over a 0.035″ straight-tipped guidewire.
2. The femoral artery sheath used is a special 14-F sheath (Schneider, Buelach, Switzerland). This sheath permits the introduction and removal of all balloon catheters with minimal trauma, resulting in fewer vascular complications. It has a proximal diaphragm, which prevents blood leakage around the guidewire when the balloon catheter is not in place. Also, the occlusive effect of the sheath in the femoral artery prevents bleeding, thus obviating the need for constant groin compression throughout the procedure.
3. The balloon catheter is passed over a 0.035″ extrastiff guidewire (Schneider, Buelach, Switzerland), a 270-cm-long exchange wire with a very stiff core, and a distal flexible curved tip.
4. The balloon catheter used is a catheter specifically designed for aortic valvuloplasty (Mansfield, Boston Scientific, Boston, MA). The balloon is configured with a proximal segment 3.5 cm long that abruptly tapers to a more narrow distal segment 2 cm long. It has a 20-mm proximal diameter and a 15-mm distal diameter (Fig. 27-1). Its pigtail tip adds stability and safety to the device. Similar catheters with single-size balloons of 15-, 18-, 20-, and 23-mm diameter are also available. The catheter has a lumen proximal and distal to the balloon, permitting monitoring of the central aortic pressure and measurement of the transaortic valvar gradient, without having to place another catheter in the contralateral femoral artery. Also, it avoids replacing the standard balloon catheter with a pigtail catheter after the dilation, for taking hemodynamic measurements and performing aortic angiograms.
5. The aortic annulus in adolescents is almost invariably the same size as in an adult, hence the initial balloon catheter size selection is not made on the aortic annulus diameter. Rather, the dilation is

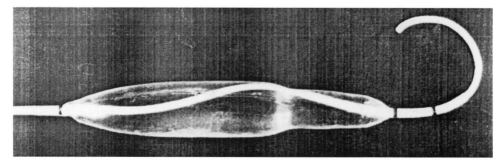

Fig. 27-1. Distal end of the double-size 9-F triple-lumen pigtail balloon catheter used for sequential percutaneous aortic valvuloplasty. The balloon has a proximal segment 3.5 cm long and 20 mm in diameter that tapers to a distal segment 2 cm long and 15 mm diameter.

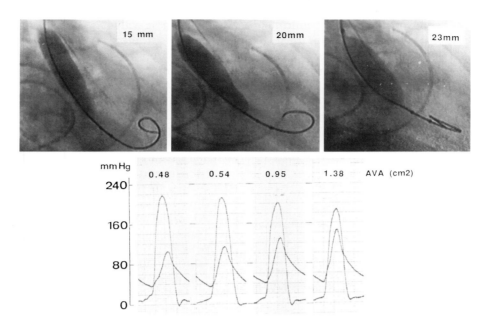

Fig. 27-2. Typical example of the sequential steps of percutaneous aortic valvuloplasty in a 38-year-old man with congenital aortic stenosis. The 0.035″ extrastiff guidewire is maintained within the pigtail end of the catheter. Initial dilation with the 15-mm distal segment (**upper panel**, *left*) is followed by dilation with the 20-mm proximal segment of the balloon (**upper panel**, *middle*). Because of suboptimal results, a single size 23-mm balloon inflation was then performed (**upper panel**, *right*). The mean transvalvular gradient decreased sequentially from 90 mmHg at basal state to 35 mmHg at the end of the procedure and the valve area increased from 0.48 to 1.38 cm².

begun with a 15-mm portion of the balloon, complemented by the 20-mm portion of the same balloon. If the result is not satisfactory, a 23-mm balloon is used (Fig. 27-2).

6. The balloon inflation is performed with a 25:75 mixture of contrast medium and saline, to make it easier deflate the balloon rapidly.

7. The balloon is initially inflated slowly with a 20-ml syringe, while the primary operator fixes the balloon in a stable position. Once proper fixation of the balloon is achieved, the balloon is rapidly inflated with a 10-ml syringe, until the hourglass shape of the balloon disappears. It is important to note that during inflation, only the flexible part of the wire should protrude beyond the balloon catheter.

RESULTS

The first series on balloon aortic valvuloplasty was performed by Lababidi and associates[51] and included 23 patients. The gradient before valvuloplasty was 113 ± 48 mmHg and was brought down to 32 ± 15 mmHg. There were no deaths. Mild aortic regurgitation was noted in 10 patients. Balloon aortic valvuloplasty has since been performed by several groups of workers. The results of some of the largest reported studies are shown in Table 27-1. Our own experience with balloon aortic valvuloplasty includes 17 young patients 12 to 49 years old with either congenital (8 of 17) or rheumatic (9 of 17) aortic valve stenosis. We used the double-balloon technique in the first four patients in this series, and thereafter the single balloon technique. The peak transvalvular gradient decreased from 81 ± 21 mmHg to 47 ± 21 mmHg, and the aortic valve area increased from 0.72 ± 0.26 cm² to 1.24 ± 0.35 cm². Aortic regurgitation was the only complication of the procedure and was seen in all patients following valvuloplasty. It was minimal in 13 patients, moderate in 3, and severe in 1, who underwent an elective aortic valve replacement 3 months later. The regurgitation was tolerated well in the other patients. No other complication was seen.

The Valvuloplasty Registry reviewed data from 204 children and infants who underwent aortic balloon valvuloplasty between 1982 and 1986. It was successful in 192 of 204 patients.[57] The peak gradient decreased from 77 ± 28 mmHg to 30 ± 14 mmHg. This decrease in peak systolic gradient was attributed to a combination of a significant decrease in left ventricular systolic pressure and a significant in-

Table 27-1. Immediate Results of Balloon Aortic Valvuloplasty

Authors	No. of Patients	Age in Years [range (mean)]	Pre-BAV Gradient in mmHg (mean ± SD)	Post-BAV Gradient in mmHg (mean ± SD)	Post-BAV Valve Area in cm²/m² (mean)	Post-BAV Regurgitation Increase[a] [no./total (%)]	Surgery Requirement
Lababidi et al., 1984[51]	23	2–17 (9)	113 ± 48	32 ± 15	NA	6/23 (25) mild	Nil
Walls et al., 1984[41]	27	1.7–17 (9)	108 ± 46	32 ± 16	NA	7/27 (25) mild, 1/27 (4) mod.	2/27 (7.5%) for residual stenosis
Helgason et al., 1987[52]	15	0.03–15 (8.8)	86 ± 21	28 ± 14	0.73	8/15 (57) mild	1 for femoral artery rupture
Mullins et al., 1987[53]	14	NA	68	24	NA	2/14 (14) mod.	Nil
Beekman et al., 1988[54]	16 (1 balloon)	0.25–17 (8)	82 ± 24	46 ± 16		3/16 (18) mild	Nil
	11 (2 balloons)	0.25–21 (10)	76 ± 16	26 ± 13	NA	2/11 (18) mild 1 mod.	
Sholler et al., 1988[47]	12	1 d–3 wk (0.03)	56 ± 34	29 ± 28	NA	3/12 (25) mild, 3/12 (25) mod.	1 each for valve leaflet avulsion and femoral artery
	68/80	0.2–39 (10.7)	79 ± 23	34 ± 19	0.79	24/68 (35) mild, 1/68 mod.	1 each for balloon removal and mitral valve repair
Vogel et al., 1989[45]	25	0.5–16.7 (9.3)	66 ± 26	24 ± 17	1.24 (10 pts.)	6/25 (25) mild, 3/25 (12) mod.	4 for valvotomy for residual stenosis and 3 for femoral artery complications
Sullivan et al., 1989[55]	34	1.3–17 (7)	71 ± 30	28 ± 19	NA	9/34 (27) mild	1 each for valvotomy and femoral artery repair
Rao et al., 1989[56]	16	0.6–16 (8)	72 ± 21	28 ± 13	NA	2/16 (12.5) mild	Nil
Valvuloplasty Registry, 1990[57]	204	1 d–20 yr (10.1)	77 ± 28	30 ± 14	NA	14/204 (7) mild 1.5% mod. 2% severe	8/204 (4%) for valvotomy
O'Connor et al., 1991[58]	33	0.3–21 (8.5)	77 ± 23	35 ± 17	0.64	6/33 (18) mild	3/33 (9%) valvotomy for residual stenosis

Abbreviations: NA, not available.

[a] Grading of post-balloon aortic valvuloplasty (BAV) increase in regurgitation: mild, increase by grade 1/5 to 2/5; moderate, increase by grade 3/5; severe increase by grade ≥4/5. Grading (in 5 grades) according to classification of Hunt et al.[61]

crease in aortic systolic pressure. The left ventricular systolic pressure decreased from 174 ± 40 mmHg to 133 ± 27 mmHg. The cardiac index remained relatively unchanged at 4.1 ± 1 to 3.9 ± 1 L/min/m². On reviewing the major trials of balloon aortic valvuloplasty, a percent reduction of peak-to-peak pressure gradient of more than 50% was achieved in most of the series,[47,51–54,56] with values ranging from 43%[54] to 71%.[51] The mean postdilation gradient ranged from 27 to 38 mmHg, with most of the series reporting values less than 35 mmHg. Values of the mean postdilation valve area ranged from 0.64 cm2/m2[58] to 0.79cm2/m2.[47] Thus, it is a relatively effective means of providing acute relief of valvar aortic stenosis in both infants and children.

Complications

Complications during and immediately after balloon valvuloplasty are minimal. Hypotension and bradycardia have been noted during inflation and these normalize following balloon deflation. Inflating the balloon for shorter periods (5 seconds)[49] or using a bifoil or a trifoil balloon[59] or double balloons[60] have all been advocated to reduce hypotension during valvuloplasty procedures. Transient left bundle branch block, ventricular ectopy, nonsustained ventricular tachycardia, and mitral valve perforation have all been reported.[57] Deaths related to the procedure have been reported (2.5% and 4% in the Valvuloplasty Registry[57] and in the series by Sholler et al.,[47] respectively). All the deaths in both the series occurred in very young infants (younger than 3 months). Postvalvuloplasty aortic regurgitation is commonly reported. The incidence of an increase in aortic regurgitation following valvuloplasty varies from 10 to 30%.[45,47,51,53–58] In the Valvuloplasty Registry, newly developed or increasing aortic regurgitation after dilation occurred in 10%.[57] However, most of the cases of regurgitation were not severe. The incidence of temporary femoral artery occlusion varies from 10 to 20%.[47,53,57] In the Valvuloplasty Registry, femoral artery thrombosis or damage occurred in 12% and was seen most commonly in children under 1 year of age; it was found to be related to the balloon-to-aortic annulus diameter ratio.[57] Permanent femoral artery pulse loss occurred in 2.5% of patients.

Intermediate Results

Long-term effectiveness studies of balloon valvuloplasty for congenital aortic stenosis have not yet been performed. However, the intermediate follow-up results have been documented in many studies and are shown in Table 27-2. The incidence of restenosis at follow-up periods up to 32 months has been negligible. At intermediate follow-up, the need for a repeat balloon valvuloplasty, surgical valvotomy, or valve replacement following dilation varies from 10 to 25%.[51,52,56,63] There was minimal or no progression of aortic regurgitation, compared with the regurgitation seen immediately after dilation. In our series, follow-up Doppler studies at an average duration of 36 months after dilation revealed no cases of restenosis or any progression in regurgitation grade.

BALLOON AORTIC VALVULOPLASTY IN INFANTS

Valvar aortic stenosis in the neonate is commonly associated with patent ductus arteriosus (60%), hypoplastic left heart (47%), coarctation of aorta (23%), and hypoplastic aortic arch (20%).[65] Critical aortic valve stenosis in the neonate is a life-threatening condition, presenting as intractable congestive heart failure with severe left ventricular dysfunction.[66] Medical therapy is only palliative, and until recently these infants underwent either a closed or open heart valvotomy. Surgery is associated with a very high operative mortality rate, with figures ranging from 9 to 86%[65,67–70] and only a few centers reporting a mortality rate less than 20%.[68,69]

Valvuloplasty in the infants is fraught with problems. In the Valvuloplasty Registry, the results were poorer in infants compared with older children.[57] Also, the risk of major complications (including death) and minor complications (such as femoral artery pulse loss) was much higher in infants compared with older children. Zeevi et al.[71] have compared balloon aortic valvuloplasty with surgical valvotomy in neonates, with 16 patients in each group. There were six early deaths and one late death after surgery five of six neonates requiring a second operation died. In six patients, at follow-up (26 ± 17 months) the peak gradient was 52.2 ± 23 mmHg and left ventricular end diastolic pressure was 18.2 ± 5.2 mmHg. Aortic regurgitation was mild in five and moderate in one patient. After balloon dilation, there were three early and two late deaths. The immediate postdilation peak gradient was 27 ± 24 mmHg, representing a more than 50% reduction in the gradient. New aortic regurgitation developed in six neonates, mild in four and severe in two. At follow-up (17.6 ± 7.8 months) the peak gradient was 46 ± 11 mmHg in five patients by catheterization studies, and 43.8 ± 22.9 mmHg in four patients by Doppler. There was mild

Table 27-2. Intermediate Results of Balloon Aortic Valvuloplasty

Authors	No. of Patients	Duration of Follow-up (months)	Gradient mmHg (mean ± SD)	Comments
Lababidi et al., 1984[51]	6	3–9	38 ± 32	2/6 (33%) valvotomy for restenosis
Walls et al., 1984[41]	14	3–13	37 ± 22	—
Helgason et al., 1987[52]	10	1.5–6	41 ± 25	3/10 (30%) increase in gradient 1, increase in regurgitation
Worms et al., 1988[62]	11	3–12	NA	No restenosis
Sholler et al., 1988[47]	29 (Doppler)	1–24	40 ± 22	Increase by 3 grades of regurgitation in 1
	16 (Catheterization)	1–25	45 ± 29	Grade 1 increase in regurgitation in 2
Vogel et al., 1989[45]	9	3–13	30 ± 17	—
Sullivan et al., 1988[55]	24	2–19	35 ± 20	1/24 (4%) restenosis
Rao et al, 1989[56]	16	3–32	35 ± 23	4/16 (25%) restenosis
Shrivastava et al., 1990[63]	13 (Catheterization)	7–15	45 ± 30	2/13 (15%) increase in regurgitation
	10 (Doppler)	2–16	54 ± 23	3/10 (30%) restenosis
O'Connor et al., 1991[58]	27	19	29 ± 16	2/19 (10%) moderate increase in regurgitation
Sandhu et al., 1993[64]	8	14–30	30 ± 13	—

aortic regurgitation in three patients. In the series by Kasten-Sportes et al.[72] on 10 neonates, balloon dilation was successful in 6 of 10 patients. The mortality rate was 30%. Dilation was successful in seven patients, with gradients coming down from 61 ± 24 mmHg to 20 ± 14 mmHg. Aortic regurgitation occurred in three patients, with one having severe and the other two mild-to-moderate regurgitation. Thus valvuloplasty results compare favorably with surgery, and it can be considered an alternative to surgery in neonates with critical valvar aortic stenosis.

BALLOON DILATION IN SUBAORTIC STENOSIS

Despite the lack of long-term studies, balloon dilation is now being accepted as a mode of treatment for discrete subaortic membranous stenosis. de Lozo et al.[73] were the first to dilate discrete subaortic stenosis successfully. The gradient was reduced from 65 ± 18 to 12 ± 9 mmHg, with follow-up studies 7 months later showing no evidence of restenosis. Many later studies reported successful dilation of membranous subaortic stenosis.[49,74,75] Our experience with discrete membranous subaortic stenosis is limited to three patients, two adolescents and one

adult (Fig. 27-3). In all three patients, there was a excellent reduction of gradient (65 to 0 mmHg, 60 to 10 mmHg, and 55 to 16 mmHg). There was no postdilation regurgitation, nor were there other complications. Doppler-calculated gradients in two patients 40 months later revealed no restenosis.

COMPARISON WITH SURGICAL VALVOTOMY

Long-term follow-up studies (more than 5 to 10 years) of balloon valvuloplasty patients should provide a better basis for comparison with surgery. The acute results of balloon valvuloplasty studies are comparable to that of surgical valvotomy. The operative mortality varies between 0 and 4%, with an average of 2%, when infants are excluded. Late mortality varies between 4 and 22%.[29–40] The early (i.e., periprocedural) mortality rate for balloon valvuloplasty, excluding infants, approaches zero.[41,45,49,51–58] In patients who have undergone surgical valvotomy, reoperation rates are 25 to 40% at 15 to 20 years.[30–40] The need for a repeat balloon valvuloplasty, surgical valvotomy, or valve replacement in patients who have undergone balloon dilation varies from 10 to 25%, at follow-up periods of up to 32 months.[51,52,56,63]

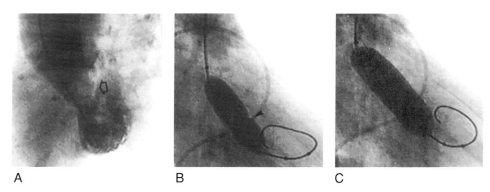

A   B   C

Fig. 27-3. (A) Balloon dilation of a discrete subaortic stenosis in a 25-year-old woman. The subaortic membrane is clearly seen on the left ventricular angiogram (*arrow*), left anterior oblique view. **(B)** 23-mm-diameter balloon is used for dilation and inflated until the waste **(C)** disappears. The mean gradient decreased from 65 mmHg at basal state to 0 mmHg after dilation. In this patient, the mean gradient was 25 mmHg on echo-Doppler control 3 years later.

The incidence of severe aortic regurgitation following valvotomy over a period of 8 to 18 years varies from 6 to 20%.[30-40] The incidence of severe postvalvuloplasty regurgitation was 2% in the Valvuloplasty Registry,[57] with all the intermediate follow-up studies showing minimal or no progression in the regurgitation grade.[45,47,51,52,55,56,58,61-63] Hence valvuloplasty compares favorably with surgery, and many authorities believe that it should be considered the treatment of choice for children with congenital valvar aortic stenosis: it is less invasive, and (more importantly) surgical valvotomy has a significant incidence of early and late mortality, late development of regurgitation, and need for reoperation. Also, valvuloplasty can be repeated in select patients should restenosis occur.[76]

FACTORS AFFECTING ACUTE AND LONG-TERM RESULTS

Sholler et al.[47] have evaluated the influence of various technical and morphological features on the acute outcome and found that patient age, past history of surgical valvotomy, number of dilating balloons (one versus two), and balloon/annulus ratio did not significantly influence the percent reduction in gradient. The valve morphology (unicommissural versus bicommissural) did not influence percent reduction in gradient. However, substantial increases in aortic regurgitation (more than 3 of 5 grades) occurred more frequently with a unicommissural valve. Balloon/annulus ratio significantly influences the increase in aortic regurgitation; a 26% incidence of significant dilation-induced aortic regurgitation is seen with a balloon/annulus ratio more than 100%, compared with an 11% incidence with a balloon/annulus ratio of 100% or less. Beekman et al.[54] claim that the double-balloon technique may be superior to single-balloon valvuloplasty in reducing the gradient, without an associated increase in the complication rate. Rao et al.[56] have evaluated the risk factors associated with restenosis and found that the valve morphology, past surgical valvotomy, number of balloons used, maximum balloon inflation pressure, number of inflations, and total duration of inflation did not influence the rate of restenosis. Age 3 years or less at the time of dilation and immediate postvalvuloplasty gradient 30 mmHg or more were the only two factors associated with restenosis.

CONCLUSIONS

The excellent acute hemodynamic results of balloon aortic valvuloplasty, the sustained hemodynamic benefit, the low mortality, the acceptable rate of complications, and the uncommon occurrence of early restenosis have made it the treatment of choice for many children and young adults with isolated valvar aortic stenosis. The technique is particularly useful in infants with critical stenosis and can be applied to subaortic stenosis and previous surgical valvotomy patients as well. However, at best, balloon valvuloplasty for congenital aortic stenosis can be regarded as a palliative therapeutic procedure, since late restenosis (after 5 to 10 years), as in surgical valvotomy, should be expected in patients undergoing the procedure. At present, we recommend balloon aortic valvuloplasty for stenosis of severe grade, (i.e, peak gradient more than 75 mm) Hg with normal cardiac output or a valve area less than 0.5 cm²/m² body surface area) regardless of symptoms and for moderate stenosis (i.e., gradient 50 to 75 mmHg or valve area 0.5 to 0.8 cm²/m²) in the presence of symptoms or left ventricular strain pattern on ECG.

REFERENCES

1. Dotter CT, Judkins MP. Transluminal treatment of arteriosclerotic obstruction. Description of a new technic and a preliminary report of its application. Circulation 1964;30:654–70
2. Gruntzig AR, Senning A, Siegothaler WE. Non-operative dilatation of coronary artery stenosis: percutaneous transluminal angioplasty. N Engl J 1979;301:61–8
3. Rashkind WJ, Miller WW. Creation of an atrial septal defect without thoracotomy. A palliative approach to complete transposition of the great arteries. JAMA 1966;196:991–92
4. Singer MI, Rowen R, Dorsey TJ. Transluminal aortic balloon angioplasty for coarctation of the aorta in the newborn. Am Heart J 1982;103:131–2
5. Lock JE, Bass JL, Amplatz K et al. Balloon dilation angioplasty of coarctation in infants and children. Circulation 1983;68:109–6
6. Lock JE, Castaneda-Zuniga WR, Fuhrman BP et al. Balloon dilation angioplasty of hypoplastic and stenotic pulmonary arteries. Circulation 1983;67:962–7
7. Kan JS, White RI, Mitchell SE et al. Percutaneous balloon valvuloplasty: a new method for treating congenital pulmonary valve stenosis. N Engl J Med 1982;307:540–2
8. Inoue K, Owaki T, Nakamura et al. Clinical application of transvenous mitral commissurotomy by a new balloon catheter. J Thorac Cardiovasc Surg 1984;87:394–402
9. Rubio V, Limon Lason R. Treatment of pulmonary valvular stenosis and of tricuspid stenosis using a modified catheter. p. 205. In: Second World Congress of Cardiology, Washington, DC, 1954, program abstracts II.
10. Semb BKH, Tijonneland S, Stake G et al. "Balloon valvulotomy" of congenital pulmonary valve stenosis with tricuspid valve insufficiency. Cardiovasc Radiol 1979;2:239–41
11. Lababidi Z. Aortic balloon valvuloplasty. Am Heart J 1983;106:751–2
12. Samanek M, Slavik Z, Zborilova B et al. Prevalence, treatment and outcome of heart disease in live born children. A prospective analysis of 91,823 live born children. Pediatr Cardiol 1989;10:205–11
13. Waller BF. Rheumatic and nonrheumatic conditions producing valvular heart disease. pp. 3–104. In Frankl WS, Brest AN (eds): Cardiovascular Clinics. Valvular Heart Disease. Comprehensive Evaluation and Management. FA Davis, Philadelphia, 1986
14. Fenoglio JJ Jr, McAllister HA Jr, DeCastro CM et al. Congenital bicuspid aortic valve after age 20. Am J Cardiol 1977;39:164–9
15. Subramanian R, Olson LJ, Edwards WD. Surgical pathology of pure aortic stenosis. A study of 374 cases. Mayo Clin Proc 1984;59:683–90
16. Passik CS, Ackermann DM, Pluth JR et al. Temporal changes in the causes of aortic stenosis. A surgical pathologic study of 646 cases. Mayo Clinic Proc 1987;62:119–23
17. Kelly TA, Rothbart RM, Cooper CM et al. Comparison of outcome of asymptomatic patients older than 20 years with valvular aortic stenosis. Am J Cardiol 1988;61:123–30
18. Frank S, Johnson A, Ross J Jr. Natural history of valvular aortic stenosis. Br Heart J 1973;35:41–6
19. Rapaport E. Natural history of aortic and mitral valve disease. Am J Cardiol 1975;35:221–7
20. Braunwald E, Goldblatt A, Aygen MM et al. Congenital aortic stenosis. Circulation 1963;27:426–62
21. Chizner MA, Pearle DL, de Leon AC Jr. The natural history of aortic stenosis in adults. Am Heart J 1980;99:419–24
22. Campbell M. The natural history of congenital aortic stenosis. Br Heart J 1968;30:514–26
23. Ross J Jr, Braunwald E. Aortic stenosis. Circulation, suppl. 1968;37:61–7
24. Pellikka PA, Nishimura RA, Bailey KR et al. The natural history of adults with asymptomatic hemodynamically significant aortic stenosis. J Am Coll Cardiol 1990;15:1012–17
25. Friedman WF, Modlinger J, Morgan JR. Serial hemodynamic observations in asymptomatic children with valvar aortic stenosis. Circulation 1971;43:91–7
26. Cohen LS, Friedman W, Braunwald E. Natural history of mild congenital aortic stenosis elucidated by serial hemodynamic studies. Am J Cardiol 1972;30:1–5
27. Wagner HR, Ellison RC, Keane JF et al. Clinical course in aortic stenosis. Circulation, suppl. I. 1977;56:47–56
28. Keane JF, Driscoll DJ, Gersony WM et al. Second natural history study of congenital heart defects. Results of treatment of patients with aortic valvar stenosis. Circulation, suppl. I. 1993;87:16–27
29. Kirklin JW, Barratt Boyes BG. Congenital aortic stenosis. pp. 972–88. In: Cardiac Surgery. John Wiley & Sons, New York, 1986
30. Jack WD, Kelly DT. Long term follow up of valvotomy for congenital aortic stenosis. Am J Cardiol 1976;38:231–4
31. Lawson RM, Bonchek LI, Manashe V et al. Late results of surgery for left ventricular outflow tract obstruction in children. J Thorac Cardiovasc Surg 1976;71:334–41
32. Stewart JR, Paton BC, Blount SG Jr et al. Congenital aortic stenosis 10 to 22 years after valvotomy. Arch Surg 1978;113:1248–52
33. Sandor GGS, Olley PM, Trusler GA et al. Long term follow up of patients after valvulotomy for congenital valvular aortic stenosis in children. A clinical and actuarial follow up. J Thorac Cardiovasc Surg 1980;80:171–6
34. Dobell ARC, Bloss RS, Gibbons JE et al. Congenital valvular aortic stenosis: surgical management and long term results. J Thorac Cardiovasc Surg 1981;81:916–20
35. Presbitero P, Sommerville J, Revel-Chion R et al. Open aortic valvotomy for congenital aortic stenosis: late results. Br Heart J 1982;47:26–34
36. Jones M, Barnhart GR, Morrow AG. Late results after operation for left ventricular outflow tract obstruction. Am J Cardiol 1982;50:569–79
37. Ankeney JL, Tzeng TS, Liebman J. Surgical therapy for congenital aortic valvular stenosis. J Thorac Cardiovasc Surg 1983;85:41–8
38. Kai-Sheng Hsieh, Keane JF, Nadas AS et al. Long term follow up of valvotomy before 1968 for congenital aortic stenosis. Am J Cardiol 1986;58:338–41
39. Brown JW, Stevens LS, Scott Holly BS et al. Surgical spectrum of aortic stenosis in children: a thirty year

experience with 257 children. Ann Thorac Surg 1988; 45:393–403

40. de Boer DA, Robbins RC, Maron BJ et al. Late results of aortic valvotomy for congenital valvar aortic stenosis. Ann Thorac Surg 1990;50:69–73
41. Walls JT, Lababidi Z, Curtis JJ et al. Assessment of percutaneous balloon pulmonary and aortic valvuloplasty. J Thorac Cardiovasc Surg 1984;88:352–6
42. Hill JA, Conti CR. Balloon valvuloplasty 1988: a review. Clin Cardiol 1989;12:113–20
43. Rao PS. Balloon dilatation in infants and children with cardiac defects. Cathet Cardiovasc Diagn 1989;18:136–49
44. Mullins CE. Transseptal left heart catheterization: experience with a new technique in 520 pediatric and adult patients. Pediatr Cardiol 1983;4:239–45
45. Vogel M, Benson LN, Burrows P et al. Balloon dilatation of congenital aortic valve stenosis in infants and children: short term and intermediate results. Br Heart J 1989;62:148–53
46. Gorlin R, Gorlin SG. Hydraulic formula for calculation of the area of the stenotic mitral valve, other cardiac valves and central circulatory shunts. Am Heart J 1951;41:1–29
47. Sholler GF, Keane JF, Perry SB et al. Balloon dilation of congenital aortic valve stenosis: results and influence of technical and morphological features on outcome. Circulation 1988;78:351–60
48. Letac B, Cribier A, Koning R et al. Results of percutaneous transluminal valvuloplasty in 218 adults with valvular aortic stenosis. Am J Cardiol 1988;62:598–605
49. Rao PS. Balloon aortic valvuloplasty in children. Clin Cardiol 1990;13:458–66
50. Cribier A, Gerber LI, Letac B. Percutaneous balloon aortic valvuloplasty: the French experience. pp. 849–67. In Topol E (ed): Textbook of Interventional Cardiology. WB Saunders, Philadelphia 1990
51. Lababidi Z, Wu J, Walls JT. Percutaneous balloon aortic valvuloplasty: results in 23 patients. Am J Cardiol 1984;54:194–7
52. Helgason H, Keane JF, Fellows KE et al. Balloon dilation of the aortic valve: studies in normal lambs and in children with aortic stenosis. J Am Coll Cardiol 1987;9:816–22
53. Mullins CE, Nihill MR, Vick GW III et al. Double balloon technique for dilation of valvular or vessel stenosis in congenital and acquired heart disease. J Am Coll Cardiol 1987;10:107–14
54. Beekman RH, Rocchini AP, Crowley DC et al. Comparison of single and double balloon valvuloplasty in children with aortic stenosis. J Am Coll Cardiol 1988;12:480–5
55. Sullivan ID, Wren C, Bain H et al. Balloon dilatation of the aortic valve for congenital aortic stenosis in childhood. Br Heart J 1989;61:186–91
56. Rao PS, Thapar MK, Wilson AD et al. Intermediate-term follow-up results of balloon aortic valvuloplasty in infants and children with special reference to causes of restenosis. Am J Cardiol 1989;64:1356–60
57. Rocchini AP, Beekman RH, Shachar GB et al. Balloon aortic valvuloplasty: results of the valvuloplasty and angioplasty of congenital anomalies registry. Am J Cardiol 1990;65:784–9
58. O'Connor BK, Beekman RH, Rocchini AP et al. Intermediate-term effectiveness of balloon valvuloplasty for congenital aortic stenosis. A prospective follow-up study. Circulation 1991;84:732–8
59. Meier B, Freedli B, Oberhansli I. Trifoil balloon for aortic valvuloplasty. Br Heart J 1986;56:292–3
60. Al Kasab S, Riberio P, Al Zaibag M. Use of double balloon technique for percutaneous balloon pulmonary valvotomy in adults. Br Heart J 1987;58:136–41
61. Hunt D, Baxley WA, Kennedy JW et al. Quantitative evaluation of cineaortography in the assessment of aortic regurgitation. Am J Cardiol 1973;31:696–700
62. Worms AM, Marcon F, Cloez JL et al. Percutaneous transluminal valvuloplasty in aortic valve stenosis in children. Arch Mal Coeur 1988;81:617–25
63. Shrivastava S, Das GS, Dev V et al. Follow up after percutaneous balloon valvuloplasty for noncalcific aortic stenosis. Am J Cardiol 1990;65:250–2
64. Sandhu SK, Lloyd TR, Crowley DC et al. Balloon valvuloplasty in young adults with congenital aortic stenosis. Abstracts from the 66th Scientific Session, American Heart Association. Circulation, suppl. I. 1993;88:341
65. Keane JF, Bernhard WF, Nadas AS. Aortic stenosis surgery in infancy. Circulation 1975;52:1138–43
66. Lakier JB, Lewis AB, Heymann MA et al. Isolated aortic stenosis in the neonate: natural history and hemodynamic considerations. Circulation 1974;50:801–8
67. Kugler JD, Campbell E, Vargo TA et al. Results of aortic valvotomy in infants with isolated aortic valve stenosis. J Thorac Cardiovasc Surg 1979;78:553–8
68. Messina LM, Turley K, Stanger P et al. Successful aortic valvotomy for severe congenital valvular aortic stenosis in the newborn infant. J Thorac Cardiovasc Surg 1984;88:92–6
69. Sink JD, Smallhorn JF, Macartney FJ et al. Management of critical aortic stenosis in infancy. J Thorac Cardiovasc Surg 1984;87:82–6
70. Edmunds LH, Wagner HR, Heymann MA. Aortic valvotomy in neonates. Circulation 1980;61:421–7
71. Zeevi B, Keane JF, Castaneda AR et al. Neonatal critical valvar aortic stenosis. A comparison of surgical and balloon dilation therapy. Circulation 1989;80:831–9
72. Kasten-Sportes CH, Piechaud JF, Sidi D et al. Percutaneous balloon valvuloplasty in neonates with critical aortic stenosis. J Am Coll Cardiol 1989;13:1101–5
73. de Lezo JS, Pan M, Herrara N et al. Percutaneous transluminal balloon dilatation of discrete subaortic stenosis. Am J Cardiol 1986;58:619–21
74. Lababidi Z, Weinhaus L, Stoeckle H et al. Transluminal balloon dilatation for discrete subaortic stenosis. Am J Cardiol 1987;59:423–5
75. Arora R, Goel PK, Lochan R et al. Percutaneous transluminal balloon dilatation in discrete subaortic stenosis. Am Heart J 1988;116:1091–2
76. Meliones JN, Beekman RH, Rocchini AP et al. Balloon valvulolasty for recurrent aortic stenosis after surgical valvotomy in childhood: immediate and follow-up results. J Am Coll Cardiol 1989;13:1106–10

28 Balloon Aortic Valvuloplasty in the Adult

Raymond G. McKay

Balloon aortic valvuloplasty was first performed in adults in 1986 for the treatment of symptomatic aortic valve stenosis. Since that time, the acute and long-term efficacy of the procedure has been described by two large multicenter registries as well as by numerous individual series. At the present time, aortic valvuloplasty is considered a palliative technique for nonoperative patients, which results in a modest improvement in hemodynamics and at least short-term amelioration of symptoms. The long-term benefit of the procedure, however, has been limited by a high valvular restenosis rate.

HISTORICAL DEVELOPMENT

The earliest reports on mechanical dilatation of the stenotic aortic valve came from the surgical literature on closed aortic commissurotomy.[1] Unlike the treatment of pulmonic and mitral stenosis, these early attempts to perform surgical aortic valvuloplasty were largely unsuccessful. In the 1950s, both Bailey and Harken[1] experimented with the transventricular and retrograde insertion of various valvulotomes that were designed to cut through the stenotic aortic valve somewhat indiscriminately. They found, however, that the procedure usually resulted in acute aortic insufficiency. Realizing that the cusps must be preserved and only commissures divided, Bailey and others worked on several aortic dilators that were inserted either through the left ventricular apex or in retrograde manner through the innominate artery. Despite these changes, mortality remained high and clinical improvement in most

patients was limited. As a result, closed aortic valvulotomy for aortic stenosis was largely abandoned soon after the development of open aortic valve surgery.

Valvulotomy under direct vision for congenital aortic stenosis was first described in 1956 and subsequently performed using both an inflow occlusion technique and cardiopulmonary bypass. Late follow-up of patients undergoing open valvulotomy has revealed a high rate of restenosis requiring aortic valve replacement, as well as a significant incidence of major complications, including aortic regurgitation, infective endocarditis, and embolization. Similar results have been noted with mechanical decalcification and debridement procedures performed in adult patients with calcific aortic stenosis.

Percutaneous balloon dilatation of the aortic valve was first performed in children with congenital aortic stenosis in 1984 by Lababidi.[2] Lababidi's results were soon confirmed by Ruprath and Nehaus who further demonstrated the efficacy of this technique in infants and adolescents.

Balloon aortic valvuloplasty for adults with calcific stenosis was first performed in 1986 by Cribier[3] using a single balloon retrograde technique from the femoral artery. Cribier's reports were soon followed by reports from our laboratory[4] and by many other centers. The earliest patients treated with aortic valvuloplasty primarily included elderly patients with severe calcific aortic stenosis in whom the procedure resulted in dramatic clinical improvement.

Several modifications of the retrograde balloon aortic valvuloplasty technique were subsequently reported. The performance of balloon aortic valvuloplasty by way of a transseptal approach involving antegrade positioning of aortic valvuloplasty balloons advanced over a guidewire from the femoral vein was described in 1987 by Block and Palacios.[5] Also in 1987, the use of a double-balloon technique for performing aortic valvuloplasty was described by Dorros and colleagues.[6]

In 1986 and 1987, two large multicenter registries, the Mansfield Scientific Aortic Valvuloplasty Registry and the National Heart Lung and Blood Institute Balloon Valvuloplasty Registry, were formed to evaluate the safety and long-term benefits of the procedure. Over 1,100 patients were enrolled in these two registries in a 2-year period. In 1991, following a review of registry data, the United States Food and Drug Administration approved the use of aortic valvuloplasty in nonsurgical candidates.

PATHOPHYSIOLOGIC MECHANISMS

Based on postmortem and intraoperative balloon dilatations of the aortic valve, three mechanisms of increased aortic valve orifice area have been identified for balloon aortic valvuloplasty: fracture of calcific nodules, splitting of fused commissures, and simple leaflet stretching.[7] The degree to which each of these mechanisms apply in a given patient depends on the underlying etiology of aortic stenosis (i.e., senile degenerative, congenital bicuspid, and rheumatic). Fracture of calcific nodules primarily occurs in calcific senile degenerative and in calcific bicuspid disease. Separation of fused commissures occurs primarily in rheumatic aortic stenosis, and, to a lesser extent, in bicuspid valves. Simple leaflet stretching presumably occurs to some degree in all forms of aortic stenosis.

The variable mechanism of aortic valvuloplasty is a partial explanation for the heterogeneous improvement in valve area that is observed with the procedure, with some patients demonstrating large increases in aortic valve area and others demonstrating little or no change. Only small increases in aortic leaflet motility are expected from fractures of calcific nodules and leaflet stretching, while larger improvements in valvular function may be expected from splitting fused commissures. Given the decreasing incidence of rheumatic disease in the general population, most large series of aortic valvuloplasty patients involve calcific disease in the elderly, in which only small increases in calculated aortic valve area have been reported.

The variation in mechanism of dilatation and etiology of valvular stenosis presumably is also an important factor in the time course of valvular restenosis in any given patient. Histologic studies of calcified valves excised after valvuloplasty have demonstrated relatively rapid healing of the fractures with active cellular proliferation in crevices of calcific nodules and even foci of ossification. Similarly, simple leaflet stretching would be expected to result in a relatively transient improvement in valvular function, since intrinsic recoil of stretched leaflets occurs in a short time period. Commissural separation, alternatively, would be expected to result in a longer improvement in valve function similar to mitral valvuloplasty.

Postmortem studies have also been predictive in illustrating the mechanical consequences of using oversized balloons to aggressively dilate the stenotic aortic valve. Leaflet tearing, leaflet avulsion, and annular rupture have all been identified in this setting. Unlike pulmonic valvuloplasty, these pathologic changes are poorly tolerated clinically and have resulted in dramatic complications in isolated patients.

RATIONALE FOR THE PROCEDURE

The major clinical benefit that is associated with aortic valvuloplasty is usually a dramatic, short-term improvement in symptoms of congestive heart failure, presyncope with exertion, and angina. Hemodynamic studies have demonstrated that the small improvement in aortic valve area that is achieved with valvuloplasty is usually associated with a mild increase in cardiac output and a significant decrease in left heart filling pressures. In addition, several studies have demonstrated a progressive increase in left ventricular ejection fraction and a progressive decrease in left ventricular chamber volumes in patients with depressed ventricular function.[8] The time course of these improvements is usually over a period of 6 weeks to 3 months following valve dilatation. Unfortunately, all these hemodynamic improvements reverse when the aortic valve restenoses.

PATIENT SELECTION

Based on the poor long-term results of aortic valvuloplasty studies, the procedure should be considered a palliative technique that is used to improve symptoms and should be reserved for patients who are deferred from aortic valve replacement. Specific patient groups that should be considered include the following clinical subsets:

1. Elderly, symptomatic patients (i.e., > 80 years of age) who are deferred from surgical intervention because of frailty, senility, or other medical conditions that would result in an unacceptably high risk of mortality and morbidity. Given the range in surgical mortality in the elderly population that has been published, each patient must be considered individually with ongoing consultation from a cardiovascular surgeon.
2. Symptomatic patients with terminal diseases or other associated illnesses that preclude surgical intervention (e.g., pulmonary disease, bleeding dyscrasias, renal failure).
3. Patients with severe left ventricular dysfunction or cardiogenic shock in whom valvuloplasty is performed to improve hemodynamics before anticipated definitive surgical intervention.
4. Patients with life-threatening noncardiac conditions that require urgent surgical intervention and general anesthesia. In this clinical setting, valvuloplasty may transiently improve the patient's hemodynamics and subsequently decrease the risk of general anesthesia and surgical intervention.
5. Patients with aortic stenosis characterized by a low cardiac output and low transaortic pressure gradient, where it is not clear whether valvular or myocardial disease is responsible for severe left dysfunction or whether ventricular function is recoverable following valvular improvement. In these patients, if aortic valvuloplasty results in hemodynamic or ventricular function improvement, there is a better indication that the patient might do well with definitive aortic valve replacement. Alternatively, a poor outcome form valvuloplasty may be used to help defer the patient from unnecessary surgery.

Apart from the appropriate selection of patients, it should be noted that there are several major contraindications to performing balloon aortic valvuloplasty. Patients with severe peripheral vascular disease who cannot tolerate placement of 12-F valvuloplasty sheath in their femoral artery without vascular compromise should be deferred. Similarly, patients with severe iliac or aortic tortuosity, abdominal aortic aneurysms, or aortic atherosclerotic disease should be avoided because of the difficulty in passing an aortic valvuloplasty balloon retrograde from the femoral artery and because of the risk of a peripheral cholesterol embolization. For all of these patients, aortic valvuloplasty using the antegrade transseptal approach may be an alternative approach.

Because aortic valvuloplasty may increase aortic insufficiency by one to two grades, patients with pre-existing moderate or severe aortic insufficiency should also not be considered candidates. Finally, patients with aortic valve vegetations or left ventricular mural thrombus should be deferred because of the risk of embolization from the heart.

SELECTION OF AORTIC VALVULOPLASTY EQUIPMENT

Aortic valvuloplasty catheters with balloon diameters ranging from 15 to 23 mm are used most commonly to dilate adult aortic valves. Commercially available catheters consist of 9-F double-lumen catheters with latex balloons that are 5 cm long (Mansfield, Boston Scientific, Watertown, MA). One lumen of the catheter is used for balloon inflation/deflation, while the second lumen accommodates a 0.038-cm guidewire. Because ventricular systole tends to eject the valvuloplasty catheter during balloon inflation, the relatively long balloon length facilitates balloon placement within the aortic valve. Balloons are initially prepped by applying negative pressure to the balloon lumen to remove air. Balloon inflation is achieved with a hand-held syringe filled with a 50:50 mixture of contrast medium and saline. This mixture may be further diluted to allow faster inflation-deflation times. Current catheter sizes up to 20 mm in diameter require insertion through a 12-F sheath, while larger 23-mm catheters require a 14-F sheath.

Several modifications of the standard aortic valvuloplasty catheter have been developed. In order to achieve a lower deflated profile, several polyethylene terephthalate (PET) balloon catheters have been investigated. PET balloons, however, have been hindered by a high incidence of rupture secondary to perforation of the balloon by calcium spicules. Letac and Cribier[9] have also developed a specialized valvuloplasty catheter that allows for simultaneous hemodynamic monitoring during valve dilatation and minimizes the need for catheter exchange. The Cribier device consists of a 9-F catheter with three lumens and a distal pigtail tip. One lumen located proximal to the balloon is used for continuous monitoring of aortic pressure. A distal lumen with multiple orifices in the pigtail tip is used for measuring left ventricular pressure and for contrast injections. The third lumen is used for balloon inflation/deflation. The balloon is double sized, with a proximal segment that is 3.5 cm long and 20 mm in diameter when inflated and a distal segment that is 2 cm long and 15 mm when inflated. A larger double-sized balloon with a proximal 23 mm segment and a distal 18 mm segment has also been developed. Use of this device allows the operator to continuously measure systemic pressure during and after balloon inflations and to measure aortic valve gradient without valvuloplasty catheter removal. The double balloon size also obviates the need for multiple catheter exchanges.

PRETREATMENT

Before balloon aortic valvuloplasty, all patients should routinely undergo right and left cardiac catheterization, left ventriculography, aortography, and coronary angiography to confirm the presence of aortic stenosis, assess prevalvuloplasty ventricular function, and rule out significant aortic insufficiency and coronary artery disease. In patients with severe ventricular dysfunction who cannot tolerate an iodinated contrast load, echocardiography can be used as an alternative technique to assess ventricular function and aortic insufficiency. In elderly and critically ill patients who cannot tolerate multiple catheterization procedures, diagnostic catheterization and aortic valvuloplasty can be performed as a single procedure. If coronary angiography indicates the presence of significant coronary artery disease that may be contributing to the patient's clinical symptoms, then consideration should be given to combined aortic valvuloplasty and coronary angioplasty. In this setting, the order in which aortic valvuloplasty and coronary angioplasty is performed should be determined by a clinical judgment as to whether the patient's valvular or coronary problem is primary.

All patients undergoing balloon valvuloplasty should be ideally pretreated with medical therapy to stabilize congestive heart failure and anginal symptoms. Supplemental oxygen, inotropic agents, and vasopressors should be used where indicated.

Routine assessment of hematocrit, electrolytes, renal function, and clotting parameters should be determined in all valvuloplasty patients. Blood should be cross-matched and four units of packed cells should be immediately available in the event of a valvuloplasty complication requiring urgent transfusion. A Foley urinary catheter is usually placed in all patients. Informed consent, ideally with the input of a cardiovascular surgeon to educate the patient on surgical alternatives, should be obtained.

OPERATIVE TECHNIQUE

In our laboratory, balloon aortic valvuloplasty is currently performed using a single-balloon advanced retrograde from the femoral artery (Fig. 28-1). The patient initially undergoes standard placement of 8-F percutaneous introducer sheaths in the femoral artery and contralateral femoral vein. Between 3,000 and 5,000 U of intravenous heparin are administered. Continuous measurement of systemic arterial pressure is made throughout the procedure from the femoral artery sidearm. Right heart catheterization is performed with a 7-F balloon-tipped catheter that has pacing capability in the event that temporary transvenous pacing is required. Left heart catheterization is performed using a 7-F pigtail catheter using a 0.038″ straight-tipped guidewire to cross the aortic valve. After placement of left and right heart catheters, measurements are made of systemic arterial, left ventricular, pulmonary artery, and pulmonary capillary wedge pressures, as well as Fick cardiac output. Aortic valve area is determined using the Gorlin formula.

Following prevalvuloplasty measurements, a 300-cm 0.038″ exchange guidewire is advanced through the left heart catheter into the left ventricle, and the left heart catheter is withdrawn. An additional curve is placed in the distal tip of the exchange guidewire to minimize trauma to the endocardium with subsequent balloon inflations and exchanges. The 8-F femoral artery sheath is then replaced with a 12 F introducer sheath. Balloon dilatation is performed subsequently with the valvuloplasty catheter inserted percutaneously and advanced retrograde over the exchange guidewire to the level of the aortic valve. The initial valvuloplasty balloon used in most patients is a 20-mm balloon, with an 18-mm balloon rarely used for extremely small patients with low body surface areas. If there is insufficient gradient reduction and if transient hypotension did not occur with inflation of the 20-mm balloon, a 23-mm balloon may be cautiously used following removal of the 20-mm catheter (Fig. 28-2). For each balloon, a total of three to five inflations is performed until full inflation of the balloon across the aortic orifice is achieved. Usually, a "waist" in the valvuloplasty balloon produced by the stenotic valve will be diminished or eliminated. The duration of each inflation of each balloon is variable (range: 20 to 60 seconds), depending on the degree of hemodynamic compromise induced by left ventricular outflow tract obstruction from the fully inflated balloon. After valve dilation, the valvuloplasty catheter is exchanged for a pigtail catheter and repeat measurements of pressures, cardiac output, and calculated aortic valve area are made.

The maximum balloon size which can be used to dilate the stenotic aortic orifice remains controversial. It has been shown in many cases that increasing balloon sizes result in progressively larger decreases

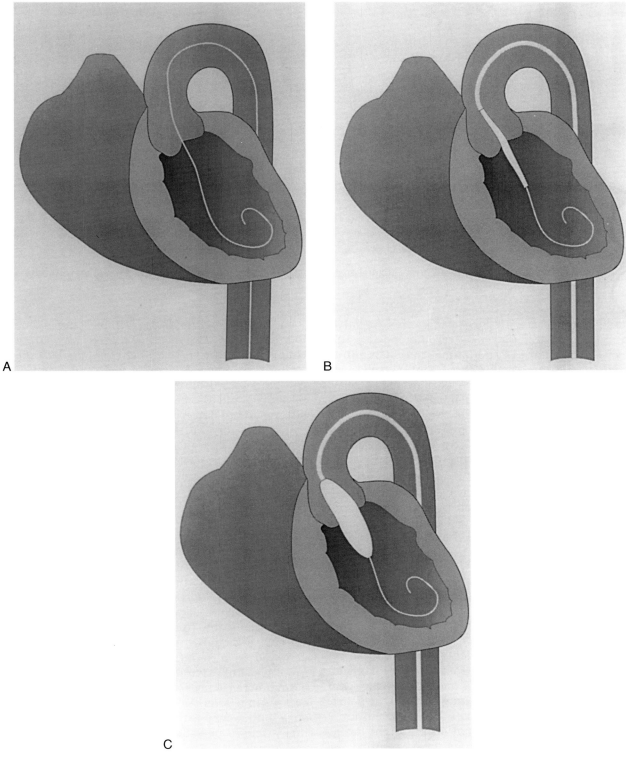

Fig. 28-1. Operative technique of balloon aortic valvuloplasty. **(A)** Following left heart catheterization, the pigtail catheter is exchanged for a 300-cm, 0.038″ guidewire in which an additional curve has been placed in the distal tip to minimize trauma to the endocardium. **(B)** The aortic valvuloplasty catheter is advanced retrograde over the 0.038″ guidewire to the level of the aortic valve. **(C)** The valvuloplasty balloon is inflated with a hand-held syringe until full inflation of the balloon across the aortic valve is achieved.

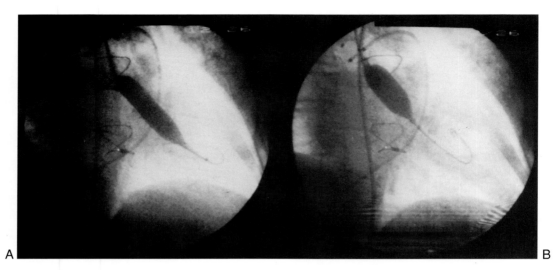

Fig. 28-2. **(A)** Angiogram of an inflated 20-mm aortic valvuloplasty balloon. **(B)** Angiogram of an inflated 23-mm aortic valvuloplasty balloon.

in valve gradients with larger increases in valve area. Some investigators have recommended using balloon sizes that are 1.2 to 1.3 times the aortic annulus diameter. Alternatively, aortic rupture and massive aortic regurgitation have been reported with oversized balloons. At the present time, it seems prudent not to oversize balloons' particularly given the poor long-term results of the procedure even in the presence of large aortic valve increases in isolated patients. One approach to balloon sizing is to measure the aortic valve annulus by using aortography or echocardiography and to use similar-sized balloons. An alternative approach used in our laboratory is to progressively increase the balloon size until transient hypotension occurs during balloon inflation.

POSTVALVULOPLASTY MANAGEMENT AND FOLLOW-UP

Following the procedure, patients are monitored in the coronary care unit for at least 24 hours. During this time period, the patient's medical therapy can be optimized with use of the indwelling right heart catheter and calculation of serial cardiac outputs. Depending on the clinical situation, the right heart catheter and indwelling vascular sheaths can be removed either immediately or up to 24 hours after the procedure. In the event of hematoma formation or bleeding from the arterial access site, heparin can be reversed with intravenous protamine. Patients can be reambulated 12 to 24 hours following sheath removal.

Following valvuloplasty, all patients should be followed with serial echocardiography to assess changes in aortic valve and left ventricular function. Progressive improvement in ventricular physiology can be detected up to 3 months after dilation. The patient should also be followed closely with noninvasive means to detect restenosis.

ACUTE CLINICAL RESULTS

Table 28-1 lists acute hemodynamic results in over 2,000 patients from five major valvuloplasty studies, including data from Hôpital Charles Nicolle (Rouen, France), Massachusetts General Hospital (Boston, MA), Beth Israel Hospital (Boston, MA), the Mansfield Scientific Aortic Valvuloplasty Registry, and the NHLBI Balloon Valvuloplasty Registries.[9–13] On average, the procedure results in approximately a 50% decrease in aortic valve gradient and a 50% increase in calculated aortic valve area (Fig. 28-3). In most patients, the final valve area is between 0.7 and 1.1 cm^2, although valve areas less than 0.7 cm^2 are achieved in a significant number of patients. All large series of valvuloplasty patients have also noted a mild increase in cardiac output, and significant decreases in left ventricular systolic and diastolic pressure, pulmonary artery pressure, pulmonary capillary wedge pressure, and pulmonary vascular resistance.

COMPLICATIONS

Table 28-2 lists major complications for aortic valvuloplasty patients from the same five centers listed in Table 28-1.[9–13] Procedural mortality ranges between

Table 28-1. Acute Hemodynamic Results Associated With Aortic Valvuloplasty

Study	No. of Patients	Preaortic Valve Gradient (mmHg)	Postaortic Valve Gradient (mmHg)	Preaortic Valve Area (cm^2)	Postaortic Valve Area (cm^2)
Hopital Charles Nicolle, Rouen, France	218	72 ± 25	29 ± 14	0.52 ± 0.18	0.93 ± 0.33
Massachusetts General Hospital, Boston, MA	310	61 ± 2	27 ± 2	0.50 ± 0.01	0.90 ± 0.02
Beth Israel Hospital, Boston, MA	170	71 ± 20	36 ± 14	0.60 ± 0.20	0.90 ± 0.30
Mansfield Registry	492	60 ± 23	30 ± 13	0.50 ± 0.18	0.82 ± 0.30
NHLBI Registry	674	55 ± 21	29 ± 13	0.50 ± 0.20	0.80 ± 0.30

Table 28-2. Aortic Valvuloplasty Complications

Complication	Hopital Charles Nicolle (n = 284)	MGH (n = 310)	BIH (n = 170)	Mansfield Registry (n = 492)	NHLBI Registry (n = 674)
Procedural death	1%	NA	0%	4.9%	3%
In-hospital death	4.5%	8.6%	3.5%	7.5%	8%
Embolic episodes	0.7%	1.2%	0%	2.2%	4%
Cardiac tamponade	1%	0.3%	1.7%	1.8%	1%
Vascular surgery	4%	9.6%	10%	5.4%	5%
Severe AI	1.6%	1.5%	1.2%	1%	0.5%
Nonfatal arrhythmia	0.5%	NA	3.5%	1%	8.7%
Myocardial infarction	0.2%	0.5%	0.5%	0.2%	1%

Abbreviations: AI, aortic insufficiency; BIH, Beth Israel Hospital; MGH, Massachusetts General Hospital; NA, not available.

1 to 4.9%, and in-hospital mortality ranges from 3.5 to 8.6%. The most common causes of death included hemodynamic compromise, cardiac tamponade, fatal arrhythmia, cerebrovascular accident, and sepsis. The most common nonfatal complication involved vascular repair of the arterial access site (range: 4 to 10%). Embolic events, massive aortic insufficiency, and ventricular perforation with tamponade all occurred in a range of 0 to 4%. Other less common complications included myocardial infarction and nonfatal arrhythmia, which occurred with an incidence of less than 1%. Total periprocedural complications ranged between 22.6 and 25% between the Mansfield Scientific and NHLBI registries. The significant incidence of complications that can occur with valvuloplasty necessitates that the procedure be performed with onsite surgical back-up.

Similar to balloon angioplasty, it is important to realize that current techniques of performing aortic valvuloplasty result in a lower incidence of complications than have been previously published. Procedural mortality in individual series currently is less than 1%, with an in-hospital mortality of less than

4%. This improvement in procedural complications is presumably related to the learning curve associated with the procedure, better patient selection, and improvement in valvuloplasty equipment.

LONG-TERM FOLLOW-UP

The long-term improvement after aortic valvuloplasty is limited by a high incidence of valvular restenosis and early mortality. Table 28-3 list survival rates and event-free survival rates in four large valvuloplasty studies.[9,11,14,15] The 1-, 2-, and 3-year overall survival rates range between 55 and 75%, 45 and 60%, and 28 and 53%, respectively. Event-free survival with freedom from death, valve replacement, repeat valvuloplasty or recurrent symptoms ranges from 38 to 50% at 1 year, from 19 to 25% at 2 years, and from 7 to 8% at 3 years.

Several studies have examined the long-term determinants of survival and event-free survival.[14] In general, the best long-term results after valvuloplasty were observed among patients who would

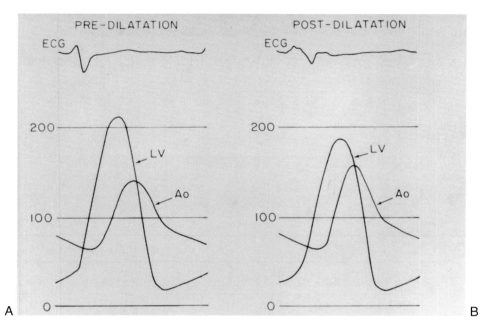

Fig. 28-3. Typical hemodynamic results following balloon aortic valvuloplasty in an elderly patient with calcific aortic valve stenosis. **(A)** Predilation: peak aortic gradient (mmHg), 66; cardiac output (L/min), 3.4; aortic valve area (cm^2) 0.4. **(B)** Postdilation: peak aortic gradient (mmHg) 32; cardiac output (L/min), 3.9; aortic valve area (cm^2), 0.6.

also have been expected to have excellent long-term results after aortic valve replacement. Significant predictors of event-free survival include left ventricular ejection fraction, left ventricular and aortic systolic pressure, and the percent reduction in the aortic valve gradient. The pulmonary capillary wedge was also inversely associated with event-free survival.

REPEAT BALLOON AORTIC VALVULOPLASTY

Repeat balloon aortic valvuloplasty can be performed if clinical and aortic valve restenosis develops and if the patient cannot undergo aortic valve replacement.[9,16] The risk of repeat valvuloplasty, usually

performed at the time of repeat catheterization, is not different from the initial procedure.[16] The degree of hemodynamic improvement for the second valvuloplasty is usually similar or sometimes less than that produced by the initial valvuloplasty, even when larger balloons are utilized. Patients who demonstrate less hemodynamic improvement with a second valvuloplasty in comparison to the first procedure tend to rapidly develop a second restenosis.

CONCLUSIONS

Balloon aortic valvuloplasty is a purely palliative procedure that results in a small improvement in aortic valve area with at least short-term palliation

Table 28-3. Clinical Follow-up of Balloon Aortic Valvuloplasty

	Hopital Charles Nicolle	Massachusetts General Hospital	Beth Israel Hospital	Mansfield Registry
No. of patients	274	310	205	492
Follow-up	16 mo	12–36 mo	12–36 mo	12 mo
% Survival	68%	55%, 1 yr	75%, 1 yr	64%
		45%, 2 yr	60%, 2 yr	
		28%, 3 yr	53%, 3 yr	
% Event-free survival	62%	38%, 1 yr	50%, 1 yr	43%
		19%, 2 yr	25%, 2 yr	
		7%, 3 yr	8%, 3 yr	

of symptoms. The procedure is associated with a high rate of restenosis, and does not improve long-term mortality. It may be useful in treating elderly and other patients who are deferred from aortic valve replacement, in patients with depressed ventricular function as preparation for cardiac surgery, in patients who require emergency noncardiac surgery, and in patients with low aortic valve gradients-low cardiac output as a predictive test for surgical intervention. The patients who have the best long-term result from the procedure are those who would have also have been expected to have excellent long-term results after aortic valve surgery.

REFERENCES

1. Bailey CP, Glover RP, O'Neill TJE, Ramirez HPR: Experiences with the experimental surgical relief of aortic stenosis. J Thorac Surg 1950;20:516–22

2. Lababidi Z, Wu JR, Walls JT: Percutaneous balloon aortic valvuloplasty: results in 23 patients. Am J Cardiol 1984;53:194–7

3. Cribier A, Savin T, Saondi N et al: Percutaneous transluminal valvuloplasty of acquired aortic stenosis: an alternative to valve replacement? Lancet 1986;1:63–7

4. McKay RG, Safian RD, Lock JE et al: Balloon diltation of calcific aortic stenosis in elderly patients: postmortem, intraoperative, and percutaneous valvuloplasty studies. Circulation 1986;74:119–25

5. Block PC, Palacios IF: Comparison of hemodynamic results of antegrade versus retrograde percutaneous balloon aortic valvuloplasty. Am J Cardiol 1987;60:659–62

6. Dorros G, Lewin RF, King JF, Janke LM: Percutaneous transluminal valvuloplasty in calcific aortic valve stenosis: the double balloon technique. Cathet Cardiovasc Diagn 1987;13:151–6

7. Safian RD, Mandell VS, Thurer RE et al: Postmortem and intraoperative balloon valvuloplasty of calcific aortic stenosis in elderly patients: mechanisms of successful dilatation. J Am Coll Cardiol 1987;9:655–60

8. Safian RD, Warren SE, Berman AD et al: Improvement in symptoms and left ventricular performance after balloon aortic valvuloplasty in patients with aortic stenosis and depressed left ventricular ejection fraction. Circulation 1988;78:1181–91

9. Letac B, Cribier A, Koning R, Bellefleur J: Results of percutaneous transluminal valvuloplasty in 218 adults with valvular aortic valve stenosis. Am J Cardiol 1988;62:598–605

10. McKay RG: The Mansfield Scientific Aortic Valvuloplasty Registry: overview of acute hemodynamic results and procedural complications. J Am Coll Cardiol 1991;17:485–91

11. Moreno PR, Jang IK, Block PC, Palacios IF: Long term follow-up of percutaneous aortic balloon valvuloplasty in the elderly: the Massachusetts general experience. Circulation 1993;88:1–340 (abst).

12. NHLBI Balloon Valvuloplasty Registry Participants. Percutaneous balloon aortic valvuloplasty: acute and 30-day follow-up results in 674 patients. Circulation 1991;84:2383–97

13. Safian RD, Berman AD, Diver DJ et al: Balloon aortic valvuloplasty in 170 consecutive patients. N Engl J Med 1988;319:125–30

14. Kuntz RE, Tosteson ANA, Berman AD et al: Predictors of event-free survival after balloon aortic valvuloplasty. N Engl J Med 1991;325:17–23

15. O'Neill WW: Predictors of long-term survival after percutaneous aortic valvuloplasty: report of the Mansfield Scientific Balloon Aortic Valvuloplasty Registry. J Am Coll Cardiol 1991;17:193–8

16. Kuntz RE, Tosteson ANA, Maitland LA et al: Immediate results and long-term follow-up after repeat balloon aortic valvuloplasty. Cathet Cardiovasc Diagn 1992;25:4–9

17. Bashore TM, Davidson CJ and the Mansfield Scientific Aortic Valvuloplasty Registry Investigators: Follow-up recatheterization after balloon aortic valvuloplasty. J Am Coll Cardiol 1991;17:1168–95

29 | Transluminal Implantation of Valves

Dušan Pavčnik

Percutaneous interventional radiology and cardiology has progressed at a breathtaking pace and there does not appear to be end in sight. This chapter describes the initial design and experimental evolution of a mechanical prosthetic aortic valve developed by Pavčnik and colleagues[1] and a biologic aortic valve developed by Andersen and colleagues[2] that can be implanted by using a transcatheter technique.

Heart valve replacement began in 1952, when Hufnagel and Harvey[3] surgically implanted the first valvular prosthesis in the descending aorta. Over 20 different mechanical and biologic cardiac valves have been developed since that time. However, placement of these prosthetic valves requires general anesthesia and major surgery, with their associated morbidity and mortality. Therefore, we need to devise a prosthetic heart valve that can be placed percutaneously by using a transcatheter technique.

MECHANICAL VALVE

Description

The prosthetic aortic valve created for transcatheter insertion was based on the caged-ball and seat design (Fig. 29-1). The cage was a barbed Gianturco self-expanding stainless steel stent[4] with four to six lengths (3.0 cm) of flat, flexible stainless steel wire attached at the cranial end to form the top of the cage (Fig. 29-2).

The seat, or ring, was constructed of two stainless steel wires coiled together in a springlike configuration and covered with an expandable nylon mesh. Barbs were located at various points around the ring for stabilization after placement. The ring was attached to the cage assembly with a length of stainless steel tubing (Fig. 29-2).

The ball was a detachable latex balloon placed at the tip of a 60-cm-long 5-F highflow catheter for delivery and placement within the cage and ring assembly (Fig. 29-3). It was filled with air, contrast material Angiovist 370, or a liquid silicone prepolymer system before detachment. This system had a low enough initial viscosity to be injected through the delivery catheter with a 1-ml syringe. Polymerization of the mixture occurred within 25 minutes after mixing, and when fully cured, the polymer had the consistency of soft rubber.

Animal Studies

Initial in vivo testing of the valve was carried out in 12 adult mongrel dogs (21 to 27 kg). After induction of general anesthesia, the right common carotid artery was surgically isolated and an 11- or 12-f Teflon sheath was introduced. Heparin sodium (100 IU/kg) was administered via a cephalic vein. The sheath was advanced into the ascending aorta under fluoroscopic monitoring.

With the animal in the left lateral position, an aortogram was obtained to determine the diameter of the sinus of Valsalva and ascending aorta (Fig. 29-4). This was necessary to select the appropriate size of prosthetic valve. For placement in dogs, the valve was made in several different sizes. The cage was 2.2. cm long (1.7-cm stent plus wire top 0.5 cm high) and was either 2.8 or 3.0 cm in diameter. The outside

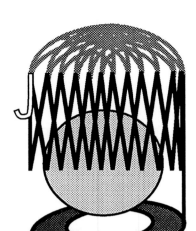

Cage

Ball

Ring

Fig. 29-1. Caged-ball valve for percutaneous transcatheter placement. The three main components of the prosthesis (cage, ring, and ball) are depicted.

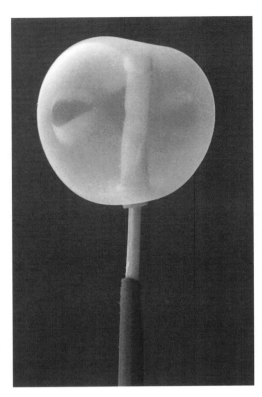

Fig. 29-3. Detachable latex balloon used as the ball. The balloon is attached to a 5-F high-flow catheter, which is passed coaxially through the Teflon introducer sheath. The balloon is filled with air in this picture.

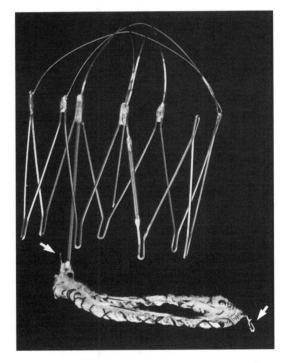

Fig. 29-2. Cage and ring assembly. Note the flat wires that form the top of the cage and the tubing that joins the ring to the stent. The ring is covered with expandable nylon mesh. Three anchoring barbs (two on ring and one on stent) can be seen (*arrows*).

diameter of the ring ranged in 2-mm increments from 2.4 to 3.4 cm. In all cases, the inside diameter of the ring was 0.8 cm less than the outside diameter. This difference was due to the width of the ring formed by the nylon mesh.

After aortography, the tip of the delivery sheath was positioned in the posterior noncoronary cusp. A small amount of contrast medium was injected to check the position of the sheath, and the tip was marked by placement of a needle in the overlying skin. The prosthetic valve (cage and ring assembly) was collapsed, loaded into the sheath, and advanced to the tip by using a 9-F pusher catheter (Fig. 29-5). As the ring exited the sheath, it opened and was anchored against the annulus by the barbs. In all cases, the ring was placed below the ostia of the coronary arteries. As the ring opened, the cusps of the aortic valve were trapped between the ring and the aortic wall. This created considerable regurgitation and an appropriate model for evaluating the efficacy of the new device (Fig. 29-6). Once the ring was positioned correctly, the entire device was extruded into the aorta. The detachable balloon was then advanced through the sheath and placed into the cage. After inflation, the balloon was detached from the delivery

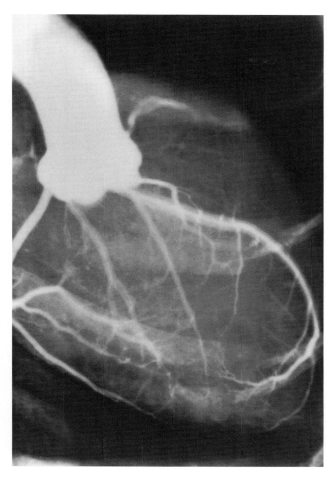

Fig. 29-4. Normal aortogram obtained before valve placement. The dog is in the left lateral position.

catheter. The movement of the ball (balloon) was checked fluoroscopically in the anteroposterior and lateral projections (Fig. 29-7). The competency of the valve and the patency of the coronary arteries were tested and documented by injecting contrast medium directly above the top of the cage (Fig. 29-8).

All dogs were followed up fluoroscopically for as long as the valve remained functional. When valve failure occurred, the animal was killed with an overdose of pentobarbital sodium administered intravenously and a complete necropsy was performed.

Results

Results obtained in these initial feasibility studies led to various design changes in the valve. Development of the final ring design allowed delivery through an 11- or 12-F Teflon sheath.

In all 12 animals, the ring assembly was successfully placed below the ostia of the coronary arteries.

Postmortem examination showed that the ring was securely anchored against the annulus of the aorta by the barbs, and no damage to the surrounding stuctures was noted. The cusps of the aortic valve were trapped between the ring and the aortic wall, resulting in complete incompetence of the natural valve (Fig. 29-6). On a scale of 4, the resulting aortic insufficiency was consistently grade 4. The entire left ventricle was opacified, and the contrast material remained in the ventricular cavity throughout sequential cardiac cycles, even after termination of injection.

The ring and cage assembly consistently reformed after being pushed from the sheath, and the unit was easily positioned and securely anchored in place. Once the assembly was in position, the detachable ball (balloon) was inserted into the valve and released between the ring and cage. In the first nine dogs, the ball was filled with air (three dogs) or contrast medium (six dogs). In the final three animals,

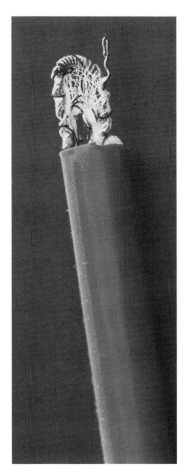

Fig. 29-5. Collapsed prosthesis being pushed out of 12-F Teflon sheath. The ring with anchoring barb is just beginning to emerge from the sheath.

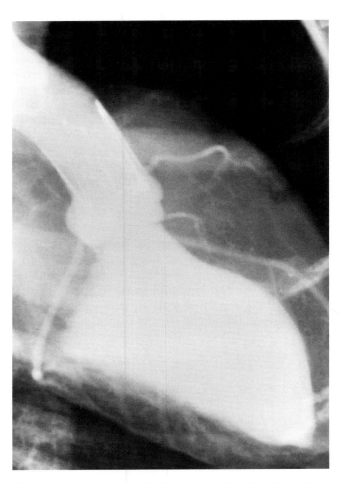

Fig. 29-6. Aortogram obtained immediately after placement of cage and ring assembly in ascending aorta. The dog is in the right anterior oblique position. Note the massive regurgitation resulting from compression of the normal cusps by the ring.

the radiopaque silicone prepolymer system was used to fill the poppet. However, a small amount of air remained trapped in the balloon.

The last three valves that were placed showed excellent functional results for up to 3 hours. However, in all three cases, the ball escaped into the aorta through the top of the cage after 1, 2.5, and 3 hours, respectively.

During the time the valve remained functional, the ring and surrounding structures were sufficiently close together to prevent leakage of blood between them, and the coronary arteries remained patent. A thin layer of clot formed on the nylon mesh immediately after valve placement. This provided a barrier that effectively channeled blood flow through the central opening of the ring during systole and prevented leakage of blood around the ball back into the left ventricle during diastole.

BIOLOGIC VALVE

Description

The new biologic heart valve was prepared by mounting a porcine aortic valve into an expandable stent. The stent was constructed of two 0.55-mm surgical stainless steel wires (monofilament), each folded in 15 loops (Fig. 29-1A). Three of the loops were 14 mm high, designed to the commissures of a porcine aortic valve. The remaining loops in the first wire and all the second wire loops were 8 mm high. Each folded wire was bent into a circle (diameter, 22 mm) which was closed end-to-end by soldering. The two circles were then stacked upon each other and interfixed by Merseline 2-0 sutures (Fig. 29-9A).

The foldable valve was a porcine aortic valve taken from a 90-kg slaughtered pig. The aortic valve was carefully dissected and cleaned manually to remove unwanted material, the diameter, thickness, and height of the cleaned valve annulus was 27 mm, 1 mm, and 2 mm, respectively. The height of each of the three commissural sites was 8 mm.

The stent-valve was prepared by mounting the cleaned aortic valve inside the stent (Fig. 29-9B, C). The aortic annulus, which included the three commissural sites, were fixed to the metallic stent by 45-50 Prolene 5-0 sutures. The external diameter of the stent-valve was approximately 12 mm when collapsed (Fig. 29-9D, E), and 32 mm when entirely expanded (Fig. 29-9F, G). After the stent-valve had been manually compressed on the carrier balloon catheter, the stiffness of the metal prevented it from uncoiling spontaneously (Fig. 29-9D, E). After expansion, the stiffness of the metal minimized spontaneous recoil, when the balloon was deflated (Fig. 29-9F, G).

The carrier balloon catheter used for implantation was a conventional 12-F three-foiled aortic valvuloplasty balloon dilatation catheter (Schneider, Zürich, Switzerland). Each of the three balloons was 70 mm long and had a diameter of 15 mm. The total diameter of the three balloons was 31 mm when inflated. Two soft rubber blocks (3 mm high) were mounted on each of the three balloons, separated by a distance of 18 mm (Fig. 29-9D, F). The blocks ensured a stable position for the stent-valve in the middle of the balloons, and avoided migration during catheter advancement and balloon inflation. The carrier balloon catheter was mounted in a self-constructed 41-F flexible introducer sheath (external diameter, 13.6 mm; internal diameter, 12.5 mm; length 75, cm). The stent-valve-loaded carrier balloon catheter was retracted into the introducer sheath during intravascular introduction and advancement to minimize friction against the vessel wall. A standard

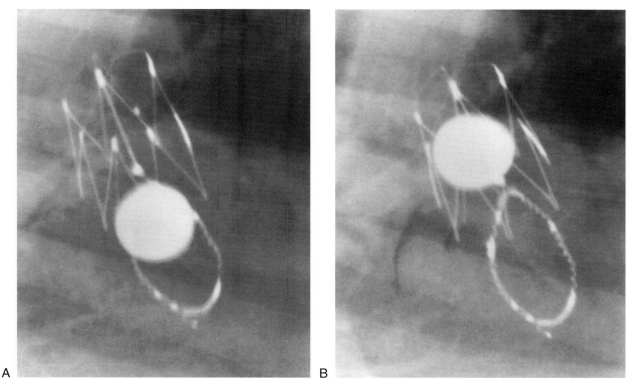

A

B

Fig. 29-7. Radiographs showing movement of the ball during the cardiac cycle: **(A)** diastole, **(B)** systole.

guidewire, 300 cm long and 0.9 mm in diameter, was used for conventional catheter-over-guidewire advancement of the carrier balloon catheter.

Animal Studies

Seven pigs weighing 70 kg were used for implantation. Because the femoral arteries of 70-kg pigs are only 3 to 4 mm in diameter, retroperitoneal access to the abdominal aorta was made through a midline laparotomy. The aorta was exposed over a distance of 6 to 7 cm cranial to the renal arteries and cross-clamped proximally and distally. During temporary cross-clamping, a 4-cm long incision enabled an 8- to 10-cm long vascular prosthesis (diameter 20 mm), to be sutured end-to-side to the aorta at an angle of 45 degrees. The prosthesis was used to gain intravascular access for the 41 F introducer sheath. The animals were given no antiplatelet or anticoagulant drugs, and after implantation, angiography, and pressure measurements, the pigs were exsanguinated under continuous anaesthesia.

The guidewire was advanced retrogradely into the left ventricle under continuous fluoroscopy, and subsequently the introducer sheath was advanced over the guidewire into the descending thoracic aorta. The carrier balloon catheter was then pushed out from the sheath and advanced further around the aortic

arch. For supracoronary implantation, the stent-valve was positioned just beneath where the right brachiocephalic artery started. For subcoronary implantation the stent-valve was positioned in the aortic root/left ventricular outflow tract beneath the coronary arteries at the level of the native aortic valve (Fig. 29-10).

When the stent-valve was placed in the right position, implantation (stent-valve expansion) was performed by balloon inflation (4 atm in 15 seconds), which overdilated (overstretched) the vessel. The elastic recoil of the vessel secured fixation and minimized periprosthetic leakage. Subsequently, the deflated balloon catheter, guidewire, and sheath were withdrawn. Two pigs were exposed to double stent-valve implantation with the first one implanted in the supracoronary position; the second stent-valve was advanced retrogradely through the first valve and implanted in the subcoronary position.

With supracoronary implantation, all five stent-valves were fixed in the ascending aorta; the aortic diameter was overstretched by 3 to 4 mm. Four of the five stent-valves were positioned more than 1.5 cm above the genuine valves; none of the valves obstructed the brachiocephalic artery. In one animal (no. 4), in which the stent-valve was implanted 3 mm above the native aortic valve, the stent-valve was competent, thus leaving only a small volume of blood

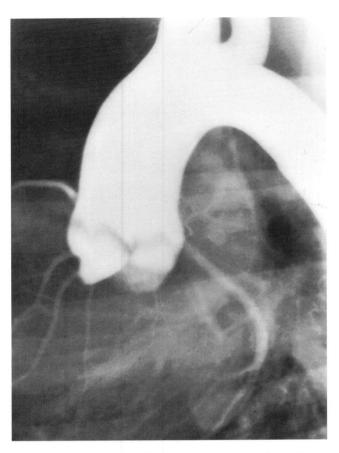

Fig. 29-8. Aortogram showing competency of prosthetic valve and patency of coronary arteries. The filling defect seen in the aortic annulus is due to the ring (same dog as in Figure 29-6).

between the native valve and the stent-valve available for coronary flow in diastole. This caused ST-segment elevation and pump failure. All the stent-valves were competent at inspection and without coagulated blood on the cusps. However, small thrombi were seen on the metal and sutures.

With subcoronary implantation, all stent-valves were implanted at the level of the genuine valves, which were completely compressed between the metal stent and the vessel/heart wall. Two of the four stent-valves were implanted beneath the origin of the coronary arteries. The other two (nos. 3 and 5) restricted coronary flow. In pig no. 3, both coronary arteries were obstructed, and the pig died due to pump failure. In pig no. 5 the left coronary ostium was free of the stent-valve, but the right coronary artery was partially obstructed. This animal was hemodynamically stable, but died suddenly from ventricular fibrillation 1.5 hours after implantation. Mild regurgitation at aortography was found in two stent-valves. This was caused by tightness of one of the

stent-valve cusps in one case (probably caused by the preparation); in the other there was a small paraprosthetic leak.

Results

All the animals survived the initial postimplant period, and pressure measurement and angiography was accomplished. None of the stent-valves caused severe stenosis, and only trivial contrast regurgitation was seen in two pigs. Left ventricular end-diastolic pressures were unchanged after stent-valve implantation in five of seven pigs, but increased in two due to left ventricular failure caused by restriction of the coronary blood flow.

All nine prosthetic valves were undamaged by the implantation procedure, and the sutures kept the biologic valves inside the stent stable. No hematoma, bleeding, or aortic dissection was seen in any of the seven pigs. Four pigs, in which no mechanical complications were seen, fulfilled the study's protocol. In three animals, the coronary flow was restricted.

DISCUSSION

Mechanical heart valves are generally of three designs: caged-ball, disk, or biologic. Catheter-mounted valves have previously been constructed by Matsubara and associates[5] for short-term treatment of acute aortic insufficiency. These devices were mounted on long catheter wires that extended out through the vessel wall. Their position in the bloodstream was secured by external fixation of the extending catheter wires to the skin. Consequently, such valves were not suitable for permanent implantation.

The mechanical prosthetic aortic valve described in this chapter, a caged-ball and seat design, functions as a simple one-way ball valve. Clinical use of this valvular design was first reported in the early 1960s by Harken and associates and Starr and Edwards. We chose this design for our work because it is practical and durable and because we believed that it could be constructed in such a way that it could be passed through a relatively small introducer system. We succeeded in formulating a self-expanding valve that could be collapsed and easily pushed through an 11 or 12-F Teflon sheath. Although this sheath size may require a cutdown for introduction, as was performed in this study, further miniaturization of the compressed valve diameter should allow consistent percutaneous delivery.

Regardless of design, all valves with a fabric-covered ring will cause hemolysis if a paravalvular leak develops. Thus, even an "ideal" valve must be posi-

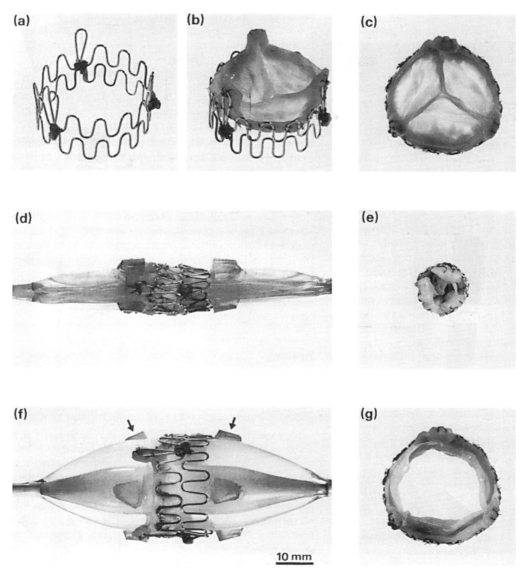

Fig. 29-9. (A) The stent was constructed with two 0.55-mm stainless steel wires folded in 15 loops. **(B,C)** A three-leaflet porcine aortic valve was mounted inside the stent and fixed to the metal by sutures to form the stent-valve. **(D)** Before implantation, the stent-valve was mounted on a deflated three-foiled balloon dilatation catheter. **(E)** The diameter of the collapsed stent-valve was 12 mm. **(F,G)** Balloon inflation expanded the stent-valve to an external diameter of 32 mm. Each of the three balloons was mounted with two elastic blocks (*arrows*), to prevent migration of the stent-valve from the middle of the balloons. (From Andersen et al.,[2] with permission.)

tioned securely in the valve annulus. Secure fixation of our cage and ring assembly was easily accomplished by use of barbs on both the stent and ring. Attachment of these two components to each other also helped prevent movement of the valve once placed. In addition, cellular overgrowth of the stent and ring should occur, which would ensure stability.

The ring was covered with a fine mesh of expandable nylon material to provide a framework for cellular overgrowth, which, in turn, would prevent possi-

ble emboli from forming on the ring. Previous work with the material has shown that neointimal encasement of the mesh occurs when it is placed in the aorta. The current experiments demonstrated that a thin layer of clot formed on the nylon mesh immediately after valve placement. This provided a barrier that effectively channeled blood flow through the central opening of the ring during systole and prevented leakage of blood around the ball back into the left ventricle during diastole. However, additional

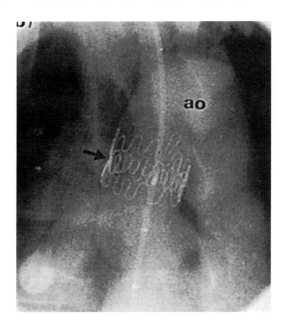

Fig. 29-10. Biologic stent valve implanted in supracoronary position. (From Andersen et al.,[2] with permission.)

studies are needed to evaluate what happens to the material over an extended period, especially with regard to possible shape changes resulting from shrinkage of the neocellular covering.

The third element of our prosthesis is the ball. Latex balloons were used for this purpose because they were readily available, inexpensive, and easily fitted with a self-sealing valve for inflation; the inflated diameter could be varied; they became spherical when filled with contrast medium or silicone, and they could be passed through the introducer sheath. The only problem we encountered was the inability to remove all the air from the balloon before inflation with the silicone prepolymer system. This resulted in a "dimpled" silicone cast. If the covering balloon ever failed, exposing this imperfection, the efficiency and hemodynamics of the valve could be compromised.

No physiologic parameters (e.g., electrocardiogram, heart rate, ventricular or systemic pressures) were assessed during these very preliminary studies because the focus of this research was feasibility and mechanical functionality.

The biologic stent devices were self-constructed from available materials. The 0.55-mm wire fulfilled the criteria of minimal spontaneous "uncoil" and "recoil" after compression and dilatation. If the metal loops were longer than 8 mm, it was much easier to dilate the stent, but this resulted in larger deformation by the opposing elastic recoil from the vessel or the heart. If the loops were smaller, the stent was too stiff to be fully expanded by the balloon. Andersen and colleagues used biologic valves, because they were easy to obtain and mount inside the stent. Other types of foldable valves may also prove suitable, for example, tricuspid polyurethane heart valve.

The extrathoracic approach was mandatory. As femoral arteries are very small in pigs we chose the abdominal aortic route for catheterization. Obviously, the femoral route should be used in humans, preferably by a percutaneous approach, alternatively by arteriotomy. Implantation was easy in both the ascending and descending aortas where small movements of the carrier balloon catheter were not critical. However, with subcoronary implantation such movements proved to be a problem. A catheter that does not obstruct the blood flow during stent-valve expansion could be the solution.

This is a very preliminary technical study, and many important questions remain to be answered about the stent-valve. Since only acute studies were performed, the long-term durability of the valve is unknown. There are still questions regarding neointimalization, calcification, thrombogenicity, and dislodgment during long-term gradual dilation or even necrosis of the portion of the aorta where the valve is implanted. Furthermore, valvular or aortic pathology, such as calcium, vegetative debris, fibrosis, and abscess formation could prevent accurate fixation or become a source of embolization. Thus, many more complex and long-term animal studies must be performed before even speculation concerning clinical use is begun.

Although a great deal of work remains to be done, these early results indicate that the development of a mechanical and biologic prosthetic aortic valve for transcatheter placement is feasible.

REFERENCES

1. Pavčnik D, Wright KC, Wallace S. Development and initial experimental evaluation of a prosthetic aortic valve for transcatheter placement: work in progress. Radiology 1992;183:151–4
2. Andersen HR, Knudsen LL, Hasenkam JM. Transluminal implantation of artificial heart valves: description of a new expandable aortic valve and initial results with implantation by catheter technique in closed chest pigs. Eur Heart J 1992;13:704–8
3. Hufnagel CA, Harvey WP. The surgical correction of aortic insufficiency. Bull Georgetown Univ Med Cent 1952;6:60
4. Wright KC, Wallace S, Charnsangavej C et al. Percutaneous endovascular stents: an experimental evaluation. Radiology 1985;156:68–72
5. Matsubara T, Yamazoe M, Tamura Y et al. Balloon vatheter with check valves for experimental relief of acute aortic regurgitation. Am Heart J 1992;124:1002–8

30 Balloon Valvotomy in Tricuspid Valve Stenosis

Peter C. Block

Rheumatic tricuspid stenosis and bioprosthetic tricuspid stenosis can be treated using percutaneous balloon valvotomy techniques. Experience in using balloon valvotomy for either indication is limited because of the relative rarity of tricuspid stenosis.[1-6] Reports show that the pressure gradient can be reduced by approximately 70%. With this reduction most calculated valve areas are doubled.

RHEUMATIC TRICUSPID STENOSIS

Description of Technique

Double-balloon valvotomy or single-balloon valvotomy for tricuspid valve stenosis is an outgrowth of pulmonic and mitral balloon valvotomy. The advantage of using balloons for right-sided lesions is that only the venous system is used and a transseptal or retrograde approach is not necessary. Therefore complications are fewer.

Both femoral regions are prepared and draped in the usual fashion. Thermodilution cardiac output and right-sided pressure measurements are first performed using a Swan-Ganz catheter or other right-sided catheters. It is of note that in the presence of significant tricuspid regurgitation, thermodilution cardiac output measurements may not be accurate. The Fick technique to calculate cardiac output is preferable and should be used in most patients if possible.

A 7-F introducer is placed in the right femoral vein or in both femoral veins if both veins are to be used.

A floating balloon (7 F) catheter is then passed antegrade across the tricuspid valve. Simultaneous measurements of the pressure in the right atrium and right ventricle should be performed. This can be done using a double-lumen balloon catheter or with two catheters if necessary—one in the right ventricle and one in the right atrium. Care must be taken to calibrate identical simultaneous right atrial pressure tracings from both catheters. One catheter is then advanced to the right ventricular cavity. This gives a more reliable pressure gradient.

It is possible to pass a 0.038″ Teflon-coated exchange wire with a curved J tip into the pulmonary artery through the tip of the floating balloon catheter if it has been advanced out the right ventricular outflow tract. Usually a guidewire in the pulmonary artery will not allow adequate placement of the dilating balloon catheter across the tricuspid valve. Therefore it is preferable to place the tip of both guidewires in the right ventricular apex. To best accomplish this a 0.038 "extra stiff" transfer guidewire is passed through the tip of the right ventricular catheter. A large curl is made in the soft tip of the transfer wire so that right ventricular irritability and the chance of perforation are minimized. Once the first transfer wire is in the right ventricular apex, the floating balloon catheter and sheath are removed and either a long sheath placed across the tricuspid valve and a second wire placed parallel to the first or a double-lumen catheter is advanced over the first guidewire into the right ventricle and the second guidewire is passed antegrade through the tip of the double lumen to the apex. The double-lumen catheter or sheath is removed, leaving both guidewires in place.

Maintenance of position across the tricuspid valve is helped by preshaping of the transfer guidewire so that a relatively large loop conforms to the pathway from the right atrium across the tricuspid valve to the right ventricular apex.

Dilating balloon catheters, usually 18 to 20 mm in diameter, are advanced percutaneously over each guidewire and positioned across the tricuspid valve under fluoroscopic control. It may be difficult to align the balloons properly across the stenotic tricuspid valve, since the valve plane may be difficult to establish with certainty. If the right ventricle is small (in the absence of any tricuspid regurgitation this is frequently the case) this adds to the problem. Inflation of the first and then the second balloon sequentially helps to certify that the balloons are across the tricuspid valve. A "waist" should be seen if the balloons are in proper position, as the balloons are inflated. With full inflation the waist should disappear as the tricuspid valve is split by the expanding balloons.

Balloons are fully inflated once or twice and then deflated and withdrawn. Repeat hemodynamic and cardiac output measurements are performed at the end of the procedure to establish improvement in tricuspid valve orifice size. Heparin is not needed during the procedure, although if there is a history of pulmonary emboli or thromboembolic disease in the past, heparinization should be performed. It need not be reversed at the end of the procedure when the balloon catheters are withdrawn if the final venous pressure is low.

Mechanism of Valvuloplasty in the Tricuspid Position

The mechanism of valvuloplasty for rheumatic tricuspid stenosis is similar to that for mitral rheumatic stenosis. The commissures of the valve, which are fused by the rheumatic process, are reopened by the expanding balloon catheters. It is likely that in tricuspid stenosis only one or two of the commissures are reopened, but the improvement in tricuspid valve function overcomes this deficiency. In general, the diminution in gradient and improvement in valve orifice size calculates to a doubling in valve opening.

Selection of Patients and Results

Isolated tricuspid stenosis is rare. Percutaneous balloon valvotomy is an alternative to surgical therapy for this condition. Tricuspid stenosis is more commonly found associated with mitral stenosis. If the mitral valve has appropriate anatomy for balloon di-

lation, both lesions can be treated by percutaneous balloon valvotomy. However, if there is associated severe regurgitant valve disease that would require surgery of the mitral, aortic, or tricuspid valve, balloon valvotomy is not indicated.

In general, the tricuspid valve gradient is decreased from approximately 6 ± 1.0 to 1.8 ± 0.06 mmHg.[1,4,5] In treatment of native valve tricuspid stenosis, valvular regurgitation does not seem to be a significant complication. Tricuspid valve area increases more than 100% from 0.75 to 1.8 cm^2. Cardiac output after tricuspid balloon valvotomy increases by approximately 1 L/min.[1]

BIOPROSTHETIC TRICUSPID STENOSIS

The issue of whether balloon valvotomy is useful for bioprosthetic tricuspid stenosis is not entirely clear. Experience with this problem is quite limited.[1,3,4–9] Rarely, bioprosthetic tricuspid stenosis is produced by commissural fusion. More commonly, it results from stiffening or thrombosis of the valve leaflets or cusp areas. If commissural fusion occurs, this may be produced by calcium deposits that "bridge" the bioprosthetic valve leaflet edges and cause fusion.[10] Most bioprosthetic tricuspid stenosis is due to thickening of the valve leaflet tissue or thrombus, which may be more or less organized on the ventricular surface of the bioprosthetic valve. When this occurs, valve motion is restricted. Fibrosis and hyalinzation of thrombus produces stiff nodules beneath the valve and restricts valve function.

The mechanism of balloon valvotomy in bioprosthetic stenosis is not clear. If there is commissural fusion, the commissures may be reopened by the expanding balloons. However, if hyalinized thrombi or fresh thrombi are present, dislodgement of thrombus with embolization into the pulmonary circulation (often associated with no clinical sequelae) might improve valve function. Microfractures of hyalinized nodules underneath the valve surface is a more likely effect of balloon dilation. This would produce improvement in valve motion, but refibrosis ("healing" of the splits in the nodule) would gradually produce restenosis. This appears to be the case clinically in most of the patients who undergo bioprosthetic tricuspid valvotomy with balloon techniques.[2,3]

Description of Technique

The technique is identical to that used for rheumatic tricuspid stenosis. The presence of a bioprosthetic valve usually makes it easier to visualize the plane of the tricuspid valve. This is not necessarily the case, and care should be taken to be certain that balloons do traverse the stenotic bioprosthetic valve as they are inflated.

If a patient has had evidence of pulmonary hypertension or thromboembolic disease in the past, the development of small pulmonary emboli from dislodgment of subvalvular thrombus may produce clinical sequelae. However, this has not been reported and it is unlikely that the thromboemboli are large enough in size in most instances to cause clinical problems. With bioprosthetic tricuspid stenosis the development of tricuspid regurgitation is a common outcome. This is usually tolerated better than tricuspid stenosis, since elevation of right atrial pressure only occurs during systole. Nevertheless, severe tricuspid regurgitation may be clinically just as significant as modest tricuspid stenosis and care should be taken to evaluate patients postvalvuloplasty for the presence of tricuspid regurgitation. Although this can be assessed by advancing a pigtail catheter across the reopened tricuspid valve to perform a right ventriculogram, assessment by echocardiographic, noninvasive means is equally helpful. The development of moderate tricuspid regurgitation in and of itself should not be considered a failure of the technique. However, most patients who have severe tricuspid regurgitation or who develop restenosis will ultimately require surgery.

REFERENCES

1. Al Zaibag M, Ribeiro P, Kasab SA. Percutaneous balloon valvotomy in tricuspid stenosis. Br Heart J 1978; 57:51–3
2. Attubato MJ, Stroh JA, Bach RG et al. Percutaneous double-balloon valvuloplasty of porcine bioprosthetic valves in the tricuspid position. Cath Card Diagn 1990; 20:202–204
3. Block PC, Smalling R, Owings RM. Percutaneous double balloon valvotomy for bioprosthetic tricuspid stenosis. Cath Card Diagn 1994;33:342–344
4. Goldenberg IF, Pedersen W, Olson J et al. Percutaneous double balloon valvoloplasty for severe tricuspid stenosis. Am Heart J 1989;118:417–419
5. Khalilullah M, Tyagi S, Yadav BS et al. Double-balloon valvuloplsty of tricuspid stenosis. Am Heart J 1987;114:1232–1233
6. Orbe LC, Sobrino N, Arcas R et al. Initial outcome of percutaneous balloon valvuloplasty in rheumatic tricuspid valve stenosis. Am J Card 1993;71:353–354
7. Chow WH, Cheung KL, Tai YT, Cheng CH. Successful percutaneous balloon valvuloplasty of a stenotic tricuspid bioprosthesis. Am Heart J 1990;119(3 Pt 1): 666–668
8. MacGregor JS, Cavero PG, McCluskey ER, Cheitlin MD. Percutaneous valvuloplsty to relieve stenosis of a bioprosthetic tricuspid valve in a patient with bacterial endocarditis. Am Heart J 1994;128:199–202
9. Slama MS, Drieu LH, Malergue MC et al. Percutaneous double balloon valvuloplsty for stenosis of porcine bioprostheses in the tricuspid valve position: a report of 2 cases. Cath Card Diagn 1993;28:142–148
10. Waller BF, McKay C, Van Tassel J, Allen . Catheter balloon valvuloplasty of stenotic porcine bioprosthetic valves. Part I: anatomic considerations. Part II: mechanisms, complications, and recommendations for clinical use. Clin Pathol Correl Clin Cardiol 1991;14: 686–91, 764–772

31 Introduction

Bernhard Meier

DEVELOPMENT OF PERCUTANEOUS TRANSLUMINAL CORONARY ANGIOPLASTY

Interventional cardiology started unobtrusively in 1966 with the introduction of balloon septostomy.[1] However, it really got off the ground with the innovation of percutaneous transluminal coronary angioplasty (PTCA) in 1977.[2] PTCA grew in less than two decades to become the most frequent major medical intervention worldwide.

The 1980s were characterized by some adjustments in indications for PTCA and by significant refinement of the conventional material consisting primarily of balloon catheters, guidewires, and guiding catheters (Fig. 31-1). The 1990s started on a comfortable level in terms of equipment and operator skills (Fig. 31-2). A considerable share of time and interest could now be devoted to alternative methods for PTCA, such as drills, lasers, stents, local delivery devices, and the new diagnostic tools, coronary angioscopy and intracoronary ultrasound and Doppler measurements. Without the reassuring background of conventional balloon angioplasty, however, clinical evaluation of such devices would not be conceivable. So far, none of the new devices has seriously challenged the dominant role of balloon angioplasty, but the stent clearly has expanded its potential.

The key attributes of balloon angioplasty have been from the start its simplicity and fairly good safety and reliability. The clinical success rate was surprisingly high from the outset, considering the somewhat primitive approach. After some additional increase in the first decade it plateaued at about 85 to 95%.

INDICATIONS AND RESULTS OF PTCA

There is a widespread tendency to diagnose and actively treat coronary artery disease in a much earlier stage. PTCA is both the major reason for this tendency and the logical answer to its consequences (Fig. 31-3). Early coronary artery disease means single or, at the most, double, vessel disease and PTCA is well suited for the treatment of these stages. In advanced multivessel disease, however, PTCA plays a secondary role at best. It may be used when it comes to recurrences after bypass surgery, palliation of inoperable patients, or acute interventions during myocardial infarction. For patients with proximal triple vessel disease involving all major coronary vessels (Fig. 31-4), bypass surgery is still the therapy of choice. An exception is illustrated in Figure 31-5, where each of the vessels showed only a single discrete lesion ideal for PTCA. Fortunately, none of these lesions recurred after a two-stage PTCA, necessitating but two nights at the hospital. In such patients, PTCA may match the results of bypass surgery at a lower price in terms of monetary expenses, hospital stays, absenteeism from gainful activity, and subjective suffering. However, we must not forget that these cases account for only about 10% of patients with multivessel disease.

The recently published randomized studies on PTCA versus bypass surgery in patients with multivessel disease[4–7] have to be seen in that light. Only less than 10% of the screened patients were included (Fig. 31-6). The draw attained by PTCA in most of these studies can only be extrapolated to patients

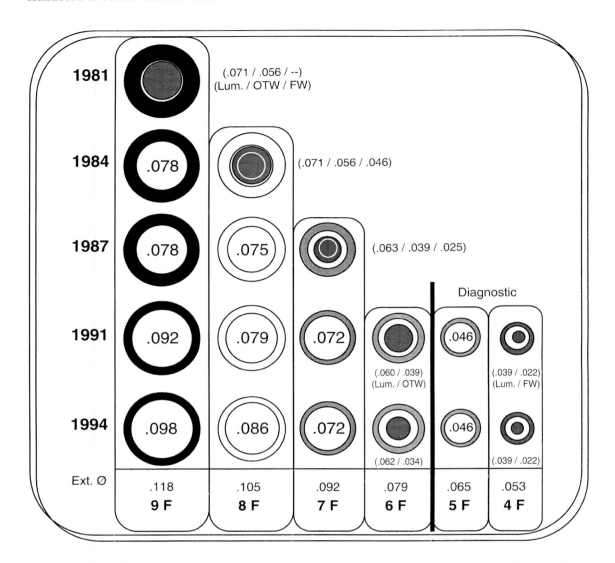

Fig. 31-1. Evolution of cross sections (diameters in inches) of guiding catheters and balloon shafts for coronary angioplasty from 1981 to 1994. There was a significant gain in lumina of guiding catheters which, together with the concurrent decrease in the diameter of balloon shafts, improved the space available for contrast medium injection so dramatically that by 1991 conventional PTCA through a 6 F catheter was more comfortable than it had been through a 9 F catheter in 1981 and PTCA through 4 F catheters had become a reality. Ø, diameter; *Ext.*, external; *F*, French; *FW*, fixed wire; *Lum.*, lumen of catheter; *OTW*, over the wire.

akin to the ones included and not to multivessel patients in general. On the other hand, PTCA patients tend to experience their problems in a front-loaded fashion. The relatively short follow-up of the studies comparing PTCA with bypass surgery in multivessel disease as well as the study comparing PTCA with medical treatment in single vessel disease[8] may therefore not give PTCA a fair deal. As shown in Fig. 31-7 on the example of the first angioplasty patients successfully treated by Gruentzig and his coworkers, recurrence and even iterative recurrence is quite common with PTCA during the first year. Patients arriving at 6 to 12 months after PTCA without recurrence, however, have a very stable course. The dilated lesion appears to be sealed and further problems commonly originate from other lesions, exclusively. In the long run, the draw of these studies may turn into a comfortable victory for PTCA, after all. However, once again, be reminded, these were highly selected patients.

Fig. 31-2. Refinements of conventional coronary angioplasty gear achieved by 1990 enabled intricate interventions such as the PTCA depicted. It was performed for a stenosis of a diagonal branch of the left anterior descending coronary artery through a tortuous right internal mammary artery bypass graft to be accessed via an elongated and ectatic aorta and right subclavian artery.

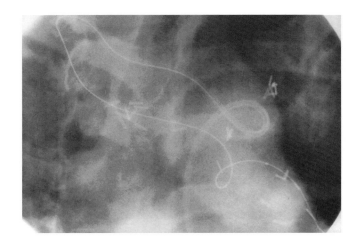

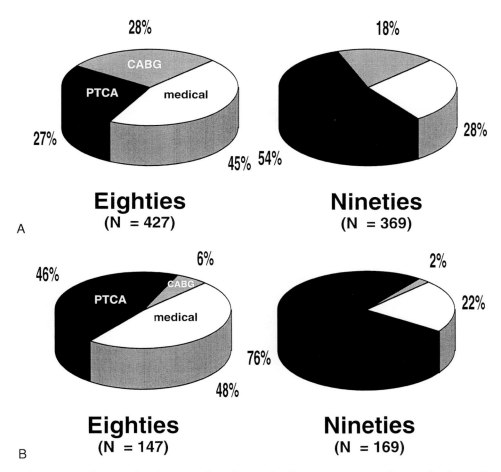

Fig. 31-3. Recommendations for therapy after diagnosis of coronary artery disease in the early eighties and the early nineties.[3] PTCA gained ground mainly on easy cases and at the cost of medical therapy. In multivessel disease, it increased its share among patients with distal and side branch involvement predominantly. Coronary artery bypass grafting (*CABG*) maintained its strong position in triple vessel disease with involvement of all major branches. **(A)** Patients with all stages. **(B)** Patients with single vessel disease. (*Figure continues.*)

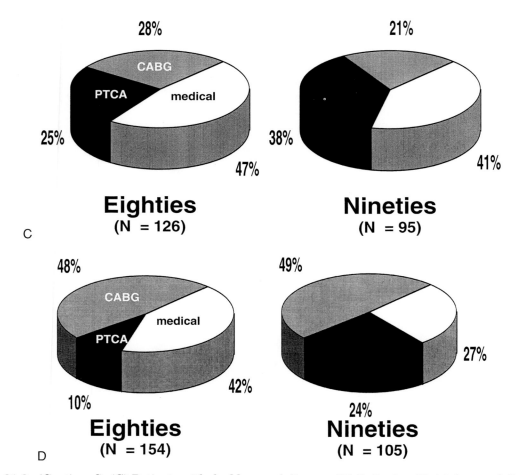

Fig. 31-3. (*Continued*). **(C)** Patients with double vessel disease. **(D)** Patients with triple vessel disease.

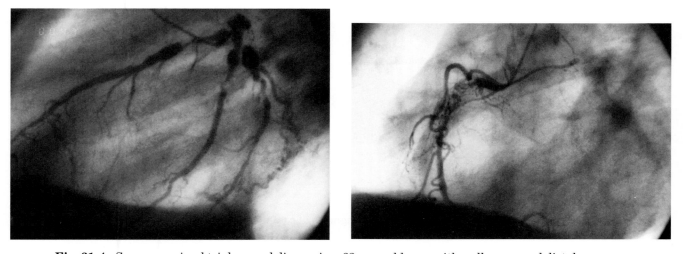

Fig. 31-4. Severe proximal triple vessel disease in a 62-year-old man with well-preserved distal coronary arteries and left ventricular function. This situation is well suited for coronary bypass surgery but not for coronary angioplasty.

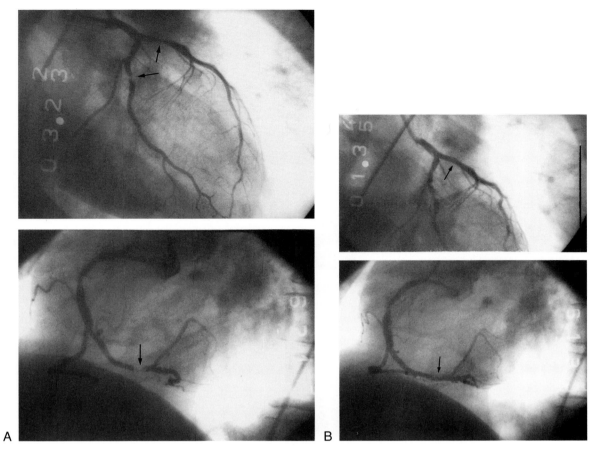

Fig. 31-5. (A) Triple vessel disease in a 55-year-old physician with discrete lesions in the proximal left anterior descending coronary artery, the proximal left circumflex coronary artery, and the major left ventricular (posterolateral) branch of the dominant right coronary artery (*arrows*). The left ventricular function was normal. **(B)** Good immediate result after simultaneous PTCA of the left anterior descending and the right coronary arteries on the first day (*arrows*). (*Figure continues.*)

CURRENT TENDENCIES OF PTCA

The fact that the major reason for the rapid growth in numbers of PTCA is its increased application to simple cases (Fig. 31-3) asks for simplified material and techniques, sometimes referred to as "PTCA Lite."[9–11] More importantly, it also emphasizes the need for combining diagnostic and therapeutic interventions whenever possible. PTCA performed during the diagnostic session[12–15] is commonly called "ad hoc PTCA," but a variety of other names are also in use (Table 31-1). "PTCA at first sight"[16] is a subgroup of "ad hoc PTCA." It includes only patients who undergo PTCA during their very first diagnostic coronary angiogram. They constitute the ultimate challenge for "ad hoc PTCA." In other ad hoc patients, for example, those who undergo a restudy for suspected restenosis, the coronary anatomy to be found can be anticipated well enough to premeditate the strategy and discuss it in advance with the patient. Even in true "PTCA at first sight," the results were competitive with those of PTCA done apart from the diagnostic study.[16] These are results generated before digitized catheterization laboratories were standard

Table 31-1. Expressions for PTCA Performed Immediately After Diagnostic Angiography

Ad Hoc PTCA	One Time PTCA
Single Session PTCA	Stop And Go PTCA
Diagnostic Session PTCA	Dessert PTCA
Follow On PTCA	PTCA At First Sight[a]

[a] Pertains exclusively to patients without a prior coronary angiogram.

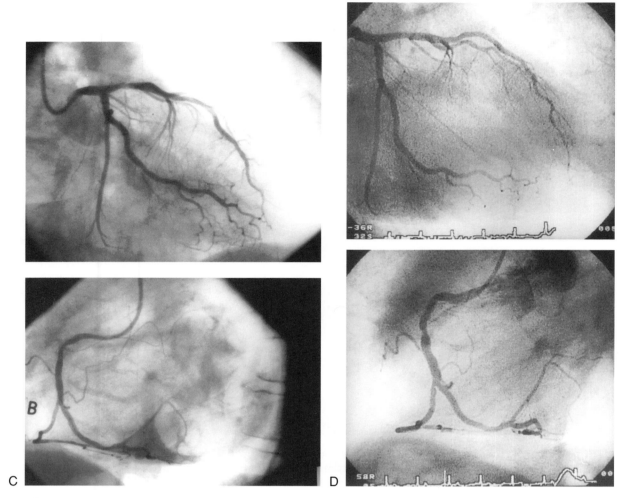

Fig. 31-5. (*Continued*). **(C)** Some deterioration in the left anterior descending coronary artery but persistently excellent result in the right coronary artery the following day allowing the additional PTCA of the left circumflex coronary artery. **(D)** Excellent long-term result 5 years later in all three arteries.

which further facilitate PTCA performed without waiting for a film to be developed and discussed. Therefore, the gain in overall time, cost, and material saved, the enhanced patient comfort, and the accelerated vocational rehabilitation come virtually free of increased risks for errors and complications. These advantages should not be foregone, even though the informed consent will have to be provisionally obtained in patients that may never go on to have a PTCA. There is an increasing awareness of the patients about the possibility of PTCA in general and "ad hoc PTCA" in particular, and PTCA teams not yet subscribing to the latter will see their hands forced to change their policy in order to stay competitive. This is bad news for hospitals offering coronary angiography, but not PTCA. They will be a thing of the past before long, which in most cases will mean that they

will take up PTCA rather than giving up coronary angiography. The most compelling argument for "ad hoc PTCA" has not even been mentioned yet. It eliminates the small but significant risk of morbidity and mortality on the waiting list that has to be added to the risk of the intervention itself in patients not taken care of immediately.

To use PTCA in patients with multivessel disease in whom bypass surgery is indicated but considered risky has been in people's mind for quite some time.[17] It has been scientifically backed up recently in a paper[18] that prompted the (premature) announcement of the "coming out of PTCA."[19] The community of interventional cardiologists seem to join this trend with a certain reluctance. They have to face mortality figures way above the 1 to 2% generally accepted in average elective PTCA patients, although the mor-

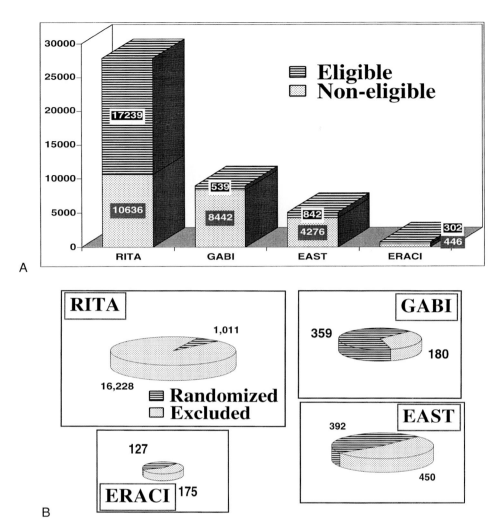

Fig. 31-6. (A) Patients found eligible among the ones screened in major randomized studies on PTCA versus bypass surgery in patients with multivessel disease. **(B)** Patients included into the randomization among the ones deemed eligible (pie size indicates the number of patients). *EAST,* Emory Angioplasty Versus Surgery Trial[7]; *ERACI,* Argentine Trial of Percutaneous Transluminal Coronary Angioplasty Versus Coronary Artery Bypass Surgery in Multivessel Disease[5]; *GABI,* German Angioplasty Bypass Surgery Investigation[6]; *RITA,* Randomised Intervention Treatment of Angina.[4]

tality is projected even higher with bypass surgery in that particular subgroup of patients. The more frequent and more cognizant use of stents is about to bring this topic into the limelight, once again.

PERSPECTIVES OF PTCA

The future of PTCA is bright. Coronary angioplasty will maintain its position in the lead of major medical interventions for many years to come with coronary artery disease still increasing in a steadily aging population. PTCA will grow to be an even more impor-

tant economic factor in industrialized countries, creating jobs and revenue not only through employed hardware and applied patient care but also through publications, teaching seminars, and medical tourism.

There are little boundaries to the human imagination when it comes to modifications of the procedure and introduction of so called new devices. They will keep the interventional cardiologists sharp and on the go. Only, we have to be careful not to find ourselves too often in the role of the emperor in Hans Christian Andersen's "The Emperor's New Clothes."[20]

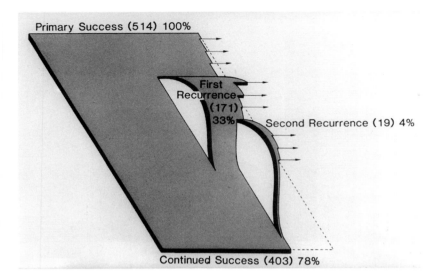

Fig. 31-7. First-year course of the initial patients with successful PTCA by Gruentzig and coworkers.[2] The roughly 80% of patients arriving at 1 year with a continued success had a remarkably stable situation, afterward proving that recurrence is only a problem within the first months after PTCA.

REFERENCES

1. Rashkind WJ, Miller WW. Creation of an atrial septal defect without thoracotomy. JAMA 1966;196:991–2
2. Grüntzig A. Transluminal dilatation of coronary artery stenosis. Lancet 1978;1:263
3. Pande AK, Meier B, Rutishauser W. Implications of coronary angiography in patients with suspected or known coronary artery disease. Int J Cardiol 1993;38:159–66
4. RITA Trial Participants. Coronary angioplasty versus coronary artery bypass surgery: the Randomised Intervention Treatment of Angina trial. Lancet 1993;341:573–80
5. Rodriguez A, Boullon F, Perez-Baliño N et al, on behalf of the ERACI group. Argentine randomized trial of percutaneous transluminal coronary angioplasty versus coronary artery bypass surgery in multivessel disease (ERACI): in-hospital results and 1-year follow-up. J Am Coll Cardiol 1993;22:1060–7
6. Hamm CW, Reimers J, Ischinger T et al, for the German Angioplasty Bypass Surgery Investigation. A randomized study of coronary angioplasty compared with bypass surgery in patients with symptomatic multivessel coronary disease. N Engl J Med 1994;331:1037–43
7. King SB III, Lembo NJ, Weintraub WS et al, for the Emory Angioplasty versus Surgery Trial (EAST). A randomized trial comparing coronary angioplasty with coronary bypass surgery. N Engl J Med 1994;331:1044–50
8. Parisi AF, Folland ED, Hartigan P, on behalf of the Veteran Affairs ACME Investigators. A comparison of angioplasty with medical treatment of single-vessel coronary artery disease. N Engl J Med 1992;326:10–6
9. Villavicencio R, Urban P, Muller T, Favre J, Meier B. Coronary balloon angioplasty through diagnostic 6 French catheters. Cathet Cardiovasc Diagn 1991;22:56–9
10. Mehan VK, Meier B, Urban P, Verine V, Haine E, Dorsaz PA. Coronary angioplasty through 4 French diagnostic catheters. Cathet Cardiovasc Diagn 1993;30:22–6
11. Urban P, Meier B, Haine E, Verine V, Mehan V. Coronary stenting through 6 French catheters. Cathet Cardiovasc Diagn 1993;28:263–6
12. Feldmann RL, McDonald RG, Hill JA et al. Coronary angioplasty at the time of initial cardiac catheterization. Cathet Cardiovasc 1986;12:219–22
13. Myler RK, Stertzer SH, Clark DA et al. Coronary angioplasty at the time of the initial angioplasty: ad hoc angioplasty possibilities and challenges. Cathet Cardiovasc Diagn 1986;12:213–4
14. Haraphongse M, Tymchack W, Rossal R. Coronary angioplasty at the time of the initial diagnostic angiography in patients with unstable angina. Cathet Cardiovasc Diagn 1988;14:73–5
15. O'Keefe JH, Reeder GS, Miller GA, Bailey KR, Holmes DR Jr. Safety and efficacy of percutaneous transluminal coronary angioplasty performed at the time of diagnostic catheterization compared with that performed at other times. Am J Cardiol 1989;63:27–9
16. Moles V, Meier B, Pande AK, Mehan V, Urban P, Dorsaz P. PTCA at first sight: angioplasty based on video only. J of Invas Cardiol 1992;4:344–8
17. Taylor GJ, Rabinovich E, Mikell FL et al. Percutaneous transluminal coronary angioplasty as palliation for patients considered poor surgical candidates. Am Heart J 1986;111:840–4
18. Morrison DA, Barbiere CC, Johnson R et al. Salvage angioplasty: an alternative to high risk surgery for unstable angina. Cathet Cardiovasc Diagn 1992;27:169–78
19. Meier B. The "coming out" of coronary balloon angioplasty. Cathet Cardiovas Diagn 1992;27:165–6
20. Meier B. New devices for coronary angioplasty: the emperor's new clothes revisited. Am J Med 1995;98(5):429–31

32 Training and Surgical Back-Up

Bernhard Meier

TRAINING

Mental Qualities

The operator's peace of mind is the ultimate proof for adequate training in coronary interventions, as in virtually all professions. This peace of mind is based on adequate prior teaching and regular practice, experienced ancillary personnel, up-to-date equipment, and sufficient time to accomplish the task. But it is also subject to specific mental qualities. The interventional cardiologist is no longer just an intellectual explorer like the more contemplative clinical colleague. He is a practical repairman. He is summoned (by himself or others) to take care of a problem. He is expected to be completely in charge once he has accepted the case. Like a surgeon, he takes a more comprehensive responsibility for the patient than a diagnostic cardiologist. He will be glorified at times if he succeeds in the therapeutic endeavor, but he will unequivocally be the culprit if he fails and the patient's situation deteriorates. In contrast to a cardiac surgeon, the interventional cardiologist disposes of an armamentarium of tools and technical possibilities that are restricted, his patient is awake, and in case of an inadvertent outcome there always was this other therapeutic option named bypass surgery that probably should have been selected in the first place. Being a lone fighter walking on dangerous paths, the interventional cardiologist exercises one of the most stressful occupations of modern medicine. Consequently, not all cardiologists and not even all invasive cardiologists qualify to become an interventional cardiologist for purely mental reasons.

Skills

Skill is another topic to address. Some argue that interventional cardiology requires minimal skill since all one can do at catheterization is advance, retract, or rotate one or, rarely, two instruments at a time. Then why should extended training periods be required to become an interventional cardiologist? It may well be true that virtually everybody qualifies to acquire the manual skills for coronary angioplasty within a reasonably short training period. These skills are much less demanding than the ones necessary to perform heart surgery, or to play a musical instrument for that matter. However, much more important than dexterity is the experience regarding indications, pitfalls, equipment, radiographic techniques (projection angles, etc.), manipulative knacks and tricks, when to insist and when to stop, and last, but not least, what to do in case of complications. This kind of knowledge does not require a particularly brilliant mind, but it cannot be gathered in a few months. It comes with close contact to hundreds of real cases under the guidance of the truly experienced.

The invasive cardiologist destined to become an interventional cardiologist likes the manual part of his profession, works in a relaxed mood during a diagnostic study—even in the elderly patient presenting technical challenges—and never loses composure in case of unexpected problems. He accepts the downsides of interventional cardiology such as unpredictable schedules, depressive moods after grave complications, and strains on his own coronary arteries, in exchange for an exciting and often extremely gratifying occupation.

383

Guidelines

Summarizing the requirements of various national and international authorities,[1-7] the interventional cardiologist embarking on independent activities should look back on about 3 years of training in internal (general) medicine, 2 years in general cardiology, 1 year in invasive cardiology, and a final year in interventional cardiology at a high-volume center (at least 300 annual procedures) with at least one (preferably two) full-time interventional cardiologists. The recommendable number of therapeutic coronary procedures assisted and performed with the assistance of an experienced colleague is difficult to determine. In a highly active environment with daily case discussions among peers, fewer cases with personal involvement (sterile participation at the table) are required than in a center with just the teacher and the disciple. Important knowledge and skills can be gleaned from discussion of cases not attended live as well as from colleagues simultaneously in the training program (shared errors and mistakes) and seasoned catheterization laboratory personnel.

Table 32-1 reflects a reasonable minimal training record to be acquired before embarking on unsupported activities in coronary catheter interventions.[8]

Table 32-1. Curriculum of Interventional Cardiologists Before Independence

Curriculum	Minimum (unofficial)	According to Authorities
Internal (general) medicine (years)	3[a]	3
Clinical cardiology (years)	2[a]	2
Invasive cardiology (years)	0.5	1
Diagnostic catheterization (cases)		
As assistant	50	200
As operator	100	100
Interventional cardiology (years)	0.5	1
Therapeutic catheterization (PTCA cases)		
As assistant	5	50
As operator	25	75
Practical courses	1	2

[a] 1 year of each can be combined.
Abbreviation: PTCA, percutaneous transluminal coronary angioplasty.

It may not suffice for "slow learners" or for activities in remote and unskilled catheterization laboratories. It will definitely not meet all the somewhat unrealistic requirements voiced by authorities, which are summarized in Table 32-1. Table 32-2 depicts some detailed national and international requirements that were published.

The required experience to use so-called "new" devices is not defined and depends on the specific characteristics of the device. A balloon expandable stent is used frequently at all busy laboratories, and its implantation is technically close to simple balloon angioplasty. Other instruments are rarely used and feature distinctly different and complex techniques. They should remain restricted to the accomplished high volume operator with a long track record in intricate procedures. Only if they unequivocally prove to be essential should they be dispersed among the less experienced operators. At present there is no such device commercially available that meets these requirements. Noncoronary interventions (valvuloplasty, shunt closure, pathway ablation, etc.), not unlike new coronary devices, need special training recommendations that are beyond the scope of this chapter.

SURGICAL BACK-UP

History, Guidelines, and Organization

The expressions surgical stand-by or surgical back-up were added to the medical vocabulary in the wake of angioplasty just like the terms restenosis, abrupt closure, chronic total occlusion, etc. The first emergency coronary bypass operation due to a failed attempt at PTCA dates back to 1978 and the seventh patient of Andreas Grüntzig. Of Grüntzig's initial 50 patients, 7 (14%) underwent emergency bypass operations, all with excellent results.[10]

Ideal prerequisites for a surgical back-up for PTCA are as follows:

1. Informed consent of the patient
2. Surgeon and anesthesiologist briefed
3. Operating room immediately available for at least 12 hours to account for out-of-laboratory subacute occlusions[11,12]
4. Transport possible with accessory equipment (cardiac monitor, intraaortic balloon pump, perfusion pump, left ventricular assist devices, percutaneous cardiopulmonary bypass, etc.)
5. Continuous resuscitation possible en route, which precludes small elevators or ambulances

Table 32-2. National and International Requirements for Interventional Cardiologists Before and After Independence

Requirements	USA[a]	WHO[b]	CH[c]	D[d]	F[e]	GB[f]
Before independence						
Coronary catheterization cases						
Diagnostic						
As assistant	100	100	50		100	
As operator	200	200	200	500	200	
Therapeutic (PTCA)						
As assistant	50	50	50	50	50	50
As operator	75	75	100		75	50
After independence						
PTCA cases per year	75	50	50	50	75	50
24-hour PTCA service	Yes				Yes	
2 physicians per case			No	Yes	Yes	
Surgical back-up						
In-house	Yes	Yes				
Close by			Yes	Yes	Yes	Yes

Abbreviations: CH, Switzerland; D, Germany; F, France; GB, Great Britain; NL, Netherlands; PTCA, percutaneous transluminal coronary angioplasty; USA, United Stated of America; WHO, World Health Organization; yes, explicitly required; no, explicity not required.

[a] Data from Cowley et al.,[4] Douglas et al.,[5] and Ryan et al.[6]
[b] Data from Bourassa et al.[2]
[c] Data from ref. 7.
[d] Data from ref. 1.
[e] Data from Monassier et al.[9]
[f] Data from Gray et al.[3]

As for the day-to-day arrangements for surgical back-up, the next room available policy is a typical pattern in institutions with a busy surgical schedule and several daily coronary angioplasty procedures. This means that interventional cardiology and cardiac surgery function independently, dealing with emergencies as they arise.

Most current guidelines for coronary angioplasty outlined in Table 32-2 require surgical back-up for all procedures. In-house back-up is usually requested—except for Germany, France, Great Britain, and Switzerland.[1,3,7,9]

Classification and Results of Emergency Coronary Bypass Surgery

Several types of emergency surgery have to be distinguished, that is, for convenience, for threatening infarction, and for ongoing infarction.

Emergency surgery for convenience pertains to patients who are operated on taking advantage of the surgical back-up for logistic reasons rather than medical. The outcome of such patients is that of elective surgery.

Emergency surgery for threatening infarction after coronary angioplasty represents an excellent utilization of surgical back-up. Again, this indication produces normal bypass surgery results.

Emergency surgery for ongoing infarction caused by an angioplasty attempt, finally yields results similar to those of surgery for spontaneously occurring infarction. The question why the latter is rarely practiced finds an answer in unsatisfactory results. In the setting of an infarction because of an angioplasty attempt, the problem is iatrogenic, the patient is already in the hospital, the coronary angiogram is available for expedite surgical revascularization, and the surgeon is dealing with a well-informed patient and a premeditated situation where frequently only a single coronary artery needs grafting. Finally, most of these events occur during regular working hours.

Nevertheless, periprocedural infarction rates of emergency bypass operations for failed PTCA range from 16[13] to 80%.[14] The large variation is explained by the influence of definitions of infarction and indications for emergent surgery. If only patients with true evidence for ongoing ischemia are sent for emergency surgery, the periprocedural infarction rate approaches 100%.[15]

In-hospital mortality rates for emergency surgery after failed PTCA range from 0[13] to 26%.[16] Only few patients transferred for surgery in cardiogenic shock let alone under cardiorespiratory resuscitation survive. However, these patients stand virtually no chance to survive if treated conservatively. Surgeons willing to operate on them are hardly to be held responsible for the high ensuing mortality.

As for the long-term outcome after emergency surgery for failed coronary angioplasty, only 20% of patients suffer a persistent decrease in ejection fraction over baseline.[17] The 5-year survival rates are at least 90% in most reports,[18–20] except for elderly patients.[21]

Outcomes of patients with emergency bypass surgery for failed angioplasty have deteriorated over the past years[14,20] in spite of perfusion systems and improved surgical techniques. The aging angioplasty population provides one explanation for this development.[22] More important is the fact that emergency surgery is increasingly being reserved for severe cases. Angioplasty operators realized that they may in fact harm patients by sending them for emergency surgery for ischemia in a small myocardial territory or simply for fear that such an ischemia might occur. As amply proved by the large studies on myocardial infarction, a small or medium-size infarction treated conservatively in a hospital environment harbors practically no mortality, and its functional outcome is good. It is preferable to perform an emergency bypass operation on top of an infarction to possibly reduce its size.

Other Measures for Acute Coronary Artery Occlusion

There are a number of measures that can and should be taken to keep the coronary artery open, which usually stabilizes the patient. The coronary stent is the most attractive of them and typically obviates the need for emergency operation altogether.[23] Perfusion balloons[24] and dedicated bailout autoperfusion catheters[25] have been widely used in the past but are about to be rendered obsolete by the stent. Active perfusion systems[26,27] and the temporary stent[28] have proved too cumbersome, which explains their poor acceptance.

There are insufficient data to support the widespread use of the intraaortic balloon pump in these situations, although its use has been repeatedly advocated.[29] Left ventricular assist devices such as the percutaneous cardiopulmonary bypass,[30] the hemopump,[31] or the left atrial/ventricular-aortic bypass,[32] however, may be lifesaving in experienced hands when used for moribund patients.

Recommendations

Personal experience and the fact that selected patients have been treated with minimal or no surgical coverage without adverse outcomes at many centers[32–40] allow recommendations that deviate from international guidelines. The conclusion of a particular study was that surgical back-up is not necessary for 80% of angioplasty patients.[38] Without contesting that timely emergency operations save myocardium or even lives of individual patients, it is unclear whether emergency surgery saves or spends human lives in a final account.

Reasonable policies for surgical back-up are summarized in Table 32-3. When determining strategies for surgical back-up, the risk profile of the patient, that is, the clinical picture expected in case of abrupt closure primes the risk profile of the lesion—the propensity for abrupt closure.

In all cases, the preliminary decision about the

Table 32-3. Risk Profiles of Coronary Angioplasty and Need for Surgical Back-up

High risk
  In-house surgery required
  Intervention schedule toward the end of routine surgical program
  Lesion risk high: high probability for occlusion(s)
  Patient risk high: severe clinical picture expected in case of occlusion(s)
Moderate risk
  In-house surgery required unless large experience with coronary stents and out-of-house surgery close by
  No special arrangement
  Lesion risk low; low probability for occlusion(s)
  Patient risk high: severe clinical picture expected in case of occlusion(s)
Low risk
  In-house surgery not required if crew is highly experienced
  No special arragement
  Lesion risk high: high probability for occlusion(s)
  Patient risk low: silent or mild clinical picture expected in case of occlusion(s)
Minimal risk
  In-house surgery not required if crew is highly experienced
  No special arrangement
  Lesion risk low: low probability for occlusion(s)
  Patient risk low: silent or mild clinical picture expected in case of occlusion(s)
High risk in "inoperable" patient
  Crashes frequent
  Possibility to ask for surgical help to be maintained but used infrequently
  In-house surgery required and staff alerted
  Thorough preliminary discussion with patient, family, referring physician, surgeon, and anesthesiologists
  Expertise with left ventricular assist devices mandatory

strategy in case of closure of the coronary artery has to be discussed with the patient. The plan to forego emergency bypass surgery and to conservatively treat the possible ischemia induced by the vessel occlusion is accepted readily by the patient most of the time, but it should be based on a diligent estimation of the patient's global risk with and without emergency surgery. Moreover, the decision has to be challenged again in the actual event of a vessel occlusion.

The high-risk inoperable patients of Table 32-3 may justify the prophylactic insertion of extracatheters before angioplasty, such as a venous and an additional arterial line to provide quick access in case of need for a pacemaker, an intraaortic balloon pump, and/or a left ventricular assist device. Hypotension or cardiac arrest are frequent sequelae of acute vessel occlusion in these patients. They render additionally needed punctures difficult and time-consuming.

The time spent for rescue maneuvers with catheters should be kept to a minimum not to further reduce the amount of salvageable myocardium in the rare patients to be sent for emergency surgery in case of an untreatable coronary occlusion. Once the decision for emergency surgery is made and accepted by patient, surgeon, and anesthesiologist, blood is ordered, the patient is shaved, and complementary catheters are introduced by the cardiologist or anesthesiologist without delaying transport. The femoral sheath is secured to prevent inadvertent extraction before, during, or after surgery. A venous pacemaker is inserted in patients with bradycardia.

Economic Considerations

Recently, the most common pattern of surgical back-up for coronary angioplasty in the United States was still an open operating room during the procedure (64%), followed by the "next room available" arrangement (24%).[41] The remainder of centers (all with in-house surgery) favored patient-adjusted back-up strategies. Offering surgical back-up according to the rules represents indisputably the ideal setting, provided the back-up is not overused. Yet there is a price to pay. The cost for surgical back-up was projected nationally at about $160,000,000 actual cost and $270,000,000 billed to patients for the year 1990 in a survey, not including the fees of the physicians involved.[40] As it serves only a few percent of angioplasty patients, the estimated cost per patient actually undergoing emergency surgery amounts to over $50,000. In addition, there is the not universally welcome incentive to create new surgical facilities to comply with the rules in hospitals with a catheteriza-

tion laboratory. These facilities are bound to divert patients from established high-volume surgical institutions while practicing bypass surgery at low-volume activity with all the intrinsic disadvantages.

In many countries, waiting lists for coronary angioplasty are common in spite of the fact that in some regions more than half of the procedures are already performed in hospitals without cardiac surgery. Strict adherence to the guidelines would prolong the waiting lists and preclude angioplasty for a significant number of good candidates for the procedure. The number of deaths on the waiting list to be expected would risk to be considerably larger than that attributable to the absence of immediate surgical back-up. Hence proscribing coronary angioplasty without proper surgical back-up is not to the advantage of mankind.

REFERENCES

1. Deutsche Gesellschaft für Herz- und Kreislaufforschung, Kommission für Klinische Kardiologie (unter Mitwirkung der Arbeitsgruppe transluminale Angioplastie). Empfehlungen für die Durchführung der Perkutanen Transluminalen Koronarangioplastie (PTCA). Z Kardiol 1987;76:382–385
2. Bourassa MG, Alderman EL, Bertrand ME et al. Report of the Joint International Society and Federation of Cardiology/World Health Organization Task Force on Coronary Angioplasty. Eur Heart J 1988;9:1034–1045 Circulation 1988;78:780–789
3. Gray HH, Balcon R, Dyet J et al. Guidelines for training in percutaneous transluminal coronary angioplasty (PTCA): report of the Council of the British Cardiovascular Society/BCIS). Br Heart J 1992;68:437–439
4. Cowley MJ, Faxon DP, Holmes DR Jr. Guidelines for training, credentialing, and maintenance of competence for the performance of coronary angioplasty: a report from the Interventional Cardiology Committee and the Training Program Standards Committee of the Society for Cardiac Angiography and Interventions. Cathet Cardiovasc Diagn 1993;30:1–4
5. Douglas JS Jr, Pepine CJ, Block BC et al. on behalf of the American College of Cardiology Cardiac Catheterization Committee. Recommendations for development and maintenance of competence in coronary interventional procedures. J Am Coll Cardiol 1993;22:629–631
6. Ryan TJ, Bauman WB, Kennedy JW et al. Guidelines for percutaneous transluminal coronary angioplasty. A report of the American College of Cardiology/American Heart Association Task Force on Assessment of Diagnostic and Therapeutic Cardiovascular Procedures (Committee on Percutaneous Transluminal Coronary Angioplasty). J Am Coll Cardiol 1983;22:2033–2054; Circulation 1993;88:2987–3007
7. Arbeitsgruppe PTCA und Fibrinolyse der Schweizerischen Gesellschaft für Kardiologie. Empfehlungen zur Qualitätssicherung in der interventionellen Kardiologie. Schweiz Ärzt Z 1994;75:1897–1898
8. Meier B. Gaining, maintaining, and surveying competence in the interventional cardiology laboratory. Int J Cardiol 1990;29:9–14

9. Monassier JP, Bertrand M, Cherrier F et al. Recommandations concernant la formation des médecins coronarographistes et angioplasticiens, l'organisation et l'équipement des centres de coronarographies et d'angioplastie coronaire transluminale. Arch Malad Coeur Vaiss 1991;84:1783–7

10. Grüntzig AR, Senning A, Siegenthaler WE. Nonoperative dilatation of coronary-artery stenosis: percutaneous transluminal coronary angioplasty. New Engl J Med 1979;301:61–68

11. Steffenino G, Meier B, Finci L et al. Acute complications of elective coronary angioplasty: a review of 500 consecutive procedures. Br Heart J 1988;59:151–158

12. Detre KM, Holmes DR Jr, Holubkov R et al. and co-investigators of the National Heart, Lung, and Blood Institute's Percutaneous Transluminal Coronary Angioplasty Registry. Incidence and consequences of periprocedural occlusion. The 1985–1986 National Heart, Lung, and Blood Institute Percutaneous Transluminal Coronary Angioplasty Registry. Circulation 1990;82:739–750

13. Levy RD, Bennett DH, Brooks NH. Desirability of immediate surgical standby for coronary angioplasty. Br Heart J 1991;65:68–71

14. Craver JM, Weintraub WS, Jones EL et al. Emergency coronary artery bypass surgery for failed percutaneous coronary angioplasty: a 10-year experience. Ann Surg 1992;215:425–434

15. Murphy DA, Craver JM, Jones EL et al. Surgical revascularization following unsuccessful percutaneous transluminal coronary angioplasty. J Thorac Cardiovasc Surg 1982;84:342–348

16. Hochberg MS, Gregory JJ, McCullough JN et al. Outcome of emergent coronary artery bypass following failed angioplasty. Circulation 1990;82(Suppl III):III-361 (abs).

17. Stark KS, Satler LF, Krucoff MW et al. Myocardial salvage after failed coronary angioplasty. J Am Coll Cardiol 1990;15:78–82

18. Lazar HL, Haan CK. Determinants of myocardial infarction following emergency coronary artery bypass for failed percutaneous coronary angioplasty. Ann Thorac Surg 1987;44:646–650

19. Tuzku M, Simpfendorfer C, Dorosti K et al. Long-term outcome of unsuccessful percutaneous transluminal coronary angioplasty. Am Heart J 1990;119:791–196

20. Buffet P, Villemot JP, Danchin N et al. Emergency coronary artery surgery after percutaneous transluminal coronary angioplasty: immediate results and long-term outcome in 100 cases. Arch Malad Coeur Vaiss 1992;85:17–23

21. Talley JD, Weintraub WS, Roubin GS et al. Failed elective percutaneous transluminal coronary angioplasty requiring coronary artery bypass surgery: in-hospital and late clinical outcome. Circulation 1990;82:1203–1213

22. Lazar HL, Faxon DP, Paone G et al. Changing profiles of failed coronary angioplasty patients: Impact on surgical results. Ann Thorac Surg 1992;53:269–273

23. Sigwart U, Urban P, Golf S et al. Emergency stenting for acute occlusion after coronary balloon angioplasty. Circulation 1988;78:1121–1127

24. Erbel R, Clas W, Busch U et al. New balloon catheter for prolonged percutaneous transluminal coronary angioplasty and bypass flow in occluded vessels. Cathet Cardiovasc Diagn 1986;12:116–123

25. Hinohara T, Simpson JB, Phillips HR et al. Transluminal catheter reperfusion: a new technique to reestablish blood flow after coronary occlusion during percutaneous transluminal coronary angioplasty. Am J Cardiol 1986;57:684–686

26. Angelini P, Heibig J, Leachman DR. Distal hemoperfusion during percutaneous transluminal coronary angioplasty. Am J Cardiol 1986;58:252–255

27. Cleman M, Jaffee CC, Wohlgelernter D. Prevention of ischemia during percutaneous transluminal coronary angioplasty by transcatheter infusion of oxygenated Fluosol DA 20%. Circulation 1986;74:555–562

28. Heuser RR, Mehta S, Strumpf RK. ACS RX flow support catheter as a temporary stent for dissection or occlusion during balloon angioplasty. Cathet Cardiovasc Diagn 1992;27:66–74

29. Murphy DA, Craver JM, Jones EL et al. Surgical management of acute myocardial ischemia following percutaneous transluminal coronary angioplasty: role of intra-aortic balloon pump. J Thorac Cardiovasc Surg 1984;87:332–339

30. Shawl FA, Domanski MJ, Punja S, Hernandez TJ. Percutaneous cardiopulmonary bypass support in high-risk patients undergoing percutaneous transluminal coronary angioplasty. Am J Cardiol 1989;64:1258–1263

31. Wampler RK, Frazier OH, Lansing AM et al. Treatment of cardiogenic shock with the hemopump left ventricular assist device. Ann Thorac Surg 1991;52:506–513

32. Babic UU, Grujicic SN, Djurisic Z, Vucinic M. Nonsurgical left-atrial aortic bypass. Lancet 1988;2:1430–1431

33. Taylor GJ, Rabinovich E, Mikell FL et al. Percutaneous transluminal coronary angioplasty as palliation for patients considered poor surgical candidates. Am Heart J 1986;111:840–844

34. Richardson SG, Morton P, Murtagh JG et al. Management of acute coronary occlusion during percutaneous transluminal coronary angioplasty: experience of complications in a hospital without on site facilities for cardiac surgery. Br Med J 1990;300:355–358

35. Renner U, Busch U, Baumann G et al. Herzchirurgische Operationsbereitschaft für die perkutane transluminale Koronarangioplastik (PTCA): Erfordernisse und derzeitige Praxis. Herz Kreislauf 1991;23:409–411

36. Iniguez A, Macaya C, Hernandez R. Comparison of results of percutaneous transluminal coronary angioplasty with and without selective requirement of surgical standby. Am J Cardiol 1992;69:1161–1165

37. Klinke WP, Hui W. Percutaneous transluminal coronary angioplasty without on-site surgical facilities. Am J Cardiol 1992;70:1520–1525

38. Meier B, Urban P, Dorsaz PA, Favre J. Surgical standby for coronary balloon angioplasty. JAMA 1992;268:741–745

39. Morrison DA, Barbiere CC, Johnson R et al. Salvage angioplasty: an alternative to high risk surgery for unstable angina. Cathet Cardiovasc Diagn 1992;27:169–178

40. Vogel JHK. Changing trends for surgical standby in patients undergoing percutaneous transluminal coronary angioplasty. Am J Cardiol 1992;69:25F–32F

41. Cameron DE, Stinson DC, Greene PS, Gardner TJ. Surgical standby for percutaneous transluminal coronary angioplasty: a survey of patterns of practice. Ann Thorac Surg 1990;50:35–39

33 Balloon Angioplasty for Unstable Angina

Pim J. de Feyter
Patrick W. Serruys

Since the introduction of percutaneous transluminal coronary angioplasty (PTCA) for single-lesion stable angina, the indications have widened and also include various subgroups of unstable angina.[1-4] Today Balloon angioplasty is considered a formidable treatment modality in the management of patients with unstable angina unresponsive to medical treatment. However, it has been recognized that balloon angioplasty for unstable angina is less safe, the immediate results are less favorable, and the procedure is associated with a higher major complication rate (death, myocardial infarction, and need for acute bypass surgery) when compared with the results obtained using elective balloon angioplasty. Angioplasty of an unstable lesion requires the availability of immediate surgical back-up during the procedure.

The introduction of new potent antithrombin or antiplatelet treatment, in addition to heparin or aspirin, appears very promising to reduce the occurrence of major procedural complications.

RATIONALE AND MECHANISM OF ACTION

The major recognized physiopathologic mechanisms underlying unstable angina include (1) plaque fissuring, which sets into action a complex interplay of (2) platelet activation, adhesion, and aggregation, (3) activation of the coagulation system with formation of a transient, labile intraluminal thrombus; and (4) local vasoconstriction by the platelet release of vasoactive products (serotonin and thromboxane A_2) and production of thrombin, which is aggravated by an abnormal vasoreactivity response associated with endothelial dysfunction.[5-8]

Platelet adhesion to the ruptured subendothelium is mediated by the expression of glycoprotein (GP) IA receptor, which binds with collagen, and GPIB receptor, which binds via the von Willebrand factor to collagen (Fig. 33-1). Platelet aggregation takes place via GPIIB/IIIA receptor, which binds with von Willebrand factor and fibrinogen, thus linking the platelets. Activation of the coagulation system results in fibrin formation, which stabilizes the platelet aggregate to form a white platelet-rich thrombus. Depending on local rheologic factors, which are predominantly determined by the severity of the pre-existing stenosis and magnitude of blood flow disturbance due to the formation of the platelet thrombus, a fibrin red cell-rich thrombus may develop that is superimposed upon the platelet-rich thrombus.

Thrombin plays a key role in these processes (Fig. 33-2). Thrombin converts fibrinogen in fibrin and cross-links fibrin, it reinforces platelet aggregation, and, once formed it greatly self-amplifies formation of thrombin. Self-amplification of thrombin formation via activation of platelets and factors V and VIII results in sufficient amounts of thrombin, which is thought to be necessary for effective hemostasis and thrombosis.

Intracoronary thrombosis formation causes perturbation of coronary blood flow. The resulting extent and duration of perturbation of blood flow, mod-

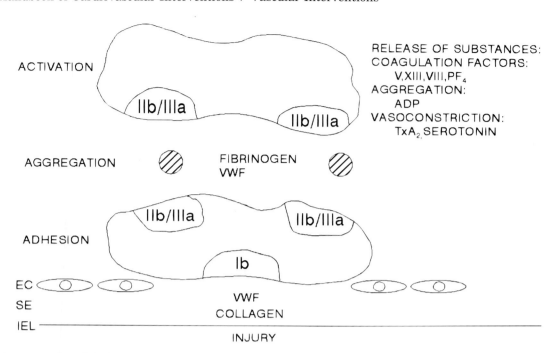

Fig. 33-1. Simplified schematic of platelet activation, adhesion, and activation. Platelet activation induces release of many substances. Platelet adhesion is mediated by platelet GPIA/IB receptors. Platelet aggregation by platelet GPIIB/IIIA receptors. VWF, von Willebrand factor; PF4, platelet factor 4; TxA$_2$, thromboxane A$_2$, EC, endothelial cells; SE, subendothelium; IEL, internal elastic lamina.

ulated by the collateral circulation, will determine the ensuing clinical syndrome, which may range from no symptoms to unstable angina, myocardial infarction, or sudden death (Fig. 33-3). In patients with unstable angina, a labile transient occlusive thrombus is formed, which may accumulate or disintegrate over time and which is the cause of the waxing and waning of ischemia in the acute phase.

The rationale for a mechanical intervention in un-

stable angina is evident. The underlying pre-existing coronary lesion is severe in most patients with unstable angina. Angioplasty effectively widens the lumen. However, angioplasty is associated with an increased risk of major complications. This may be related to the induction of further damage of the already ruptured thrombogenic plaque, which may re-trigger or intensify ongoing intracoronary thrombosis formation.

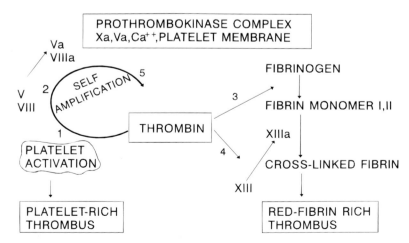

Fig. 33-2. Key role of thrombin in hemostasis and thrombosis. 1 platelet activation; 2, activation factors V and VIII; 3, conversion of fibrinogen into fibrin; 4, cross-linking fibrin; 5, self-amplification of thrombin. (Adapted from Webster et al.,[70] with permission.)

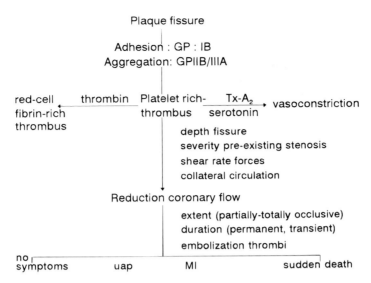

Fig. 33-3. Schematic of paradigm of acute ischemic syndromes. GP, glycoprotein receptor; Tx-A$_2$, thromboxane A$_2$; UAP, unstable angina pectoris; MI, myocardial infarction.

INSTRUMENTATION

From the early beginning of percutaneous intervention, unstable lesions have been treated with balloon angioplasty. New techniques such as excimer laser, high-speed rotablation, or stenting have not been considered suitable for unstable angina. Directional coronary atherectomy may offer some advantages, because this technique makes it possible to remove the total "thrombogenic" plaque and may thus overcome the problem of abrupt vessel occlusion by thrombosis formation.[9,10] In a study performed in the Thorax Center, we compared the success and complication rates of directional coronary atherectomy in 82 patients with stable and 68 patients with unstable angina.[11] The overall success rate was 91% for stable and 88% for unstable angina. The in-hospital major complication rate was not significantly different when the stable and the unstable groups were compared (9 vs 12%). Abdelmeguid et al.[12] performed directional atherectomy in stable patients (group I, n = 77) and in two subgroups of patients with unstable angina; those with progressively worsening angina (group II, n = 110) and those with angina at rest or postinfarction angina (group III, n = 100). They reported a higher major complication rate of 7.0% in group III versus 1.3% in group I and 0.9% in group II.

These results indicated that the pathophysiology of unstable angina rather than the intervention is responsible for the increase of complications. Thus balloon angioplasty continues to be the mainstay of intervention for unstable angina. Directional atherectomy may have some advantages in ulcerated, thrombotic lesions.

PATIENT POPULATION

Patients with unstable angina may be classified into three distinct subgroups. Although is some overlap exists between the subgroups, there are differences in prognosis and management.[13,14]

Progressive Angina

Braunwald IB includes, patients with (1) new-onset angina of a progressive nature or (2) chronic angina who experience a change in their anginal pattern involving an which has now increase in frequency or severity. These patients do not have angina at rest. This subgroup appears to have a rather benign clinical course and may often only require medical treatment. Only in case of failure under medical treatment do they require revascularization (PTCA or bypass surgery).

Angina at Rest

Braunwald IIB and IIIB includes patients with (repeated periods of) angina at rest with or without ST-segment or T-wave changes on a baseline electrocardiogram (ECG). These patients appear to have a worse prognosis, which requires more aggressive intervention. If they are refractory to medical treatment these patients require emergency revascularization.

Early Postinfarction Angina

Braunwald IIC and IIIC compress patients with (1) early (within 30 days) postinfarction angina at rest with or without ST segment or T-wave changes or (2) angina pectoris induced by minimal exercise. These patients appear to have a high likelihood of recurrent myocardial infarction and mortality, which requires more aggressive interventions.

PRETREATMENT TO REDUCE MAJOR PROCEDURAL COMPLICATIONS

Since the inception of PTCA, heparin and aspirin administered before the procedure have been considered cornerstone treatments to prevent acute complications during balloon angioplasty. However, in particular in patients undergoing balloon angioplasty for unstable angina, the occurrence of major complications is high.

Prolonged pretreatment with anticoagulants or thrombolytic agents might reduce the occurrence of major complications during angioplasty for unstable angina. Four recent nonrandomized studies have demonstrated that prolonged heparinization (3 to 6 days preceding the intervention) in patients with unstable angina scheduled for PTCA improved the safety of the procedure and markedly decreased the occurrence of abrupt vessel closure during angioplasty[15-18] (Table 33-1). The efficacy of pretreatment with thrombolytics to reduce the occurrence of complications during angioplasty has been disappointing. Three randomized trials, studying the efficacy of tissue plasminogen activator (t-PA) or intravenous urokinase did not demonstrate a clear beneficial effect; thus pretreatment with thrombolytics is currently not recommended.[19-21]

The preventive role of thrombolytic treatment, routinely given during balloon angioplasty, is not established either. Four studies have addressed this issue.[22-25] Zeiher et al.[22] showed that in a randomized study of 251 consecutive patients concomitant intracoronary infusion of urokinase during the procedure did not significantly reduce the frequency of acute complications. Ambrose et al.[23] performed a double-blind randomized pilot study of intracoronary urokinase 150,000 IU or placebo in 93 unstable angina patients (66 patients had pain at rest and 27 patients postinfarction angina). They could not demonstrate a difference in the incidence of abrupt occlusion between both groups; however, urokinase decreased the number of intracoronary filling defects at 15 minutes after angioplasty. Data from the TAUSA trial showed that adjunctive urokinase given during angioplasty for ischemic rest pain was associated with an increase of adverse angiographic and clinical events.[24] Also, the data from the Thrombolysis in Myocardial Infarction Phase IIIB (TIMI-IIIB) trial clearly demonstrated that addition of recombinant (r)t-PA during PTCA for patients with unstable angina and non-Q-wave infarction is not beneficial and in fact may even be harmful.[25] Therefore, adjunctive treatment with a thrombolytic agent during PTCA is not indicated and may even be detrimental.

It may be concluded that only prolonged pretreatment with heparin is currently recommended, in particular if there is angiographic evidence of the presence of intracoronary thrombus. Prolonged pretreatment with more potent drugs, such as GPIIb/IIIa receptor inhibitors or direct antithrombins, might prove to be more efficacious to reduce abrupt occlusion during balloon angioplasty.

In a recently performed placebo-controlled pilot study, the efficacy of chimeric 7E$_3$ was studied in 30 patients given placebo and 30 treated patients; all had refractory unstable angina and were scheduled for balloon angioplasty.[26] All patients were also treated with heparin, aspirin, and nitroglycerin. Treatment was started and continued for 16 to 24 hours until the scheduled angioplasty of the culprit lesion. The end points of the study were recurrent ischemia or major events (death, myocardial infarc-

Table 33-1. Pretreatment With Prolonged Heparinization to Reduce PTCA Complications in Patients With Unstable Angina

Author	Total No.	Heparin/ No Heparin (no.)	Duration of Heparin (days)	Occurrence of Abrupt Vessel Closure (%)	
				Heparin	No Heparin
Hettleman et al.[15]	188	62/126	3	1.6	10.3
Laskey et al.[16]	53	35/18	6	5.7	33
Pow et al.[17]	110	41/69	4	0	10
Lukas et al.[18]	304	135/169	5.7	1.5	8.3

tion, and urgent angioplasty/bypass surgery), before, during, or within 24 hours following angioplasty. Seventy-three percent of the randomized patients were male, and the mean age was 61 years. A previous myocardial infarction had occurred in 19% within the preceding 7 days. A total of 12 major events occurred in seven patients in the placebo group, whereas only one adverse event occurred in the chimeric 7E$_3$ group (Table 33-2). The Evaluation of Chimeric 7E$_3$ Fab in the Prevention of Ischemic Complications (EPIC) trial tested the efficacy of chimeric 7E$_3$ Fab in 2,099 patients undergoing high-risk PTCA.[27] High-risk PTCA was defined as angioplasty in patients with acute myocardial infarction, unstable angina, or high-risk anatomic or clinical characteristics. All patients received aspirin and high-dose heparin, and they were randomized into three treatment arms: placebo (696), c7E$_3$ Fab bolus (695), and c7E$_3$ Fab bolus followed by continuous infusion for 12 hours (708). The primary efficacy was tested with a composite end point: death, myocardial infarction, and urgent intervention. The results are summarized in Table 33-3(A). A single bolus of 7E$_3$ Fab appeared not to be effective, whereas a bolus followed by infusion markedly reduced complications during PTCA. This benefit was immediate and sustained throughout the 30-day follow-up. This beneficial effect was achieved at the price of increased bleeding complications, which occurred primarily at the vascular puncture sites. The patients were followed prospectively for 6 months, and the overall adverse coronary event rate at 6 months is tabulated in Table 3(B).[28] In a subanalysis it appeared that the clinical benefit with platelet GPIIb/IIIa inhibition was striking in patients with unstable angina[29] (Table 33-3C). The data support the notion that acute-phase administration of c7E$_3$ bolus plus infusion reduces the need for target vessel repeat revascularization, suggesting that profound platelet inhibition during the initial procedure may be associated with reduction of late restenosis.

Direct antithrombins have a potent anticoagulant effect and may be more effective than heparin in reducing adverse events during angioplasty. A recent study demonstrated that hirulog, in place of heparin during coronary angioplasty, was associated with a low rate (3.9%) of abrupt vessel closure.[30] The bleeding complications were minimal. Topol et al.[31] performed a multicenter, randomized angiographic trial to investigate the efficacy of recombinant hirudin for unstable angina. The study recruited patients with rest ischemic pain, an abnormal ECG, and angiographic visual appearance of thrombus. They compared the efficacy of heparin versus hirudin. Overall the patients treated with hirudin showed better angiographic improvement with regard to increase in cross-sectional area and minimal luminal diameter. In a pilot study, designed as a double-blind trial with two allocations to hirudin and one to heparin, the safety and efficacy of hirudin was tested in patients undergoing angioplasty for stable angina.[32] All patients received aspirin during the procedure. The end points were periprocedural ischemic events, bleeding complications, and early angiographic outcome. A total of 113 patients was randomized. The mean age was 58 years, 78% were males, 38% had previous myocardial infarction, and 83% had single-vessel disease. It appeared that patients given hirudin had fewer periprocedural complications and a lesser incidence of postprocedural ischemia (Table 33-4). The occurrence of major bleeding at the puncture site was increased. No significant difference was seen in early angiographic outcome between both groups.

The preliminary results of the Helvetica trial showed that hirudin reduced the incidence of major adverse coronary events within the first 96 hours after angioplasty of patients with unstable angina who were on pretreatment with heparin.[33] Major adverse events occurred in 17.4% of the patients treated with heparin only versus 6.4% of the patients who were treated with hirudin ($P = 0.007$). This favorable effect was achieved without a significant increase in major bleeding complications.

However, the potency of these new drugs is highlighted by the increase in the occurrence of cerebrovascular bleeding in the TIMI-9 trial,[34] HIT-III Study,[35] and GUSTO-II-A,[36] trial which were terminated prematurely. Apparently the dosage of antithrombin used in combination with thrombolytic agents was too high. The adjusted dosage of hirudin will be further studied in the GUSTO-II-B trial, and the results of that and other studies should be awaited before definitive conclusions can be drawn about the safety of the novel direct antithrombins.

Table 33-2. Randomized Trial of Chimeric 7E$_3$ Versus Placebo: Number of Periprocedural Clinical Events

	Chimeric (n = 30)	Placebo (n = 30)
Death	0	1
Myocardial infarction	1	4
Urgent PTCA	0	3
Urgent stent	0	1
Late PTCA/CABG	0	3
Patients with major complications	1	7

Abbreviations: CABG, coronary artery bypass graft.

Table 33-3. Results of the EPIC Trial (%)

	Placebo (n = 696)	Bolus (n = 695)	Bolus + Infusion (n = 708)	P Value vs. Placebo
A. First 30 days				
Composite end points				
Death	1.7	1.3	1.7	
Myocardial infarction	8.6	6.2	5.2	0.013
Urgent intervention	7.8	6.4	4.0	0.003
Total events	12.8	11.4	8.3	0.009
Bleeding complications				
Stroke	0.6	0.7	0.7	
Major bleeds	7.0	11.0	14.0	
Thrombocytopenia	3.0	4.0	6.0	
B. Events at 6 months				
Death	3.4	2.6	3.1	
Myocardial infarction (%)	10.5	8.0	6.9	
Composite end points (death, myocardial infarction, CABG, PTCA)	35.1	32.6	27.0	0.001
Target vessel repeat revascularization	22.3	21.0	16.5	0.007

End Points at 30 days	Placebo (n = 156)	Chimeric 7E$_3$ Bolus (n = 168)	Chimeric 7E$_3$ Bolus + Infusion (n = 165)
C. Subanalysis of patients with unstable angina pectoris			
Death	3.2	0.6	1.2
Myocardial infarction	9.0	4.2	1.8
CABG/PTCA	5.8	4.2	3.6
Composite end point	12.8	7.8	4.8

Table 33-4. Randomized Double-Blind Trial of Recombinant Hirudin Versus Heparin: Clinical Events During Angioplasty[a]

	Hirudin (n = 74)	Heparin (n = 39)
Cardiac complications		
Death	0	0
Myocardial infarction	0	2 (5)
Emergency CABG	1 (1)	3 (8)
Other complications		
Major bleeding at puncture site	4 (5)	0
24-hr ECG ST-segment displacement[b]	3 (4)	3 (8)

[a] Data are number of patients, with percent in parentheses.
[b] Excluding subjects with cardiac events.

OPERATIVE TECHNIQUES

In most patients with unstable angina scheduled for percutaneous intervention, balloon angioplasty is considered the preferred technique and in only few lesions might directional atherectomy be preferable. Because of the high likelihood of abrupt occlusion in unstable angina, it is wise to anticipate and take the necessary precautions. This should also be done in unstable patients with an occluded ischemia-related vessel, because (contrary to common opinion) this also might turn out to be a dangerous procedure.[37] Ensure the availability of immediate surgical back-up. Use guiding catheters and guidewires that allow the use of perfusion balloons or bail-out stent implantation. Determine the activated clotting time (ACT) before and during intervention and adjust heparin to achieve an ACT, above 300 seconds. In general, it is wise to dilate only the ischemia-related vessel in patients with refractory unstable angina who have multivessel disease. Necessary subsequent dilations can be performed at a later stage under safe, stable conditions. Wait 10 to 15 minutes after successful dilation in the catheterization laboratory and repeat the angiogram. If the result is still satisfactory the patient is referred to a medium care unit, where ECG monitoring is possible.

If an abrupt occlusion occurs during the procedure, immediate redilation with the same balloon or a larger size balloon may remedy the problem. Again, wait 10 to 15 minutes and repeat the angiogram. If the abrupt occlusion is refractory to repeat angioplasty, attempt to establish its cause: occlusive thrombus formation or occlusive dissection. Occlusive thrombus formation is suspected in cases of abrupt occlusion where after (repeated) dilation an immediate satisfactory result is obtained, without visible dissection, but gradually "haziness" appears and blood flow becomes less. In this situation adjunctive thrombolytic treatment may be effective.[38–42] The result of a strategy consisting of a combination of thrombolytic treatment and redilation to manage abrupt occlusion is listed in Table 33-5. Although this strategy reduces the need for acute surgery, it could not prevent progression to myocardial infarction in 25 to 50% of the patients. However, there appears to be a rebound effect after stopping the thrombolytic treatment. Gulba et al.[38] demonstrated that after initial angiographic success the reocclusion rate was 55% during repeat angiography 24 to 36 hours later. In most patients these reocclusions were associated with the development of a myocardial infarction.

In situations of refractory occlusive dissection and coronary anatomy, suitable for stent implantation, bail-out stenting may solve the immediate problem. It remains difficult in these situations to decide whether stent implantation should be considered as definitive treatment or as a bridge until later surgery. We now refer patients to semielective surgery if (1) after stent implantation the result still is not satisfactory; (2) significant other coexisting coronary lesions are present; (3) left main stem occlusion threatened; (4) life-threatening severe left ventricular-dysfunction in case of subacute stent occlusion; (5) is present a high likelihood of severe bleeding complications during subsequent intense anticoagulant therapy exists; or (6) a contraindication to anticoagulation exists. Depending on the situation, bypass surgery should be performed immediately or within 24 hours after stent implantation.

Emergency surgery is indicated in refractory abrupt occlusions not suitable for stent implantation. In general, bail-out stent implantation is not indicated in patients with extreme tortuosity and small occluded coronary vessel segments (less than 2 mm in diameter). If possible, perfusion balloons should be placed to relieve ischemia. An intra-aortic balloon pump should be inserted in case of hemodynamic instability.

POSTOPERATIVE TREATMENT

After percutaneous intervention of an unstable lesion the patient is usually kept under heparin treatment for 4 to 6 hours. After stopping the heparin the sheaths are removed either 4 hours later or (for logistic reasons) the next morning. Calcium channel blockers are given during a period of 12 to 24 hours following the procedure and then stopped. Nitrates and β-adrenergic blockers are discontinued after the procedure, except in early postinfarction patients, who will continue their β-blocker medication. Patients are discharged 24 to 36 hours after the procedure. Aspirin 80 mg/d is given during the next 6 months.

SHORT- AND LONG-TERM RESULTS

Patients with new-onset of angina or with worsening of pre-existing angina, but without symptoms of chest pain at rest (class I according to recently proposed classification of Braunwald), should initially be treated pharmacologically only if this treatment fails should they be referred for revascularization (coronary angioplasty or bypass surgery). This deferred strategy gives this category of initially unstable patients the opportunity to progress to a lower risk group. They will now be stabilized, so that at the time they undergo revascularization the immediate results of balloon angioplasty will be similar to the results achieved with elective balloon angioplasty.[43–47] The success rate is well above 90%, the procedural mortality rate is less than 1%, the procedural myocardial infarction rate is less than 2%, and the need for acute surgery is less than 3%.

Patients who present with angina at rest and who have been stable for more than 48 hours (similar to a IIb, IIc Braunwald classification) appear to have an unfavorable prognosis, in particular when the anginal attacks were accompanied with reversible ST segment or T-wave changes and the coronary angiogram demonstrated a severe proximal lesion. These patients often require revascularization.

Patients who present with angina at rest or who have early postinfarction angina, refractory to pharmacologic treatment (similar to a IIIb, IIIc Braunwald classification) appear to have a worse prognosis, which dictates urgent revascularization.

Table 33-5. Outcome of Treatment of Abrupt Occlusion With Intracoronary or Intravenous Thrombolytics and Redilation

Author	No. of Patients	Clinical Success No.	Clinical Success %	Failure With Major Complications (no.) Death	MI	Em/CABG	Failure Without Major Complications (no.)	Thrombolytic Treatment
Gulba et al.[38,a]	27	13	48	0	14	2	0	t-PA
Schiemann et al.[39,b]	48	43	90	0	0	1	5	Urokinase
de Feyter et al.[40,a]	34	18	53	2	13	5	0	Streptokinase
Verna et al.[41,a]	23	15	65	1	5	3	0	Urokinase
Vaitkuss et al.[42,b]	27	14	52	0	8	4	0	Urokinase

a Abrupt occlusion during PTCA of patients with stable and unstable angina.
b All patients had PTCA for acute ischemic syndromes.

Table 33-6. Coronary Angioplasty for Initially Stabilized Unstable Angina Pectoris[a]

Author	Year	No. of Patients	Success Rate (%)	Major Complication Rate (%) Death	Myocardial Infarction	Acute Surgery	Coronary Events After Successful Angioplasty Death (%)	Myocardial Infarction (%)	Angina Pectoris (%)	Follow-Up (mo, mean)
Quigley et al.[48]	1986	25	81	4	12	12	0	0	32	14
de Feyter et al.[49]	1987	71	87	0	10	12	2	2	23	12
Steffenino et al.[50]	1987	89	90	0	5	5	0	1.5	23	10
Myler et al.[51]	1990	220	85	0	6.6	6.1	1	2.5	29	37
Stammen et al.[52]	1992	631	91	0.3	3.6	4.7	0.4	1.0	29	6
Total (no.)		1,036								
Average (%)			89	0.3	5.1	5.8	0.7	1.4	27	13.2

a Definitions of unstable angina: (1) Quigley et al.: new-onset angina, coronary insufficiency, changing pattern of pre-existing angina, angina at rest or variant angina: (2) de Feyter et al.: chest pain at rest accompanied by ST-T changes; (3) Steffenino et al.: worsening in the frequency or severity of chest pain or severe episodes of prolonged pain at rest; (4) Myler et al.: onset 1–2 weeks before PTCA; (5) Stammen et al.: PTCA after 15 days after hospitalization.

Table 33-7. Coronary Angioplasty for Refractory Unstable Angina Pectoris

Author	Year	No. of Patients	Success Rate (%)	Major Complication Rate (%)			Coronary Events After Successful Angioplasty			
				Death	Myocardial Infarction	Acute Surgery	Death (%)	Myocardial Infarction (%)	Angina Pectoris (%)	Follow-Up (mo, mean)
Timmis et al.[53]	1987	56	70	5.4	7.1	12.5	3.3	3.3	39	6
de Feyter et al.[54]	1988	200	89.5	0.5	8	9	2.5	4	25	24
Plokker et al.[55]	1988	469	88	1	4.9	3	1.5	0.1	21	19.3
Sharma et al.[56]	1988	40	88	0	0	12	0	0	34	11
Perry et al.[57]	1988	105	87	2	9	4	—	—	—	—
Myler et al.[51,a]	1990	310	79	0.3	6.5	9.4	5.8	6.3	33	37
Morrison[58,b]	1990	56	84	3.6	7.2	9	1.8	1.8	32	10
Rupprecht et al.[59]	1990	202	83	2.0	6.5	7.9	4.5	3.0	29	36
Total (no.)		1,438								
Average (%)			85	1.3	6.3	6.8	2.7	2.9	28	25.3

a Unstable angina pectoris defined as onset less than 1 week before PTCA.
b Patients were managed with intra-aortic balloon counterpulsation.

Table 33-8. Coronary Angioplasty for Early Postinfarction Angina Pectoris

Author	Year	No. of Patients	Success Rate (%)	Major Complication Rate (%)			Coronary Events After Successful Angioplasty			
				Death	Myocardial Infarction	Acute Surgery	Death (%)	Myocardial Infarction (%)	Angina Pectoris (%)	Follow-Up (mo, mean)
de Feyter et al.[60]	1986	53	89	0	8	8	0	4	26	9
Holt et al.[61]	1986	70	76	2	5	12	2	4	21	27
Gottlieb et al.[62]	1987	47	91	2	4	2	3	3	18	16.3
Safian et al.[63,a]	1987	68	87	0	1.5	1.5	0	2	41	17
Hopkins et al.[64]	1988	54	81	0	0	4	0	2	25	11
Suryapranata et al.[65,a]	1988	60	85	0	5	7	0	5	23	20
Morrison[66]	1990	66	88	3	3	3	5	0	20	14
TIMI-II[67]	1989	216	92	1.0	11	7.9	—	—	—	—
Total (no.)		634								
Average (%)			88	1.1	6.3	6.5	1.3	2.5	22	16.6

a Coronary angioplasty of patient with non-Q-wave myocardial infarction.

The immediate success rate, the major complication rate, and the coronary event rate after successful balloon angioplasty are listed for balloon angioplasty for initially stabilized unstable angina[48–52] (Braunwald classification IIb, IIc; Table 33-6), for refractory unstable angina[51,53–59] (Braunwald classification IIIb; Table 33-7), and for early postinfarction unstable angina[60–67] (Braunwald classification IIIc; Table 33-8). The inmediate success rate for the various subgroups varies from 85 to 89%. The immediate success rate is lower than the immediate success rate of approximately 92% achieved in patients undergoing elective balloon angioplasty today.[43–48] The lower success rate in unstable angina is primarily due to the higher major complication rate during coronary angioplasty. Coronary angioplasty is associated with a much higher occurrence of abrupt coronary occlusion (approximately 10% of the cases), which is often refractory to repeated, longer lasting inflations with the same sized or bigger balloons.

The higher incidence of major complications in unstable angina is probably related to the additional balloon injury of the already ruptured unstable lesion. The fissure may enlarge, thereby exposing the deeper, more thrombogenic arterial wall layers to the streaming blood. The additional damage may intensify the processes of platelet activation, adhesion and aggregation, and activation of blood coagulation, which are often refractory to heparin and may require the use of more potent antiplatelet drugs, direct antithrombins, or even fibrinolytic treatment. The prognosis after successful coronary balloon angioplasty is favorable. The late mortality and late nonfatal myocardial infarction rates are low (Tables 33-6 to 33-8).

IMMEDIATE INVASIVE STRATEGY FOR UNSTABLE ANGINA

It would be of great interest to demonstrate that an early invasive strategy could prevent progression to myocardial infarction or cardiac death, in patients with symptoms and signs suggestive of unstable angina early after admission into the hospital. In TIMI-IIIB trial, which addressed this issue, it was disappointing to note that demonstrated early invasive strategy compared with early conservative strategy was not more effective in preventing progression to myocardial infarction or cardiac death.[25] However, an early invasive strategy reduced the number of days in-hospital and the number of readmissions, as well as the need for intensive antianginal medication.

CURRENT INDICATIONS

At present, randomized studies that have established the merits of pharmacologic treatment, balloon angioplasty, and bypass surgery among various subgroups of patients with unstable angina are not available. Today, it is established practice that patients with unstable angina should initially receive adjusted and individualized pharmacologic treatment to achieve a prompt, satisfactory anti-ischemic response. Possible treatments are as follows:

- Bed rest (cardiac care unit) and sedation
- Treatment of precipitating factors (anemia, hypertension, tachycardia)
- Anticoagulant (heparin) or antiplatelet treatment (aspirin)
- Stepwise intensification, with individual tailoring of a pharmacologic regimen including adequate administration of β-adrenergic blockade to achieve a resting pulse of less than 60 bpm
- Calcium antagonists and nitroglycerin (long-acting or intravenous) to reduce preload vasodilation and afterload (systolic aortic pressure less than 110 mmHg) and induce coronary vasodilation

Individualization and adjustment of treatment are based on (1) the history of unstable angina; (2) the time interval between the last attack of chest pain and initiation of treatment; (3) the presence of ECG changes of ST and T-wave changes; (4) the antiischemic response on pharmacologic treatment; (5) the presence of ischemia during stress testing; and (6) the coronary anatomy and left ventricular function. Accordingly, a practical management approach is proposed (Figs. 33-4 through 33-6). Pharmacologic treatment is usually effective in most patients. However, early angiography and revascularization (PTCA or bypass surgery) is indicated if this initial approach fails and ischemic episodes continue despite "full" anti-ischemic treatment. The interval of watchful waiting should not exceed 48 hours.

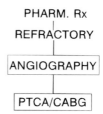

Fig. 33-4. Triage approach to the patients who present with new-onset or accelarated angina pectoris. New onset of severe AP. Accelerated AP (no rest pain) (IB, IC).

PAIN AT REST (IIB, IIC)

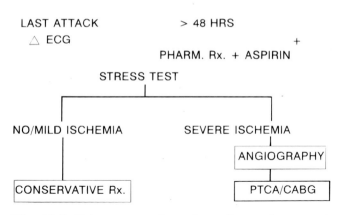

Fig. 33-5. Triage approach to the patients who present with recent-onset angina or with a worsening pattern of angina.

Patients with unstable angina who initially stabilize but who exhibit severe ischemia during stress testing or who have high-risk lesions (left main or three-vessel disease or a severe lesion of proximal ramus descendens anterior) should be referred for a revascularization procedure. The indications to proceed either with PTCA or bypass surgery in unstable angina unresponsive to pharmacologic treatment are still controversial. In general, bypass surgery is indicated if the following conditions are present: (1) significant left main disease, (2) significant three-vessel disease, (3) ischemia-related lesion not amenable to balloon angioplasty, and (4) severely depressed left ventricular function. Balloon angioplasty is indicated if an ischemia-related lesion suitable for balloon angioplasty exists in patients with single-vessel or two-vessel disease. In selected patients with multivessel disease, one might, to enhance safety, prefer dilation of the ischemia-related vessel only, rather than attempting to achieve complete revascularization by multiple dilations.

CURRENT OUTLOOK AND POTENTIAL DEVELOPMENTS

Intracoronary thrombosis appears to play a keyrole in unstable angina; henceforth cornerstone treatment should be directed against platelets to inhibit their activation, adhesion, and aggregation against coagulation to inhibit thrombin, which plays a major role in hemostasis and thrombosis.

The currently used combination treatment of heparin and aspirin during balloon angioplasty does not appear to be potent enough to prevent the occurrence of major complications. The introduction of new antiplatelet drugs and direct thrombin inhibitors may be more effective in stabilizing the unstable lesion and preventing abrupt coronary occlusion during a percutaneous intervention. Platelet GPIIb/IIIa receptor blockers, which effectively block the final common pathway of platelet aggregation, appear very promising. Soon a new class of GPIIb/IIIa receptor blockers, the disintegrins, will become available for clinical testing. The disintegrins are isolated from viper venoms, they have a low molecular weight, and they inhibit the RGD sequence located on the ligand. The RGD sequence is recognized by the GPIIb/IIIa receptor and is essential for binding with the ligand. The disintegrins bind to the RGD recognition site on the platelet GPIIb/IIIa receptor and thereby effectively block the GPIIb/IIIa receptor.[68] The direct anti-

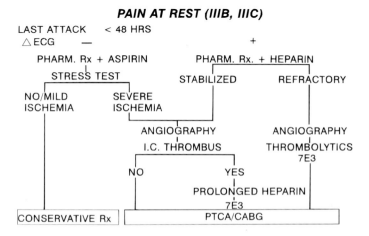

Fig. 33-6. Triage approach to the patients who present with angina at rest or with early postinfarction angina.

thrombins, such as hirudin, or Hirulog, have several potential advantages as anti-coagulants when compared with heparin. Direct antithrombins, in contradistinction to heparin, do not need antithrombin III to inactivate thrombin. Heparin is inactivated by specific antiheparin proteins such as platelet factor 4 or nonspecific heparin-binding proteins, which does not occur with hirudin. Hirudin, contrary to heparin, also inactivates fibrin-bound thrombin. This latter effect may be extremely important because inhibition of the conversion of fibrinogen to fibrin in an evolving clot may more effectively stop ongoing thrombosis.[69]

The introduction of new interventional techniques in the near future may reduce the major complication rate. Directional atherectomy guided by ultrasound imaging may more completely remove the thrombogenic components of the plaque and thus may prevent abrupt coronary occlusion. Heparin-coated stents effectively inhibit the adhesion and aggregation of platelets, as has been shown in animal experiments. Primary heparin-coated stent implantation may be a foreseeable option within the near future to treat unstable lesions. Local delivery of plaque "passivating" substances (antithrombins, GPIIb/IIIa blockers) may reduce the major complications associated with percutaneous intervention of unstable lesions. Finally, the use of intracoronary ultrasound or angioscopy may facilitate the prediction of lesions likely to cause abrupt occlusions and may better guide the management of abrupt occlusions.

REFERENCES

1. Williams DO, Riley RS, Singh AK et al. Evaluation of the role of coronary angioplasty in patients with unstable angina pectoris. Am Heart J 1981;102:1–9
2. Meyer J, Schmitz HJ, Kiesslich T et al. Percutaneous transluminal coronary angioplasty in patients with stable and unstable angina pectoris: analysis of early and late results. Am Heart J 1983;106:973–80
3. Faxon DP, Detre KM, McGabe CH et al. Role of percutaneous transluminal coronary angioplasty in the treatment of unstable angina: report from the National Heart, Lung and Blood Institute Percutaneous Transluminal Coronary Angioplasty and Coronary Artery Surgery Study Registries. Am J Cardiol 1983;53:131C–5C
4. de Feyter PJ, Serruys PW, Brand van den M et al. Emergency coronary angioplasty in refractory unstable angina. N Engl J Med 1985;313:342–7
5. Fuster V, Badimon L, Badimon JJ et al. The pathogenesis of coronary artery disease and the acute coronary syndromes. N Engl J Med 1992;326:242–50 and 310–8
6. Ludmer PL, Selwijn AP, Shook TL et al. Paradoxical vasoconstriction induced by acctylcholine in atherosclerotic coronary arteries. N Engl J Med 1986;315:1046
7. Falk E. Morphologic features of unstable atherothrombotic plaques underlying acute coronary syndroms. Am J Cardiol 1989;63:114E–20E
8. Davies MJ, Thomas AC. Plaque fissuring—the cause of acute myocardial infarction, sudden ischemic death and crescendo angina. Br Heart J 1985;53:363–73
9. Safian RD, Gelbfish JS, Erny RE et al. Coronary atherectomy: clinical, angiographic and histologic findings and observations regarding potential mechanisms. Circulation 1990;82:69–79
10. Hinohara T, Rowe M, Robertson GC et al. Effect of lesion characteristics on outcome of directional coronary atherectomy. J Am Coll Cardiol 1991;17:1112–20
11. Umans VAWM, de Feyter PJ, MacLeod D et al. Acute and long-term outcome of directional coronary atherectomy for stable and unstable angina. Am J Cardiol 1994;74:641–6
12. Abdelmeguid AE, Ellis SG, Sapp SK et al. Directional coronary atherectomy in unstable angina. J Am Coll Cardiol 1994;24:46–54
13. Braunwald E. Unstable angina: a classification. Circulation 1989;80:410–4
14. Betriu A, Heras M, Cohen M et al. Unstable angina: outcome according to clinical presentation. J Am Coll Cardiol 1992;19:1659–63
15. Hettleman BD, Aplin RA, Sullivan PR et al. Three days of heparin pretreatment reduces major complications of coronary angioplasty in patients with unstable angina, abstracted. J Am Coll Cardiol 1990;15:154
16. Laskey MAL, Deutsch E, Barnathan E et al. Influence of heparin therapy on percutaneous transluminal coronary angioplasty outcome in unstable angina pectoris. Am J Cardiol 1990;65:1425–9
17. Pow TK, Varricchione TR, Jacobs AK et al. Does pretreatment with heparin prevent abrupt closure following PTCA? J Am Coll Cardiol 1988;11:238A
18. Lukas MA, Deutsch E, Hirschfeld JW et al. Influence of heparin on percutaneous transluminal coronary angioplasty outcome in patients with coronary arterial thrombus. Am J Cardiol 1990;65:179–82
19. Topol EJ, Nicklas JM, Kander N et al. Coronary revascularization after intravenous tissue plasminogen activator for unstable angina pectoris: results of a randomized placebo-controlled trial. Am J Cardiol 1988;62:368–71
20. van den Brand M, van Zijl A, Geukens R et al. Tissue plasminogen activator in refractory unstable angina. A randomized double blind placebo controlled trial in patients with refractory unstable angina and subsequent angioplasty. Eur Heart J 1991;12:1208–14
21. Haine E, Urban P, Dorsaz PA. Double-blind randomized evaluation of urokinase prior to angioplasty. Early and late outcome, abstracted. Circulation, suppl. 1. 1992;86:1–652
22. Zeiher AM, Kasper W, Gaissmaier C et al. Concomitant intracoronary treatment with urokinase during PTCA does not reduce acute complications during PTCA: a double-blind randomized study, abstracted. Circulation, suppl. III. 1990;82:189
23. Ambrose JA, Torre SR, Sharma SK et al. Adjunctive thrombolytic therapy for angioplasty in ischemic rest angina: results of a double-blind randomized pilot study. J Am Coll Cardiol 1992;20:1197–204
24. Ambrose JA, Almeida OD, Sharma SK et al. Adjunctive thrombolytic therapy during angioplasty for is-

chemic rest angina. Results of the TAUSA-trial. Circulation 1994;90:69–77

25. TIMI-III-B Investigators. Effects of tissue plasminogen activator and a comparison of early invasive and conservative strategies in unstable angina and non-Q-wave myocardial infarction. Results of the TIMI-III-B trial. Circulation 1994;89:1545–56

26. Simoons ML, de Boer MJ, van den Brand MJBM et al. Randomized trial of a GPIIb/IIIa platelet receptor blocker in refractory unstable angina. Circulation 1994;89:596–603

27. EPIC Investigators. Use of a monoclonal antibody directed against the platelet glycoprotein IIb/IIIa receptor in high-risk coronary angioplasty. N Engl J Med 1994;330:956–61

28. Topol EJ, Califf RM, Weisman HF et al. Randomized trial of coronary intervention with antibody against platelet IIb/IIIa integrin for reduction of clinical restenosis: results at 6 months. Lancet 1994;343:881–6

29. Lincoff AM, Califf RM, Anderson K et al. Striking benefit with platelet GPIIb/IIIa inhibition by c7E3 among patients with unstable angina: outcome in the EPIC trial, abstracted. Circulation 1994;90:1–21

30. Topol EJ, Bonan R, Jewitt D et al. Use of direct antithrombin, hirulog, in place of heparin during coronary angioplasty. Circulation 1993;87:1622–9

31. Topol EJ, Fuster V, Harrington RA et al. Recombinant hirudin for unstable angina pectoris. A multicenter, randomized angiographic trial. Circulation 1994;89: 1557–66

32. van den Bos AA, Deckers JW, Heyndrickx GR et al. Safety and efficacy of recombinant hirudin (CGP 39 393) versus heparin in patients with stable angina undergoing coronary angioplasty. Circulation 1993;88: 2058–66

33. Serruys PW, Fox KAA, Herrman JP et al. R-Hirudin reduces the incidence of major adverse cardiac events reported within the first 96 hours post angioplasty in unstable patients pre-treated by heparin, abstracted. J Am Coll Cardiol 1995;25:80A

34. Antman EM. Hirudin in acute myocardial infarction. Circulation 1994;90:1624–30

35. Neuhaus KL, van Essen R, Tebbe U et al. Safety observations from the pilot phase of the randomized r-Hirudin for Improvement of Thrombolysis HIT-III Study. Circulation 1994;90:1638–42

36. GUSTO-II-A Investigators. Randomized trial of intravenous heparin versus recombinant hirudin for acute coronary syndromes. Circulation 1994;90:1631–7

37. Planté S, Laarman GJ, de Feyter PJ et al. Acute complications of percutaneous transluminal coronary angioplasty for total occlusion. Am Heart J 1991;121: 417–26

38. Gulba DC, Daniel W, Simon R et al. Role of thrombolysis and thrombin in patients with acute coronary occlusion during percutaneous transluminal coronary angioplasty. J Am Coll Cardiol 1990;16:563–8

39. Schieman G, Cohen BM, Kozina J et al. Intracoronary urokinase for intracoronary thrombus accumulation complicating percutaneous transluminal coronary angioplasty in acute ischemic syndromes. Circulation 1990;82:2052–60

40. de Feyter PJ, van den Brand M, Laarman GJ et al. Acute coronary artery occlusion during and after percutaneous transluminal coronary angioplasty: fre-

quency, prediction, clinical course, management and follow-up. Circulation 1991;83:927–36

41. Verna E, Repetto S, Boscarini M. Management of complicated coronary angioplasty by intracoronary urokinase and immediate reangioplasty. Cathet Cardiovasc Diagn 1990;19:116

42. Vaitkus PT, Herrmann HC, Laskey WK. Management and immediate outcome of patients with intracoronary thrombus during percutaneous transluminal coronary angioplasty. Am Heart J 1992;124:1–8

43. Bredlau CE, Roubin GS, Leimgruber PP et al. In-hospital morbidity and mortality in patients undergoing elective coronary angioplasty. Circulation 1985;72: 1044–52

44. Hartzler G. Complex coronary angioplasty: multivessel/multilesion dilatation pp. 250–67. In Ischinger T (ed): Practice of Coronary Angioplasty. Springler-Verlag, New York, 1986

45. Holmes DR, Holubkov R, Vlietstra RE. Comparison of complications during PTCA from 1977 to 1981 and from 1985 to 1986: the NHLBI-PTCA Registry. J Am Coll Cardiol 1988;12:1149–55

46. Tuzcu EM, Simpfendorfer C, Badhwar K et al. Determinants of primary success in elective PTCA for significant narrowing of a single major coronary artery. Am J Cardiol 1988;62:873–5

47. Feyter PJ, van den Brand M, Serruys PW et al. Increase of initial success and safety of single-vessel PTCA in 1371 patients: a seven-years experience. J Interv Cardiol 1988;1:1–9

48. Quigley PJ, Erwin J, Maurer BJ et al. Percutaneous transluminal coronary angioplasty in unstable angina; comparison with stable angina. Br Heart J 1986; 55:227–30

49. de Feyter PJ, Serruys PW, Suryapranata H et al. PTCA early after the diagnosis of unstable angina. Am Heart J 1987;114:48–54

50. Steffenino G, Meier B, Finci L et al. Follow-up results of treatment of unstable angina by coronary angioplasty. Br Heart J 1987;57:416–9

51. Myler RK, Shaw RE, Stertzer SH et al. Unstable angina and coronary angioplasty. Circulation, suppl. II. 1990;82:88–95

52. Stammen F, De Scheerder I, Glazier JJ et al. Immediate and follow-up results of the conservative coronary angioplasty strategy for unstable angina pectoris. Am J Cardiol 1992;69:1533–7

53. Timmis AD, Griffin B, Crick JCP et al. Early percutaneous transluminal coronary angioplasty in the management of unstable angina. Int J Cardiol 1987;14: 25–31

54. de Feyter PJ, Suryapranata H, Serruys PW et al. Coronary angioplasty for unstable angina: immediate and late results in 200 consecutive patients with identification of risk factors for unfavorable early and late outcome. J Am Coll Cardiol 1988;12:324–33

55. Plokker HWT, Ernst SMPG, Bal ET et al. Percutaneous transluminal coronary angioplasty in patients with unstable angina pectoris refractory to medical therapy. Cathet Cardiovasc Diagn 1988;14:15–8

56. Sharma B, Wyeth RP, Kolath GS et al. Percutaneous transluminal coronary angioplasty of one vessel for refractory unstable angina pectoris: efficacy in single and multivessel disease. Br Heart J 1988;59:280–6

57. Perry RA, Seth A, Hunt A et al. Coronary angioplasty

in unstable angina and stable angina: a comparison of success and complications. Br Heart J 1988;60:367–2

58. Morrison DA. Percutaneous transluminal coronary angioplasty for rest angina pectoris requiring intravenous nitroglycerin and intra-aortic balloon counterpulsation. Am J Cardiol 1990;66:168–71

59. Rupprecht HJ, Brennecke R, Kottmeyer M et al. Short- and long-term outcome after PTCA in patients with stable and unstable angina. Eur Heart J 1990;11:964–73

60. de Feyter PJ, Serruys PW, Soward A et al. Coronary angioplasty for early postinfarction unstable angina. Circulation 1986;54:460–5

61. Holt GW, Gersh BJ, Holmes DR et al. The results of percutaneous transluminal coronary angioplasty (PTCA) in post infarction angina pectoris, abstracted. J Am Coll Cardiol 1986;7:62

62. Gottlieb SO, Brim KP, Walford GD et al. Initial and late results of coronary angioplasty for early postinfarction unstable angina. Cathet Cardiovasc Diagn 1987;13:93–9

63. Safian RD, Snijder LD, Synder BA et al. Usefulness of PTCA for unstable angina pectoris after non Q-wave acute myocardial infarction. Am J Cardiol 1987;59:263–6

64. Hopkins J, Savage M, Zaluwski A et al. Recurrent ischemia in the zone of prior myocardial infarction: results of coronary angioplasty of the infarct related artery. Am Heart J 1988;115:14–9

65. Suryapranata H, Beatt K, de Feyter PJ et al. Percutaneous transluminal coronary angioplasty for angina pectoris after a non-Q-wave acute myocardial infarction. Am J Cardiol 1988;61:240–3

66. Morrison DA. Coronary angioplasty for medically refractory unstable angina within 30 days of acute myocardial infarction. Am Heart J 1990;120:256–61

67. TIMI Study Group Phase II trial. Comparison of invasive and conservative strategies after treatment with intravenous tissue plasminogen activator in acute myocardial infarction. N Engl J Med 1989;320:618

68. Coller BS. Inhibitors of the platelet glycoprotein IIb/IIIa receptor as conjunctive therapy for coronary artery thrombolysis. Coronary Artery Dis 1992;3:1016–9

69. Zoldhelyi P, Fuster V, Chesebro JH. Antithrombins as conjunctive therapy in arterial thrombolysis. Coronary Artery Dis 1992;3:1003–9

70. Webster MWI, Chesebro JH, Fuster V: Antithrombotic therapy in acute myocardial infarction: enhancement of thrombolysis, reduction of reocclusion and prevention of thromboembolism. p. 333. In Gersh BJ, Rahintoola SH (eds): Acute Myocardial Infarction. Elsevier, New York, 1991

34 Direct Angioplasty

Joel K. Kahn
William W. O'Neill

The use of coronary interventions, predominantly balloon angioplasty, without preceding thrombolytic therapy for the acute reperfusion of patients with evolving myocardial infarction is referred to as direct angioplasty. We have been involved in the clinical care and investigation of patients treated in this manner for over a decade. The validation of this approach in recent randomized trials comparing direct angioplasty with intravenous thrombolytic therapy has been gratifying, and we anticipate that the numbers of these procedures will increase. We discuss the history, rationale, technique, clinical outcome, indications, and limitations of this topic.

HISTORY

The origins of catheter-based treatments for acute myocardial infarction date back to the early 1970s when emergency bypass surgery was being evaluated for this condition in a few centers. Emergency cardiac catheterization was necessary to evaluate the coronary anatomy. Once it was established from these studies that the sudden and complete thrombosis of a coronary atherosclerotic lesion was present in most patients with acute myocardial infarction, guidewires and intracoronary thrombolytic agents were used to re-establish antegrade coronary flow. By the beginning of the 1980s, proficiency in coronary angioplasty was developing, including the treatment of intracoronary thrombus in patients with unstable angina. The use of a balloon angio-

plasty catheter to reperfuse the infarcted myocardium was a logical but bold extension of this work. Probably the first direct infarct angioplasty to be performed was described in detail by Geoffrey Hartzler, of the Mid America Heart Institute.[1] The patient described had a subsequent event-free survival for 7 years until his death of noncardiac causes. Hartzler's group continued to investigate the effects of direct angioplasty and reported on a series of 41 patients treated with angioplasty for acute myocardial infarction.[2] Twelve of the patients were treated with direct angioplasty and the procedure was successful in 11 patients. Potential limitations of slow coronary flow and acute reocclusion were identified in a small number of patients, and the investigators concluded by calling for randomized trials of this technique in acute myocardial infarction. The Mid America Heart Institute series of direct angioplasties was increased to 29 patients in 1984, with an overall 92% hospital survival.[3] Soon thereafter, small observational series of patients treated with direct angioplasty at the University of Florida[4] the Mayo Clinic,[5] the University of Michigan and Beaumont Hospitals,[6] Toulouse,[7] and St. Vincent's Hospital in Indianapolis[8] confirmed that arterial patency could be achieved with balloon angioplasty in acute myocardial infarction. The only randomized trial of direct angioplasty at that time was the study we reported in 1986 comparing direct angioplasty with intracoronary streptokinase in 56 patients with a first myocardial infarction.[6] Reperfusion was achieved in 83% of angioplasty and 85% of thrombolytic patients, but the residual stenosis was significantly less for angioplasty patients (43 vs 83%). Repeat catheterization at 7 to 10 days after the myocardial infarction demonstrated a greater rise in left ventricular ejection fraction in the angioplasty group (8 vs 1%). Thus, by the mid-1980s, direct angioplasty appeared to be a promising method of reperfusion for acute myocardial infarction, supplanting intracoronary thrombolytic administration.

Simultaneous with increasing experience using direct angioplasty for acute myocardial infarction was the growing experience with intravenous thrombolytic agents. Publication of the Grupo Italiano per lo Studio della Streptochinasi Infarto Miocardio (GISSI) trial results demonstrated a survival advantage using this approach.[9] A number of trials results published the following year demonstrated that the routine use of angioplasty after intravenous thrombolytic therapy with tissue plasminogen activator was detrimental compared with a more conservative approach. A swing in enthusiasm away from angioplasty for acute myocardial infarction was voiced by many authorities, although the difference between direct angioplasty and routine sequential thrombolysis with angioplasty was not sufficiently emphasized.[10]

Renewed interest in direct angioplasty developed after publication of the results in 500 patients from the Mid America Heart Institute[11] followed soon thereafter by an analysis from the same institution of contemporary results with the procedure.[12] An accompanying editorial by Bernhard Meier[13] titled "Balloon angioplasty for acute myocardial infarction. Was it buried alive?" suggested that direct angioplasty was preferable to intravenous thrombolysis for large infarctions when a catheterization laboratory was readily available. The controversy that followed led to the organization and initiation of several randomized trials of direct angioplasty versus intravenous thrombolysis (discussed in detail below) that have led to an acceptance of direct angioplasty as the most effective method of infarct artery reperfusion.

RATIONALE AND MECHANISM OF ACTION

The rationale for direct infarct angioplasty is to apply "catheter lysis" locally within the coronary arterial tree with the aim of disrupting the thrombotic and atherosclerotic components of a complex plaque mechanically to achieve rapid, sustained, and nearly complete patency and flow in the infarct vessel. Compared with intravenous thrombolysis, several potential advantages were recognized even in the early

experience with direct angioplasty.[2,6] These included contraindications to emergency catheterization and angioplasty in only a small minority of patients without vascular access or with an untreated life-threatening contrast allergy (less than 1% of patients), rapid confirmation of the diagnosis of arterial thrombosis, rapid assessment of other prognostically significant coronary stenoses such as left main trunk disease, recanalization rates of over 90%, residual lumens of typically less than 40% diameter stenosis, low rates of complicating strokes and cardiac rupture, low rates of recurrent ischemic events in the hospital, and the potential for early discharge in low-risk patients.

The morphologic consequences of direct angioplasty have been examined in a limited number of patients dying of their infarct and may not be representative of the larger population of survivors. Residual coronary stenosis, intimal hemorrhage and plaque disruption, and distal embolization of plaque elements have been seen.[14,15]

PATIENT POPULATION

Patients selected for direct infarct angioplasty and those entered into randomized trials generally demonstrate the following symptoms: ischemic chest pain of greater than 30 minutes, present within 12 hours of the onset of pain, although if pain is ongoing patients are considered up to 24 hours after the onset of symptoms; 1 mm or greater ST segment elevation in contiguous electrocardiographic (ECG) leads or 2 mm or greater ST segment depression in contiguous leads; left bundle branch block or nonspecific ST changes if the clinical history is compatible with acute myocardial infarction and a circumflex territory myocardial infarction is being considered; palpable femoral pulses; and no history of life-threatening contrast reactions.[16–18] Patients with prior bypass surgery, those on chronic warfarin anticoagulation, those with exclusions for thrombolytic therapy such as recent stroke, and those with cardiogenic shock are not excluded. Patients over age 75 who are in cardiogenic shock rarely survive, however, and are not considered candidates for aggressive therapy.

Patients with somewhat confusing and atypical symptoms and abnormal ECG findings that might indicate myocardial infarction also might indicate pericarditis, aortic dissection, prolonged angina without infarction, or noncardiac causes of chest pain can be considered for emergency catheterization without full systemic heparinization; angioplasty can be applied only in those patients in whom an infarction is confirmed by ventriculography and arteriography.

PRETREATMENT

Patients with suspected myocardial infarction in the emergency center or coronary care unit are administered chewable aspirin (325 mg), intravenous heparin in a 10,000-U bolus, and intravenous nitroglycerin and morphine sulfate to initiate pain control. We no longer routinely administer intravenous lidocaine or intravenous magnesium to patients. After informed consent is obtained, sedation with benzodiazepines is given since it is our impression that the emergency procedure can be quite stressful for the patient. In the past a major question existed as to whether pretreatment with intravenous thrombolytic agents is beneficial before infarct angioplasty. We performed a trial randomizing patients to emergency room administration of intravenous streptokinase or placebo before infarct angioplasty and found an overall detrimental effect using pretreatment with agent; we prefer to perform direct infarct angioplasty without thrombolytic agents whenever possible.[19]

PROCEDURAL TECHNIQUE

Patients are mobilized to the catheterization laboratory as quickly as possible and optimally within 30 minutes of arrival in the emergency center. Both groins are prepared while ECG is initiated. Continuous ST segment monitors are applied when available. We routinely place 8-F arterial and 6-F venous sheaths unless a pulmonary artery flotation catheter is indicated, in which case an 8-F venous sheath is inserted. A single wall puncture is attempted. Occasionally a Doppler needle is used for access when pulses are poor or the blood pressure is low. An additional 10,000 U of intravenous heparin is generally given after access is completed. The patient's hemodynamic status may need to be optimized with fluids or pressor agents before initiating angiography. In patients with cardiogenic shock an intra-aortic balloon pump will be inserted from the opposite femoral access site. Oxygenation should be assessed and intubation will occasionally be necessary.

We recommend contrast ventriculography in nearly all patients at the initiation of the procedure. The exception would be patients in pulmonary edema or cardiogenic shock. It is possible to perform a ventriculogram in over 90% of patients and the information achieved is indispensible in regard to the site and severity of wall motion abnormalities and global left ventricular function, mitral regurgitation, true and pseudoaneurysms of the ventricle, and (rarely) documentation of frank cardiac rupture.

Adequate views of all coronary arteries and bypass grafts, if present, are obtained. The infarct vessel must be identified. Usually this poses no problems, but on occasion (particularly in post-bypass patients), it may be impossible to determine the infarct vessel, and gentle probing of the most likely candidate with a coronary guidewire is required.

Certain patients may not require immediate angioplasty after angiography. Patients with minimal disease may be found after complete reperfusion with heparin or because of erroneous diagnosis. Patients with arterial reperfusion who have an underlying coronary stenosis of less than 70% and brisk coronary flow are treated medically. It is uncertain whether patients rendered free of chest pain who have infarct arteries with 70 to 99% residual stenoses and brisk coronary flow should be dilated immediately or, alternatively, transferred to the coronary care unit on intravenous heparin for a procedure at a later date. We have generally performed angioplasty at the time of presentation for fear of arterial reclosure if the patient is left untreated. Patients with critical left main narrowing or critical proximal three-vessel coronary disease and good target vessels are considered for emergency coronary bypass grafting rather than immediate angioplasty. In the Primary Angioplasty for Myocardial Infarction (PAMI) trial, 9 of 195 patients (5%) were referred for emergency bypass surgery.[16] Multivessel disease itself, however, is not a contraindication to immediate angioplasty, although in-hospital mortality is higher compared with a group of patients with single-vessel coronary disease, and the residual narrowings may have to be addressed with subsequent angioplasty or bypass surgery prior to discharge.[20] Angioplasty therapy is most likely to be beneficial in patients with high clinical risk (shock, elderly, anterior or second myocardial infarction) who have low-risk angiographic findings (one- or two-vessel disease, ejection fractions greater than 25%).[21]

When angioplasty is pursued, an additional bolus of 10,000 U is administered and and activated clotting time (ACT) is determined and kept in excess of 350 seconds. We generally select a 0.014″ floppy guidewire with a compatible balloon catheter sized to match the proximal portion of the occluded or stenosed vessel. We do not usually select perfusion balloons as the trade-off in profile hampers ease of crossing, and we have not found a few extra minutes of

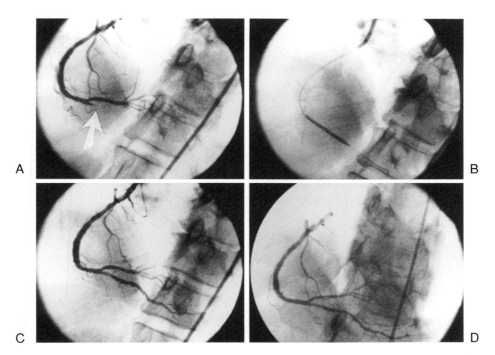

Fig. 34-1. Left anterior oblique projections of the right coronary artery in a 67-year-old man with an acute inferior myocardial infarction. **(A)** The posterior descending artery branch is totally occluded. **(B)** A 30-mm-long 2.5-mm balloon is inflated. **(C)** Patency is restored to the artery. **(D)** Recatheterization at 6 months demonstrates sustained patency.

vessel occlusion to be problematic. We often select longer balloon catheters (30 to 40 mm) for infarct angioplasty and have found that we rarely observe the squirting "watermelon seed" motion sometimes found with shorter balloon catheters (Fig. 34-1). The floppy guidewire will usually traverse the recently occluded artery to a distal position. Rarely, the catheter must be brought up to the stenosis to provide additional guidewire support to cross, or stiffer wires will be needed. Once across the occlusion, contrast and often nitroglycerin injections are performed to assess distal guidewire position, with adjustments to the main lumen performed if needed. We have found that low pressure inflations of 2 to 4 atm will result in complete balloon expansion in most cases. We generally dilate two to three times for up to 2-minute inflations.

Intense spasm is occasionally seen in the distal vessel. With time this will usually resolve spontaneously ("naturolysis"), but intracoronary nitroglycerin or verapamil may be needed on occasion. Dissection can occur from the guidewire passage or balloon trauma. We handle these like elective cases with prolonged, low-pressure inflations, occasionally using a perfusion balloon and a catheter with at least a 1:1 balloon/artery ratio. Residual and persistent thrombus is an occasional problem. Most clots will respond

to repeated and prolonged balloon inflations. We are using fewer intracoronary thrombolytics than in previous years but sometimes they seem to assist the procedure. In extreme cases we have aspirated thrombi directly from the artery through multipurpose guiding catheters to achieve sustained antegrade flow.[22] We have also had experience with the transluminal extraction catheter (Interventional Technologies, Inc.), which is discussed in Chapter 70. In our center and at Northwestern University we treated 70 patients in this manner with promising results, although larger studies will be needed.[23]

Slow or absent antegrade coronary flow with a patent vessel at the end of the procedure has been observed occasionally since the earliest days of infarct angioplasty.[2] This may involve showers of atherothrombotic debris to the microcirculation or more likely represents intense vasoconstriction in the precapillary bed from platelet active mediators. Intracoronary nitroglycerin may be tried and will often relieve this finding. Alternatively, intracoronary verapamil can be administered, although a temporary transvenous pacemaker should be in place in the event of transient heart block. Finally, we have observed cases in which an intra-aortic balloon pump seems to facilitate recovery of brisk antegrade flow (Fig. 34-2).

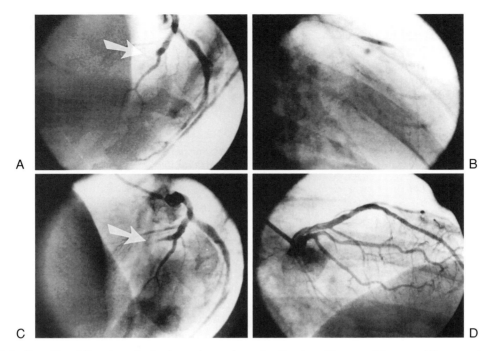

Fig. 34-2. Results of direct angioplasty and counterpulsation in a 51-year-old man with an acute anterior myocardial infarction. **(A)** Left anterior oblique projection demonstrating an occluded anterior descending artery after a diagonal branch (*arrow*). **(B)** Right anterior oblique projection with guidewire postioned in artery and full balloon inflation. **(C)** Left anterior oblique projection showing no-reflow of contrast material to the distal artery despite multiple balloon inflations (*arrow*). **(D)** Repeat angiography on day 7. The patient had been treated with intra-aortic counterpulsation for 48 hours after the direct angioplasty. Wide patency and brisk flow were present.

POSTOPERATIVE MANAGEMENT

Once adequate arterial results are achieved, the patient's overall status is assessed. A pulmonary artery catheter or transvenous pacemaker may be placed if indicated. In larger infarcts, in cases complicated by residual thrombus or slow coronary flow, or in patients with poor left ventricular function or multivessel disease, an intra-aortic balloon pump is placed through the original arterial access site. We are investigating the value of routine balloon pumping in higher risk infarctions treated with direct angioplasty in the ongoing PAMI 2 trial. The preliminary results of a multicenter trial of routine intra-aortic balloon augmentation following direct angioplasty reported a reduction in vessel reocclusion from 18 to 4% and vessel restenosis from 27 to 18% when a balloon pump was inserted for 48 hours.[24]

Most patients are transported to the coronary care unit, although we are investigating the safety of monitoring low-risk patients with good procedural results in a step-down telemetry unit. Intravenous nitroglycerin and heparin are generally continued for 24 hours. In higher risk cases, we may choose 36 to 48 hours of continuous anticoagulation before

interruption. At that point, the patient is either weaned off heparin completely or heparin is reduced to one-fourth to one-half of its infusion rate and sheaths are removed when the ACT is less than 150 seconds. In moderate- or high-risk cases, full-dose anticoagulation will be resumed 2 to 4 hours later.

Patients are ambulated as soon as feasible and maintained on aspirin and β-blockers along with oral nitrates. We discharge most patients by the sixth hospital day, but the PAMI 2 trial is investigating the safety of discharge on the fourth hospital day in low-risk patients.

SHORT- AND LONG-TERM RESULTS

Completion of the PAMI and Zwolle randomized trials of thrombolytic agents versus direct infarct angioplasty provides a contemporary international multicenter experience of the clinical results with these techniques.[6,17] There were some differences in study design. The PAMI study used tissue plasminogen activator and enrolled patients up to 12 hours from the onset of symptoms, whereas the Zwolle trial

Table 34-1. Baseline Clinical Characteristics in the PAMI and Zwolle Trials of Direct Angioplasty Versus Thrombolytics for Acute Myocardial Infarction

	PAMI	Zwolle	P Value
No. of patients	395	142	
Mean age (yr)	60	60	0.92
Male (%)	73	85	0.003
Time of onset to admit (min)	234	211	0.13
Angioplasty	49	49	0.99
Heart rate (bpm)	76	73	0.04
Anterior infarction (%)	35	39	0.42
Killip class (%)			
I	86	80	0.07
II	12	14	0.51
III	2	6	0.03
IV	0	0	1.0
Multivessel disease (%)	54	62	0.11

Table 34-3. Pooled Comparison of the In-Hospital Outcome in the PAMI and Zwolle Trials of Direct Angioplasty Versus Thrombolytics for Acute Myocardial Infarction

	PTCA	Thrombo-lytics	P Value
No. of patients	265	272	
Survival (%)	98	93	0.004
No stroke (%)	99.7	97	0.006
No reinfarction (%)	96	87	0.001

Abbreviation: PTCA, percutaneous transluminal coronary angioplasty.

administered streptokinase up to 6 hours from the onset of pain. The Zwolle trial also excluded patients over age 75 years. Because of similarities in baseline clinical characteristics in the two study populations, however (Table 34-1), the results of these two trials have been pooled to analyze larger numbers of patient events. The overall results of the two trials are compared in Table 34-2. When the pooled data were used to compare angioplasty with thrombolytic therapy in 696 patients, a very low rate of hospital death, reinfarction, and stroke was seen in the angioplasty patients compared with those who received thrombolytics (Table 34-3). Also striking was the achievement of early patency with Thrombolysis in Myocar-

dial Infarction Trial TIMI grade 3 flow in 96% of patients treated with direct angioplasty compared with 54% of patients in the angiographic substudy of the GUSTO trial treated with front-loaded tissue plasminogen activator and heparin.[25]

The pooled analysis of the degree of risk reduction with angioplasty for major adverse events is impressive (Table 34-4), particularly when compared with the results of other accepted interventions for myocardial infarction such as intravenous β-blockers or aspirin (typically a 25% risk reduction). Subgroup analysis indicated that patients most likely to benefit from angioplasty included those with anterior myocardial infarction, a heart rate over 100 bpm at presentation, age more than 70 years, and an increased risk of stroke.

The participants in the Zwolle trial were restudied with coronary angiography at a mean of 82 days after infarction. The infarct-related artery was patent in 68% of patients treated with streptokinase and 91% of those assigned to angioplasty. Restenosis, defined as more than 50% narrowing, was present in 17% of the patients restudied in the angioplasty group.[17]

Table 34-2. Overall In-Hospital Outcome Comparisons in the PAMI and Zwolle Trials of Direct Angioplasty Versus Thrombolytics for Acute Myocardial Infarction

	PAMI	Zwolle	P Value
No. of patients	395	142	
Stroke (%)	2	1	0.77
Death (%)	5	3	0.37
Reinfarction (%)	5	6	0.41
Death/ reinfarction (%)	9	8	0.75

Table 34-4. Pooled Analysis of the Risk Reduction for Events in the PAMI and Zwolle Trials of Direct Angioplasty Versus Thrombolytics for Acute Myocardial Infarction (%)

	Risk PTCA	Risk Thrombo-lytics	Risk Reduction
Death	2.3	6.9	67
Stroke	0.3	2.9	90
Death or reinfarction	4.3	13.5	68

Participants in the PAMI trial were assessed clinically at 6 months after their myocardial infarction. Death had occurred in 3.7% of patients in the angioplasty group compared with 7.9% in the thrombolytic group, and either death or nonfatal reinfarction had developed in 8.5 and 16.8% of these groups, respectively.[16]

The Zwolle trial was extended to recruit additional patients and was enlarged from 142 to 301 patients.[26] Comparing streptokinase with direct angioplasty, in-hospital mortality was observed in 7 versus 2% of patients, recurrent in-hospital infarction was reduced from 10 to 1%, and predischarge left ventricular ejection fraction measured by radionuclide techniques was 44 versus 50%, respectively.

CURRENT INDICATIONS

The major limitation of angioplasty therapy for myocardial infarction is a logistic one. If no angioplasty facilities and operators exist in an institution, this therapy will not be immediately available to patients. At William Beaumont Hospital, angioplasty therapy for acute myocardial infarction is used to treat all patients at all times of day and night with the rare exception of an anticipated excessive (longer than 1-hour) delay in the availability of an open cardiac catheterization laboratory. This has been facilitated by a dedicated Chest Pain Emergency Center that has shortened the time to identification and recruitment of myocardial infarction patients to the interventional laboratory. We feel that it is mandatory for patients with an acute anterior myocardial infarction to proceed to the interventional catheterization laboratory for angiography and angioplasty, if available, because of the *dramatic reduction in the risk of death and reinfarction compared with lytic therapy* (1.4% vs. 15%) observed in the pooled PAMI and Zwolle study groups (Fig. 34-3).

Hospitals without cardiac catheterization laboratories will continue to rely on intravenous thrombolytic agents in eligible patients. In patients with absolute contraindications to thrombolytic therapy, excellent results with angioplasty have been observed, and patients with larger infarctions or with hemodynamic compromise should be considered for transfer to an angioplasty center.[27]

In United States, angioplasty at hospitals with cardiac catheterization facilities but without cardiac surgical teams has been proscribed. The selective use of angioplasty for acute myocardial infarction in these hospitals is currently being re-examined. In the Myocardial Infarction, Triage, and Intervention Registry, 441 patients were treated with direct angioplasty, half at hospitals with no on-site surgery.[28] Patency was established in 88% of patients regardless of the type of hospital, and overall survival was 93%. Of patients treated with direct angioplasty, six (1.4%) underwent cardiac surgery within 6 hours of catheterization. Only one patient was from a hospital without on-site surgery. Survival at 1 year did not differ for patients treated with angioplasty at surgical or nonsurgical centers. These results suggest that in hospitals without on-site surgery, direct angioplasty may be an option if experienced interventional cardiologists are available and a liaison with a nearby surgical facility is established. This might be particularly beneficial to patients with contraindications to thrombolytic therapy and with hemodynamic compromise or large infarctions.

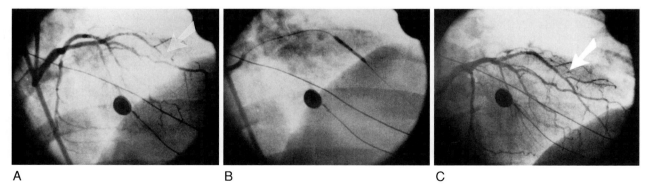

A   B   C

Fig. 34-3. Right anterior oblique projections with cranial angulation during a direct infarct angioplasty in a 28-year-old diabetic woman with an acute anterior myocardial infarction. **(A)** The mid-left anterior descending, artery is totally occluded (*arrow*). **(B)** Full balloon inflation is shown. **(C)** Wide patency with brisk flow was achieved (*arrow*). The patient had excellent salvage of ventricular function and has had no cardiac events in over 2 years of follow-up.

FUTURE DIRECTIONS

Ongoing and future research will focus on adjunctive therapies that may further improve the outcome with acute intervention in myocardial infarction. Adjunctive pharmacologic therapies such as antiplatelet regimens, hirudin, and fluorochemical emulsions are being studied. The role of routine adjunctive hemodynamic support with intra-aortic balloon pumping is being examined in the PAMI 2 trial and at Duke University. Strategies for managing no-reflow in the setting of acute intervention for myocardial infarction must be realized. Methods of reducing vascular complications and transfusion rates, perhaps with vascular sealing devices, will require investigation. Protocols for reducing hospital stay and costs in appropriate selected low-risk patients have been developed. Currently, the results of the randomized trials of direct angioplasty indicate to us that when appropriately applied, the diagnostic and prognostic information acute intervention provides, the ability to achieve high rates of sustained recanalization, and the feasibility of providing immediate hemodynamic support or emergency cardiac surgery if needed make direct angioplasty the optimal method of managing an acute myocardial infarction.

REFERENCES

1. Kahn JK, Rutherford BD, Hartzler GO. Direct angioplasty for acute MI. Cardio 1990;102–36
2. Hartzler GO, Rutherford BD, McConahay DR et al. Percutaneous tranluminal coronary angioplasty with and without thrombolytic therapy for treatment of acute myocardial infarction. Am Heart J 1983;106: 965–73
3. Hartzler GO, Rutherford BD, McConahay DR. Percutaneous transluminal coronary angioplasty: application for acute myocardial infarction. Am J Cardiol 1984;53:117C–21C
4. Pepine CJ, Prida X, Hill JA. Percutaneous transluminal coronary angioplasty in acute myocardial infarction. Am Heart J 1984;107:820–2
5. Holmes DR, Smith HC, Vlietstra RE et al. Percutaneous transluminal coronary angioplasty, alone or in combination with streptokinase therapy, during acute myocardial infarction. Mayo Clin Proc 1985;60:449–56
6. O'Neill WW, Timmis GC, Bourdillion PD et al. A prospective randomized clinical trial of intracoronary streptokinase versus coronary angioplasty for acute myocardial infarction. N Eng J Med 1986, 314:812–8
7. Marco J, Caster L, Szatamary LJ, Fajadet J. Emergency percutaneous transluminal coronary angioplasty without thrombolysis as initial therapy in acute myocardial infarction. Int J Cardiol 1987;15:55–63
8. Rothbaum DA, Linnemeier TJ, Landin RJ et al. Emergency percutaneous transluminal coronary angioplasty in acute myocardial infarction: a 3 year experience. J Am Coll Cardiol 1987;10:264–72
9. GISSI Investigators. Effectiveness of intravenous thrombolytic treatment in acute myocardial infarction. Lancet 1986:1:397–401
10. Salem DN, Desnoyers MR, Berman AD, Konstam MA. Coronary angioplasty and thrombolysis for acute myocardial infarction: is two a crowd? Am J Med 1989;86: 259–61
11. O'Keefe JH, Rutherford BD, McConahay DR et al. Early and late results of coronary angioplasty without antecedent thrombolytic therapy for acute myocardial infarction. Am J Cardiol 1989;64:122–30
12. Kahn JK, Rutherford BD, McConahay DR et al. Catheterization laboratory events and hospital outcome with direct angioplasty for acute myocardial infarction. Circulation 1990;82:1910–5
13. Meier B. Balloon angioplastly for acute myocardial infarction. Was it buried alive? Circulation 1990;82: 2243–5
14. Colavita PG, Ikeder RE, Reimer KA et al. The spectrum of pathology associated with percutaneous transluminal coronary angioplasty during acute myocardial infarction. J Am Coll Cardiol 1986 8:855–60
15. Waller BF, Rothbaum DA, Pinkerton CA et al. Status of the myocardium and infarct related coronary artery in 19 necropsy patients with acute recanalization using pharmacologic, mechanical or combined types of reperfusion therapy. J Am Coll Cardiol 1987, 9: 785–801
16. Grines CL, Browne KF, Marco J et al. A comparison of immediate angioplasty with thrombolytic therapy for acute myocardial infarction. N Engl J Med 1993; 328:673–9
17. Zijlstra F, Jan de Boerr M, Hoorntje JCA et al. A comparison of immediate coronary angioplasty with intravenous streptokinase in acute myocardial infarction. N Engl J Med 1993;328:680–4
18. Gibbons RJ, Holmes DR, Reeder GS et al. Immediate angioplasty compared with the administration of a thrombolytic agent followed by conservative treatment for myocardial infarction. N Engl Med 1993;328: 685–91
19. O'Neill WW, Weintraub R, Grines CL et al. A prospective, placebo controlled, randomized trial of intravenous streptokinase and angioplasty versus lone angioplasty therapy of acute myocardial infarction. Circulation 1992;86:1710–7
20. Kahn JK, Rutherford BD, McConahay DR et al. Results of primary angioplasty for acute myocardial infarction in patients with multivessel coronary disease. J Am Coll Cardiol 1990;16:1089–96
21. O'Neill WW. Angioplasty therapy for acute myocardial infarction: current status and future directions. pp. 359–66. In Vogel JKH, King SB (eds): The Practice of Interventional Cardiology. Mosby YearBook St. Luisa 1993
22. Kahn JK, Hartzler GO. Percutaneous thrombus aspiration in acute myocardial infarction. Cathet Cardiovasc Diagn 1990;20:54–7
23. Larkin TJ, Grines CL, Safian RD. A prospective pilot study of transluminal extraction atherectomy in acute myocardial infarction. (in preparation)
24. Ohman EM, George BS, White CJ et al. Reocclusion of the infarct related artery after primary or rescue angioplasty: effect of aortic counterpulsation, abstracted. Circulation 1993;88:I-106
25. GUSTO Angiographic Investigators. The effects of tissue plasminogen activator, streptokinase, or both on

coronary-artery patency, ventricular function, and survival after acute myocardial infarction. N Engl J Med 1993;329:1615–22

26. Jan de Boer M, Hoorntje JCA, Ottervanger JP et al. Immediate coronary angioplasty versus intravenous streptokinase in acute myocardial infarction: left ventricular ejection fraction, hospital mortaliy and reinfarction. J Am Coll Card 1994;23:1004–8

27. Himbert D, Juliard JM, Steg PG et al. Primary coronary angioplasty for acute myocardial infarction with contraindication to thrombolysis. Am J Cardiol 1993; 71:377–81

28. Weaver WD, Litwin PE, Martin JS. Use of direct angioplasty for treatment of patients with acute myocardial infarction in hospitals with and without on-site cardiac surgery. Circulation 1993;88:2067–75

35 Elective Coronary Intervention

Anthony C. De Franco
Eric J. Topol

Four general strategies are used in percutaneous transluminal coronary angioplasty (PTCA) following myocardial infarction: direct, rescue, empiric, and elective. These are distinguished according to their timing and principal purpose (Table 35-1). *Direct angioplasty,* which is discussed in Chapter 34, refers to immediate percutaneous mechanical revascularization of the infarct artery as soon as possible after the patient's initial presentation as an alternative to thrombolytic therapy or conservative management. *Rescue angioplasty,* discussed in Chapter 36, refers to intervention when intravenous thrombolytic therapy has failed to reperfuse the culprit vessel and is performed as soon as possible after the clinical diagnosis is suspected. *Empiric angioplasty* is defined as the routine use of the procedure as prophylaxis against recurrent ischemia, *in the absence of actual ischemia documented by clinical criteria or functional testing.* Empirical angioplasty can be either *immediate* (performed as soon as possible, usually within 18 hours, after the acute infarction or successful thrombolysis) or *deferred* (performed from 18 hours to 1 week after the event, without provocative testing). Although each of the randomized trials that have studied empiric angioplasty soon after thrombolytic therapy has limitations, overall their results have been remarkably consistent: in the absence of hemodynamic compromise or ischemia, empiric angioplasty does not improve global left ventricular function nor does it reduce morbidity or mortality when compared with the *selective* use of PTCA for hemodynamic complications or spontaneous or provokable ischemia.

In this chapter we evaluate elective coronary angioplasty following thrombolytic therapy for acute myocardial infarction. We review the data from prospective, randomized trials that have led to the current recommendations for angioplasty after the acute phase of infarction. Although new developments in the therapy of acute coronary syndromes will almost certainly modify the applicability of these data (some of the trials were concluded over 6 years ago), the data they provide can nevertheless guide the physician to the appropriate use of post-thrombolytic coronary interventions.

IMMEDIATE ANGIOPLASTY

Historical Perspective and Rationale

In the early 1980s, two small, nonrandomized studies first reported the use of revascularization after thrombolytic therapy. In 1982 Meyer et al.[1] described the utility of PTCA in dilating residual stenoses in 21 patients after successful intracoronary streptokinase for acute myocardial infarction, later referred to as "strep and stretch." In the 17 patients in whom the procedure was successful, no in-hospital reocclusions were seen, and only patients had evidence of recurrent ischemia during the follow-up period. In the 18 patients treated medically, 4 developed recurrent ischemia in-hospital and 3 died during follow-up. Mathey et al.[2] reported similarly favorable results in a group of patients treated with

Table 35-1. Coronary Angioplasty Strategies for Acute Myocardial Infarction

Strategy	Thrombolytic Therapy	Goal	Timing
Direct (primary)	No	Recanalization	As soon as possible
Rescue	Yes	Recanalization when thrombolysis fails	As soon as possible
Empirical	Varies	Prophylactic for recurrent ischemia	Immediate Deferred: either Early (18–48 hours) Late (48 hours or more)
Elective	Varies	Treatment of angina or documented ischemia	Often after 7 days or more

surgical revascularization after thrombolytic therapy. These initial favorable reports supported the notion that coronary revascularization soon after thrombolytic therapy might lead to an overall reduction in adverse clinical events.

The rationale for the strategy of balloon dilation as soon as possible after thrombolytic therapy for acute myocardial infarction was that the occlusive lesion in the infarct vessel was known to consist of both underlying atherosclerotic plaque and overlying thrombus. Compared with treating only the thrombus, compressing the plaque with an angioplasty balloon would presumably lead to less recurrent ischemia, improved myocardial perfusion, and an improvement in the patient's functional status. The designs of these trials are summarized in Table 35-2; and the incidence of death in three of these is illustrated in Figure 35-4.

Immediate Angioplasty (Within 18 Hours) After Thrombolytic Therapy

In the Thrombolysis and Angioplasty in Myocardial Infarction-1 (TAMI-1) trial, 386 patients who presented within 4 hours of symptom onset were treated with intravenous tissue plasminogen activator (t-PA) and underwent emergency angiography at 90 minutes.[3] This study is important because randomization took place at the time that the coronary anatomy was known. Of the total, 93 patients (25%) had contraindications to angioplasty, such as left main trunk obstruction or extensive multivessel disease. In 96 additional patients (25%) the infarct vessel was totally occluded. Of the remaining patients, 99 were assigned to immediate PTCA (at 90 minutes) and 98 to a strategy of delayed PTCA (7 to 10 days after thrombolytic therapy). There were no differences in

Table 35-2. Summary of Randomized Trials of Intravenous Thrombolysis Followed by Empiric Angioplasty Performed Immediately (Most often at 90 minutes) After Thrombolytic Therapy

Study	Randomized No. of Patients PTCA	Control	Thrombolytic Strategy (if applicable)	Timing of PTCA	Control Group	Major Finding
For open or for all infarct vessels						
TAMI-1[3]	99	98	t-PA	Immediately	Lysis + delayed PTCA	No advantage of immediate PTCA
ECSG[71]	183	184	t-PA	Immediately	No PTCA	No advantage of immediate PTCA
TIMI-IIA[4]	195	194	t-PA	Immediately	No PTCA	No advantage of immediate PTCA
O'Neill et al.[7]	63	58	SK	Immediately	Lysis + PTCA	Direct PTCA superior, less complicated, less expensive
For closed vessels						
TAMI-5[72]	287	288	t-PA, UK or t-PA + UK	Immediately	Lysis + delayed cath. (5–7 days)	Aggressive strategy had less recurrent ischemia, improved regional vessel motion and patency

Abbreviations: SK, streptokinase; t-PA, tissue plasminogen activator; UK, urokinase; PTCA, percutaneous transluminal coronary angioplasty. (Modified from Topol,[70] with permission.)

the primary study end point, predischarge left ventricular function, or mortality (4 vs. 1%) between the immediate and deferred PTCA groups. The incidence of in-hospital reocclusion was also similar between the two groups.

In the Thrombolysis in Myocardial Infarction-IIA (TIMI-IIA) trial, 389 patients who received intravenous t-PA were randomized prior to 90-minute angiography to receive one of three treatment strategies; either immediate (within 2 hours) or delayed (18 to 48 hours) balloon angioplasty of the infarct artery or a conservative strategy of predischarge angiography and angioplasty only in those with exercise-induced ischemia and suitable coronary anatomy.[4] All patients underwent emergency angiography at 90 minutes. The primary end point was left ventricular function assessed by radionuclide ventriculography; no significant differences were found between the two groups at hospital discharge or at 6 weeks. was also similar between the two groups. Most importantly, patients randomized to undergo immediate angioplasty had a higher incidence of transfusion, of coronary bypass surgery, and of the combined end point of major adverse events [death, recurrent myocardial infarction, emergency coronary artery bypass graft (CABG), and transfusion].

In the European Cooperative Study Group (ECSG) trial, 367 patients who received t-PA were randomized either to immediate angioplasty or to conservative management, in which only patients with spontaneous or provokable ischemia underwent PTCA 10 to 20 days after initial presentation.[5] Immediate angioplasty did not reduce myocardial infarct size, nor did it reduce the incidence of reinfarction. However, patients randomized to immediate PTCA had a significantly higher incidence of recurrent ischemia (17 vs. 3%) bleeding complications (41 vs. 23%), and blood transfusions (10 vs. 4%). The study was terminated prematurely because patients who had immediate angioplasty had a higher mortality at 2 weeks (7 vs. 3%, respectively). This difference in mortality persisted at 1 year (9.3 vs. 5.4%, respectively).[6]

The studies discussed thus far examined the role of adjunctive angioplasty in a population of patients treated with thrombolytic therapy. O'Neill et al.[7] examined the role of adjunctive thrombolytic therapy in patients treated with immediate angioplasty. In a group of 122 patients who presented within 4 hours of symptom onset treated with intravenous heparin and oral aspirin, one-half were randomized to streptokinase (1.5 million U) administered intravenously over 30 minutes and one-half were randomized to placebo. All patients went to angiography immediately; 106 had coronary anatomy suitable for angioplasty and underwent the procedure; 58 patients actually received both streptokinase and PTCA. Angioplasty was successful in 95% of patients, The combination of intravenous streptokinase and immediate PTCA did not improve outcome compared with PTCA alone. There were no differences in 24-hour or 6-week radionuclide ejection fraction values, and at 6 months there were no differences in infarct artery patency (87% overall) or restenosis (38% overall). However, for patients randomized to the combination of thrombolytic therapy and immediate angioplasty, the need for emergency CABG was greater (10.3 vs. 1.6%), the transfusion rate was higher (39 vs. 8%), and the hospital course was longer and more expensive.

Current Indications for Immediate Angioplasty

In aggregate, these trials conclusively demonstrate that the combination of thrombolytic therapy and immediate angioplasty for acute myocardial infarction does not enhance early or late ventricular function, does not improve arterial patency rates, and does not lower long-term reocclusion or restenosis rates. Instead, these data indicate that this strategy often leads to a higher incidence of adverse events, including recurrent ischemia and infarction, bleeding and transfusion, emergency bypass, or death. Thus, in patients with a significant but subtotal stenosis (minimum luminal diameter 50 to 90% of normal) but *without evidence of ischemia,* immediate angioplasty after thrombolysis is unnecessary and often dangerous. Furthermore, these patients are at low risk *without* intervention, particularly if they have single-vessel disease, as we discuss later.

Histopathology studies and intravascular ultrasound have suggested a potential mechanism by which these adverse events may occur[8,9] (Fig. 35-1). These target lesions have recently ruptured and caused a thrombotic occlusion; they often have a higher lipid content or a less thick fibrous cap than more fibrotic (and thus more stable) plaques. It is the lipid content that is thought to be the most thrombogenic constituent.[10] Angioplasty causes additional mechanical disruption and may expose even more of the thrombogenic "lipid core," further stimulating platelet aggregation and the release of clot-bound thrombin, both of which propagate the thrombus. The end result is an increased risk of abrupt closure. Angioplasty soon after thrombolytic therapy may also cause hemorrhage into the vessel wall, perhaps more extensively than with either therapy alone. These additional forms of injury may tip the balance of hemostasis toward rethrombosis.

thrombus, or of the constituents of the underlying plaque, may significantly affect the way the lesion responds to intervention or the likelihood of postprocedure reocclusion. New methods of tissue characterization—such as angioscopy (which can detect angiographically occult thrombus), high-frequency ultrasound (which may distinguish thrombus from other tissue), and spectroscopy guidewires (which may identify the extent of lipid within the plaque)—may successfully stratify lesion risk far more accurately than we can by angiography alone.

Second, new methods of local drug delivery may allow more complete resolution of thrombus after thrombolytic therapy. For example, new catheters are capable of delivering thrombolytic drugs or pharmacologic adjuncts such as hirudin directly to the thrombus or plaque rupture site. The Dispatch catheter (Fig. 35-5) is an over-the-wire balloon device designed for local drug delivery. A spiral-shaped coil of balloon material creates a chamber between the device and the vessel wall; pharmacologic agents can be infused into the chamber via the catheter. Isolation from the arterial circulation (while the coils are inflated) allows the drug to have prolonged contact with the wall; in addition, the central lumen within the device allows antegrade blood flow to the distal circulation.

New antiplatelet agents may reduce the incidence of abrupt vesssel closure. Compared with newer antiplatelet agents, aspirin is a relatively weak inhibitor of platelet aggregation. Recent data from the evaluation of chimeric 7E$_3$ Fab in the Prevention of Ischemic Complications (EPIC) trial demonstrate that an antibody to the glycoprotein (GP)IIb/IIIa receptor could reduce the ischemic complications of interventional procedures (death, acute myocardial infarction, urgent PTCA, or CABG) in patients with high-risk target lesions; this agent was particularly helpful in decreasing the vessel reclosure rate in the subgroup of patients who required intervention soon after thrombolytic therapy for acute myocardial infarction. Integrilin is an oligopeptide inhibitor of the GPIIb/IIIa receptor that has a rapid onset of action and a short half-life. The Integrelin to Manage Platelet Aggregation to Prevent Coronary Thrombosis (IMPACT) trial is a multicenter, double-blind, randomized trial that will enroll 3,500 patients to test the effect of this agent in routine angioplasty. Although this trial will primarily enroll patients undergoing elective procedures, patients with recent thrombolytic therapy are not specifically excluded. Finally, direct thrombin inhibitors such as hirudin may also decrease the rate of reocclusion in this setting. However, these devices and drugs will need to be proved to improve survival or left ventricular

function in prospective, randomized trials before their use in *empiric* angioplasty can be recommended.

ELECTIVE ANGIOPLASTY

Elective angioplasty following myocardial infarction refers to the performance of the procedure to treat spontaneous postinfarction ischemia or ischemia provoked by functional testing. A complete review of the indications for elective angioplasty versus medical therapy or surgical revascularization is beyond the scope of this chapter.

TRIALS OF ANGIOPLASTY AFTER THROMBOLYTIC THERAPY: IMPLICATIONS FOR RISK STRATIFICATION

Several authors have extrapolated data from the trials of immediate angioplasty to reach conclusions about the utility of angiography after thrombolytic therapy. However, clinical application of these conclusions requires care, because these trials were not designed to test the utility of angiography apart from the intervention. This distinction has important implications for risk stratification after thrombolytic therapy.

Elective Angiography After Acute Myocardial Infarction

For uncomplicated acute myocardial infarction patients (those who do not require angiography as a prelude to direct revascularization or whose condition occurred a result of shock or hemodynamic or mechanical complications) there are two approaches to elective angiography, *routine* and *selective*. In the *routine approach*, coronary angiography is a standard component of the postinfarction risk assessment of all (or nearly all) patients. In the *selective* approach, catheterization is performed only for spontaneous ischemia or for a functional test that suggests ischemia. Which of these approaches is most appropriate following thrombolytic therapy is still controversial. Our usual strategy is to recommend coronary angiography routinely early (on days 1 to 2) in the hospital course; however, the available data can support both approaches after thrombolytic therapy, for which several in-depth reviews are available.[38–40]

Accepted Indications for Angiography

Several high-risk clinical characteristics almost always indicate prompt coronary angiography. Recurrent ischemia or hemodynamic instability or mechanical complications (such as suspected papillary muscle or septal rupture) are several examples. Unfortunately, clinical variables do not predict which patients will ultimately require urgent angiography for these indications. In the TIMI-II trial, symptom-driven angiography was required in 24% of 33% of patients randomized to the "conservative" strategy during the initial hospitalization. Other trials have documented similar cross-over rates. Other clinical events may often lead the clinician to recommend angiography. For example, complex or frequent ventricular dysrhythmias may be an indicator of residual ischemia and may correlate with an increased risk of late cardiac morbidity and mortality.[38,41-44] Patients with an ejection fraction less than 45% and those spared from potentially large infarcts (such as a threatened anterior infarct successfully treated with thrombolytics) are also often recommended for "selective" angiography. Patients who have had a prior myocardial infarction have a higher mortality rate during long-term follow-up. At the end of 1 year, 60% of patients randomized to the conservative arm of TIMI-II for "watchful waiting" ultimately had angiography within the first 12 months of the index infarction.[16] Therefore, even a "selective" strategy often requires angiography in a substantial number of patients after thrombolytic therapy.

Routine Angiography After Thrombolytic Therapy

The rationale for advocating routine angiography is to define location and severity of the responsible lesion, to identify patients with severe coronary artery disease (who may warrant bypass surgery) promptly and accurately, and to expedite early hospital discharge and return to work in selected patients. The most important reason we usually recommend angiography routinely after thrombolytic therapy is that it provides important prognostic information incremental to the clinical history and functional test. On the basis of data from several trials, routine angiography can separate post-thrombolysis patients into five categories (Fig. 35-6) with very different prognoses and treatment requirements.[3,5,12,45-48] For example, two- or three-vessel coronary disease (defined as stenosis of more than 70%) markedly worsens the short-term prognosis after thrombolytic therapy.[49]

In the TAMI trials, 236 of 855 patients (27.6%) had multivessel disease; these patients had an in-hospital mortality of 11.4%, nearly three times higher than patients with single-vessel disease (4.2%).[49] The strongest independent predictors of in-hospital mortality were regional wall motion in the noninfarct zone ($P = 0.0057$) and the number of diseased vessels ($P = 0.04$). The second of these variables, the number of diseased vessels, is most accurately determined by angiography. Lee and colleagues[50] combined data from several of the TAMI trials[3,45,51] and used a regression model to predict mortality based on angiographic findings. This analysis led these investigators to the conclusion that each diseased coronary vessel increases mortality to the same extent as a 16-year increase in age or a 13-point reduction in ejection fraction. In summary, angiography accurately stratifies post-infarction risk; when this information is combined with clinical data and data from functional testing, it can identify those patients for whom revascularization should be recommended. These data are particularly important given the uncertainties about the validity of functional testing after thrombolysis, discussed below.

Angiographic data from post-thrombolysis angioplasty trials *underestimate* the severity of underlying coronary disease in the population of patients with acute myocardial infarction who are eligible for thrombolytic therapy. For example, patients in the TIMI-II trial had a much *lower* incidence of multivessel disease compared with patients in studies done in the prethrombolytic era, probably because TIMI-II (and other early trials of thrombolytic therapy) specifically excluded the types of patients with the highest prevalence of multivessel disease, such as the elderly, those with severe hypertension or previous cerebrovascular events.[52-54] Thus, we cannot readily apply the conclusions regarding the incidence of multivessel disease and the utility of angiography derived from trials such as TIMI-II trial to all patients with AMI.

Selective Angiography After Thrombolytic Therapy

Clinicians who advocate the selective use of angiography after thrombolytic therapy argue that it is practical, because the procedure is expensive and often unavailable without hospital transfer. At least in theory revascularization would be performed only when symptoms or the results of functional testing documented ischemia. Furthermore, advocates of a selective approach argue that in post-thrombolysis patients both strategies lead to the same clinical out-

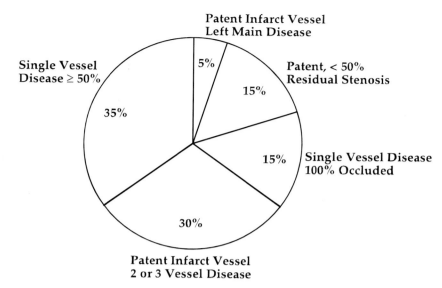

Fig. 35-6. Proportion of patients in each of the five anatomic subsets distinguished after thrombolytic therapy. Current noninvasive methods have limitations and may not accurately identify reliably the 5% of patients with left main stenosis or its equivalent. Approximately 15% of patients have an occluded infarct artery at elective angiography; these patients must be distinguished from those with an occluded vessel and ongoing ischemia. Patients with minimal residual stenosis of the infarction-related vessel account for approximately 15%; these patients have an excellent prognosis. Approximately 35% of patients at angiography have single-vessel disease with a residual stenosis of more than 50%; the optimal treatment of these patients is the subject of this chapter. Routine angiography provides accurate definition of the coronary anatomy and prompt triage of patients to the appropriate form of therapy. (From Topol et al.,[73] with permission; data extrapolated from references.[5,12,45,72,74–76])

come with respect to death, reinfarction, and ventricular function. Rogers et al.,[12,47] in a retrospective analysis, compared the TIMI-IIA strategy of predischarge catheterization without angioplasty to the conservative strategy of selective catheterization from TIMI-II and found that routine angiography did not reduce acute or 1-year adverse outcomes. As we have discussed, patients randomized to a "conservative" strategy in the both the TIMI-II trial[12,47] and the SWIFT trial[14] had outcomes identical to those in the "invasive" strategy (Figs. 35-1 and 35-3). However, these trials were not designed to test routine angiography per se; instead, they tested a strategy of angiography *coupled* with angioplasty. The implications of this important difference are discussed below.

Noninvasive testing is the alternative to identify patients with residual ischemia, left ventricular dysfunction, or exercise-induced dysrhythmias; these patients would then warrant angiography. In our opinion, there are three major problems with noninvasive testing as the *primary* method of risk stratification after thrombolytic therapy (Table 35-5). First, several studies have questioned the validity of functional testing after thrombolytic therapy.[55–59] Data on functional testing from the prethrombolytic era is

not readily applicable to post-thrombolysis patients, because patients who have received thrombolytic therapy are a fundamentally different population, as we have discussed. However, proponents of stress testing would emphasize that there is empiric validation of noninvasive risk stratification, because of the excellent 1-year outcome of conservatively treated, "low-risk" patients such as those in TIMI-II and SWIFT.

Second, functional tests can be difficult to interpret after thrombolytic therapy. For example, noninvasive studies in this setting have had a poor sensitivity and specificity for noninfarct vessel anatomy.[57] In addition, one cannot assume that the *absence* of ischemia after thrombolytic therapy is due to significant myocardial salvage and the absence of a significant residual stenosis, because a high-grade stenosis *without* a perfusion abnormality is often due to *more* extensive myocardial necrosis *despite* thrombolytic therapy.[60] In this study, the higher the patient's creatinine phosphokinase value, the more likely a negative thallium scan.

Third, in several studies, the percentage of patients who simply cannot perform the test has ranged from 20 to 45%;[61–63] this is a strong predictor of a poor prognosis, with a 10 to 15% mortality rate

Table 35-5. Studies of Functional Testing After Intravenous Thrombolysis

Study	No. of Patients	Study Design	Test	Major Finding
Simoons et al.[55]	533	Streptokinase compared with conventional therapy	Predischarger treadmill exercise	Functional test not predictive of reinfarction or death during 5-year follow-up
Chaitman et al.[56]	1,958	t-PA, t-PA compared with catheterization and angioplasty (if suitable)	Predischarge and 6-week postdischarge supine bicycle ergometry and electrocardiogram	Functional test not predictive of reinfarction or death during 6-month follow-up
Burns et al.[57]	47	t-PA compared with placebo	Exercise SPECT; thallium on day 8	Sensitivity of detecting substantial stenosis in the infarction-related vessel, 95%; specificity, 14%, for stenosis of a noninfarction-related vessel: sensitivity, 35%; specificity, 79%
Touchstone et al.[58]	21	Streptokinase	Exercise thallium on day 10	Only 25% of patients with preserved regional wall motion have provocable ischemia
Weiss et al.[59]	37	Streptokinase	Exercise-gated blood pool scintigraphy at 7 weeks	46% of patients with early therapy and a significant residual stenosis had a negative test, correlated with reduced evidence of salvage

Abbreviations: SPECT, single-photon emission computerized tomography.
(Modified from Topol et al.,[73] with permission; data from references 55–59.)

within 2 years.[38,64–67] Other reservations (modified from De Franco and Topol,[40] with permission) regarding the use of exercise testing as the primary risk stratification method may be summarized as follows:

1. Nearly all reported data are derived from patients who did not have myocardial reperfusion therapy; no study has correlated functional tests and long-term clinical outcome following pharmacologic reperfusion.
2. The testing may not allow diagnosis of viable, noninfarcted tissue.
3. Simple exercise electrocardiographic markers are often difficult to interpret after thrombolysis due to persistent abnormalities.
4. Positive predictive accuracy and sensitivity in detecting multivessel coronary disease are lower than in chronic stable angina.
5. Reported series in both the prethrombolytic era and more recent studies exclude certain subgroups (the elderly, patients unable to exercise, and so forth) that have a high long-term risk of recurrent ischemic events and mortality.
6. Follow-up duration is short in most reported studies; when follow-up is adequate, predictive value falls dramatically.
7. Submaximal testing may not attain sufficient workload to exclude myocardial ischemia reliably.

It is critically important to uncouple the diagnostic angiogram from the interventional procedure. The randomized trials of immediate, empiric angioplasty studied the combination of diagnostic angiography and angioplasty; these trials cannot be used to proscribe the diagnostic portion of the procedure in those cases in which it is clinically indicated. Rather than coupling angiography to angioplasty, as in the early trials, *angiography should be coupled to functional testing*—the former most rapidly identifies patients at the highest and lowest risk; the latter determines the physiologic significance of lesions in patients at intermediate risk (such as those with one- or two-vessel disease). Combined data from both noninvasive tests and angiography are often invaluable for reassuring the patient and for prescribing an exercise program as part of an aggressive risk factor reduction program.[1]

Cost

Many clinicians assume a priori that a routine approach to angiography in most patients would be more expensive than a selective strategy; however, this assumption has been seriously challenged. Early routine angiography can shorten the hospital stay of selected patients[3,68] (such as the 10 to 15% with minimal residual stenoses or those with single-vessel

Table 36-1. Partial List of Potential Mechanisms by Which "Late" Reperfusion may Result in a Mortality Reduction in Patients with Acute Myocardial Infarction

---

I. Reduction in infarct size
II. Mechanical factors
    Improved healing
    Less expansion
        Less aneurysm formation (arrhythmia, thrombus)
        Lower wall stress
        Improved diastolic function
    Prevention of rupture
    Scaffolding
III. Electrophysiologic milieu
    Arrhythmia protection
    Prevention of late after-depolarizations
    Preservation of sympathetic fibers and heart rate variability
IV. Potential to provide collateral flow
V. Patient selection

(Modified from Cardiff et al.[99] with permission.)

months. Patients randomized to late PTCA demonstrated a trend toward a higher rate of infarct artery patency (43 vs. 19%). Patients with a patent infarct artery had a higher ejection fraction than did those with a closed infarct artery (9.4 ± 6.2% vs. 1.6 ± 8.8%, $P = 0.0096$). However, the efficacy of late PTCA was somewhat limited by a high reocclusion rate by 4 months (40%)

In aggregate, these data and data from other trials suggest that it is possible to achieve late reperfusion with either thrombolytic therapy or angioplasty in patients who present relatively late after infarction and that late reperfusion can result in a measurable improvement in ventricular function[41,42] (Table 36-1).

RESULTS OF RESCUE PTCA

Nonrandomized Trials

In the late 1980s and early 1990s, several nonrandomized series defined the angiographic success rates, reocclusion rates, and relative mortality rates of patients treated with rescue angioplasty. These data were the subject of a meta-analysis by Ellis et al.[43] (summarized in Table 36-2) that led these authors to several conclusions. First, rescue PTCA had a high angiographic success rate, ranging from 71 to 100%. Although this range is impressive, it is considerably lower than in trials of direct PTCA, probably because patients who fail thrombolytic therapy are a more difficult subset in whom to perform angioplasty.[43-49] These patients may have anatomic reasons for resistance to therapy, such as very extensive plaque rupture, a large plaque burden, or a heavy clot burden. Second, in these early studies, reocclusion rates after successful rescue PTCA averaged 18%, with a high of 29%.[2] Third, patients who required rescue angioplasty and in whom the procedure was *successful* had a higher mortality (7 to 9%) than patients who initially reperfused with either direct PTCA (1 to 5%)[44-48] or thrombolytic therapy (6 to 7%).[9] The additional time (and myocardial necrosis) that elapses prior to recanalization with rescue angioplasty is probably a major factor in this higher mortality rate. Finally, there was little *overall* improvement in systolic function by the time of hospital discharge.

That all but one the studies in this meta-analysis were nonrandomized limits the implications for clinical practice. Although these studies demonstrate that patients who fail thrombolytic therapy can achieve a high infarct vessel patency rate with rescue angioplasty, they do not prove that this improved patency rate results in improved survival. In several of these series, patients in whom rescue PTCA failed to achieve patency had much higher mortality rates (35 to 40%)[13] than those in whom the procedure was successful.[50-53] If this were a cause-and-effect relationship, it would imply that a failed *attempt* at rescue angioplasty might be harmful, and that, on balance, the overall effect of failed rescue could outweigh any the benefit from successes. However, in a nonrandomized series there may be an unintentional selection bias to refer for the procedure primarily those patients most critically ill or at highest risk. Thus, this data creates a dilemma: Is the higher mortality rate for patients who *fail* rescue angioplasty due to the clinical features of the population under study, or is it the direct result of the procedure itself? Randomized trials would be necessary to investigate this issue.

Randomized Trials

Three recent, randomized trials provide the most important data on the outcome of patients treated with a strategy of rescue angioplasty. Belenkie et al.[54] studied 28 patients who presented 3 to 6 hours after symptom onset; 16 were randomized to rescue PTCA. Angioplasty was successful in reestablishing vessel patency in 13 of the 16 patients. Rescue PTCA re-

Table 36-2. Meta-Analysis of Series of Rescue PTCA Prior to the TAMI-5 and RESCUE Trials

Study	No. of Patients	Thrombolytic Regimen	Success (%)	Reocclusion (%)	ΔEF	Mortality (%)
Topol	86	rt-PA	73	29	− 1	10.4
Califf	15	rt-PA	87	15	+ 1	NR
	25	UK	84	12	+ 1	NR
	12	rt-PA + UK	92	0	+ 2	NR
Belenkie	16	SK	81	NR	+ 2	6.7
Fung	13	SK	92	16	+ 10	7.6
Topol	22	rt-PA + UK	86	3	+ 5	0
Grines	12	rt-PA + SK	100	8	NR	NR
Holmes	34	SK	71	NR	− 11	11
Grimes	10	rt-PA + SK	90	12	+ 5	10
O'Connor	90	SK	89	14	− 1	17
Baim	37	rt-PA	92	26	NR	5.4
Whitlow	26	rt-PA	81	29	− 2	NR
	18	UK	89	25	+ 1	NR
Ellis et al.[43]	109	rt-PA	79	20	+ 1	10.1
	5	rt-PA + UK	80	20	+ 2	20
	59	SK	76	18	+ 4	10.2
Pooled SK, UK or combination	308[a]		260/308 (84%)[b]	31/223 (14%)	− 1	11.2
Pooled rt-PA only	252[c]		191/252 (76%)[b]	38/157 (24%)	− 1	9.5
Total	560[c]		451/560 (80%)	69/380 (18%)	− 1	10.6

Abbreviations: ΔEF, the change in left ventricular ejection fraction from baseline to the measurement before hospital discharge; NR, not reported; rt-PA, recombinant tissue-type plasminogen activator; SK, streptokinase; UK, urokinase.

[a] Five patients included in both the series of Topol et al. and this series are counted separately.

[b] $P = 0.01$.

[c] 21 patients included in both the series of Califf et al. and this series are counted separately.

sulted in a trend toward a lower in-hospital mortality rate when compared with patients not randomized to rescue PTCA (7 vs. 33%, $P = 0.13$). At follow-up, however, there was no difference in mean left ventricular systolic performance. On average, the hospital mortality was 10.6%.

Although the TAMI-5 trial was not specifically a study of rescue angioplasty, it did test the strategy of angioplasty for infarct vessels with TIMI 0 or 1 flow after thrombolytic therapy. This trial (Fig. 36-3) was a 3×2 factorial design in which 575 patients were first randomized to either t-PA, urokinase, or a two-drug combination; thereafter, patients were again randomized to one of two catheterization strategies. Within each lytic arm, one-half of the patients were assigned to an emergency angiogram and rescue PTCA if the infarct artery was occluded (TIMI flow grade 0 or 1) or to a strategy of delayed coronary angiography 5 to 7 days later. The strategy of rescue PTCA resulted in a high immediate patency rate of 96% and a high predischarge patency rate of 94%. The deferred angiography group had a discharge patency rate of only 90% ($P = 0.065$). In addition, the aggressively treated group had fewer episodes of recurrent ischemia (35 vs. 25%, respectively, $P < 0.005$)

and thus needed less emergency intervention. Wall motion indices within the infarct zone also improved. Note that one group of patients who received particular benefit from an aggressive strategy of early angiography and rescue PTCA when indicated were those with a prior myocardial infarction.

The most important study of rescue angioplasty to date is the RESCUE trial[49] (Fig. 36-4). Patients were eligible for enrollment if, despite any standard thrombolytic regimen, they had angiographic confirmation of persistent left anterior descending artery occlusion (TIMI flow grade 0 or 1) within 8 hours of the onset of chest pain and greater than 90 minutes from the start of thrombolytic therapy. This study limited enrollment to patients with left anterior descending artery occlusions to test the strategy of rescue angioplasty in the subset at highest risk (and thus the easiest in which to demonstrate a benefit and the smaller the sample size required). One-hundred fifty-one patients were randomly assigned to two treatment groups. Patients in the conservative arm were treated with vasodilators, aspirin, and heparin; patients in the PTCA arm received these therapies plus angioplasty and additional intracoronary thrombolytics, as indicated. Major exclusionary

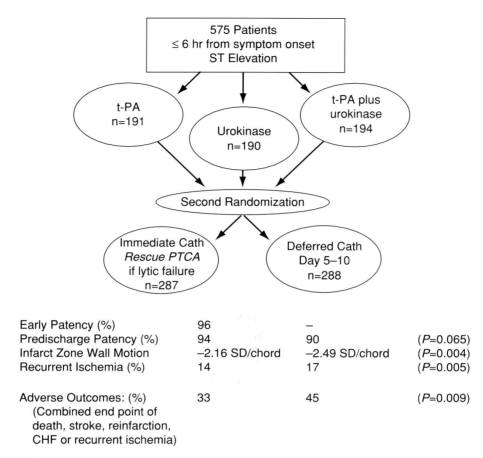

Early Patency (%)   96   –
Predischarge Patency (%)   94   90   (*P*=0.065)
Infarct Zone Wall Motion   –2.16 SD/chord –2.49 SD/chord (*P*=0.004)
Recurrent Ischemia (%)   14   17   (*P*=0.005)

Adverse Outcomes: (%)   33   45   (*P*=0.009)
  (Combined end point of
  death, stroke, reinfarction,
  CHF or recurrent ischemia)

Fig. 36-3. Schematic diagram of the TAMI-5 trial. This study was a 3 × 2 factorial design in which patients were randomized to one of the thrombolytic regimens shown. Patients in each arm were then randomized again to a strategy of either an emergency angiogram and rescue PTCA if the infarct artery was occluded (TIMI flow grade 0 or 1) or to a strategy of delayed coronary angiography 5 to 7 days later. Rescue PTCA resulted in a higher immediate patency rate and a higher predischarge patency rate Note that the aggressively treated group had fewer episodes of recurrent ischemia and a lesser need for acute intervention. Wall motion within the infarct zone were also improved. (Modified from Califf et al.,[17] with permission.)

criteria were cardiogenic shock before randomization, prior myocardial infarction, and left main stenosis of 50% or more. The overall technical success rate of 92% compares favorably with previously reported nonrandomized series. Most importantly, rescue angioplasty significantly reduced the incidence of the combined end point of death and severe heart failure (6% in the PTCA group versus 17% in the conservatively treated group). In addition, the PTCA group had a higher mean exercise ejection fraction at 30 days (43 vs. 38%, *P* <0.04), although resting mean ejection fractions were not significantly different.

As noted above, an important issue that previous, nonrandomized series could not address was the high mortality rate for patients in whom rescue PTCA failed. In one series, the mortality rate for this group of patients was as high as 39%.[13] However, on the

basis of these studies, it was unclear whether failed rescue was the *cause* of the higher mortality rate, or whether this group of patients was simply more ill at the time of catheterization and thus at high risk of death regardless of therapy. The RESCUE trial does not settle this dilemma because, in this study, the procedural success rate was a remarkably high 92%. This is probably due to improvements in technique and equipment compared with studies performed in an earlier era as well as the commitment and experience of the participating centers. Thus, although the number of patients enrolled in the RESCUE trial did not allow it to demonstrate a mortality advantage for rescue PTCA, the study does not indicate a mortality disadvantage for those in whom the procedure fails.

Finally, it is important to note that the RESCUE

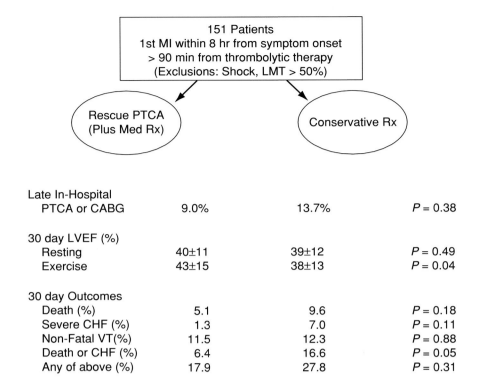

Late In-Hospital			
PTCA or CABG	9.0%	13.7%	*P* = 0.38
30 day LVEF (%)			
Resting	40±11	39±12	*P* = 0.49
Exercise	43±15	38±13	*P* = 0.04
30 day Outcomes			
Death (%)	5.1	9.6	*P* = 0.18
Severe CHF (%)	1.3	7.0	*P* = 0.11
Non-Fatal VT(%)	11.5	12.3	*P* = 0.88
Death or CHF (%)	6.4	16.6	*P* = 0.05
Any of above (%)	17.9	27.8	*P* = 0.31

Fig. 36-4. Schematic diagram of the RESCUE trial. Rescue angioplasty significantly reduced the incidence of the combined end point of death and severe heart failure. In addition, the PTCA group had a higher mean exercise ejection fraction at 30 days. CHF, congestive heart failure; LVEF, left ventricular ejection fraction. (From Ellis et al.,[49] with permission.)

trial may actually underestimate the potential benefit of rescue angioplasty in some subsets of patients. Patients who underwent angiography within the shortest time from the onset of symptoms tended not to be randomized in the trial. All patients eligible for randomization at participating hospitals were followed in the registry portion of the study. Whereas the mean time to angiography in the study patients was hours, the mean time to angiography in the registry was 3.1 hours. Thus, there was a bias against randomizing the earliest patients. As a group, these "early" patients might have been more likely to demonstrate myocardial salvage and thus display a greater absolute improvement in systolic function. Data from the registry portion of the study will be available in 1995.

CURRENT INDICATIONS

Currently available data support the strategy of rescue angioplasty for patients with TIMI grade 0 or 1 infarct vessel flow despite thrombolytic therapy. Patients who are likely to derive the greatest benefit

from an aggressive strategy of early angiography and rescue PTCA are those at highest risk (such as those with prior myocardial infarctions, as demonstrated in TAMI-5) and those with anterior infarctions (as demonstrated in RESCUE). Although the RESCUE trial did not include patients with circumflex or right coronary occlusions, these patients may benefit if the infarct artery supplies a large myocardial territory. The TAMI-5 trial demonstrates that patients appropriately treated with rescue angioplasty have fewer episodes of recurrent ischemia and that wall motion indices within the infarct zone can improve. The RESCUE trial demonstrates that for patients with anterior infarction, rescue angioplasty reduces the incidence of the combined end point of death and severe heart failure and increases mean exercise ejection fraction at 30 days.

Although these recent trials have provided scientific support for the application of rescue angioplasty, two important issues remain unresolved. First, although the data support the use of rescue angioplasty for patients with TIMI flow grades of 0 or 1, limited data are available on the use of rescue angioplasty for patients with TIMI grade 2 flow. In a recent subgroup analysis of 108 patients from the

TAMI-1 study who had TIMI grade 2 infarct vessel flow at immediate catheterization, Ellis et al. compared 49 patients who underwent rescue PTCA with 59 patients who were initially treated with medical therapy only. Patients who underwent rescue PTCA had a *higher* mortality rate (6.1 vs. 1.7%); however, the rescue PTCA group had a modest but statistically significant improvement in ejection fraction (an increase of 2.4% in those who had rescue versus a loss of 0.7% in those who did not). Thus, in the absence of overt ischemia, the routine use of rescue angioplasty for patients with TIMI grade 2 flow cannot be sanctioned.

Second, although the RESCUE trial supports rescue angioplasty within 8 hours of symptom onset, in the absence of overt ischemia it is unclear at what time *beyond* 8 hours physicians should exclude patients from this invasive (and expensive) form of therapy. This issue is quite important because more than 30% of patients with acute myocardial infarction present beyond 6 hours from symptom onset.[55] As we have discussed, data from other trials suggest that late reperfusion with either thrombolytic therapy or angioplasty in patients who present relatively late can result in a measurable, albeit transient, improvement in ventricular function.[12,41,42] In the absence of definitive data, treatment decisions are best made on an individual patient basis.

IDENTIFICATION OF THROMBOLYTIC FAILURES: THE "RATE-LIMITING" STEP

The rapid and accurate diagnosis of failed thrombolysis is a requirement for the strategy of rescue angioplasty to be truly applicable to patients most likely to benefit; however, a major limitation to date has been the inaccuracy of clinical criteria in determining the patency status of the infarct vessel. Recent studies have demonstrated that continuous ST-segment monitoring (with or without vector analysis) identifies patients who fail intravenous thrombolysis with a reasonable level of sensitivity and specificity. Krucoff et al.[56] studied this technique in 144 patients treated with thrombolytic therapy. All patients were studied acutely with angiography; 27% had an occluded infarct vessel on first injection. ST recovery analysis had a sensitivity of 64%, a specificity of 90%, and a positive predictive value of 71% for identifying infarct vessels with TIMI flow grades of 2 or 3. The only more accurate clinical indicator of reperfusion after thrombolysis is rapid and complete ST-segment normalization.[57,58] Although this finding was associated with a patent infarct artery in 96% of cases in the TAMI-1 trial, it occurred in only 6% of patients with an open artery at acute catheterization.[58] Several traditional "markers" of reperfusion, such as ventricular dysrythmias, have recently been shown to be associated with persistent occlusion.[59]

Until a more reliable noninvasive technique to determine the status of the infarct vessel is established, urgent angiography is the only definitive method to triage patients to rescue angioplasty. However, several other noninvasive techniques appear promising. Rapid analysis of creatine kinase isoforms[60–66] and measurement of myoglobin release, particularly the difference between the washout of these two proteins,[67,68] may also prove to be of value, as may bedside determination of troponin T release.[69–75] To be of greatest clinical utility, a noninvasive technique will need to have a high enough sensitivity to identify the vast majority of patients whose infarct vessels are closed and yet have a high enough specificity to minimize the number of patients sent for urgent angiography whose infarct vessels are actually open.

TECHNICAL ASPECTS

Clinical Assessment

A rapid but complete evaluation of the patient's clinical status is essential prior to rescue angioplasty. Central venous cannulation is essential in case fluids or medications are required rapidly. Right heart catheterization to determine pulmonary artery and "wedge" pressures is often valuable, and occasionally this procedure should be performed first if the patient is hypotensive or if a mechanical complication (such as rupture of a papillary muscle or the ventricular septum) is suspected. Left ventricular pump failure may improve with diuresis, inotropic medications, or intra-aortic balloon counterpulsation; hypotension due to right ventricular infarction, hypovolemia, or tamponade may benefit from volume expansion.

In the absence of a specific contraindication, the physician should place an intra-aortic balloon pump (IABP) in virtually all rescue angioplasty candidates, especially in patients with ongoing ischemia, hypotension, or pulmonary edema, and in patients with left ventricular dysfunction (especially in the presence of multivessel disease).[76,77] If a relative contraindication to an IABP is present (such as severe iliofemoral or aortic disease), the physician should consider placing a 5-F sheath in the contralateral femoral artery in the event that the patient requires an IABP urgently. This is especially important in the patient with known or suspected left ventricular dysfunction; contralateral arterial access can be lifesaving if hemodynamic compromise or collapse occurs during the procedure. In the patient with tenuous hemodynamics, respiratory compromise, or frank pulmonary edema, elective intubation before rescue angioplasty is preferable to urgent intubation during the procedure. A temporary pacemaker placement should be placed emergently if signs of intermittent heart block exist or any bradycardia with rate-responsive hypotension is present.

Often the most important piece of information before urgent angiography is a review of any prior angiogram (or a report if the film is unavailable). This is invaluable in patients with bypass grafts and in those with a totally occluded culprit vessel ostium; in the latter situation, a "stump" may be difficult to identify despite multiple angiographic projections. Knowledge of the anatomy before urgent angiography is also useful when the target vessel makes an abrupt angulation after the occluded segment; angulated segments can make definite confirmation of intraluminal wire position difficult.

Medical Adjuncts

Once vessel patency is re-established, inhibiting the platelet and fibrin response is essential to prevent reocclusion.[78–80] Although many patients who present with a myocardial infarction and who subsequently require rescue angioplasty should have received aspirin at the time of initial thrombolytic administration, it is essential that the interventional cardiologist confirm this. We administer a total dose of 650 mg of soluble aspirin before attempted rescue. It is imperative that the aspirin *not* be enteric coated and that it be *chewed* to facilitate rapid gastric absorption. Intravenous heparin should be started (if the patient is not already receiving it) and titrated to an activated clotting time of at least 300. Heparin is usually maintained for 24 hours after rescue PTCA, especially if a large intimal dissection or intraluminal filling defect is present. Nitrates may provide some antiplatelet activity along with vasodilation.[81] Although dextran may have some additional benefit in the patient who was not previously taking aspirin, its antiplatelet effect is not maximal until 4 to 6 hours after infusion.[82] Therefore, there is probably little clinical benefit even when dextran is administered 30 minutes before angioplasty.[83] Dextran also poses a significant hemodynamic burden that these patients may tolerate poorly. For those patients who have received a fibrin-specific thrombolytic agent such as t-PA as the initial treatment at presentation, additional adminstration of a non-fibrin-specific agent provides no advantage when rescue angioplasty is required.

Equipment Selection

Although elective angioplasty warrants ionic contrast in the vast majority of cases to minimize both cost and the risk of exacerbating thrombosis, the hemodynamic instability and potential for arrythmias justify the use of nonionic media for most rescue PTCA candidates. After inserting an 8-F arterial sheath, it is our preference to perform angiography first with an 7-F diagnostic catheter; if the patient is a candidate for rescue PTCA the sheath is exchanged for an 8-F and the appropriate guiding catheter is advanced to the target vessel. Interestingly, in the TAMI trials, the hydrostatic force transmitted to the thrombus during diagnostic angiography resulted in recanalization of the target vessel in 8% of cases.[2,57,58,86]

The cardiologist should select a highly flexible guidewire and then progress to a stiffer type only after the former fails to cross the lesion. In the setting of acute infarction, an over-the-wire system is preferable to a fixed-wire system (unless the vessel is small or extremely difficult to maneuver), because the operator can maintain guidewire position across the stenosis during the entire procedure. An over-the-wire balloon will also allow contrast injection into the distal vessel beyond the obstruction, confirming the intraluminal placement of the device. As in elective PTCA, target lesion location and morphology often influence the operator's choice of wire type and diameter. An 0.018 wire may provide more forward support for tracking a balloon across a tortuous segment proximal to the target site; rarely, a severe, distal stenosis may be easier to cross with a 0.010 mm wire. The use of continuously tapered guidewires (without a discrete transition zone) may be especially useful in very tortuous vessels or angulated segments; however, these wires are usually radiopaque and may obscure the status of the target lesion during the procedure. Regardless of the specific wire chosen, the operator must try to avoid forceful probing and must keep the guidewire tip free within the vessel lumen during crossing of the target lesion, to avoid additional trauma to the target vessel and subintimal dissection.

Balloon catheter selection depends primarily on artery size and balloon material requirements; these factors are similar to the considerations during elective PTCA, as discussed in Chapter 35. However, in the setting of acute infarction, there are three situations in which some operators prefer to begin with a small diameter (1.5 to 2.5 mm) balloon: (1) if accurate vessel sizing is impossible due to complete occlusion; (2) if the operator questions whether the guidewire is truly in the lumen distal to the total occlusion; and (3) if crossing the target stenosis is expected to be difficult (due to tortuosity, calcification, and other factors) and initial dilation with a balloon that can readily cross is necessary. Once this predilation is successful and flow is re-established, the operator can estimate the arterial size more accurately and can proceed to a balloon artery ratio closer to 1:0. Due to the "soft" nature of the underlying plaque and superimposed thrombus, rarely will high-inflation pressures (<8 atm) be necessary to achieve adequate dilation.

Although proper equipment selection influences the speed and success rate of rescue angioplasty, the experience and judgment of the operator are the most important factors that influence procedural success.[87] If a target vessel has a stenosis of less than 70% and TIMI grade 3 flow, PTCA is contraindicated.[88] During rescue PTCA, the experienced operator will often accept a slightly greater residual stenosis (25 to 30%) than he or she would for an elective procedure. Since no conclusive data have yet proved that a larger postprocedure influences restenosis, the risk of striving for an "optimal" lumen rarely, if ever, outweighs the need to avoid causing an extensive dissection with an aggressive inflation strategy. As a rule, the operator should attempt PTCA of *only the culprit vessel*. Rare exceptions might include patients with *two* potential culprit lesions in whom it is impossible to determine which is responsible for the acute coronary syndrome, or the patient with continued hemodynamic instability despite successful rescue PTCA of the presumed target lesion. Perhaps the most difficult patient is one with multivessel disease who will ultimately require bypass surgery; if transportation to a ready operating suite will not be available for 30 to 45 minutes or more, the experience and judgment of the operator must determine whether PTCA should be attempted as a "bridge" to surgery. In summary, the checklist in Table 36-3 should be consulted before attempting rescue angioplasty.

OTHER MANAGEMENT ISSUES

Besides the usual technical difficulties that can complicate elective angioplasty, several problems are particularly common in the setting of rescue angioplasty.

Table 36-3. Checklist Before Attempting Rescue Angioplasty

I. Clinical assessment
   Prior angiogram reviewed?
   Hemodynamic assessment completed?
   Venous cannulation/pulmonary artery catheter indicated?
   Intra-aortic balloon pump/contralateral arterial access indicated?
   Elective intubation indicated?
II. Medical adjuncts
   Two soluble aspirin
   Nitrates, heparin, and other routine medications
   H_2 antagonists
III. Equipment selection
   Flexible guidewire, if possible
   Over-the-wire, 0.018 system when feasible
IV. Troubleshooting
   Obvious thrombus: use non-fibrin-specific agent, when feasible
   Recurrent closure: consider thrombus, dissection, and/or spasm
   Right coronary target: beware of unexpected hypotension, bradycardia, and dysrhythmias

Role of Adjunctive Intracoronary Thrombolytics

If an infarct vessel remains persistently occluded despite intravenous thrombolysis, most interventional cardiologists would proceed directly to mechanical intervention. Despite successful rescue PTCA, some patients have a large amount of residual thrombus, and *intracoronary* thrombolytics may be indicated. In such cases, the interventionist should choose a non-fibrin-specific agent (such as 100,000 to 500,000 U of urokinase) for direct coronary infusion. In addition to infusion via the coronary guiding catheter, two newer, more selective techniques are now available. The Dispatch catheter (Scimed Life Systems, Minneapolis, Min) is a local drug delivery catheter that allows the administration of a drug directly to the site of a coronary thrombus site; by means of a chamber design, the device allows a high local concentration of the agent with a relatively small total dose. A central core allows perfusion of the distal coronary bed during drug administration. This device may be most useful in proximal, large, and relatively accessible coronary segments. For smaller and more distal target sites (particularly those beyond very tortuous segments), direct intracoronary administration via a Tracker catheter (Target Therapeutics, San Jose, CA) or via the lumen of a balloon probably provides higher concentration of the lytic agent at the target site than does nonspecific intracoronary instillation via the guiding catheter.

Recurrent Closure

Occasionally, despite initially successful vessel dilation, reclosure occurs after each inflation. The differential diagnosis in this situation includes vessel spasm, occult dissection, or recurrent thrombosis; in some cases, more than one mechanism may be responsible. Angiographically apparent thrombus may respond to either intracoronary thrombolytics or repeat inflations. If no obvious evidence of residual thrombus or dissection exists and if systolic pressure is adequate, we administer intracoronary nitroglycerin or verapamil, or both, because the initial rescue PTCA may have released potent vasoconstrictors.[89] If drugs fail, prolonged inflations with a standard balloon or perfusion catheter may succeed. Some operators prefer to "upsize" the balloon by 0.5 mm, aiming for a balloon artery ratio of 1–1.2:1. If these measures fail, the cardiologist faces the dilemma of whether to place a stent in the setting of acute myocardial infarction. Although some operators consider acute infarction a relatively strong contraindication, others will deploy a stent as long as no gross evidence of thrombus exists angiographically (G. S. Roubin, personal communication). If a stent is necessary in the setting of acute infarction, many interventionalists will place a coronary infusion catheter proximally and infuse urokinase for 6 to 12 hours (G. S. Roubin, personal communication). No data are available on the use of temporary or removable stents in this situation. In the future, newer medical adjuncts, such as hirudin or glycoprotein IIb/IIIa inhibitors, may help in those situations in which recurrent thrombosis is the cause of repeated reclosure.

Other Devices

Although directional atherectomy[90] and laser angioplasty[91] have been reported to be useful in acute infarction angioplasty, the data are insufficient to justify their routine use. A trial of the transluminal atherectomy device in patients with acute infarction is currently in progress. Ultrasound atherectomy may have a unique role in thrombus dissolution.[92] A preliminary investigation of a thrombus aspiration catheter is currently under way in Europe.[93] Emergency percutaneous cardiopulmonary bypass should be considered in patients with profound hypotension unresponsive to IABP or refractory ventricular arrhythmias.[94]

Table 36-4. Potential Technical Problems During Rescue Angioplasty

Inability to identify the culprit vessel or lesion
Large amount of residual thrombus
Inability to cross lesion
Recurrent closure after initially successful rescue PTCA
    Recurrent thrombosis
    Dissection
    Spasm

Right Coronary Rescue: An Additional Risk

A disproportionate percentage of patients undergoing rescue PTCA of the right coronary artery have periprocedural complications. Several investigators have noted a relatively high incidence of dysrhythmias, including severe sinus bradycardia, Mobitz type 2 and type 3 atrioventricular block, ventricular fibrillation, and cardiac arrest.[13,95] These reactions may be poorly responsive to fluids, atropine, and dopamine and may require intravenous norepinephrine for successful treatment. In addition, the risk of abrupt closure and subsequent reclosure is twice as high in the right coronary artery compared with the left. Most of these patients were stable before the attempted rescue, and the procedure itself was usually technically uncomplicated. Thus, the interventional cardiologist must be even more alert to potential complications when attempting right coronary rescue.

The potential technical problems may be summarized in Table 39-4.

POST-RESCUE MANAGEMENT

Immediate postoperative care is directed toward hemodynamic status and the prevention of reocclusion. At the conclusion of successful but suboptimal rescue PTCA, the elective use of intra-aortic balloon counterpulsation may help to maintain target vessel patency by increasing coronary diastolic pressure and flow.[77,96] In the unusual patient who did not receive an IABP at the start of the procedure, the operator should consider this form of support at the procedure's conclusion, particularly if the target site has a significant dissection or other features suggesting a higher rate of early reocclusion.[76,77]

Femoral sheaths are usually left in place for 24 hours in the absence of severe hemorrhage. This ob-

relatively low-frequency operators: 1986–1987 experience. Am J Cardiol 1988;61:1229–31

88. The SWIFT (Should We Intervene Following Thrombolysis) Trial Study Group. The SWIFT trial of delayed elective intervention versus conservative treatment after thrombolysis with anistreplase in acute myocardial infarction. BMJ 1991;302:555–60

89. Kahn JK, Hartzler GO. Evidence for dynamic coronary vasoconstriction in the early minutes of acute myocardial infarction. Am Heart J 1990;121:188–90

90. McKeever L, Marek J, Kerwin P et al. Bail-out directional atherectomy for abrupt coronary artery occlusion following conventional angioplasty. Cathet Cardiovasc Diagn 1993;1:31–6

91. de Marchena E, Mallon S, Posada J et al. Direct holmium laser assisted angioplasty in acute myocardial infarction. Am J Cardiol 1993;71:1223–5

92. Harpaz D, Chen X, Francis C et al. Ultrasound enhancement of thrombolysis and reperfusion in vitro. J Am Coll Cardiol 1993;21:1507–11

93. Fajadet J, Marco J. Case presentation at the Sixth Annual Washington Hospital Center Transcatheter Cardiac Therapeutics Course, Washington, DC, February 1994

94. Teirstein PS, Vogel RA, Dorros G et al. Prophylactic versus standby cardiopulmonary support for high risk percutaneous transluminal coronary angioplasty. J Am Col Cardiol 1993;21:590–6

95. Gacioch GM, Topol EJ. Sudden paradoxic clinical deterioration during angioplasty of the occluded right coronary artery in acute myocardial infarction. J Am Coll Cardiol 1989;14:1202–9

96. Ishihara M, Sto H, Tateishi H et al. Intraaortic balloon pumping as the postangioplasty strategy in acute myocardial infarction. Am Heart J 1991;122:385–9

97. Homeister JW, Hoff PT, Fletcher DD et al. Combined adenosine and lidocaine administration limits myocardial reperfusion injury. Circulation 1990;82:595–608

98. Kitakaze M, Hori M, Kamada T. Role of adenosine and its interaction with alpha adrenoceptor activity in ischaemic and reperfusion injury of the myocardium, review Cardiovasc Res 1993;27:18–27

99. Califf R, Topol E, Gersh B. From myocardial salvage to patient salvage in acute myocardial infarction: the role of reperfusion therapy. J Am Coll Cardiol 1989;14:1382–8

37 Percutaneous Coronary Intervention After Bypass Surgery

John S. Douglas, Jr.

Andreas Gruentzig[1] clearly recognized the value of percutaneous transluminal coronary angioplasty (PTCA) in the postsurgical coronary artery bypass graft (CABG) patient; such patients accounted for 16% of the first large series he reported. Although early reports from the National Heart, Lung, and Blood Institute (NHLBI) registry indicated that PTCA in post-CABG patients was associated with increased risk, subsequent experience was contradictory. In the early 1980s, no procedural mortality and procedural success rates approaching 90% were reported in over 100 consecutive procedures with Q-wave infarction in a single patient.[2] In the mid 1990s, patients with prior CABG account for 15 to 25% of percutaneous coronary intervention in many angioplasty centers, and it is in these patients that new nonballoon approaches to percutaneous myocardial revascularization have the most applicability.

RATIONALE

Palliation of recurrent ischemic symptoms with repeat CABG is associated with perioperative mortality and Q-wave infarction rates three to five times that of first operations, angina relief is less complete, and graft patency is reduced.[3] These factors and the consequent narrowing of therapeutic options after each surgical procedure have led cardiologists to avoid reoperation when safe and effective percutaneous strategies can be applied.[4] Additionally, many symptomatic patients with absolute (or relative) contraindications to surgery are candidates for PTCA. The safety and effectiveness of percutaneous methods depend on a host of factors, the foremost being location of target lesion(s) and extent of coronary disease and left ventricular dysfunction.

INSTRUMENTATION

Although balloon angioplasty remains the dominant percutaneous interventional strategy (Fig. 37-1), the second decade of coronary intervention has witnessed an increasing application of nonballoon devices, especially in patients with prior CABG. Those patients with older fibrocalcific native vessel lesions are frequently selected for rotational atherectomy, directional atherectomy (DCA) or excimer laser angioplasty (ELCA). Maintenance of familiarity with this new technology and its nuances, selection criteria, and optimal application place considerable demands on the invasive cardiologist. The Gianturco-Roubin stent, approved for treatment of suboptimal or failed PTCA, has become a valuable strategy, especially in post-CABG patients in whom surgical relief of ischemia is not readily available. This stent is used primarily in native vessels, in 2 to 3% of patients in our experience. Saphenous vein graft lesions, shown to have high recurrence rates with balloon angioplasty, have lower complication and recurrence rates with Palmaz-Schatz stenting of mid-graft sites. The place of transluminal extraction atherectomy (TEC) in the treatment of saphenous vein grafts has not been clearly determined. Observational studies suggest that TEC is a valuable adjunct in some patients with lesion-associated thrombus.

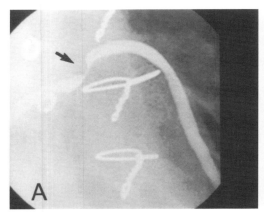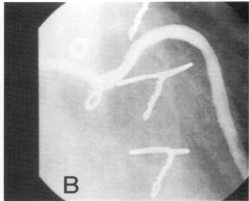

Fig. 37-1. Severe stenosis of a saphenous vein graft to the left anterior descending artery **(A)** causing unstable angina 10 years postoperatively in a 66-year-old woman judged unsuitable for reoperation. She had contraindications to Coumadin, and stenting was therefore ruled out; severe iliac disease prevented consideration of DCA. **(B)** Balloon angioplasty using an AL-1 guide catheter and 3-mm balloon was successful, and symptoms have been relieved for 16 months. Restenosis in our experience occurs in over 50% of mid-saphenous vein graft lesions following balloon angioplasty, but significant palliation is frequently possible.

PATIENT POPULATION

The increasing frequency of clinical application of repeat revascularization strategies is related to the large number of postsurgical patients, the progressive nature of atherosclerosis, and the shortened longevity of veins interposed in the arterial circulation. Of 3,481 patients who underwent a first coronary bypass operation between 1978 and 1981 at Emory University Hospital and were followed for 12 years, 30% required reoperation, whereas freedom from PTCA at 5, 10, and 12 years was 98, 88, and 78%, respectively.[5] In 1992, 467 patients with prior CABG underwent PTCA at Emory University Hospital, accounting for 27% of percutaneous coronary interventions. In one-half of the patients, the site treated was in a saphenous vein graft. The youngest patient was 5 and the oldest almost 90 years of age.

PRETREATMENT

Measures for optimal preparation and performance of percutaneous interventional procedures have been described in detail.[6,7] In general, patients with prior CABG are handled in standard fashion. Exceptions are those in whom intravascular stenting is planned (where ticlopidine is added to aspirin pretreatment) or when extreme left ventricular dysfunction or possible cardiogenic shock mandate intra-aortic balloon pumping or standby. We have not found in-laboratory cardiopulmonary bypass to be necessary in a broad spectrum of patients undergoing PTCA following coronary bypass surgery.

PROCEDURAL TECHNIQUE AND TIPS

Native Vessel Intervention

Angioplasty or atherectomy of native coronary artery lesions in post-CABG patients may present unique challenges. In approaching the protected left main coronary lesion, or ostial right coronary stenosis, the interventional operator frequently encounters a rigid lesion that responds poorly to balloon angioplasty (Fig. 37-2). Elastic recoil may also be a significant factor. We have found rotational atherectomy to be particularly helpful at these sites as an initial strategy, but adjunctive DCA or balloon angioplasty is usually required if the artery is large. ELCA is also effective as initial therapy unless heavy calcification is present. Palmaz-Schatz stenting of left main coronary lesions has been reported to be lifesaving in the setting of perioperative graft closure and cardiogenic shock.

Recanalization of chronic occlusions may be required when conduits are occluded or too diffusely diseased for intervention. In the presence of chronic occlusions with bridging collaterals but fine recanalized tracts (you have to look carefully to see them), we have found 0.010″ diameter steerable wires to be particularly effective. When bridging collaterals are

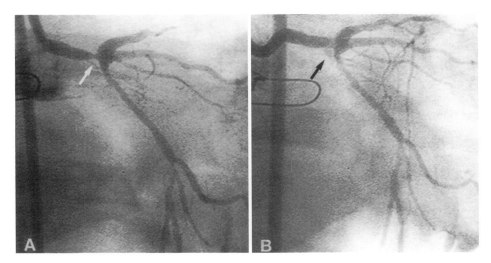

Fig. 37-2. A 69-year-old man developed disabling angina 12 years after CABG. **(A)** Recatheterization revealed a patent saphenous vein graft to the left anterior descending artery and severe stenosis of the left main with moderate calcification. Saphenous vein grafts to the right coronary artery and **(B)** Obtuse marginal were occluded. Following predilation to 17 atm, directional atherectomy with a 7-F atherocatheter was successful (residual stenosis 24%). Histology revealed calcified atheroma. Three years later symptoms recurred. The graft to the left anterior descending artery was found to be occluded, the left main was widely patent, and reoperation was required. Currently, in heavily calcified left main lesions, we believe rotational atherectomy is the initial procedure of choice.

present with no evidence of a recanalized tract, more aggressive strategies with stiffer wires or hydrophilic wires or new devices are usually required. We have found the Jagwire (Mansfield, Watertown, MA), a 0.016″ diameter nitinol wire with 0.025″ diameter hydrophilic-coated 2-cm tip, to be useful in this situation. A 300-cm wire is used to permit catheter changes since the 0.025″ tip prevents wire removal through the dilation catheter and wire changes.

To reach distal native coronary lesions, dilation catheters or other interventional devices are frequently passed through graft conduits. When very long venous grafts have been implanted that wrap the heart (snake grafts), an extra long balloon catheter shaft (or shortened guide catheter) may be required to reach the lesion. Extra length may also be needed when the right internal mammary is inserted quite distally in the right or circumflex system and when a very redundant arterial graft is present. One easy technique for shortening the guide catheter without sacrificing wire position requires only that unneeded guide catheter length be amputated with a scalpel and then the open catheter end be closed by sliding a flared, short sheath 1 F size smaller over the wire onto the stub of the guide catheter.[8] If retrograde passage is required from graft insertion into more proximal segments of native coronary arteries, special guidewire strategies may be necessary: a soft steerable guidewire without transition points (Cordis Reflex wire, for example) is passed retrograde as far as possible; then the tip of a very flexible low-profile balloon catheter is advanced around the corner into the proximal native vessel. The soft wire is replaced by a stiffer wire, which is advanced retrograde as far as possible, followed by advancing the balloon catheter.[9] This incremental strategy is frequently effective, but high-performance balloon catheters and optimal guide catheter backup become important.

Saphenous Vein Graft Intervention

For saphenous vein graft angioplasty, a 7- or 8-F guide catheter is commonly used. A multipurpose shape is selected for most vein grafts to the right coronary artery, a multipurpose or right Judkins shape for horizontal or inferiorly directed saphenous vein grafts to the left anterior descending artery (LAD), and a left Amplatz 1.5 or 2 (or hockey-stick) for superiorly oriented saphenous vein grafts to the LAD (Fig. 37-1) and for virtually all diagonal and circumflex grafts. Guide catheters with side holes are frequently used and are particularly helpful for smaller vein grafts and ostial saphenous vein graft lesions. For ostial stenoses where guide catheter

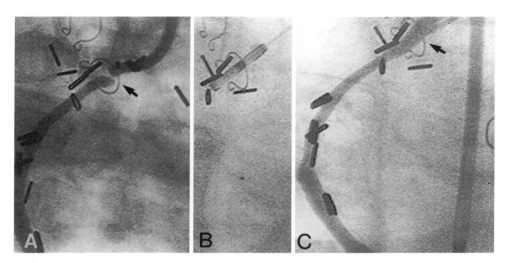

Fig. 37-3. Unstable angina occurred in a 65-year-old man 7 years following CABG. **(A)** High-grade stenosis was present at the ostium of the saphenous vein graft to the right coronary artery. A LIMA graft to the left anterior descending artery and two grafts to the circumflex coronary were widely patent. A multipurpose guide catheter was used to advance a 7-F atherocatheter across the lesion **(B)** over an extra support 0.014″ diameter guidewire, and **(C)** an excellent angiographic result was obtained. In our experience, restenosis rates following DCA and Palmaz-Schatz stents are similar at this site (approximately 50 to 60%).

seating is difficult or impossible, a sharper tip diagnostic catheter and a balloon-on-a-wire may be required. Because of high restenosis rates with balloon angioplasty of aorto-ostial graft lesions, directional atherectomy is frequently used, either after PTCA with a 2-mm balloon or as a primary strategy (Fig. 37-3). Restenosis rates following Palmaz-Schatz stenting or ELCA at this site are similar to that following DCA in our experience.

Lesions in the mid-portion of saphenous vein grafts occurring within 3 years of CABG frequently respond favorably to balloon angioplasty and rarely cause distal embolization, but restenosis rates exceed 50%. Slight balloon oversizing is safe in this time period, but, as vein grafts age, the risk of perforation increases and balloon oversizing has an increased risk. In general, we size the balloon 1:1 for the vein graft and reserve oversizing for suboptimal results. The long-term results with DCA and ELCA are similar, but DCA is usually preferred over balloon angioplasty or ELCA for eccentric or shelf-like lesions. The most favorable results reported for mid-saphenous vein graft lesions are with multicenter use of the Palmaz-Schatz stent where 98.7% of 626 deployments were successful, subacute stent thrombosis occurred in only 1.3% of patients, and restenosis occurred in 18% of de novo and 38% of restenotic lesions.[10] Keys to procedural success include excellent guide catheter backup, predilation of severe stenoses, and use of a high-pressure inflation to expand the stent fully to achieve 0% residual stenosis.

In angioplasty of saphenous vein grafts in place more than 3 years, embolic events are more common with all interventions. A relatively low rate of coronary atheroembolization has been observed with the Wall stent and the Palmaz-Schatz stent, however, perhaps due to trapping of atherosclerotic debris between the stent and graft wall. Intragraft thrombus is a strong predictor of embolic complications, and a number of marginally effective strategies have been reported. We favor pretreatment with intragraft urokinase (500,000 to 1,000,000 U over 2 to 8 hours) followed by heparinization for several days prior to intervention. Although prolonged urokinase infusion can recanalize even chronically occluded saphenous vein grafts, the long-term gain relative to risk, discomfort, and cost is usually small overall. A rare patient, however, may obtain quite good long-term results. In the largest reported series, in-hospital complications occurred in one-third of patients.[11] While use of DCA and TEC devices has permitted broadening of indications in aging saphenous vein grafts, complications and late cardiac events are common and this should engender a conservative approach. Conversely, intervention with balloon angioplasty at distal anastomotic lesions in saphenous vein grafts is associated with very low complications and restenosis rates. Consequently , when these lesions appear within a few years of surgery, they should not be treated with nonballoon devices unless refractory restenosis occurs.

Internal Mammary Artery Graft Intervention

Most lesions in either left internal mammary artery (LIMA) or right internal mammary artery (RIMA) grafts can be successfully treated from a femoral approach using 7- or 8-F guide catheters. A brachial artery approach may be preferred if it is difficult to seat the femoral catheter and especially if poor guide catheter support is noted in the presence of severe graft tortuosity or distal location of the targeted lesion (Fig. 37-4). A novel guide catheter shape for a brachial approach to internal mammary angioplasty has been reported.[12] In patients with significant subclavian artery stenosis (or occlusion), dilation or stenting has been performed before CABG to permit use of the LIMA and following CABG to improve symptoms in patients with LIMA in place.[13,14] In general, a balloon-on-a-wire dilation catheter is favored for internal mammary artery PTCA, but an over-the-wire system is used when maximal steerability is required, for recanalization of total occlu-

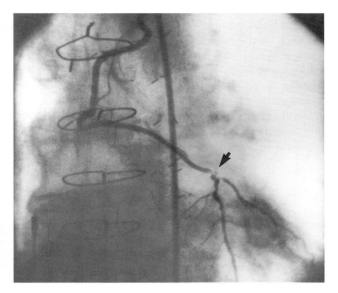

Fig. 37-4. A 73-year-old man developed recurrent angina 2 to 3 months following CABG and was found to have high-grade stenosis at the junction of LIMA and left anterior descending artery, a patent saphenous vein graft to the obtuse marginals, and a normal right coronary artery. Because of severe LIMA tortuosity, he was treated medically for 18 months, but symptoms worsened and an attempt at PTCA at this site from a femoral approach was unsuccessful (8-F internal mammary angioplasty guide catheter and 20-mm balloon-on-a-wire) due to inadequate backup. An attempt from the left brachial approach was successful using an internal mammary angioplasty guide catheter, probe sheath, and 20-mm balloon-on-a-wire. Use of the probe sheath enhanced both backup and steerability.

sions, or if passage retrograde into the proximal native coronary artery is required. Perfusion catheters and stents are useful to improve results of internal mammary artery PTCA, but these strategies are rarely needed for anastomotic lesions, the most common and the most favorable IMA lesions for PTCA.[15,16] Patient comfort is enhanced by usage of a low-osmolar contrast agent and a recent blinded study suggested that ioxaglate, a low-osmolar ionic dimer, was better tolerated than iopamidal, a nonionic monomer.[17]

POSTPROCEDURAL MANAGEMENT

Post-CABG patients undergoing successful uncomplicated PTCA receive routine management and are discharged from the hospital within 24 hours.[6] Postprocedural heparinization is used in patients with documented or suspected thrombus, stent implantation, native vessel rotational atherectomy, or at the operator's discretion. Coumadin anticoagulation is rarely utilized (stents, definite thrombus, occasional saphenous vein graft) and then usually along with aspirin therapy, which is ubiquitous unless contraindicated. Coumadin therapy in stented patients is usually continued for 3 months. Patients receive instruction in low-fat diet, cessation of smoking, and exercise, and lipid lowering agents are prescribed as indicated.

FOLLOW-UP

Patients receive recommendations for follow-up evaluation that are tailored to their probability of restenosis (or occlusion) and possible consequences. Most patients are advised to undergo a functional evaluation at 3 to 4 months or sooner if symptoms recur, and patients judged to be at high risk are advised to have repeat coronary arteriography.

RESULTS OF INTERVENTION

Patient selection factors largely determine procedural success and complication rates of coronary intervention in patients with prior CABG. Over a decade ago, in 129 consecutive post-CABG patients, the success rate approached 90%, 1 patient had Q-wave infarction, 4 had non-Q-wave infarction, and no in-hospital deaths occurred.[2] In more than 2,000 reported saphenous vein graft angioplasties, procedural success was 90%, emergency CABG was required in 0.3 to 5%, Q-wave infarction occurred in 0 to 2.5%, and 0.8% died.[18] The most frequent complication of saphenous vein graft intervention, non-Q-wave myocardial infarction, was noted in 13% of 672 vein graft angioplasties at Emory, with most infarctions occurring in saphenous vein grafts in place for over 3 years.[19] The highest success rate and lowest complication rates occurred in angioplasty of lesions at the distal anastomosis (graft-native vessel junction). The most common cause of in-hospital mortality in early series was embolic myocardial infarction following recanalization of totally occluded saphenous vein grafts. Intervention in older grafts has been associated with a higher complication rate, especially when thrombus was associated. In a recently published series of saphenous vein graft interventions, directional and extraction atherectomy yielded a procedural success in 76% when thrombus was present, but in-hospital mortality was over 3%, and 24% of patients with diffuse saphenous vein graft disease had myocardial infarction even though one-half of patients were pretreated with urokinase.[20] Preliminary results from the CAVEAT II comparison of DCA with balloon angioplasty in saphenous vein grafts indicate better angiographic results with DCA, but more Q-wave infarctions and similar restenosis. Although the use of atherectomy devices may have permitted expansion of indications for intervention in aging saphenous vein grafts, complications and late cardiac events are relatively common.

Initial results of multicenter use of the Palmaz-Schatz coronary stent in saphenous vein grafts have been quite favorable. In 626 patients, stent deployment was successful in 98.7%; myocardial infarction occurred in 1.9%, CABG occurred in 3.9%, and in-hospital mortality was 2.3%. Only 1.3% of patients experienced stent thrombosis.[10] Angiographic follow-up in 299 patients at 6.6 months revealed restenosis in 27%, 18% in de novo lesions, and 38% in those with prior PTCA. A randomized comparison of the use of this stent with balloon angioplasty is currently in progress. A recently published review summarized the less favorable results of the use of other stents in saphenous vein grafts.[21] Multicenter use of the excimer laser in vein grafts has produced initial success, complication, and restenosis rates comparable to those reported for balloon angioplasty.[22]

Results of intervention for internal mammary artery graft lesions have been published in 17 reports totaling 177 patients; success was achieved in 164 (93%), and complications were infrequent (1 Q-wave infarction, 5 dissections, and no deaths).[18] Restenosis occurred in only 6 of 33 patients who had follow-up angiography. Although most of the reported cases had lesions at the anastomosis of graft to native coronary artery, 12 of 32 lesions in one report were at the ostium or extremely proximal portion of IMA grafts. Although restenosis at the anastomosis site is uncommon following balloon angioplasty (probably less common than at any other site), the long-term outcome following PTCA at the other sites is unknown.

The long-term prognosis of patients who have undergone PTCA after CABG is dependent on multiple clinical factors (age, extent of native vessel and graft disease, left ventricular function) as well as the probability of restenosis of the site(s) instrumented. In over 1,500 patients who had native vessel PTCA, actuarial survival at 6 years was 81% and event-free survival 55%.[23] Multivariate predictors of survival were ejection fraction less than 40%, age greater than 70, unstable angina, and multivessel disease. In approximately 600 patients who underwent balloon angioplasty of saphenous vein grafts at Emory University, 5-year survival was 81% and myocardial infarction-free survival 62%.[19] Myocardial infarction-free, repeat revascularization-free survival was 31% at 5 years. Restenosis occurred in 45% of lesions at the distal anastomosis, 61% of mid-vein graft lesions, and 68% at the proximal anastomosis. Survival at 5 years was 92% for distal lesions, 72% for mid-vein lesions, and 67% for proximal lesions ($P < 0.0001$). Unfortunately, development of lesions in older grafts, particularly at ostial and mid-vein sites, predicts late cardiac events in at least 20 to 30% of patients within 6 months irrespective of the percutaneous revascularization strategy applied.[24]

CURRENT INDICATIONS

Recurrence of ischemia after CABG may be related to lesions in native coronary arteries or bypass grafts, or both. Selection for intervention must be based on a careful analysis of factors such as the likelihood of a successful procedure, risk of complications, and probability of long-term symptomatic benefit compared with medical therapy and repeat CABG.[2,7,18] In patients experiencing recurrence of angina soon after CABG, coronary arteriography is indicated. Graft occlusion and perianastomotic lesions are common, and angioplasty of native vessels or anastomotic lesions of vein or arterial grafts can often be attempted with reasonable risk and good long-term benefit. Recanalization of thrombosed vein grafts within a month of CABG is probably unwarranted due to risks of thrombolytic therapy and low probability of long-term patency. We have however, been able to recanalize short-segment occlusions in internal mammary angioplasty grafts with documented late patency. Focal lesions in grafts appearing within 3 years of CABG can be treated with balloon angioplasty, atherectomy, excimer laser, or stents with very small procedural morbidity or mortality; lesion characteristics, however, frequently influence the choice of interventional strategy. We believe that stenting will be the treatment of choice for mid-saphenous vein graft lesions when it becomes generally available. We commonly use DCA for ostial lesions and some very eccentric or bulky vein graft lesions when reoperation does not seem justified. In grafts in place for more than 3 years, atherosclerotic lesions increase relative to age of graft, and the threat of coronary atheroembolization restricts intervention to relatively focal disease.

The status of the LAD and its graft should influence the choice of revascularization strategies. Reoperation is frequently advised when a vein graft to a large LAD is severely diseased, whereas a patent arterial graft to the LAD favors nonsurgical therapy. Angioplasty is generally not preferred for thrombus-laden grafts, although prolonged thrombolytic therapy or TEC, or both, may be considered in selected patients in whom reoperation is not a good option. Recanalization of totally occluded saphenous vein grafts not associated with acute myocardial infarction is controversial and rarely justified in our experience.

COSTS

Detailed analysis of the costs of repeat revascularization strategies in post-CABG patients has not been published. Recent analysis, however, of hospital costs in a broad range of patients undergoing coronary intervention indicates that a number of preprocedural clinical factors are associated with increased cost (unstable angina, cardiogenic shock, elective stent placement, angiographic thrombus, age 70 years).[25] Because of the frequent use of more costly new devices in post-CABG patients and the higher late cardiac event rate, assessment of clinical benefit relative to cost is particularly important in this patient subgroup.

CONCLUSIONS

The interventional cardiologist's array of strategies for percutaneous coronary therapy (balloon, laser, atherectomy, stents) has its greatest application in the postoperative patient with recurrent angina. In selecting treatment, the clinician must carefully weigh the options with the aim of obtaining the most cost-effective and long-lasting revascularization possible at the lowest risk. Patients most likely to benefit are those with focal lesions of native coronary arteries, arterial grafts, or distal vein graft anastomotic sites. The most difficult problems in patients with prior bypass surgery are vein graft atheroembolism and restenosis. Palmaz-Schatz stenting, as promising as it appears for reducing restenosis, does not obviate atheroembolism. Patients best suited for repeat surgery have multiple complex lesions or degenerated saphenous vein grafts (or both) and adequate left ventricular function.

REFERENCES

1. Gruentzig AR, Senning A, Siegenthaler WE. Nonoperative dilatation of coronary-artery stenosis. Percutaneous transluminal coronary angioplasty. N Engl J Med 1979;301:61–8
2. Douglas JS Jr, Gruentzig AR, King SB III et al. Percutaneous transluminal coronary angioplasty in patients with prior coronary bypass surgery. J Am Coll Cardiol 1983;2:745–54
3. Loop FD, Lytle BW, Cosgrove DM et al. Reoperation for coronary atherosclerosis. Ann Surg 1990;212:378–86
4. Mills RM, Kalan JM. Developing a rational management strategy for angina pectoris after coronary bypass surgery: a clinical decision analysis. Clin Cardiol 1991;14:191–7
5. Weintraub WS, Jones EL, Craver JM et al. Incidence of repeat revasularization after coronary bypass surgery. J Am Coll Cardiol 1992;19:98A
6. Douglas JS Jr, King SB III. Techniques of percutaneous transluminal angioplasty and atherectomy of the coronary arteries. pp. 1345–58. In Alexander RW, Schlant RC (eds): Hurst's The Heart. 8th Ed. McGraw-Hill, New York, 1994
7. Ryan TJ, Bauman WB, Kennedy JW et al. Guidelines for percutaneous transluminal coronary angioplasty. J Am Coll Cardiol 1993;22:2033–54
8. Stratienko AA, Ginsberg R, Schatz RA et al. Technique for shortening angioplasty guide catheter length when therapeutic catheter fails to reach target stenosis. Cathet Cardiovasc Diagn 1993;30:331–3
9. Kahn JK, Hartzler GO: Retrograde coronary angioplasty of isolated arterial segments through saphenous vein bypass grafts. Cathet Cardiovasc Diagn 1990;20:88–93.
10. Leon MB, Wong SC, Pichard AD. Balloon-expandable stent implantation in saphenous vein grafts. p. 11. In Henmann HC, Hirshfeld JW (eds): Clinical Use of the Palmaz-Schatz Intracoronary Stent. Futura, Mount Kisco, NY, 1993
11. Hartmann JR, McKeever LA, Stamato NJ et al. Recanalization of chronically occluded aortocoronary saphenous vein bypass grafts by extended infusion of urokinase: initial results and short-term clinical follow-up. J Am Coll Cardiol 1991;18:1517–23
12. Brown RIG, Gilligan L, Penn IM et al. Right internal

mammary artery graft angioplasty through a right brachial artery approach using a new custom guide catheter: a case report. Cathet Cardiovasc Diagn 1992; 25:42–5

13. Ernst S, Bal E, Plokker T et al. Percutaneous balloon angioplasty (PBA) of a left subclavian artery stenosis or occlusion to establish adequate flow through the left internal mammary artery for coronary bypass purposes. Circulation 1991;84:II-591

14. Shapira S, Braun S, Puram B et al. Percutaneous transluminal angioplasty of proximal subclavian artery stenosis after left internal mammary to left anterior descending artery bypass surgery. J Am Coll Cardiol 1991;18:1120–3

15. Almagor Y, Thomas J, Colombo A. Balloon expandable stent implantation of a stenosis at the origin of the left internal mammary artery graft. Cathet Cardiovasc Diagn 1991;24:256–8

16. Bajaj RK, Roubin GS. Intravascular stenting of the right internal mammary artery. Cathet Cardiovasc Diagn 1991;24:252–5

17. Miller RM, Knox M. Patient tolerance of ioxaglate and iopamidol in internal mammary artery arteriography. Cathet Cardiovasc Diagn 1992;25:31–4

18. Douglas JS Jr. Percutaneous intervention in patients with prior coronary bypass surgery. pp. 339–54. In Topol EJ (ed): Text Book of Interventional Cardiology. WB Saunders, Philadelphia, 1994

19. Douglas JS Jr, Weintraub WS, Liberman HA et al. Update of saphenous vein graft (SVG) angioplasty: restenosis and long term outcome. Circulation 1991;84: II-249

20. Guzman LA, Villa AE, Whitlow P. New atherectomy devices in the treatment of old saphenous vein grafts: are the initial results encouraging? Circulation 1992; 86:I-780

21. DeFeyter PJ, Van Suylen RJ, DeJaegere PPT et al. Balloon angioplasty for the treatment of lesions in saphenous vein bypass grafts. J Am Coll Cardiol 1993; 22:1539–49

22. Untereker WJ, Palacios IF, Hartzler G et al. Excimer laser coronary angioplasty of saphenous vein grafts. Circulation 1992;86:I-780

23. Miranda CP, Rutherford BD, McConahay DR et al. Elective PTCA in post-bypass patients: comparison between those undergoing native artery dilatations and those undergoing bypass graft dilatations. Circulation 1992;86:I-457

24. Sketch MH Jr, Davidson CJ, Schatz RA et al. Predictors of clinical outcome with new device usage in saphenous vein grafts. Circulation 1993;88:I-645

25. Ellis SG, Grierson J, Brown KJ et al. Correlates of increased hospital cost of coronary intervention. Circulation 1993;88:I-602

38 Angioplasty Alternatives

Douglass A. Morrison

In the United States, more than 500,000 patients are admitted to the hospital annually with a diagnosis of unstable angina,[1] which is frequently cited as the reason for performing coronary angiography,[2] coronary artery bypass graft surgery (CABG),[3] and percutaneous transluminal coronary angioplasty (PTCA).[4,5] Among patients undergoing these procedures, adverse outcomes are consistently more frequent in patients with unstable angina compared with patients who have stable angina or no symptoms.[3–6]

UNSTABLE ANGINA IS A HETEROGENEOUS GROUP OF DISORDERS

Unstable angina is composed of a spectrum of clinical entities.[7] At one end are patients with relatively mild symptoms, which may be infrequent or difficult to elicit, or both; most of these patients have a favorable prognosis. At the other end are patients with more frequent symptoms that are easy to elicit. These patients appear to have a less favorable prognosis, at least over the short term. Among the least favorable prognostic subsets are "medically refractory" unstable angina patients.[7,8] Two empiric observations from the surgical literature regarding patients with medically refractory rest angina are that

1. Medically refractory patients with acute ischemic syndromes, *as a group,* benefit from surgical revascularization.[9–18]
2. The risk of adverse outcomes (morbidity and mortality) with surgical revascularization is significantly higher when surgery is performed on medically refractory than medically stabilized patients.[9–22]

These points are tempered by both the lack of uniformity and the lack of precision with which the terms unstable angina, medically refractory, medically stabilized, acute ischemic syndrome, and high risk have been defined.[22]

MEDICALLY REFRACTORY UNSTABLE ANGINA

The following concepts are relevant to the discussion of medically refractory unstable angina.[8]

Prospective, randomized trial data suggest that a medical regimen *must* include aspirin and probably aspirin and heparin (directed at a therapeutic target such as 1 partial thromboplastin time 60 to 80 seconds) for the patient to be considered "refractory."[23–26]

Simply specifying that the patient is on an antianginal regimen including drugs of various categories (β-blockers, nitrates, calcium blockers) *or* above arbitrary doses is not adequate. There are large individual variances in response. A more reasonable concept is to use enough of one or more drugs to lower heart rate and blood pressure to some target levels.[8,27–29]

It is clear that different physicians have highly variable "thresholds" for the use of either intravenous nitroglycerin or intra-aortic balloon counterpulsation. Nevertheless, in the Veterans Administration Surgical Registry, regardless of threshold or justification, to CABG on both of these therapies (prior to CABG) have emerged as powerful independent risk factors.[21] Thus they point toward "medically refractory."

The questions of how long a patient must be on a regimen, how many episodes of symptoms are necessary, and whether reversible electrocardiographic (ECG) changes are required to be labeled refractory are unsettled.[8,19,20,30] These issues appear to be individual and require clinical judgment that is difficult to codify.

There are strong feelings and relatively few objective data relevant to which drugs should be used first and whether one drug should be titrated to maximum before a second or third category of antianginal is added.[31] Many excellent clinicians extrapolate from data obtained in acute myocardial infarction and chronic stable angina cohorts to recommend β-blockers first, titrated toward resting bradycardia. The frequency of severe left ventricular dysfunction, chronic obstructive pulmonary disease with a reversible component, and diabetes (among other co-morbidities) can clearly impact on this approach. Conversely, many other excellent clinicians use intravenous nitroglycerin as first-line therapy. Finally, much of the registry and prospective trial data that we have all used to guide our thinking were obtained before many of the currently used drugs (including aspirin and intravenous nitroglycerin) were either recognized as effective or commercially available.

"HIGH RISK" FOR ADVERSE OUTCOMES WITH CABG

Extent of coronary disease, defined as one, two, or three vessels with a more than 70% luminal diameter narrowing has consistently emerged from data registries and trials as a risk factor.[3,9–22] Left main coronary narrowing is also a recognized risk factor.[3,9–22]

Ventricular dysfunction defined as left ventricular ejection fraction (LVEF) less than 0.55 is a risk factor. LVEF less than 0.35 or 0.30 is a stronger risk factor; patients with this "severe" left ventricular dysfunction category have been systematically excluded from most randomized trials.[3,9–22] Accordingly, extrapolation from data obtained in patients with LVEF measures between 0.30 and 0.55 to recommend CABG for patients with LVEF less than 0.30 is intuitive but not necessarily valid.

Almost every practicing cardiac surgeon "knows" that extent of coronary disease in terms of diffuse disease is highly predictive of adverse outcomes with CABG.[3] To my knowledge, no surgeon knows how to

define or codify rigorously "diffuse disease." Accordingly, how patients with "diffuse disease" have been identified and excluded from randomized trials is difficult to say. What is abundantly clear is that this factor is among the most important used by surgeons to turn down cases (see section on Prohibitive Risk below).[22,32]

The VA Surgical Registry, among other data bases, has provided much important information on univariate clinical factors that predict risk of adverse outcomes with CABG.[3,21] The following factors have been identified as among the predictors of high risk:

1. Prior heart surgery
2. Age greater than 70 years
3. Recent myocardial infarction (various definitions most commonly, <7 days or <30 days)
4. LVEF less than 0.35
5. Coming to CABG on intravenous nitroglycerin
6. Coming to CABG on intra-aortic balloon pump (IABP)
7. Emergency CABG (<24 hours) after catheterization
8. Rales on physical examination
9. Coming to CABG on diuretics

The following co-morbidities are among those recognized to confer additional risk with CABG[21]:

1. Peripheral vascular disease by history or examination
2. Chronic obstructive pulmonary disease
3. Diabetes, especially requiring insulin
4. Hypertensive cardiovascular disease (i.e., with left ventricular hypertrophy)
5. Hepatic dysfunction
6. Cerebrovascular insufficiency

Multivariate models have been developed to refine further the assessment of risk of adverse outcomes with CABG.[3,19–22]

An important corollary of this brief review of CABG risk factors should be apparent: the symptomatic patients presenting for revascularization appear to be weighted toward higher risk with each passing year. There are more older patients as the "baby boom" population ages (risk 2). There are more post-CABG patients coming back with angina after their surgeries in the 1970s and 1980s (risk 1). The success of thrombolysis and vasodilators and diuretics has produced more myocardial infarction survivors with severe ventricular dysfunction (risk 4). Therapeutic advances in other specialties have been accompanied by more survivors with advanced co-morbidities who then develop symptomatic myocardial ischemia. Accordingly, for most clinicians, the treatment of high risk-unstable angina is becoming a larger part of our practice every year.

"PROHIBITIVE RISK"

At the extreme end of the high-risk medically refractory unstable ischemia spectrum one can find patients who are so "high risk" that surgery does not seem reasonable[32-34] (Table 38-1). This is a painful reality for most cardiac surgeons who have worked diligently to become proficient, and accordingly they rarely write about it. Two reports *have* evaluated patients with "prohibitive risk," including seriously demented or metastatic cancer patients.[19,20] Nearly every other patient becomes "individualized" to the point that teasing out the underlying concepts becomes difficult. The undisputed reality is that there are objectively documented patients with medically refractory rest angina (reversible ECG changes, with pain despite medication, to the point of resting bradycardia or early heart failure) who are refused surgical revascularization.[32] In the past, this has meant it would be inconsistent to use a balloon pump (a bridge to revascularization) or even perform coronary angiography (since surgery was the only revascularization option). Such patients are usually moved out of the unit and given narcotics. I am unaware of any systematic study, but my experience is that, although the long-term outlook is grim, some patients can be admitted multiple times before they die.[32]

THE SALVAGE ANGIOPLASTY HYPOTHESIS

Balloon angioplasty is an alternative revascularization strategy for medically refractory rest angina patients who have been refused surgery on the basis of "prohibitive risk."[22,32] We have reported our early experience with 34 consecutive patients who were admitted to our hospital with medically refractory rest angina, refused surgical revascularization, and then given salvage angioplasty[32] (Table 38-1). Our results have been encouraging enough to continue, and we have currently performed salvage angioplasty on more than 150 patients with discharge from index hospitalization in more than 90%.[35,36]

The rationale for salvage angioplasty is straightforward.[32] Unstable high-risk patients are less able to tolerate physiologic perturbations than stable patients. Bypass surgery involves several major physiologic perturbations that need not accompany angioplasty such as (1) general anesthesia, (2) cardiopulmonary bypass, (3) ventricular fibrillation and defibrillation, (4) cardioplegia, (5) large volume shifts and frequent transfusion of blood products, and (6) opening of the pleural and pericardial spaces.

High-Risk Angioplasty: The Denver VA Experience

In the 5-year period from May 1988 through June 1993, 6,342 patients were admitted to the intensive care units of the Denver VA; Medical Center 1,020 (16%) had a diagnosis of unstable angina and 813 (13%) patients were admitted with a diagnosis of "rule out" myocardial infarction.[35] (Table 38-2). Presumably, many of the "rule outs" ruled out, and some of these became unstable angina; similarly, many of

Table 38-1. The Denver VA Salvage PTCA Experience

	No. %
Patients estimated 30-day CABG mortality	34 23.8
Actual 30-day mortality	4/34 11.8
Acute myocardial infarction	4/34 11.8
Went home	30/34 89

(From Morrison et al.,[32] with permission.)

Table 38-2. Demographics of Patients With Unstable Angina at Denver VA Medical Center Between May 1988 and June 1993

Category	No. (%)
Admission to intensive care	
Total	6,342 (100)
With diagnosis of unstable angina	1,020 (16)
With diagnosis, rule out myocardial infarction	813 (13)
Underwent coronary arteriography	2,144 (100)
Underwent coronary angiography with presumptive diagnosis of unstable angina	1,136 (53)
Underwent CABG	578
Underwent PTCA	624 (100)
Subsets among 624 PTCA patients	
Unstable angina	441 (71)
Rest angina	288 (46)
Medically refractory	225 (36)
Medically refractory with ≥ risk factors	207 (33)

the unstable patients were stabilized and some were found to be noncardiac. During the same time frame, 2,144 patients came to coronary angiography; 1,136 (47%) of these were for unstable angina. During this period 578 patients underwent CABG and 624 patients underwent PTCA.

Components of "High-Risk" Unstable Angina in the Denver Experience

Among the 624 patients who underwent PTCA, 441 (71%) had unstable angina, 288 had rest angina, and 225 had medically refractory rest angina where medically refractory was defined as pain despite:

1. Bed rest in an intensive care unit
2. Low flow oxygen
3. Intravenous heparin
4. Oral aspirin
5. Enough nitrate and or β-blocker or calcium blocker so that heart rate was less than 70 bpm or blood pressure less than 140 mmHg

From the VA Surgical Registry, six univariate factors associated with a 9% or greater risk of perioperative (30-day) mortality were identified:

1. Prior CABG
2. Age greater than 70 years

Table 38-4. Outcome of 207 Medically Refractory Patients With Unstable Angina at High Risk for Mortality at PTCA

Characteristics	No. (%)
Discharged after PTCA	196 (95)
Discharged angina-free	186 (90)
Emergency CABG	2 (1)
In-hospital infarction	9 (4)
Late infarctions	17 (8)
Late CABG	8 (4)
Late PTCA	44 (21)

3. Left ventricular ejection fraction less than 0.35
4. Recent myocardial infarction ($\leq$ 30 days)
5. Intravenous nitroglycerin
6. IABP

Among the 207 patients with medically refractory rest angina and at least one "risk factor" who underwent angioplasty, the numbers and proportions with each risk factor are as shown in Table 38-3. Of these 207 medically refractory rest angina patients, 196 (95%) went home and 186 (90%) went home angina free. There were 11 in-hospital deaths (5.1%). Nine patients (4.2%) had periprocedural infarctions and two (.9%) went to emergency CABG (Table 38-4).

In late follow-up (from 3 to 60 months; average, 24 months), have been nine patients (4%) were lost and

Table 38-3. Patient Population: Denver VA High-Risk PTCA

Patient Risk Characteristic	No.	%
Coronary anatomy		
one-vessel	67	32
two-vessel	49	24
three-vessel	91	44
LVEF (measured in 129 patients)		
$\geq$0.55	66	51
0.35–0.55	33	26
Under 0.35	30	23
"High-risk" factors for CABG		
Age >70 years	34	17
Prior CABG	85	41
Prior myocardial infarction	108	52
IV nitroglycerin	126	61
IABP	31	15
"Prohibitive risk"		
Refused CABG	55	26
Hemodynamic compromise	29	14

Table 38-5. CABG and PTCA Survival (Estimates in %) for Registry (1987–1988) and Denver CABG (1987–1993) and Denver PTCA (1988–1993) Patients

Months After Surgery	CABG Registry	CABG Denver	PTCA Denver
1	88	92	93
6	85	89	90
12	82	88	87
18	81	86	84
24	79	85	82
30	77	83	82
36	75	83	77
42	73	81	76
48	71	80	—
60	68	77	—
Number	1,043	222	207
Person years of follow-up	3.8	3.2	2.0

Table 38-6. Specific High-Risk Factor Percentage Among Unstable Angina High-Risk Registry (1987–1988) and Denver CABG and Denver PTCA Patients 1987–1993

Risk Factor	CABG Registry	CABG Denver	PTCA Denver
Age 70+	17	18	17
Prior CABG	28	21	41
Recent myocardial infarction	54	35	52
IV nitroglycerine	44	62	61
IABP	13	15	15
LVEF <0.35	19	7	23[a]

a LVEF measured in 129 of 207 PTCA patients.

3. Shock or hemodynamic compromise
4. Coronary anatomy unfavorable for PTCA
5. Co-morbidity

Multivessel Disease Revascularization

Multivessel angioplasty was a paradigm shift from the role proposed for PTCA by its founder, Andreas Gruntzig.[38] The first issue to be confronted was an increased risk of acute occlusive syndromes by virtue of multiple vessel dilation. The nightmare of this strategy would be the acute occlusion of a single vessel, leading to hypotension and thus to occlusions of other diseased or dilated vessels. A second potential problem with multivessel angioplasty that had not been confronted with single-vessel angioplasty had to do with vessels that were significant (i.e., flow limiting) but not amenable to dilation, such as old total occlusions. This led to the concept of "incomplete revascularization," which had proved problematic for surgical revascularization.[3-5]

A third issue in the multivessel paradigm is that of restenosis; with multiple dilations, the risk of at least one lesion restenosing and resulting in subsequent procedures appeared to increase at least in an additive fashion.[4,5]

For unstable angina patients, a breakthrough concept was that of the culprit lesion, (i.e., the ischemia-producing artery).[39] If the vessel causing the symptoms could be identified, single-lesion angioplasty could potentially provide stabilization even in a patient with multivessel disease.[39]

Enthusiasm for culprit lesion angioplasty must be balanced not only by awareness of incomplete revascularization, but also by the realization that unstable lesions are much more likely to clot and occlude acutely. The empiric data regarding (1) higher rates of acute occlusive syndromes and (2) benefits of predilation treatment with heparin are widely acknowledged.[4,5] Procedural use of thrombolytics, anticoagulants, and antispasmodics are more controversial.

The recently reported United Kingdom Randomized Intervention Treatment of Angina (RITA) trial compared mortality and infarction rates between cohorts treated with CABG versus PTCA.[40] In that study, 55% of patients had multivessel disease and 59% had experienced rest angina.[40] The combined death and infarction rates were not different between the two strategies at 2 1/2 years. Reports of other randomized trials, specifically the Emory Angioplasty Surgery Trial and the German Angioplasty Bypass Investigation, support the notion that mul-

follow-up, there were 27 additional deaths, giving a total of 38 deaths or 19% long-term mortality. Late CABG was performed in 8 patients (4%) and repeat PTCA was performed in 44 (21%), with late infarction in 17 (8%). The mortality of 220 "high-risk" patients who underwent CABG at the Denver VA Medical Center is contrasted with the mortality of the 207 Denver VA PTCA patients and a cohort of 2,570 patients who underwent CABG nationwide (high-risk VA Surgical Registry; Table 38-5 and 38-6).

In a large consecutive case cohort of patients who "needed" revascularization by virtue of medically refractory rest angina, all of whom had at least one univariate factor associated with short-term CABG mortality of 9% or more, angioplasty provided an alternative revascularization strategy. Which strategy (PTCA or CABG) is preferred to stabilize "high-risk" medically refractory rest angina patients can only be definitively answered by a prospective randomized clinical trial.

PARADIGM SHIFT IN REVASCULARIZATION STRATEGY

To effect a major change in the way one attempts to solve a problem, Thomas Kuhn[31] has suggested that we must first effect a change in thinking about the problem, which he has called a "paradigm shift." To develop angioplasty as a viable alternative to surgery for "high-risk" patients, a paradigm shift is required. The revascularization paradigm is made up of several components, which may be considered separately:

1. Multivessel disease
2. Severe left ventricular dysfunction

tivessel disease patients have comparable rates of death and infarction by 1 year whether they are revascularized by PTCA or CABG.[41,42] Repeat revascularization rates and relief of symptoms appear to favor CABG for multivessel disease. More importantly, all three of these trials excluded more than 92% of screened patients, with most angiographic exclusion being done by the interventionists.[40–42] Consecutive retrospective case reports from numerous centers have documented the feasibility and safety of PTCA as an alternative revascularization strategy for unstable angina patients with multivessel disease.[28,29,43–46] Nevertheless, acute complications and restenosis rates are higher for PTCA in multivessel-disease patients than in single-vessel disease patients.[4,5] Similarly, the data from prospective trials suggest that late procedures (coronary angiography, PTCA, and CABG) are performed significantly more frequently for multivessel-disease patients who undergo an initial PTCA as opposed to initial CABG.[40–42]

None of the trials or consecutive case studies focuses on medically refractory rest angina. In our series, 155 of 212 patients (73%) had two- or three-vessel disease. We performed two-vessel angioplasty in 55 patients, three-vessel angioplasty in 6 patients, and one-vessel angioplasty in 151 patients.

Severe Left Ventricular Dysfunction

Patients with severe left ventricular dysfunction (defined as LVEF < 0.35) have been excluded from PTCA versus CABG trials just as they were excluded from the older CABG versus medical therapy trials.[3–5,40–42]

Several retrospective, consecutive case series have supported the feasibility of performing PTCA in selected cases.[47–50] These series consistently document higher rates of adverse outcomes than seen when PTCA was performed in patients with normal systolic left ventricular function.[47–50] These series were not focused on refractory rest angina.

Our series includes 30 patients with measured LVEF less than 0.35 and 29 additional patients with sustained blood pressure less than 100 mmHg. (We do not routinely perform contrast ventriculography on patients with unstable ischemia and sustained hypotension). Of the 30 patients with reduced LVEF, 29 went home; 25 of these were angina free and 9 completed negative treadmill exercise testing.

Hemodynamic Instability

A number of retrospective consecutive case series in the literature support revascularization (most often by angioplasty) attempts in acute infarction compli-

cated by cardiogenic shock.[51–53] These studies do not address the issue of PTCA versus CABG. Clearly the distinction between infarction and unstable angina is blurred in the presence of shock.

Our series includes 29 patients who arrived with sustained hypotension and underwent PTCA. Mortality in this cohort was 21% (6 of 29) by the end of index hospitalization. Accordingly, 23 of these patients were discharged from the hospital. Whether CABG could have been performed on these 29 patients with a lower mortality is not known.

Coronary Anatomy Unfavorable for PTCA

Our ongoing trial diverts most clearly from contemporary practice when it comes to coronary anatomy.

The American College of Physicians/American College of Cardiology/American Heart Association (ACP/ACC/AHA) guideline lists the following types of anatomy as "type C lesions"[4,5]:

- Diffuse (>20 mm)
- Excessive tortuosity of proximal segment
- Extremely angulated segments (90°)
- Total occlusions (>3 months old)
- Inability to protect major side branches
- Degenerated vein grafts with viable lesions

The guidelines goes on to state that success can be expected less than 60% of the time and that complications are "high" with C lesions. Accordingly, the guideline concludes that "type C are not considered suitable for PTCA."[4,5]

By contrast, both Goudreau et al.[54] and Brymer et al.[55] have reported success rate of more than 90% with the diffuse (>20 mm) subset.

In our study, most cases involved type C lesions.[35] Clinical success in pain-free (patients sent home) was 90%.[35] This is similar to our report of 89 vein graft lesions in 75 consecutive cases.[36]

Perhaps equally important, all the cases reported here were done with conventional balloon angioplasty. Adjunctive pharmacotherapy was used, but atherectomy, lasers, or stents were not employed.

Co-morbidity

Clinically significant co-morbidity is prevalent in an elderly population. Specific co-morbidities that cause surgeons to consider refusing CABG include:

1. Metastatic cancer
2. Severe dementia
3. Chronic obstructive pulmonary disease severe enough to necessitate chronic systemic corticosteroid use or chronic home oxygen therapy, or both
4. Chronic systemic corticosteroid use for another medical condition (i.e., rheumatoid disease)
5. Chronic renal failure (i.e., chronic serum creatinine, >2.0 or necessitating chronic dialysis, or both)
6. Peripheral vascular disease significant enough to preclude femoral access for IABP or cardiopulmonary support (we have percutaneously used femfem bypass grafts as access for PTCA or IABP without complication)
7. Cardiogenic shock (most of these revascularization attempts are currently done by PTCA in our hospital)
8. Acute pulmonary edema or noncardiac respiratory failure necessitating intubation and mechanical ventilation (patients whose ischemia is ongoing usually receive PTCA)

VETERANS AFFAIRS COOPERATIVE STUDY 385

In October of 1993 the Cooperative Studies Evaluation Committee approved VA Cooperative Study 385, Angina With Extremely Serious Operative Mortality Evaluation (AWESOME). In February 1995 this study began to enroll patients with unstable angina defined by any one of the following:

1. Recurrent rest angina
2. Rest angina with reversible ECG changes
3. Rest angina without ECG change, but occurring in a patient with prior infarct or angiographically documented coronary artery disease
4. Postinfarction angina
5. Unstable angina medically stabilized, but followed by an abnormal low-level exercise test

From this unstable angina cohort, a medically refractory cohort are identified. These patients continue to have angina or angina equivalent despite

1. Bed rest
2. Low-flow oxygen
3. Oral aspirin
4. Intravenous heparin
5. Enough nitrate or β-blocker or calcium blocker such that resting heart rate is less than 70 bpm or resting blood pressure is less than 140 mmHg, or both

From among these medically refractory angina patients, "high-risk" for adverse outcome with CABG patients are identified by virtue of having two or more of the following risk factors:

1. Prior CABG
2. Age greater than 70 years
3. LVEF less than 0.35
4. Recent (30 days) infarction
5. Intravenous nitroglycerin
6. Intra-aortic balloon counterpulsation

Coronary arteriograms are performed in a standard fashion and reviewed by both cardiothoracic surgeons and interventional cardiologists to assess revascularization potential using either CABG or PTCA. Patients accepted by both the surgeons and the cardiologists are approached for voluntary participation in the randomized trial. Patients who are rejected by either surgeons or interventionists or who refuse randomization are being followed in a registry. Patients who are accepted by both surgeons and cardiologists and who sign voluntary informed consent forms are being randomized to either initial CABG or PTCA. Co-morbidities are being noted but are not part of the randomization or stratification in AWESOME.

Randomized patients are being prospectively followed for survival, myocardial infarction, repeat hospitalization, repeat coronary angiograms, subsequent revascularization by either PTCA or CABG, symptoms, exercise tolerance, and quality of life. Patients are enrolled for 4 years and an additional year of follow-up is planned. Because uniform enrollment over time is anticipated, an average follow-up of 3 years is planned.

The study plan calls for 14 centers to enroll 14 patients a year for 4 years, or a total of 784 patients, which is above the 740 needed to detect a 6% difference in 3-year survival at an 80% level of confidence. The VA Medical Centers currently enrolling randomized and registry patients are as follows:

- *Cardiology Principal Investigator:* Douglass A. Morrison, M.D., Denver
- *Surgery Principal Investigator:* Stewart Scott, M.D., Asheville
- *Biostatistician:* Jerome Sacks, Ph.D., Chicago
- Albuquerque VA Medical Center
- Ann Arbor VA Medical Center
- Asheville VA Medical Center

- Dallas VA Medical Center
- Denver VA Medical Center
- Durham VA Medical Center
- Lexington VA Medical Center
- Little Rock VA Medical Center
- Memphis VA Medical Center
- New York VA Medical Center
- Portland VA Medical Center
- Tucson VA Medical Center
- West Los Angeles VA Medical Center
- West Roxbury (Boston) VA Medical Center

This study will provide a firm clinical foundation for or refute the application of coronary angioplasty as an alternative revascularization strategy to bypass surgery in "high-risk" medically refractory unstable angina.

CONCLUSIONS

1. Unstable angina is frequent and important.
2. Among the most difficult unstable angina patients to manage are patients with medically refractory ischemia.
3. Although it is an imperfect definition, a patient on aspirin and heparin and enough nitrate, β-blocker, or calcium blocker to achieve resting bradycardia and or hypotension (or both) who continues to have ischemia is probably "refractory". One can infer more emphatically that the patient is refractory if (a) the clinician perceives a need for intravenous nitroglycerin or intra-aortic balloon counterpulsation; (b) the drug regimen has been in place a long time; (c) episodes of ischemia are frequent; and (d) the patient has more symptoms that are objective (i.e., with ECG changes).
4. Medically refractory patients benefit from CABG in terms of symptoms and cardiac events, but
5. CABG is associated with more frequent and more severe adverse outcomes in medically refractory patients.
6. In addition to "medically refractory" a number of other harbingers of adverse outcomes with CABG exist that can be easily identified to categorize "high-risk" patients. These include:
   a. Prior heart surgery
   b. age more than 70 years
   c. Recent myocardial infarction
   d. LVEF less than 0.35
   e. Coming to CABG on LABP
   f. Coming to CABG on intravenous nitroglycerin

   g. Coming to CABG on diuretics
   h. Rales
   i. Major co-morbidity
7. Other factors for high risk of adverse outcomes with CABG are difficult to define. Among the most widely recognized is the presence of "diffuse coronary disease."
8. Based on some combination of factors, cardiac surgeons perceive "prohibitive risk" of CABG-associated mortality and refuse to revascularize some patients. The numbers and proportions of patients refused for CABG cannot be expected to diminish when:
   a. More "high-risk" patients are presenting for revascularization
   b. Government and third-party payers are insisting on greater and greater scrutiny of adverse outcomes such as operative mortality
   c. Operative mortality statistics are being "published" in the lay media and on the Internet
9. The Denver VA high-risk angioplasty consecutive case experience supports the hypothesis that angioplasty is an alternative for some high-risk as well as some prohibitive-risk medically refractory unstable angina patients.
10. VA Cooperative Study 385 (AWESOME) is designed to test the angioplasty alternative against coronary bypass surgery for the treatment of high-risk, medically refractory unstable angina. AWESOME began enrollment and randomization at 14 VA Medical Centers in February 1995 and is proceeding apace.

REFERENCES

1. Graves EJ. National Hospital Discharge Survey: Annual Summary, 1990. DHHS publication (PHS) 93-1775:4. National Center for Health Statistics Bethesda, MD, 1991
2. Ross J Jr, Brandenburg RO, Dinsmore RE et al. ACC/AHA guidelines for coronary angiography: a report of the American College of Cardiology/American Heart Association Task Force on Assessment of Diagnostic and Therapeutic Cardiovascular Procedures. J Am Coll Cardiol 1987;10:935–950; Circulation 1987;76:963A–77A
3. Kirklin JW, Akins CW, Blackstone EH et al. ACC/AHA Task Force Report: Guidelines and Indications for Coronary Artery Bypass Graft Surgery. J Am Coll Cardiol 1991;17:543–89
4. Ryan TJ, Klocke FJ, Reynolds WA and the ACP/ACC/AHA Task Force on Clinical Privileges in Cardiology Clinical competence in percutaneous transluminal coronary angioplasty. J Am Coll Cardiol 1990;15:1469–74
5. Ryan TJ, Bauman WB, Kennedy JW et al. Guidelines for Percutaneous Transluminal Coronary Angio-

plasty: a report of the American College of Cardiology/American Heart Association Task Force on Assessment of Diagnostic and Therapeutic Cardiovascular Procedures (Committee on Percutaneous Transluminal Coronary Angioplasty). J Am Coll Cardiol 1993; 22:7:2033–54

6. Faxon DP, Detre KM, McGabe CH et al. Role of percutaneous transluminal coronary angioplasty in the treatment of unstable angina: report from the National Heart, Lung and Blood Institute Percutaneous Transluminal Coronary Angioplasty and Coronary Artery Surgery Study Registries. Am J Cardiol 1983;53: 131C–5C

7. Braunwald E. Unstable angina; a classification. Circulation 1989;80:410–4

8. Morrison DA. What constitutes medically refractory? pp. 105–18. In Morrison DA, Serruys PW (eds). Medically Refractory Rest Angina. Marcel Dekker, New York, 1992

9. Luchi RJ, Scott SM, Deupree RH and the Principal Investigators and their Associates of Veterans Administration Cooperative Study No 28: Comparison of medical and surgical treatment for unstable angina pectoris. N Engl J Med 1987;316:977–84

10. Scott SM, Luchi RJ, Deupree RH and the Veterans Administration Unstable Angina Cooperative Study Group: Veterans Administration Cooperative Study for Treatment of Patients with Unstable Angina. Circulation, suppl. I. 1988;78:I-113–21

11. Parisi AF, Khuri S, Deupree RH et al. Medical compared with surgical management of unstable angina: 5 year mortality and morbidity in the Veterans Administration Study. Circulation 1989;80:1176–89

12. Russell RO, Moraski RE, Kouchoukos N et al. Unstable angina pectoris: National Cooperative Study Group to Compare Medical and Surgical Therapy. I. Report of protocol and patient population. Am J Cardiol 1976;37:896–902

13. Russell RO, Moraski RE, Kouchoukos N et al. Unstable angina pectoris: National Cooperative Study Group to Compare Surgical and Medical Therapy. II. In-hospital experience and initial follow-up results in patients with one, two, and three vessel disease. Am J Cardiol 1978;42:839–48

16. Pugh B, Platt MR, Mills LJ et al. Unstable angina pectoris: a randomized study of patients treated medically and surgically. Am J Cardiol 1978;41:1291–8

17. Brown CA, Hutter AM Jr, DeSanctis RW et al. Prospective study of medical and urgent surgical therapy in randomizable patients with unstable angina pectoris: results of in-hospital and chronic mortality and morbidity. Am Heart J 1981;102:959–64

18. Booth DC, Hultgren HN, Scott S et al. and the Investigators of Cooperative Study No. 28: Quality of life after bypass surgery for unstable angina: 5-year follow-up results of a Veterans Administration Cooperative Study. Circulation 1991;83:87–95

19. Edwards FH, Bellamy R, Burge JR et al. True emergency coronary artery bypass surgery. Ann Thorac Surg 1990;49:603–11

20. Golding LAR, Loop FD, Sheldon WC et al. Emergency revascularization for unstable angina. Circulation 1978;58:1163–6

21. Grover FL, Hammermeister KE, Burchfiel C and the VA Surgeons: Initial report of the Veterans Administration Surgery. Ann Thorac Surg 1991;50:12–28

22. Morrison DA. Summary of "high risk" and "prohibitive risk" for surgery or angioplasty in unstable angina. pp. 385–401. In Morrison DA, Serruys PW, (eds): Medically Refractory Rest Angina. Marcel Dekker, New York, 1992

23. Lewis HD Jr, Davis JW, Archibald DG et al. Protective effects of aspirin against acute myocardial infarction and death in men with unstable angina. N Engl J Med 1983;309:396–403

24. Cairns JA, Gent M, Singer J et al. Aspirin, sulfinpyrazone, or both in unstable angina. N Engl J Med 1985; 313:1369–75

25. Telford AM, Wilson C. Trial of heparin vs. Atenolol in prevention of myocardial infarction in intermediate coronary syndrome. Lancet 1981;1:1225–8

26. Theroux P et al. Aspirin, heparin, or both to treat acute unstable angina. N Engl J Med 1988;319:1105–11

27. Grambow DW, Topol EJ. Effect of maximal medical therapy on refractoriness of unstable angina pectoris. Am J Cardiol 1992;70:577–81

28. deFeyter PJ, Serruys PW, van den Brand M et al. Emergency coronary angioplasty in refractory unstable angina. N Engl J Med 1985;313:342–7

29. DeFeyter PJ, Serruys PW, Suryapranata H et al. Coronary angioplasty early after diagnosis of unstable angina. Am Heart J 1987;114:48–54

30. Ouyang P, Brinker JA, Mellits ED. Variables predictive of successful medical therapy in patients with unstable angina. Selection by multivariate analysis from clinical, electrocardiographic and angiographic evaluations. Circulation 1984;70:367–76

31. Agency for Health Care Policy and Research Clinical Practice Guideline X. Unstable Angina: Diagnosis and Management. US Department of Health and Human Services, Washington, DC, 1994

32. Morrison DA, Barbiere CC, Johnson R et al. Salvage angioplasty: an alternative to high risk surgery for unstable angina. Cathet Cardiovasc Diagn 1992;27: 169–78

33. Feldman RL, Carmichael M, Domingo M et al. Coronary angioplasty in patients who were considered poor bypass surgery candidates. J Invasive Cardiol 1991;3: 170–4

34. Colle JP, Delarche N. Clinical factors affecting the immediate outcome of PTCA in patients with unstable angina and poor candidates for surgery. Cathet Cardiovasc Diagn 1991;23:155–63

35. Morrison DA, Sacks J, Grover F, Hammermeister KE. Effectiveness of percutaneous transluminal coronary angioplasty for patients with medically refractory rest angina pectoris and high risk of adverse outcomes with coronary artery bypass grafting. Am J Cardiol 1995; 75:237–40

36. Morrison DA, Crowley ST, Veerakul G et al. Percutaneous transluminal angioplasty of saphenous vein graft lesions for medically refractory rest angina. J Am Coll Cardiol 1994;23:1066–70

37. Kuhn T. The Structure of Scientific Revolutions. 2nd Ed. pp. 10–52. University of Chicago Press, Chicago. 1970

38. Gruentzig AR, Senning A, Siegenthaler WE. Nonoperative dilatation of coronary-artery stenosis: percutaneous transluminal coronary angioplasty. N Engl J Med 1979;301:61–8

39. Wohlgelernter D, Cleman M, Highman HA, Zaret ABL. Percutaneous transluminal coronary angio-

plasty of the "culprit lesion" for management of unstable angina in patients with multivessel coronary artery disease. Am J Cardiol 1986;58:460–4

40. RITA Trial Participants. Coronary angioplasty versus coronary artery bypass surgery: the Randomized Intervention Treatment of Angina (RITA) trial. Lancet 1993;341:573–80

41. Hamm CW, Reimers J, Ischinger T et al. German Angioplasty Bypass Surgery Investigation. A randomized study of coronary angioplasty compared with bypass surgery in patients with symptomatic multivessel coronary disease. N Engl J Med 1994;331:1037–43

42. King SB III, Lembo NJ, Weintraub WS et al. For the Emory Angioplasty Surgery Trial. Randomized trial comparing coronary angioplasty with coronary bypass surgery. N Engl J Med 1994;331:1044–50

43. deFeyter PJ, Serruys PW, Arnold A et al. Coronary angioplasty of the unstable angina related vessel in patients with multi-vessel disease. Eur Heart J 1986; 7:460–7

44. Timmis AD, Griffin B, Crick JCP, Sowton E. Early percutaneous transluminal coronary angioplasty in the management of unstable angina. Int J Cardiol 1987;14:25–31

45. Plokker HWT, Ernst SMPG, Bal ET et al. Percutaneous transluminal coronary angioplasty in patients with unstable angina pectoris refractory to medical therapy. Cathet Cardiovasc Diagn 1988;14:15–8

46. Myler RF, Shaw RE, Stertzer SH et al. Unstable angina and coronary angioplasty. Circulation, suppl. II. 1990;82:II-88–II-95

47. Serota H, Deligonol U, Lee WH et al. Predictors of cardiac survival after percutaneous transluminal coronary angioplasty in patients with severe left ventricular dysfunction. Am J Cardiol 1991;67:367–72

48. O'Keefe JH, Allan JJ, McCallister BD et al. Angioplasty versus bypass surgery for multivessel coronary artery disease with left ventricular ejection fraction <40%. Am J Cardiol 1993;71:897–901

49. Anwar A, Mooney MR, Stertzer SH et al. Intra-aortic balloon counterpulsation support for elective coronary angioplasty in the setting of poor left ventricular function—a two center experience. J Invasiv-Cardiol 1990; 2:175–80

50. Kohli RS, DiSciascio G, Cowley MS et al. Coronary angioplasty in patients with severe left ventricular dysfunction. J Am Coll Cardiol 1990;16:807–11

51. Goldberg RJ, Gore JM, Albert JS et al. Cardiogenic shock after acute myocardial infarction N Engl J Med 1991;325:1117–22

52. Bengston JR, Kaplan AJ, Pieper KS et al. Prognosis in cardiogenic shock after acute myocardial infarction in the interventional era. J Am Coll Cardiol 1992;19: 907–14

53. Lee L, Erbel R, Brown TM et al. Multicenter Registry of Angioplasty Therapy of Cardiogenic Shock: initial and long-term survival. J Am Coll Cardiol 1991;17: 599–35

54. Goudreau E, DiSciascio G, Kelly K et al. Coronary angioplasty of diffuse coronary artery disease. Am Heart J 1991;121:12–1

55. Brymer JF, Khaja F, Kraft PL. Angioplasty of long or tandem coronary artery lesions using a new longer balloon dilation catheter. Cathet Cardiovasc Diagn 1991;23:84–8

39 | **Puncture Site Management**

David Ho
Gary Roubin

Because of the evolution of coronary interventional technology, the incidence of groin and vascular complications has increased over the last few years. High-dose anticoagulation, adjunctive thrombolytic therapy, and new interventional devices that require large-diameter arterial sheaths have all contributed to the rising number of vascular complications requiring medical or surgical intervention.[1] To reduce the incidence of puncture site complications, meticulous attention to detail is important, from the time of vascular puncture to removal of the vascular sheath and from the application of mechanical compression devices to the ambulation of the patient.

TIMING OF SHEATH REMOVAL

After diagnostic catheterization or valvuloplasty during which only low-dose heparin is given, sheaths can be removed at the end of the procedure. It should be emphasized that groin complications are generally reduced if sheaths are removed sooner rather than later. After angioplasty, sheaths are generally removed in 4 hours or when the activated clocking time (ACT) is less than 150 seconds. In patients requiring intra-aortic balloon pump (IABP) support overnight or in those with suboptimal results in whom urgent access may be required, heparin is restarted 3 to 4 hours after percutaneous transluminal coronary angioplasty (PTCA) or when ACT has fallen below 150 seconds. In these patients, heparin is stopped the next morning and sheaths and IABP removed 3 to 4 hours later.

When IABP is used for support during PTCA and is not required afterward, the intra-aortic balloon together with the sheath can be removed over a long wire and replaced with a larger (0.5 to 1.0 F larger) sheath. This will prevent bleeding, and the larger sheath can be removed later together with the angioplasty sheaths. In patients with sheaths in both groins, we generally remove all the sheaths at the same time except in patients who have undergone cardiopulmonary support (CPS) angioplasty. In this group of patients the large arterial cannula (17 to 19 F) and venous cannula (19 to 21 F) are removed 4 to 6 hours after angioplasty or when the ACT falls below 150 seconds. Cautious use of protamine for stepwise reduction in ACT levels can assist in early sheath removal, especially in CPS patients. Heparin is then recommended and maintained while the patient is supported by IABP. If the patient is stable the following morning, heparin is ceased and the IABP and sheaths removed 4 hours later.

PATIENT PREPARATION

The patient should be connected to a monitor for heart rate, rhythm, and blood pressure monitoring. Good intravenous access to the patient should be available so that any pain-induced vasovagal reaction may be treated promptly by atropine and bolus intravenous fluids. Midazolam (1 to 2 mg) or diazepam (2 to 4 mg) is given intravenously for sedation. The groin area is then locally infiltrated with 20 ml

1 to 2% lidocaine. Three to 5 ml of blood should be withdrawn from the side arms of the sheaths prior to removal so that any thrombus around the sheath may be removed. The operator should palpate the pedal pulses just before sheath removal to form a fresh mental picture of the location and volume of the distal pulses.

MANUAL COMPRESSION

The index, middle, and ring fingers of the left hand are positioned 1 cm cranial to the skin puncture site. The venous sheath is first pulled and a light-to-medium pressure applied. The arterial sheath is then firmly held at the hub and slowly withdrawn while increasing pressure is applied to maintain hemostasis. At this stage the operator confirms that pressure is being applied directly on the anterior wall of the artery by rolling the fingers around the artery to search for the maximum upward impulse. A medially displacing impulse on one's fingertips would suggest that the finger position is too medial, whereas a laterally displacing impulse would suggest that one is too lateral to the artery. Sufficient pressure is now applied to prevent any bleeding from the arterial puncture site into the subcutaneous tissue while ensuring distal flow. The skin puncture site should be exposed at all times so that any underlying bleeding caused by insufficient pressure may manifest itself by bleeding through the skin incision site. The duration of compression depends on the degree of anticoagulation, any underlying hypertension, and the diameter of the sheath. After a diagnostic catheterization during which only low-dose heparin is given, 5 to 15 minutes of manual pressure is usually enough to achieve hemostasis. In patients with hypertension, in those with aortic incompetence with wide pulse pressure, in chronic renal failure patients with a high-output state, and in elderly patients with sclerotic arteries, manual compression may have to be applied for a longer period.

MECHANICAL COMPRESSION

Mechanical compression devices are invaluable since most interventional procedures these days involve the use of large diameter sheaths, anticoagulation, or thrombolytic agents; thus a long compression time is often necessary. Intravenous analgesics such as morphine (2 to 4 mg IV) or meperidine hydrochloride (25 to 50 mg IV) may be required in addition to the sedatives described above. Several mechanical compression devices are available. One such device is the C-clamp (Clamp Ease, Pressure Products, Malibu, CA). The base of the C-clamp is first placed posterior to the hip of the patient. The plastic compression disc is then snapped onto the C-arm and the C-arm attached to the frame of the C-clamp. The C-arm is then swung in a clockwise or counterclockwise direction until the compression disc is 1 cm cranial to the arterial puncture site. The C-arm is then slid forward or backward until the compression disc is directly anterior to the artery. At this stage, both sheaths are grabbed by the hubs and withdrawn by 1″. The whole C-arm is then lowered until a medium pressure is applied on a gauze square on top of the sheaths at the skin incision site. The venous sheath is first removed with the right hand. With the left hand applying further downward pressure on the C-arm, the arterial sheath is then removed by firmly grabbing the hub of the sheath with the right hand. Once the arterial sheath is removed, further pressure is applied and the C-arm locked into position by turning the vertical knob clockwise. Fine adjustment to the pressure can be performed by turning the horizontal knob clockwise or counterclockwise. It is recommended that enough pressure be applied initially to arrest bleeding as well as to occlude distal pulses. Pressure is then slowly reduced until distal perfusion resumes. Prior documentation of the location and volume of the pedal pulses by the operator is important, since the presence of a distal pulse earlier would now give the operator the confidence to reduce pressure further to restore distal flow. The groin area should be observed for any bleeding or enlarging hematoma. The operator should have a low threshold for reapplying manual pressure if necessary so that the C-arm can be repositioned. In patients with no palpable distal pulses, a Doppler machine may be used to document distal flow. When in doubt, one should err on the side of high pressure and observe the lower limb for 5 to 10 minutes. If a blue blotchy color develops in the lower limb, pressure can be reduced by rotating the knob on the C-arm 180 degrees every 30 seconds until the blotching disappears.

Heart rate and blood pressure should be monitored every 5 to 10 minutes and the groin area inspected frequently. Automatic blood pressure cuff devices (e.g., Dynamap, Critikon, Tampa, FL), which inflate automatically at preset intervals and trigger an alarm if the blood pressure should fall below a preset limit, are invaluable for this purpose.

Pneumatic Compression

A more sophisticated compression device, the FemoStop (USCI, Billerica, MA), consists of a hand-held pump that inflates a transparent pressure bubble attached to a pressure arch made of hard plastic (Fig.

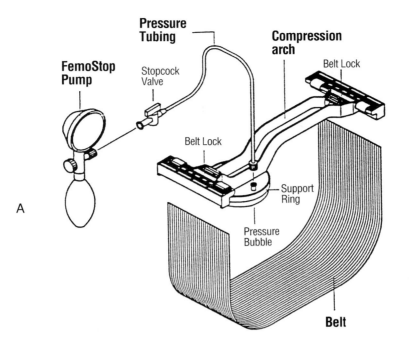

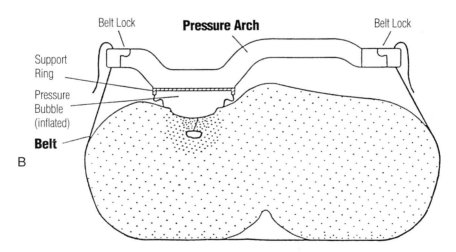

Fig. 39-1. **(A)** Components of the femoral compression arch and pump (FemoStop). **(B)** Cross-sectional view of the patient's hip with the compression arch attached to the belt and pressure applied by the inflated transparent pressure bubble over the femoral puncture site.

39-1). A polyester belt is positioned around the patient's hip; this can be done either on the catheter table, before the patient is prepped for the procedure if immediate sheath removal is planned, or in bed at the time of sheath removal. The belt is then attached to the arch with the center of the deflated bubble positioned 1 cm cranial to the skin puncture site (somewhat higher in obese patients), and the belt is then tightened firmly. One must insist on a firm attachment of the belt to prevent tilting of the arch. Adequate compression of the puncture site should be

achieved while the bubble is only partially inflated. If the bubble is overinflated, the inside pressure may reflect excessive stretching of the bubble and not the accurate pressure transmitted to the tissue. The bubble is then inflated while the sheath is gradually withdrawn. If bleeding still occurs the pressure is further increased until hemostasis is obtained. The optimal initial pressure can easily be ascertained by palpating the pedal pulse and ensuring that distal perfusion is maintained while hemostasis is still achieved. Normally after about 5 minutes the pressure can be reduced by another 20 mmHg, and even in heavily anticoagulated patients after 30 minutes it is also advisable to reduce the pressure further to moderate values (e.g., 50 to 60 mmHg). It may be advisable to leave a pressure of some 40 mmHg for the first 3 hours following sheath removal. There is no reason to detach the apparatus before the patient is allowed to ambulate; in case of recurrent bleeding the bubble can just be inflated again. In very prolonged compressions (in the case of systemic thrombolysis, for example) it is advisable to reduce the pressure briefly every 30 to 60 minutes to allow skin perfusion and avoid the development of blisters. In such cases it may be preferable to place a gauze pad between the plastic material of the bubble and the skin.

This device is more comfortable than the solid mechanical devices and allows pressure controlled compression. In patients undergoing simple diagnostic catheterization it can be attached while the patient is still on the catheter table immediately after the procedure; it thus allows relatively free transfer of the patient to the bed and reduces staff time. Male and female patients may be able to urinate with the device in place, and male patients can even stand up without risk of hemorrhage. In patients with bleeding around sheaths in whom anticoagulation is not fully reverted, this device may provide a comfortable means of temporary compression to control bleeding. No further treatment with sandbags or adhesive tape (or both) is required after use of the FemoStop.

Duration

The duration of mechanical compression depends on the diameter of the sheath, degree of anticoagulation, and any underlying clinical conditions mentioned earlier. For diagnostic catheterization, 15 to 20 minutes of mechanical compression is often adequate. For angioplasty using an 8-F sheath, 30 to 60 minutes of compression are required. Patients who have received an intracoronary stent, who are treated with ticlopidine and aspirin, and who have a 9 to 11-F sheath often require 60 to 90 minutes of compression. Those with an IABP may require 90 to 120 minutes of compression. In patients with a systolic blood pressure of more than 150 mmHg, intravenous nitroglycerin may be used in an attempt to shorten the duration of compression and reduce the chance of bleeding. However, one should ensure that hypotension secondary to sedation, analgesics, and pain-induced vasovagal reactions do not occur before commencing nitroglycerin infusion.

Patients with large arterial cannula (17 to 19 F) following CPS angioplasty generally require 3 hours or more to achieve hemostasis. These patients are often anticoagulated for IABP in the contralateral groin. They are often anesthetized and ventilated, so more prolonged mechanical compression is usually well tolerated. However, pressure should be reduced after 3 to 4 hours since pressure necrosis of the skin due to prolonged compression may occur. In patients receiving prolonged compression, the pressure should be lessened every 30 to 60 minutes to allow perfusion of the skin.

Removal of Compression Devices

The FemoStop may be left in place for a prolonged period (i.e., several hours) without undue discomfort. Low pressure between 20 and 40 mmHg may be adequate to maintain hemostasis once the initial compression has been successful. The C-clamp should be slowly released over 1 to 2 minutes to allow the tissue to expand slowly. It is then removed and the groin observed for 2 to 3 minutes. Gradual release in pressure over 20 to 60 minutes prior to C-clamp removal is not recommended. Any underlying bleeding during this period will be masked since the skin incision site is often compressed and no surface bleeding is allowed. Inadequate compression over a prolonged period before hemostasis is achieved is a precursor of pseudoaneurysm development.

By contrast, the FemoStop should always be left at low pressures as long as the patient is comfortable with it even after the pressure has been reduced to zero. It is advisable to leave the device in place for several hours, for two reasons: first, patient movement is automatically restricted as long as the patient feels the device in place and second, nothing is easier in case of recurrent bleeding than simply inflating the bubble again. No further sandbag or pressure dressing is required afterward.

If any surface bleeding or swelling suggests an underlying enlarging hematoma, pneumatic or mechanical pressure should be reapplied. Occasionally a small amount of bleeding may persist from the venous puncture site. This is best managed by light pneumatic or manual compression. Bleeding from small arteries at the edge of the skin incision may be persistent but is usually of small volume; it is automatically eliminated once prolonged pneumatic pressure is applied. Before the patient is mobilized a simple transparent dresssing or bandage is placed over the skin incision. A so-called pressure bandage is not recommended since this only provides a false sense of security. The vertical resultant force (F) exerted on the arterial puncture site is trivial compared with the tangential tension (T) applied to the bandage (F = T × sine angle between bandage and skin, which is nearly 0 degrees). Any underlying bleeding may be masked and treatment often delayed until the gauze under the bandage is heavily soaked with blood. The other disadvantage is the potential for cutaneous blistering and excoriation as a result of allergies to these bandages. In patients who are confused or uncooperative, pressure bandages or sandbags may be applied as a reminder to the patient to minimize lower limb movement. After 2 to 4 hours, the patient is allowed to sit up to 30 degrees or turn and lie on the side. The patient is kept on bed rest until the next day, when ambulation is allowed.

GROIN COMPLICATIONS

Following PTCA, the overall local vascular complication rate requiring surgical repair is around 1.5%. In a prospective study of 2,107 consecutive patients undergoing interventional procedures over a 12-month period, serious bleeding requiring transfusion occurred in 7.3%. The most common site of bleeding was at the puncture site and occurred in 5.8% of the patients. Other common sites include gastrointestinal (1.8%) and retroperitoneal (0.9%). Predictors of need for transfusion include female sex, low body weight, age, urgent procedures, low baseline hemoglobin, long duration of procedure, large sheath size, heparin dose/weight, thrombolytic use, and multivessel disease. In another study of over 2,000 high-risk angioplasty patients, clinical predictors of bleeding complications included old age, light weight, female sex, baseline hematocrit, history of hypertension, total heparin dose, and duration of procedure.

The use of urokinase in the catheterization laboratory has also been shown to be associated with a high rate of bleeding. A recent multicenter retrospective study of 210 patients showed an overall rate of bleeding in 28% of patients given urokinase therapy in the catheterization lab; 63% of bleeding incidents occurred in the groin, 17% in the gastrointestinal tract, 2% retroperitoneally, and 0.5% intracranially. Blood transfusion was required in 83% of the patients who bled. Age 70 years or older was the only factor correlated with bleeding. Intravenous administration of urokinase was associated with a higher incidence of bleeding compared with intracoronary administration.

Hematoma and Pseudoaneurysm

Hematoma is by far the most common of all puncture site complications. Not uncommonly, significant blood loss results, requiring transfusion or even re-suscitation. A hematoma may become encapsulated and remain in communication with an artery via a patent tract, resulting in a pseudoaneurysm. The reported incidence of pseudoaneurysm varies widely. A recent report on 2,400 consecutive patients undergoing diagnostic catheterization (n = 1,519) or interventional procedures (n = 881) showed an overall incidence of pseudoaneurysm of 0.3%.[2] The incidence may be as high as 10% after complex PTCA, when large sheaths are used and in anticoagulated patients following stent placement, especially if routine color flow Doppler study is performed since Doppler study is more sensitive than physical examination in detecting small pseudoaneurysms. Those who are female, elderly, or hypertensive and those who are anticoagulated are at increased risk. Low arterial puncture sites (superficial femoral artery or profundus artery) may also increase the likelihood for pseudoaneurysm development because of their deep anatomic location. The diagnosis is made by ultrasound in the patient with a tender pulsatile mass and a systolic bruit following recent arterial puncture. Treatment depends on size and whether the patient requires long-term anticoagulation. In patients who do not require anticoagulation, a pseudoaneurysm less than 2 to 3 cm in size may be followed clinically. The swelling, tenderness, and systolic bruit often resolve, and repeat ultrasound in 1 to 2 weeks often demonstrates spontaneous thrombosis.[3] In fact, 10 to 15 minutes of simple finger compression will often result in closure of small pseudoaneurysms in patients who are not anticoagulated. For pseudoaneurysms 3 cm or larger in size and for patients who require anticoagulation, ultrasound-guided external compression is the treatment of choice.[4,5] Surgical repair is rarely required and should be reserved for very painful or expanding pseudoaneurysms that do not respond to external compression.

Arteriovenous Fistula

The incidence of arteriovenous (AV) fistula following diagnostic and therapeutic cardiac catheterization combined is around 0.1 to 1.0%. AV fistulae are more common when the arterial and venous puncture sites are on the same side, when the femoral puncture site is inappropriately low, when the puncture extends through the posterior arterial wall, or in patients with multiple procedures and in those receiving anticoagulation. Most AV fistulae are relatively asymptomatic and rarely require intervention. The diagnosis is made by ultrasound in the patient with a continuous murmur. Most such fistulae will close spontaneously, requiring only clinical follow-up. They rarely result in claudication unless the patient has underlying peripheral vascular disease. Treatment of persistent AV fistula includes ultrasound-guided external compression or surgical division of the fistula.

Thrombotic Occlusion

The reported incidence of arterial thrombosis is less than 1% following PTCA and comprises only 5% of all vascular complications. The elderly and those with underlying peripheral vascular disease, cardiomyopathy, or hypercoagulation states are at increased risk, and ischemia, amputation, and death may result. The diagnosis is obvious in the patient with sudden onset of severe pain, anesthesia, paresthesia with a cold, pale, or cyanotic distal extremity, and absence of distal pulses. Similar symptoms may be due to arterial spasm or compromise in flow (or both) due to the physical presence of the arterial sheath. In these situations removal of the arterial sheath will often relieve symptoms and restore flow to the lower extremities. Most patients will respond to conservative management with intravenous heparin for several days. In patients with persistent or severe symptoms, surgical exploration of the occluded artery and evacuation of thromboembolic debris may be required.

CLOSURE OF FEMORAL PSEUDOANEURYSM AND ARTERIOVENOUS FISTULA BY EXTERNAL COMPRESSION

The principle cause of pseudoaneurysm and AV fistula is inadequate compression following sheath removal. Thus, the mouth of the fistula or tract is actually the point where the sheath once entered the vessel. By applying external compression, the communicating tract between the artery and the pseudoaneurysmal cavity (in the case of a pseudoaneurysm) or between the artery and vein (in the case of an AV fistula) becomes apposed, arresting any through-flow (Fig. 39-2). Subsequent thrombosis within the pseudoaneurysmal cavity and the tract leads to closure of the tract.

Techniques

Heparin should be stopped for at least 4 hours prior to mechanical compression for closure of pseudoaneurysms or AV fistula. Sufficient sedation and anal-

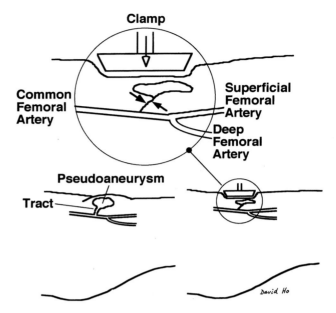

Fig. 39-2. A femoral pseudoaneurysm formed as a result of inadequate compression following removal of sheaths or dishesion of the arteriotomy wound. The pseudoaneurysmal sac remains in communication with the superficial femoral artery via a patent tract. The mouth of the tract is therefore the point where the arterial sheath once entered the vessel. By applying external compression (*open arrow*), the communicating tract between the artery and the pseudoaneurysmal cavity becomes apposed (*closed arrows*), arresting any through-flow. Subsequent thrombosis within the pseudoaneurysmal cavity and the tract leads to closure of the pseudoaneurysm.

gesics are given and the patient monitored as described for mechanical compression. Color flow Doppler is used to identify the pseudoaneurysmal tract or AV communication tract. It is useful for the operator to exert pressure on the ultrasound probe so an idea of the amount of pressure required to occlude flow across the communicating tract may be obtained. Once adequate pressure is applied, the color flow across the communicating tract should be arrested. The ultrasound probe is now replaced by the compression bubble of the FemoStop or the disc of the C-clamp and adequate pressure applied to occlude the communicating tract. Distal perfusion can be monitored either manually or by Doppler. Compression for 60 minutes is often required to close pseudoaneurysms and AV fistulae. Pseudoaneurysms that are more than 5 cm in diameter may require more prolonged compression and often require a second or third compression to achieve closure. This is often performed on separate days for patient comfort or logistic reasons. Persistent femoral bruit usually indicates failure of closure of the AV fistula or pseudoaneurysm. For patients who failed one or two mechanical compression attempts, especially those who tolerate mechanical compression poorly, surgical closure should be considered.

Following successful closure of the pseudoaneurysm or AV fistula, a small dressing is applied and the patient kept on bed rest overnight. The patient is ambulated the next day and a repeat ultrasound examination performed prior to hospital discharge. Since the success rate of closure by mechanical compression is reduced with chronicity of the pseudoaneurysm, closure by external compression should be attempted as soon as the diagnosis is made. Contraindications include impending femoral compartment syndrome, groin infection, ischemia of tissue overlying the pseudoaneurysm, and ischemia of the limb during effective compression.

BRACHIAL AND RADIAL ARTERY PUNCTURE SITES

For percutaneous brachial puncture sites, sheaths are also removed within 4 hours or when ACT is less than 150 seconds. The principles of sheath removal are similar to the femoral technique described earlier. The brachial artery is compressed manually to achieve hemostasis while ensuring adequate distal flow. Pressure is generally applied for 20 to 30 minutes. A small dressing and splint are then applied to immobilize the arm until the next day, when gentle movement is allowed. The arterial puncture site should be observed for development of hematoma, change in sensation, or loss in distal pulses. Complications associated with percutaneous brachial puncture are rare. Occasionally, thrombosis and distal embolization may occur, requiring surgical repair of the artery or embolectomy. These complications can be minimized with proper arterial puncture technique, adequate anticoagulation, use of a small-sized sheath, and early removal of the sheath.

The radial artery approach using a 6-F sheath for PTCA and stenting has recently been used in some centers. Sheaths are removed immediately at the end of the procedure and a tourniquet applied over a folded gauze square over the radial artery puncture site for 15 to 60 minutes. These centers only use aspirin and ticlopidine, with or without low molecular weight heparin in their anticoagulation regime for their stent patients and have a low incidence of stent thrombosis or bleeding complications. Patients can ambulate at the end of the procedure and be discharged the next day.

MANAGEMENT OF PUNCTURE SITE BLEEDING FOLLOWING STENT PLACEMENT

Nowadays, most centers use only antiplatelet agents (aspirin and ticlopidine) following stenting. This has significantly reduced the incidence of bleeding and puncture site complications. The following discussion is applicable to those who require full anticoagulation following stenting, for example, those with suboptimal angiographic results, acute stent thrombosis, or those with residual thrombus burden. Although puncture site complications may be reduced by using a graduated ambulation protocol, meticulous attention to puncture techniques, and careful anticoagulation monitoring, many bleeding complications are unpredictable and occur when anticoagulation is not excessive.

In the event of aggressive anticoagulation following stenting, bleeding complications have been reported in 8 to 40% of cases. The puncture site is the most common site of bleeding among stent patients. In a series of 83 patients requiring transfusion after stent placement, most (69%) of the bleeding complications involved the femoral arterial puncture site. Most puncture site bleeding occurs within the first few days while the patient is still in hospital. Once bleeding is diagnosed, heparin should be stopped. When bleeding is not life threatening, anticoagulation may be reinstituted once hemostasis is achieved. When bleeding is life threatening (e.g., large groin hematoma resulting in hypovolumic shock and renal failure), anticoagulation should be stopped and the patient left on antiplatelet therapy only. Most pseudoaneurysms and AV fistulae in stented patients can be closed by external compression after heparin infusion has been interrupted for 4 to 6 hours. AV fistulae and small pseudoaneurysms can also be managed conservatively until anticoagulation is discontinued at 1 or 2 months, when spontaneous closure may occur. Elective external compression or surgical repair can be performed on those persisting after cessation of anticoagulation.

Bleeding complications in most stent series appear to have a learning curve. For those patients in whom full anticoagulation is deemed necessary, a graduated mobilization protocol is useful in reducing the incidence of bleeding. An example of such a protocol includes keeping the patient at complete bed rest on the first day following stenting. On day 2, the patient may move and sit up in bed. On day 3, the patient may begin to ambulate cautiously but is not allowed to ambulate fully until day 4. In female patients, a Foley catheter during the first 2 days will reduce excessive movement, which may disrupt the puncture

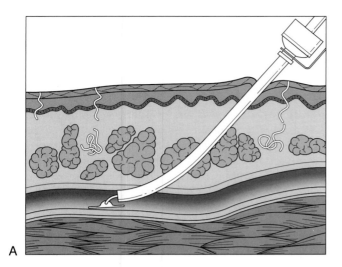

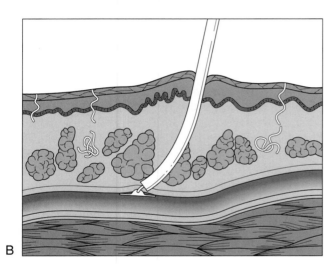

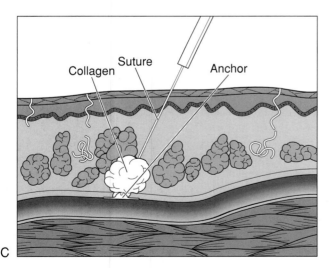

Fig. 39-3. The Angio-Seal hemostatic puncture closure device. **(A)** Bioresorbable anchor deployed into arterial lumen via an introducer sheath (which replaces the angio-

site. The importance of careful monitoring of anticoagulation, use of a flow sheet to document anticoagulation results, and the current dose of heparin and Coumadin, cannot be overemphasized. Prior to discharge, patients should be seen by a nurse coordinator who provides education on the stent and anticoagulation treatment. Patients are also advised to avoid heavy lifting for 2 weeks. More liberal mobilization may be used with less stringent anticoagulation regimes.

NEW TECHNIQUES AND DEVICES

Vascular Plugging Devices

The VasoSeal (Datascope, Oakland, NY) uses a highly thrombogenic, purified, biodegradable, bovine collagen cylinder delivered by a guidewire system to plug the arteriotomy site. These collagen plugs have been shown to reduce the duration of manual compression despite full-dose anticoagulation. Typically only 3 to 5 minutes of manual pressure is required. They have also been shown to shorten duration of immobilization and hospital stay. However, two recent large studies with over 1,000 patients each have shown a relatively high incidence of vascular complication requiring surgical repair. Collagen inadvertently introduced into the femoral artery may result in local obstruction, complete occlusion, and loss of distal pulses. Peripheral embolization of collagen or other thrombogenic material may also occur. Major bleeding resulting in hematoma, aneurysm, or AV fistula also appears to be a problem in up to 5% of the patients. In 0.5 to 1.0% of the patients, protrusion of the collagen plug into the femoral artery results, necessitating surgical repair. Thus, although the use of collagen plugs can reduce the duration of bed rest and hospital stay, the method requires further refinement to reduce complications.

A new device, the Kensey-Nash hemostatic puncture closure device (HPCD) (Angio-Seal, Quinton, Seattle, WA), seems to hold promise in achieving immediate hemostasis without the complication rate of previous collagen plug devices and is currently under

plasty sheath at the end of the PTCA procedure). **(B)** The anchor is secured at the arterial puncture site as the introducer sheath and suture are drawn back, keeping the anchor apposed to the sheath. **(C)** Collagen is deployed immediately outside the arterial wall. The suture keeps the compressed collagen plug and anchor apposed, forming a secure seal.

clinical evaluation. The Angio-Seal has three bioresorbable components: a small anchor, a collagen sponge, and a suture (Fig. 39-3). The anchor is deployed inside the artery, and the collagen sponge is positioned on the outside of the artery. The suture links the anchor to the collagen plug to achieve hemostasis. All components are absorbed by the body in 60 to 90 days. In a recent randomized study of 142 patients (91 diagnostic catheterization, 51 PTCA), the HPCD was successfully deployed in 69 of 73 patients (94%) randomized to HPCD. Hemostasis was achieved in 58 of 69 patients (84%) within 1 minute. Only three hematomas and one pseudoaneurysm occurred in the HPCD group compared with six hematomas and two pseudoaneurysms among 69 patients randomized to receive manual compression ($P =$ NS). In another randomized study of 63 patients, HPCD inserted immediately after PTCA or coronary angiogram allowed hemostasis to be achieved within 4 minutes. Patients were mobilized 4 hours later without any complications, resulting in a short hospital stay.

Biodegradable collagen has also been used to close pseudoaneurysms and AV fistulae. Collagen was applied subcutaneously into the aneurysm to provoke clotting so that closure was achieved. A recent study reported success in all 56 aneurysms attempted (diameter 2 cm or more). One patient developed infection as a complication. Closure of AV fistulae using spring coils applied within the fistula introduced via an intra-arterial delivery system has also been reported. Femoral puncture closure using percutaneous suture devices are also under investigation. These devices allow a purse string-like suture to be inserted and secured using an innovative technique.

REFERENCES

1. Oweida SW, Roubin GS, Smith RD III, Salam AA. Post-catheterization vascular complications associated with percutaneous transluminal coronary angioplasty. J Vasc Surg 1990;12:310–5
2. Muller DWM, Shamir KJ, Ellis SG et al. Peripheral vascular complications after conventional and complex percutaneous coronary interventional procedures. Am J Cardiol 1992;69:63–8
3. Kotval PS, Khoury A, Shah PM, Babu SC. Doppler sonographic demonstration of the progressive spontaneous thrombosis of pseudoaneurysms. J Ultrasound Med 1990;9:185–90
4. Fellmeth BD, Roberts AC, Bookstein JJ et al. Postangiographic femoral artery injuries: nonsurgical repair with US-guided compression. Radiology 1991;178:671–5
5. Agrawal SK, Pinheiro L, Roubin GS et al. Nonsurgical closure of femoral pseudoaneurysms complicating cardiac catheterization and percutaneous transluminal coronary angioplasty. J Am Coll Cardiol 1992;20:610–5

40 Magnum Wire

Bernhard Meier

Total occlusion was added to the list of indications for coronary angioplasty shortly after its introduction. The main components of a chronic total coronary occlusion are an atherosclerotic plaque and an organized thrombus. The texture of the thrombus is instrumental for success. The older and the more fibrosed it is, the smaller the chance to cross it with the recanalization device.

INDICATIONS

Indications have to be balanced between the technical difficulties expected and the clinical risks projected on the one side and the likely subjective benefit on the other side. The indication threshold is low for a recanalization attempt that is part of the diagnostic coronary angiogram since it means little additional inconvenience and cost. The threshold is intermediate if the patient is still hospitalized, but it should be high in case long-distance travel is involved.

The typical candidates have effort angina but no rest angina. A well-collateralized total occlusion functionally imitates a significant stenosis without its risk for acute infarction. Noncontracting myocardium appears to be a logical contraindication to a revascularization attempt of the occluded culprit vessel. However, noncontracting myocardium may be hibernating[1] or stunned[2] rather than irreversibly damaged. Hibernation (stalled function to preserve viability during marginal oxygen supply) is a more obvious reason for noncontracting myocardium than stunning (delayed resumption of function after re-

flow) to support a recanalization attempt. Left ventricular recuperation after successful coronary recanalization is inconsistent, slow, and hard to document by crude assessment of global left ventricular ejection fraction.[3,4] This relegates it to the secondary goals for recanalization of chronic total coronary occlusions.

Indications should be heavily based on the projection of success derived from duration, length, and aspect of the occlusion. An occlusion flush at the orifice of the vessel or tapering into a small side branch is a contraindication for angioplasty. Adequate visualization of the distal part of the occluded artery via collaterals is a mandatory prerequisite. First, there is little hope of reconstructing a vessel that appears obliterated over its entire length. Second, myocardial areas of occluded vessels completely devoid of collateral blood flow are always akinetic and hardly hibernating.

RESULTS

Success rates are largely dependent on the indications.[5] In recent short occlusions with a funnel-shaped stump, they approach those of angioplasty of nontotal lesions. In old, long, and nipple-free occlusions, they are close to zero.

The risk pattern, however, is favorable irrespective of the indications. Reocclusion after recanalization generally does not cause harm, in contrast to an acute closure after angioplasty of a stenosed vessel. It only reinstitutes the preintervention status. Of course, the risk of angioplasty for chronic total occlusion is still higher than that of diagnostic coronary angiography. Vessels on the way to the occlusion may be damaged. In case of a very important vessel this may well jeopardize the patient's life. Collaterals may be impeded by subintimal channels. This may cause infarctions even in the setting of chronically occluded coronary arteries. There is a minute but definite risk of coronary perforation by the guidewire (probably more frequent than detected) or rupture by a subintimally placed balloon (Fig. 40-1).

A long subintimal pathway is a relatively frequent reason for failure with more vigorous attempts of recanalization. Generally, it goes clinically unrecognized, and the true distal lumen is reestablished by blood inflow through the collaterals. Of course, this still leaves the occluded segment unrecanalized and the procedure a failure. A blunt tip on the recanalization wire should reduce the risk of a subintimal path but does apparently not eliminate it.

Techniques and materials for angioplasty have to

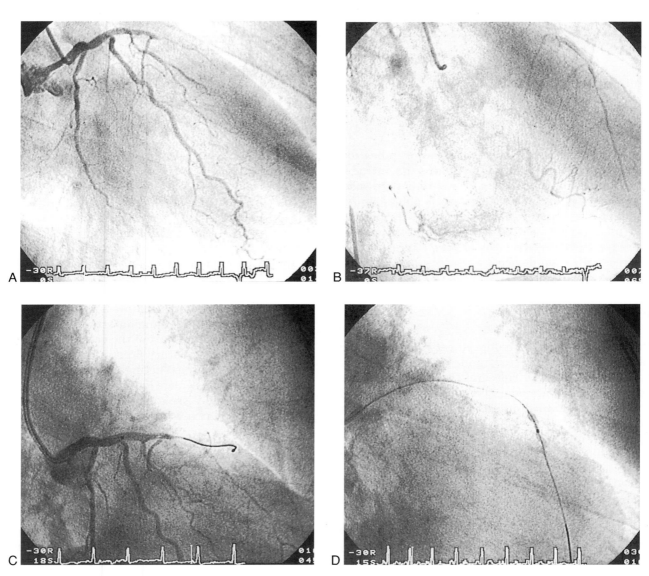

Fig. 40-1. Rupture of a left anterior descending coronary artery of a 68-year-old woman secondary to a recanalization attempt of a chronic total occlusion **(A).** The occlusion was relatively short, as evidenced by the collateralization from the right coronary artery but the distal vessel was tortuous and small of caliber due to long-standing disease **(B).** The recanalization with the Magnum proved difficult **(C),** and a subintimal path beyond the occlusion is likely. The 3-mm Magnarail balloon could be passed relatively easily, but upon inflation it showed several indentations and failed to straighten the vessel **(D).** These are indirect signs of a subintimal position. At 16 bar, the balloon was fully expanded (*Figure continues.*)

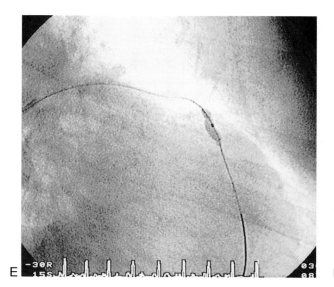

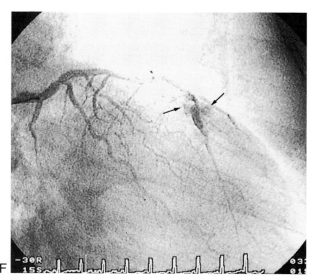

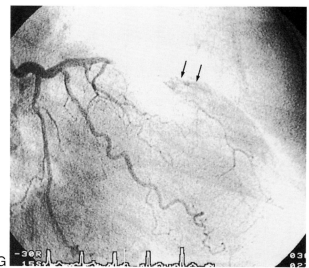

Fig. 40-1. (*Continued*). (**E**) but apparently had caused a rupture of the vessel with extravasation of contrast medium (**F,** *arrows*). There were no clinical sequelae because the leak remained contained in the surrounding tissue. However, no further dilations to the proximal part of the recanalized artery were done for fear of increasing the inflow into the leak. The vessel reoccluded promptly, leaving but a faint cloud of contrast medium at the site of the rupture (**G,** *arrows*).

be modified also for other reasons when it comes to chronic total coronary occlusions. Floppy coronary guidewires may easily negotiate tight and eccentric nontotal lesions, but they tend to buckle when used for chronic total occlusions. Stiffer wires succeed where floppy wires fail. Since even the most rigid conventional coronary guide wires are still quite flexible, bracing of the guidewire by advancement of the balloon catheter close to the tip is needed to provide adequate stiffness. These aspects have led to the Magnum technique for chronic occlusion angioplasty described in this chapter.

MAGNUM SYSTEM

The Magnum wire features a Teflonized solid-steel shaft with a diameter of 0.021″ in its original version and 0.018″ and 0.014″ in more recent versions.[6] It has a flexible, shapeable distal part, and an olive tip of 1-mm diameter (0.7 mm in the smaller versions). The 0.021″ version is compatible with Magnum and Magnarail balloons of Schneider and necessitates at least a 7-F guiding catheter. The smaller versions work with most commercialized over-the-wire balloons and Monorail balloons, most of which fit through modern 6-F guiding catheters. In cases with a poor chance of success, plain support catheters can be used rather than balloon catheters to stiffen the wire. For the 0.021″ wire there is the Magnarail Probing catheter and for the smaller Magnum wires the Multifunctional Probing catheter (both from Schneider, Zurich, Switzerland).[7]

Figure 40-2 demonstrates the different salient aspects of the Magnum technique using a particularly intricate case, for an example.

A randomized study on patients with total coronary occlusions, unassociated with acute infarction and devoid of antegrade flow, compared the performance of the Magnum 0.021″ system with that of a variety of conventional systems.[8] A total of 100 consecutive patients were randomized in the catheterization laboratory to the Magnum system or a conventional system. A cross-over was imposed if the balloon could not be placed properly within 20 minutes of fluoroscopy time. The alternate system had

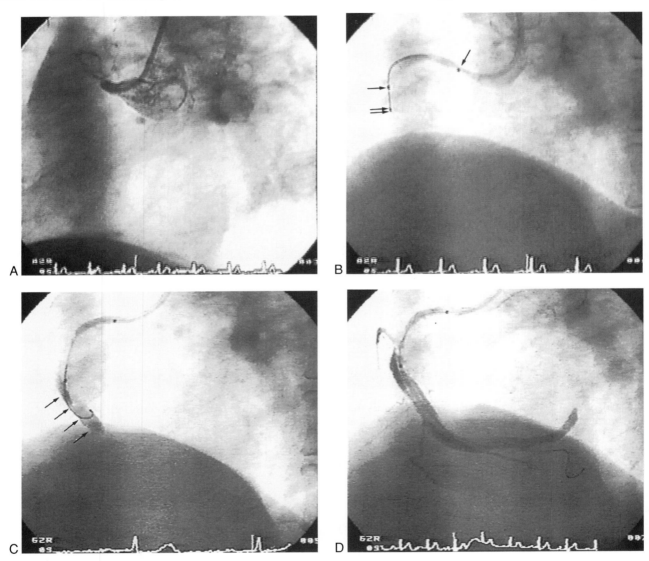

Fig. 40-2. Recanalization of a chronically occluded right coronary artery (**A**) of a 48-year-old patient using a 0.014 Magnum wire with a long Goldie balloon (3.5 mm in diameter) through a 6-F Amplatz left 3 Pink Power guiding catheter (Schneider). The occlusion could be entered only after supporting the Magnum wire with the balloon catheter advanced maximally to the ball tip (**B;** *double arrow,* ball tip of the Magnum wire; *single arrow,* balloon markers). A contrast medium injection through the guiding catheter revealed a subintimal pathway (**C**). The contrast medium travels through the Monorail lumen of the balloon catheter providing a faked distal injection revealing the subintimal cul de sac (*arrows*). Further contrast medium injections and the search for the true lumen with the wire extended the subintimal channel first to the beginning of the posterolateral branch (**D**) (*Figure continues.*)

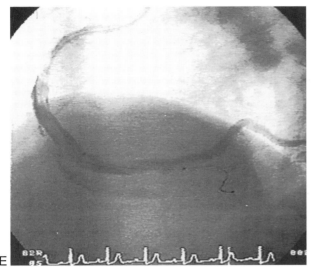
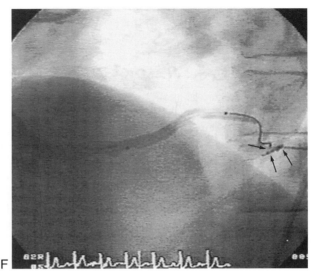
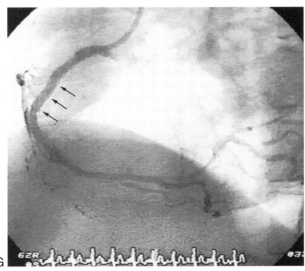

Fig. 40-2. (*Continued*). and then to its very end **(E)**. The subintimal lumen opacified by the contrast medium is quite apparent. There was no flow. The wire resides in the subintimal space of the posterior descending coronary artery. The balloon is in the proximal segment of the right coronary artery in Fig. D and in the distal segment in Fig. E. After withdrawing the wire and reshaping its tip, the true lumen could be found at the proximal end of the dissection. The proof of the correct positioning of the wire in the distal true lumen of the posterolateral branch is provided by the flow beyond the tip of the wire (**F,** *arrows*). Several dilations with the long balloon over the entire length of the common right coronary artery and well into the posterolateral branch led to an angiographically acceptable result that had been improved by the implantation of an 18-mm Palmaz stent (Johnson & Johnson) into the proximal part of the vessel (**G,** *arrows*).

to be tried for an equal amount of time. There were 52 occlusions in the Magnum group and 51 in the conventional group. Baseline characteristics were comparable, such as age, sex, angina class, stress test, prior infarction or coronary intervention, and left ventricular function of the patients, as well as site, diameter (mean, 3.0 mm), duration (6 weeks), and length (1.4 cm) of the occlusions. Primary suc-

cess was superior in the Magnum group (Table 40-1). The Magnum system was more successful independent of the coronary artery. A clear-cut decline of primary success with increasing duration of occlusion was demonstrated for the conventional group over the initial 3 months but not for the Magnum group. There were no significant differences between the groups regarding fluoroscopy time or number of

Table 40-1. Randomized Results of Magnum System Versus Conventional Systems for Chronic Total Occlusions

	Magnum (n = 52)	Conventional (n = 51)	P
Success as first device	67%	45%	<0.05
Success as cross-over device	39% (11/28)	13% (2/16)	<0.05

(From Pande et al.,[8] with permission.)

guiding catheters and balloons used per lesion. None of the Magnum wires had to be exchanged during the procedure (most were even resterilized and reused), in contrast to an average consumption of 1.4 conventional wires per occlusion. There was one complication in the Magnum group (nontransmural infarction) and one in the conventional group (death at sheath removal due to protamine allergy).

To date, we have performed coronary angioplasty with the Magnum system in 804 patients, attempting almost 820 occlusions (Table 40-2). The vast majority of these procedures were performed with the 0.021″ version of the Magnum wire as the primary instrument. The Magnum wire proved universally applicable with advantages over conventional systems, particularly in difficult cases.

Other centers have had similar results. One institution underscores the advantages of the Magnum wire for angioplasty for acute occlusions, be they spontaneous or induced by an angioplasty with a conventional guidewire.[9]

The higher price of the Magnum wire compared with conventional wires is compensated for by a reduced need for wire replacement during the case and, if consistent with local policies, by reutilization. In addition, the initial passage of the 1-mm olive tip and the sturdy rail provided by the Magnum wire obviate the need for predilation with small balloons, which may amount to substantial savings for operators used to predilating tight lesions. The relative stiffness of the wire is advantageous in cases where the balloon does not track properly over a conventional, more flexible wire around a sharp bend (e.g., acute take-off of the left circumflex coronary artery). Retraction of the guiding catheter from a wedging position or deep intubation of the coronary artery for backup, also appears easier and safer with the Magnum wire.

The following disadvantages of the largest version of the Magnum system are of note: First, it requires balloons with a large central lumen and thus a less ideal deflated profile. This problem is largely overcome by the increased pushability of the system. Second, the presence and high radiopacity of the Magnum wire and the olive tip occasionally hamper the distal runoff or its assessment in small vessels. This has been somewhat amended by making the wire radiolucent except for the very tip. Nevertheless withdrawal of the wire partially for assessment of the result may be required. Readvancing the wire, if necessary, is rarely a problem since the Magnum wire is unsurpassed in terms of steerability and maneuverability. Third, the use of this Magnum system with 6 F or smaller guiding catheters is impossible. Yet, it can be used comfortably with 7-F guiding catheters with an internal lumen of 0.070″ or more.

The smaller versions of the Magnum wire are free of these shortcomings, but they do provide significantly less power to cross tough occlusions. Their smaller ball tip produces less resistance in the occlusive tissue. This facilitates progress through the occlusion, but it also increases the risk of subintimal passage or perforation.

Overall, the Magnum system is a helpful adjunct not only for angioplasty of chronic total occlusions but also for routine cases. It needs minor adjustments from conventional techniques but facilitates several basic maneuvers such as wire steering, guiding catheter placement and stabilization for backup, and balloon advancement.

OUTLOOK

Even if primary success of angioplasty of chronic total coronary occlusions can be improved by new technologies and skills, the clinical yield will never

Table 40-2. Magnum System for Chronic Total Occlusions

	Number	%
Procedures	804	100
Success	535	67
after failure of other device		27
Perforation	2	0.2
Death	5	0.6

compare with that of coronary angioplasty of stenoses. Recanalization angioplasty, a low-yield procedure, has to remain low-risk and low-cost. This sets limits to new tools and techniques. Laser instruments (e.g., the recently introduced bare excimer laser wire [Spectranetics]) hold the highest potential for passing old occlusions, yet, they are disqualified for risk and cost reasons. Mechanical means hold a lower potential for recanalization (unless solid wires that act like needles are considered), but they are simpler to handle, fraught with less risk, and far less costly. Blunt and sturdy wires, such as the Magnum wire, are likely to remain the mainstay of revascularization gear.

REFERENCES

1. Rahimtoola SH. The hibernating myocardium. Am Heart J 1989;117:211–21
2. Braunwald E, Kloner RA. The stunned myocardium: prolonged, postischemic ventricular dysfunction. Circulation 1982;66:1146–9
3. Serruys PW, Umans V, Heyndrickx GR et al. Elective PTCA of totally occluded coronary arteries not associated with acute myocardial infarction; short-term and long-term results. Eur Heart J 1985;6:2–12
4. Melchior JP, Doriot PA, Chatelain P et al. Improvement of left ventricular contraction and relaxation synchronism after recanalization of chronic total coronary occlusion by angioplasty. J Am Coll Cardiol 1987;4:763–8
5. Meier B. Chronic total occlusion. pp. 318–38. In Topol EJ (ed): Textbook of Interventional Cardiology. 2nd Ed. WB Saunders, Philadelphia, 1994
6. Meier B, Carlier M, Finci L et al. Magnum wire for balloon recanalization of chronic total coronary occlusions. Am J Cardiol 1989;64:148–54
7. Meier B. Magnarail probing catheter: new tool for balloon recanalization of chronic total coronary occlusions. J Invasive Cardiol 1990;2:227–9
8. Pande AK, Meier B, Urban P et al. Magnum/Magnarail versus conventional systems for recanalization of chronic total coronary occlusions: a randomized comparison. Am Heart J 1992;123:1182–6
9. Seggewiss H, Fassbender D, Gleichmann U et al. Recanalisation of occluded coronary arteries. Dtsch Med Wochenschr 1992;17:1543–9

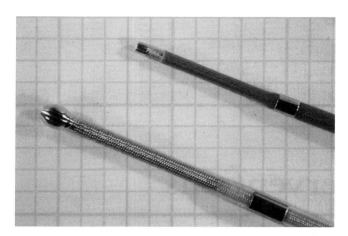

Fig. 41-1. Rotacs catheter for peripheral (2.2 mm) and coronary arteries (1.3 mm).

sel wall,[11] and (3) through the thrombus occluding the last patent lumen (transluminally).

Our working hypothesis was that a relatively large blunt and flexible catheter meeting the occcluded area under slow rotation with only a slight axial thrust would search the route of least resistance. Based on this principle, our group developed low-speed rotational angioplasty (Rotacs, Osypka GmbH, Grenzach-Wyhlen, Germany).[8–10] This catheter should detect the thrombotically occluded formerly patent lumen and find its way through, expressing fluid instead of removing material, with only a minor tendency toward entering the plaque or some of the pre-existing dissections. After experimental investigations in postmortem human arteries,[9] the first clinical procedure was performed in peripheral arteries in December 1986[10,21] and in coronary arteries in September 1987.[22,23]

TECHNIQUE

Peripheral System

The electrically driven rotating catheter (outer diameters, 1.8 and 2.2 mm) consists of four V$_2$A steel coiled wires of 0.2 mm each with an inner lumen that allows the introduction of exchange wires and injection of contrast agents. The catheter is covered with a highly flexible Teflon shrinking tube and has an olive-shaped blunt tip (Fig. 41-1). The motor unit (the same as that used in the coronary system), offering a continously variable speed ranging between 0 and 500 rpm is battery operated with a high level of electrical safety (Fig. 41-2).

After antegrade puncture of the femoral artery and

subsequent intra-arterial injection of 5,000 U of heparin, a conventional 7-F sheath is introduced, and angiography of the entire extremity is performed. A frozen picture of the occluded area is obtained via digital subtraction angiography, used as a road map to mark the obstructed area from behind the live radiographic image.

In patients with an occlusion of the iliac artery, an initial retrograde puncture of the contralateral femoral artery is performed; a 4-F pigtail catheter is placed into the abdominal aorta and a frozen picture selected that subsequently helps—via road mapping—with retrograde puncture of the femoral artery at the distal end of the occlusion. This procedure has proved to facilitate finding the artery with absent pulsation in the groin as well as careful insertion of the sheath into a relatively short distal vessel stump.

The Rotacs catheter is introduced directly through the plastic seal into the conventional hemostatic sheath and advanced, under fluoroscopic control to the obstructed area. When the occlusion is reached, the small motor unit, placed in the right hand of the operator, is started and the obstructed area slowly passed using a low rotational speed of 100 to 200 rpm under slight axial thrust and continous fluoroscopic monitoring. Once the occlusion is passed, blood is aspirated and disposed of, and contrast material is injected through the Rotacs catheter to document the intraluminal localization distal to the occlusion. A 0.35″ exchange wire, on standby in the rotating catheter approximately 2 cm behind the tip during the rotation procedure, is then reintroduced and advanced into the distal vessel. After retraction of the Rotacs catheter, the new channel is documented by angiography and further dilated using a conventional balloon catheter.

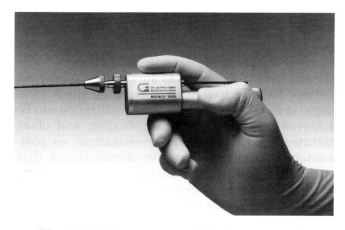

Fig. 41-2. Rotacs motor unit (battery operated).

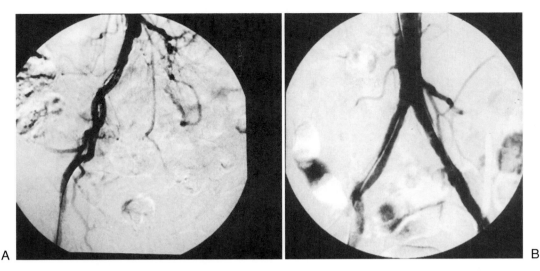

Fig. 41-3. Chronic occlusion of the left common iliac artery before **(A)** and after **(B)** reopening with the Rotacs catheter.

Coronary System

The coronary catheter, available in diameters of 1.3 and 1.6 mm, is equipped with a nonrotating outer shielding catheter made of polyethylene to protect the proximal vessel during rotation. This seems to be of importance especially in the left main coronary artery. The shielding catheter can be moved back and forth, changing the stiffness of the rotating catheter. The closer the shielding catheter is advanced toward the tip, the stiffer the rotating catheter. Using the different lengths available, the procedure can be performed via either the femoral (Judkins) or brachial (Sones) approach.

RESULTS

Peripheral Vessels

From December of 1986 to the present, more than 500 patients with chronic occlusions of peripheral vessels have been treated in Frankfurt; the procedure is now carried out in our center, as in several other centers, on a routine basis.

Acute Success Rates

In occluded superficial and popliteal arteries with an estimated duration of occlusion between 5 and 48 months (angiographically documented duration of up to 36 months) and occlusion lengths between 4 and 35 cm (mean, 12.5 cm) the acute success rate using Rotacs as the first attempt was more than 80%.

In patients in whom Rotacs was used after failure of conventional techniques, the acute success rate was still over 60%.[21] In occlusions of the iliac artery, which so far have not been considered indications for conventional balloon angioplasty,[7] low-speed rotational angioplasty has been successful in 62% of patients (Fig. 41-3).

Complications

No penetrations or perforations of the vessel wall have been observed. In 8% of the patients, there was angiographic evidence of dissections, comparable with conventional balloon angioplasty[6,24,25]; in 90% of these cases, the vessels were heavily calcified. No clinical consequences were seen. In 0.8%, a small distal embolization was detected angiographically but caused no further problems. In one iliac occlusion, balloon dilation after successful reopening resulted in a displacement of plaque material into the contralateral common iliac artery that was removed by the surgeon. In 4.8% of the patients a hematoma occurred at the puncture site, findings comparable to the results of conventional balloon angioplasty.[25-28] No patient died.

Limitations and Angiographic Preconditions

Vessels with fluoroscopically evident plaque-shaped calcifications in the occluded area more or less regularly obstructing the entire vessel lumen along the cross-sectional diameter (the respective resistances can be felt by the operator) are not likely to be suc-

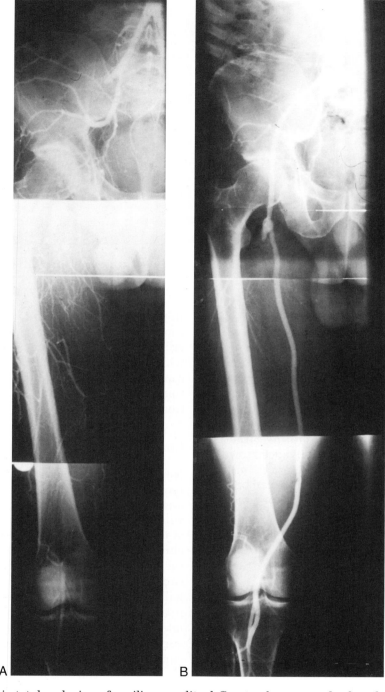

Fig. 41-4. Chronic total occlusion of an iliaco-popliteal Goretex bypass graft after the third operation **(A)** and after reopening with the Rotacs catheter, balloon dilation and implantation of a 6 mm stent into the distal anastomosis **(B)**.

cessfully reopened. By contrast, calcifications along the vessel wall in a longitudinal direction marking the path of the vessel do not restrict the chances of success even in cases of substantial stenosis. In a total of four patients with very old occlusions, major proximal collaterals had developed with a min-

imum angular distance that paralleled the native vessel. Since there was no definite proximal vessel stump, both the rotating catheter and the conventional guidewires kept slipping into the respective collateral, without inflicting any damage to the collateral.

First Long-Term Results

Angiographic long-term controls in femoral and popliteal arteries (mean, 4.4 months after reopening) showed a lasting good result without significant stenoses in 48%, relevant restenoses in 17%, and complete reocclusions in 35%; these data are comparable to conventional balloon angioplasty.[6,26] However, the total number of open vessels (65%) was significantly higher than in conventional angioplasty.

Evolving New Indications

Besides reopening chronic occlusions of bypass grafts (Fig. 41-4), several other new indications including occlusions of the subclavian artery (Fig. 41-5) are under investigation with encouraging early results.[29] A multicenter questionnaire, gathering results from the learning curves of 74 centers, already includes 1,252 patients and shows comparable good results.[30]

Coronary Arteries

From September 1987 to the present, more than 400 patients with chronic coronary occlusions in whom an attempt to reopen the artery with a conventional guidewire had failed were treated with the rotating catheter. The indication was based on documented ischemia in the vast majority of patients; in some patients (especially younger ones) without signs of ischemia the procedure was done for prognostic reasons.[31–33]

Acute Success Rate

After a learning curve, essentially influenced by a better understanding of morphologic preconditions and consequent further technical development, the acute success rate has now reached 70% (Fig. 41-6).[34,35] The age of occlusion turned out to be one of the most important factors: in occlusions with durations from 1 to 3 months the acute success rate was 93%, from 4 to 6 months it was 74%, from 6 to 12 months it was 52%, and in occlusions with durations of more than 12 months it was 8%.[23]

Complications

There were no deaths or arterial perforations. In two patients (nos. 23 and 30) dissection of a second large vessel occurred, which hindered the flow, and successful bypass surgery was performed. In both cases, the proximal stump of the occluded artery (left anterior descending artery) had been very short. This anatomic precondition should be considered a contraindication for reopening procedures. In 10% of the patients, dissections without impedement of flow were detected, results comparable with conventional balloon angioplasty. In three patients with relatively fresh occlusions, balloon angioplasty following the recanalization procedure resulted in distal embolization and caused infarction in one case.[23,35,36]

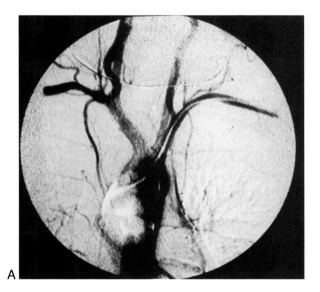 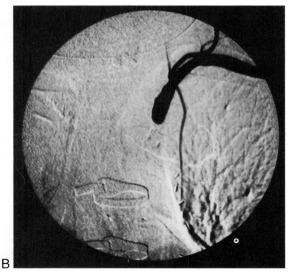

A   B

Fig. 41-5. Chronic occlusion of the left subclavian artery **(A)** in a patient after coronary bypass surgery (using the left inferior mesenteric artery) and the result after reopening with the Rotacs catheter and balloon dilation **(B)**.

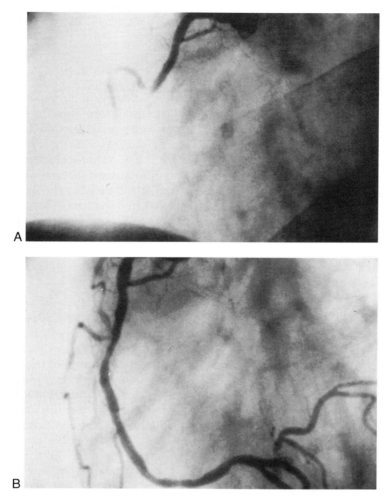

Fig. 41-6. Chronic occlusion of the right coronary artery **(A)** and the result after reopening with the Rotacs catheter and balloon dilation **(B)**.

First Long-Term Results

Angiographic follow-up in 76 of 84 consecutive patients after successful reopening (mean, 4 months after the intervention) documented an open vessel in 74%. In 45% good results were obtained without significant narrowing. Restenosis was found in 29% and was successfully redilated in 21 of these 22 patients. In 26% of the patients complete reocclusion turned out to be hard to reopen a second time.

DISCUSSION

Chronic arterial vessel occlusions are likely to be caused in most cases by ulcerating atherosclerotic plaques that cause stenoses of the vessel lumen subsequently occluded by thrombotic deposition.[15,37] Two major consequences may be derived from this

type of pathophysiologic process. First, a clear risk of dissection, and even wall perforation, is involved in the attempt to reopen occlusions mechanically due to preformed rupturing, a risk that rises with increasing occlusion length. Second, there is a soft point, a point of least resistance among concentrated obstructions in the occluded area that may persist for a yet unknown longer period. This soft point is the final occluding thrombus that indicates the last patent lumen and might help in pioneering through the occlusion.

The relatively thin and straight wires commonly used in conventional recanalization techniques may therefore easily enter such preformed dissections. Even with successful re-entry into the vessel lumen and ensuing neolumen, there are unsatisfactory acute and long-term results. The risk of wall perforation is especially high when such a wire is advanced through a vessel bend and approaches a delicate portion of wall. Thin wires therefore seem to be more dangerous than the relatively large and flexible catheter with an ideally blunt tip applied in the Rotacs technique. Low-speed rotation is associated with minimum adhesive friction, thus facilitating forward movement, passage through the vessel bends, and an especially sensitive transmission of any distal-to-proximal resistance.

These properties may be responsible for the definitively low tendency toward dissection observed so far in all our experimental and clinical studies, as a result of which we may conclude that there is virtually no risk of vessel wall perforation deriving from this procedure.

High-speed rotation techniques are not comparable with our technique: they differ fundamentally and technically, namely, with regard to the mechanism of recanalization.[38,39] Abrasive catheters rotating at high speeds of up to 150,000 rpm, some with diamond-covered sharp drilling heads, are geared to remove obstructive material by abrading. Inversely, low-speed rotational angioplasty aims at gently displacing or compressing the vessel-occluding material and consequently reducing volume as a result of fluid expression. The procedure can be compared with exposing without cutting.

Once the olive-shaped blunt tip has approached the obstructing material by slight axial thrusts, low-speed rotation leads the catheter to search the path of least resistance. Since the final occluding thrombus lags behind the other obstructive components in its organization and calcification, it represents and remains the softest part of the obstruction, offering easy penetration for a long time, possibly for years. It can be assumed that the rotating catheter will thus pass the obstruction through the last real lumen, as is also indicated by the often astonishing smooth channel surfaces achieved with subsequent balloon dilation, which is always performed.

Our experimental and clinical studies, which have now been under way for more than five years, demonstrate that reopening occluded vessels by means of low-speed rotational angioplasty has proved to be a particularly gentle and safe procedure with a low complication rate.[40] In peripheral arteries, the acute success rate with primary intervention exceeds 80%; even the very long occlusions were successfully reopened. In case conventional attempts fail, successful recanalization of formerly nontreatable occlusions can be achieved in more than 60% of cases by applying low-speed rotational angioplasty at a minimum time interval of 4 weeks from the primary intervention. This time period seems necessary for the sites of predilection and dissections to close following unsuccessful conventional reopening procedures. In chronic coronary occlusions that failed to be re-

opened with a conventional guidewire, the acute success rate of the Rotacs catheter is now around 70%.

In conclusion, both in peripheral and coronary arteries the new technique seems to expand the option of nonsurgical revascularization. Indeed, several large centers in Europe have taken over the technique as a routine procedure.[41–44] Randomized trials are needed to assess finally the relative importance of this technique; first results are encouraging.[44]

REFERENCES

1. Dotter CT, Judkins MP. Transluminal treatment of arteriosclerotic obstruction: description of a new technique and a preliminary report of its application. Circulation 1964;30:654
2. Grüntzig A, Hopff H. Perkutane Rekanalisation chronischer arterieller Verschlüsse mit einem neuen Dilatationskatheter. Modifikation der Dottertechnik. Dtsch Med Wochenschr 1974;99:2502
3. Kober G, Wochenschr Vallbracht C, Lang H et al. Transluminale koronare Angioplastik 1977–1985. Erfahrungen bei 1000 Eingriffen. Radiologe 1985;25:346
4. Simpson JB, Blain DS, Robert E, Harrison DC. A new catheter system for coronary angioplasty. Am J Cardiol 1982;49:1216
5. Faxon DP, Kelsey S, Kellet MA et al. Predictors of a successful angioplasty (PTCA registry). Circulation 1986;74:768
6. Zeitler E. Die perkutane transluminale Rekanalisation chronischer Stenosen und Verschlüsse peripherer Arterien. Wien Med Wochenschr 1985;135:384
7. Graziani L. Percutaneous recanalization of total iliac and femoropopliteal artery occlusions. Eur J Radiol 1987;7:91
8. Vallbracht C, Kress J, Schweitzer M et al. Rotationsangioplastik—ein neues Verfahren zur Gefäßwiedereröffnung und -erweiterung. Z Kardiol 1987;76:608
9. Kaltenbach M, Vallbracht C. Rotationsangioplastik—ein neues Katheterverfahren Fortschr Med 1987; 105:412
10. Vallbracht C, Liermann D, Prignitz I et al. Results of low speed rotational angioplasty for chronic peripheral occlusions. Am J Cardiol 1988;1:935
11. Baroldi G. Distribution of arterio-atherosclerotic obstructive lesions in coronary arteries. Vasc Surg 1974; 8:53
12. Freudenberg H, Knierim HJ, Möller C, Janzen CH. Qualitative morphologische Untersuchungen zur Koronarsklerose und Koronarinsuffizienz. Basic Res Cardiol 1974;69:161
13. Hangartner JRN, Charleston AJ, Daries MJ, Thomas AC. Morphological characteristics of clinically significant coronary artery stenosis in stable angina. Br Heart J 1986;56:501
14. Vlodaver ZJ, Edwards JE. Pathology of coronary atherosclerosis. Prog Cardiovasc Dis 1974;14:256
15. Schmitt W, Wack HO, Benecke G. Das Substrat chronischer arterieller Stenosen und Okklusionen. Dtsch Med Wochenschr 1971;86:1522
16. Alexander K, Buhl V, Holsten D, Poliwoda H, Wagner HH. Fibrinolytische Therapie des chronischen Arterien-verschlusses. Med Klin 1968;63:2067

17. Beck A. Perkutane Angioskopie: erste Erfahrungsberichte der PTA und der lokalen Lyse unter angioskopischen Bedingungen. Radiologe 1987;27:55

18. Ehringer H, Fischer M, Lechner K, Mayrhofer E. Thrombolytische Therapie nicht akuter arterieller Verschlüsse. Dtsch Med Wochenschr 1970;95:10

19. Hey D, Benecke G, Sandritter W. Die fermentative Löslichkeit von Fibrin in Thromben und bei fibrinösen Entzündungen. Klin Wochenschr 1966;44:770

20. Martin M, Schoop W, Zeitler E. Thrombolyse bei chronischer Arteriopathie. Verlag H. Huber, Bern 1970

21. Vallbracht C, Liermann D, Prignitz I et al. Low speed rotational angioplasty in chronic peripheral artery occlusions. Experience in 83 patients. Radiology 1989; 172:32

22. Kaltenbach M, Vallbracht C. Reopening of chronic coronary artery occlusions by low speed rotational angioplasty. J Interv Cardiol 1989;2:137

23. Kaltenbach M, Vallbracht C, Hartmann A. Wiedereröffnung chronischer Kranzgefäßverschlüsse durch ROTACS. Fortschr Med 1991;109:331

24. Grüntzig A. Die perkutane transluminale Rekanalisation chronischer Arterienverschlüsse mit einem neuen Dilatationskatheter. Verlag Witzstrock, Baden-Baden, 1977

25. Roth FJ, Heinig TH, Berliner P et al. Perkutane Rekanalisation peripherer Gefäße. In Günther RW, Thelen M (eds): Interventionelle Radiologie. Vol. 20. Georg-Thieme-Verlag, Stuttgart, 1988

26. Schneider E, Grüntzig A, Bollinger A. Die perkutane transluminale Angioplastie (PTA) in den Stadien II und IV der peripheren arteriellen Verschlußkrankheit. VASA 1982;11:336

27. Seyferth W, Ernsting M, Grosse-Verholt R, Zeitler E. Complications during and after Percutaneous Transluminal Angioplasty. p. 161. Springer-Verlag, Berlin, 1983

28. Zeitler E, Schmidtke I, Schoop W et al. Ergebnisse nach perkutaner Angioplastie bei über 700 Behandlungen. Röntgenpraxis 1976;29:78

29. Vallbracht C, Kollath J, Liermann D et al. Erfolgreiche Wiedereröffnung eines iliaco-poplitealen Goretex-Bypasses mit der Rotationsangioplastik. Fortschr Röntgenstr 1991;154:566

30. Vallbracht C, Kämpf AH, Liermann D et al. Low speed rotational angioplasty in chronic peripheral occlusions. Experiences in 1252 patients. Radiology 1992; 185:743

31. Vallbracht C, Stock M, Oster H et al. Wiedereröffnung chronischer Koronararterienverschlüsse—erste Hinweise auf eine prognostische Indikation. Herz 1994; 19:162

32. Kadel C, Burger W, Hartmann A et al. Langfristige Prognose nach erfolgreicher und erfolgloser PTCA chronischer Koronararterienverschlüsse. Z Kardiol, suppl. I. 1994;83:126

33. Kadel C, Schertel B, Vallbracht C, Schräder R. Klinische Bedeutung von Kollateralen, die von mittels PTCA rekanalisierten Koronarverschlüssen ausgehen. Z Kardiol, suppl. 1. 1995;84:58

34. Vallbracht C, Sittler B, Scheffler E et al. Chronische Koronararterienverschlüsse—alter Morphologie und Chance der Wiedereröffnung. Z Kardiol 1992;81:664

35. Kaltenbach M, Hartmann A, Vallbracht C. Procedural results and patient selection in recanalization of chronic coronary occlusions by low speed rotational angioplasty. Eur Heart J 1993;14:826

36. Burger W, Kadel C, Keul HG, Vallbracht C, Kaltenbach M. A word of caution: reopening chronic coronary occlusions. Cathet Cardiovasc Diagn 1992;27:35

37. Fulton WFM. Koronaratherosklerose, Fissurbildung der Plaques und Thrombose. In De Bono DP, Brodier ML et al (eds): Thrombolytische Therapie des akuten Herzinfarktes. Springer-Verlag, Berlin, 1987

38. Kensey RK, Nash JE, Abrahams C et al. Recanalization of obstructed arteries with a flexible rotating tip catheter. Radiology 1987;165:387

39. Ritchie JL, Hansen DD, Vracko H, Auth D. In vitro rotational thrombectomy—evaluation by angioscopy. Circulation 1986;74:1822

40. Vallbracht C, Liermann D, Landgraf H et al. Recanalization of chronic arterial obstructions: low-speed rotational angioplasty. 5 years experience in peripheral and coronary vessels. Eur J Med 1993;2:232

41. Nase-Hüpmeier S, Uebis R, Vallbracht C et al. Rekanalisation chronischer Koronararterienverschlüsse mit der Rotationsangioplastik. Akutergebnisse bei 20 Patienten. Z Kardiol 1991;80:62

42. Nase-Hüpmeier S, Uebis R, Vallbracht C et al. Low speed rotational angioplasty to recanalize chronic coronary artery occclusions: acute results and 6 months follow-up in 25 patients. Eur Heart J 1992;13:1219

43. Rieser R, Vallbracht C, Roth FJ. Indikationen zur Rotationsangioplastie der A. femoralis und A. poplitea. Fortschr Rötgenstr 1991;155:545

44. Danchin N, Julliere Y, Cassagnes J et al. Randomized multicenter study of low speed rotational angioplasty versus standard angioplasty for chronic total coronar occlusion. Circulation, suppl. 1. 1992;86:3110

42 Laser Guidewire

Jaap N. Hamburger
Patrick W. Serruys

Since the introduction of percutaneous transluminal coronary angioplasty (PTCA) in the late 1970s, this technique has increasingly been utilized as an alternative to coronary artery bypass surgery in the treatment of coronary artery disease. The continuing development of techniques and hardware for percutaneous interventions has promoted an ever expanding range of suitable indications. As a result, the number of PTCAs performed annually is about to surpass the number of bypass graft operations.[1] However, as a consequence of its dependency on guidewires for the guidance of any device into the coronary artery, the treatment of chronic total occlusions has always been the "stepchild of PTCA."

The first reports on the application of PTCA in the treatment of totally occluded coronary arteries were published by Savage et al.,[2] and Heyndrickx et al.[3] In recent years several centers have published data on large series of patients with totally occluded coronary arteries. The major issue in most of these studies was the description of those variables considered to be predictive of procedural success, such as lesion morphology, site of occlusion, experience of the interventional cardiologist performing the angioplasty, and, most importantly, amount of time elapsed since occlusion.[4–9] As could be expected, the old adage "the better the selection, the better the result" was certainly applicable and might explain the wide variety of reported success rates, ranging from 18 up to 80%. Considering the high success rates of PTCA for treatment of coronary stenoses, it is readily understood why the frustration due to frequent failure in the setting of total occlusion usually leads to referral for bypass grafting. However, in the light of the promising results in recent publications on cineangiographic[10] and clinical[9,11,12] late outcome of successfully treated patients, further exploration and improvement of techniques, aimed at the treatment of this potentially large group of patients,[13] seems justifiable.

XeCl EXCIMER LASER IN THE TREATMENT OF TOTAL CORONARY OCCLUSION

As stated above, the major limitation of PTCA for coronary occlusions is the inability of the operator to pass a guidewire through the occlusion into the distal bed; failure is secondary either to the inability to traverse through the occluded area or to subintimal tracking of the guidewire. Failure to traverse a total occlusion might result from failure to direct adequate force into the lesion, while subintimal wire tracking probably results from the guidewire finding a "path of least resistance."

A technique that seems explicitly qualified for treating total occlusions is forward debulking using a XeCl excimer laser, emitting invisible ultraviolet laser light at a wavelength of 308 nm. The basic mechanism of tissue ablation at this wavelength is considered to be a combination of photochemical dissociation of lipids and vaporization of tissue water.[14] It has been shown that the magnitude of this mecha-

493

nism is related to the energy density at the tip of the catheter and the catheter tip diameter.

Since its introduction in 1988, several thousand patients with symptomatic coronary artery disease have been treated by excimer laser coronary angioplasty, both in the United States and in Europe.[15–21]

THE LASER GUIDEWIRE

The Spectranetics Prima Coronary Total Occlusion System (model 018-003; Spectranetics, Colorado Springs, CO), consisting of an 0.018″ laser guidewire and a support catheter, has been designed to combine the mechanical attributes of a typical coronary guidewire with the ablative energy of the CVX-300 excimer laser to ease the initial crossing of total coronary occlusions (Fig. 42-1). The wire consists of optical fibers with a 45-μm diameter encased within a 0.018″ diameter shaft. The distal 30 cm of the wire is relatively floppy and is treated with a lubricious coating. The distal coil tip is radiopaque for visualization under fluoroscopy. The wire tip is shapable and, if required, reshapable during a procedure to meet specific anatomic circumstances.

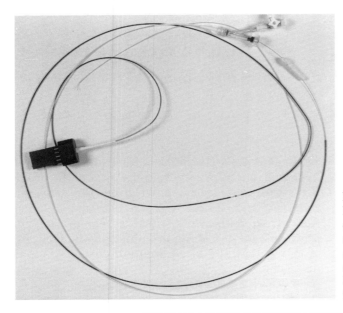

A

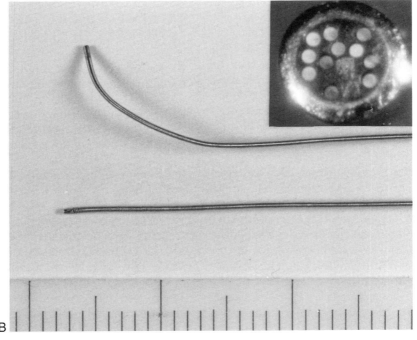

B

Fig. 42-1. The Prima Total Occlusion System. **(A)** The laser wire inside the support catheter. Note the proximal coupler and the premounted torque device. **(B)** The straight nonshapeable, nonsteerable tip of the first-generation laser wire (*bottom*) and the shapeable, steerable tip of the second-generation laser wire (*top*). (**Insert** *top right*) Magnification of the laser wire tip showing the 45-μm multifiber configuration.

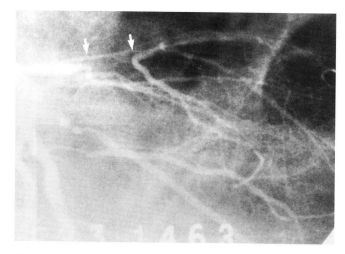

Fig. 42-2. Total occlusion of a proximal left coronary artery. Bilateral simultaneous injection of contrast medium, showing the occlusion stump and the distal lumen.

Furthermore, it has a torque device mounted on the proximal shaft. The support catheter that comes with the laser guidewire is 135 cm long and has a single 0.018″ wire-compatible lumen. It has a radiopaque marker mounted 1 mm proximal to a 2.5-F tapered tip. Finally, the system is supplied with a 15-cm-long tapered "peel-off" introducer to assist insertion of the laser guidewire into the support catheter.

The laser parameters typically used for the laser wire are an energy density of 60 mJ/mm^2 and a pulse repetition rate of 25 Hz. The pulse energy at this fluence is approximately 1.2 mJ.

Procedure

Since the laser guidewire is designed to ablate tissue, it is likely to advance through any type of vascular tissue once the laser has been activated. As a result, the proper alignment of the laser wire during laser activation is obviously the most critical issue involved in this procedure. Therefore, to allow for proper steering through a missing segment, both a proximal entry point and a clear distal (anatomic) entry point leading into a visible true distal lumen are absolute prerequisites (Fig. 42-2).

Making use of the intercoronary collateral circulation, most laser wire procedures are thus performed using simultaneous bilateral and (whenever available) biplane coronary angiography (Fig. 42-3). A monoplane system could be used provided frequent views from different angles are made prior to each advancement of the laser guidewire.

We currently use the following approach to optimize the chances of a successful procedure. A guiding catheter with an enlarged inner lumen and a minimum size of 8 F providing good coaxial alignment

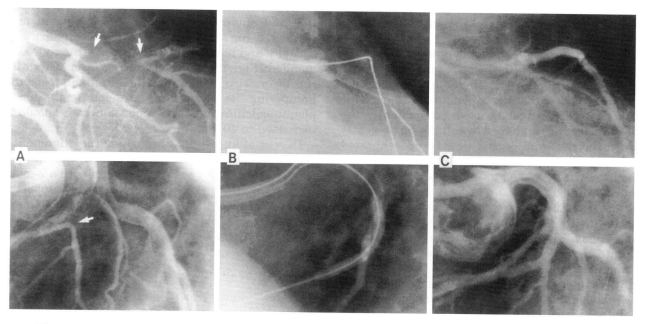

Fig. 42-3. Total occlusion of the left anterior descending artery (LAD) and the first diagonal branch. *Top row,* right anterior oblique view; *bottom row,* left superior oblique view. **(A)** The laser wire was used to recanalize both the occlusion in the LAD and the proximal diagonal branch. **(B)** Two long kissing balloons. **(C)** Final result.

artery. Contralateral injection of contrast medium showing the intraluminal position of the laser wire tip.

498 • Handbook of Cardiovascular Interventions / Vascular Interventions

502 • Handbook of Cardiovascular Interventions / Vascular Intervention

cost effectiveness of primary angioplasty as opposed to primary thrombolysis. In this regard one should consider not only the costs of the procedure itself, but the implications for the community if primary angioplasty becomes accepted as the preferred procedure over thrombolysis. This would entail the establishment of cardiac catheterization laboratories and most probably cardiac surgical programs (see below) with their attendant costs in large numbers of institutions that currently do not have that capability. Moreover, all the studies of primary angioplasty have been carried out in centers that have had extensive experience with elective angioplasty, and it is questionable whether these results can be extrapolated to the community at large. In the Myocardial Infarction, Triage, and Intervention (MITI) Registry, 1-year mortality in patients undergoing primary angioplasty and thrombolysis was virtually identical. Even among centers without on-site cardiac surgical programs, those individuals performing primary PTCA in the MITI Registry of hospitals in Seattle had extensive prior PTCA experience based on frequent activity at other large centers, and this may account for eqivalent survival figures[31] (Fig. 43-4). Currently, for most patients in the United States and other countries, the only reasonable initial approach is that of intravenous thrombolytic therapy (followed by careful observation with prompt intervention in the event of recurrent ischemia). Using this strategy, a substantial proportion of patients (the majority) will not require any subsequent intervention. Sicker patients, including those with cardiogenic shock, pulmonary edema, or other manifestations of hemodynamic compromise, should undergo primary angioplasty if at all feasible. It remains to be seen whether this will also be the preferred approach for other high-risk patients.

PTCA IN ANGINA PECTORIS

PTCA was originally developed for the treatment of symptomatic patients with angina pectoris and primarily single-vessel disease in whom the "culprit" lesion was technically suitable.[32] The widespread popularity of PTCA warrants a critical evaluation of its appropriate utilization in relation to medical therapy and its role in comparison with CABG, particularly in patients with multivessel disease. It is well established that the initial success rate of PTCA is high and in the intermediate term mortality and myocardial infarction rates are low.[33] Whereas, PTCA *may* indeed be the treatment of choice compared with medical therapy, particularly in patients with a high-grade proximal left anterior descending artery stenosis or in patients with severely symptomatic angina, it has taken almost 10 years after introduction of the technique before it was subjected to the rigorous scrutiny of randomized clinical trials. The need for such trials is particularly cogent in the light of advances in both medical and cardiac surgical care and the current appropriate focus upon costs.

A recent analysis of a large private insurance claims database of patients under the age of 65 in the United States introduces concerns about the appropriate utilization of PTCA in clinical practice (Table 43-1). Approximately 96% of procedures were single-vessel angioplasties (most of the patients had a diagnosis of stable angina pectoris) yet in only approximately 30% of patients was there documenta-

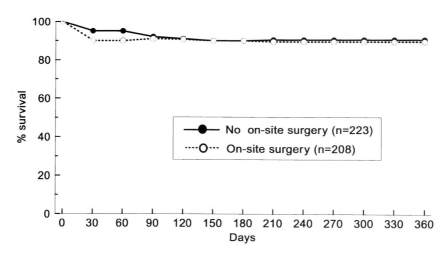

Fig. 43-4. One-year survival curves for patients with acute myocardial infarctions treated with primary angioplasty at centers with and without on-site cardiac surgical programs. (Modified from Weaver et al.,[31] with permission.)

Table 43-1. PTCA Practices in the United States Based on an Insurance Claims Database of 2,101 Patients[a]

Practices	%
Single-vessel PTCA	96
Stable angina pectoris	72
No prior exercise stress test	66
No prior exercise stress test, after myocardial infarction	91

[a] Only 29% of the study cohort had exercise testing before angioplasty and single-vessel procedures were performed in approximately 95% of all procedures.
(Modified from Topol et al.,[34] with permission.)

tion of an exercise test prior to the procedure.[34] The recent American College of Cardiology/American Heart Association (ACC/AHA) guidelines state very clearly that among patients with mild or no symptoms there should be "objective evidence of myocardial ischemia during laboratory testing."[35] Moreover, in a recent analysis of *all* PTCA procedures performed in the state of California during 1989, it is disturbing to note that among institutions performing PTCA, fewer than 200 procedures per year were done in 50% of these institutions. The complications at these low-volume institutions (as assessed by the emergency bypass surgery and mortality rates) are correspondingly higher than the published figures for institutions performing more than 200 cases per year[36] (Fig. 43-5).

SINGLE-VESSEL DISEASE

No randomized trial to date has demonstrated a *survival* benefit from coronary revascularization (CABG or PTCA) over medical therapy in patients with single-vessel disease. The Veterans Affairs Angioplasty Compared to Medicine (ACME) trial evaluated "softer" end points such as exercise tolerance and symptoms at 6 months, in 212 patients with single-vessel disease randomized to medical therapy or PTCA.[37] The patients in the PTCA arm were more likely to be free of angina, and improvement in exercise tolerance on a treadmill at 6 months compared with entry was greater than among those treated medically (Fig. 43-6) It should be kept in mind, however, that approximately 25% of patients in the PTCA arm had a repeat PTCA or bypass surgery in the intervening 6 months. There was no difference in terms of death or myocardial infarction between the two groups. Given that approximately half of the medically treated patients were free of angina at 6 months and that the improvement in treadmill performance on exercise testing was achieved at a cost of 7 bypass operations and 18 repeat PTCAs in the angioplasty group, a reasonable conclusion would advocate that a medical approach should be initially undertaken for all patients, reserving PTCA for those who "fail" due to persistent symptoms or severe ischemia.

A strong case could be made for a randomized trial of angioplasty versus CABG surgery for patients with single-vessel disease involving the proximal left anterior descending coronary artery, particularly given the high rate of restenosis following angio-

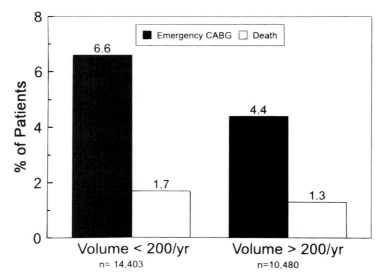

Fig. 43-5. Emergency CABG and death rates at institutions in California where less than or greater than 200 angioplasties per year are performed. (Modified from Ritchie et al.,[36] with permission.)

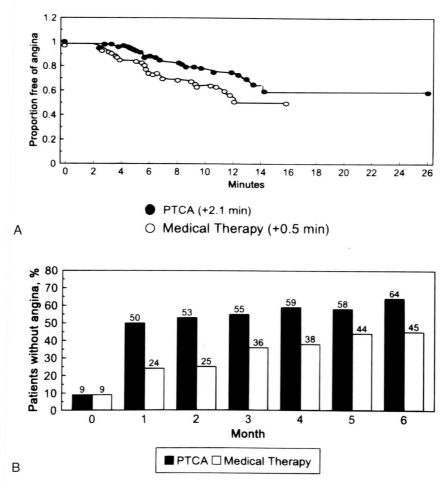

Fig. 43-6. (A) Duration of angina-free exercise on the treadmill. The proportion of patients who were free of angina is plotted as a function of the duration of exercise time until the onset of angina. **(B)** Percentage of patients free of angina at each month after randomization. 0, month prior to randomization. Subsequent bars refer to the six clinic visits in the months after randomization. (Modified from Parise et al.,[37] with permission.)

plasty, but no such trials are in progress. Although angioplasty in patients with this lesion is safe and associated with a high initial success rate, restenosis rates are higher than in PTCA at other sites, and the late prognosis is consequently characterized by a higher rate of recurrent symptoms and the need for repeat revascularization.[38–42]

MULTIVESSEL DISEASE

The randomized trials of coronary bypass surgery and medical therapy highlighted the benefits of surgical revascularization over medical therapy in patients with multivessel disease and left ventricular dysfunction.[6,7] It is evident that the "sicker" the patient in terms of left ventricular dysfunction, severity of ischemia, and number of diseased vessels, the

greater the benefit from revascularization. Ischemia, rather than angina, is the current target of therapy, and impaired left ventricular function (in the setting of documented ischemia) is an important indication rather than a contraindication to surgery. Although these trials of bypass surgery compared with medical therapy provided a wealth of information about the indications for coronary revascularization, the data cannot be universally extrapolated to the results of angioplasty in comparison with medical therapy.

Difficulties in Comparing PTCA With CABG Using the Published Literature

There are difficulties in using the published literature to draw comparisons between the two forms of revascularization.

Technical Advances

Whereas the technical advances related to CABG and medical therapy probably began to plateau a decade or so ago, in the case of percutaneous revascularization, techniques continue to improve and the learning curve is on a steeply "ascending limb." This has expanded the pool of patients who are amenable to percutaneous techniques including patients with complex anatomy and those with multivessel disease. Unfortunately, because of this rapid growth in percutaneous technology, randomized trials will always be vulnerable to criticism on the basis of a "moving target," as current therapeutic modalities become outdated or even invalid in the face of newer techniques.

Patient Heterogeneity

A compounding complicating factor in using the published literature for comparison of PTCA and CABG in patients with multivessel disease is the marked variability in clinical profiles between the two groups, including the stability of ischemia or angina, the amount of myocardium at jeopardy, and left ventricular function. Studies performed to date would suggest that patients, who do undergo PTCA have less severe disease and better left ventricular function as compared with those undergoing CABG surgery.[43,44] If one examines the Collaborative Study in Coronary Artery Surgery (CASS) database, 62% of patients with multivessel disease undergoing surgery had triple-vessel disease.[45] Likewise, 62% in the Emory University series had triple-vessel disease.[46] By contrast, the National Heart, Lung, and Blood Institute (NHLBI) PTCA registry shows that of the patients with multivessel disease who undergo angioplasty, only 41% had triple vessel disease.[47] The percentage of patients with triple-vessel disease who underwent angioplasty was even lower in the study by Deligonul et al.[39] (26%), the Emory University series[46] (21%), the Mayo Clinic series[48] (38%), and the Duke University report[49] (10%) (Fig. 43-7). In most PTCA series, patients with left ventricular dysfunction (i.e., ejection fraction <50%) comprise only 15 to 20% of the population.[47,48]

Angioplasty for multivessel disease appears to have a high initial success rate with a relatively low complication rate.[43,44] On the other hand, the results among patients with left ventricular dysfunction the are disappointing. The 2-year mortality in patients who underwent PTCA with ejection fractions of 40% or less has been shown to be as high as 25%.[50] Other retrospective studies would suggest that predictors of poor long-term results with multivessel PTCA include an age greater than 70 years, an ejection fraction less than 40%, or prior CABG surgery.[51]

Duration of Follow-Up

Other factors that need to be taken into account include the much shorter duration of follow-up after PTCA compared with bypass surgery, which is now

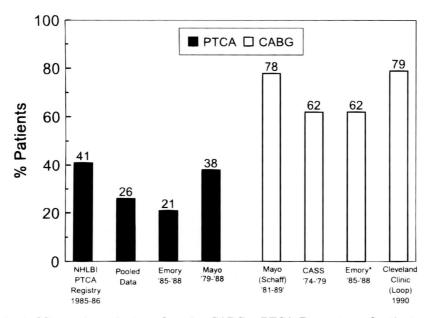

Fig. 43-7. Extent of disease in patients undergoing CABG or PTCA. Percentage of patients with multivessel disease who have triple-vessel disease. *, excludes left main coronary artery disease; NHLBI, National Heart, Lung, and Blood Institute. (Data from Kennedy et al.,[45] Weintraub et al.,[46] Detre et al.,[47] and Bell et al.[48])

well into its third decade.[33,42,43,52,53] The incidence of hard end points such as myocardial infarction and death are relatively infrequent after PTCA; consequently, softer, more subjective criteria are used as surrogate end points including exercise tolerance, symptoms, and repeat revascularization (including repeat PTCA).

Completeness of Revascularization

Another area of uncertainty is the importance of complete revascularization for long-term survival and morbidity. The CASS data would suggest that for bypass surgery, complete revascularization is preferable, particularly among patients with severe ischemia and or left ventricular dysfunction.[54] Among patients undergoing PTCA, an early study by Vandormael et al.[55] showed that the short-term event-free survival was significantly better in those patients who had complete revascularization. The experience from the Mayo Clinic was similar, since the 5-year event-free survival rate was 62% in those patients who underwent complete revascularization as opposed to 37% in those who did not (including patients with single-vessel disease).[48] By contrast, the NHLBI (PTCA) Registry for patients with multivessel disease did not show a difference at 26 months in the rates of myocardial infarction or death, but there was an increased rate of repeat revascularization among patients incompletely revascularized initially.[56] This was supported by a retrospective study of O'Keefe et al.,[51] which also revealed a higher rate of subsequent CABG surgery in those patients not completely revascularized at the time of their initial procedure.

Using currently available technology, complete revascularization is obtainable only in a minority of patients with multivessel disease; this is partly the result of chronically completely occluded vessels. Only 23 and 9% of patients with double- and triple-vessel disease, respectively, were able to be completely revascularized according to the NHLBI PTCA registry cohort.[58] While "culprit" angioplasty may be sufficient in terms of relieving symptoms and the functional ischemic burden, particularly in patients with unstable angina and multivessel disease, prospective long-term studies have yet to be performed.[59] Whereas complete revascularization remains a desirable goal, differences in attitudes exist toward PTCA and coronary bypass surgery that influence the choice of the procedure. PTCA is easily repeatable and there is no need to treat all lesions at once. The major objective of angioplasty is to treat all "functionally significant" lesions, as opposed to

coronary bypass surgery, in which the impetus is to bypass all anatomically obstructive lesions. Incomplete revascularization after PTCA is therefore often the result of a strategic decision or its technical limitations, due to the presence of complete occlusions or complex anatomy. By contrast, incomplete revascularization after surgery is primarily due to the presence of severe diffuse disease and small-caliber vessels, or prior myocardial infarction with vessels supplying areas of akinetic myocardium. These different therapeutic approaches may have implications on the long-term results of incomplete revascularization following both procedures.

Impact of Restenosis

Restenosis remains the "Achilles' heel" of PTCA. The impact of restenosis on the late outcome after angioplasty is profound and is the major reason for the recurrence of symptoms and repeat revascularization procedures. In this respect, the completeness of revascularization may act as a double-edged sword in that the advantages of complete percutaneous revascularization may be nullified to some extent by the higher frequency of restenosis and the necessity for repeat diagnostic or therapeutic procedures. This is a complex issue that also has a major effect on the economic impact of PTCA compared with bypass surgery. Relative costs are the focus of ancillary analyses of the randomized trials (see below) in addition to decision analysis models aimed at evaluating the cost effectiveness of repeat PTCA.[60]

RECENT RANDOMIZED TRIALS

PTCA Versus Medical Therapy

The Veterans Administration ACME trial (see above) is the only published trial of its kind to date comparing medical therapy with PTCA in patients with single-vessel coronary artery disease. In patients with double-vessel disease who were randomized in the ACME trial, the exercise time was no different at 6 months in the PTCA group as compared with the medical treatment group, although the numbers were too small to draw any definitive statistic conclusions.

PTCA Versus CABG

In 1993, the preliminary results of several randomized trials comparing PTCA with bypass surgery were published. Despite significant differences in the patient populations and designs of these trials, the results are reasonably consistent and concordant with the data collected from previous nonrandomized comparative studies in individual series. In essence, rates of death and myocardial infarction are similar in the two groups, whereas, as expected, patients undergoing PTCA undergo more recurrent revascularization procedures and are more frequently symptomatic than their surgical counterparts.

The preliminary results of the United Kingdom's Randomized Intervention of Angina trial (RITA) showed that after 2.5 years of follow-up no significant difference was seen in the incidence of death or nonfatal myocardial infarction when comparing PTCA with CABG surgery in patients with one- to three-vessel coronary artery disease[61] (Fig. 43-8). Patients had to be deemed eligible for equivalent revascularization by either PTCA or CABG surgery according to a cardiologist and a cardiac surgeon. Approximately one-third of patients enrolled had single-vessel disease. The PTCA group, however, did have a higher frequency of repeat diagnostic and therapeutic procedures, were more symptomatic, and required more antianginal medications at 2.5 years.

Preliminary data from the even smaller Argentine Randomized Trial for PTCA versus CABG Surgery in multivessel disease (ERACI) also showed no difference between the two groups with respect to in-hospital or 1-year mortality, although the CABG group was more asymptomatic, free from repeat interven-

tions, and had fewer combined cardiac ischemic events at 1 year.[62] "Complete" revascularization was more frequently achieved in the CABG group (88 vs. 51%, $P < 0.001$).

The German Angioplasty-Bypass Intervention (GABI) trial is a similar trial in which 358 patients with a minimum of two-vessel coronary disease were randomized to be revascularized by PTCA or CABG, if amenable for both.[63] The results are consistent with other studies in that there has been no significant difference in in-hospital or 6-month follow-up with respect to death or myocardial infarction. There were, however, more repeat interventions performed on the PTCA group (46.5 vs. 6.7%). The 6-month angiographic restenosis rate was 34%, whereas among patients undergoing CABG, 22% had grafts that were either occluded or stenosed by greater than 50%.

The Coronary Angioplasty Bypass Revascularization Investigation (CABRI) is a similar European-based, international trial comparing these two strategies in patients over a 5-year time span.[64] The end points, in addition to those mentioned above, include new cardiovascular events and changes in left ventricular function. A total of 1,054 patients was entered in this study in 1992, and follow-up is currently being compiled. The 1-year follow-up data were presented at the 15th Congress of the European Society of Cardiology and demonstrated no significant difference with respect to mortality, myocardial

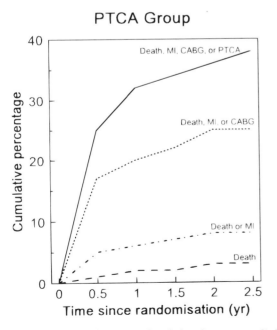

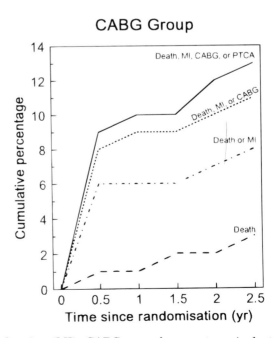

Fig. 43-8. Cumulative risk of death, myocardial infarction (MI), CABG, or subsequent angioplasty (PTCA) in patients randomized to PTCA or CABG in the RITA Trial.

infarction, or degree of symptoms, but a greater frequency of repeat interventions in the PTCA group.[64]

At Emory University, the Emory Angioplasty versus Surgery Trial (EAST) is a single-center comparison of these two techniques in 379 patients with multivessel disease.[65] In addition to death and myocardial infarction, primary end points include large thallium imaging defects. Secondary end points include angiographic follow-up, anginal status, exercise tolerance, need for repeat revascularization, quality of life, and cost analyses. Preliminary data were presented at the 66th Scientific Sessions of the AHA, and again no significant difference was seen between the two groups at 3 years with respect to the major primary end points, although the frequency of revascularization was significantly higher in the PTCA group. An unexpected finding was the absence of any difference in quality of life or overall 3-year costs between the groups, despite the greater in-hospital cost for the surgical group.

In North America, the largest of these trials, under the auspices of the NHLBI, is the Bypass Angioplasty Revascularization Investigation (BARI).[66] This is a 14-center trial in which approximately 2,000 patients were enrolled on entry completion in 1991. Patients were required to have unstable angina, a recent myocardial infarction, severe angina or severe ischemia with a history of previous angina or myocardial infarction, and at least a 50% stenosis in two or more major coronary arteries. Revascularization could be performed by either procedure as assessed by a BARI cardiologist and surgeon. End points are similar to those mentioned for the CABRI and EAST studies.

Although much of the data presented to date is preliminary, consistent and interesting trends are discernable. In regard to the hard end points of death and myocardial infarction, results are similar between PTCA and bypass surgery (at least in the short term), but this is achieved at the cost of a higher (yet acceptable) rate of repeat revascularization in the PTCA group (half of whom will undergo coronary bypass surgery) and more frequent recurrence of symptoms. Nonetheless, several caveats have to be born in mind. The numbers entered into these trials are still relatively small, and data from BARI, which is the largest trial, are not yet available. *Moreover, the results cannot be extrapolated to subsets of patients who were not entered into these randomized trials.* The trial population consists of highly selected patients with *good* ventricular function and lesions that were deemed to be technically suitable; in many of the studies revascularization had to be deemed equivalent by both techniques. For most patients with multivessel disease, the incidence of complete revascularization is markedly less with PTCA compared with CABG due to the presence of chronic complete occlusions; left ventricular dysfunction is present in a substantial proportion and it is likely that coronary bypass surgery will still be the treatment of choice in such patients. By contrast, for the selected patient whose clinical and angiographic characteristics are similar to those included in the randomized trials, it is reasonable to use PTCA as the initial therapeutic strategy followed by surgery for patients who fail. This is a decision that must be individualized according to patient preference, physician expertise, age, and the presence of other co-morbid conditions.

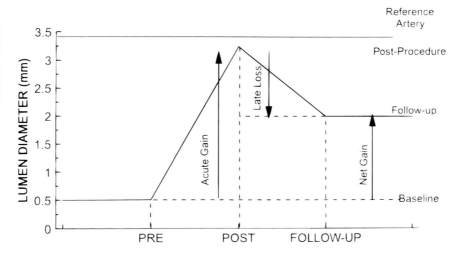

Fig. 43-9. Schematic diagram demonstrating that the late procedural outcome after coronary intervention is determined by the offsetting effects of "acute gain" immediately after the procedure and the "late loss" that occurs over the ensuing 4 to 6 months. (Modified from Kuntz and Baim,[67] with permission.)

An important determinant of the role of PTCA compared to CABG in patients with multivessel disease is cost, and this is currently under investigation in several studies. Any potential benefit of percutaneous revascularization may be nullified if multiple angioplasty procedures or if bypass surgery is subsequently performed. Approaches to reducing the high incidence of restenosis are pivotal, and if successful will have profound implications for the place of PTCA in patients with multivessel disease. If one believes in the "bigger is better" hypothesis and that achieving the best acute result possible results in a lower restenosis rate, new techniques such as directional coronary atherectomy and intracoronary stenting may improve upon the "acute gain" of PTCA and decrease the "late loss," therefore decreasing the long term restenosis rates[67] (Fig. 43-9). All new devices which have different primary mechanisms of action from PTCA should be critically assessed in prospective trials. The basic mechanisms for and prevention of restenosis are a focus of intense investigation at the cellular and molecular level, but in the interim clinical interest is focused upon the potential for new devices to modify restenosis.

CONCLUSIONS

It is hoped that randomized trials of angioplasty versus medical therapy or bypass surgery will provide us with greater insight and information to guide us in the selection of the optimal form of therapy. Outcomes in patients with single-vessel coronary disease are excellent when patients are treated medically, and to date no therapy has been shown to be better. Whether the improvement in symptoms and exercise performance will ultimately justify both the short- and long-term cost of angioplasty as opposed to medical therapy remains to be seen. Currently, PTCA is clearly indicated for persons with single-vessel disease who are refractory to medical therapy, although the potential for overutilization remains a concern.

Bypass surgery will likely remain the treatment of choice for most patients with triple-vessel disease and left ventricular dysfunction, left main coronary artery disease, and diffusely diseased vessels. Among patients with multivessel disease, PTCA is likely to play a prominent role in patients with two-vessel disease, good left ventricular function, or in advanced age, or in those in whom it is considered a salvage procedure. The likelihood of angioplasty superceding bypass surgery as the treatment of choice for patients with multivessel disease and left ventricular systolic dysfunction depends on the ability to treat most if not all total chronic occlusions and

on the ability to eliminate restenosis—this remains in the future. Currently, PTCA and CABG are traditionally thought of as competitive procedures, but it is appropriate to consider them as complementary in that increasingly PTCA is being performed in patients with previous bypass surgery, and in the face of a continued high rate of restenosis, CABG is performed in approximately 25% of patients within 1 to 2 years of angioplasty.

REFERENCES

1. Lytle BW, Cosgrove D, Loop FD. Future implications of current trends in bypass surgery. Cardiovasc Clin 1991;21:265
2. Holmes DR Jr, Vlietstra RE. Balloon angioplasty in acute and chronic coronary artery disease. JAMA 1989;261:2109
3. Feinleib M, Havlik RJ, Gillum RF et al. Coronary heart disease and related procedures: National Hospital Discharge Survey data. Circulation, suppl. I 1989; 79:I-13
4. Takaro T, Hultgran HN, Lipton M et al. The VA Cooperative Randomized Study of Surgery for Coronary Arterial Occlusive Disease. II. Subgroup with significant left main lesions. Circulation, suppl. III. 1976;51: III-107
5. European Coronary Surgery Study Group. Long-term results of prospective randomised study of coronary artery bypass surgery in stable angina pectoris. Lancet 1982;2:1173
6. Alderman EL, Bourassa MG, Cohen LS et al. Ten-year follow-up of survival and myocardial infarction in the randomized Coronary Artery Surgery Study. Circulation 1990;82:1629
7. The VA Coronary Artery Bypass Surgery Cooperative Study Group. Eighteen-year follow-up in the Veterans Affairs Cooperative Study of Coronary Artery Bypass Surgery for stable angina. Circulation 1992;86:121
8. Mock MB, Fisher LD, Holmes DR Jr et al. Comparison of effects of medical and surgical therapy on survival in severe angina pectoris and two-vessel coronary artery disease with and without left ventricular dysfunction: a Coronary Artery Surgery Study Registry study. Am J Cardiol 1998;61:1198
9. Kaiser GC, Davis KB, Fisher LD et al. Survival following coronary artery bypass grafting in patients with severe angina pectoris (CASS): an observational study. J Thorac Cardiovasc Surg 1985;89:513
10. Subcommittee on Coronary Artery Bypass Surgery: ACC/AHA guidelines and indications for coronary artery bypass graft surgery. Circulation 1991;83:1125
11. Topol EJ, Cliff RM, George BS et al. A randomized trial of immediate versus delayed elective angioplasty after intravenous tissue plasminogen activator in acute myocardial infarction. N Engl J Med 1987;317: 581
12. Simoons ML, Arnold AER, Betriu A et al. Thrombolysis with tissue plasminogen activator in acute myocardial infarction: no additional benefit from immediate percutaneous coronary angioplasty. Lancet 1988;1: 197

13. The TIMI Research Group: Immediate versus delayed catheterization and angioplasty following thrombolytic therapy for acute myocardial infarction: TIMI-II A results. JAMA 1988;260:2849

14. The TIMI Study Group. Comparison of invasive and conservative strategies after treatment with intravenous tissue plasminogen activator in acute myocardial infarction: results of the Thrombolysis in Myocardial Infarction (TIMI) II Trial. N Engl J Med 1989;320:618

15. SWIFT Trial Study Group. SWIFT trial of delayed elective intervention *v* conservative treatment after thrombolysis with anistreplase in acute myocardial infarction. BMJ 1991;302:555

16. Barbash GI, Roth A, Hod H et al. Randomized control trial of late in-hospital angiography and angioplasty versus conservative management after treatment with recombinant tissue-type plasminogen activator in acute myocardial infarction. Am J Cardiol 1990;66:538

17. Terrin ML, Williams DO, Kleiman NS et al. Two- and three-year results of the Thrombolysis in Myocardial Infarction (TIMI) phase II clinical trial. J Am Coll Cardiol 1993;22:1763

18. Mueller HS, Cohen LS, Braunwald E et al. Predictors of early morbidity and mortality after thrombolytic therapy of acute myocardial infarction. Analysis of patient subgroups in the Thrombolysis in Myocardial Infarction (TIMI) trial, phase II. Circulation 1992;85: 1254

19. Ellis SG, Van de Werf F, Ribeiro-daSilva E et al. Present status of rescue coronary angioplasty: current polarization of opinion and randomized trials. J Am Coll Cardiol 1992;19:681

20. Braunwald E. Myocardial reperfusion, limitation of infarct size reduction of left ventricular dysfunction, and improved survival. Should the paradigm be expanded? Circulation 1989;79:441

21. Califf RM, Topol EJ, Gersh BJ. From myocardial salvage to patient salvage in acute myocardial infarction: the role of reperfusion therapy. J Am Coll Cardiol 1989;14:1382

22. Ritchie JL, Davis KB, Willims DL et al. Global and regional left ventricular function and tomographic radionuclide perfusion: the Western Washington Intracoronary Streptokinase in Myocardial Infarction Trial. Circulation 1984;70:867

23. Gersh BJ, Anderson JL. Thrombolysis and myocardial salvage: results of clinical trials and the animal paradigm: paradoxic or predictable? Circulation 1993;88: 296

24. ISIS-2 (Second International Study of Infarct Survival) Collaborative Group. Randomised trial of intravenous streptokinase, oral aspirin, both, or neither among 17,187 cases of suspected acute myocardial infarction: ISIS-2. Lancet 1988;2:349

25. Krucoff MW, Croll MA, Pope JE, et al. Continuous 12-lead ST-segment recovery analysis in the TAMI 7 Study. Performance of a noninvasive method for real-time detection of failed myocardial reperfusion. Circulation 1993;88:437

26. Ellis AK, Little T, Zaki Masud AR et al. Early noninvasive detection of successful reperfusion in patients with acute myocardial infarction. Circulation 1988;78: 1352

27. Grines CL, Browne KF, Marco G et al. A comparison of immediate angioplasty with thrombolytic therapy for acute myocardial infarction. N Engl J Med 1993; 328:673

28. O'Neill WW, Zijlstra F, Suryapranata H et al. Meta-analysis of the PAMI and Netherlands randomized trials of primary angioplasty versus thrombolytic therapy of acute myocardial infarction, abstracted. Circulation, suppl. I. 1993;88:1–106

29. Gibbons RJ, Holmes DR, Reeder GS et al. Immediate angioplasty compared with the administration of a thrombolytic agent followed by conservative treatment of myocardial infarction. N Engl J Med 1993; 328:685

30. Zijlstra F, Jan de Boer M, Hoorntje JCA et al. A comparison of immediate coronary angioplasty with intravenous streptokinase in acute myocardial infarction. N Engl J Med 1993;328:680

31. Weaver WD, Litwin PE, Martin JS. Use of direct angioplasty for treatment of patients with acute myocardial infarction in hospitals with and without onsite cardiac surgery. The Myocardial Infarction, Triage, and Intervention Project Investigators. Circulation 1993;88:2067

32. Grüntzig AR, Senning A, Siegenthaler WE. Nonoperative dilatation of coronary-artery stenosis: percutaneous transluminal coronary angioplasty. N Engl J Med 1979;301:61

33. Talley JD, Hurst JW, King SB III et al. Clinical outcome 5 years after attempted percutaneous transluminal coronary angioplasty in 427 patients. Circulation 1988;77:820

34. Topol EJ, Ellis SG, Cosgrove DM et al. Analysis of coronary angioplasty practice in the United States with an insurance-claims data base. Circulation 1993; 87:1749

35. Ryan TJ, William BB, Kennedy JW et al. Guidelines for percutaneous transluminal coronary angioplasty. J Am Coll Cardiol 1993;22:2033

36. Ritchie JL, Phillips KA, Luft HS. Coronary angioplasty: statewide experience in California. Circulation 1993;88:2735

37. Parisi AF, Folland ED, Hartigan P, for the Veterans Affairs ACME Investigators. A comparison of angioplasty with medical therapy in the treatment of single-vessel coronary artery disease. N Engl J Med 1992; 326:10

38. Dorros G, Stertzer SH, Cowley MJ et al. Complex coronary angioplasty: multiple coronary dilatations. Am J Cardiol 1984;53:126C

39. Deligonul U, Vandormael MG, Kern MJ et al. Coronary angioplasty: a therapeutic option for symptomatic patients with two and three vessel coronary disease. J Am Coll Cardiol 1988;11:1173

40. Gersh BJ, Holmes DR Jr. Coronary angioplasty as the preferred approach to treatment of multivessel disease: promising, appealing but unproved. J Am Coll Cardiol 1990;16:1104

41. O'Keefe JH Jr, Rutherford BD, McConahay DR et al. Multivessel coronary angioplasty from 1980 to 1989: procedural results and long-term outcome. J Am Coll Cardiol 1990;16:1097

42. Faxon DP, Ruocco N, Jacobs AK. Long-term outcome of patients after percutaneous transluminal coronary angioplasty. Circulation, suppl. IV. 1990;811:IV-9

43. Henderson RA, Raskino C, Karani S et al. Comparative long-term results of coronary angioplasty in single and multivessel disease. Eur Heart J 1992;13:781

44. Hartzler GO. Coronary angioplasty is the treatment of choice for multivessel coronary artery disease. Chest 1986;90:877

45. Kennedy JW, Kaiser GC, Fisher LD et al. Clinical and angiographic predictors of operative mortality from the Collaborative Study in Coronary Artery Surgery (CASS). Circulation 1981;63:793

46. Weintraub WS, Jones EL, King SB III et al. Changing use of coronary angioplasty and coronary bypass surgery in the treatment of chronic coronary artery disease. Am J Cardiol 1990;65:183

47. Detre K, Holubkov R, Kelsey S et al. Percutaneous transluminal coronary angioplasty in 1985–1986 and 1977–1981: the National Heart, Lung, and Blood Institute Registry. N Engl J Med 1988;318:265

48. Bell MR, Bailey KR, Reeder GS et al. Percutaneous transluminal angioplasty in patients with multivessel coronary disease: how important is complete revascularization for cardiac event-free survival? J Am Coll Cardiol 1990;16:553

49. Mark DB, Nelson CL, Califf RM. Hanell FE Jr et al. Continuous evolution of therapy for coronary artery disease. Initial results from the era of coronary angioplasty. Circulation 1994;89:2015

50. Ellis SG, Cowley MJ, DiSciascio G et al. Determinants of 2-year outcome after coronary angioplasty in patients with multivessel disease on the basis of comprehensive preprocedural evaluation: implications for patient selection. Circulation 1991;83:1905

51. O'Keefe JH Jr, Allan JJ, McCallister BD et al. Angioplasty versus bypass surgery for multivessel coronary disease with left ejection fraction < or = 40% ventricular dysfunction. Am J Cardiol 1993;71:897

52. Detre K, Holubkov R, Kelsey S et al. One-year follow-up results of the 1985–1986 National Heart, Lung, and Blood Institute's Percutaneous Transluminal Coronary Angioplasty Registry. Circulation 1989;80:421

53. Gruentzig AR, King SB II, Schlumpf M et al. Long-term follow-up after percutaneous transluminal coronary angioplasty: implications for patient selection. Circulation 1991;83:1905

54. Bell M, Gersh BJ, Schaff HV et al. Effect of completeness of revascularization on long-term outcome of patients with three-vessel disease undergoing coronary artery bypass surgery: a report from the Coronary Artery Surgery Study (CASS) Registry. Circulation 1992;86:446

55. Vandormael MG, Chaitman BR, Ischinger T et al. Immediate and short-term benefit of multilesion coronary angioplasty: influence of degree of revascularization. J Am Coll Cardiol 1985;6:983

56. Reeder GS, Holmes DR Jr, Detre K et al. Degree of revascularization in patients with multivessel coronary disease: a report from the National Heart, Lung, and Blood Institute Percutaneous Transluminal Coronary Angioplasty Registry. Circulation 1988;77:638

57. O'Keefe JH Jr, Rutherford BD, McConahay DR et al. Early and late results of coronary angioplasty without antecedent thrombolytic therapy for acute myocardial infarction. Am J Cardiol 1989;64:1221

58. Bourassa MG, Holubkov R, Yeh W et al. Strategy of complete revascularization in patients with multivessel coronary artery disease (a report from the 1985–1986 NHLBI PTCA Registry). Am J Cardiol 1992;70:174

59. Diver DJ, McCabe CH, McKay RG et al. Coronary angioplasty of a "culprit" lesion in patients with multivessel coronary disease, abstracted. J Am Coll Cardiol 1987;9:16A

60. Cohen DJ, Breall JA, Ho KKL et al. Evaluating the potential cost-effectiveness of stenting as a treatment for symptomatic single-vessel coronary artery disease: use of a decision-analytic model. Circulation 1994;89:1859–74

61. RITA Trial Participants. Coronary angioplasty vs. coronary artery bypass surgery in the Randomized Intervention Treatment of Angina (RITA) Trial. Lancet 1993;341:573

62. Rodriguez A, Boullon F, Perez-Baliño N et al. Argentine randomized trial of percutaneous transluminal coronary angioplasty versus coronary artery bypass surgery in multivessel disease (ERACI): in-hospital results and 1-year follow-up. J Am Coll Cardiol 1993;22:1060

63. Hamm CW, Ischinger T, Reimers J et al. A randomized study of coronary angioplasty compared with bypass surgery in patients with symptomatic multivessel coronary disease. German Angioplasty, Bypass Surgery Investigation (GABI). N Engl J Med 1994;331:1037

64. Coronary Artery Bypass Revascularization Investigation (CABRI). Presented at the 15th Congress of the European Society of Cardiology, 1993

65. King SB 3rd, Lembo NJ, Weintraub WS et al. A randomized trial comparing coronary angioplasty with coronary bypass surgery. Emory Angioplasty versus Surgery Trial (EAST). N Engl J Med 1994;331:1044

66. Williams DO, Baim DS, Bates E et al. Coronary anatomic and procedural characteristics of patients randomized to coronary angioplasty in the Bypass Angioplasty Revascularization Investigation (BARI). Am J Cardiol 1995;75:27C–33C

67. Kuntz RE, Baim DS. Defining coronary restenosis: newer clinical and angiographic paradigms. Circulation 1993;88:1310

68. Grossman W, Baim DS. Cardiac Catheterization, Angiography and Intervention. 4th Ed. Lea & Febiger, Philadelphia, 1991

44 Acute Complications

David R. Holmes, Jr.

The frequency of interventional coronary artery procedures has increased dramatically since the introduction of percutaneous transluminal coronary angioplasty (PTCA) in 1977. This increase is related to (1) improvements in equipment that have facilitated access to a variety of lesions and arterial segments, (2) expanding operator experience, and (3) significant expansion in patient and angiographic lesion selection criteria. In addition to conventional angioplasty, new techniques have also developed such as atherectomy, laser, and intracoronary stents. Success rates have improved significantly. In the initial National Heart, Lung, and Blood Institute (NHLBI) PTCA Registry, which included 3,248 patients and 3,567 procedures performed from September 1977 to September 1992, the initial success rate (defined as ≥ 20% decrease in luminal diameter stenosis) was 61%.[1,2] Failure was usually related to the inability to cross the lesion with the limited equipment available at that time. The mortality rate in this group of patients, the majority of whom (72%) had single-vessel disease, was 1.9%; acute myocardial infarction occurred in 5% and emergency coronary bypass graft surgery (CABG) in 7%. In the subsequent 1985 to 1986 NHLBI Registry, 1,802 patients undergoing their initial angioplasty without having had an infarction within 10 days prior to the procedure were enrolled from August 1985 to May 1986 with an angiographic success rate of 91% (one or more with lesions improved by ≥ 20%) and complications of death in 1.0%, acute myocardial infarction in 4.3%, and need for emergency CABG in 1.8%.[1–3] These improvements occurred even though baseline demographics had changed and more higher risk patients were being treated; 53% had two- or three-vessel disease, and 49% had unstable angina. The success rates have continued to improve into the present time—single and multicenter experiences are documenting success rates of approximately 95%. Success rates depend on how the outcome is assessed. In the past, most studies used visual assessment of lesions before and after intervention. More recently, quantitative coronary angiography (QCA) has been used for more reproducible assessment. Using these techniques, success rates have been significantly lower than when visual estimates were used. In the coronary angioplasty venous excisional atherectomy trial (CAVEAT)-1, a visual success rate of 96.4% was seen for both PTCA and directional coronary atherectomy (DCA).[4] When core laboratory-blinded QCA analysis was performed, success rates fell to 89% for DCA and 80% for PTCA (P <0.001). These differences relate not to complications of the procedure, which could theoretically have been more reliably detected by QCA, but rather to assessment of the final postprocedure angiographic result.

During the phase of increased success rates, complication patterns have also changed. Some new complication patterns have emerged with new technology, for example, coronary perforation, whereas other complication patterns have remained the same, occurring irrespective of which specific device is used.

The major complications of percutaneous revascularization procedures are death, myocardial infarction, emergency CABG, and hemodynamic instabil-

515

ity.[2,3] These may result from a number of specific events but are the final end result.

MORTALITY

Mortality depends in large measure on the baseline demographics of the patient population, clinical presentation, degree and extent of coronary artery disease, and left ventricular function.[5,6] The complex inter-related relationships between these variables makes "score card" assessment difficult. Mortality rates have been reported in several ways. In some studies, mortality is limited to procedural mortality. In others, mortality is defined by death within 24 hours. Finally, in some studies, all in-hospital deaths are considered. These differing time considerations for capturing mortality also make comparisons of studies difficult.

In general, patients with more hemodynamic instability have higher mortality rates. In three recent randomized trials of PTCA versus lytic therapy for acute myocardial infarction, the in-hospital mortality in the patients undergoing PTCA was 2.2%, ranging from 0 to 4.3%.[7] Perhaps the highest risk patients are those with acute myocardial infarction and cardiogenic shock. In these patients, in-hospital mortality rates of 15 to 40% have been reported. The mortality in this setting may have nothing to do with PTCA per se but may reflect the degree of irreversible left ventricular dysfunction. In patients with unstable angina, mortality rates are lower than in those with acute myocardial infarction but still somewhat increased compared with stable angina. In the thrombolysis and angioplasty in unstable angina (TAUSA) trial of 469 patients with unstable angina and coronary arterial thrombus, there was no in-hospital mortality.[8] The Evaluation of Chimeric 7E₃ Fab in the Prevention of Ischemic Complications (EPIC) trial has recently been reported.[9] In this trial of unstable high-risk patients undergoing percutaneous revascularization procedures, even in the patients in the control arm treated with heparin alone, the in-hospital mortality was 1.7%. The patients with stable angina can be expected to have an improved outcome with mortality rates less than 1 to 1.5%. The effect of new devices on mortality in-hospital is difficult to ascertain. These new devices are usually used in higher risk patients and higher risk lesions. In the New Approaches to Coronary Intervention (NACI) Registry experience of 3,201 lesions in 2,835 patients treated from November 1990 to November 1992, mortality was 1.6% but ranged from 0.6 to 5.7% depending on the specific device.[10,11] Much of the variability relates to baseline clinical and angiographic features.

In-hospital mortality also depends on the severity and extent of coronary artery disease and left ventricular function.[12] In the 1985 to 1986 NHLBI PTCA Registry, the mortality for single-vessel disease was 0.2%.[3] The mortality for two-vessel disease was 0.9% and for three-vessel disease 2.8%. In the same registry in patients with an ejection fraction of 45% or less, the in-hospital mortality was 0.8%.

Multivariate correlates of mortality have been studied.[5,6] In a series of 8,052 consecutive patients without evolving acute myocardial infarction, death occurred in 32.[6] It was directly related to arterial closure in 26 of these cases. Left ventricular failure was the most common cause of death and was independently correlated with female gender ($P <0.001$), a myocardial jeopardy score ($P <0.001$), and PTCA of a proximal right coronary artery.

MYOCARDIAL INFARCTION

The incidence of myocardial infarction as a complication of percutaneous procedures has varied widely. This variability is related to differences in definition. For example, non-Q-wave versus Q-wave myocardial infarction, the screening procedure used, as with measurement of enzymes in all patients or just in those with recurrent chest pain and the subset of patients undergoing treatment, for instance for vein graft disease or native coronary lesions. The incidence also depends on the specific device used. In the NACI Registry, the incidence of Q-wave myocardial infarction was 1.3%, and the incidence of non-Q-wave myocardial infarction was 4.5%, and ranging from 2.5 to 7.7% depending on the specific device used.[11] In the CAVEAT-1 and -2 trials, the incidence of myocardial infarction, particularly non-Q-wave, was highest in patients treated with DCA, particularly in vein graft lesions.[4,13] Rotablator has also been associated with an increased incidence of non-Q-wave myocardial infarction compared with historical cohorts of patients undergoing PTCA.

Non-Q-wave myocardial infarctions have the most variability, occurring with greater frequency than Q-wave infarctions. The long-term follow-up of these patients is not clear. Some non-Q-wave infarctions appear to have little clinical relevance, while others are associated with recurrent events and even mortality. This variability may in part depend on the etiology of the infarction. A small side branch may occlude during treatment with no sequelae but only a minor enzyme elevation. This should not prolong hospital stay nor should it affect long-term outcome. Occlusion of a large side branch or distal embolization of atherothrombotic material obstructing flow to the target vessel may have major complications with

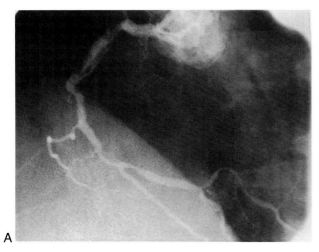

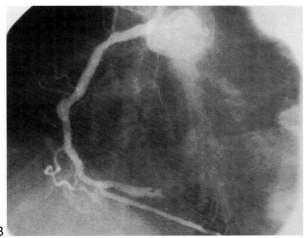

Fig. 44-1. Left anterior oblique view of the right coronary artery. **(A)** At baseline there is a large proximal thrombus. **(B)** During the procedure, the thrombus was dislodged distally.

larger infarction, hemodynamic instability, and even death (Fig. 44-1).

EMERGENCY CORONARY BYPASS GRAFT SURGERY

The need for emergency surgery has decreased significantly from approximately 7% in the initial PTCA Registry to approximately 2 to 3% at the present time.[1] Emergency surgery is usually the result of acute or threatened closure. Since the introduction and widespread use of perfusion balloons for prolonged inflation, as well as (even more importantly) intracoronary stents, the frequency of emergency surgery has decreased.[14–17] With these new devices, even if surgery is required, improved outcome may

result. In the past, there was a strong relationship between emergency CABG and myocardial infarction, and even death. In patients with emergency CABG, myocardial infarction rates ranged up to 40 to 60%. In addition, patients going to emergency CABG in the past usually did not receive an internal thoracic artery graft because of hemodynamic instability. With the use of stents, even if surgery is required, the stents can be used as a bridge to surgery, improving flow and hemodynamics and decreasing the incidence of procedural-related myocardial infarction. In the Cook Registry of patients with abrupt closure, the incidence of emergency CABG was 3.2%, and an additional 4.3% required elective CABG. In this high-risk group of 94 patients, the in-hospital mortality was 2.1% and the incidence of Q-wave myocardial infarction was 4.3%. These are substantial improvements compared with earlier patients treated without stents.[14–17]

HEMODYNAMIC INSTABILITY

There is limited information on periprocedural hemodynamic instability. In the past, this was usually the result of acute closure of a dilated segment that supplied most of the viable myocardium or occurred during PTCA for acute myocardial infarction. Partial cardiopulmonary assist devices were developed for this setting and in selected cases were very helpful.[18] Unfortunately, the equipment required very large arterial and venous cannulae, limiting widespread use. In selected patients at very high risk, these devices may be placed prophylactically; more commonly, a small sheath is placed in the contralateral femoral artery and vein to facilitate placement should hemodynamic compromise occur. Expanded use of perfusion balloons has helped substantially. One risk of hypotension is that if it occurs during dilation of a second lesion, the first lesion may also occlude because of low perfusion pressure.

Hemodynamic instability may become more common with the increasingly widespread use of Rotablator atherectomy. No reflow or slow flow is relatively common with this device and may result in severe and even prolonged hypotension, requiring intravenous pressors and pacing. Careful case selection and meticulous attention to detail with slow passes and sequential burr sizes may help to obviate this problem.

POTENTIAL CARDIAC EVENTS

The aforementioned complications of death, myocardial infarction, emergency CABG, and hemodynamic stability are the end result of a number of potential cardiac events of percutaneous revascularization procedures. Cardiac complications can be subdivided into those related to the target lesion and those in the coronary artery but remote from the target lesion. In addition, as previously mentioned, hemodynamic compromise may occur. Noncardiac vascular complications most frequently include peripheral vascular complications but may involve the central nervous system. Finally, numerous nonvascular complications may occur, the most important of which is renal dysfunction. This, however, occurs after leaving the catheterization laboratory and will not be discussed further as an acute complication. These events may be summarized as follows:

Cardiac target lesion
• Acute closure
• Threatened closure
• Dissection
• Perforation
• Side branch occlusion
Cardiac vascular bed remote from target lesion
• Acute closure
• Threatened closure
• Dissection
• Perforation
• Branch vessel occlusion
• Compromise collaterals
Noncardiac vascular, peripheral vascular
• Thrombosis
• Thromboembolism
• Pseudoaneurysm
• Laceration, bleeding
• Dissection
Cerebrovascular
• Thromboembolism
Nonvascular
• Renal dysfunction

Target Lesion Complications

Acute closure syndromes remain the major complication of percutaneous revascularization.[16–22] Acute closure defined as Thrombolysis in Myocardial Infarction (TIMI) 0 or 1 flow in a previously patent arterial segment may be abrupt in onset or may be preceded by threatened closure defined as a reduction in TIMI flow of at least 1 grade in association with ischemic pain or electrocardiographic changes or both. Abrupt closure complicates 4 to 8% of interventional procedures. This incidence has not changed markedly over time. Typically, abrupt clo-

sure manifests while the patient is in the catheterization laboratory, although in 25 to 30% of patients, it may occur after leaving the laboratory. Usually, in the latter situation, some features such as a dissection or residual filling defect were present during the procedure. In many laboratories, following the initial dilation or treatment, the patient is kept in the laboratory for 10 to 15 minutes and then repeat angiography of the treated segment is performed. If flow remains excellent and the angiographic result is stable, the procedure is then terminated. Using this protocol, abrupt closure following the procedure is uncommon.

Abrupt or threatened closure can be the result of several factors: dissection, intracoronary thrombus,

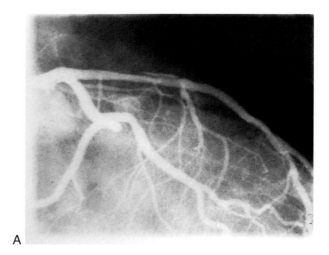

A

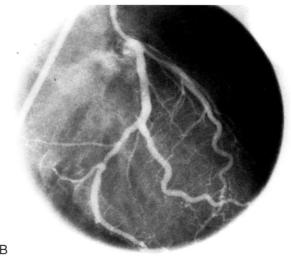

B

Fig. 44-2. (A) Dissections vary widely from small discrete flaps that do not limit flow and are often associated with excellent long-term outcome to **(B)** large dissections that go on to acute closure.

spasm, or recoil. Dissection is the most common single cause of acute or threatened closure[15,20–22] (Fig. 44-2). Often two factors are present—typically, dissection and thrombus.[19] In the setting of dissection that limits flow and may cause hypotension, there is stasis in the treated segment that has been damaged by balloon inflation, and this is the substrate for thrombus formation and platelet deposition, which can further impede flow. Usually, the dissection is evident angiographically, although in some patients, it may be identified only with angioscopy or intravascular ultrasound. In distinguishing the thrombus from dissection as the most important mechanism of acute closure in a specific patient, angioscopy is more reliable. Local spasm of the treated segment may also play a role, particularly with some of the new technology, such as Rotablator. Recoil may also occur in very rigid lesions or elastic ostial lesions. Typically, however, recoil does not result in acute closure.

Prediction of acute closure based on pretreatment angiography is an imperfect science.[21–23] Some of the associated factors are as follows:

Procedural
• Oversized balloons
• Inappropriate deep guide catheter intubation

• Stiff guidewires
• Failure to ensure adequate antiplatelet and anticoagulation treatment
Angiographic
• Coronary artery thrombus
• Unprotected significant side branch
• Bulky vein graft lesion
• Lesion eccentricity
• Diffuse disease
• Lesion calcification

Angiographic features most prominently include intracoronary thrombus. Other lesions are also at risk. In these lesion subsets, percutaneous revascularization procedures can still be performed, but it is essential to match the specific technology with the specific lesion to optimize the result. Such a process of matching technology and the specific lesion has been enhanced by the increasing use of new imaging technology such as intravascular ultrasound (Table 44-1). By matching technology and specific lesion type, the initial outcome may be improved. This may become more important if the concept of having to achieve an ideal result to decrease restenosis rates ("bigger is better") is validated in well-controlled series and is achievable without excess risk.

Despite treatment of ideal lesions or matching

Table 44-1. Type of Lesion and Appropriate Technology for Optimal Result

	PTCA	DCA	Rotablater	TEC	ELCA	Holmium Yag	Stent[a]
Concentric type A lesions	+						
Chronic total occlusions	+				+		
Long lesions							
Calcified			+				
Mild or no calcification			+		+	+	
Eccentric lesions							
Large vessels		+					+
Smaller vessels			+			+[b]	
Calcified lesions			+				
Thrombus-containing lesions							
Large vessels		+		+			
Smaller vessels						+	
Vein graft disease							
Focal de novo	+	+					+
Focal restenotic	+						+
Diffuse disease				+	+		
Ostial location		+		+	+		
Angulated lesions							
Large vessels	+						
Smaller vessels	+		+				

Abbreviations: PTCA, percutaneous transluminal coronary angioplasty; DCA, directional coronary atherectomy; TEC, transluminal extraction catheter; ELCA, excimer laser coronary angioplasty.
[a] Expanding indication in large vessels to treat acute or threatened closure or prevent restenosis.
[b] DELCA, directional excimer laser coronary angioplasty.

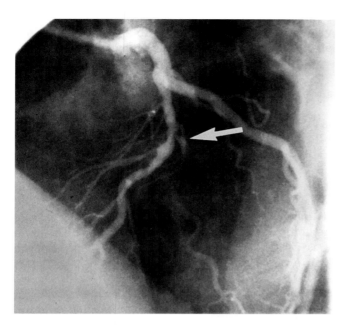

Fig. 44-4. Left anterior oblique view of the left coronary artery. Prior to treatment of the left anterior descending lesion, there is a large diagonal with an ostial stenosis that arises out of the lesion. Following initial intervention, the diagonal is compromised.

the planned procedure. Factors assessed include the size of the side branch, the degree of ostial narrowing, the angulation of the branch takeoff, and the location of the plaque in the target lesion. If the plaque is on the contralateral side of the branch, there may not be compromise of the branch lumen. In addition to the potential for side branch occlusion, ostial lesions have the tendency toward more elastic recoil, making potential dilation more problematic.

Several approaches have evolved, including both conventional balloon technology and new technology:

Conventional balloon technology
- Simultaneous: both segments
- Sequential dilation: both segments
- Guidewire placed: branch vessel for access should dilation of target lesion compromise branch
- Observation of effect of target lesion: dilation of branch vessel only if compromise of branch vessel recurs

New approaches
- Direction atherectomy with short catheter
- Eccentric laser
- Rotablator atherectomy

None of these without problems, but they can be used in specific cases to optimize the result. For small side

branches, often no measures are taken. Even if these occlude, they usually do not result in any clinical consequences.

Perforation

The final complication of treatment of the target lesion is perforation[24] (Fig. 44-5). Limited information is available on perforation with conventional technology because it is so rare. With new technology, perforation is still uncommon, but it occurs more frequently compared with conventional PTCA. The incidence varies depending on case selection, operator experience, and specific device used. With Excimer laser coronary angioplasty, the incidence was 1.3% but declined to 0.4% over time. Perforation has also been reported with the Rotablator and DCA. Typically, it is an acute event occurring during the proce-

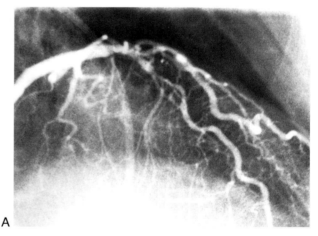

A

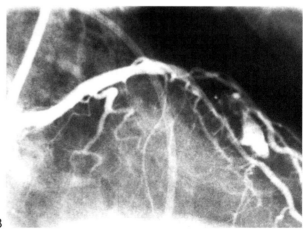

B

Fig. 44-5. Right anterior oblique view of the left anterior descending prior to (**A**) and after (**B**) excimer laser coronary angioplasty that resulted in a discrete vessel perforation.

dure. The extent and severity vary substantially from a small amount of periaventitial staining to hemopericardium and tamponade. If the perforation is large, emergency surgery is usually required. During this time, a perfusion balloon can be used to seal the perforation but maintain distal flow. If the perforation is limited and stable, observation is usually chosen with discontinuation of anticoagulation. If the Excimer Laser Coronary Angioplasty (ELCA) Registry of 2,759 patients, as previously mentioned, perforation occurred in 1.3%.[24] Among these 36 patients, 36.1% required CABG, 16.7% experienced myocardial infarction, and 5.6% had a fatal outcome.

Perforation results from excessive ablation at one part of the circumference of the arterial wall. Whether this is the location of the more normal tissue that is ablated is not certain. Identification of lesions at increased risk of perforation has been difficult. It has been felt that highly angulated lesions or branch lesions may be at increased risk, although even with these lesions, the risks of perforation are low. Careful patient selection, sizing of the device selected, slow careful ablation, and assessment of the results after treatment with the ablative device are important to prevent this complication.

Cardiac Vascular Bed Remote From Target Lesion

The complications that occur in the coronary arterial tree remote from the target lesion are similar and may have similar outcomes. The mechanism of the complications, however, may be considerably different.

Acute or Threatened Closure

Acute or threatened closure may occur either proximal or distal to the target lesion. Proximal acute or threatened closure may be the result of guide catheter dissection (Fig. 44-6); this has been a particular problem with DCA involving the right coronary artery. With the large guiding catheters, particularly if some ostial disease is present, proximal dissection may occur. Although it is uncommon with conventional PTCA, if a deep-seating maneuver is required, guide catheter dissection may also occur. There are two other potential mechanisms of acute or threatened closure proximal to the target lesion: (1) a dissection of the target vessel site, which propagates retrogradely, and (2) guidewire-induced dissection during attempts at intubating the arterial segment. The latter was more frequent with the earlier gener-

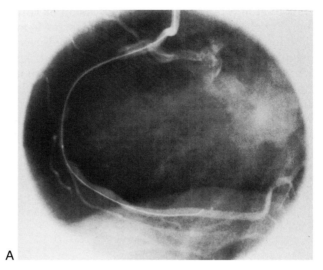

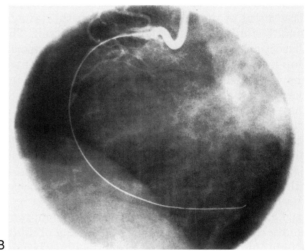

Fig. 44-6. Left anterior oblique view of right coronary artery prior to intervention (**A**) and following intervention (**B**) that resulted in a guide catheter dissection and vessel occlusion.

ation of stiffer guidewires. With increasing operator experience and improved guidewire design, this latter is less of a problem. Irrespective of the mechanism of acute or threatened closure, it requires a similar treatment strategy to that outlined for target vessel closure. If the mechanism is a dissection that starts at the target site and has propagated retrogradely, the entire length of the dissection should be covered with a stent.

Thromboembolism

Acute or threatened closure may also occur downstream from the target site.[19] This may result from a dissection that propagates downstream, thromboembolism of a bulky atheromatous lesion or thrombus (Fig. 44-1), or intense spasm. The latter is most common with rotational atherectomy procedures but usually can be treated with intracoronary nitroglycerin or intracoronary verapamil, or both. Thromboembolism can be suspected if there is no evidence of dissection and yet a distal abrupt cutoff is apparent on angiography. Mechanical disruption of the distal thromboembolism with low-pressure balloon inflations may be successful in restoring flow. If the amount of material is large, however, intracoronary lytic therapy, usually urokinase, may also be effective. If the occluded vessel is very distal and supplies little myocardium, the occlusion can be treated just with heparin.

Dissection

Treatment of dissection remote from the target lesion is similar to dissection at the site itself. These dissections tend to be longer, which has important implications because any treatment should involve the entire length of the dissection. Recently, longer perfusion balloons have become available, which may enhance outcome. These longer dissections are rarely well treated with DCA, and more commonly stents are required unless the dissection is very long and cannot be fully covered. Such a dissection may occlude a branch vessel. In this setting, successful dilation of the branch vessel is uncommon because the orifice may not be able to be identified or engaged. A proximal dissection may also compromise collaterals. This may occur in the setting of dilation for chronic total occlusion and can result in ischemia in the distribution of the chronic occlusion. When dissection proximal to occlusion occurs, the chances of a successful procedure decrease markedly.

Perforation

Perforation remote from the target lesion is uncommon. In the ELCA Registry, it was seen in only 8 of 36 patients with perforation.[24] This related to sudden and more rapid advancement of the catheter than was optimal, with subsequent ablation of the more normal arterial wall distal to the target lesion. With optimal device manipulation, it should be extremely uncommon. Great care should be taken to treat the target lesion alone and no other portions of the vessel. In the event that perforation occurs, remote from the target lesion, it can be managed in the same fashion with prolonged inflation and discontinuation of the anticoagulation if the patient and the lesion are stable, or emergency surgery if the perforation is large or hemodynamic instability exists.

Noncardiac Vascular Complications

The most common complication of interventional procedures are noncardiac, usually peripheral vascular (Plate 44-1). The incidence of these complications has increased with the use of larger devices, older patients, and more intensive antiplatelet and anticoagulant regimens. The complications increase even further when interventional procedures are combined with systemic thrombolytic therapy such as in the setting of acute myocardial infarction. With conventional PTCA, reported vascular complication rates range from 0.7 to 9%. This variability in reported frequency is a function of patient population undergoing treatment as well as the means used to ascertain the specific complications. For example, routine duplex scanning of the femoral artery may document an increased incidence of pseudoaneurysm. Directional atherectomy with its larger sheaths has the potential for increased complications, although in the CAVEAT-1 trial, there was no difference between DCA and PTCA; both had a 6.6% incidence of vascular complication.[4] Of all 1,012 patients in this study, 67 had a complication; 15 of these required a blood transfusion for excess bleeding, and 14 required vascular surgery. Patients undergoing stent implantation have the highest incidence of peripheral vascular complications—this is related to the intensive anticoagulant and antiplatelet regimens required to prevent subacute closure. Although increased experience with stent patients and earlier sheath removal has resulted in decreased incidence, it remains a significant problem that increases hospital stay, procedural costs, and total charges. In a recent experience of stent implantation for focal vein graft stenosis, vascular surgery was required in 8.5% of 164 procedures, and an additional 14% of patients required transfusions alone for excess bleeding.

Assessment of risk factors associated with increased peripheral vascular complications is difficult because of the relatively nonspecific nature of these risk factors. Potential baseline risk factors include female gender, older age, severe obesity, and peripheral arterial disease. Procedural risk factors include the sheath size, the degree and duration of heparin anticoagulation, and the length of time the sheath is maintained in place. Other factors that may be as (or even more) important have not been qualified. These include the location of the arterial puncture. The inguinal crease is often used as a landmark for femoral arterial puncture, whereas, in fact, the landmark that should be used is the inguinal ligament. In older, heavy patients the crease may be substantially caudad to the ligament. Puncture using the crease as a guideline may be too low to allow for adequate hemostasis. In patients coming to vascular surgical repair for continued bleeding, the arterial puncture site is often too low, making compression difficult. Another important variable is sheath placement. There may be "burring" of the dilator or sheath on initial placement, which can create an irregular tear in the femoral artery (Fig. 44-7). Because of these bleeding concerns, particularly in stent patients, there is an increase in the use of brachial or even radial approaches. A final factor also deals with multiple catheterizations from the same site. On occasion, bleeding occurs at the initial site from the diagnostic angiogram and not from the subsequent arterial puncture used for the interventional procedure.

Avoidance of these vascular problems requires meticulous attention to detail. The location of the arterial puncture should be optimal, using the inguinal ligament as a guideline. If possible, front wall puncture should be achieved. Sheath or dilator burring should be avoided. This is a particular problem in patients with multiple previous procedures and in whom there may be fibrous tissue present at the site. Anticoagulation and antiplatelet therapy should be enough to prevent thrombosis but should be monitored to avoid excessive treatment effect. This is particularly true of stent patients, in whom bleeding is now more common than subacute closure. Wide swings in anticoagulation should be avoided. The sheath should be removed as early as possible using activated clotting time for guidance, with the sheath pulling out at an activated clotting time of less than 180 seconds. Heparin can then be reinstituted if required. In patients who do not have an indication for continued heparin, it should not be used. The site must be held long enough for hemostasis. A variety of devices are available including a C-clamp and Femostop; all of these require specific attention to detail. Patient mobilization, particularly with large sheaths, should be slow and cautious. If a significant hematoma is present, consideration should be given to duplex scanning to assess for the presence of a pseudoaneurysm. If this is identified, ultrasound-guided compression may be very effective, particularly if the neck of the aneurysm is small and can be compressed. In the future, vascular plugs and other means of closing the arterial puncture should be very important and will substantially decrease patient morbidity after interventional procedures.

It must be kept in mind that widespread adjunctive use of new medical approaches to complement interventional procedures may impact on vascular complications. Potent antithrombin and antiplatelet approaches such as hirudin and glycoprotein IIb/IIIa receptor blockers when administered concurrently may cause a marked increase in bleeding. In the EPIC trial, the frequency of major bleeding in patients receiving glycoprotein IIb/IIIa receptor blocker was twice that seen in the control group at 14%.[9]

Cerebrovascular events as a complication of interventional procedures are extremely rare. This has been a definite advantage of the primary dilation approach to acute myocardial infarction compared with thrombolytic therapy. Both thromboembolic and hemorrhagic events may occur, however. The former may result from manipulation of the guiding catheter in a shaggy ascending aorta or from a thrombus in the catheter that is inadvertently flushed out into the systemic circulation. Hemorrhagic events may result from excessive anticoagulation with heparin. Although they are very uncommon, careful evaluation is required if symptoms occur.

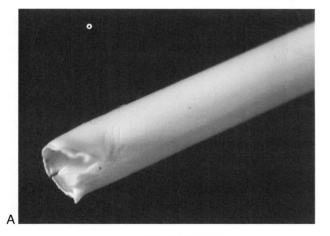

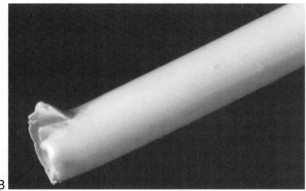

Fig. 44-7. Burring of the tip of the introducer. This may result from inadequate dilation with the introducer, fibrosis of the subcutaneous and periadventitial tissue, or arterial wall calcification at the entry site. The burring may result in arterial wall damage.

SUMMARY

The field of interventional cardiology continues to change. The limitations and complications of conventional balloon dilation technology are increasingly widely understood. Improved technology has dramatically increased success rates with PTCA. Complications still occur and may be unpredictable; fortunately, new technology offers a substantial number of bailout options to optimize the initial result. New approaches have also developed to solve the limitations of PTCA. These new approaches as primary therapy can be extremely effective in selected patients. They carry with them some of the same complications (such as acute closure or dissection) as conventional PTCA but in addition have other complications, for example, coronary perforation. Knowledge of the complication patterns is essential in planning the optimal treatment strategy for the specific patient and lesion to be addressed.

REFERENCES

1. Detre K, Holubkov R, Kelsey S et al. Percutaneous transluminal coronary angioplasty in 1985–1986 and 1977–1981: the National Heart, Lung, and Blood Institute Registry. N Engl J Med 1988;318:265–70
2. Holmes DR Jr, Holubkov R, Vlietstra RE et al. Comparison of complications during percutaneous transluminal coronary angioplasty in 1977–1981 and 1985–1986: the National Heart, Lung, and Blood Institute Percutaneous Transluminal Coronary Angioplasty Registry. J Am Coll Cardiol 1988;12:1149–55
3. Detre KM, Holmes DR Jr, Holubkov R et al. Incidence and consequences of periprocedural occlusion: the 1985–1986 National Heart, Lung, and Blood Institute Percutaneous Transluminal Coronary Angioplasty Registry. Circulation 1990;82:739–50
4. Topol EJ, Leya F, Pinkerton CA et al. A comparison of directional atherectomy with coronary angioplasty in patients with coronary artery disease. N Engl J Med 1993;329:221–7
5. Ellis SG, Roubin GS, King SB et al. In hospital cardiac mortality after acute closure after coronary angioplasty: analysis of risk factors from 8,207 procedures. J Am Coll Cardiol 1988;11:211–6
6. Ellis SG, Myler RK, King SB et al. Causes and correlates of death after unsupported coronary angioplasty: implication for use of angioplasty and advanced support techniques in high risk settings. Am J Cardiol 1991;68:1447–51
7. Simari RD, Berger PB, Bell MR et al. Coronary angioplasty in acute myocardial infarction: primary, immediate adjunctive, rescue, or deferred adjunctive approach? Mayo Clin Proc 1994;69:346–58
8. Ambrose JA, Almeida OD, Sharma SK. Adjunctive thrombolytic therapy during angioplasty for ischemic rest pain. Results of the TAUSA trial. Circulation 1994;90:69–77
9. EPIC Investigators. Use of a monoclonal antibody directed against the platelet glycoprotein IIb/IIIa receptors in high risk coronary angioplasty. N Engl J Med 1994;330:956–62
10. Detre KM, Baim D, Buchbinder M et al. Baseline characteristics and therapeutic goals in the New Approaches to Coronary Intervention (NACI) registry. Coronary Artery Dis 1993;4:1013–22
11. Baim DS, Kent KM, King SB III et al. Evaluating new devices. Acute (in-hospital) results from the New Approaches to Coronary Intervention Registry. Circulation 1994;89:471–81
12. Holmes DR Jr, Detre KM, Williams DO et al. Long-term outcome of patients with depressed left ventricular function undergoing percutaneous transluminal coronary angioplasty. The NHLBI PTCA Registry. Circulation 1993;87:21–9
13. Holmes DR Jr, Topol EJ, Califf RM et al. A multicenter, randomized trial of coronary angioplasty versus directional atherectomy for patients with saphenous vein bypass graft lesions. Circulation 1995;91:1966–74
14. Roubin GS, Cannon AD, Agrawal SK et al. Intracoronary stenting for acute and threatened closure complicating percutaneous transluminal coronary angioplasty. Circulation 1992;85:916–27
15. Lincoff AM, Popma JJ, Ellis SG et al. Abrupt vessel closure complicating coronary angioplasty: clinical, angiographic and therapeutic profile. J Am Coll Cardiol 1992;19:926–35
16. deFeyter PJ, vanden Brand M, Jaarman G et al. Acute coronary artery occlusion during and after percutaneous transluminal coronary angioplasty. Frequency, prediction, clinical course, management and follow-up. Circulation 1991;83:927–36
17. Hearn AJ, King SB, Douglas JS et al. Clinical and angiographic outcomes after coronary artery stenting for acute or threatened closure following percutaneous transluminal coronary angioplasty: initial results with a balloon expandable stainless steel design. Circulation 1993;88:2086–96
18. Lincoff AM, Popma JJ, Ellis SG et al. Percutaneous support devices for high risk or complicated coronary angioplasty. J Am Coll Cardiol 1991;17:770–80
19. Mabin TA, Holmes DR, Smith HC et al. Intracoronary thrombus: role in coronary occlusion complicating percutaneous transluminal coronary angioplasty. J Am Coll Cardiol 1985;5:198–202
20. Popma JJ, Topol EJ, Hinohara T et al. Abrupt vessel closure after directional coronary atherectomy: the US Directional Atherectomy Investigative Group. J Am Coll Cardiol 1992;19:1372–9
21. Sinclair IN, McCabe CH, Sipperly ME, Baim DS. Predictors, therapeutic options and long-term outcome of abrupt closure. Am J Cardiol 1988;61:61G–6G
22. Ellis SG, Roubin GS, King SB. Angiographic and clinical predictors of acute closure after native vessel coronary angioplasty. Circulation 1988;77:372–9
23. Bell MR, Reeder GS, Garratt KN et al. Predictors of major ischemic complications after coronary dissection following angioplasty. Am J Cardiol 1993;71:1402–7
24. Holmes DR Jr, Reeder GS, Ghazzal ZMB et al. Coronary perforation after excimer laser coronary angioplasty: the Excimer Laser Coronary Angioplasty Registry experience. J Am Coll Cardiol 1994;23:330–5

45 Restenosis

Stanley K. Lau
David P. Faxon

Percutaneous transluminal coronary angioplasty (PCTA), first performed by Dr. Andreas Gruentzig in September of 1977, is now widely used and commonly accepted.[1] However, the problem of restenosis continues to trouble angioplasty,[2] resulting in reoccurrence of symptoms and the need for another procedure in 12 to 50% of patients within 6 months (Figure 45-1). Recent reports demonstrate that despite the problem of restenosis, angioplasty has increased from 100,000 procedures in 1985 to more than 350,000 procedures in the United States over the past 5 years alone.[3] If one assumes a 30% restenosis rate, the incidence of restenosis has risen from 30,000 patients in 1985 to more than 105,000 patients in 1992. Recent cost estimates suggest that a coronary angioplasty in the United States costs nearly $10,000 and thus results in at least a billion dollars in direct costs to the United States health care system. In addition, the expense in medication and loss of work contributes substantially to the cost burden. Various strategies have been formulated to reduce the incidence of restenosis, but none have been successful to date despite improved angioplasty equipment, adjunctive pharmacologic therapy, and new interventional devices. In fact, as interventional techniques have improved along with increased operator experience, more complex anatomy and multivessel disease are undergoing angioplasty, and the incidence of restenosis is rising.

DEFINITIONS

One of the major problems in studying restenosis is its definition. It is recognized that restenosis is a complex medical problem that results in renarrowing of the treated coronary lesion. Restenosis can be defined by angiographic, clinical, or functional testing definitions.

Angiographic Definition

At least 13 definitions of restenosis have been recorded in the literature (Table 45-1) and there have led to more confusion than to greater clarity. The lack of a uniform definition imposes difficulties in comparing different studies and in understanding the true natural history of this phenomenon.

Not only do the definitions overlap considerably, but there are patients who have been defined with restenosis by one definition who did not have it by other definitions. More than a 50% luminal diameter at the time of follow-up has become the standard angiographic definition of restenosis in clinical trials, as this appears to relate more closely to reoccurrence of symptoms and the need for repeat angioplasty. In addition, this definition does not rely on a comparison with baseline angiography. However, it does imply that restenosis is an dichotomous event, (i.e., it happens or it does not). Whereas this type of defini-

527

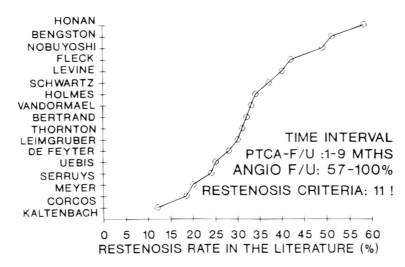

Fig. 45-1. Restenosis rates found by different authors, applying 11 different restenosis criteria, different angiographic follow-up (F/U) times (1 to 9 months), and different analysis techniques (visual or quantitative). (From Serruys et al. [55] with permission.)

Table 45-1. Angiographic Definitions of Restenosis Used in Various Clinical Trials

1. Diameter stenosis ≥50% at follow-up
2. Return to within 10% of the pre-PTCA diameter stenosis
3. Immediate post-PTCA diameter stenosis <50% that increases to ≥50% at follow-up
4. Same as no. 3, but a diameter stenosis ≥70% at follow-up
5. Loss during follow-up of at least 50% of the initial gain at PTCA
6. Loss ≥20% diameter stenosis from post-PTCA to follow-up
7. Loss ≥30% diameter stenosis from post-PTCA to follow-up
8. Area stenosis ≥85% at follow-up
9. A diameter stenosis ≥70% at follow-up
10. Loss ≥1 mm² in stenosis area from post-PTCA to follow-up
11. Loss ≥0.72 mm in minimal luminal diameter from post-PTCA to follow-up
12. Loss ≥0.5 mm in minimal luminal diameter from post-PTCA to follow-up
13. Diameter stenosis >50% at follow-up with >10% deterioration in diameter stenosis since PTCA of a previously successfully dilated lesion (defined as diameter stenosis <50% with a gain of >10% at PTCA)

(Modified from Serruys et al.[55] with permission.

---

tion is useful for making clinical decisions, it does not accurately reflect the biologic process. Also, measurement of percent stenosis depends on accurate measurement of a reference diameter, as well as a stenotic diameter. Physicians commonly use the visual assessment method, which has important limitations. The visual method has been shown to overestimate stenoses before intervention and to underestimate their severity after intervention. The greatest range of inaccuracy is in the 25 to 50% range, where most restenosis definitions operate. Electronic caliper assessments tend to overestimate noncritical stenoses and underestimate critical stenoses, and the measurement is not reproducible.[6] Whereas quantitative coronary angiography (QCA) can be helpful in determining the percent stenosis, changes in the reference diameter can also change the percent stenosis during follow-up. The QCA technique measures stenosis less severely than visual methods. Rensing et al.[7] indicated that when QCA was used the average preintervention diameter stenosis was 60 to 70%. This is significantly lower than the typical 90% lesion read by visual assessment. The postintervention diameter stenosis was 35 to 40% which is higher than usually reported at less than 25% by visual assessment.[8] QCA provides, however, an accurate method of measurement that is more reproducible than visual assessments. More importantly, QCA can measure the absolute minimal lumen diameter, which is highly reproducible and correlates well with symptoms and funtional testing. In addition, studies measuring mean luminal diameter have shown that restenosis is a continuous process, not a dichotomous one.

The concept of restenosis as a continuous process is not a new one. In the National Heart, Lung, and Blood Institute (NHLBI) PTCA. Registry Report on Restenosis of 1984, Holmes et al.[9] illustrated that the change in percent lumen diameter from immediately after PTCA to follow-up angiography was a continuous parametric distribution. This observation was incorrectly attributed to an artifact of the visual measurement era. In 1990, Kuntz et al.[10] reported that a histogram of late loss in 184 lesions treated with the Palmaz-Schatz stent, atherectomy, or laser balloon angioplasty followed a gaussian distribution. This is supported by the Rensing et al.[7] 1992 study that reported a near gaussian distribution of luminal diameter after angioplasty in 1,445 successfully dilated lesions. The concept of restenosis as a continuous process has the following features:

1. Nearly all treated coronary lesions exhibit some degree of luminal renarrowing, and this is in agreement with the biologic process of restenosis.
2. It is also possible to use parametric rather than less powerful, categoric statistical tests.
3. The gaussian phenomenon depends on the accuracy and reproducibility of quantitative angiographic measurement.

Kuntz et al.[11] recently advocated the use of the "loss index" to define restenosis. The loss index measures the ratio of absolute late loss to absolute gain (Fig. 45-2). A steep loss slope (0.5 or more) is unfavorable. This binary concept is quite similar to the original definition of restenosis proposed by Dr. Gruentzig more than 15 years ago, namely, that restenosis should be defined as the loss of 50% of the initial gain.

The use of intravascular ultrasound as an adjunct to angiography has been proposed as an alternative means of assessing postangioplasty results. However, when one compares the image of a vessel acquired by ultrasound to the silhouette of a dye column by angiography, dimensions measured by ultrasound such as minimum lumen diameter correlate poorly with QCA, particularly following angioplasty.[12] Currently, there are no accepted definitions of restenosis using an intravascular ultrasound.

Clinical Definition

Restenosis can be defined by clinical end points such as recurrent angina, myocardial infarction, need for revascularization, and death.

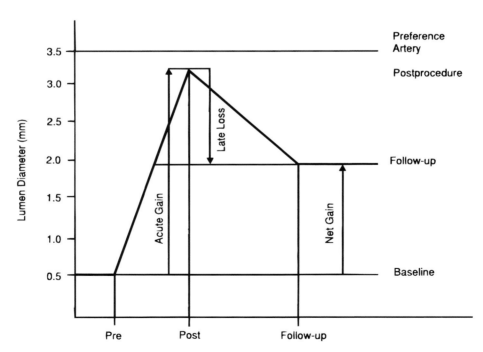

Fig. 45-2. Schematic showing drawing changes in luminal dimension over time after coronary intervention. Late procedure outcome is influenced by both the acute gain provided by the intervention (pre > post) and the subsequent late loss that occurs over 4 to 6 months after the intervention (post > follow-up). The net gain is thus the sum of the offsetting effects of acute gain and late loss. (From Kuntz et al.,[57] with permission.)

Recurrent Angina

Recurrent angina after intervention is the common clinically used definition of restenosis. In 102 patients studied by Joelson et al.,[13] repeat angiography for recurrent angina after PTCA demonstrated restenosis in 61%, new significant stenosis in 15%, no narrowing in 15%, and incomplete revascularization in 9%. In the NHLBI Registry, the incidence of restenosis was highest within the first 5 months, and as many as 81% of patients with restenosis were symptomatic.[9] Angiographic restenosis was present in 56% with definite or probable angina and in 14 % of asymptomatic patients.

Myocardial Infarction

Myocardial infarction after coronary intervention is a rare event. Acute myocardial infarction during the same hospitalization represents abrupt closure and occurs in 1 to 8% of patients.[9] Later restenosis almost always presents with recurrent angina and in less than 1% with myocardial infarction. This may suggest that restenotic lesions tend to be more fibromuscular than lipid laden and are rarely associated with plaque rupture and infarction.

Need for Repeat Revascularization

It is generally accepted that stenoses of less than 50% diameter rarely require a subsequent revascularization procedure and that repeat revascularization may be an adequate surrogate for angiographic restenosis. In the NHLBI PTCA Registry, repeat revascularization was necessary in 20% of patients by 6 months, and by 5 years 30% had had a repeat angioplasty. The overwhelming majority of the repeat PTCAs were for restenosis when performed within the first year. However, after the first year, the most common reason for a repeat procedure was the need to treat a new stenosis or a previously undilated stenosis. More current randomized clinical trials have utilized repeat revascularization of the index vessel (target lesion angioplasty) as a surrogate for angiographic restenosis.[14]

Silent Ischemia

Silent ischemia is common, with 4 to 25% of asymptomatic patients having angiographic restenosis at routine follow-up angiography. However, approximately 25% of patients with silent restenosis will have ischemia on exercise testing.[15] Such patients (with exercise testing performed within 1 month of angioplasty) have a similar prognosis when compared with those who have ischemia and symptoms.[16] A recent report also suggests that silent restenosis may be associated with regression of the stenosis, if the patients are followed for more than 1 year, and that the long-term outcome of silent restenosis is excellent even without repeat PTCA.

Detection of Restenosis by Functional Testing

Although functional testing is frequently used to detect restenosis, a number of significant limitations have been noted from previous trials. First, many studies have had incomplete angiographic follow-up. Withdrawal bias and patient selection have been significant, and the studies have been unable to distinguish ischemia in the index vessel from other unrelated significant lesions. Finally, not all patients can exercise or perform at an inadequate level of stress, which makes interpretation difficult.

Treadmill Exercise Test

A review of the value of exercise testing in predicting restenosis by Hillegass et al.[17] indicated that the positive predictive value was only 57% and a negative predictive value of 75% (Table 45-2). This low positive predictive value is most likely related to incomplete revascularization, which occurs in the vast majority of patients with multivessel disease.[16,18] Some studies have also shown that even in patients with single-vessel disease, the exercise test is not highly predictive. In the Glaxo Restenosis and Symptoms Project (GRASP), 706 patients had a predischarge, symptom-limited, modified Bruce treadmill test after successful angioplasty. However, the results did not predict subsequent clinical events nor angiographic restenosis at 6-month follow-up.[14]

Nuclear Exercise Test

Radionuclide angiography has also been shown to be poorly predictive, with positive and negative predictive values of 39 and 85%, respectively, from pooled studies (Table 45-2). The pooled positive and negative predictive values for the prediction of restenosis by ^{201}Th scintigraphy are reported as 66 and 81%, respectively. The negative predictive value of the nuclear exercise test provides adequate assurance that significant restenosis is unlikely to be present in a patient who has a low pretest probability and a negative test result, but it is not very helpful in determining the presence of restenosis. The use of early ^{201}Th scintigraphy may be misleading. In one study of 43 patients who had a successful angioplasty and no evi-

Table 45-2. Summary of Trials to Detect Restenosis Through Functional Testing

Type of Testing	No. of Studies	No. of Patients	No. of Patients with Angiographic Follow-Up	Positive Predictive Value (%)	Negative Predictive Value (%)
Exercise treadmill	10	1,679	1,452	57 ($\pm$2)	75 ($\pm$1)
Radionuclide angiography	5	203	178	39 ($\pm$4)	85 ($\pm$2)
²⁰¹Th scintigraphy	8	499	415	66 ($\pm$2)	81 ($\pm$2)

(Modified from Hillegass et al.,[39] with permission.)

dence of clinical or angiographic restenosis, 28% had an abnormal scan that did not return to normal immediately after the procedure (4 to 18 days). This raises concern about the usefulness of ²⁰¹Th in following patients after angioplasty.

PATHOPHYSIOLOGY

Clinical studies by Serruys et al.[4] and Nobuyoshi et al.[19] have clearly demonstrated that restenosis is a "time-related phenomenon," with its greatest inci-

dence in the first 4 months following a procedure. Long-term clinical studies also indicate that with favorable vessel healing during the initial 6 months, a successful angioplasty result appears to be stable for many years after the procedure.

Restenosis has been compared with the generalized wound healing process (Fig. 45-3). Numerous studies have demonstrated that angioplasty results in severe arterial damage with removal of the endothelium, stretching of the artery, and creation of local tears through the neointimal plaque and media. The healing process that results from this severe degree of vascular injury can be divided into three phases:

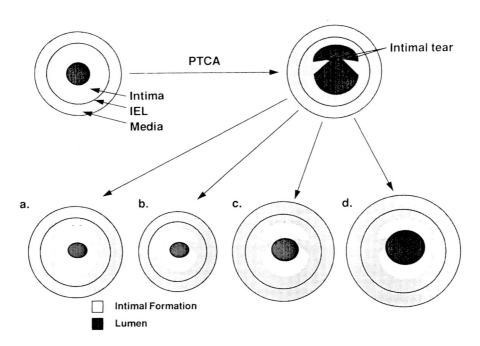

Fig. 45-3. Expanded paradigm of restenosis after angioplasty. Several possible responses to balloon injury are illustrated. The classical paradigm (a) is intimal formation with no remodeling. If vascular constriction occurs (b), even minimal amounts of neointima may result in restenosis. A moderate amount of compensatory enlargement (c) may accommodate neointima with less lumen narrowing. Augmented compensatory enlargement (d) may result in a widely patent artery despite significant intimal formation. (From Currier et al.[56] with permission.)

an initial phase, a granulation phase, and a remodeling phase.

Initial Events of Restenosis

De-endothelialization

De-endothelialization after angioplasty injury is almost unavoidable, with exposure of the subendothelial structures to circulating blood elements.

Platelet Deposition and Thrombus Formation

With exposure of lipid and collagen to circulating blood, platelet adhesion and aggregation occur almost immediately and to a much greater extent than occurs from mild forms of vascular injury. Adhesion and aggregation are mediated by platelet glycoprotein receptors Ia, Ib, and IIb/IIIa, which bind to collagen, von Willebrand factor, and fibrinogen. Platelets release a number of active factors, as well as platelet-derived growth factor (PDGF). The accumulation of fibrin onto aggregated platelets results in thrombus formation, often within the neointimal tears. Thrombin is also recognized to be a growth stimulant.

Growth Factors Activation of Smooth Muscle Cells

A number of growth factors are released from platelets or infiltrating monocytes and macrophages, as well as polynuclear lymphocytes. In addition, smooth muscle cells that are damaged in the process of vascular stretching also release growth factors, particularly fibroblast growth factor.[21] The most important growth factors are believed to be PDGF, fibroblast growth factor, insulin-like growth factor, and transforming growth factors-β.

Phenotypic Modulations of Smooth Muscle Cells

After balloon injury, smooth muscle cells that are in the quiescent contractile phenotype within the media and intima are converted by growth factor stimulation into a synthetic phenotype. Activation of these cells then leads to the second phase of wound healing, which is granulation.

Granulation

During the granulation phase, activated smooth muscle cells move into the damaged intima and proliferate as soon as 2 to 3 days after balloon injury.

About 50% of the cells that migrate into the media never divide, but do continue to form extracellular matrix and may compose up to 10% of the final intimal population. After 2 weeks in experimental studies, the amount of smooth muscle cells in the neointima appears to remain constant. Synthesis of extracellular matrix may continue for months, and in experimental studies it counts for 50% of the intimal thickening that finally results from vascular injury. Smooth muscle cells under the stimulation of various growth factors produce collagens, proteoglycans, elastin, fibronectin, and laminin. Transforming growth factor-β is important in the regulation of matrix production and degradation.

Remodeling

The final healing phase of restenosis is heralded by the regrowth of the endothelial barrier over the injured arterial segment.[23] Regeneration occurs at a rate of 0.2 mm/d for 8 to 12 weeks in the rat carotid artery. Endothelial regeneration can be incomplete and has been observed in human vascular grafts. Following stenting, however, endothelial regeneration and coverage appear to be complete by 4 weeks following injury.[24] Smooth muscle cells gradually revert back to their contractile phenotype by 6 months.[25] This is comparable to the observation that restenosis almost always is completed in the same time period. During this phase, extracellular matrix undergoes a change, with collagen replacing the proteoglycans as the major component of the matrix. Organization of the collagen fibrils into a more compact scar with contraction, as occurs in wound healing, may also occur in restenosis.

Recent studies from our laboratory would suggest that increased intimal hyperplasia is also associated with generalized compensatory enlargement of the arterial wall (remodeling). As the wall thickness increases, compensatory dilation is capable of limiting the narrowing of the lumen. In experimental studies, animals that developed restenosis had an inadequate degree of geometric remodeling compared with animals who had no evidence of angiographic restenosis. Remodeling in these studies was the primary determinant of restenosis. Even small changes in overall vessel size have profound effects on lumen size, given the geometric factors involved. Recent studies using intravascular ultrasound also indicate that geometric remodeling with dilation or contraction occurs in humans, and preliminary studies suggest it may be a major mechanism of restenosis, contributing 60% to late loss.[26] The processes that lead to compensatory dilation or constriction of the artery have not yet been clearly defined.

Table 45-3. Summary of Clinical Restenosis Trials (Meta-analysis)

Study	No. of Studies	No. of Patients	Follow-up Cath [No. (%)]	Odds Ratio	95% Confidence Interval
Aspirin vs. placebo	3	573	389 (68)	1.0	0.7–1.4
High- vs. low-dose aspirin	4	923	504 (55)	1.3	0.8–1.8
Ticlopidine vs. placebo	3	612	552 (90)	1.1	0.7–1.7
Thromboxane A_2 inhibitor or blocker	3	1673	1,544 (92)	0.9	0.6–1.3
Prostacyclin/analogues vs. placebo	3	693	576 (83)	0.7	0.5–1.0
Calcium antagonist vs. placebo	5	919	752 (82)	0.7	0.5–0.9
Heparin vs. placebo	2	446	277 (62)	1.4	0.8–2.4
Steroid vs. placebo	3	890	624 (70)	1.0	0.8–1.2
Angiotensin-converting enzyme inhibitor vs. placebo	2	2129	1,672 (79)	1.1	0.9–1.3
Fish oil vs. placebo	9	1358	926 (68)	0.6	0.5–0.8

(Modified from Hillegass et al.,[39] with permission.)

PHARMACOLOGIC PREVENTION

The pharmacologic prevention of restenosis has been directed toward the early components of the process, namely, platelet deposition and thrombosis and smooth muscle cell proliferation. It is noteworthy that little attention has been paid to the particularly important aspect of late remodeling, which may be more critical in determining eventual lumen size than the early events following vascular injury. Antiplatelets, anticoagulants, calcium antagonists, cholesterol-lowering agents, anti-inflammatory agents, and antiproliferatives have all been tried in more than 50 major clinical trials that randomized more than 15,000 patients (Table 45-3). The types of drugs studied and their mechanisms are summarized in Table 45-4. Overall, no category has been clearly shown to be of benefit in reducing restenosis.

Antiplatelet Agents

Acetylsalicylic Acid (Aspirin)

The first major clinical trials in the prevention of restenosis used aspirin, since prevention of platelet deposition and release of PDGF was thought to be important in the ultimate development of intimal hyperplasia and lumen narrowing.[27] Aspirin has the ability to inhibit thromboxane A_2 and to block the enzyme cyclooxygenase irreversibly. However, in high doses it appears to be less effective, since it inhibits the production of prostacyclin, which prevents platelet aggregation. Trials using different doses of aspirin ranging from 320 mg/d to 1,500 mg/d, starting at least 1 day before angioplasty and continuing throughout, have not shown benefit in the reduction of restenosis either clinically or angiographically. In the trials combining aspirin and dipyridamole versus

Table 45-4. Pharmacologic Agents for Restenosis Prevention and Their Relation to Proposed Mechanisms of Restenosis

Agent	Mechanism
Calcium antagonists	Recoil and spasm
Aspirin, dipyridamole, thromboxane A_2 receptor antagonists, thromboxan A_2 synthetase inhibitor, prostacyclin, ticlopidine, Ω-3 fatty acids	Platelet activation
Warfarin, heparin, low molecular weight heparins	Thrombus formation
PDGF antagonist	Growth factors
Angiotensin-converting enzyme inhibitors, lovastatin, angiopeptin, low molecular weight heparins, colchicine	Smooth muscle cell proliferation
Steroids	Inflammation

(Modified from Franklin and Faxon,[54] with permission.)

placebo, the rate of acute complications was lower, but the rate of restenosis was not reduced. Schwartz et al.[28] showed that periprocedural myocardial infarctions were reduced in the treatment group. Chesebro et al.[29] confirmed these results in a recent trial in the United States. Thromboxane A_2 is a potent platelet inhibitor; however, three randomized, double-blind, placebo-controlled trials (CARPORT, M-HEART, and GRASP) evaluating two thromboxane A_2 receptor blockers showed no reduction in restenosis. Recently, the platelet glycoprotein IIb/IIIa receptor antibody (7E3) was shown to reduce significantly 1-month and 6-month clinical events in the multicenter Evaluation of Chimesic 7E$_3$ Fab in the Prevention of Ischemic Complictions (EPIC) trial.[30] Further studies with other potent glycoprotein antagonists are under way.

Anticoagulants

Anticoagulants have also failed to show any benefit. A prospective trial by the M-HEART group suggests an inverse relationship between the duration of heparin therapy and the incidence of restenosis.[31] However, Ellis et al.[22] found no difference in short-term use of intravenous heparin started before and continued for 18 to 24 hours after PTCA. A study by Faxon et al.[33] evaluating enoxaparin, a low molecular weight heparin, versus placebo failed to demonstrate any significant benefit. Recently, the EMPAR and FACT trials evaluating low molecular weight heparin were also negative. The anticoagulant warfarin has also been evaluated by Thorton et al.[34] and Urban et al.[35]; no clinical benefit was demonstrated. Also, the potent direct antithrombin hirudin was evaluated in the Helvetica Trial, again without demonstration of long-term clinical or angiographic benefit.[36]

Fish Oils

Seven randomized trials have evaluated fish oils, but the results have been conflicting. Four studies showed a reduction in restenosis whereas three did not, and only one study had at least 94% follow-up.[37] A recent report from the large multicenter trial (FORT) conducted by the National Institutes of Health failed to demonstrate any benefit, with at least 2 weeks of pretreatment at the highest dose of fish oil previously studied. These results all demonstrate limited benefits for fish oils in preventing restenosis.

Other Agents

Other agents that have been tried in the prevention of restenosis include calcium channel blockers, angiotensin-converting enzyme inhibitors, cholesterol-

Table 45-5. Limitations of Previous Randomized Restenosis

Inadequate drug therapy
  Single agent studied
  Inadequate drug administration, no pretreatment, low dose, inadequate duration
  Therapeutic effect of agent studied not measured
Study design flaws
  Small sample size (inadequate power)
  Inadequate follow-up
  Variable end points and definitions of restenosis

(Modified from Franklin and Faxon,[54] with permission.)

lowering agents, and anti-inflammatory agents. Calcium antagonists may play an important role in mediating elastic recoil and coronary spasm immediately after angioplasty; however, several clinical trials have failed to demonstrate benefit.[38] In the meta-analysis performed by Hillegas et al.[39] modest benefit was demonstrated. The European MERCATOR Trial using cilazapril[40] and the recently reported American counterpart MARCATOR,[41] which used various doses of cilazapril, both failed to show benefit in angiographic evidence of restenosis or reduction in clinical events. Likewise, other growth inhibitors such as angiopeptin, a somatostatin analogue, have also failed to show angiographic benefit, although a reduction in clinical events was evident.[42] The only antiproliferative agent to date shown to reduce restenosis is Trapidil, an antiplatelet drug that inhibits PDGF. However, the two reported studies are small, and confirmation is necessary.[43]

Limitations of Restenosis Trials

It is difficult to interpret restenosis trials meaningfully because of numerous problems with previous studies. Inadequate dosages of drugs and study design flaws have limited many clinical trials (Table 45-5). A lack of consensus on end points and the definition of restenosis also make it difficult to compare one study with another. Nevertheless, the current findings of clinical trials suggest that, despite a great deal of effort in this area, the current strategies to prevent restenosis have not been effective and newer directions need to be undertaken.

PREDICTORS OF RESTENOSIS

Whereas numerous clinical trials have failed to demonstrate benefit in reduction of restenosis by pharmacologic agents, a great deal has been learned about the restenosis process and the factors responsible for it. Several clinical trials have examined the clinical and angiographic predictors have subsequent late lumen loss. A recent report from the CARPORT, MARCATOR, and MERCATOR trials indicated that few clinical variables are predictive. Most importantly, the usual risk factors for coronary artery disease, such as hypertension, hyperlipidemia, and cigarette smoking, do not appear to have a significant relationship with late lumen loss.[44,45] However, the presence of unstable angina or recent myocardial infarction do.[46] These findings would suggest that unstable plaque, particularly rapidly progressing plaques with thrombus, may be more susceptible to restenosis.[47,48]

The principle predictors of restenosis are angiographic and include the lumen diameter following the procedure, the change in lumen diameter (before and after the procedure) or acute gain, and to a lesser degree, the morphology of the coronary stenosis. These observations lend credence to the concept that a large lumen diameter following the procedure is desirable and can result in a lower incidence of restenosis. The difficulty with balloon angioplasty is that it cannot achieve a large lumen without a significantly increased risk of complications. This has led to the suggestion that the new interventional devices may be useful in combating restenosis.

PREVENTION OF RESTENOSIS: THE USE OF NEW DEVICES

The use of new interventional devices, particularly directional atherectomy (DCA) and coronary stenting, can result in large initial gain without a signifi-cant increase in acute complications. Quantitative angiographic studies indicate that irrespective of the device, the ratio of late loss to acute gain averages 0.5 and thus, the more acute gain achieved, the more late loss there is. However, since the ratio is less than 1, there are advantages to a larger acute gain and a larger lumen at the end of the procedure, because there is a lower incidence of restenosis using the definition of a late percent stenosis of more than 50% (Fig. 45-4). Whereas these generalizations appear to hold true in many studies, there are concerns that they may not be applicable to all situations. For instance, it may not be true that bigger is better for specific lesion morphologies, and it does not take into account variable tissue response to injury in different lesion locations and in different patients.[49] It is also known that larger vessels have a lower restenotic rate and thus, the size of the reference diameter may be important in determining the ultimate restenosis rate. In fact, the use of atherectomy and stenting is preferred in vessels larger than 3 mm in diameter, and this may also impact on the final restenosis rate (Fig. 45-5).

Randomized Trials on New Devices and the Prevention of Restenosis

Directional Atherectomy

The CAVEAT trial was the first randomized comparison between DCA and PTCA.[14] A total of 1,012 patients was randomized to DCA (n = 512) or PTCA (n = 500). Two-thirds of the patients presented with unstable angina. DCA produced a greater increase in vessel diameter, but was associated with a higher rate of early complications (11 vs. 5%). DCA achieved

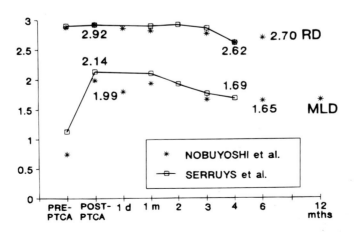

Fig. 45-4. Minimal luminal diameter (MLD) and reference diameter (RD) values found in the studies by Nobuyoshi et al. and Serruys et al. Results are remarkably similar. (From Serruys et al.[55] with permission.)

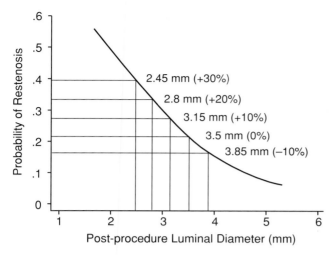

Fig. 45-5. Multivariate logistic modeling of the probability of restenosis (defined as late stenosis >50%) as a function of postprocedure luminal diameter, as illustrated for a hypothetical 3.5-mm artery. A 2.45-mm (30%) residual stenosis typical of conventional angioplasty would have a 40% probability of restenosis. By contrast, a 3.5-mm (0%) residual stenosis typical of a stent would have an 18% probability of restenosis, whereas a 3.15-mm (10%) residual stenosis obtainable with directional atherectomy would have a 23% probability of restenosis. (From Kuntz et al.[57] with permission.)

a better acute gain compared with PTCA (median 1.05 vs. 0.86 mm). At 6 months, the rate of restenosis defined as greater than 50% stenosis at follow-up was 50% for atherectomy and 57% for angioplasty. The probability of death or myocardial infarction was higher in the DCA group (8.6 vs. 4.6%). In summary, the CAVEAT trial demonstrated a small reduction of restenosis when compared with balloon angioplasty, but at the expense of a higher complication rate during the initial hospital stay and a greater financial cost. No clinical benefits were demonstrated for atherectomy at 6 months.

The Canadian Coronary Atherectomy Trial (CCAT) is a multicenter study randomized 274 patients with de novo lesions in the proximal third of the left anterior descending artery to either DCA or PTCA.[50] While half the patients had unstable angina, there was no significant difference in acute outcome for both groups. With atherectomy there was a larger acute gain, but a larger late loss, resulting in similar minimal lumen diameters in both groups during follow-up. At 6-month follow-up, the DCA group had a restenosis rate of 46%, and the PTCA group had a rate of 43%, with a reference diameter of 3.13 vs. 3.23 mm. The results of this study are in contrast to a subgroup analysis in the CAVEAT trial showing that for proximal left anterior descending

artery lesions, the DCA group had a lower restenosis rate. In both studies there was a trend toward a higher incidence of periprocedural myocardial infarction and a need for emergency bypass surgery in the atherectomy group.

The CAVEAT II trial compared DCA with PTCA in saphenous vein grafts and showed no difference in angiographic restenosis, but a lower rate of subsequent revascularization.[51] These studies have been criticized for failing to perform DCA optimally by reducing the residual stenosis to less than 10%. As a result, two additional trials (BOAT and OARS) are endeavoring to evaluate the more aggressive use of DCA.

Stents

Two randomized trials using the Palmaz-Schatz tubular slotted stent have evaluated the influence of stenting on restenosis. The Stress Restenosis Study (STRESS; n = 410 patients) and the Belgium and Netherlands Stent trial (BENESTENT; n = 520 patients) compared late angiographic and clinical outcomes of elective stent placement versus balloon angioplasty in patients with focal lesions (<15 mm in length) in large native vessels (>3 mm in diameter).[28,52] In patients assigned to the stent group, acute angiographic results were better; both acute gain and procedural minimal luminal diameter were increased compared with PTCA. The difference persisted at angiographic follow-up, resulting in a reduction of restenosis rate. Restenosis was defined as more than 50% diameter stenosis at follow-up. The rate was reduced by 33% in STRESS and by 39% in BENESTENT. This reduction was at the expense of subacute stent thrombosis (3.5% in both studies) and a higher frequency of vascular and bleeding complications in the stent patients (9.3% for STRESS and 14.6% for BENESTENT). These two studies represent the first positive impact of new devices on restenosis and again validate the concept that a large, postprocedural lumen diameter is of benefit in reducing the rate of restenosis.

NEW DIRECTIONS

To date, pharmacologic therapy has been extremely disappointing. However, recent experimental studies suggest that one possible explanation for the failure of pharmacologic studies is that we have been aiming at the wrong target; more attention needs to be paid to evaluating the role of remodeling in the restenosis process. Remodeling is a complex biologic process that involves matrix deposition and organi-

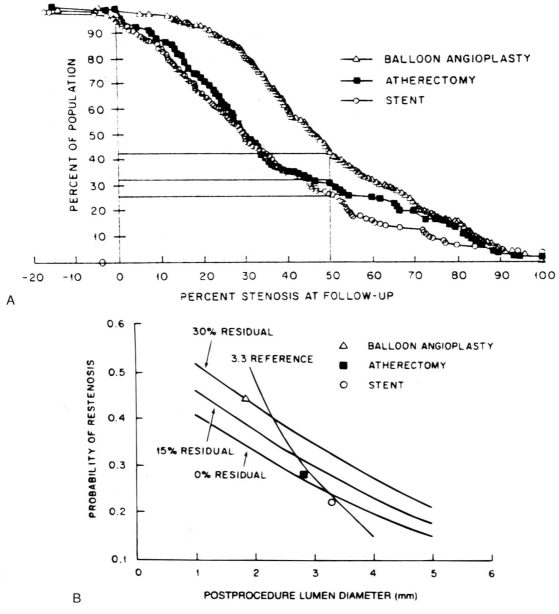

Fig. 45-6. **(A)** cumulative distribution curves of percent stenosis at 6 months in cohorts of conventional angioplasty, atherectomy, and Palmaz-Schatz stent patients, showing the somewhat lower incidence of restenosis (>50% diameter stenosis) for stenting and atherectomy. **(B)** multivariate logistic modeling of the probability of restenosis as a function of postprocedure luminal diameter and percent residual stenosis (0, 15, and 30% respectively). The single (curved) crossing line corresponds to a 3.0-mm reference artery. The particular device used was not a determinant of restenosis, but the different diameters and residual stenoses obtained with each device accurately predicted the probability of restenosis actually observed. (From Kuntz et al.[11] with permission.)

zation of matrix components, as well as re-endothe-liazation and return of the smooth muscle cells to a quiescent phenotype. These changes in vessel diameter may be the most important factor and may ultimately determine the final lumen size. The results of recent studies showing by intravascular ultrasound

that remodeling occurs in de novo atherosclerosis and that restenotic lesions show constriction, suggests that this late phenomenon may play an important role in determining restenosis. New pharmacologic agents directed toward matrix deposition, composition, and crosslinking of collagen should all be explored as new avenues in be prevention of restenosis.

In addition, experimental studies have suggested that high drug dosage is necessary to reduce restenosis experimentally. A large number of agents have been successful in experimental trials, but none have shown clinical benefit. One possible explanation for this difference is that the drug dosages used in clinical trials have been inadequate. However, in clinical trials, many of the drugs (such as colchiline or angiotensin-converting enzyme inhibitors), cannot be given at doses similar to animal studies without significant toxicity. Thus, many investigators are evaluating the role of local delivery as a means of achieving high drug concentration at the site of angioplasty. Local drug delivery catheters, such as the hydrogel balloon catheter, Wolinsky porous balloon, perfusion balloon, sheathed balloon, channel balloon, and drug injection catheters, have been shown to be able to deliver drugs locally to the site of vascular injury. Coated stents and biodegradable stents have also been shown to be effective in releasing sufficient quantities of drug locally, to help prevent restenosis (theoretically). Whereas animal studies have shown feasibility, clinical trials have not yet been conducted.

Molecular biologic approaches to preventing restenosis have a number of distinct advantages. Antisense oligonucleotides to c-*myc* and c-*myb,* which block cell reproduction and cell function, have been shown to be effective in in vitro and in vivo models. Local delivery is essential, but questions remain about the ability to deliver high enough concentrations or long enough duration of oligonucleotides locally in order to inhibit restenosis. The specificity of antisense oligonucleotides has also been questioned. Nevertheless, clinical trials are currently being undertaken. In addition, investigators such as Nabel and colleagues have demonstrated that transfer of genes via adenovirus or retrovirus can be done in vascular tissue and that vascular cells express the marker genes as part of the genetic code. Recently, this group also demonstrated that introduction of a retinoblastoma gene product inhibited neointimal formation.[53] Again, one of the major limitations of gene transfer is an adequate uptake of genetic material by the target cell, but newer techniques have shown substantial improvement in labeling index through use of adenoviral vectors. Local delivery would be mandatory for adequate delivery of genetic material to the angioplasty site. Finally, some investigators have demonstrated the ability to target cells selectively using specific receptor-binding toxins. These fusion toxins are capable of attaching to cells expressing a certain receptor and then killing the cell by introduction of the toxin inside the cell, without disturbing surrounding tissue. Studies using a fusion toxin containing a growth factor such as fibroblast growth factor or a cytokine such as interleukin-2 have been successfully accomplished in vivo, with mixed results to date. One of the disadvantages of this approach is that cell necrosis itself may be a further stimulus to cell proliferation and may counteract the benefits of this technique. Further investigation is necessary to evaluate the benefit fully of any newer molecular biologic approach.

While at present we have a limited ability to prevent restenosis clinically, armed with a greater understanding of the process, it seems likely that a means of preventing this problem will be developed. Stents will probably gain greater acceptance. Through a reduction in geometric remodeling, drug therapy could be focused on the single process of neointimal thickening. Alternatively, drugs (probably locally delivered) aimed at both intimal proliferation and remodeling may provide the therapeutic benefit that has been so elusive to date.

REFERENCES

1. Gruentzig AR, King SB, Schlumpf M, Siegenthaler W: Long-term follow-up after percutaneous transluminal coronary angioplasty: the early Zurich experience. N Engl J Med 1987;1127–1102
2. Leimgruber PP, Roubin GS, Hollman J et al. Restenosis after successful coronary angioplasty in patients with single vessel disease. Circulation 1986;73:710–7
3. Califf RM, Fortin DF, Harlan WR et al. Restenosis after coronary angioplasty: an overview. Circulation 1991;17:2b
4. Serruys PW, Luijten HE, Beatt KJ et al. Incidence of restenosis after successful angioplasty: a time related phenomenon. A quantitative angiographic study in 342 consecutive patients at 1, 2, 3 and 4 months. Circulation 1988;77:361–71
5. Fleming RM, Kirkkeeide RL, Smalling RW, Gould KL. Patterns in visual interpretation of coronary arteriograms as detected by quantitative coronary artiography. J Am Coll Cardiol 1991;18:945
6. Kalbfleisch SJ, McGillem MJ, Pinto IM et al. Comparison of automated quantitative coronary angiography with caliper measurements of percent diameter stenosis. Am J Cardiol 1990;65:1181
7. Rensing BJ, Hermans WR, Deckers JW et al. Luminal narrowing after percutaneous transluminal balloon angioplasty following a near Gaussian distribution: a quantitative angiographic study in 1,445 successfully dilated lesions. J Am Coll Cardiol 1992;19:939
8. Fleck E, Dacian S, Kirschinger J, Hall D, Rudolph W. Quantitative changes in stenotic coronary artery lesions during follow-up after PTCA, abstracted. Circulation, suppl. II. 1984;70:11
9. Holmes DR, Vliestra RE, Smith HC et al. Restenosis after percutaneous transluminal coronary angio-

plasty: a report from the PTCA Registry of the National Heart, Lung and Blood Institute. Am J Cardiol 1984;53:77

10. Kuntz RE, Schmidt DA, Levine MJ et al. Importance of postprocedure luminal diameter on restenosis following new coronary interventions. Circulation, suppl. III. 1990;82:III-45

11. Kuntz RE, Gibson MC, Nobuyoshi M, Baim DS. Generalized model of restenosis after conventional balloon angioplasty, stenting and directional atherectomy. J. Am Coll Cardiol 1993;21:15–25

12. St. Goar FG, Pinto FJ, Alderman EL et al. Intravascular ultrasound imaging of angiographically normal coronary arteries: an in vivo comparison with quantitative angiography. J Am Coll Cardiol 1991;18:952

13. Joelson JM, Most AS, Williams DO. Angiographic findings when chest pain recurs after successful percutaneous transluminal coronary angioplasty. Am J Cardiol 1987;60:792

14. Topol EJ, Califf RM et al. for the CAVEAT Study Group. A comparison of directional atherectomy with coronary angioplasty in patients with coronary artery disease. N Engl J Med 1993;329:221

15. Bengtson JR, Mark DB, Honan MB et al. Detection of restenosis after elective coronary angioplasty using the treadmill exercise test. Am J Cardiol 1990;65:28–34

16. Deligonul U, Vandormael MG, Shah Y et al. Prognostic value of early exercise testing after successful coronary angioplasty: importance of the degree of revascularization. Am Heart J 1989;117:509

17. Hillegass WB, Bengtson JR, Ancukiewcz M et al. for the GRASP Investigators. Predischarge exercise testing does not predict clinical events or restenosis after successful angioplasty. Circulation, suppl. I. 1992;86:I-137

18. Vandormael MG, Deligonul U, Kern MJ et al. Multilesion coronary angioplasty: clinical and angiographic follow-up. J Am Coll Cardiol 1987;10:246–52

19. Nobuyoshi M, Kimura T, Nosaka H et al. Restenosis after successful percutaneous transluminal coronary angioplasty: serial angiographic follow-up of 299 patients. J Am Coll Cardiol 1988;12:616–23

20. Myler RK, Bell W. Thrombogenesis and thrombolysis in acute ischemic syndromes. Pathophysiological and pharmacological rationales for and limitations of thrombolytics, antithrombin, antiplatelet therapy and angioplasty. J Am Coll Cardiol 1991;3:95–114

21. Barbul A, Pines E, Caldwell M. Growth factors and other aspects of wound healing: biological and clinical implications. Prog Clin Biol Res 1988;266:161–75

22. Cloves AW, Schwartz SM. Significance of quiescent smooth muscle cell migration in the injured rat carotid artery. Cir Res 1985;56:139

23. Reidy MA, Clowes AW, Schwartz SM. Endothelial regeneration: inhibition of endothelial regeneration in arteries of rat and rabbit. Lab Invest 1983;49:569

24. Anderson PG, Bajaj RK, Baxley WA, Roubin GS. Vascular biology of balloon-expandable flexible coil stents in humans. J Am Coll Cardiol 1992;19:372

25. Nobuyoshi M, Kimura T, Ohishi H et al. Restenosis after percutaneous transluminal coronary angioplasty: pathologic observations in 20 patients. J Am Coll Cardiol 1991;17:433–9

26. Mintz GS, Kovach JA, Javier SP, Ditrano CJ, Leon MB. Geometric remodelling in the predominant mech-

27. Schwartz L, Bourassa MG, Lesperance J et al. Aspirin and dipyridamole in the prevention of restenosis after percutaneous transluminal coronary angioplasty. N Engl J Med 1988;318:1714

28. Fishman DL, Leon MB, Baim DS et al. A randomized comparison of coronary stent placement and balloon angioplasty in the treatment of coronary artery disease. New Engl J Med 1994;331:496–501

29. Chesebro JH, Webster MW, Reeder GS et al. Coronary angioplasty: antiplatelet therapy reduces acute complications but not restenosis, abstracted Circulation 1989;80:II-64

30. The EPIC Investigators. Use of a monoclonal antibody directed against the platelet glycoprotein IIb/IIIa receptor in high-risk coronary angioplasty. N Engl J Med 1994;33:956–61

31. Hirshfeld JW, Goldberg S, MacDonald R et al. Lesion and procedure related variables predictive of restenosis after PTCA: a report from the M-HEART study, abstracted. Circulation, suppl. 4. 1987;76:215

32. Ellis SG, Roubin GS, Wilentz J, Douglas JS, King SB. Effect of 18- to 24-hour heparin administration for prevention of restenosis after uncomplicated coronary angioplasty. Am Heart J 1989;117:777–82

33. Faxon DP, Spiro T, Minor S et al. Enoxaparin, a low molecular weight heparin, in the prevention of restenosis after angioplasty: results of a double blind randomized trial, abstracted. J Am Coll Cardiol 1992;318:549–57

34. Thorton MA, Gruntzig AR, Hollman J, King SB, Douglas JS. Coumadin and aspirin in prevention of recurrence after transluminal coronary angioplasty: a randomized study. Circulation 1984;69:721–7

35. Urban P, Buller N, Fox K et al. Lack of effect of warfarin on the restenosis rate or on clinical outcome after balloon coronary angioplasty. Br Heart J 1988;60:485–8

36. Serruys PW, Deckers J. A double-blind randomized heparin-controlled trial evaluating acute and long-term efficacy of r-hirudin (CGP39343) in patients undergoing coronary angioplasty. Circulation, suppl. 1994;90:I-394

37. Reis GJ, Boucher TM, Sipperly ME et al. Randomized trial of fish oil for prevention of restenosis after coronary angioplasty. Lancet 1989;2:177–81

38. Corocos T, David PR, Val PG et al. Failure of diltiazem to prevent restenosis after percutaneous transluminal coronary angioplasty. Am Heart J 1985;109:926–31

39. Hillegass WB, Ohman EM, Califf RM. Restenosis: the clinical issues. p. 415. In Topol EJ (ed): Textbook of Interventional Cardiology. WB Saunders, Philadelphia, 1990

40. MERCATOR Study Group. Does the new angiotensin converting enzyme inhibitor cilazapril prevent restenosis after percutaneous transluminal coronary angioplasty. Results of the MERCATOR study: a multicenter, randomized, double-blind, placebo-controlled trial. Circulation 1992;86:100–10

41. Faxon DP on behalf of the MARCATOR Study Group. Effect of high dose angiotensin-converting enzyme inhibition on restenosis: final results of the MARCATOR study, a multicenter, double-blind, placebo-controlled trial of cilazapril. J Am Coll Cardiol 1995;2:362–9

42. Emanuelsson H, Beatt KJ, Bagger J-P et al. Long-term

effects of angiopeptin treatment in coronary angioplasty. Circulation 1995;91:1689–96

43. Maresta A, Balducelli M, Cantini L et al. Trapidil (triazolopyrimidine), a platelet-derived growth factor antagonist, reduces restenosis after percutaneous transluminal coronary angioplasty. Results of the randomized, double-blind STARC study. Circulation 1994;90:2710–5

44. Bourassa MG, Lesperance J, Eastwood C et al. Clinical, physiologic, anatomic, and procedural factors predictive of restenosis after percutaneous transluminal coronary angioplasty. J Am Coll Cardiol 1991;18:368–76

45. Hirshfeld JW, Schwartz SS, Jugo R et al. and the M-HEART Investigators. Restenosis after coronary angioplasty: a multivariate statistical model to relate lesion and procedural variables to restenosis. J Am Coll Cardiol 1991;18:647–56

46. Meyer J, Schmitz HJ, Kiesslich T et al. Percutaneous transluminal coronary angioplasty in patients with stable and unstable angina pectoris: analysis of early and late results. Am Heart J 1983;106:973–80

47. Potkins BN, Roberts WC. Effects of coronary angioplasty on atherosclerotic plaques and relation of plaque composition and arterial size to outcome. Am J Cardiol 1988;62:41–50

48. Waller BF. Coronary luminal shape and the arc of disease-free wall: morphologic observations and clinical relevance. J Am Coll Cardiol 1985;6:1100

49. Garratt KN. Bigger is not neccessarily better: in search of an optimal (not maximal) atherectomy result. J Interv Cardiol 1992;6:107–12

50. Alderman AG, Cohen EA, Kimball BP, Schwartz L et al. A comparison of directional atherectomy with balloon angioplasty for lesions of the left anterior descending coronary artery. N Engl J Med 1993;329:228–33

51. Holmes DR, Topol EJ, Califf RM et al. A multicenter, randomized trial of coronary angioplasty versus directional atherectomy for patients with saphenous vein bypass graft lesions. Circulation 1995;91:1966–74

52. Serruys PW, de Jaegere P, Kiemereij F et al. A comparison of balloon expandable stent implantation with balloon angioplasty in patients with coronary artery disease. New Engl J Med 1994;331:489–95

53. Chang MW, Barr E, Seltzer J et al. Cytostatic gene therapy for vascular proliferative disorders with a constitutively active form of the retinoblastoma gene product. Science 1995;267:518–22

54. Franklin SM, Faxon DP. Pharmacologic prevention of restenosis after coronary angioplasty: review of the randomized clinical trials. Coronary Artery Dis 1993;4:232–42

55. Serruys PW, Rensing BJ, Hermans LURM, Beatt KJ. Definition of restenosis after percutaneous transluminal coronary angioplasty: a quickly evolving concept. J Invest Cardiol 1989;4:265–76

56. Currier JW, Faxon DP. Restenosis after percutaneous transluminal coronary angioplasty: have we been aiming at the wrong target? J Am Coll Cardiol 1995;24:516–20

57. Kuntz RE, Safian RD, Carrozza JP et al. The importance of acute luminal diameter in determining restenosis after coronary atherectomy or stenting. Circulation 1992;86:1827

46 Vocational Rehabilitation After Coronary Interventions

Nicolas Danchin

The present development of myocardial revascularisation procedures [coronary artery bypass graft (CABG) and percutaneous transluminal coronary angioplasty (PTCA)] has increased health costs. However, these procedures, which improve both functional status and physical capacity, might help initially disabled patients retain or resume their employment, thereby partially or totally covering their own cost. In addition, for many patients (particularly young patients), work resumption is one of the components of an adequate psychological response to the occurrence of a heart condition. Therefore it is no surprise that vocational rehabilitation after myocardial revascularization has been recognized as an important issue very early in the development of both CABG[1] and PTCA,[2,3] especially since a vast majority of patients undergoing myocardial revascularization at that time were young and active. At present, however, with an increasing proportion of elderly (and therefore retired) patients undergoing myocardial revascularization, it might be thought that work resumption is no longer clinically and socially relevant. This is not the case, however; because of the major increase in the numbers of revascularization procedures, the absolute number of active people undergoing CABG or PTCA has certainly not decreased over the years.

In the present chapter, the factors expected to prevent return to work after myocardial revascularization procedures are analyzed and the actual figures of vocational outcome after CABG or PTCA as well as the place of cardiac rehabilitation discussed.

THEORETIC AND METHODOLOGIC CONSIDERATIONS

Four main factors are theoretically involved in determining the working capacity of a patient after myocardial revascularization: left ventricular function; degree of myocardial revascularization (complete versus incomplete); presence of concurrent illnesses; and psychosocial factors. The first two factors represent major determinants of the patients' exercise capacity.

Left Ventricular Function

Left ventricular function determines the capacity of the left ventricle to provide an adequate cardiac output in most circumstances of everyday life, particularly during work. In the absence of previous myocardial infarction, myocardial revascularization avoids the development of left ventricular dysfunction during exercise and consequently should permit virtually any kind of work. By contrast, in case of previous myocardial infarction, there may be an imbalance between myocardial function and the physical requirements of the previous employment of the patient, independent of the procedure. Therefore, the problem of the working capacity becomes the same as after myocardial infarction.

Extent of Revascularization

Although complete myocardial revascularization is the goal of most therapeutic interventions, incomplete revascularization has become fairly common, particularly after PTCA in patients with multivessel coronary disease. In practice, incomplete revascularization of the myocardium may be found if minor narrowed vessels or vessels supplying an infarcted area are not bypassed or submitted to angioplasty, or in case of partial failure of the revascularization procedure (early occlusion of a bypass graft, restenosis after PTCA). In the first two instances, the amount of myocardium that is potentially ischemic during exercise is small and is not likely to impair the working capacity of the patients. In the third instance, the amount of myocardium jeopardized during exercise may be larger and may constitute a true hindrance to work resumption by limiting the physical capacity of the patients.

Concurrent Illnesses

Concurrent illnesses correlate with a poorer long-term prognosis after revascularization; obviously, the presence of such diseases will also constitute an obstacle to work resumption.

Social Parameters

Lastly, return to work after myocardial revascularization may be limited by specific social parameters. Some occupations are prohibitive for cardiac patients for medical-legal considerations (bus drivers, airplane pilots, fire-fighters, and so forth). The local rate of unemployment also has a bearing on vocational outcome. However, although all these factors are of theoretic importance in determining the working capacity of a patient after myocardial revascularization, they do not always coincide with the factors actually impeding return to work, as evidenced by many clinical studies.

In addition, a word of caution is necessary for interpreting the rates of return to work reported after CABG or PTCA, which may vary widely according to the methodology used. When studying overall return to work at any time, or rate of patients actually employed at a given time after the procedure, the rates obtained with the former method are higher than those obtained with the latter. Other authors may study vocational outcome in all patients below the age of retirement at the time of revascularization or only those patients previously employed.

RETURN TO WORK AFTER CABG

Return to work after CABG is variable according to country. In the United States and Canada return to work is usually higher than 60% and may be as high as 85%.[1] In Europe, similar results have been reported in Great Britain during the early 1980s; however, in Germany, France, or Switzerland, the rates are usually more disappointing and rarely exceed 50%.

Several studies have analyzed the factors likely to influence work resumption. Most have found little predictive value regarding work resumption for medical preoperative and operative parameters: in most studies, left ventricular function, a major determinant of exercise capacity, is not related to subsequent re-employment.[4,5] The extent of coronary artery disease (number of diseased vessels) is usually not related to work resumption.[4,6] More importantly, the number of grafts placed and the completeness of revascularization, which may determine the presence or absence of postoperative myocardial ischemia, are unrelated to return to work.[4] Among the other medical variables, previous myocardial infarction or functional class of preoperative angina are related to work resumption in all but a few studies. Lastly, we showed that the presence of a noncardiovascular illness and a longer duration of symptoms of coronary artery disease before surgery had a negative influence on return to work.[4]

In contrast to preoperative medical variables, a strong relation exists between postoperative health status and work resumption. Physical capacity during postoperative exercise tests and the presence of postoperative angina are directly related to work resumption.[7]

Many nonmedical parameters have been studied in relation to the vocational outcome after coronary bypass surgery. Many of them are of primary importance, in that they are likely to influence a patient's capacity or willingness to resume the previous occupation. Age at the time of surgery, educational level, type of preoperative occupation, or annual income before surgery are related to the postoperative working status. Lastly, work resumption is related to the length of preoperative unemployment, which is the most important preoperative predictor of subsequent employment in multivariate analyses.[4]

RETURN TO WORK AFTER PTCA

The rates of return to work after PTCA in previously active patients range from 61%[8] to 84%.[9] With the changing pattern of populations undergoing PTCA since the early 1980s, involving more patients with multivessel disease, previous myocardial infarction, or previous myocardial revascularization, return to work has tended to decline, in spite of the higher clinical success rates of the procedure; in our experience, work resumption in previously employed patients who had a successful PTCA decreased from 85% in the 1980–1982 period to 69% in 1985, a difference mainly explained by the older age of the patients in the second time period and by the general socioeconomic context in our region at that time (the level of unemployment rose from 7.2 to 12.3% from 1980 to 1985).[10]

As for coronary bypass surgery, work resumption is largely influenced by the results of the procedure; in our experience, work resumption increased from 40% in case of acute failure of the procedure to 85% in patients with a primary success.[3] Similar findings were reported in 1985 by Boulay et al.[9] in a series from the Montreal Heart Institute. As with CABG, there was a strong association between functional status after the procedure, presence of residual angina, or presence of restenosis and re-employment.[10] Interestingly, the other medical or social parameters do not seem to greatly influence return to work, except age, which was found to have a negative influence on work resumption in several studies,[3,8,10] and the level of physical activity involved in the pre-PTCA occupation.[10] Other factors likely to influence the working status of patients with ischemic heart disease (emotional disturbances, overprotection by the family, attending physician attitude, or lack of cooperation by the employer) have not been specifically evaluated in clinical studies of PTCA patients.[11]

The time period from PTCA to work resumption ranges from 14 days[2] to 132 days.[3] This exceedingly long delay before work resumption in our early experience emphasized the influence of postprocedural medical management on return to work; indeed, it was explained by the finding that many patients, informed of the risk of restenosis, waited for the results of thallium exercise testing, which was routinely scheduled 3 months after the initial procedure, before resuming work.

There are no specific data about vocational outcome after coronary angioplasty using new devices. Among those, however, only the use of intracoronary stents might have an influence on vocational outcome. On the one hand, they might result in a prolongation of the time before work resumption, because it may be preferable in some professions to avoid return to work while the patients still receive oral anticoagulant therapy (a period usually lasting 1 to 2 months). On the other hand, since stents decrease the restenosis rate and reduce the need for re-PTCA, their use might avoid subsequent work interruption in some patients.

COMPARISON OF WORK RESUMPTION AFTER PTCA WITH CABG OR MEDICAL TREATMENT

PTCA offers the advantage over CABG of a hospital stay often limited to just a few days, theoretically permitting a prompt return to work. However, although PTCA was initially carried out mainly in patients with single-vessel coronary disease, therefore providing complete revascularization, most patients presently undergoing PTCA have multivessel disease, for which complete revascularization is less often achieved, and many have already suffered a myocardial infarction. On the whole, compared with coronary surgery, left ventricular function is usually not different from that of patients undergoing coronary bypass operations, and the "less invasive" profile of the PTCA procedure might be counterbalanced by a lesser efficacy in terms of completeness of revascularization.

Few studies have been specifically devoted to a comparison of return to work in patients treated with CABG or PTCA at the same institution, and none of those are randomized comparisons of the two revascularization procedures[3,8,12–14] (Table 46-1). Most do not find large differences in the rates of re-employment, but the figures after PTCA tend to be slightly higher, despite higher levels of residual angina in the PTCA groups. In the study by McGee et al.,[14] return to work in patients without postprocedural angina was significantly higher for PTCA patients (73% versus 55%).

In the Randomized Intervention Treatment of Angina (RITA) trial, comparing PTCA and CABG in patients in whom equivalent revascularization was deemed achievable by either procedure, the percentage of patients not working due to coronary disease was higher at 1 month after CABG (79%, compared with 54% after PTCA), but the difference was no longer significant from 6 months to 2 years after randomization (at 2 years: 23 and 25%, respectively).[16]

In the ACME study (randomized comparison of PTCA and medical treatment in patients with single-vessel coronary artery disease), PTCA did not seem to improve work resumption, compared with medical treatment: in the PTCA group, 42% were employed at baseline and 43% at follow-up; in the medical therapy group, the respective figures were 29 and 29%.[17]

CARDIAC REHABILITATION AND RETURN TO WORK AFTER PTCA

Cardiac rehabilitation has proved to be beneficial regarding functional status and exercise capacity in many subsets of coronary patients. Little is known,

Table 46-1. Comparison of Return to Work After CABG and PTCA[a]

Study	Return to Work (%)			Main Study Features
	CABG	PTCA	P Value	
Jang et al., 1982[12]	69 (151)	79 (163)	<0.02	Prospective
Danchin et al., 1984[3]	38 (27)	73 (73)	<0.05	Retrospective; CABG = single bypass
Meier et al., 1985[13]	87 (113)	81 (83)	ns	Retrospective
Vallbracht et al., 1985[8]	25 (54)	61 (52)	<0.001	Retrospective
Allen et al., 1990[15]	71 (106)	70 (64)	ns	Prospective
McGee et al., 1993[14]	58 (112)	69 (119)	ns	Retrospective
RITA trial, 1993[16] (% not working due to CAD)	25 (208)	23 (188)	ns	Prospective, randomized

Abbreviations: CABG, coronary artery bypass grafting; CAD, coronary artery disease; ns, not significant; PTCA, percutaneous transluminal coronary angioplasty.

[a] Only the RITA trial constitutes a randomized comparison of patients undergoing CABG or PTCA. Sizes of populations in which the working status was investigated appear in parentheses.

however, about the specific effect of rehabilitation on return to work after myocardial revascularization. After PTCA, cardiac rehabilitation may prove useful in patients with incomplete revascularization or impaired left ventricular function, to improve functional capacity. Ben Ari et al.[18] reported increased exercise capacity and favorable lipid changes in patients participating in a comprehensive rehabilitation program after PTCA, whereas no influence on restenosis, subsequent myocardial infarction, or coronary bypass surgery was found. There is no definite evidence, however, that cardiac rehabilitation can increase work resumption. For patients participating in a rehabilitation program, and in order not to hinder return to work, it is essential that overprotection by the patient's family not be replaced by overprotection by the "medical environment" available during the rehabilitation period. Indeed, when such patients are below the age of retirement, work resumption should be considered one of the goals of comprehensive care, and, whenever needed, the rehabilitation team should not hesitate to work in conjunction with occupational medicine specialists.

CONCLUSIONS

Working status after CABG or PTCA depends on two main types of parameters: (1) the final success of the revascularization procedure, which determines a patient's postoperative functional status and physical capacity and (2) preoperative nonmedical factors, the most important being age at the time of revascularization and length of the preoperative period of unemployment.

In patients with complete revascularization after PTCA and with preserved left ventricular function, cardiologists should encourage very early (1 to 2 weeks after the procedure) return to work. It is also important that the factors negatively affecting return to work after myocardial revascularization be recognized, so that proper attention can be given to the patients especially needing it; in these patients, postprocedural counseling and reorientation, with the help of a specialized rehabilitation team working in conjunction with occupational physicians, might prove helpful.

REFERENCES

1. Barnes GK, Ray MJ, Oberman A, Kouchoukos NT. Changes in working status following coronary bypass surgery. JAMA 1977;238:1259–1263
2. Holmes DR Jr, Vlietstra RE, Mock MB et al. Employment and recreation patterns in patients treated by percutaneous transluminal coronary angioplasty: a multicenter study. Am J Cardiol 1983;52:710–713
3. Danchin N, Cuilliere M, Mathieu P, Cherrier F, Faivre G. Réinsertion socio-professionnelle après angioplastie transluminale coronaire. Arch Mal Coeur 1984;77: 993–997
4. Danchin N, David P, Bourassa MG, Robert P, Chaitman BR. Factors predicting working status after aortocoronary bypass surgery. Can Med Assoc J 1982;126: 255–260
5. Johnson WD, Kayser KL, Pedraza PM, Shore RT. Employment patterns in males before and after myocardial revascularization surgery: a study of 2229 consecutive patients followed for as long as 10 years. Circulation 1982;65:6–14
6. Hammermeister KE, DeRouen TA, English MT, Dodge HT. Effect of surgical versus medical therapy on re-

turn to work in patients with coronary artery disease. Am J Cardiol 1979;44:105–111

7. Gohlke H, Schnellbacher K, Steinrûcken H, Samek L, Roskamm H. Postoperative exercise performance determines return to work pp. 102–107. In Walter PJ (ed): Return to Work after Coronary Artery Bypass Surgery. Psychosocial and Economic Aspects. Springer-Verlag, New York, 1985

8. Vallbracht C, Kober G, Scherer D, Kaltenbach M. Return to work after coronary angioplasty pp. 177–185. In Walter PJ (ed): Return to Work after Coronary Artery Bypass Surgery. Psychosocial and Economic Aspects. Springer-Verlag, New York, 1985

9. Boulay F, David P, David PR, Bourassa MG. Work status and percutaneous transluminal coronary angioplasty pp. 183–190. In Walter PJ (ed): Return to Work after Coronary Artery Bypass Surgery. Psychosocial and Economic Aspects. Springer-Verlag, New York, 1985

10. Danchin N, Juillière Y, Selton-Suty C et al. Return to work after percutaneous transluminal coronary angioplasty: a continuing problem. Eur Heart J, suppl. G. 1989;10:54–57

11. Guillette W, Judge RD, Koehn E et al. Committee report on economic, administrative and legal factors influencing the insurability and employability of patients with ischemic heart disease. J Am Coll Cardiol 1989;14:1010–1015

12. Jang GC, Gruentzig AR, Block PC et al. Work profile following coronary angioplasty or coronary bypass surgery: results from a national cooperative study. Circulation, suppl. II. 1982;66:II-123

13. Meier B, Chaves V, Segesser LV, Faidutti B, Rutishauser W. Vocational rehabilitation after coronary angioplasty and coronary bypass surgery pp. 171–176. In Walter PJ (ed): Return to Work after Coronary Artery Bypass Surgery. Psychosocial and Economic Aspects. Springer-Verlag, New York, 1985

14. McGee HM, Graham T, Crowe B, Horgan JH. Return to work following coronary artery bypass surgery or percutaneous transluminal coronary angioplasty. Eur Heart J 1993;14:623–28

15. Allen JK, Fitzgerald ST, Swank RT, Becker DM. Functional status after coronary artery bypass grafting and percutaneous transluminal coronary angioplasty. Am J Cardiol 1990;65:921–925

16. RITA trial participants. Coronary angioplasty versus coronary artery bypass surgery: the Randomised Intervention Treatment of Angina (RITA) trial. Lancet 1993;341:573–580

17. Parisi A, Folland ED, Hartigan P. A comparison of angioplasty with medical therapy in the treatment of single-vessel coronary artery disease. N Engl J Med 1992;326:10–16

18. Ben Ari E, Rothbaum MD, Linnemeier TJ et al. Benefits of a monitored rehabilitation program versus physician care after emergency percutaneous transluminal coronary angioplasty: follow-up of risk factors and rate of restenosis. J Cardiopulm Rehabil 1989;7: 281–285

47 Introduction

Ulrich Sigwart

Stents have been used in clinical practice for the last decade. The concept of scaffolding tubular structures that fail to perform adequately in the human body is so convincing and simple that almost a century ago doctors contemplated using this principle and even tried it in animals. Meanwhile, stents have revolutionized a number of therapeutic modalities. In particular, transluminal coronary angioplasty has become predictable through the use of stents. The results of several randomized trials have highlighted the role of stents in the prevention of restenosis and in the reduction of clinical events. Stents have also expanded the scope of transluminal angioplasty considerably.

Stents are not only used in blood vessels; they now form an integral part of a number of keyhole techniques in the domain of the urinary tract, the biliary ducts, the esophagus, and the bronchial system. Stent technology, however, is clearly limping behind clinical ambitions. It has become clear from experimental work and clinical trials that all stents that have been used over the last few years have important shortcomings.

The stent with the longest clinical track record, Wallstent, acquired the reputation of difficult use because of its shortening during expansion. On the other hand, this stent, which is now in the process of being revived, has some important advantages, which are flexibility and the potential for stenting long segments in a homogenous fashion. This makes it particularly suitable for degenerated bypass grafts and diffuse disease of the right coronary artery.

Precise deployment is easier with the very popular balloon expandable stents. The Johnson & Johnson Palmaz-Schatz stent has been sold in numbers exceeding a quarter of a million. This most popular of all stents is generally stiff and can be used in tortuous anatomy only if short segments are deployed, either individually placed or connected via an articulation. Side branch access is difficult or impossible after placement of this stent, as it is with the Wallstent. Balloon expansion of the stent causes important stress at the bend points and may result in uneven deployment. Embolization from the carrier balloon is a dreaded hazard with this and other balloon-expandable stents. The balloon-expandable coil stents (Gianturco-Roubin, Wiktor, Strecker, Freedom, Angiostent, and so forth) suffer from limited resistance to external radial force, which may lead to recoil after placement and requires a higher strut profile with the inherent problems of turbulence.

The Boston Scientific Strecker stent adds to these problems the feature of wire crossings, which may increase the turbulence to flow and the thrombogenic potential. The AVE microstent combines the stiffness of the individual segments of the Palmaz-Schatz with important strut thickness and has no particular advantages from the hemodynamic standpoint. On the other hand, it is relatively user friendly, and recrossing is easy.

Recent experimental and clinical data support the concept that stent designs have a crucial impact on thrombosis and hyperplasia. Variations of the design without alteration of metal mass and material may be associated with significant differences in the amount of thrombosis and restenosis. This concept had been applied to newer stents like the ACS Multi-Link stent and the NIR stent. Data primarily from

Japan and Europe, have shown restenosis rates between 3% and 13% for the ACS Multi-Link stent. These figures are lower than previously seen with other stent models. Similar restenosis rates seem to emerge from the trials using heparin-coated Palmaz-Schatz stents. The combination of biologically active surfaces and optimal stent design appears to be the direction of the future. When these principles are correctly applied, even small vessels may be amenable to stenting.

The management of stents has greatly changed over the last 5 years. Vascular stents are now being used without anticoagulation. This has dramatically reduced morbidity and cost. Outpatient stenting of blood vessels is within reach. The proliferation of this technique has resulted in a much more liberal use of stents, which are being used in more than half of all angioplasty procedures in some centers already.

In 1986 I predicted that 60% of our angioplasty procedures would use stents after a decade of experience. This prediction has proved correct, and it is now our duty to reduce the number of complications associated with stenting to a level at which they become insignificant.

48 The Self-Expanding Mesh Stent

U. Sigwart
P. Serruys

The use of percutaneous transluminal coronary angioplasty (PTCA) has grown extraordinarily, and its indications have greatly expanded.[1-5] PTCA is more effective than medical treatment in terms of symptom relief[6] and compares favorably with coronary artery bypass surgery regarding symptoms,[7] cost,[8] and return to work.[9] Randomized studies comparing angioplasty with either bypass surgery or medical treatment have shown PTCA to be effective.[10,11] However, despite improvements in technical equipment and the growing experience of operators, the two major limitations of balloon angioplasty remain. Abrupt postangioplasty closure complicates 5% of procedures,[12] and restenosis occurs in 30% to 40% of patients.[13-16] Only one mechanical device, the coronary stent, shows promise for modifying the rates of both acute occlusion and restenosis. Stents provide a "scaffolding" to support the vessel wall, tack down intimal flaps, smooth the luminal surface (thereby improving blood flow), and prevent vessel wall recoil. In 1986, the self-expanding mesh stent was the first of these devices deployed in a coronary vessel.[17] Over the following years, we have examined the role of the self-expanding mesh stent (Fig. 48-1) under circumstances of abrupt closure,[18] restenosis of native coronary vessels,[19] and restenosis of bypass graft vessels.[20] The self-expanding mesh stent has also been studied by others around the world. This chapter describes this stent and its potential advantages.

HISTORY OF CORONARY STENTING

Carrel[21] was the first to describe the experimental surgical implantation of intravascular tubing, and in 1969 Dotter[22] reported on experimental percutaneous intravascular stenting, using both plastic tubing and stainless steel coilspring prostheses. While the impervious plastic tube grafts could be reliably positioned in normal dog femoral or popliteal arteries through a left carotid arteriotomy, all stents clotted within 24 hours after implantation. This was partially overcome by the use of a stainless steel coilspring design together with the administration of heparin for 4 days, but stability of the stents remained a problem.

Variations of the metal coil design, made either of stainless steel or of nitinol (a temperature-dependent shape-memory nickel and titanium alloy) were used in experimental animals by the same group and others.[23,24] Cragg et al.[24] reported the percutaneous implantation of four nitinol coil stents in dog aortas through a 10-F catheter using a continuous cold flush (10°C) prior to stent release. Expanded coil diameter ranged from 5 to 11 mm and coil length from 1 to 6 cm. All stents remained patent at 4 weeks without anticoagulant medication. There was a tendency for closer wound stents to have greater thrombogenicity, probably because more metal was involved for a given length of stented aorta.

Self-Expanding Stents

Following Senning's suggestions, Maass et al.[25] in Zürich described the experimental use of several different self-expanding stents that could be elongated by torsion onto an ad hoc introducing device and then released into the vascular lumen, where they expanded due to their elastic properties. One hundred

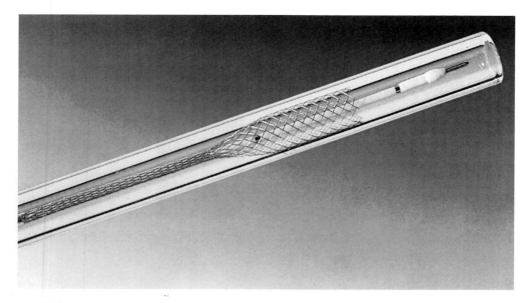

Fig. 48-1. Self-expanding mesh stent during implantation in a glass tube. The *classic* Wallstent depicted here has a doubled-over constraining membrane that has been partially retracted (unidirectional action) in this illustration. The *new (Magic)* Wallstent uses a simple sheath that can be brought forward again to reposition or retrieve the partially deployed stent.

and eighty stents were implanted into the peripheral arteries or veins of 75 dogs. Tilting (11%), migration (5%), or thrombosis (10%) of the prosthesis remained a problem with the early stent design, but marked improvement was noted when the "double helix" stent was used, since this proved more stable (tilting 6%, no migration), and no occlusive thrombus formation was observed. However, the design required a bulky introducing system and was thus unsuitable for small arteries. All stents were made of surgical stainless steel (Mediloy, Medinvent, Lausanne, Switzerland), either wire (0.3 to 0.5 mm diameter) or metal bands (0.08 to 0.30 mm thick and 1.5 mm wide). Positioning of such prostheses could be achieved without inducing pressure necrosis, and endothelial covering in previously normal arteries was complete within 6 weeks. A combination of parietal intimal proliferation and microthrombi was observed more frequently in veins than in arteries.

Gianturco's group[26,27] described a spring-loaded stainless steel stent with a zigzag pattern that was implanted into large vessels, but stent migration was observed in some cases, and prosthesis stability appeared to be suboptimal. The stent's design also restricted its use to the covering of short vascular segments.

MECHANISM OF ACTION

Several of the initial problems of self-expanding stents were solved when the coil concept was further developed and led us to the use of a mesh design with several interwoven strands (Fig. 48-1). This device, later termed the Wallstent (Medinvent) was the first to be used for clinical purposes, and a large part of the early clinical information on clinical coronary stenting was obtained with it.[17,18] The stent now consists of 20 strands of 0.06 to 0.09-mm diameter arranged into a self-expanding mesh design. The material is a nonferromagnetic cobalt-base alloy, and a 5 mm-diameter stent typically weighs about 1.4 mg/mm of length. The stent is flexible along its long axis and for coronary implants its length varies between 15 and 30 mm and its diameter between 3.0 and 6.5 mm in the fully expanded state. For any given lesion, a stent is selected so that its fully expanded diameter is somewhat larger than the estimated normal lumen of the recipient vessel; it will then be stable once positioned and exert a residual radial pressure on the arterial wall. For implantation, the stent is compressed and thereby elongated on a delivery system. This is introduced via a standard 8-F guiding catheter over an exchange guidewire after completion of balloon angioplasty. The delivery system used for coronary arteries has an outer diameter of 1.57 mm and can accommodate stents of up to 6.5 mm in diameter. A doubled-over membrane maintains the stent constrained in an elongated state. The space between the inner and outer layers of the membrane is filled with contrast medium at approximately 3 bars of pressure to ensure both lubrication and radiographic visualization. Trapped air may escape through a distally located microscopic pinhole. Retraction of the membrane allows the stent to be progressively released into the vascular lumen. Recent modifications of the stent design have brought the braiding angle from 130° to 110°. This has reduced the exerted radial force by about 30% and the amount of metal per millimeter of stented vessel by about 7%. The stent shortens significantly less compared with the classic design. Advances in polymer technology have also allowed a simple retractable sleeve without the somewhat cumbersome and (from the operator's standpoint) delicate banana-skin principle. The stent has been made more radiopaque through incorporation of a platinum core into the wires (see Fig. 48-4).

HISTOLOGY

Experimental evidence from several different animal studies shows that a thin fibrin and platelet layer is deposited on a metallic stent within minutes following implantation.[28–31] The stent slowly becomes embedded in thickened intima, and the endoluminal surface is eventually covered by neoendothelium. The neoendothelial covering is completed within 1 to 8 weeks, depending on the type of stent and the animal model studied. Using a balloon-expandable stent in the rabbit model, Palmaz et al.[32] observed an immature endothelial cover with a "crazy-paving" appearance after 1 week, and normal-appearing endothelium with flat, elongated cells at 8 weeks. Using the same stent deployed in a dog's peripheral artery,

these investigators observed that the development of neoendothelium took 3 weeks.[33]

We have made similar observations with the self-expanding stent.[17,28] Forty-seven stents were inserted in dogs (Fig. 48-2) and sheep. They were covered within the first few hours of deployment by a thin fibrin and platelet layer. Complete endothelial covering was observed at 3 weeks. The mesh design allowed islands of endothelium to grow between the stainless steel strands and eventually coalesce. The thickness of the neointima varied between 50 and 500 μm. Pressure necrosis was not seen, but thinning and slight fibrosis of the underlying media was observed with all stent devices.[29,32] All side branches covered by stents remained patent (Fig. 48-2).

The deposition of platelets and fibrin almost certainly occurs within the first hours of deployment, but the endothelial covering may be a much more protracted process.[18] In animal models intravascular stents rarely stimulate marked fibrointimal hyperplasia. Fibrointimal proliferation, however, does occur around stent struts in human arteries, perhaps due to the presence of various growth factors also found after angioplasty procedures.[34]

TECHNIQUE

During elective stenting procedures, angioplasty of the target lesion is carried out using standard procedures with any 8-F guiding catheter. Since no rapid exchange system exists for the deployment of this

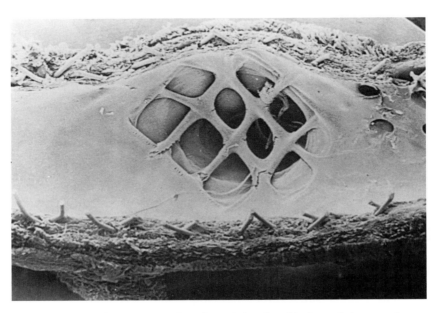

Fig. 48-2. Self-expanding mesh stent covering the origin of a side branch in a canine coronary artery. (From Sigwart et al.,[17] with permission.)

stent, the balloon catheter is withdrawn over an exchange guidewire (300 cm) or a magnetic wire. The stent is sized such that its unconstrained diameter is 10% to 20% larger than the reference diameter. This size differential not only exerts some residual radial force on the vessel wall, but also ensures that the stent will be in intimate contact with the wall. The stent length ought to exceed the length of the diseased segment or cover the entire dissection.

The introducing system is prepared by aspiration prep of the space between the outer and inner membrane of the doubled-over constraining system. When undiluted contrast under 3 to 4 bar pressure arrives at the distal pinhole, the side-arm stopcock may be closed and the wire lumen flushed with saline. A number of side openings in the shaft underlying the stent allow for rinsing of the stent itself, especially if the distal wire lumen is temporarily occluded by gentle finger pressure. The stent so prepared is then advanced over the guidewire with the stent carefully positioned across the predilated area. Since the stent contracts along its long axis as its diameter expands, the operator must estimate visually where the fully expanded stent will finally be positioned; considerable experience usually is required for this maneuver. The constraining membrane is inflated under a pressure of 4 bars and is then withdrawn slowly under fluoroscopic guidance. This action releases the stent into the vascular lumen. The position of the constraining membrane can be estimated by virtue of the undiluted contrast used to fill the space, but superior digital fluoroscopy is required. Three markers on the delivery catheter also help at deployment: the distal and proximal markers indicate the end of the elongated stent on the deployment instrument, and the middle marker helps to predict the extremity of the expanded stent. The new system is back to the original design with two markers only. Following successful deployment, the carrier catheter jumps slightly forward and can easily be moved back and forth. To minimize trauma, it is important not to try to correct the stent position once the stent has begun to open distally and starts to be in contact with the vessel wall. This precaution does not apply to the use of the new deployment system, which allows repositioning by advancing the sheath over the partially opened stent, thus recapturing it for another deployment. Finally a balloon catheter is reintroduced over the guidewire into the stented segment and a final full inflation is done to expand the stent to its desired size and embed the metal struts as thoroughly as possible into the arterial wall (sometimes termed the *Swiss kiss*). Several angiographic and ultrasonic studies have shown that the improved appearance after stenting correlates with an abolition of the translesional gradient and correlates with a reduction in postoperative events like subacute thrombosis and restenosis.[35] The introducing system can negotiate tortuous segments and deploy stents in distal locations without difficulty because of its flexibility and tapered tip design. The latter facilitates primary stenting in friable vein grafts without prior balloon dilation. Large-diameter arteries or vein grafts can be treated with the same 1.57 mm diameter introducing catheter used for small vessels since the expansion ratio of the stent is excellent (2 to 4.1, corresponding to 3.0 to 6.5 mm). We have not had problems of stent migration or premature stent release, and embolization has not occurred.

INDICATIONS

Abrupt Closure

Abrupt occlusion probably arises from major intimal flaps, which reduce flow and promote thrombus formation, as well as from vessel wall recoil.[38–43] The standard management of this complication involves repeated balloon dilations, often with prolonged, low-pressure inflations and the use of a slight increase in balloon size.[44] In earlier series, emergency surgical revascularization was necessary for approximately half the cases of abrupt closure.[45] The operation is associated with increased morbidity and mortality when compared with elective procedures.[46,47] The incidence of myocardial infarction varies between 31% and 71%[45,48] due to the unavoidable delay between vessel occlusion and surgical revascularization, and in-hospital mortality has been reported to be as high as 15%.[45] The risks of abrupt closure and its associated morbidity and mortality limit the patients for whom angioplasty is an acceptable alternative to bypass surgery.

Other approaches to the problem of abrupt closure have been evaluated. The laser balloon has successfully treated this complication, but follow-up angiography suggests an unacceptably high rate of late restenosis.[49,50] Temporary intravascular stents are intended to tack up an intimal flap and ensure normal flow for a brief period, but thus far they have been used successfully only in a minority of patients.[51] We will discuss the role of the self-expanding mesh stent in abrupt closure later in the chapter.

Coronary Artery Restenosis

The mechanism of restenosis is under intense investigation, but our knowledge is still limited. Pathologic studies in animals and humans have shown that angioplasty-involves fissuring of plaque material, sometimes not only to the level of the internal elastic membrane but also deep into the media.[42,52] The initial plaque disruption and the rheologic consequences of a suboptimal balloon dilation lead to the deposition of platelets and fibrin along the vessel wall. Mitogens are released by both the vessel wall and platelets, which causes migration of smooth muscle cells to the damaged area.[53] The compromised flow and the amount of intimal and medial damage may be among the early triggers that initiate the fibromuscular proliferation leading to restenosis.[52,54,55] Early restenosis typically occurs in the first 6 weeks after the procedure and usually is due to vascular recoil at the site of the original balloon dilation, coronary spasm, or a major intimal flap limiting flow, which is further compromised by fresh thrombus. Standard balloon dilations with variously sized balloons inflated with either low- or high-pressure inflations, for short or prolonged durations, have not altered the incidence of restenosis.[56–58] Adjunctive medical therapy also has had little effect on rates of restenosis.[59] Investigators have therefore turned to mechanical alternatives to balloon angioplasty.[60–66] There is a growing consensus that achieving the largest possible lumen diameter at the time of the procedure (acute gain) will decrease the incidence of clinically significant lumen reduction even if the unavoidable fibrointimal proliferation (late loss) is more pronounced.[67,68]

We have deployed self-expanding mesh stents for coronary artery restenosis and will discuss these results later in the chapter. Depending on its design, a stent can produce a smooth surface and normal flow and will prevent elastic recoil, making it a logical device for this problem. However, any intravascular foreign body may contribute to smooth muscle cell proliferation. The stent could act as a mechanical irritant, causing the release of mediators from the adjacent endothelium and stimulating coronary spasm or intimal hyperplasia. Perhaps most worrisome, the device can become a nidus for the development of thrombus.

Saphenous Vein Graft Stenosis

It has been well documented that balloon angioplasty within venous bypass grafts has a higher restenosis rate than in native coronary arteries. If the lesion is in the body of the graft, rates as high as 60% have been reported.[69] Stenting grafts appears to be an attractive alternative to these high restenosis rates. It is especially appealing since repeat coronary artery bypass surgery has a lower likelihood of success and an increased morbidity and mortality when compared with a first operation.[70]

CLINICAL RESULTS

Abrupt Occlusion

We reported our early experience from Lausanne using the intracoronary stent for situations of abrupt closure.[17,18] In the early days of this experimental procedure we did not have stents available in the hospital. Each situation for which a stent was indicated required us to call the company and have a device brought to the catheterization laboratory. The time delay led us to the use of intracoronary urokinase in hopes of preventing the formation of thrombus along the guidewire, which remained across the occluded area. Once the procedure became more routine, a supply of stents was kept in the laboratory, decreasing the time between occlusion and stent implantation. At that time we stopped using intracoronary urokinase.

The median hospital stay after stent deployment for abrupt closure was 7 days. The initial angiographic follow-up of this patient subgroup suggested that the combined restenosis and late occlusion rate was lower after emergency stenting than after angioplasty alone. The angiographic rate of restenosis was 3 of 17 (18%) for the patients who underwent late control angiography. During a mean follow-up period of 7 months, two patients suffered a myocardial infarction, and there were two noncardiac deaths.

Since that original report, we have deployed the self-expanding mesh stent for abrupt closure in more patients.[72] Mean stent length was 23 ± 5 mm, and mean unconstrained diameter was 3.8 ± 0.7 mm (range, 3 to 6 mm). Acute or subacute thrombosis of the stent occurred in five patients (13%): there was one death and one Q-wave myocardial infarction, and two patients required surgical bypass grafting. Thirty-four (89%) of these patients underwent control angiography at 5 to 23 months, and stent restenosis was present in 4 patients (12%).

The European multicenter experience with self-expanding mesh stents for abrupt occlusion comprised 56 patients in whom 63 devices were implanted in 57 sites from March 1986 to December 1989. Eleven cases (20%) were complicated by in-hospital stent thrombosis, but five of these were successfully recanalized using balloon angioplasty, thrombolytic treatment, or a combination of both. There were seven cases of myocardial infarction (13%), and two patients died (4%). The approach in the acute setting was not uniform in bypass surgery. Seven of the 56 patients underwent surgical revascularization within 24 to 48 hours after the procedure, although they remained clinically stable and myocardial infarction had been prevented. There was considerable variability in the rate of acute stent thrombotic complications between Lausanne (12%) and the other sites (20%). These differences probably reflect differing anticoagulation regimens, patient selection criteria, and an important learning curve effect.[73] At the present time, the data suggest that abrupt occlusion constitutes one of the best documented indications for coronary stenting.

Restenosis

The initial 50 elective stenting procedures of native coronary arteries for restenosis in Lausanne were performed in patients with a mean of 1.6 previous angioplasties at the same site (range, 1 to 4).[19] In 46 cases, a single stent was deployed, and in four cases two or more stents were implanted. All implants were technically successful. Temporary thrombotic occlusion occurred in two cases (4%), and permanent occlusion was observed in two additional cases (4%) during the hospital stay. Two of these patients underwent emergency surgery, and one of them died postoperatively from surgical complications (unrecognized tamponade). The major complication rate (Q-wave infarction, emergency surgery, or death) was 6% in-hospital. After a mean follow-up period of 8 months, angiography was repeated in 34 patients from the study group. Restenosis within the stented segment occurred in 4 patients (12%), and stent occlusion was documented in three other patients

(9%).[74] There were three late deaths (6%). Two of these deaths occurred in patients who did not adhere to their anticoagulant drug regimen. One death occurred during elective surgery for a new left main stem coronary lesion, which occurred proximal to a stent placed near the origin of the left anterior descending artery. Two patients from this group required elective surgery for restenosis within the stent.[75]

In the multicenter experience with the self-expanding stent the overall results were not optimal, but it should be kept in mind that they represent the very early learning curve of several centers, at a time when indications, technique, and postimplantation management were still not well defined.[76] The appropriate selection of patients for intracoronary stenting remains central to success and probably represents the largest portion of the learning curve.[73] The importance of anticoagulants is now again under discussion, but during the early days in Lausanne we gave each patient a card outlining their anticoagulation medications in three languages, requesting that any proposed changes be discussed with us before implementation.

Saphenous Vein Grafts

In the initial Lausanne-London series 56 patients received stents for stenosis within a saphenous vein bypass graft.[20,77] On several occasions stenting was done in old grafts that were diffusely diseased and would not have been considered appropriate targets for balloon angioplasty alone (Figs. 48-3 and 48-4). The implantation procedure for bypass grafts sometimes varied from the one we described for native

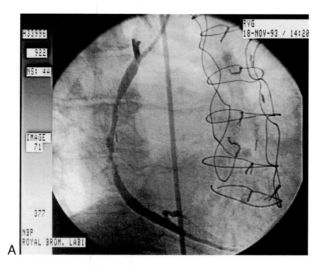
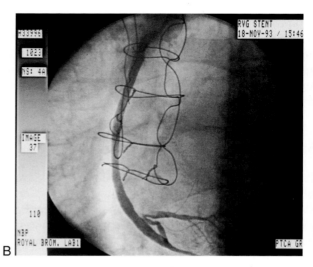

Fig. 48-3. Degenerated saphenous vein graft before **(A)** and after **(B)** stenting with a very long (8 cm) peripheral Wallstent.

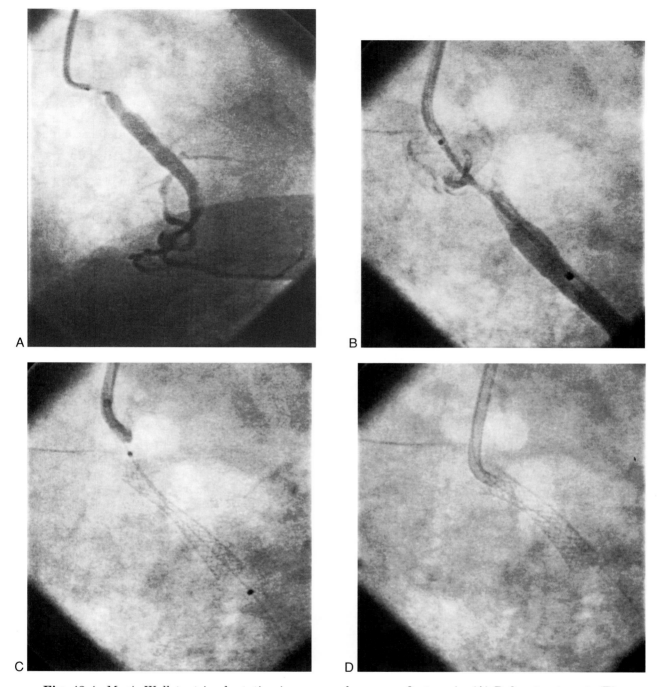

Fig. 48-4. *Magic* Wallstent implantation in a severe bypass-graft stenosis. **(A)** Before treatment. **(B)** Crossing of the lesion with a 6 mm diameter stent on its delivery system (note the two markers indicating the stent position). **(C)** After stent release (note the central indentation). **(D)** Following the *Swiss kiss* with a 5.5 mm angioplasty balloon. (*Figure continues.*)

coronary arteries. To avoid the potential embolization of friable plaque material or thrombus, the stent was inserted before any dilations were made with a standard balloon catheter. In this early series (the cases shown in Figs. 48-3 and 48-4 were done later), we attempted implantation of 78 self-expanding stents in bypass grafts of 56 patients during 60 separate procedures. The stent diameter ranged from 3.5 to 6 (mean, 4.7) mm, and the length from 15 to 30 (mean, 24) mm. Angiographic success was achieved in 59 procedures (98%). There was one case of subacute stent occlusion, and one in-hospital death.

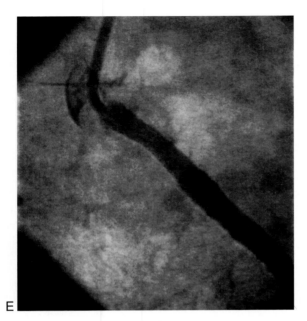

Fig. 48-4 (*continued*). (**E**) Final result.

required for six. The overall early clinical success was 87%, and the restenosis rate was 47%.

The immediate and long-term results for elective stenting of venous bypass grafts with the self-expanding device are better than the results of stenting native coronary vessels. This is probably due to the larger diameter of vein grafts, which allows larger stents to be implanted. Perhaps the lack of vasomotor tone and generally higher compliance of venous bypass grafts also play a role. The large expansion rate is of course most useful in big grafts, and the new delivery system makes ostial stenting safe and precise (Fig. 48-4). Anecdotal observations from explanted grafts with stents seem to indicate fewer degenerative changes in the stented segment compared with the rest of the vessel (Fig. 48-5). The combination of an acceptably low complication rate and the low rate of restenosis makes elective stenting of venous bypass grafts probably the best indication for the use of the self-expanding mesh stent at this time.

Transfusion or surgical repair of the vascular access site was required for five procedures (8%) because of bleeding. At follow-up, restenosis was documented in four patients (7%), with myocardial infarction for one case. There were two late deaths.

The Rotterdam experience with the self-expanding stent in saphenous vein grafts (78) comprised 69 patients with a 100% implantation success rate. There were four deaths, seven patients suffered a myocardial infarction, and coronary artery bypass graft was

CONTRAINDICATIONS

We have developed a list of contraindications to coronary stenting with the self-expanding device, which should be observed whenever possible:

- Markedly funnel-shaped segments (currently available stents are cylindrical)
- Very tight bend in the target segment

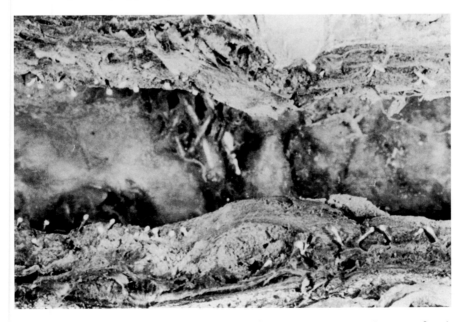

Fig. 48-5. Moderate stenosis of a vein graft in the gap between two stents 4 years after implantation. The stented segments were free from stenoses at the time of reoperation.

(since it would promote important shearing forces at both stent extremities)
- Insufficient flow anticipated through the prosthesis after implantation due to either poor distal runoff or extensive collateralization (stasis at stent level will favor thrombus formation)
- Anticipated difficulty with the antiplatelet/anticoagulation regimen

Restenosis After Stenting

Experimental animal data, histology from percutaneous atherectomy,[65,79] and surgical material excised from stented segments[80] have all documented that stent restenosis is due to excessive fibrointimal proliferation. One predictor for stent restenosis appears to be the timing of the deployment after the original angioplasty procedure. In a group of patients treated for restenosis in Lausanne, the recurrence rate was 6% in patients stented more than 3 months after their initial angioplasty, but it was 41% for those stented within 3 months.[34] Similar observations have been made with other stents and other devices such as percutaneous directional atherectomy.[81] These findings and the well-known time course for restenosis after standard balloon dilation suggest that the process of fibrointimal proliferation may have a period of hyperactivity, which will be difficult to alter with mechanical interventions alone.

Restenosis in the area covered by a self-expanding stent cannot be dealt with as successfully as in the case of balloon-expandable stents. The reason for this difference lies in the fact that a firmly embedded self-expanding stent cannot easily be enlarged any further: if the stent has reached its nominal (i.e., maximal) diameter (either passively by intrastent balloon inflation at the time of implantation or actively through its self-expanding property during the first weeks of follow-up), further expansion is impossible; if the stent is imbedded in the arterial wall in an incompletely expanded state further passive expansion would automatically shorten the device, which will be hindered by the lack of axial elasticity of the arterial wall. High-pressure balloon inflations sometimes requiring 20 bars or more may effectively enlarge the lumen by pressing the fibromuscular encroachment through the metal skeleton. On the other hand, coronary stenting does not jeopardize the patient's chances of benefiting from elective surgical revascularization should it become necessary.[80]

COMPLICATIONS

The process of inserting the self-expanding mesh stent normally is not a source of complications. The stent deployment only adds a few minutes to the procedure's time. Removing the retaining membrane that holds the self-expanding stent on the introducer catheter occasionally can be difficult. In most situations this problem responds to increasing the pressure beyond 3 bars between the membranes, but rarely the position of the guide catheter must also be changed before the membrane can be fully withdrawn. The new hydromer-coated membrane should contribute to making the retraction process smoother. Although it is not recommendable, partially deployed stents have been removed without important sequelae. Investigators have not seen evidence of side branch occlusion (Fig. 48-2), except when a stent was placed in an area of fresh thrombus that involved a side branch. There have been no cases of coronary perforation, stent erosion, or infectious complications.

The major morbidity associated with stent implantation is the potential for a thrombotic event occurring acutely or, unpredictably, in the first 4 weeks (or even longer) after the procedure. This is in contradistinction to balloon angioplasty, in which complications generally are not seen beyond the first 24 hours after the procedure. A short-term combined anticoagulant and/or antiplatelet regimen is mandatory. Unfortunately, conventional anticoagulation leads to local bleeding complications at the arterial puncture site (8% of cases in Lausanne). These patients may require blood transfusions, and some will require surgical repair of the femoral artery before bleeding problems can be controlled. Optimal femoral compression after the procedure is crucial. A pneumatic compression device (FemoStop Radi Medical, Uppsala, Sweden), which allows prolonged pressure without compromising arterial flow, is now being used. Hopefully, this device will help overcome arterial bleeding problems. The combination of aspirin and ticlopidin appears to reduce subacute stent thrombosis without an apparent increase in puncture site complications.

Several risk factors for acute stent thrombosis have become apparent. Small-diameter stents carry a greater risk of thrombosis than do large ones.[74] This observation probably explains the lower complication rate observed when vein gratis are stented. Generally bypass grafts are at least 3.5 mm in diameter and allow placement of stents of at least 4 mm in unconstrained diameter. We do not recommend stenting arteries that are smaller than 3 mm in diameter as measured by quantitative coronary angiography or intravascular ultrasound with self-expanding mesh stents.

Certain clinical situations promote thrombotic complications. Investigators have noted that patients with increased platelet counts are more likely to experience thrombotic complications.[82] Systemic hypotension, poor distal runoff, untreated significant proximal lesions, uncovered dissection flaps proximal or distal to the stent, and well-developed collateral vessels can all cause decreased flow through the stented vessel and therefore potentiate thrombus formation.

With increasing experience and better patient selection, acute thrombotic events have become less frequent. During the first half of the Lausanne series we observed thrombotic events in 14% of the procedures versus 6% for the last 49 cases.[73] Provided a catheterization laboratory is immediately available, acute stent thrombosis can often be treated effectively by balloon angioplasty and thrombolytic agents. When it is reversed, it does not appear to compromise the long-term results.[73] The procedure is fairly straightforward if thrombosis occurs during the first hours after implantation when the femoral sheath is still in place. The situation is more complex after the sheath has been removed because a second arterial puncture becomes necessary in a patient who is anticoagulated. If a thrombotic event occurs more than 2 days after stent deployment, systemic thrombolysis can be beneficial in our experience; a pneumatic compression device, however, must be placed on the puncture site.

A grossly oversized Wallstent with a diameter mismatch (ratio more than 1.5) between the self-expanding stent and the recipient vessel may be associated with thrombotic occlusion. The turbulent flow induced at the stent's extremities could contribute to thrombus formation. This makes optimal sizing an important factor, especially since good impaction of the stent struts into the vessel wall is probably equally important for preventing thrombus formation. The lesser radial force of the new Wallstent may lessen the risk of clinically important diameter mismatch.

ADJUNCT MEDICATION

Early experimental evidence showed that heparin significantly decreased the rate of acute thrombotic occlusions when it was given perioperatively for stenting of normal canine arteries.[17] Other workers using balloon-expandable stents in animals showed that aspirin was superior to warfarin in preventing subsequent stent thrombosis.[29] The evidence favoring the use of low molecular weight dextran during the implantation procedure together with aspirin, dipyridamole, and heparin is debatable.[30] At present no study has been done proving a beneficial effect of low molecular weight dextran in this context.

The drug regimen employed with Wallstents has been largely empirical; over a number of years heavy anticoagulation was used, requiring a high degree of patient compliance. Before the stent procedure, patients receive aspirin in addition to their usual medication. In the catheterization laboratory, intravenous heparin, normally 15,000 units, is administered. The activated clotting time should be at least 300 seconds at all times. After the procedure is completed, the arterial sheath is removed as soon as possible (i.e., normally after 5 hours) and a Femostop placed onto the puncture site for some 6 hours at low pressure. In the past heparin was reinstituted 12 hours after the procedure and continued until oral anticoagulation was effective (international normalized ratio for prothrombin time 2.3 or more). Aspirin 100 mg daily and dipyridamole 100 mg three times daily were prescribed for all patients. Medications were usually continued for 3 to 6 months, until control angiography was performed. All patients received calcium blocking agents to prevent the possibility of stent-induced coronary spasm. This stringent regime is now the exception. Most patients receive aspirin and ticlopidin only and leave the hospital after one night of observation.

CONCLUSIONS

The concept of peripheral vascular stenting was introduced over 20 years ago. Major interest in these devices was rekindled when the limitations of coronary balloon angioplasty resisted conventional therapy. Now, after 10 years of clinical study, coronary stenting has given us good reason for optimism. The procedure has lived up to our initial expectations in terms of its technical feasibility. Stents can be inserted under circumstances of abrupt closure and in almost all coronary segments. It is simple to implement and constitutes the best current alternative to emergency surgery for abrupt postangioplasty closure. The data obtained with self-expanding devices suggest that restenosis may be favorably influenced by stent implantation in selected subgroups, particularly for patients with saphenous vein graft lesions. The "Achilles heel" of coronary stenting remains the problem of acute or subacute thrombosis. Although its incidence appears to be decreasing as our learning curve progresses, it still makes a complex drug regimen desirable, increasing the risks of the procedure. Late stent restenosis rates are encouraging, but the data are somewhat confounded by the rates of early thrombotic complications seen in previous years. it is unclear what effect might be achieved on late restenosis rates if early thrombotic complications could be avoided, or substantially decreased.

We consider coronary stents to be one of the most promising developments in the field of interventional cardiology. Many researchers now believe that the fight against restenosis will have to include the use of pharmacologic weapons, not only mechanical means.[7,83,84] Whether a combination of these two approaches will finally prove optimal is an unresolved issue, but it does seem likely that new devices will be forthcoming that will be less thrombogenic and less likely to stimulate intimal hyperplasia.

REFERENCES

1. Dotter CT, Judkins MP. Transluminal treatment of atherosclerotic obstruction: description of a new technique and preliminary report of its application. Circulation 1964;30:654–660
2. Grüntzig A. Transluminal dilatation of coronary artery stenoses. Lancet 1978;1:263
3. De Feyter PJ, Serruys PW, van den Brand M et al. Emergency coronary angioplasty in refractory unstable angina. N Engl J Med 1985;313:342–346
4. Detre K, Holubkov PH, Kelsey S et al. Percutaneous transluminal coronary angioplasty in 1985–1986 and 1977–1981. N Engl J Med 1988;318:265–270
5. Myler RK, Topol EJ, Shaw RE et al. Multiple vessel coronary angioplasty: classification, results, and patterns of restenosis in 494 consecutive patients. Cathet Cardiovasc Diagn 1987;13:1–15
6. Parisi AF, Folland E, Hartigan P et al. A comparison of angioplasty with medical therapy in the treatment of single vessel coronary artery disease. N Engl J Med 1991;326:10–16
7. Traisnel G, Lablanche JM, Fournier JL et al. Etude comparative des résultats à court et moyen terme de l'angioplastie et du pontage dans l'angor sévère ou instable par sténose isolée de l'IVA. Arch Mal Coeur 1986;10:1430–1436
8. Reeder GS, Krishan I, Nobrega FT et al. Is percutaneous transluminal coronary angioplasty less expensive than bypass surgery? N Engl J Med 1984;311:1157–1162
9. Laird-Meeter K, Erdman RAM, van Domburg R et al. Probability of return to work after either coronary balloon dilatation or coronary bypass surgery. Eur Heart J 1989;10:917–922
10. Kramer JR, Proudfit WL, Loop FD et al. Late follow-up of 781 patients undergoing percutaneous transluminal coronary angioplasty or coronary artery bypass grafting for an isolated obstruction in the left anterior descending coronary artery. Am Heart J 1989;118:1144–1153
11. RITA trial participants. Coronary angioplasty versus coronary artery bypass surgery. The Randomised Intervention Treatment of Angina. Lancet 1993;341:573–580
12. Ellis SG, Roubin GS, King SB et al. In-hospital cardiac mortality after coronary angioplasty: analysis of risk factors from 8207 procedures. J Am Coll Cardiol 1988;11:211–216
13. Leimgruber PP, Roubin GS, Hollman J et al. Restenosis after successful coronary angioplasty in patients with single-vessel disease. Circulation 1986;73:710–717
14. Meier B. Restenosis after coronary angioplasty: review of the literature. Eur Heart J, suppl. C. 1988;9:1–6
15. Anderson HV, Roubin GS, Leimgruber PP et al. Primary angiographic success rates of percutaneous transluminal coronary angioplasty. Am J Cardiol 1985;56:712–716
16. Urban P, Meier B, Finci L et al. Coronary wedge pressure: a predictor of restenosis after angioplasty. J Am Coll Cardiol 1987;10:504–509
17. Sigwart U, Puel J, Mirkovitch V, Joffre F, Kappenberger L. Intravascular stems to prevent occlusion and restenosis after transluminal angioplasty. N Engl J Med 1987;316:701–70
18. Sigwart U, Urban P, Golf S et al. Emergency stenting for acute occlusion following coronary balloon angioplasty. Circulation 1988;78:1121–1127
19. Sigwart U, Kaufmann U, Goy JJ et al. Prevention of coronary restenosis by stenting. Eur Heart J, suppl. C. 1988;9:31–37
20. Urban P, Sigwart U, Golf S et al. Intravascular stenting for stenosis of aorto-coronary venous bypass grafts. J Am Coll Cardiol 1989;13:1085–1091
21. Carrel A. Results of the permanent intubation of the thoracic aorta. Surg Gynecol Obstet 1912;15:245–248
22. Dotter CT. Transluminally-placed coiled endarterial tube grafts. Invest Radiol 1969;4:329–332
23. Dotter CT, Buschmann RW, McKinney MK et al. Transluminal expandable nitinol stent grafting: preliminary report. Radiology 1983;147:259–260
24. Cragg A, Lund G, Rysavy J et al. Nonsurgical placement of arterial endoprostheses: a new technique using nitinol wire. Radiology 1983;147:261–263
25. Maass D, Demierre D, Deaton D et al. Transluminal implantation of self-adjusting expandable prostheses: principles, techniques and results. Prog Artif Org 1983;27:979–987
26. Wright KC, Wallace S, Charnsangavej C et al. Percutaneous endovascular stents: an experimental evaluation. Radiology 1985;156:69–72
27. Charnsangavej C, Carrasco CH, Wallace S et al. Stenosis of the vena cava: preliminary assessment of treatment with expandable metallic stents. Radiology 1986;161:295–298
28. Rousseau H, Puel J, Joffre F, Sigwart U et al. Self-expanding endovascular prosthesis: an experimental study. Radiology 1987;164:709–714
29. Roubin GS, Robinson KA, King SB et al. Early and late results of intracoronary arterial stenting after coronary angioplasty in dogs. Circulation 1987;76:891–897
30. Palmaz JC, Garcia OJ, Kopp DT et al. Balloon expandable intra-arterial stents: effect of anticoagulation on thrombus formation, abstracted. Circulation, suppl. IV. 1987;45.
31. Schatz RA, Palmaz JC, Tio FO et al. Balloon-expanda-

ble intracoronary stents in the adult dog. Circulation 1987;76:450–457

32. Palmaz JC, Sibbitt RR, Tio FO et al. Expandable intraluminal vascular graft: a feasibility study. Surgery 1956;99:199–205

33. Palmaz JC. Balloon-expandable intravascular stents. Am J Radiol 1988;150:1263–1269

34. Urban P, Sigwart U, Kaufmann U, Kappenberger L. Restenosis within coronary stents: possible effect of previous angioplasty, abstracted. J Am Coll Cardiol 1989;13:107A

35. Sigwart U, Kaufmann U, Goy JJ, Kappenberger L. Suppression of residual transstenotic pressure gradient after PTCA by implantation of self expanding stents, abstracted. Circulation, 76 suppl. IV. 1987;76:186

36. Puel J, Juillière Y, Bertrand M, Rickards A et al. Early and late assessment in stenosis geometry after coronary arterial stenting. Am J Cardiol 1988;61:546–553

37. Serruys PW, Juillière Y, Bertrand M et al. Additional improvement of stenosis geometry in human coronary arteries by stenting after balloon dilation. Am J Cardiol 1988;61:71G–76G

38. Simpfendorfer C, Belardi J, Bellamy G et al. Frequency, management and follow-up of patients with acute coronary occlusions after percutaneous transluminal coronary angioplasty. Am J Cardiol 1987;59:59:267–269

39. Mabin TA, Holmes DR, Smith HC et al. Intracoronary thrombus: role in coronary occlusion complicating percutaneous transluminal coronary angioplasty. J Am Coll Cardiol 1985;5:198–202

40. Roubin GS, Douglas JS, King SB et al. Influence of balloon size on initial success, acute complications and restenosis after percutaneous transluminal coronary angioplasty. A randomized study. Circulation 1988;78:557–565

41. Waller BF. Crackers, breakers, stretchers, shavers, burners, welders and melters. The future treatment of atherosclerotic coronary artery disease? A clinical and morphological assessment. J Am Coll Cardiol 1989;13:969–987

42. Cragg A, Amplatz K. Vascular pathophysiology of transluminal angioplasty. pp. 145–155. In Jang GD (ed): Angioplasty. McGraw-Hill, New York, 1986

43. Block PC. Mechanism of transluminal angioplasty. Am J Cardiol 1984;53:69C–78C

44. Leitshuh ML, Mills RM, Jacobs AK et al. Outcome after major dissection during coronary angioplasty using the perfusion balloon catheter. Am J Cardiol 1991;67:1056–1060

45. Meier B. *Coronary Angioplasty.* Grune & Stratton, Orlando, 1988

46. Page US, Okies JE, Colburn LQ et al. Percutaneous transluminal coronary angioplasty. A growing surgical problem. J Thorac Cardiovasc Surg 1986;92:847–852

47. Satter P, Krause E, Skupin M. Mortality trends in cases of elective and emergency aorto-coronary bypass after percutaneous transluminal angioplasty. Thorac Cardiovasc Surg 1987;35:2–5

48. Reul GJ, Cooley DA, Hallman GL et al. Coronary artery bypass for unsuccessful percutaneous transluminal coronary angioplasty. J Thorac Cardiovasc Surg 1984;88:685–690

49. Spears JR, Reyes VP, Sinclair N et al. Percutaneous coronary laser balloon angioplasty: preliminary results of a multicenter trial, abstracted. J Am Coll Cardiol 1989;13:61A

50. Spears JR, Reyes VP, Plokker HWT et al. Laser balloon angioplasty: coronary angiographic follow-up of a multicenter trial, abstracted. J Am Coll Cardiol 1991;15:26A

51. Gaspard PE, Didier BP, Delsanti GL. The temporary stent catheter: a nonoperative treatment for acute occlusion during coronary angioplasty, abstracted. J Am Coll Cardiol 1990;15:118A

52. Liu MW, Roubin GS, King SB. Restenosis after coronary angioplasty. Potential biologic determinants and role of intimal hyperplasia. Circulation 1989;79:1374–1387

53. Steele PM, Chesebro JH, Stanson AW et al. Balloon angioplasty: natural history of the pathophysiological response to injury in a pig model. Circ Res 1995;57:105–112

54. Reidy MA, Silver M. Endothelial regeneration. Lack of intimal proliferation after defined injury to rat aorta. Am J Pathol 1985;118:173–177

55. Lyon RT, Zarens CK, Lu CJ et al. Vessel, plaque, and human morphology after transluminal balloon angioplasty: quantitative study in distended human arteries. Arteriosclerosis 1987;7:306–314

56. Roubin GS, Douglas TJ, King SB et al. Influence of balloon size on initial success, acute complications, and restenosis after percutaneous transluminal coronary angioplasty: a prospective randomized study. Circulation 1988;78:557–565

57. Meier B, Gruentzig A, King SB et al. Higher balloon dilation pressure in coronary angioplasty. Am Heart J 1984;107:619–622

58. Garrahy PJ, Nath H, Anderson JC et al. Does balloon inflation duration influence the angiographic result in coronary angioplasty? abstracted. J Am Coll Cardiol 1989;13:58A

59. Blackshew JL, O'Callaghan WG, Califf RM. Medical approaches to the prevention of restenosis after coronary angioplasty. J Am Coll Cardiol 1987;9:834–848

60. Hansen DD, Auth DC, Hall M, Ritchie JL. Rotational endarterectomy in normal canine coronary arteries: preliminary report. J Am Coll Cardiol 1988;11:1073–1077

61. Vallbracht C, Liermann D, Prignitz I et al. Results of low speed rotational angioplasty for chronic total occlusions. Am J Cardiol 1988;62:935–940

62. Abela GS, Seeger JM, Barhieri E et al. Laser angioplasty with angioscopic guidance in humans. J Am Coll Cardiol 1986;8:184–192

63. Crea F, Davies G, McKenna WJ et al. Laser recanalisation of coronary arteries by metal-capped optical fibres: early clinical experience in patients with stable angina pectoris. Br Heart J 1988;59:168–174

64. Karsch KR, Haase KK, Voelker W et al. Percutaneous coronary excimer laser angioplasty in patients with stable and unstable angina pectoris. Circulation 1990;81:1849–1859

65. Isner JM, Kearney M, Berdan L et al. Core pathology laboratory findings in 425 patients undergoing directional atherectomy for a preliminary coronary artery stenosis, and relationship to subsequent outcome. The CAVEAT study, abstracted. J Am Coll Cardiol 1993;21:380A

66. Stertzer SH, Rosenblum J, Shaw R et al. Coronary

rotational ablation: initial experience in 302 procedures. J Am Coll Cardiol 1993;21:287–295

67. Kuntz RE, Safian RD, Carrozza JP et al. The importance of acute luminal diameter in determining restenosis after coronary atherectomy or stenting. Circulation 1992;86:1827–1835

68. de Jaegere PP, Strauss BH, Morel MA et al. Critical appraisal of quantitative coronary angiography and endoluminal stent implantation. In Serruys PW, Foley D, de Feyter PJ (eds): Kluwer Academic Publishers. 1993 (in press)

69. Côté G, Myler RK, Stertzer SH et al. Percutaneous transluminal angioplasty of stenotic coronary artery grafts: 5 years' experience. J Am Coll Cardiol 1987;9: 8–17

70. Loop FD, Cosgrove DM, Kramer JR. Late clinical and arteriographic results in 500 coronary artery reoperations. J Thorac Cardiovasc Surg 1981;81:675–685

71. Sigwart U, Vogt P, Goy JJ et al. Creatinine kinase levels after bail-out stenting for post-angioplasty coronary occlusion, abstracted. Circulation 1989;80: 11–258

72. Nordrehaug JE, Priestley KA, Chronos NAF et al. Self-expanding stents for emergency treatment of abrupt closure following PTCA: immediate and long-term results, abstracted. Br Heart J 1993;69:20

73. Sigwart U, Urban P, Sadeghi H et al. Implantation of 100 intracoronary stents. Learning curve effect on the occurrence of acute complications, abstracted. J Am Coll Cardiol 1989;13:107A

74. Sigwart U, Golf S, Kaufmann U et al. Analysis of complications associated with coronary stenting, abstracted. J Am Coll Cardiol 1988;11:66A

75. Goy JJ, Sigwart U, vogt P et al. Long term follow-up of the first 56 patients treated with intracoronary self-expanding stents (the Lausanne experience). Am J Cardiol 1991;67:569–572

76. Serruys PW, Strauss BH, de Feyter P et al. The Wallstent, a self-expanding stent. J Inv Cardiol 1991; 3:127–134

77. Stewart JT, Williams MG, Goy JJ et al. The use of self-expanding stents for coronary graft stenoses, abstracted. Eur Heart J, suppl. 1991;12:243

78. de Scheerder IK, Strauss BH, de Feyter PJ et al. Stenting of venous bypass grafts: a new treatment modality for patients who are poor candidates for reintervention. Am Heart J 1992;123:1046–1054

79. Strauss BH, Umans VA, van Suylen RJ et al. Directional atherectomy for treatment of restenosis within coronary stents: clinical angiographic, and histological results. J Am Coll Cardiol 1992;20:1465–1473

80. Sigwart U, Kaufmann U, Golf S et al. L'incidence et le traitement de la resténose coronarienne malgré l'implantation d'une endoprothèse. Schweiz Med Wochenschr 1988;118:1715–1718

81. Selmon M, Robertson G, Hinohara T et al. Factors associated with restenosis following successful peripheral atherectomy, abstracted. J Am Coll Cardiol 1989; 13:13A

82. Nath FC, Muller DWM, Ellis SG et al. Thrombosis of a flexible coil coronary stent: frequency, predictors and clinical outcome. J Am Coll Cardiol 1993;21:622–627

83. Serruys PW, Beatt KJ, van der Giessen WJ. Stenting of coronary arteries: are we the sorcerer's apprentice? Eur Heart J 1989;10:774–782

84. King SB. Vascular stents and atherosclerosis. Circulation 1989;79:460–462

49 The Palmaz-Schatz Stent

John C. Harrington
Richard A. Schatz

The potential advantage of intravascular mechanical support during angioplasty was first recognized by Dotter and Judkins in 1964.[1] Despite significant improvements in technique since the advent of percutaneous transluminal coronary angiography (PTCA), as reflected in the National Heart, Lung and Blood Institute (NHLBI) PTCA Registry data from 1979 to 1983 and 1985 to 1986, reporting an improvement in primary success from 61 to 78%, significant limitations remain.[2] Specifically, the incidence of acute complications and chronic restenosis remain vexing in conventional PTCA. Restenosis rates remain at 30 to 57% within the first 3 to 6 months of the index procedure as well as subsequent balloon angioplasties.[3,4] Lesion-specific characteristics such as saphenous vein bypass grafts, ostial lesions, and proximal left anterior descending artery lesions are associated with significantly higher rates of restenosis.[5-9] The pathogenesis of restenosis is multifactorial and, to date, refractory to any significant pharmacologic manipulation. Abrupt vessel closure persists as well, with an incidence of 3 to 8%[10-12] and an accompanying mortality of 4 to 10%.[13,14]

These phenomena share mechanical obstruction of the lumen as a common feature, by medial hyperplasia limiting late minimal lumen diameter (MLD) in restenosis and by exuberant recoil/spasm or extensive dissection of the media, with or without associated thrombus limiting acute luminal diameter in abrupt vessel closure.[14]

In this context the design and development of the Palmaz-Schatz stent has evolved, to provide a more effective mechanical intervention than that given by conventional PTCA.

This chapter provides a clinical review of (1) design evolutions of the Palmaz-Schatz stent; (2) stent deployment technique; (3) the pharmacologic regimen required for implantation; (4) complications associated with stent deployment; (5) restenosis in native coronaries and saphenous vein grafts, as well as management; (6) review of randomized trials; and (7) future developments.

HISTORICAL PERSPECTIVE

The first balloon-expandable stent prototype designed by Palmaz in 1981 was constructed as a continuous woven stainless surgical steel wire with silver-soldered cross points. The 6- and 8-mm stents were configured out of wire 0.15 mm in diameter, while the 10-mm stent was configured out of 0.20-mm wire. This was the first vascular prosthesis designed to be deployed by a conventional expandable balloon angioplasty catheter, as opposed to a self-expanding device.[15]

This design proved easily deployed and resistant to radial collapse.[16] Stent patency in canine arteries was reported in 1986 and appeared dependent on heparin anticoagulation and the presence of adequate distal runoff, and demonstrated an inverse relationship between intimal hyperplasia and prestented vessel lumen.[17] Although the stent demonstrated excellent biocompatibility when im-

563

The results from the first 213 nonrandomized patients to receive Palmaz-Schatz stents implanted electively in native coronary arteries were reported variable MLD and a dichotomous variable >50% diameter stenosis) versus 32% in the PTCA group. The

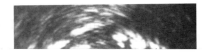

Table 49-2. Major Cardiac Events From the Stress Trial[a]

Variable	Stent (n = 205) (%)	Angioplasty (n = 202) (%)	P Value
Early events (0–14 days)			
Death	0	1.5	NS
Myocardial infarction (Q-wave)	5.4 (2.9)	5.0 (3.0)	NS
Coronary bypass surgery	2.4	4.0	NS
Stent bailout	—	6.9	—
Repeat angioplasty	2.0	1.0	NS
Any event	5.9	11.4	0.047
Late events (15–240 days)			
Death	1.5	0	NS
Myocardial infraction (Q wave)	1.5 (1.0)	2.0 (0.5)	NS
Coronary bypass surgery	2.4	4.5	NS
Repeat angioplasty	9.8	11.4	NS
Any event	15.1	15.8	NS
Cumulative events (0–240 days)			
Death	1.5	1.5	NS
Myocardial infarction (Q-wave)	6.3 (3.4)	6.9 (3.5)	NS
Coronary bypass surgery	4.9	8.4	NS
Stent bailout	—	6.9	
Repeat angioplasty	11.2	12.4	NS
Any event	19.5	26.7	NS

Abbreviation: NS, not significant.

[a] With the exception of 6.9% of angioplasty patients requiring stent bailout, there is no significant difference in major cardiac events either during acute hospitalization or in the 8-month follow-up period between patients receiving a stent versus patients receiving conventional PTCA.

incidence of clinical events at 6 months (myocardial infarction, death, CABG, or repeat PTCA) was also significantly decreased among stent patients (21%) relative to control PTCA patients (32%). The incidence of subacute thrombosis was not statistically different between stent patients (3.5%) and PTCA patients (2.7%); however, the incidence of bleeding complications was 10% among the stent recipients and only 1.6% among PTCA patients.[34] This finding may be associated with an anticoagulation regimen more potent than that employed previously (Table 49-2).

The Stent Restenosis Study (STRESS) is a randomized trial of 407 patients analyzed by intention to treat comparing conventional PTCA with the Palmaz-Schatz stent. The inclusion criteria include (1) de novo lesions, (2) native coronary arteries, (3) lesions less than 15 mm in length, and (4) lesions more than 3 mm in diameter, with (5) objective evidence of ischemia. Of 207 patients randomized to stent, the primary success rate, evaluated by core laboratory QCA, was 96.1% compared with only 83% in the 203 patients randomized to PTCA. The 4.0% incidence of emergency CABG in the PTCA group was offset by 3.5% incidence of subacute thrombosis in the stent group. Cross-over from intended to alternative ther-

apy was 3.9% in the stent group. None of these cross-over patients, however, were the result of ischemic complications. In the PTCA group, 9.9% of patients resulted in cross-over to alternative therapy, and 6.9% resulted in cross-over to stent implantation due to an ischemic event in the catheterization laboratory. Restenosis defined as more than 50% diameter stenosis was demonstrated in 29.1% of the stent group versus 42.7% of patients randomized to PTCA, representing a 33% reduction. This result appears to be largely due to a greater postprocedure MLD achieved with stent placement (2.47 to 0.44 mm) versus PTCA (1.92 to 0.51 mm) (Fig. 49-4). Multivariate analysis identified this acute gain as the most powerful predictor of angiographic follow-up MLD. Patients assigned to receive stent replacement also demonstrated a 39% reduction in target lesion revascularization (Fig. 49-5). The secondary end point of late clinical events (myocardial infarction, death, CABG, or repeat PTCA) was not significantly different between the two groups (Table 49-2). The secondary end point of vascular complications requiring surgical repair was 3.9% in the stent group and 2% in the PTCA group. Bleeding requiring blood transfusion was 4.9% in the stent group and 2.5% in the PTCA group. Whereas these end points did not reach

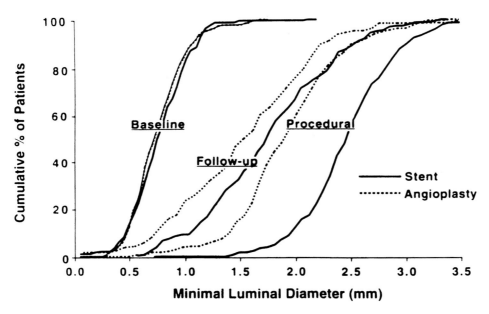

Fig. 49-4. The cumulative frequency distribution of MLD results by intention to treat. There is no preprocedure difference in lesion severity (*left*). The acute gain in patients receiving stents versus PTCA is demonstrated at the far *right*. This MLD advantage is preserved at follow-up angiography. Both curves are shifted to the left; however, the stent group maintains a larger MLD despite late loss. (Modified from Fischman et al.,[25] with permission.)

statistical significance, a trend toward increased vascular complications is noted.[35]

The conclusions offered by these trials demonstrate an increased primary success rate, fewer ischemic complications, and a significant advantage in terms of reduced restenosis in patients in whom de novo lesions are optimally dilated (less than 0% residual stenosis), with a single stent in native coronary arteries. The mechanism of this effect is identified in studies by Kuntz et al.[36] and Kimura et al.[37]

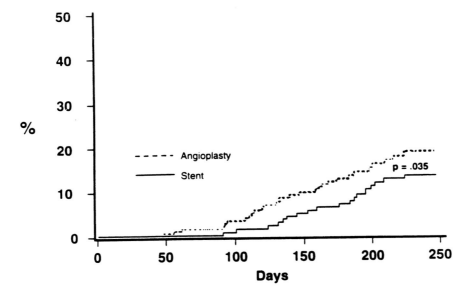

Fig. 49-5. Kaplan-Meier curve demonstrating target lesion revascularization between patients in the stent group and conventional PTCA from the STRESS trial. Patients randomized to receive stents had a lower requirement for ischemia-driven revascularization. (Modified from Fischman et al.,[25] with permission.)

Serial angiographic follow-up of stented lesions demonstrates a greater late loss of lumen diameter at 6 months; however, this is offset by a significantly greater acute gain (acute luminal diameter) at the time of stent implantation. The acute gain is markedly superior in stented lesions due to the marked reduction of lesion recoil. The late loss of lumen diameter occurs because the stent does not appear to limit intimal hyperplasia significantly; however, this synthetic reaction of the vessel wall, largely complete by 6 months, does not compromise the vessel lumen due to greater acute gain afforded by the stent.

Saphenous Vein Graft Restenosis

Restenosis in saphenous vein aortocoronary bypass grafts appears to be particularly advantageous with respect to stent versus PTCA. Leon et al.[38] reported an angiographic restenosis rate of 26% of 192 patients with a primary success rate. More recently, Piana et al.[39] reported a procedural success rate of 98%, with 80% 6-month angiographic follow-up demonstrating a 16% restenosis rate. Diaz et al.[40] reported Saphenous vein graft stent results in 63 patients (59 men) with a median graft age of 8.6 years. The 6-month angiographic follow-up in 70% of patients demonstrates a restenosis rate (>50% narrowing) of 20%.[40] Wong et al.[41] presented the 6-month angiographic follow-up in 74% of 312 consecutive patients in a multicenter registry. Saphenous vein grafts successfully stented demonstrated a restenosis rate of 29%. Multivariate analysis identified reference vessel diameter less than 3.0 mm and lesions previously dilated by PTCA and subsequently restenosed as predictors of stent restenosis. This last finding was again confirmed in a study by Fenton et al.[42] Overall restenosis in 103 consecutive patients with 72% 6-month angiographic follow-up was 35%, with de novo lesions demonstrating 26% and restenotic lesions demonstrating 47%.

These figures for restenosis in Palmaz-Schatz stenting of saphenous vein aortacoronary bypass grafts must be viewed in context against historical controls for restenosis with conventional PTCA. In a large series, Douglas et al.[43] reported in 1991 restenosis rates in similar grafts (>5 years old) of 64% and up to 80% in aorto-ostial lesions.

Management of Palmaz-Schatz restenosis has been reported by Baim et al.[44] Between 1988 and 1991, 1,189 patients underwent successful stent implantation in a multicenter registry. Only 32.5% of patients who developed restenosis (>50% residual diameter) demonstrated moderate or severe angina. Of the patients with angiographic restenosis, 30.3%

were referred for medical therapy. These patients demonstrated a 69% mean diameter stenosis. Thirty-six patients (13.6%) were referred for elective CABG. These patients demonstrated an 80% mean diameter stenosis and were on average more symptomatic. Repeat balloon angioplasty within the stented segment was the most common treatment option in 39.7% of patients with an 80% mean diameter stenosis and moderately severe angina (46% > Canadian Cardiovascular Society [CCS] class II). The redilation was uniformly successful without evidence of abrupt closure and did not require prolonged heparin or Coumadin administration. The mechanism of in-stent restenosis has been evaluated by both serial angiographic and ultrasound analysis and confirms the theory that restenosis is secondary to neointimal proliferation through the stent slots as opposed to compression of the stent.[45,46]

FUTURE DEVELOPMENTS

Optimal stent deployment contributes to an enhanced MLD and secondarily to improvement in restenosis. Routine ultrasound examination of stent contour post deployment frequently reveals an elliptical cross-sectional area and suboptimal stent and vessel dilation in up to 80% of cases despite optimal stent geometry by standard angiographic evaluation.[47] Maximizing stent geometry may translate into further improvement in restenosis rates or limit the requirements for anticoagulation. Prospective studies are currently under way to assess this theory.

Custom stents with a change in stent design to include a spiral articulation, a distal bulbous element on the SDS balloon to prevent pistoning of the outer sheath, and variable stent lengths are meant to improve flexibility, catheter trackability, and geometry with respect to different lesion characteristics. Efforts continue to identify in advance patients at risk for stent thrombosis to focus anticoagulant therapy on these patients. Initially promising results employing the evaluation of prothrombin fragment F1 + 2 have not been reproducible.[48] Heparin-coated stents may limit the need for prolonged systemic anticoagulation, as well as improve the suitability of stents for use in vessels less than 3 mm in diameter.[49] This option is to be evaluated in the BENESTENT II trial currently under way in Europe. Synthetic antithrombin agents may prove superior to heparin for post-stent anticoagulation. Biologic coatings such as seeding stents with tissue plasminogen activator secreting endothelial cells offer similar promise.[50]

In conclusion, the use of the Palmaz-Schatz stent in properly selected patients represents a safe and effective method of dealing with the most vexing constraints of conventional PTCA, specifically, an improved procedural success with fewer acute ischemic complications. Significantly, the incidence of restenosis, long the Achilles' heel of percutaneous revascularization techniques, has for the first time been reduced in a clinically meaningful manner. Relative to conventional PTCA techniques, the Palmaz-Schatz stent appears to be most useful in de novo lesions of the native coronary arteries as a primary therapy, as opposed to restenotic lesions, and in salvage of saphenous vein grafts. The efficacy of stent implantation is further enhanced by the finding that clinical restenosis is substantially less than angiographic rates of restenosis, translating into improved symptom relief. As with any evolving clinical technique, refinements in the current design may improve these results even further, perhaps ultimately justifying the routine use of these devices in all patients.

REFERENCES

1. Dotter CT, Judkins MP. Transluminal treatment of arteriosclerotic obstruction. Circulation 1964;30: 654–70
2. Detre K, Holubkov R, Kelsey S et al. and coinvestigators of the National Heart, Lung, and Blood Institute's Percutaneous Transluminal Coronary Angioplasty Registry. One-year follow-up results of the 1986–1986 National Heart, Lung, and Blood Institute's Percutaneous Transluminal Coronary Angioplasty Registry. Circulation 1989;80:421–8
3. Holmes DR, Vliestra RE, Smith HC et al. Restenosis after percutaneous transluminal coronary angioplasty (PTCA): a report from the Coronary Angioplasty Registry of the National Heart, Lung, and Blood Institute. Am J Cardiol 1984;53:77C–81C
4. Topol EJ, Leya F, Pinkerton CA et al. for the CAVEAT Study Group. A comparison of directional atherectomy with coronary angioplasty in patients with coronary artery disease. N Engl J Med 1993;329:221–7
5. Fleck E, Regitz V, Lehnert A et al. Restenosis after balloon dilatation of coronary stenosis: multivariant analysis of potential risk factors. Eur Heart J 1988;9: 15–8
6. Popma JJ, Topol EJ. Factors influencing restenosis after angioplasty. Am J Med 1990;88:16N–24N
7. Cote G, Myler RK, Stertzer SH et al. Percutaneous transluminal angioplasty of stenotic coronary artery bypass grafts: 5 years' experience. J Am Coll Cardiol 1987;9:8–17
8. Topol EJ, Ellis EG, Fishman J et al. Multicenter study of percutaneous transluminal angioplasty for right coronary artery ostial stenosis. J Am Coll Cardiol 1987;9:1214–8
9. Nobuyoshi M, Kimura T, Nosaka H et al. Restenosis after successful percutaneous coronary angioplasty: serial angiographic follow-up of 229 patients. J Am Coll Cardiol 1998;12:616–23

10. Detre KM, Holmes DR Jr, Holubkov R et al. and coinvestigators of the National Heart Lung, and Blood Institute's Percutaneous Transluminal Coronary Angioplasty Registry. Incidence and consequences of periprocedural occlusion. The 1985–1986 National Heart, Lung, and Blood Institute Percutaneous Transluminal Coronary Angioplasty Registry. Circulation 1990;82:739–50
11. Kuntz RE, Piana R, Pomerantz RM et al. Changing incidence and management of abrupt closure following coronary intervention in the new device era. Cathet Cardiovasc Diagn 1992;27:183–90
12. Gaul G, Hollman J, Simpfendorfer C, Franco I. Acute occlusion in multiple lesion coronary angioplasty: frequency and management. J Am Coll Cardiol 1989;13: 283–9
13. Dorros G, Crowley MJ, Janke L et al. In-hospital mortality rate in the National Heart, Lung, and Blood Institute Percutaneous Transluminal Coronary Angioplasty Registry. Am J Cardiol 1984;53:17C–21C
14. Lincoff AM, Popma JJ, Ellis SG, Hacker JA, Topol EJ. Abrupt vessel closure complicating coronary angioplasty: clinical, angiographic therapeutic profile. J Am Coll Cardiol 1992;19:926–35
15. Palmaz JC, Sibbitt RR, Reuter SR et al. Expandable intraluminal vascular graft: preliminary study. Radiology 1985;156:73–7
16. Palmaz JC, Sibbitt RR, Tio FO et al. Expandable intraluminal vascular graft: a feasibility study. Surgery 1986;99:199–205
17. Schatz RA, Palmaz JC, Tio FC et al. Balloon-expandable intracoronary stents in the adult dog. Circulation 1987;76:450–7
18. Palmaz JC, Windelar S, Garcia F et al. Atherosclerotic rabbit aortas: expandable intraluminal grafting. Radiology 1986;160:723–6
19. Palmaz JC, Garcia O, Kopp DB et al. Balloon-expandable intra-arterial stents: effect of antithrombotic medication on thrombus formation. pp. 125–31. In: Seither C, Seyferth W (eds): Pros and Cons in PTA and Auxiliary Methods. Springer-Verlag, Berlin, 1989
20. Schatz RA, Palmaz JC, Tio FC et al. Report of a new articulated balloon-expandable intravascular stent (ABEIS). Circulation, suppl. 3. 1988;78:1789
21. Schatz RA, Baim DS, Leon M et al. Clinical experience with the Palmaz-Schatz™ coronary stent. Initial results of a multicenter study. Circulation 1991;83: 148–61
22. Urban P, Sigwart U, Golf S et al. Intravascular stenting for stenosis of aortocoronary venous bypass grafts. J Am Coll Cardiol 1989;13:1085–91
23. Pan M, Medina A, Enrique H et al. Follow-up patency of side branches covered by a Palmaz-Schatz™ stent, abstracted. Circulation 1993;88:I-640
24. Fischman DL, Savage MP, Leon MB et al. Fate of lesion-related side branches following coronary artery stenting. J Am Coll Cardiol 1991;18:1445–51
25. Fischman DL, Savage MP, Leon MB et al. Angiographic predictors of subacute thrombosis following coronary artery stenting, abstracted. Circulation, Suppl. II. 1991;84:II-588
26. Nakamura S, Columbo S, Gaglione A et al. Coronary stenting guided by intravascular ultrasound, abstracted. Circulation 1993;88:I-598
27. Carrozza JP, Kuntz RE, Levine MJ et al. Angiographic and clinical outcomes of intracoronary stenting: imme-

for the indication of acute or threatened closure after PTCA.

proved by the Ethical Committee of each participating institution.

mostly, but not necessarily, associated with angina,

proximal artery of the vessel to be treated.

with anticoagulation alone. To answer this question, prospective randomized studies with predefined technologic strategies will be needed.

The study population consisted of 210 patients, with either suboptimal result (25%) or threatened (54%) or total (21%) vessel closure after coronary an-

the first 70 patients, all during stenting attempts of the left circumflex artery. However, the investigators soon felt that this problem was largely eliminated with the correct choice of guiding catheter (Amplatz-type) and guidewire. In the remaining patients, suc-

diate and long-term results from a large single-center experience. J Am Coll Cardiol 1992;20:328–37

28. Muller DW, Shamir KJ, Ellis SG, Topol EJ. Peripheral

for stenotic saphenous vein grafts—single center experience, abstracted. Circulation 1993;88:I-308

40. Diaz L, Fajadet J, Bar O, Cassagneau B, Marco J.

Stents intended for placement

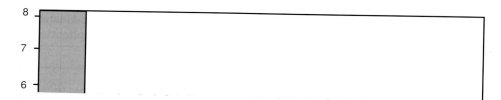

cess rate for circumflex artery lesions increased to

which made it more difficult to distinguish residual

- Cardiology Hospital C.H.R. Lille, Lille, France (9): M.M. Bertrand, MD
- CHUV Centre Hospitalier Universitaire Vaudois, Lausanne, Switzerland (8): J.J. Goy, MD
- Centre Hospitalier Régional de la Citadelle, Liège, Belgium (8): J. Boland, MD
- Hospital de la Princesa, Madrid, Spain (7): L.M. Elbal, MD
- Catharina Clinic Eindhoven, Eindhoven, The Netherlands (7): M. El Gamal, MD
- St. Mary's Hospital, London, England (6): D.W. Davies, MD

- C.H.U. Rangueil, Toulouse, France (6): J. Puel, MD
- Sahlgrenska Sjukhuset, Göteborg, Sweden (5): H. Emanuelsson, MD
- University Hospital Rotterdam, Rotterdam, The Netherlands (4): P.W. Serruys, MD
- Clinico-Universitario de Valadolid, Valadolid, Spain (4): F. Aviles, MD
- U.C.V. Hospital La Casamance Marseille, Marseille, France (3): P. Labrunnie, MD

51 | Restenosis After Wiktor Stent Implantation

Peter P. de Jaegere
Marie-Angèle Morel
Pim J. de Feyter
Patrick W. Serruys

Despite increased operator experience, improved catheter technology, and a better understanding of the mechanisms of coronary balloon angioplasty, restenosis remains the most vexing problem complicating this procedure. It has been reported to occur in 20 to 57% of patients, depending on the study population, definition of restenosis, and time to and completeness of angiographic follow-up.[1,2] Approximately 25% of these patients require repeat percutaneous transluminal coronary angioplasty (PTCA) or eventually bypass surgery during the follow-up period.[2-8] Restenosis, therefore, not only poses a medical burden on the patient but also poses an economic burden on society, already confronted with spiraling health-care costs.[9] So far, pharmacologic interventions have failed to reduce the restenosis rate, most likely reflecting our lack of knowledge of the basic pathophysiologic mechanisms of the restenosis process.[10,11] As a result, there has been a quest for new technologies, which has brought an assortment of new devices to help deal with coronary atheroma, assisting, supplanting, or integrating with PTCA.[12-15] One of these is the intracoronary stent.[12] Although it is clear from histologic studies that any kind of injury applied to the vessel wall, whatever its nature, will invariably be associated with neointimal hyperplasia as a nonspecific tissue reaction leading to restenosis when excessive, intra-

coronary stenting may reduce the angiographic restenosis rate by optimizing the immediate angiographic results.[16-18] This in turn should reduce the need for repeat revascularization.

Because some evidence from observational studies indicates that patients with restenotic lesions are at a higher risk for recurrence of restenosis after repeat PTCA, a multicenter investigational study designed to evaluate the feasibility, safety, and efficacy of Wiktor stent implantation in patients with documented restenosis of a previously dilated coronary artery was started in January 1990.[19-22] This chapter summarizes the immediate and long-term clinical and angiographic results of the first 120 consecutive patients entered in the study. In addition, the device, implantation technique, and anticoagulation protocol are described.

DESCRIPTION OF THE STENT

The Medtronic Wiktor stent was originally designed by Dominik Wiktor. It is a balloon-expandable device constructed of a single loose interdigitating tantalum wire (0.125 mm in diameter), which is formed into a sinusoidal wave and wrapped into a helical coil structure (Fig. 51-1). The sinusoidal helix design ensures that metal never touches metal, so that the potential

Table 51-2. Clinical Events Following Successful and Elective Wiktor Stent Implantation in 118 Patients With Restenosis[a]

Event	In-Hospital (n = 14 Patients)		After Hospital Discharge (n = 29 Patients)		Total (n = 43 Patients)	
	Total Count	Ranking	Total Count	Ranking	Total Count	Ranking
Death	0	0	1 (0.8%)	1 (0.8%)	1 (0.8%)	1 (0.8%)
AMI	9 (8%)	9 (8%)	0	0	9 (8%)	9 (8%)
CABG	3 (3%)	0	8 (7%)	8 (7%)	11 (9%)	8 (7%)
re-PTCA	7 (6%)	3 (3%)	21 (18%)	21 (18%)	28 (24%)	24 (20%)
Total	19 (16%)	12 (10%)	30 (25%)	30 (25%)	49 (42%)	42 (36%)

[a] In the left column of each phase of the study, all events were calculated (mutually nonexclusive). In the right column, a ranking of the events according to the highest category on a scale ranging from death, acute myocardial infarction (AMI), (emergency) bypass surgery (CABG), and repeat PTCA is shown (mutually exclusive).

All in-hospital events were related to (sub)acute stent thrombosis, which occurred in 14 patients (12%, Table 51-2). However, the overall incidence of (sub)acute stent thrombosis was 13% (15 patients), because in one additional patient, subacute stent thrombosis was documented 7 days after hospital discharge. The interval between stent implantation and the occurrence of this thrombotic event was as follows: day 0 = 5 patients, day 4 = 2 patients, day 5 = 2 patients, day 6 = 3 patients, day 10 = 1 patient, day 11 = 1 patient, day 15 = 1 patient. No deaths occurred, but 9 patients sustained an acute myocardial infarction with a creatine phosphokinase (CPK) elevation of 1,782 ± 1,370 U/L. Recanalization was performed by means of repeat PTCA in 2 patients, 2 other patients underwent emergency bypass surgery following repeat PTCA, 1 patient was directly referred for bypass surgery, and 3 patients were treated with thrombolytic therapy. The remaining patient received conventional medical therapy. Six other patients who sustained a (sub)acute stent thrombosis had an uneventful course. They were treated with repeat PTCA in combination with thrombolytic therapy (2 patients), PTCA (1 patient), and thrombolytic therapy (2 patients). One other patient suffered from chest pain associated with reversible ST-segment depression after successful stent implantation. Pain was quickly relieved after intravenous administration of nitroglycerine. Although a moderate CPK elevation up to 272 U/L was noted, no electrocardiographic evidence of myocardial necrosis was found.

A major bleeding complication necessitating blood transfusion or surgery occurred in 8 patients (7%). They all were access site-related bleedings, except in 1 patient who sustained both a groin hematoma and gastrointestinal bleeding. Three months after implant, one patient presented with an infected pharyngeal hematoma caused by Coumadin therapy.

The hospital stay (mean ± SD) of the total study population was 10.2 ± 6.5 days (range, 3 to 38). Patients with a complicated postoperative course (occlusion of the stent, bleeding complication) remained significantly longer in the hospital (17.4 ± 9.2 days, range 5 to 38) compared with the patients with an uneventful course (8.5 ± 4.2 days, range 3 to 22).

During follow-up, 1 patient (0.8%) died 3 months after stent implantation following prostate surgery (Table 51-2). Although necropsy was not performed, death was determined not to be stent related. Seven patients underwent bypass surgery between 7 days (the patient who sustained subacute stent thrombosis after hospital discharge) and 9 months following implantation (1 at 7 days, 3 at 4 months, 2 at 6 months, and 1 at 9 months). One other patient redeveloped angina 2 days following successful stent implantation in the mid left anterior descending artery. Repeat coronary angiography disclosed a left main stem stenosis, which had not been recognized on the angiogram before stent implantation; the patient was then referred for semielective bypass surgery. Another 21 patients (18%) underwent repeat dilation within the stented segment. The functional class be-

Table 51-3. Functional Class According to the Canadian Cardiovascular Society

	Baseline	Follow-up
I	15 (13%)	80 (68%)
II	34 (28%)	17 (15%)
III	36 (30%)	10 (9%)
IV	33 (28%)	7 (6%)
Unknown	2 (2%)	3 (3%)
Total	120	117[a]

[a] Failure to cross the lesion with the stent catheter occurred in two patients, another patient died during follow-up.

fore stent implantation and at follow-up is shown in Table 51-3.

Angiographic Results

Detailed angiographic data are available on 91 of the 99 patients with successful stent implantation and show no evidence of (sub)acute stent thrombosis (2 unsuccessful implantations, 15 patients with stent thrombosis, 1 death during follow-up, and 3 refusals). The results of quantitative coronary angiography are shown in Table 51-4. The incidence of restenosis according to the 50% diameter stenosis was 30% (27/91 patients). Of note, the number of balloon angioplasty procedures performed before stent implantation did not influence the risk for subsequent restenosis after stenting. The odds for restenosis in case of stent implantation for a second, third, or fourth restenosis compared with stent implantation for a first restenosis was 0.8 (95% confidence interval, 0.4 to 1.8) and 1.5 (95% confidence, 0.6 to 3.7) according to the 0.72-mm criterion and 50% diameter stenosis criteria, respectively.[23] This is in agreement with a recent study assessing the recurrent restenosis rate after repeated balloon angioplasty disclosing that the probability of recurrent restenosis after successive angioplasty procedures is similar to that reported after a first angioplasty.[24] The only statistically significant predictor of recurrence of restenosis was the relative gain when it exceeded 0.48 (odds ratio 2.7; 95% confidence interval, 1.1 to 6.4) according to the 0.72-mm criterion.[23] Furthermore, a weak but positive linear correlation was found (coefficient of 0.38, $P < 0.001$) between the relative gain (as an index of vessel wall injury) and relative loss (as an index of late neointimal hyperplasia) (Fig. 51-3).[23] These angiographic data underscore previous animal, postmortem human pathologic, and angiographic studies indicating that deep arterial injury is associated with more extensive intimal proliferation (Fig. 51-4).[25-27]

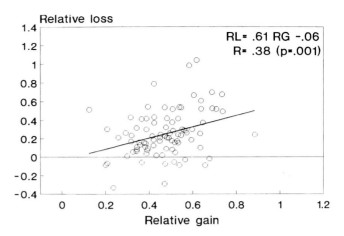

Fig. 51-3. Graphic display of the relation between the relative gain (RG = increase in minimal luminal diameter immediately after stent implantation normalized to the vessel wall) and relative loss (RL = decrease in minimal luminal diameter at follow-up normalized to the vessel wall). A positive linear relation was found with a correlation coefficient of 0.38 ($P < 0.001$) with a slope of 0.61 and an intercept on the Y-axis of -0.06. (From de Jaegere et al.,[23] with permission.)

All these findings potentially carry far-reaching clinical implications. Clearly, the greater the improvement in minimal luminal diameter achieved by intervention, the greater the magnitude of subsequent luminal narrowing will be. Unfortunately, what cannot be drawn from the data is how much damage the clinician may inflict on the vessel wall. On one hand, a suboptimal angiographic result is associated with a higher risk of subacute occlusion as a result of rheologic factors and platelet deposition and a higher need for repeat balloon angioplasty, but on the other hand, improvement of the initial result may be at the price of more extensive late neointimal thickening.[25-29] This indistinctness can be circumvented by proper matching of the balloon size or device with the vessel wall using on-line quantitative

Table 51-4. Changes in Minimal Luminal Diameter After Wiktor Stent Implantation

	Before PTCA	After PTCA	After Stent Implantation	At follow-up	
				All Patients	Patients Without Subacute Occlusion
Minimal luminal diameter (mm)	1.15 ± 0.34	1.78 ± 0.35	2.45 ± 0.33	1.51 ± 0.85	1.73 ± 0.67
Diameter stenosis (%)	60 ± 10	36 ± 11	19 ± 7	49 ± 28	42 ± 21

All parameters are expressed as mean ± SD.

Table 51-5. Relation Between Acute Recoil (mm) and Late Restenosis[a]

	Restenosis Criteria					
	0.72 mm			50% Diameter Stenosis		
	Yes n = 33	No n = 44	Difference	Yes n = 21	No n = 54	Difference
Acute recoil 1	0.26 ± 0.26	0.25 ± 0.29	−0.02 ± 0.30	0.28 ± 0.42	0.24 ± 0.28	0.04 ± 0.32
95% CI	(0.13; 0.39)	(0.16; 0.34)	(−0.14; 0.16)	(0.09; 0.47)	(0.16; 0.31)	(−0.12; 0.21)
Acute recoil 2	0.58 ± 0.27	0.70 ± 0.30	−0.12 ± 0.29	0.63 ± 0.28	0.64 ± 0.31	−0.01 ± 0.30
95% CI	(0.48; 0.67)	(0.61; 0.79)	(−0.25; 0.01)	(0.51; 0.76)	(0.56; 0.73)	(−0.16; 0.14)

[a] All values are expressed as mean ± SD. Acute recoil 1 = difference between mean final balloon diameter and mean diameter stented segment. Acute recoil 2 = difference between mean final balloon diameter and minimal luminal diameter post stent implantation.
Abbreviations: CI, confidence interval.

CONCLUSIONS

The data of the observational study with the Wiktor stent indicate that this stent can be implanted with a high technical success rate. This may be, among other factors, due to its high degree of flexibility and radiopaque features. Although the Wiktor stent was expected to be less thrombogenic, stent thrombosis occurred in 13% of the patients. The multicentric character of this study and therefore differences in stent experience between the participating centers may partially explain this. With respect to the long-term angiographic outcome, the lack of randomized comparisons precludes any firm conclusion. However, the observed recurrent restenosis rate compares favorably with historical data of balloon angioplasty. Although it is has been hypothesized that the Wiktor stent has less scaffolding properties than stents with a mesh architecture, only a minimal amount of recoil was noted, which did not contribute to late luminal renarrowing. Late luminal renarrowing was mainly caused by stent oversizing. However, this does not necessarily result in a higher restenosis rate when using dichotomous restenosis criteria. This underscores the concept that improved initial angiographic results and not lessened neointimal hyperplasia after stent implantation are responsible for a reduced restenosis rate.

ACKNOWLEDGMENT

We greatly acknowledge the editorial assistance of Dr. P. Ruygrok and Claudia Sprenger de Rover for typing the manuscript.

REFERENCES

1. Serruys PW, Luijten HE, Beatt KJ et al. Incidence of restenosis after successful coronary angioplasty: a time-related phenomenon. Circulation 1988;77: 361–71

2. Topol EJ, Leya F, Pinkerton CA et al. for the CAVEAT Study Group: A comparison of directional atherectomy with coronary angioplasty in patients with coronary artery disease. N Engl J Med 1993;329:221–7

3. Serruys PW, Rutsch W, Heyndrickx GR et al. Prevention of restenosis after percutaneous transluminal coronary angioplasty with thromboxane A2 receptor blockade. A randomized, double-blind, aspirin-placebo controlled trial. Circulation 1991;84:1568–80

4. Anonymous. Does the new angiotensin converting enzyme inhibitor cilazapril prevent restenosis after percutaneous transluminal coronary angioplasty? Results of the Mercator Study. Circulation 1992;86: 100–10

5. Serruys PW, Klein W, Tijssen JPG et al. Evaluation of ketanserin in the prevention of restenosis after percutaneous transluminal coronary angioplasty; the Post-Angioplasty Restenosis Ketanserin (PARK) trial. Circulation 1994;88:1588–601

6. Adelman AG, Cohen EA, Kimball BP et al. A comparison of directional atherectomy with balloon angioplasty for lesions of the left anterior descending coronary artery. N Engl J Med 1993;329:228–33

7. Anonymous. Coronary angioplasty versus coronary artery bypass surgery: the Randomized Interventional Treatment of Angina (RITA) trial. Lancet 1993;341: 573–80

8. Serruys PW, de Jaegere PPT et al. for the Benestent Study Group. A comparison of balloon expandable stent implantation with balloon angioplasty in patients with coronary artery disease. N Engl J Med 1994;331:489–95

9. Califf RM, Ohman EM, Frid DJ et al. Restenosis: the clinical issues. pp. 363–74. In Topol EJ (ed): Textbook of Interventional Cardiology. WB Saunders, Philadelphia, 1990

10. Herrman JPR, Hermans WRM, Vos J, Serruys PW. Pharmacological approaches to the prevention of restenosis following angioplasty. Part I. Drugs 1993;46: 18–52

11. Herrman JPR, Hermans WRM, Vos J, Serruys PW. Pharmacological approaches to the prevention of restenosis following angioplasty. Part II. Drugs 1993;46: 249–62

12. Sigwart U, Puel J, Mirkovitch V et al. Intravascular stents to prevent occlusion and restenosis after transluminal angioplasty. N Engl J Med 1987;316:701–6

13. Safian RD, Gelbfish JS, Erny RE et al. Coronary ather-

ectomy: clinical angiographic, and histologic findings and observations regarding potential mechanism. Circulation 1990;82:69–79

14. Bertrand ME, Lablanche JM, Leroy F et al. Percutaneous transluminal coronary rotary ablation with Rotablator (European experience) Am J Cardiol 1992;69:470–4

15. Margolis JR, Mehta S. Excimer laser angioplasty. Am J Cardiol 1992;69:3F–11F

16. van der Giessen WJ, Serruys PW, van Beusekom HMM et al. Coronary stenting with a new, radiopaque, balloon-expandable endoprosthesis in pigs. Circulation 1991;83:1788–98

17. Schwartz RS, Murphy JG, Edwards WD et al. Restenosis after balloon angioplasty. A practical proliferative model in porcine coronary arteries. Circulation 1990;82:2190–200

18. de Jaegere PPT, Hermans WR, Rensing BJ et al. Matching based on quantitative coronary angiography. A surrogate for randomized studies? Comparison between stent implantation and balloon angioplasty of a native coronary artery lesion. Am Heart J 1993;125:310–4

19. Williams DO, Gruentzig AR, Kent KM et al. Efficacy of repeat percutaneous transluminal coronary angioplasty for coronary restenosis. Am J Cardiol 1984;53:32C–5C

20. Meier B, King SB III, Gruentzig AR et al. Repeat coronary angioplasty. J Am Coll Cardiol 1984;4:463–6

21. Black AJ, Anderson VH, Roubin GS et al. Repeat coronary angioplasty: correlates of a second restenosis. J Am Coll Cardiol 1988;11:714–8

22. Teirstein PS, Hoover CA, Ligon RW et al. Repeat coronary angioplasty: efficacy of a third angioplasty for a second restenosis. J Am Coll Cardiol 1989;13:291–6

23. de Jaegere PPT, Serruys PW, Bertrand ME et al. Angiographic predictors of recurrence of restenosis after Wiktor stent implantation in native coronary arteries. Am J Cardiol 1993;72:165–70

24. Bauters C, Fadden EP, Lablanche JM, et al. Restenosis rate after multiple percutaneous transluminal coronary angioplasty procedures at the same site. A quantitative angiographic study in consecutive patients undergoing a third angioplasty procedure for a second restenosis. Circulation 1993;88:969–74

25. Schwartz RS, Huber KC, Murphy JG et al. Restenosis and the proportional neointimal response to coronary artery injury: results in a porcine model. J Am Coll Cardiol 1992;19:267–74

26. Nobuyoshi M, Kimura T, Ohishi H et al. Restenosis after percutaneous transluminal coronary angioplasty: pathologic observations in 20 patients. J Am Coll Cardiol 1991;17:433–9

27. Beatt KJ, Serruys PW, Luijten HE et al. Restenosis after coronary angioplasty: the paradox of increased lumen diameter and restenosis. J Am Coll Cardiol 1992;19:258–66

28. Nichols AB, Smith R, Berke A et al. Importance of balloon size in coronary angioplasty. J Am Coll Cardiol 1989;13:1094–100

29. Liu MW, Roubin GS, King SB, III. Restenosis after coronary angioplasty. Potential determinants and role of intimal hyperplasia. Circulation 1989;79:1374–87

30. de Jaegere PPT, Serruys PW, van Es GA et al. Recoil following Wiktor stent implantation for restenotic lesions of coronary arteries. Cathet Cardiovasc Diagn 1994;32:147–56

31. van Beusekom HMM, van der Giessen WJ, van Suylen RJ et al. Histology after stenting of human saphenous vein bypass grafts. Observations from surgically excised grafts 3–320 days after stent implantation. J Am Coll Cardiol 1993;21:45–54

32. White CJ, Ramee SR, Banks AK et al. A new balloon-expandable tantalum coil stent: angiographic patency and histologic findings in an atherogenic swine model. J Am Coll Cardiol 1992;19:864–9

33. Haude M, Erbel R. Coronary stenting for the treatment of restenosis after percutaneous transluminal coronary angioplasty. J Intervent Cardiol, in press

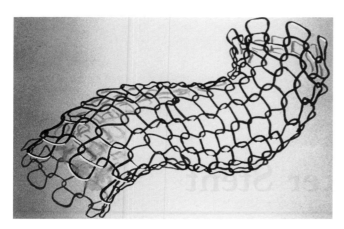

Fig. 52-1. The Strecker stent consists of a mesh tube of a single tantalum wire (diameter of filament 0.07 mm) knitted into a series of loosely interconnected loops that provide a high degree of longitudinal and radial flexibility.

(Fig. 52-1). The stent is available in 2- to 14-mm diameters with a maximum length of 8 cm for intravascular use and in 3- to 4.5-mm diameters with 15 or 25 mm lengths for coronary arteries. The prothesis is mounted on a conventional polyethylene coronary balloon angioplasty catheter (Outsider, Boston Scientific, Watertown, MA) and can be expanded to approximately six times its collapsed diameter, which is defined by the delivery system. In the unexpanded state, the proximal and distal ends of the prothesis are secured by thin-walled silicone sleeves at both ends of the delivery balloon. During full balloon expansion, the sleeves shorten in the longitudinal direction and retract from the stent by expanding in

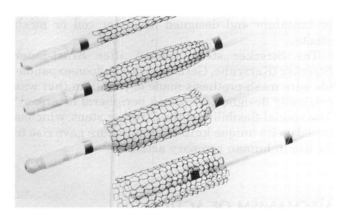

Fig. 52-2. In the unexpanded state, the proximal and distal end of the Strecker stent is secured by thin-walled silicone sleeves at both ends of the delivery balloon. During full balloon expansion, the sleeves shorten in the longitudinal direction and retract from the stent by expanding in the radial direction, thus releasing the stent from the delivery system.

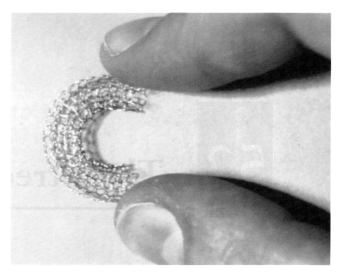

Fig. 52-3. Following full expansion of the delivery balloon, the struts become distended and locked at their intersections. Due to this change in mesh configuration, the shape of the Strecker stent remains flexible as well as widely resistant to external compression.

the radial direction, thus releasing the stent from the delivery system (Fig. 52-2). While the wire meshes remain in a tight position with the struts overlapping at their intersections in the unexpanded state, the struts become distended and locked at their intersections following full expansion of the delivery balloon. Due to this unique change in mesh configuration during expansion, the shape of the expanded Strecker stent remains flexible as well as widely resistant to external compression (Fig. 52-3).

The potential superiority of tantalum over stainless steel is based on the higher radiopacity, biocompatibility, and the absence of ferromagnetism.[16] The tantalum wire of the Strecker stent is covered by a thin layer of tantalum pentoxide, which creates an electrically negative surface charge. This negative surface charge is supposed to reduce adhesion of negatively charged platelets.

EXPERIMENTAL STUDIES

The safety of the deployment technique and the biocompatibility of the Strecker stent were demonstrated by experimental implantation of the prothesis in normal canine aortas and iliac and femoral arteries.[12,14] It has been shown by these experiments that no excessive neointimal reaction occurred during 6 months, and stent patency was documented over a period of 12 months.[12] Within 6 to 8 weeks a complete layer of endothelial cells covered the prothesis, and all side branches within the stented segments remained open.[14]

An in vitro model to test the thrombogenicity of Strecker tantalum stents in comparison with Palmaz-Schatz stainless steel stents showed no difference between the materials with respect to time of thrombotic stent occlusion, which means that the hypothesis of reduced thrombogenicity by electronegative surface charge was not supported in this model.[17]

CLINICAL EXPERIENCES IN PERIPHERAL VASCULAR DISEASE

The Strecker stent has been used in a large number of patients with peripheral vascular disease. Stents of 5 to 10 mm in diameter and 3 to 8 cm in length were successfully implanted in the femoropoliteal and iliac arteries when preceding percutaneous balloon angioplasty resulted in occlusive dissections or suboptimal results.[13,18] These stents are wrapped around 5-F balloon catheters and can be directly introduced through 8- to 10-F sheaths. The standard medical therapy following stent implantation consisted of aspirin (325 mg/d), and an additional treatment with coumadin proved to be unneccessary. In a series of more than 300 stent implantations in peripheral arteries, the initial success rate was close to 100% and the incidence of complications was less than 2%, with a long-term patency rate of 95% (3 years) for iliac artery stents and 80% (1 year) for femoropopliteal stents. Strecker stents have also been implanted successfully in patients with nonostial renal artery stenoses[19] as well as in various locations like trachea, bronchus, esophagus, biliary duct, and dialysis fistula.[20,21]

CLINICAL EXPERIENCES WITH INTRACORONARY IMPLANTATION

This section reports the experience of the Red Cross Hospital and Heart Center (Frankfurt, Germany) with implantation of Strecker stents in bail-out situations following unsuccessful prolonged balloon inflations. To assess potential advantages of the Strecker stent in the setting of bail-out stenting, a randomized study was performed in which Strecker stents were compared with Palmaz-Schatz stents with respect to procedural outcome, complication rate, and follow-up.[15]

Patient Population

Dissections requiring treatment with prolonged balloon inflations occur in about 25% of our percutaneous transluminal coronary angioplasty (PTCA) population. In 1.5 to 2%, abrupt or threatened closure is treated with stents. Fifty of these patients were randomized to either Strecker or Palmaz-Schatz stents. We excluded patients with a reference segment of the target vessel less than 3 mm in diameter, dissections longer than 30 mm, diffuse disease distal to the target lesion, and acute take-off or marked tortuosity of the vessel to be stented. Prior to stenting, 22% of the patients presented with thrombolysis in myocardial infarction (TIMI) flow 0 or 1, and in 78% the dissection caused residual narrowing of more than 75% with persistent chest pain or ischemia. The clinical data for the patients receiving either Strecker or Palmaz-Schatz stents are given in Table 52-1.

Methods

All patients were treated according to our regular PTCA protocol: acetylsalicylic acid 1,000 mg/d PO (started 1 day before the procedure); discontinuation of β-blockers; oral nitrates (2 × 20 mg isosorbide-dinitrate); heparin 5,000 U intravenously and 20,000 U intracoronarily; and intracoronary nitroglycerin for suspected vasospasm. Coronary angiograms were carried out using 8-F guiding catheters, and balloon angioplasty was performed using 0.014″ high-torque floppy guidewires and monorail balloons sized to match normal vessel diameter as assessed by visual estimation. Perfusion balloons were sized 0.5 mm larger in diameter than the previously used balloon and inflated at lower pressure (3 to 6 bar).

Balloon inflations were repeated three to five times at 30 to 60 seconds using increasing pressures up to full expansion. When angina or ST-segment elevation persisted due to occlusive dissection, additional balloon inflations of at least 10 minutes in total were carried out. In 78% of the population, perfusion balloons were used because of intolerable chest pain or marked ischemic reaction. When the operator decided to use a stent as a bail-out device, the patient was randomized to receive either the Strecker or the Palmaz-Schatz stents.

Medication

Following randomization, each patient received an additional bolus of intracoronary heparin (5,000 U) as well as intracoronary aspirin (500 mg), and an intravenous infusion of 500 ml low molecular dex-

Table 52-2. Early Results and Complications

	Palmaz-Schatz (n = 25) [no. (%)]	Strecker (n = 25) [no. (%)]	P Value
Technical success	24 (96)	23 (92)	NS
Acute stent thrombosis ≤24 hr	2 (8)	2 (8)	NS
Subacute stent thrombosis	1 (4)	2 (8)	NS
Successful re-PTCA	3/3	4/4	NS
Bleeding complications	3 (12)	4 (16)	NS
CABG during in-hospital stay	3 (12)	4 (16)	NS
Non Q-wave myocardial infarction	1 (4)	2 (8)	NS
Q-wave myocardial infarction	1 (4)	2 (8)	NS
Death	1 (4)	2 (8)	NS
No complications	12 (48)	11 (44)	NS

Abbreviation: NS, not significant.

guiding catheter as a scaling device. Quantitative geometric measurements at the coronary artery segment receiving one or more stents were performed using hand-held calipers. The nonautomated approach was chosen to circumvent the potential impact of differences in radiodensity as introduced by various stent materials on automated contour detection.[22] The following parameters were assessed: reference diameter of the stented vessel defined as the mean value from vessel diameters proximal and distal to the dissection, length of stenosis, length of dissection, minimal luminal diameter (MLD) at the inflated balloon, MLD at the deployed stent, and percent residual stenosis.

Results

Twenty-three Strecker stents (92%) and 24 Palmaz-Schatz stents (96%) could be successfully implanted. Early results and complications are listed in Table 52-2. In the Strecker group, four patients received a stent of 25 mm and two patients received two stents of 15 mm length.[17] Patients of the Strecker group received one stent of 15 mm length. In the Palmaz-Schatz group, four patients received two stents.

In the Strecker group, stent deployment was un-

successful in two cases. In one, the stent had to be retrieved together with the delivery system due to insufficient deployment despite full expansion and deflation of the balloon. In the Palmaz-Schatz group, one stent could not be advanced to the lesion in the right coronary artery. Subsequently a Streaker stent was successfully implanted.

Stent thrombosis during in-hospital stay occurred in 16% of the Streaker group and in 12% of the Palmaz-Schatz group. All thrombotic occlusions could be successfully reopened with a Magnum wire and balloon catheters. Residual thrombi were visible in one patient of each group and were successfully dissolved by intracoronary thrombolysis. Bleeding complications occurred in four patients of the Strecker group (16%) and in three patients of the Palmaz-Schatz group (12%). Q-wave infarction occurred in two patients of the Streaker group (8%) and in one patient of the Palmaz-Schatz group (4%). Two patients of the Strecker group and one patient of the Palmaz-Schatz group died during in-hospital stay.

After 4 months, five additional patients had CABG, so that 39 patients were eligible for angiographic follow-up, 37 of whom could be recatheterized. None of the patients experienced further cardiovascular events or bleeding complications (Table 52-

Table 52-3. Angiographic Follow-Up

	Palmaz-Schatz (n = (19) [no. (%)]	Strecker (n = 18) [no. (%)]	P Value
No recurrence	13 (68)	11 (62)	NS
Restenosis	6 (31)	4 (22)	NS
Reocclusion	2 (10)	3 (16)	NS

Abbreviation: NS, not significant.

Table 52-4. Quantitative Analysis

	Palmaz-Schatz (n = 24)[a]	Strecker (n = 23)[a]	P Value
Reference diameter (mm)	3.0 ± 0.5	3.03 ± 0.59	NS
Length of stenosis (mm)	15.5 ± 8.0	11.4 ± 5.0	NS
Length of dissection (mm)	25.1 ± 8.6	20.3 ± 9.6	NS
MLD at the inflated balloon (mm)	3.0 ± 0.4	3.5 ± 0.6	NS
MLD at the deployed stent (mm)	2.6 ± 0.4	3.0 ± 0.6	NS
Residual stenosis (%)	12.6 ± 11.3	8.7 ± 13.5	NS
Residual luminal narrowing <30% (%)	80	76	NS

Abbreviation: NS, not significant.
[a] n, number of stents.

3). All restenotic stents were successfully redilated. Overall, 19 (76%) of the patients with Strecker stents and 21 (84%) of the Palmaz-Schatz group were alive and had not experienced myocardial infarction.

Quantitative geometric measurements at the segment of the lesion and at the position of the implanted stents(s) are listed in Table 52-4. The cinefilms of three patients (two Strecker stents, one Palmalz-Schatz stent) were not suitable for quantitative analysis.

No significant difference was found between the mean values for length of stenosis and length of dissection in both groups of stents. The mean values of reference diameters obtained in both groups were almost identical. Since a higher degree of recoil was suspected in the Strecker group, an oversizing of Strecker stents was performed, resulting in a mean MLD of 3.5 ± 0.6 mm at the inflated balloon in contrast to the 3.0 ± 0.4 mm obtained during implantation of the Palmaz-Schatz stents. However, as illustrated in Figure 52-5, a similar degree of recoil

following stent implantation was found with the Strecker stent (14%, $P < 0.0001$) as with the Palmaz-Schatz stent (11%, $P < 0.0001$).

DISCUSSION

Whereas intracoronary stenting is performed with initial success rates comparable to those of conventional balloon angioplasty[3,4] and whereas recent reports suggest a reduced restenosis rate,[23,24] the high incidence of acute and subacute thrombosis as well as other severe complications has limited its use as an adjunct to balloon angioplasty.[6,7,9,25] Nevertheless, intracoronary stenting has been shown to be an effective technique to seal occlusive dissections and to restore coronary blood flow in the setting of acute or threatened closure following PTCA.[2,5,26,27]

Although the flexibility of the Strecker stent might suggest a higher primary success rate due to immediate adaption of the prothesis to vessel tortuosity, our randomized comparison did not show any superiority with respect to successful stent deployment. However, since only lesions suitable for both types of intracoronary stents were randomized, the potential superiority of one stent design may remain undetected by our comparison. The flexible Strecker stent appears to be suitable for coronary arteries with acute take-off, for tortuous vessels, and, since it is available at a length of 25 mm, for lesions with long dissections. Due to its length and profile, the Strecker stent is preferably implanted in rather proximally located coronary lesions.

The Palmaz-Schatz stent, on the other hand, seems to be suitable for short lesions (less than 15 mm), venous bypass grafts (diameter more than 4 mm), and more distally located lesions in which the process of stent positioning is facilitated by a relatively short and low-profile prothesis. When additional stenting distal to a previously implanted stent

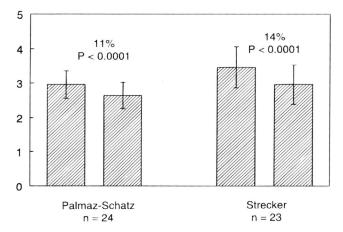

Fig. 52-5. Recoil following stent implantation. Both the Palmaz-Schatz and the Strecker stent show a similar degree of recoil after deployment.

is required, the Palmaz-Schatz stent appears to be superior because of more secure adhesion to the vessel wall, whereas the Strecker stent tends to telescope and migrate when passage with a second stent is tried. It was suspected that, because of the woven architecture and flexibility, the implantation of Strecker stents could be associated with a higher degree of recoil when compared with the Palmaz-Schatz stents. Despite the differences in design, however, our randomized comparison revealed a similar degree of recoil for both types of stents (Fig. 52-5). In addition, it can be assumed on the grounds of the present study that negative surface charge, which should reduce platelet adhesion, does not affect the incidence of thrombotic occlusion in the setting of bail-out stenting.

In contrast to elective stenting of de novo coronary lesions, for which recent studies suggest a substantially lower risk of thrombotic complications,[28] bail-out stenting remains associated with a high incidence of acute and subacute thrombosis.[8,29] Whereas the overall rate of subacute stent thrombosis ranges between 3% and 30% for stents with various designs and materials, our randomized comparison revealed no significant difference between the Strecker and the Palmaz-Schatz stents.[3,4,6,8,9,25,29] Furthermore, no difference was found in the rate of additional severe complications such as bypass surgery, myocardial infarction, or death.

With regard to the high incidence of stent thrombosis as reported in this study, it has to be pointed out that bail-out stenting was restricted to patients with failed prolonged balloon inflations in the setting of acute and threatened closure following PTCA and thus represents the worst scenario for coronary stenting in a very small high-risk subgroup of the total PTCA population (1.5 to 2%). In this subgroup, stents are implanted in the presence of severely damaged endothelium, which may explain that despite a favorable angiographic result following stent deployment and a rigorous anticoagulant regimen, stent thrombosis and associated complications remain an important limitation.

A more liberal use of intracoronary stenting in bail-out situations may reduce this high complication rate. Randomized comparative studies (GRACE) are necessary to prove whether liberal or restrictive stenting is superior and more cost effective. The postprocedural regimen of anticoagulation may also influence the complication rate. The use of second-generation antiplatelet agents[30] (eventually in conjunction with the introduction of heparin-coated stents[31,32]) might dramatically reduce the rate of acute and subacute stent thrombosis and fundamentally alter our approach to intracoronary stenting.

At the present time, the procedural success rate and the incidence of stent thrombosis as well as other severe complications have been shown to be largely unaffected by stent design and physical properties of the protheses. The Strecker and Palmaz-Schatz stents appear to be equally effective in sealing occlusive dissections and restoring coronary blood flow in the setting of bail-out stenting following prolonged balloon inflations. The individual selection of each device should be oriented to actual vessel morphology and length of the lesion to be stented. In this regard, the Strecker stent appears especially suitable for coronary arteries with acute take-off, for tortuous vessels, and for the sealing of long intimal dissections.

REFERENCES

1. Dotter CT. Transluminally placed coilspring endarterial tube grafts: long-term patency in canine popliteal artery. Invest Radiol 1969;4:329
2. Sigwart U, Puel J, Mirkovitch V, Joffre F, Kappenberger L. Intravascular stents prevent occlusion and restenosis after transluminal angioplasty. N Engl J Med 1987;316:701
3. Levine MJ, Leonhard BM, Burke JA et al. Clinical and angiographic results of balloon expandable intracoronary stents in right coronary artery stenoses. J Am Coll Cardiol 1990;16:332
4. Schatz RA, Baim DS, Leon M et al. Clinical experience with the Palmaz-Schatz coronary stent: initial results of a multicenter study. Circulation 1991;88:148
5. Roubin GS, Cannon AD, Subodh KA et al. Intracoronary stenting for acute and threatened closure complicating percutaneous transluminal coronary angioplasty. Circulation 1992;3:916
6. Serruys PW, Strauss BH, Beatt KJ et al. Angiographic follow-up after placement of a self-expanding coronary artery stent. N Engl J Med 1991;324:13
7. Serruys PW, Strauss BH, van Beusekom HM, van der Giessen WJ. Stenting of coronary arteries: Has a modern Pandora's box been opened? J Am Coll Cardiol 1991;17:143B
8. Reifart N, Langer A, Störger H et al. Strecker stent as a bailout device following percutaneous transluminal coronary angioplasty. J Interv Cardiol 1992;5:79
9. Haude M, Erbel R, Hassan J. Subacute thrombotic complications after intracoronary implantation of Palmaz-Schatz stents. Am Heart J 1993;126:15
10. van der Giessen WJ, Serruys PW, van Beusekom HMM. Coronary stenting with a new, radiopaque, balloon-expandable endoprothesis in pigs. Circulation 1992;83:1788
11. van der Giessen WJ, van Beusekom HMM, van Houten CD. Coronary stenting with polymer-coated and uncoated self-expanding endoprotheses in pigs. Coronary Artery Dis 1992;3:631
12. Barth KH, Virmani R, Strecker EP et al. Flexible tantalum stents implanted in aortas and iliac arteries: Effects in normal canines. Radiology 1990;175:91
13. Hausegger KA, Lammer J, Hagen B. Iliac artery sten-

ting—clinical experience with the Palmaz-Schatz stent, Wallstent, and Strecker stent. Acta Radiol 1992; 33:292

14. Strecker EP, Liermann D, Barth KH et al. Expandable tubular stents for treatment of arterial occlusive disease—experimental and clinical results. Radiology 1990;175:97

15. Reifart N, Haase J, Massa T et al. Randomized trial comparing two devices: the Palmaz-Schatz and the Strecker stent bailout situations. J Interv Cardiol 1994;6:539–47

16. Sawyer PN, Stanczewski B, Srinivasan S, Stempak JG, Kammlott GW. Electron microscopy and physical chemistry of healing in prothetic heart valves, skirts and struts. J Thorac Cardiovasc Surg 1974;67:25

17. Beythien C, Hamm CW, Terres W et al. In vitro model to test the thrombogenicity of coronary stents. J Am Coll Cardiol, suppl. A. 1992;19:294A

18. Osterhues HH, Vogelpohl M, Felder C et al. Implantation von Strecker-Stents in der Iliakal- und Femoropoplitealregion. Z Kardiol 1990;79:783

19. Kuhn FP, Kutkuhn B, Torsell G et al. Renal artery stenosis: preliminary results of treatment with the Strecker stent. Radiology 1991;180:367

20. Breyer G, Hässlinger K. Tracheobronchiale Stents—Indikationen und Möglichkeiten. Pneumologie 1991;45:997

21. Mohnke M, Freitag L, Greschuchna G. Endobronchiale Prothesen—Erfahrungsbericht. Pneumologie 1991;45:148

22. Strauss BH, Escaned J, Foley DP et al. Technologic considerations and practical limitations in the use of quantitative angiography during percutaneous coronary recanalization. Prog Cardiovasc Dis 1994;5:343

23. Serruys PW, Macaya C, de Jaegere P et al. Interim analysis of the Benestent trial. Circulation 1993;88:I-594

24. Colombo A, Goldberg SL, Almagor Y, Maiello L, Finci L. A novel strategy for stent deployment in the treatment of acute or thretened closure complicating balloon coronary angioplasty. J Am Coll Cardiol 1993;22:1887

25. de Jaegere PP, Serruys PW, Bertrand M et al. Wiktor stent implantation in patients with restenosis following balloon angioplasty of a native coronary artery. Am J Cardiol 1992;69:598

26. de Feyter PJ, DeScheerder I, van den Brand M et al. Emergency stenting for refractory acute coronary artery occlusion during coronary angioplasty. Am J Cardiol 1990;66:1147

27. Haude M, Erbel R, Straub U et al. Results on intracoronary stents for management of coronary dissection after balloon angioplasty. Am J Cardiol 1991;67:691

28. Schatz RA, Penn IM, Baim DS et al. Stent Restenosis Study (STRESS): analysis of in-hospital results. Circulation 1993;88:I-594

29. Jackman JD, Zidar JP, Tcheng JE. Outcome after prolonged balloon inflation of greater than 20 minutes for initially unsuccessful percutaneous transluminal coronary angioplasty. Am J Cardiol 1992;69:1417

30. Chignard M, Lalau KC, Delautier D et al. Reduced sensitivity of human platlets to PAF-acether following ticlopidine intake. Haemostasis 1989;19:213

31. Stratienko AA, Zhu D, Lambert CR et al. Improved thromboresistance of heparin coated Palmaz-Schatz coronary stents in an animal model. Circulation 1993;88:I-596

32. van der Giessen WJ, Hårdhammar PA, van Beusekom HMM. Reduction of thrombotic events using heparin-coated Palmaz-Schatz stents. Circulation 1993;88:I-661

53 | The Cordis Stent

I. M. Penn
S. G. Ray
M. Nobuyoshi
T. Kimura
C. E. Buller
M. Moscovich
D. R. Ricci

Coronary artery stenting has recently been demonstrated to be safe and effective in the setting of failed percutaneous transluminal coronary angioplasty (PTCA)[1] as well as in reducing the rate of late renarrowing in two major randomized studies.[2,3] Modifications of intra- and postprocedure techniques have resulted in a lower complication rate with a reduced need for anticoagulation. Currently available stents represent an intermediate stage in the evolution of device technology, and further development is needed to address their shortcomings and allow stenting to achieve its full potential. Areas where improvement is needed are radiographic visibility, flexibility and deliverability, and retrieveability. Stainless steel stents are difficult to visualize during fluoroscopy, and although more precise stent placement can be facilitated by the use of a double-marker balloon, there are major potential advantages in the use of a stent that can be easily visualized, particularly when stent migration is suspected. Vessel tortuosity is a major problem in stent placement and decreased trackability caused by the stiffness of the

stent on the delivery system may require deep engagement of the guide catheter and considerable force to allow passage of the stent to the target area with an attendant risk of proximal vessel trauma and stent slippage. These limitations are particularly important in the setting of failed PTCA, in which stent visibility and reliable delivery are of critical importance. The difficulty and risks of stent placement may be reduced by the use of a highly flexible stent better able to track through tortuous vessels.

DEVELOPMENT

The Cordis stent was developed as a collaborative effort between the Cordis Corporation and the Duke University Interventional Cardiac Catheterization program.[4] The basic design is a single 0.005″ diameter tantulum wire in a zigzag pattern wound into a helical coil (Fig. 53-1). This design has the advantages of flexibility and radiopacity. Not only is it easy to visualize, but its single-strand construction allows it to be unraveled, facilitating extraction in the case of stent embolization. The basic design has undergone a series of refinements in response to the results of extensive animal testing at Duke University. Between August 1988 and October 1991 131 stents were implanted into the left coronary tree of 90 healthy mongrel dogs. All animals received 5,000 to 10,000 U of heparin during the procedure and aspirin 325 mg/d thereafter. Stent size was chosen to give an initial postdeployment stent-to-artery ratio of 1.1 to 1.2. The earliest version (Early P Stent) was mounted on a noncompliant coaxial Atlas balloon using a hand crimping process. The loose ends were tied to the adjacent turn at either end of the stent. Major problems were encountered with stretching of the stent coils during balloon removal following deployment. In an attempt to solve this problem the stent was redesigned with interlocking coils (the HS stent), but this modification increased the incidence of stent migration and substantially reduced trackability. It was therefore abandoned in favor of fur-

ther development of the P design. The next version (Basic P Stent) was initially mounted on an Atlas balloon, but this was subsequently changed to a more compliant Helix balloon with a lower postdeflation profile that substantially improved catheter withdrawal following deployment. Tracking problems persisted related to the tied ends of the stent, which could become unraveled during deployment, traumatizing the vessel wall. This led to development of the Enhanced P Stent. In this version the solvent cleaning process that removes adhesive residues of fabrication was improved, the loose ends were welded rather than tied (Fig. 53-2), and a specialized crimping tool developed to lower the profile of the unexpanded stent. In addition, a process was developed to allow covalent heparin bonding of the stent. The Enhanced P Stent was associated with substantially fewer deployment problems than the Basic P Stent. All the last 28 stent deployments following final modification of the technique were completed without substituting balloon catheters and with only one minor stent migration (1 to 2 mm) on balloon withdrawal.

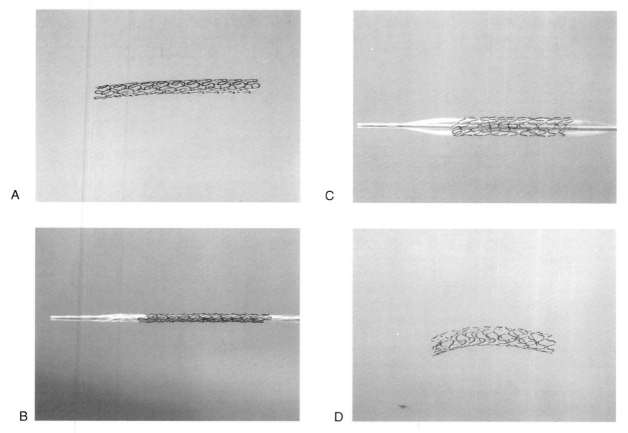

Fig. 53-1. **(A)** The unexpanded stent. **(B)** Stent crimped on the delivery balloon. **(C)** Stent expanded on the delivery balloon. **(D)** Configuration of the deployed stent.

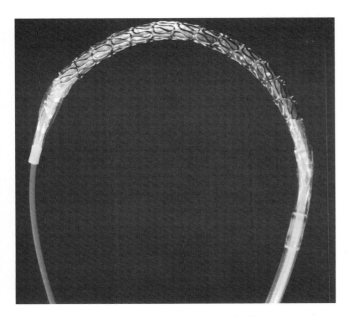

Fig. 53-2. Flexibility of the stent on a balloon catheter.

FOLLOW UP EXPERIENCE IN THE DOG MODEL

Fifty-three Enhanced P Stents mounted on Helix balloons were implanted in dogs between November 1990 and October 1991.[4] These studies were designed to examine the effects of both the heparin-coated and noncoated stents after 14 days, 28 days, and 6 months of implantation. All stents were evenly expanded or only slightly uneven with a widely patent lumen, and no evidence of stent recoil was seen after deployment. Endothelialization was complete in most stents at 14 days and in all at 28 days. By 28 days the intima was mildly thickened, covered the stent wires, reducing the lumen by 20 to 40%, and was composed mainly of smooth muscle cells and collagen. The media below the stent wires was moderately thinned and the internal elastic lamina moderately disrupted, more so when the stent was relatively oversized. The adventitia overlying the stent was mildly thickened. The proximal and distal nonstented portions of the vessels were normal even under electron microscopy. All successfully implanted stents remained patent in the long term, and no difference was seen in the angiographic or pathologic findings between the heparin coated and uncoated stents.

CLINICAL EXPERIENCE WITH THE ENHANCED P STENT

The Enhanced P Stent is now completing initial implant trials. The stent is precrimped and mounted on a 2-cm coaxial Sleuth XT Duralyn balloon and has

been available initially in 3 and 3.5 mm sizes. The nominal undilated stent length is 18 mm, decreasing to approximately 15 mm on inflation. Nominal stent sizing is achieved at 8 atm, and rated burst pressure of the delivery balloon is 10 atm. The delivery system will accept an 0.018″ guidewire and requires a guide catheter with a minimal internal diameter of 0.072″.

The first 45 implants were performed at Kokura Memorial Hospital, Kokura, Japan (n = 34) and at Vancouver Hospital, Canada (n = 11) in early 1994.

Table 53-1. Cordis Stent Implants at Kokura Memorial Hospital and Vancouver Hospital to April 1994

	Kokura	Vancouver
No.	34	11
Male	27	8
Female	7	3
Age (yr)	63 ± 8	64
Elective	28	11
Suboptimal	6	0
Restenosis	16	11
De novo	18	0
Delivery failure	3	1
Stented vessel		
Left anterior descending artery	19	7
Left circumflex artery	3	0
Right coronary artery	12	4
Stenosis characteristics		
Eccentric	11	7
Calcified	7	0
Dissection	1	0
Bend >45	7	1
Ostial (not aortic)	4	0
Stent characteristics		
3.0 mm	20	8
3.5 mm	11	7
Single	30	11
Double	3	0
Triple	1	0
Balloon atm (range)	12 ± 2 (6–16)	12 ± 2 (8–14)
Complications		
Acute/subacute occlusions	0	0
Q/non-Q myocardial infarction	0	0
Coronary artery bypass graft	0	0
Death	0	0
Major hematoma	1	0
Pseudoaneurysm	1	2
Blood transfusion	2	0

The patient and stenosis characteristics of the initial implants are outlined in Table 53-1 and the antiplatelet and anticoagulant regimen in Table 53-2.

All stenoses were predilated with an undersized balloon, either 2.5 or 3 mm with a 0.014″ or 0.018″ wire. The stent was advanced into position with the balloon under neutral pressure. A minor degree of play of the crimped stent is present on the delivery balloon, but this was not evident during stent placement, probably because of the protective effect of slight winging of the proximal and distal ends of the folded balloon, which prevents significant movement. In most cases inflation of the delivery balloon to 10 to 14 atm for 1 to 2 minutes successfully expanded the stent, but in two cases an additional high-pressure noncompliant balloon was used.

The initial clinical experience with the Cordis stent has been highly favorable, in both elective placement and placement for suboptimal results. In our experience visualization is excellent (Fig. 53-3) and trackability appears to be superior to that of the Palmaz-Schatz and Gianturco-Roubin devices. The delivery balloon is low profile, may be inflated to high pressures, and can be inserted through an 8-F guiding catheter. Withdrawal of the balloon from the expanded stent is smooth, and no problems have occurred with stent migration. The relationship of side branches to the stent structure is particularly well

Table 53-2. Antiplatelet and Anticoagulant Regimens

24–48 hours prior to implant (minimum of 1 day)
  Aspirin (uncoated) 320 mg/day.
  Dipyridamole 75 mg tid
  Calcium channel blocker
2–3 hours prior to implant
  Dextran 40 IV: 100 ml/hr for 2 hours then 50 ml/hr to 1000 ml
During procedure
  Heparin 10,000 to 15,000 U IV to obtain activated clotting time (ACT) >300 sec and further boluses as necessary to maintain ACT >300 sec
Post procedure
  Remove sheaths when ACT <150 sec
  Recommence heparin 4 hr after sheath removal
  Warfarin loading until international normalized ratio (INR) in range 2.5–3.5
  Heparin IV until INR in target range
  Continue warfarin and dipyridamole for 1–3 months
  Aspirin indefinitely
  Gastrointestinal prophylaxis while on warfarin and aspirin
  Calcium channel blocker for 1–3 months

visualized. The stent struts appear to "fish mouth" around the openings of side branches, leaving them widely patent (Fig. 53-3). In some cases there has been partial separation of the stent coils during balloon inflation, but this is not associated with loss of lumen diameter. Difficulty in visualizing the stent lumen and hence residual thrombus or plaque is a potential handicap with radiodense devices, but in practice this has not been a problem.

The one case in which stent delivery failed at Vancouver Hospital was a tight restenotic lesion in the distal right coronary artery. The proximal and mid-parts of the vessel were noncritically diseased, and the stent could not be passed through an area of stenosis in the proximal vessel even after dilation of this segment (Fig. 53-4A & B). It proved difficult to withdraw the mounted stent into the guiding catheter (8 F 4RJ), and the stent was displaced distally on the balloon. Despite repeated attempts the balloon and partially displaced stent could not be drawn back into the guiding catheter. The guide and balloon were then withdrawn into the descending aorta. While the operator was attempting to withdraw the stent in the femoral arterial sheath, the stent became completely dislodged from the balloon. However, it was easily retrieved from the guidewire by removing the mounting balloon over the wire and passing a 1.5-mm ACS Edge balloon along the guidewire through the undilated stent and inflating it distally (Fig. 4C). The inflated balloon was then used to withdraw the stent back into the guiding catheter. The excellent visualization of the stent made this much easier than it would have been with a stainless steel device.

Clinical and Angiographic Follow-up

Periprocedural complications are listed in Table 53-1. Three patients needed surgical repair of a femoral pseudoaneurysm, and two required a blood transfusion. All patients receiving Cordis stents during the initial pilot implantation program will be followed up at 2, 6, and 12 months. At 2 months patients will undergo a stress test, and the 6 month follow-up will include an exercise thallium scan and repeat angiography. Follow-up is so far at an early stage, with no patient having a stent implanted for longer than 4 months (as of May 1994), but there have been no episodes of acute or subacute stent thrombosis, myocardial infarction, or symptomatic recurrent ischemia in stented patients. Ten patients have undergone quantitative angiographic follow-

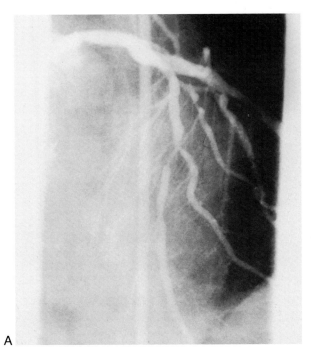

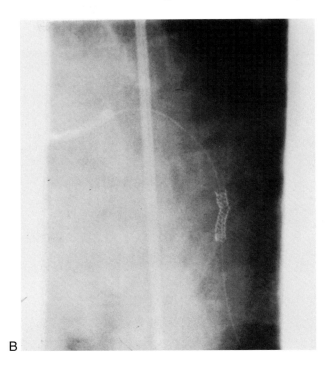

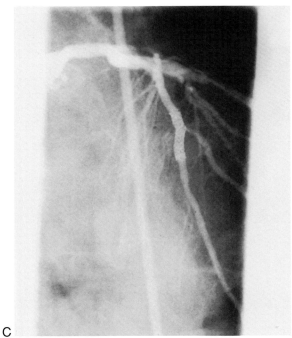

A

B

C

Fig. 53-3. Successful stent delivery. **(A)** Tight stenosis in the left anterior descending artery overlapping the origin of a large diagonal branch. **(B)** Expanded stent in position showing "fish mouthing" of the coils into the origin of the diagonal branch. **(C)** Post-stent angiogram with a widely patent stent lumen and persisting flow in the diagonal branch.

up at Kokura Memorial Hospital 1 month after stent implantation. Mean residual stenosis in the stented segment was 9.3 ± 7.5% at 1 month. This compares with 8.7 ± 7.2% for all 34 patients immediately after stent implantation. On the basis of this limited information stent recoil does not appear to be a problem, but it is impossible to draw conclusions about restenosis.

CONCLUSIONS

The limited initial experience suggests that the Cordis stent may be an improvement on current technology, at least in terms of its visibility and trackability, but its handling characteristics will be put to greater test in the forthcoming trial of failed angioplasty.

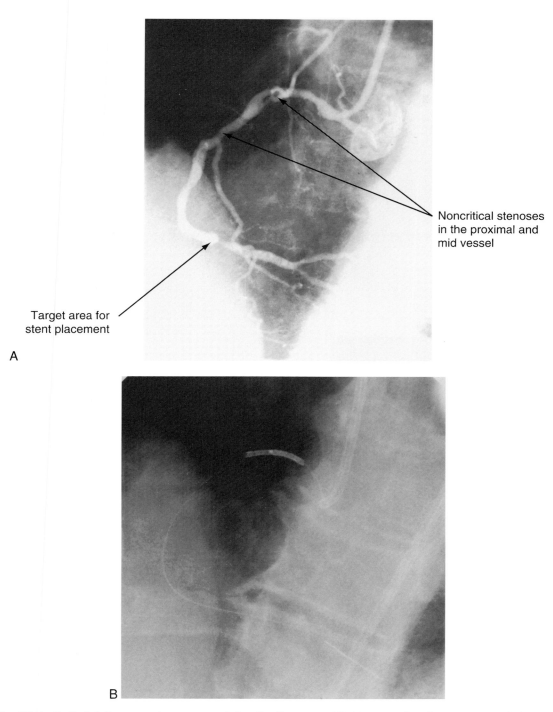

Fig. 53-4. Failed delivery and recovery of the Cordis stent. **(A)** Preprocedural angiogram of the right coronary artery in the 60° left anterior oblique view showing the tight distal restenotic segment that was the target for stent placement and noncritical proximal and mid-vessel disease. **(B)** Cordis stent stuck in the proximal diseased segment despite considerable guide catheter push. (*Figure continues.*)

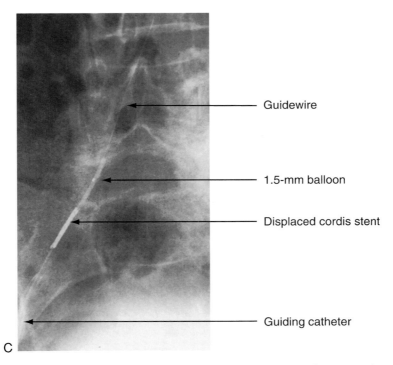

Guidewire

1.5-mm balloon

Displaced cordis stent

Guiding catheter

C

Fig. 53-4 *(Continued).* **(C)** Retrieval of the displaced stent from the guidewire in the abdominal aorta using a 1.5-mm balloon passed through the stent.

One area of particular concern during long-term angiographic follow-up must be whether a tendency exists to restenosis at sites of partial coil separation, analogous to restenosis at the articulation with the Palmaz-Schatz stent. If this is the case then further modification of the stent structure may be necessary.

REFERENCES

1. Penn IM, Ricci DR, Brown RI et al. Randomized study of stenting versus prolonged balloon dilation in failed angioplasty (PTCA): preliminary data from the Trial of Angioplasty and Stents in Canada (TASC II), abstracted. Circulation 1993;88:3231

2. Fischman D, Savage M, Leon M et al. Acute and late angiographic results of the Stent REStenosis Study (STRESS), abstracted. J Am Coll Cardiol Feb 1994; Special Issue;61A

3. Serruys PW, Macaya C, de Jaegere P et al. Interim analysis of the Benestent Trial, abstracted. Circulation 1993;88:3195

4. Bauman RP, Muhlestein JB, Stack RS. Development of a closed-coil metallic stent. pp. 913. In Roubin GS et al. (ed): Interventional Cardiovascular Medicine: Principles and Practice. Churchill Livingstone, New York, 1994

Gianturco-Roubin Coronary Flexible Coil Stent

54

David Ho

Gary Roubin

Work on the Gianturco-Roubin coronary flexible coil stent, which is balloon expandable, began in 1979 when Cesar Gianturco, a radiologist, investigated its use in peripheral vessels. The device was adapted for coronary use in 1985 when collaborative work with Gary Roubin was instigated.

Initial experiments demonstrated ease of deployment and long-term patency in the coronary artery of dogs. By 2 to 4 days, light and electron microscopy showed layers of platelets, red cells, and fibrin covering the stent coils. Endothelialization began by the fourth day and was confluent by 14 days. At 6 months, normal-appearing flow-directed endothelium had appeared. Additional studies done in the peripheral vessels of atherosclerotic rabbits and in swine coronaries confirmed the canine findings and demonstrated the stent's ability to improve the luminal appearance of dissected vessels.

In 1987, the U.S. Food and Drug Administration (FDA) gave permission for a Phase I study in humans under an investigator-sponsored (Gary S. Roubin) investigational device exemption. In this study, the stent was used as a bail-out device in the setting of acute closure complicating percutaneous transluminal coronary angioplasty (PTCA). Following stenting, all patients underwent coronary artery bypass grafting (CABG). In study patients, none had a Q-wave myocardial infarction, and all left the hospital within 8 days. These data led to FDA approval for an ongoing study, using the stent to treat acute and threatened closure complicating PTCA. The device has been under critical multicenter evaluation since this time under sponsorship of the manufacturer and patent holder. The device was the first stent approved by the FDA for coronary use and was released for clinical application on June 1, 1993.

RATIONALE

Balloon angioplasty suffers from three limitations: (1) a significant number of patients have unsuitable coronary anatomy; (2) in those suitable for, and who undergo PTCA, 5 to 10% will develop acute or threatened coronary closure; and (3) restenosis occurs in 30 to 40% of dilated vessels. The flexible coil stent, originally developed specifically for deployment in patients with acute or threatened closure, appears to have an impact on all three problems. Once used as a bridge to preserve myocardium while awaiting emergency surgery, this stent is now commonly used to avoid surgery totally.

Acute Closure

Despite the advent of new devices for coronary angioplasty such as directional arthrectomy, rotational arthrectomy, transluminal extraction arthrectomy, and the laser, the incidence of acute closure remains high. This is due partly to the complex coronary anatomy that is now attempted and partly to the inherent trauma associated with passage of these new devices. Despite various methods of salvage, such as pro-

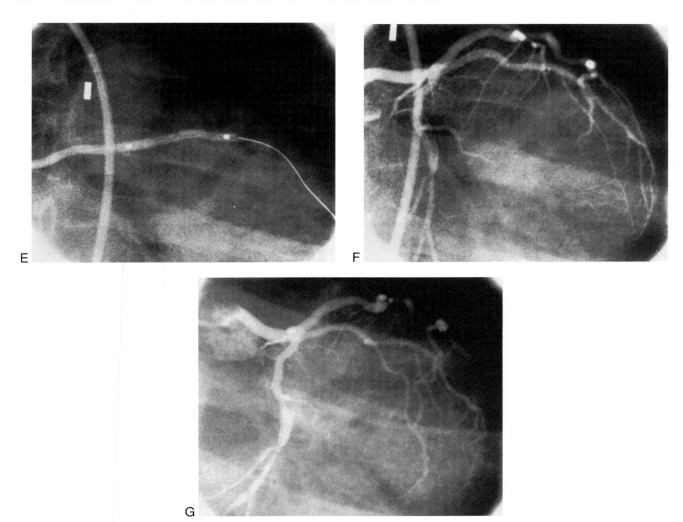

Fig. 54-2. (*continued*)

to standard measures: (1) residual stenosis of 50% or more, (2) significant dissection (10 mm or more in length with or without extraluminal contrast), or (3) ongoing angina or electrocardiographic (ECG) changes. A case of threatened closure treated by the flexible coil stent is shown in Figure 54-3.

Contraindications

Contraindications include recent gastrointestinal or cerebral hemorrhage, bleeding diathesis, or other disorders that limit the use of antiplatelet or anticoagulant therapy or both. Relative contraindications include thrombocytopenia or other platelet disease, significant anemia of unknown origin, symptoms of or active peptic ulcer disease, active menstruation, a history of recent gastrointestinal or genitourinary bleeding, diabetic proliferative retinopathy, chronic

pulmonary or gastrointestinal inflammatory disease, and disseminated neoplasia. The risk of bleeding needs to be balanced against the risks of acute closure and the likely outcome of emergency surgery. If necessary, the device may still be placed, although subsequent bleeding complication rates will be higher.

Other contraindications include extreme proximal vessel tortuosity, particularly in the presence of severe calcification. In addition, vessels that have poor distal runoff, due to either residual unstentable dissection, distal occlusion, or supplying nonfunctioning myocardium, are poor risks for stenting. Use of the device in acute myocardial infarction is not specifically contraindicated, but the placement of the device in a vessel with a large burden of thrombus must be accompanied by adjunctive local urokinase administration.

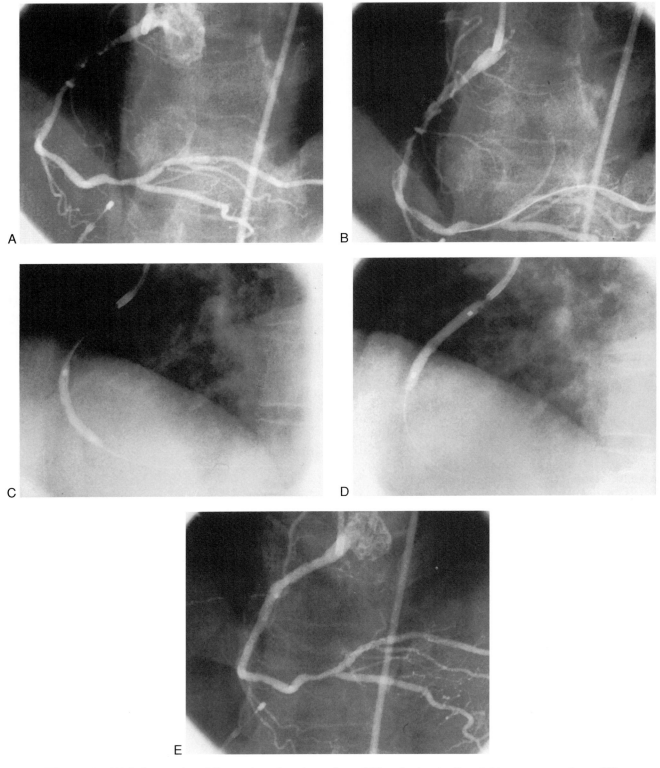

Fig. 54-3. (A) left anterior oblique view showing a long diffuse lesion in the right coronary artery. **(B)** Long spiral dissection extending to the crux following PTCA. **(C)** A 4.0 × 20-mm stent was deployed to cover the distal limit of the dissection. **(D)** A second 4.0 × 20-mm stent was deployed to cover the proximal extent of the dissection, overlapping the distal stent by around one-fifth of the length. **(E)** Final angiogram showed no residual dissection or filling defect.

PRETREATMENT

Since acute closure is unpredictable, patients are routinely given soluble aspirin (325 mg bid) and ticlopidine (250 mg bid) on the evening before PTCA. The importance of antiplatelet therapy (at least 500 mg of soluble aspirin) prior to stenting cannot be overemphasized. At the beginning of the angioplasty, patients routinely receive 7,000 to 10,000 units of intra-arterial heparin. Supplement bolus doses are given as necessary to maintain an activated clotting time (ACT) of 250 to 350 seconds. Dipyridamole and dextran are no longer recommended.

STENTING TECHNIQUE AND TIPS

Guiding Catheters

An appropriately sized guiding catheter must be selected at the beginning of the procedure to ensure that an adequately sized stent can be placed if needed. For deployment of stent sizes 3.0 mm or less in diameter, standard 8-F guiding catheters with an internal diameter of 0.077″ or more are adequate. For stent sizes 3.5 and 4.0 mm, superlarge lumen 8-F guiding catheters with internal diameters 0.086″ or more (e.g., Lumax, Cook, Cordis, GuideZilla, Schneider, Big-Max, Scimed), or large lumen 9-F guiding catheters with internal diameters of 0.089″ or more are required. It is recommended that a nominal stent size of 0.5 mm larger than the normal vessel size be used to ensure optimal outcome. Hence, angioplasty to a 3.0-mm artery should commence with a superlarge lumen 8-F or large lumen 9-F guiding catheter. Large lumen Tuohy-Borst adapters (at least 6-F internal diameter; USCI, ACS, Medtronic) are needed to allow passage of the stent (Fig. 54-4).

Routine use of these adapters is recommended for all PTCA procedures. Superlarge Tuohy-Borst adapters (e.g., Microvena, Cook) allow use of the peel-away introducer sheath that is recommended for operators not familiar with the use of the stent.

One can generally begin cases with a right Judkin's or a short-tipped left Judkin's guide catheter. If the preprocedural angiogram shows severe proximal tortuosity or unusual vessel takeoff and the likelihood of stenting is high, an Amplatz-shaped catheter may be used to begin the coronary angioplasty. Amplatz-shaped catheters are also used for left-sided vein grafts. A multipurpose guiding catheter is used for down-sloping takeoff, right-sided vein grafts. Strong guiding catheter support and good guiding catheter technique is essential for placement of this stent. Guiding catheters that soften with time or do not fit well in the ostium should be avoided, especially for distal lesions in tortuous and diffusely diseased vessels. Prior to stent placement, the push-pull technique is useful in testing adequacy of guiding catheter support. In this test, one gently advances the guiding catheter while the balloon catheter is withdrawn to test if the tip of the guiding catheter will intubate the ostium. If the tip falls out of the ostium easily, support may be inadequate, and a different guiding catheter may be required.

Guidewires

Routine use of a 0.016″ or 0.018″ system is recommended. This allows the operator to exchange the guidewire through the balloon catheter for an 0.018″ extra-support wire (Cook, ACS, Microvena) or 0.017″ hyperflex wire (USCI) if necessary. This is achieved by placing the balloon catheter tip distal to the dissection and then exchanging the wire. If a 0.014″ sys-

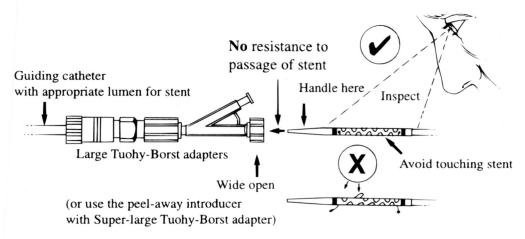

Guiding catheter with appropriate lumen for stent

No resistance to passage of stent

Handle here

Inspect

Avoid touching stent

Large Tuohy-Borst adapters

Wide open

(or use the peel-away introducer with Super-large Tuohy-Borst adapter)

Fig. 54-4. Equipment inspection. See text.

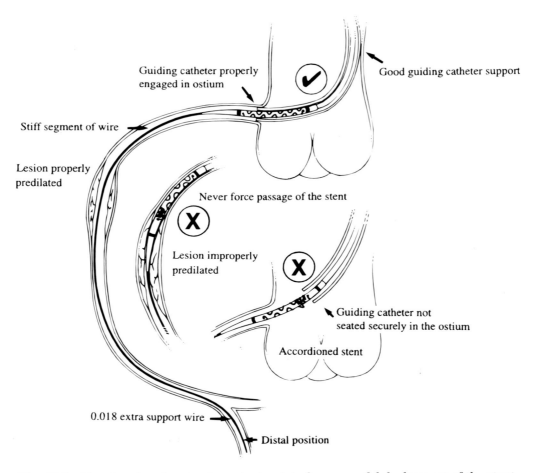

Fig. 54-5. Line drawing showing important points for successful deployment of the stent.

tem is used, inexpensive exchange catheters (Cook) are available for changing to a 0.018″ extra support wire. The extra support wire tends to straighten the proximal vessel and allows better tracking during stent balloon advancement. The tip of the wire should be placed as distally as possible to ensure that the stiff shaft of the wire is across the lesion (Fig. 54-5). In straightforward anatomic situations, the usual 0.016″ or 0.018″ wires, or the new 0.014″ extra support wire from ACS may be adequate, although this is not recommended for the inexperienced operator.

Angioplasty Balloon

Use of the 0.018″ wire requires 0.018″ compatible balloon catheters for routine PTCA to avoid laborious changes of wires and balloons when stenting becomes necessary. A number of manufacturers produce suitable over-the-wire as well as monorail balloons with excellent crossing profiles.

Roadmap

Angiography is first repeated in orthogonal views after intracoronary nitroglycerin (200 μg) to assess the size of the vessel and the extent of dissection. A suitable freeze frame image is then selected to serve as the roadmap for stent placement. The extent of extraluminal contrast staining, filling defects and their relative positions to side branches, and other markers are used for subsequent fine positioning of the stent. It is important that the extent of a dissection be defined and that at least transient good distal runoff be identified. Placement of a stent into a vessel with poor distal flow or failing to cover the entire dissection is a significant risk factor for stent thrombosis.[3]

Equipment Check

The angioplasty equipment is then evaluated for compatibility and adequacy of support. Will the existing guide catheter provide sufficient backup? Will the current guidewire provide a suitable rail for the stent or will a 0.018″ support wire be required? If doubt exists, it is best to consider changing the guidewire or the guide catheter (or both) at the outset rather than fail to deploy the stent. If a smaller Y-adapter is used, it should be replaced by a large-bore adapter before stenting.

Sizing and Length

The appropriate choice of stent diameter size is essential for successful stenting. The balloon material is relatively bulky, but the design markedly decreases the risk of stent dislodgement and embolization. The balloon is relatively compliant compared with conventional PTCA balloons. Thus, low-pressure deployment is recommended. Characteristically, this stent undergoes a slight (on average, 15%) elastic recoil. To compensate for this recoil, the delivering balloon is 0.5 mm larger than the stent. Thus, a 3.5-mm stent is delivered on a 4.0-mm balloon, but this balloon does not reach this "nominal" size at low pressures within an atherosclerotic artery and "potential balloon size" should not be considered in choosing the correct stent size.

In vivo quantitative angiographic study showed that at low inflation pressures the flexible coil stent and its compliant deployment balloon are both considerably constricted by the vessel wall. The diameters achieved are substantially less than the nominal diameter.[4] Accordingly, one should choose a stent of a nominal size 0.1 to 0.5 mm larger than the reference diameter of the vessel to be stented. It is recommended that vessels 2.0 to 2.4 mm in diameter be supported by a 2.5-mm stent, vessels 2.5 to 2.9 mm

Table 54-1. Change in Pattern of Usage of the Gianturco-Roubin Stent Following Recommendation of the New Sizing Strategy

Stent Diameter (mm)	Stents Implanted (%)	
	Clinical Trial[a]	University of Alabama[b]
2.0	1.4	0
2.5	20.4	3.7
3.0	44.6	34.0
3.5	21.3	27.3
4.0	12.3	35.0

[a] The multicenter clinical trial.
[b] Over a recent 9-month period at the University of Alabama (March 1993 to November 1993; number of stents = 297).

Table 54-2. Patients Receiving Single and Multiple Stents at the University of Alabama Over a Recent 9-Month Period (March 1993 to November 1993; Number of Patients = 231)

No. of Stents	No. of Patients (%)
1	186 (80.5)
2	30 (13.0)
3	13 (5.6)
4	2 (0.9)
5	1 (0.4)

in diameter by a 3.0-mm stent, vessels 3.0 to 3.4 mm in diameter by a 3.5-mm stent, and vessels 3.5 to 4.0 mm in diameter by a 4.0-mm stent. The stent should then be deployed at the lowest possible pressure that completely expands the stent. This is usually between 3 and 5 atm. The extra metal from a slightly larger stent appears to translate to better circumferential support and improved angiographic results. Supplemental dilation with a noncompliant balloon at higher pressures (14 to 16 atm) should be routinely performed to optimize stent placement. The noncompliant balloon should be sized to the diameter of adjacent "normal" segments. The pattern of stent usage following the change in sizing strategy is shown in Tables 54-1 and 54-2.

Since the extent of a dissection is often poorly visualized angiographically, a 20-mm stent is recommended to ensure that the extent of the dissection is "bracketed" by the end coils of the stent. Shorter 12-mm stents are used for discrete intimal flap or localized restenosis. They are more trackable than the 20-mm length.

Paving the Way

It is crucial that the target lesion be fully dilated before the device is placed (Fig. 54-5). The next step is to ensure that the proximal vessel will accommodate passage of the stent. Depending on the tortuosity, it may be necessary to predilate even modest stenosis in the proximal vessel to allow a smooth passage for the stent. Disease and tortuosity in the segment 10 to 20 mm distal to the lesion also need to be considered since this may hinder fine positioning of the stent. To avoid any significant recoil from hindering stent advancement, a series of short inflations to any significant disease at or proximal to the lesion immediately prior to withdrawing the initial balloon and changing out to the stent balloon is recommended.

Stent Placement

The stent balloon is prepared in the standard negative pressure fashion. The operator's gloves should be washed cleaned of thrombus and the metal coils handled as little as possible. The stent balloon catheter is then advanced over the extra-support wire to the Y-adapter. After inspecting to ensure that the coils and, especially, the end loops have not been accidentally lifted up from the balloon, the stent is advanced through the widely opened Tuohy-Borst Y-adapter (Fig. 54-4). Inexperienced users can use the peel-away introducer sheath provided. There should be no resistance to the passage of the stent through the Y-adapter or the guiding catheter. The stent balloon is then advanced to the distal guide catheter. It is important that the guide be seated securely inside the coronary ostium before advancing the stent out of the guide catheter into the coronary artery (Fig. 54-5). With the assistant applying a gentle traction on the guidewire, the operator advances the stent balloon catheter into the vessel while maintaining a forward pressure on the guide catheter. Repeated small injections of contrast are given to position the stent finely. The stent wires cannot be visualized but can be positioned precisely by using the proximal and distal balloon markers. Complete stent coils begin approximately 2 to 3 mm inside the markers. If the operator is in doubt about the extent of a dissection, the stent should be placed a little distally and an additional proximal stent added if necessary.

Inflating the Stent Balloon

Once the stent is placed optimally in the coronary artery, the balloon is rapidly inflated to 4 atm. The stent is often fully expanded by simply maintaining pressure at 4 atm for 30 seconds. Occasionally, 5 or 6 atm for 60 to 90 seconds may be required. The balloon is deflated once the stent is fully expanded (Fig. 54-6). When the balloon is fully deflated, the operator gently removes the balloon catheter while the assistant advances the guidewire. At this stage, the guide catheter should be pulled back slightly to avoid inadvertent deep intubation and dissection of the vessel.

It is important to remember that the stent balloon is very compliant and at high pressure, the balloon diameter is 0.5 mm greater than the nominal stent diameter. Inflating the balloon to higher pressures can result in dissection proximal and distal to the stent where the balloon is not constrained by the stent coils. Undersizing stents should be avoided at all times. Undersizing and overexpansion may open the stent like a clamshell so the loops no longer interdigitate, allowing arterial tissue and plaque to prolapse into the lumen.

Supplemental Inflations

One should consider the stent balloon simply as a vehicle for reliable delivery of the stent to the lesion and for initial deployment of the stent at low pressure (4 atm). Indentation of the stent balloon is often evident during deployment at low pressure. Following removal of the stent balloon, a high-pressure noncompliant balloon sized to the vessel should be advanced into the stent and inflated to high pressure (14 to 16 atm) for several minutes if tolerated. This supplemental inflation is particularly useful if the stented lumen appears hazy and irregular after initial stent deployment and will fully expand the stent and smooth out the vessel lumen (Fig. 54-6). A relatively low-profile balloon should be used for this purpose. Previously inflated balloons with a large residual profile should be avoided due to potential dislodgement of the stent. To avoid distal dissection, it is important to restrict high-pressure inflations to within the stent coils. If the distal limit of the stent is in doubt and the balloon potentially in the uncovered distal vessel, lower pressure inflations should be initially used.

With this stent in situ, the risk of dissection or vessel perforation is reduced. Each protruding plaque fragment between the stent coils is somewhat equivalent to a small discrete lesion and often responds favorably to high-pressure angioplasty with a noncompliant balloon. We term this stent assisted high pressure balloon angioplasty.

A Second Stent

Placing a second stent proximal to the first is straightforward, whereas placing a second stent distally through a deployed stent is more difficult and sometimes impossible. Passage of the second stent through the first stent may contort both stents, resulting in acute or subacute thrombosis. It is thus important to ensure that the distal dissection is covered with the first stent. Having deployed a stent to cover the distal extent of dissection, a second stent may be required to cover the proximal dissection (Figs. 54-2 and 54-3). This stent should be positioned to overlap partially the proximal portion of the first stent so any potential prolapse of atheromatous material between the two stents is avoided. By taking freeze-frame images of the first stent during full inflation and using side branches as landmarks, the position of the second stent can be finely controlled to ensure a degree of overlap, bearing in mind again that the first complete loop is 2 to 3 mm inside the marker. The use of multiple Gianturco-Roubin Flexi-

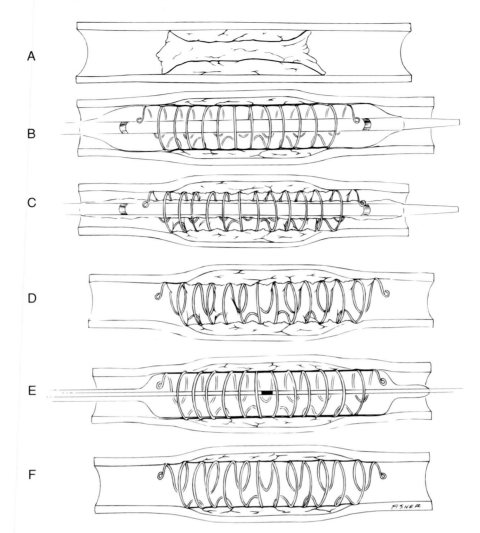

Fig. 54-6. **(A)** Line drawing of a lesion that had been predilated. **(B)** The stent was deployed at low pressure over 30 to 60 seconds. Adequate time was given for full deflation of the balloon **(C)** before it was carefully withdrawn. **(D)** Note the presence of a small amount of luminal irregularity and residual stenosis caused by plaques protruding between the struts of the stent. Following supplemental dilation with a noncompliant balloon inflated to 14 to 16 atm **(E),** optimal luminal diameter was achieved with minimal luminal irregularity or residual stenosis **(F).**

ble Coil stents during a single procedure has not been associated with increased incidence of stent thrombosis[2,3] or restenosis.[2]

Stenting Distal to a Deployed Stent

On occasion, despite careful assessment before stenting, it will become apparent that residual dissection is present distal to the first stent deployed. A small degree of residual dissection may respond to a prolonged inflation. Failing this, an attempt to deploy a second stent through the existing stent can be made. Careful angiography is again performed to deter-

mine the length of residual dissection that must be covered. If possible, a 12-mm stent is preferred, since it will track more easily through the deployed stent. Care must be taken when passing the second stent through the existing stent. If the already stented segment is relatively straight, passing a second stent should pose little difficulty. If the already stented segment is tortuous, the coils may clutch one another, contorting both stents and occluding the vessel. Before placing the second stent, it is critical to "postdilate" the first stent at high pressures. Excellent guide support and extra support wires also facilitate this maneuver.

Stenting Within a Stent

A residual flap of plaque or dissection may sometimes prolapse into the vessel lumen between the coils of the stent. This situation often responds to prolonged supplemental inflations as described above. When this fails to resolve the problem, a second stent of equal diameter can be placed within the first. This technique is useful in optimizing the luminal result in some patients. The use of two overlapping stents in this manner has not been associated with increased incidence of stent thrombosis or restenosis. After placement of the second stent, high-pressure supplemental balloon inflations are essential.

Multivessel Stenting

In patients with significant stenoses in multiple vessels, one can generally proceed to angioplasty of the second vessel after the first vessel is stented. Since the patient is committed to antiplatelet with or without anticoagulation therapy, one should have a low threshold for placing additional stents if indicated.

Stenting at Side Branches

Since there are gaps between the loops of this stent, flow in major side branches is seldom compromised. If necessary, it is possible to pass a wire and balloon into a side branch and perform PTCA through the stent. A fixed wire device is the most convenient. The "kissing balloon" technique can be used within a stent to optimize the luminal result. Care must be taken in advancing or withdrawing the balloon catheter through the side branch. It is also possible to place a stent in a side branch followed by stenting of the main vessel. In this situation, the side branch should be stented first before the main vessel.

Stenting at Ostial Sites

A clear and precise profile view of the origin of the vessel must be obtained. The stent is first advanced well into the vessel. The guide is then withdrawn and the stent carefully pulled back until the proximal marker is 4 to 5 mm outside the vessel to ensure that the first complete coil of the stent is adjacent to the aortic wall (in the case of aorto-ostial lesions) or the origin of the vessel (e.g., origin of the left circumflex). Leaving part of the stent in the aorta or the distal left main coronary artery does not appear to be a problem. However, care must be taken with subsequent engagements of the ostium (even months later)

so as not to damage the stent. Soft-tipped or diagnostic catheters should be used. Similarly, care must be taken in passing a balloon catheter through the left anterior descending artery if the ostia of the left circumflex or the first diagonal have previously been stented.

Tapering Vessels

This stent can also be fashioned to "fit" tapering vessels. This is done by deploying the stent initially at the lowest inflation pressure possible to expand the coils. The balloon is then withdrawn proximally and inflated at higher pressure to increase the diameter of the stent in the larger, more proximal vessel. When a large-diameter difference is encountered (e.g., vein graft to distal vessel or left main stem to left anterior descending) the large proximal segment should be well compressed against the wall with a large balloon.

Intracoronary Urokinase Infusions

Intracoronary urokinase infusion is occasionally required in vessels with residual thrombus stented in the context of acute myocardial infarction. The urokinase infusion (80,000 to 100,000 U/hr) can be maintained for 12 to 24 hours. To infuse intracoronary urokinase, an infusion catheter (Tracker 18, Target Therapeutics or the Cook perfusion catheter) is placed over the guidewire into the coronary artery. Using the proximal and distal markers, the infusion holes are placed proximal to and covering the length of the stent. To make up the infusion solution, 1,000,000 U of urokinase are mixed with 250 ml of half-normal saline solution and infused through an air filter at 20 ml/hr (80,000 U/hr). Higher initial infusion rates can be used for a large thrombus burden. The guide catheter is then backed out of the coronary ostia and connected to a heparin infusion (again through an air filter) via an infusion pump. The infusion is continued for 12 to 24 hours until the next day when repeat angiography and supplemental angioplasty can be performed as necessary.

Occasionally, haziness and ill-defined lucencies may persist after stent placement in patients with a thrombogenic vessel who present with unstable angina or recent myocardial infarction. If this does not respond to supplemental balloon inflations, intracoronary urokinase infusions for 16 to 24 hours may also be useful in producing a good angiographic result.

Intra-aortic Balloon Pump

The intra-aortic balloon pump is invaluable in patients with poor left ventricular function, in those with difficult anatomy with poorly tolerated flow occlusion, and in those with diffuse disease or proximal tortuosity in whom a long stent placement time is anticipated. This will often allow the operator enough time for proper positioning and deployment of the stent. In patients stented in the setting of acute myocardial infarction, in those with suboptimal poststent angiographic results and reduced distal flow, and in those with poor ventricular function, use of the intra-aortic balloon pump for 24 to 48 hours following stenting has also been useful in augmenting coronary diastolic flow and maintaining stent patency.

COMPLICATIONS, PITFALLS, AND TIPS TO AVOID THEM

With proper guide catheter and guidewire support and appropriate push-pull technique, it is relatively easy to deploy this stent. On occasion, the device may not cross the area to be stented. If an extra support guidewire is not being used, the guidewire should be replaced with such a wire. If guiding catheter support is inadequate, a new guide with a different curve may be tried. Occasionally, such failure to cross is due to proximal or distal disease, the severity of which has been underestimated. If this is the case, the proximal vessel should first be dilated with a high-pressure balloon.

Changing to a 0.018″ Extra Support Wire

The balloon catheter is first advanced distally beyond any dissection flap. The existing guidewire is then withdrawn and replaced by the 0.018″ extra support wire. If the initial balloon used was not compatible with a 0.018″ wire or is a monorail system, the balloon should first be removed over an extension wire (or with the use of the "trapper balloon" if the ID of the guide is less than 0.079″). A 0.018″ compatible, noncompliant balloon (which can be used later for supplemental inflation after stent deployment) or exchange catheter (Cook, Target Therapeutics) is then advanced across the lesion before the original wire is removed and replaced by the extra support wire. The Cook exchange kit also comes with a low friction exchange catheter that allows simple advancement over the existing wire along its length inside the

guiding catheter (without inadvertent advancement of the wire). Once the proximal end of the wire exits this catheter, the assistant holds the wire while the exchange catheter is advanced across the lesion. The original wire is then removed and replaced by the extra support wire.

Changing the Guide Catheter

If the guide catheter diameter will not permit the passage of a suitably sized stent or if better guiding catheter support is required, the guiding catheter can be exchanged over an extra support coronary guidewire. To avoid the risk associated with recrossing a dissected vessel, the extra support 0.018″ wire is first placed distally in the coronary vessel. If the extra support wire used was not the long exchange variety, the wire should first be extended. The guide catheter is then exchanged with the help of an assistant in a similar fashion to the exchange of balloon catheters. A small loop of guidewire should be left in the aortic root to allow for guide catheter rotation as it comes across the aortic arch and enters the ascending aorta. This is important to prevent inadvertent loss of guidewire position, particularly when positioning right Judkins and Amplatz guide catheters. To reduce blood loss, the replacement guide should be flushed and made ready with a large-bore Tuohy-Borst adapter attached.

Ensuring Excellent Coaxial Guide Support

When stenting the right coronary artery, it is important to check the right anterior oblique view to ensure that the guide is coaxial with the plane of the proximal vessel. If not, clockwise rotation will seat the guide snugly into the coronary ostia. When using Amplatz-shaped catheters, especially in the right coronary artery, one with side perfusion holes is preferred. This will avoid the need to disengage and reengage the ostium repetitively due to flow occlusion, potentially dissecting the vessel. In the left coronary artery the short-tipped JL4 guiding catheter should be seated securely in the ostium of the left main coronary artery prior to advancing the stent. In tortuous, diffusely diseased, or calcified left circumflex or left anterior descending vessels, consider changing out to an AL1 or AL2 catheter before attempting to place a stent.

In difficult situations, the assistant may have to pull back on the extra support wire while the operator applies constant forward pressure to advance the stent balloon. This may need to be repeated several times, with the operator pausing to allow the assistant to readvance the guidewire again before traction is reapplied. Asking the patient to take deep inspirations to straighten the proximal vessels is also useful. If there is marked tortuosity, a 12-mm instead of a 20-mm stent may be considered. Occasionally, one may need to intubate the vessel deeply to obtain adequate backup support. In these situations, it is important that the guiding catheter does not encroach the stent balloon since this may contort the stent. If the patient is likely to become ischemic during this sometimes prolonged maneuver, the prior placement of an intra-aortic balloon pump will allow time to position the stent.

Retrieving Stents

In the event that a stent cannot be deployed in the desired location or when a stent has been contorted during passage, the stent balloon with the undeployed stent is slowly withdrawn to the mouth of the guide catheter. Using an extension wire, a loop is formed at the aortic root as the guide catheter and stent balloon are withdrawn as one unit through the arterial sheath. If the stent gets caught in the valve of the sheath, the sheath should be removed together with the stent balloon/guide catheter as one unit over the intracoronary guidewire. Care must be taken to ensure that the stent balloon is inside the sheath. With smaller stents and superlarge lumen 8-F or above guiding catheters, it is possible to remove the stent through the guide. Undue force must never be used since the stent may become degloved off the balloon. The stent is usually warped by the time it is retrieved and should be discarded. A new sheath is then inserted carefully over the extra support wire. By leaving the coronary guidewire in place as the guide catheter and stent balloon are removed, one can ensure that the stent will remain on the guidewire even if it is inadvertently sleeved off the balloon. The stent can then be retrieved by grabbing the stent wire with an endomyocardial bioptome or a special removal device (Cook) or by threading a balloon through the stent and inflating to low pressure within or distal to the stent before withdrawal.

POSTSTENT MANAGEMENT

A dramatic change has occurred in poststent management over the last 2 years. Recent studies have shown that anticoagulation can be safely withheld when adequate stent expansion is achieved and flow optimized in the stented and adjacent segments. To ensure even and proper stent strut expansion, supplemental high-pressure balloon dilation is vital. The poststent antithrombotic protocol, which used to consist of aspirin, persantin, dextran, heparin, and warfarin, has been reduced to simply aspirin with or without ticlopidine in many centers. This regimen has led to a reduction in bleeding complications and hospital stay. Nevertheless, patients should preferably be managed in a specialized unit manned by nurses skilled in the management of poststent patients. Because of a small risk of coronary spasm, patients routinely receive a calcium channel blocker and intravenous nitroglycerin for at least 24 hours following stenting.

Poststent heparin infusion is no longer routinely used in many centers including ours. Sheaths are removed within 6 hours or when the ACT has fallen to lower than 150 seconds. Where heparin infusion is considered necessary, heparin is held for several hours to allow the ACT to fall to 150 to 170 seconds when the sheaths are removed and pressure applied with a mechanical compression device (e.g., Clamp Ease, Pressure Products, Malibu, CA) for 1 hour or until hemostasis is achieved. Heparin is restarted at 800 to 1,000 U/hr without a bolus 2 to 3 hours after hemostasis is achieved. The activated partial thromboplastin time (PTT) is kept between 55 and 75 seconds.

Coumadin is also no longer used in many centers including ours. Uncomplicated patients are discharged the next day. Patients stented during or soon after acute myocardial infarction or those with markedly suboptimal results after stenting are put on subcutaneous low molecular weight heparin 30 mg bid for 10 days. For patients in whom anticoagulation with heparin and coumadin are deemed necessary, a 3- to 4-day gradual mobilization program in which the patients spend the first 2 days in bed is recommended to reduce bleeding complications. Soluble aspirin (325 mg bid) and ticlopidine (250 mg bid) are continued throughout this time together with an H_2 receptor antagonist and a stool softener.

Bleeding

The reported incidence of bleeding complications in the anticoagulation era was around 6%. This figure is expected to decrease further with current protocols using no anticoagulation. The puncture site is the most common site of bleeding among stent patients. In the multicenter registry, of 83 bleeding complications (in 79 patients) requiring transfusion after stent placement, most (69%) of the bleeding complications involved the femoral arterial puncture site.[2] Gastrointestinal bleeding requiring transfusion occurred in 1.8%, genitourinary bleeding in 0.8%, retroperitoneal bleeding in 0.8%, and intracranial bleeding in 0.2%. In patients receiving anticoagulation, careful monitoring with the use of flow sheets to document anticoagulation results and a graduated mobilization protocol is useful in reducing the incidence of bleeding. Most puncture site bleeding occurs within the first few days, while the patient is still in hospital. In clinical situations where bleeding is not life threatening and may be related to high-dose heparin given at the time of the procedure (e.g., epitaxis, hematuria, or mild hemoptysis within the first 24 hours), anticoagulation, if deemed necessary, may be reinstituted once hemostasis is achieved. Where bleeding is significant and related to anticoagulation (e.g., large groin hematoma or retroperitoneal bleed), anticoagulation should be stopped while leaving the patient on antiplatelet therapy only, especially if a large stent was used and there was a good poststent angiographic result. When bleeding is life threatening (e.g., upper gastrointestinal tract bleed or hemoptysis causing respiratory distress), all anticoagulation and antiplatelet therapy should be stopped and the patient observed carefully over 7 to 10 days for ischemic symptoms suggesting stent thrombosis.

Management of Stent Thrombosis

In the Gianturco-Roubin stent registry series, in which 38% of the patients received a stent 2.5 mm or less in size, the incidence of stent thrombosis was 5% for the 1990 to 1991 cohort. In a more recent series of 300 vessels stented with the Gianturco-Roubin stent, the incidence of stent thrombosis was only 2% when the stent used was more than 3 mm in diameter.[3] Stent thrombosis is invariably related to complex anatomy and dissections that cannot be completely controlled with stenting. Improved implantation techniques of the Gianturco-Roubin stent and optimal sizing may further reduce the incidence of stent thrombosis.[4] Bolus intravenous heparin (5,000 to 10,000 U), especially when APTT is subtherapeutic, may be useful in stabilizing the patient while preparing for urgent recatheterization. Stent thrombosis can be managed by redilation with or without bolus thrombolytic therapy. In patients with a large thrombus burden despite bolus thrombolytics, overnight intracoronary infusion of urokinase may be considered either before or after redilation. Occasional bleeding from the previous puncture site can be managed by using the FemoStop or C-clamp. In patients who are not deemed ideal candidates for

redilation or in those for whom thrombolytic therapy is contraindicated, emergency bypass surgery should be considered.

FOLLOW-UP

Stent or anticoagulation education (or both) are given to all patients before discharge to their referring physician for follow-up. Aspirin (325 mg bid), ticlopidine (250 mg bid), nitrates, calcium channel blocker, and H_2 receptor antagonists are continued for 4 weeks. Since the stent is fully endothelialized by 3 weeks, ticlopidine with or without anticoagulation may be stopped at this time or earlier if the patient experiences side effects or bleeding complications. By 4 weeks, the patient is left on only 325 mg or 1 enteric-coated aspirin per day unless residual disease is present. Repeat angiography at 2 months is recommended for those with suboptimal results, especially when large amounts of myocardium are at risk. Angiographic follow-up is also recommended for patients with extensive dissections requiring multiple stents and patients stented for long (>20 mm) dissections. Restenosis within the stent should be treated by balloon dilation. Laser and directional athrectomy are not recommended. These patients do not require additional anticoagulation at the time of the second procedure.

RESULTS: SHORT AND LONG-TERM

In the multicenter registry, from September 1988 to June 1991, 518 patients underwent attempted stenting with the 20-mm-long Gianturco-Roubin stent (indication for stenting was acute closure in 31% and threatened closure in 69%).[2] Successful deployment was achieved in 494 patients (95.4%). Despite the indications for stent placement and patient population, overall in-hospital results showed a patient mortality of 2.2%, Q-wave myocardial infarction in 3.0%, and non-Q-wave myocardial infarction in 2.5%. Emergency CABG was performed in 4.3%, and a further 3.0% had CABG before hospital discharge. Except for CABG, no significant difference was seen in the incidence of adverse events between the acute closure group and the threatened closure group. Table 54-3 lists the incidence of death, CABG, and myocardial infarction for the acute closure group, threatened closure group, and the group as a whole from the registry. Results from the 1985 to 1986 National Heart, Lung, and Blood Institute (NHLBI)

Table 54-3. Incidence of Adverse Events due to Acute and Threatened Closure Complicating PTCA: Stenting (2) Compared with NHLBI PTCA Registry (5)

	1985–1986 NHLBI PTCA Registry (n = 122)	Stenting (%)		
		Threatened Closure (n = 337)	Acute Closure (n = 156)	Overall (n = 493)
CABG				
Emergency	35.0	2.7	7.7	4.3
Nonemergency	5.0	2.1	5.1	3.0
Within 6 months of discharge	5.8	8.3	3.8	6.9
Cumulative at 6 months	45.8	13.1	16.6	14.2
Myocardial infarction				
In-hospital	40.2	4.5	7.6	5.5
Within 6 months of discharge	0.8	1.5	1.9	1.6
Cumulative at 6 months	41.0	6.0	9.5	7.1
Death				
In-hospital	5.0	2.1	2.6	2.2
Within 6 months of discharge	1.6	1.2	1.9	1.4
Cumulative at 6 months	6.6	3.3	4.5	3.6

PTCA registry are listed alongside for comparison.[5] In the NHLBI report, of 122 patients with periprocedural occlusion, 60 patients (49%) were successfully redilated with PTCA. Of those who were not successfully redilated, 43 (35%) were managed by CABG, and 19 (16%) were managed medically. In-hospital mortality was 5% in each of these treatment groups. Incidence of myocardial infarction was 27% for the PTCA group, 49% for the medically managed group, and 56% for the emergency CABG group. Another 10% of the initially redilated group eventually underwent CABG before hospital discharge. These data are representative of many such studies done over the last 10 years. Taking into consideration that one is comparing with historical controls or across different cohorts, results from the stent series compare favorably with those reported in all previous studies, both in-hospital and at 6 months. These studies reported the need for in-hospital CABG in 33 to 41% of cases and an incidence of myocardial infarction from 28 to 54%.

Stent Thrombosis

In the registry series, stent thrombosis occurred in 8.7%.[2] Of 300 vessels (288 patients) stented at our institution from October 1989 to February 1992, stent thrombosis developed in 22 patients (22 vessels, 7%) at 6 ± 3 days (range, 0 to 11 days) after stenting.[3] The most significant predictors of stent thrombosis were (1) poststenting residual dissection and (2) use of a stent with a diameter of 2.5 mm

or less. Poststent residual dissection was associated with a thrombosis rate of 29% compared with 5% when dissection was absent. Use of stents 2.5 mm or smaller was associated with a thrombosis rate of 13% compared with 2% when stents 3.0 mm or more were used. Vessels with a residual filling defect were associated with a thrombosis rate of 12% compared with 7% when residual filling defect was absent. Twenty-one of the 22 patients (95%) with stent thrombosis had either stents 2.5 mm or less, residual dissection, or a residual filling defect. When both residual dissection or luminal filling defect and a small stent were present, the incidence of thrombosis was 9 of 30 (30%). When none of these characteristics were present, the incidence of thrombosis was only 1 of 125 (1%, $P <$ 0.001). The learning curve appears to play a part. As the operators became more experienced, stents were sized more generously, greater care was taken to cover all dissection adequately, and anticoagulation was managed more meticulously. In that series of patients stented with severe dissection, threatened closure, or established closure, our incidence of stent thrombosis was 12% for the first 50 vessels stented, 8% for the next 50 vessels, and 6% for the last 200 vessels stented. A parallel fall has also been observed in the multicenter registry.

Bleeding

The problem of bleeding in stented patients has followed a similar course. Initially, both the University of Alabama and the multicenter registry had a 25%

incidence of bleeding, requiring a transfusion of 2 units or more. This has progressively fallen to 6% in the last 6 months of the registry. It should be noted that more mortality and morbidity arise from bleeding complications than from stent thrombosis. In our series of 288 stented patients, three deaths were related to major bleeding (one from pulmonary hemorrhage and two from multiorgan failure following surgical repair for ongoing groin bleeding), whereas only one death was related to stent thrombosis. The incidence of bleeding and vascular complications has fallen dramatically with the current practice of using only antiplatelet agents and no anticoagulation in the poststent protocol.

Restenosis

In the multicenter registry, angiographic follow-up in 338 patients at 181 ± 47 days showed a restenosis rate of 39% (defined as >50% stenosis).[2] Importantly, 37.7% of the patients stented had a 2.5 mm or less stent placed, and the indication for stenting was usually severe vessel wall disruption. Restenosis rates of 50 to 70% have been reported in similar populations of patients treated medically. Recent practice of the new sizing strategy, increased attention to the technical details of stent placement, and supplemental inflations to achieve a smooth lumen appears to reduce further the incidence of stent thrombosis and restenosis.[4] In a recent controlled study, 66 patients with class B or C lesions who had more than 0.3-mm minimal luminal diameter loss at 24-hour angiography were randomized to medical therapy or the Gianturco-Roubin stent.[6] At 4 (±1) months' follow-up, restenosis (≥50% stenosis) was present in 76% of the medical group whereas the stented group had a restenosis rate of only 21% ($P < 0.001$).

Experience with the use of this stent for acute or threatened closure in saphenous vein grafts is also encouraging. Of 54 stents deployed in the vein grafts of 46 patients, angiographic follow-up at a mean time of 5 ± 1.8 months in 40 patients (87%) showed a restenosis rate of 30%. Larger stents (3.5 mm or more) appeared to be associated with a lower rate of restenosis.

CURRENT INDICATIONS

The flexible coil stent is currently indicated in acute and threatened closure following angioplasty. Although the FDA-approved indication is limited to the above clinical situations, a recent study suggests that the flexible coil stent may also be useful in situations of recurrent restenosis where elastic recoil may be a predisposing factor.[6]

COSTS

Hospital Stay

In the days of routine anticoagulation, the main additional cost was the extra 3 to 4 days of hospital stay, which amounted to a total of $1,500 to $2,000 plus laboratory charges. This extra cost is no longer relevant in this "no-anticoagulation" era.

Equipments and Drug Costs

Large-bore Tuohy-Borst adapters, guiding catheters, and 0.018″ compatible balloon catheters are similar in price to those used in standard angioplasty procedures. They should not add to the cost of the procedure if this equipment was chosen at the outset of the case. The current cost of the stent is around $1,000. If an additional high-pressure balloon is required, this adds around $600. An extra support wire or an "exchange" catheter (or both) costs around $100. Ticlopidine and H_2 receptor antagonist cost around $60 and $90, respectively, for 4 weeks of therapy.

A previous study (in the anticoagulation era) at our institution on cost savings from using the stent instead of emergency CABG for acute closure complicating PTCA showed that the mean individual patient cost for PTCA, PTCA with stent, and PTCA with emergency CABG was $8,061, $13,787, and $39,310, respectively. Thus, although stenting for acute closure would add around $5,700 to the procedure, the savings compared with emergency CABG were over $25,000. When we add the reduced incidence of myocardial infarction, far less discomfort, and earlier return to work, stenting is clearly a more attractive solution. This cost savings is more marked now that most patients are discharged the next day.

CURRENT OUTLOOK AND FUTURE DEVELOPMENTS

The flexible coil stent is an indispensable tool in our center and others. It has largely reduced the complications associated with acute vessel closure and the need for urgent CABG. In the past, stent thrombosis and bleeding had resulted in significant morbidity and mortality. With experience in deployment techniques, patient selection, sizing, and supplemental high-pressure balloon inflations to ensure proper embedment of the stent struts, the incidence of stent thrombosis has been reduced. This has allowed a reduction in the degree of anticoagulation and even eliminated the need for anticoagulation in most patients, resulting in less bleeding complications and a shortened hospital stay.

A new generation flexible coil stent (GR II) is currently under clinical evaluation. The architecture is based on the current stent's design, and the stent is constructed of a flat wire and strengthened with an additional backbone. The stent has a lower profile, is more trackable, and can be delivered through a 6-F guiding catheter for stent sizes 4.0 mm or less. Ultra radiopaque gold markers at each end of the stent ensures accurate placement. Mounted on a 0.014″ high-pressure, noncompliant balloon, it obviates the need for an additional high-pressure balloon for postdeployment dilation. It is available in sizes up to 4.5 and 5.0 mm (delivered through a 7-F guiding catheter) and lengths up to 40 mm. To target the problem of stent thrombosis, research is being done on prototypes coated with antiplatelet agents and thrombin inhibitors such as heparin, hirudin, and hirulog.

REFERENCES

1. Roubin GS, Cannon AD, Agrawal SK et al. Intracoronary stenting for acute and threatened closure complicating percutaneous transluminal coronary angioplasty. Circulation 1992;85:916–27
2. George BS, Voorhees WD, Roubin GS et al. Multicenter investigation of coronary stenting to treat acute or threatened closure after percutaneous transluminal coronary angioplasty: clinical and angiographic outcomes. J Am Coll Cardiol 1993;22:135–43
3. Agrawal SK, Ho DSW, Liu MW, et al. Predictors of thrombotic complications following placement of the flexible coil stent. Am J Cardiol 1994;73:1216–9
4. Ho DSW, Liu MW, Iyer S, Parks JM, Roubin GS. Sizing the Gianturco-Roubin coronary flexible coil stent. Cathet Cardiovasc Diagn 1994;32:242–8
5. Detre KM, Holmes Jr DR, Holubkov R et al. Incidence and consequences of periprocedural occlusion: the 1985–1986 National Heart, Lung, and Blood Institute's Percutaneous Transluminal Coronary Angioplasty Registry. Circulation 1990;82:739–50
6. Rodriguez A, Santaera O, Larribau M et al. Coronary stenting decreases restenosis in lesions with early loss in luminal diatmeter 24 hours after successful PTCA. Circulation 1995;91:1397–1402

55 The ACS Multi-Link Stent System

Ulrich Sigwart

Stenting of arteries with adequate devices produces better primary results than any other angioplasty technique.[1,2] The results of randomized trials have highlighted the role of stents in the prevention of restenosis and in the reduction of clincal events.[3,4] Stent technology is still in its infancy. From experimental work and clinical trials it has become clear that all stents used over the last few years exhibit important shortcomings. The stent first used in humans, the Wallstent, soon acquired a reputation of being difficult to handle.[5] Although it is very flexible, the deployment of this stent indeed requires training.[6,7] The shortening of the stent during deployment makes the implanted length difficult to predict. Side branch access is impossible after placement of this stent, and the wire crossings may promote a higher rate of thrombosis compared with stents that are composed of one layer of material only. The Palmaz-Schatz stent is generally stiff, and only short segments, individually placed or connected via an articulation, can be used in tortuous arteries.[8] Side branch access is virtually impossible after placement of this stent, as it is with the Wallstent. The balloon expansion of the stent causes significant stresses at the bend points and results in twisting of the struts, thus augmenting the stent profile and the degree of turbulence. Expansion is uneven in most cases, and embolization from the carrier balloon has also been reported.[9]

The flexible balloon-expandable stents (Gianturco-Roubin, Wiktor, Strecker) suffer from reduced resistance to external radial force, leading to recoil after placement, and higher wire profile, with its inherent problems related to turbulence and large gap size.

The Strecker stent adds to these problems the feature of wire crossings.[10–12]

Clinical observations confirm these concerns. The thrombosis rate is still unacceptably high for vessels under 3-mm diameter,[13] embolization of friable atheroma cannot always be prevented by stents with a large gap size, and restenosis figures differ substantially between different stents.[14] Our aim was to develop a metallic stent combining the most desirable positive features while avoiding the negative features of currently available stents.

DESIGN GOALS

A stent used for the treatment of vascular dissections as well as the prevention of restenosis should be strong enough to withstand some radial pressure, should have a relatively small gap size, to tack up even smaller dissections or friable material, should have a low profile, not creating excessive turbulence to the blood stream, and should be flexible. It should also allow easy delivery without the danger of embolization of the stent. A low metal surface ought to be one of the essentials of such a stent. It should not shorten with expansion, should be available in various diameters and lengths to avoid placement of multiple stents, and should allow side branch access in case of need. A stent is described below in which these design goals were observed as much as possible.

MECHANISM OF ACTION

Balloon expansion was chosen for its reliable and precise positioning. Balloon expansion also allows for embedding of the stent structures and smoothing of the internal arterial surface (Swiss Kiss) without further manipulation. The drawbacks of balloon expansion reside in the danger of balloon rupture; therefore the internal stent surface must be adequately smooth and the balloon possibly be protected by a safety membrane. A layer of silicone-based elastic material can be used for this purpose. This membrane also tends to prevent dislocation of the stent before deployment and a more even distribution of forces during balloon expansion.

Stainless steel was selected for its physical properties. It has never been shown that tantalum, which is more brittle, attracts less thrombus compared with stainless steel. Different 316L stainless steel manufacturing processes were evaluated until appropriate tensile and microstructural properties were found. The stent structure is comprised of polished corrugated rings interconnected by small bridges (Fig. 55-1). The thickness of each individual ring is approximately 50 μm. This makes the strut thickness significantly less compared with any other stent design. The generously spaced interconnecting struts do not interfere with its flexiblity and thereby allow for virtually unlimited stent length. The gaps are smaller compared with the stents described above, thus creating a smoother vascular surface and reducing the amount of turbulence. Smaller gaps create a uniform support, which is able to tack up small flaps and dissections. By refining the mesh, the metal-to-air ratio of the stent surface could be reduced by 35% compared with the Palmaz-Schatz stent. To control the amount of stress and avoid fractures during expansion, the expansion ratio must be keep within certain limits. For this reason different stents with 0.25-mm-diameter increments are being used. The stent was tested in a purposely built pulse duplicator that not only mimics the cyclic changes of systolic and diastolic arterial diameter but also the contraction and relaxation movements imposed by the beating heart, which produce bending. The pulse duplicator testing verified the structural integrity of the stent design after 380 million cycles, corresponding to 10 years of actual life.

The collapse pressure of this stent is slightly lower than that of the Palmaz-Schatz stent but higher compared with the original and revised version of the self-expanding mesh stent, the Gianturco-Roubin stent, and the Wiktor stent. The structure of the stent allows easy side branch assess and even dilation of bifurcations. In this respect it resembles the Gianturco-Roubin and Wiktor stents without comprising on structural integrity.

Uneven expansion remains a major challenge for all balloon-expandable stents. An innovative balloon wrapping technique consisting of multiple small folds arranged in a spiral pattern was developed to guarantee even expansion of all segments. The stent, which is crimped on a stretchable elastic membrane covering the entire delivery balloon, is protected externally by a tubular sleeve of 5 F outer dimensions. The distal end of this sleeve is tapered. A metal radiopaque marker allows identification of the sleeve position in relation to the two balloon markers, which indicate the stent position on the delivery balloon. Sleeve withdrawal can be performed with one hand with the help of a specially designed manipulator. The sheath is lubricated with saline using a syringe. A push-button action on the manipulator is initiated to unblock the safety mechanism. after which the stent is exposed on the delivery balloon. Once the desirable position is confirmed, the aspiration-prepped balloon is inflated to a pressure of 8 bar and then deflated. The system is withdrawn without further manipulation.

TESTING

Rabbit Experiments

The first prototypes of the stent were implanted in rabbit aortas and iliac arteries. Insertion was performed via the carotid artery. There were no deployment failures, with the stent crimped onto the early prototype delivery balloon without any sheath protection. When the stent was implanted in the common iliac artery, the internal iliac artery leaving from the stented area could invariably be catheterized using the delivery balloon. We have not observed any thrombotic occlusions and the stent was typically imbedded in new intimal lining after the third week.

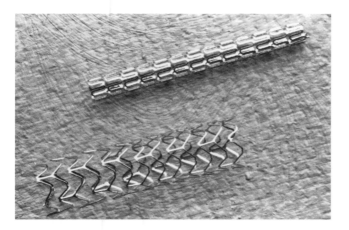

Fig. 55-1. Metallic stent composed of multiple corrugated rings individually bridged.

Canine Experiments

The final stent design was used in coronary arteries in 28 dogs.[15] Due to its flexibility the stent could be easily delivered and precisely deployed in all cases. Thirteen 3.0-mm and 15 3.5-mm stents were deployed in 11 left anterior descending coronary arteries and in 17 circumflex coronary arteries. The dogs were pretreated with Aspirin and dipyridamole and received heparin and dextran 40 during the implantation procedure.

Angiographic follow-up revealed thrombolysis in myocardial infarction (TIMI) grade 3 angiographic patency at 3 days in 5 cases, at 2 weeks in 5 cases, at 1 month in 5 cases, and at 6 months in 10 cases; one animal was kept for 1 year follow-up.

There were no deaths and no acute thrombotic events. At 2 weeks and 1 month the stent surface was endothelialized from 80 to 100%. At 6 months and 1 year the stents were all 100% endothelialized. There was no evidence of thrombus formation or excessive neointimal hypoplasia.

Human Experience

The stent was first used at the Royal Brompton Hospital in suboptimal results and abrupt closure after percutaneous transluminal coronary angioplasty in 10 pilot cases.[16] It has been used in a multicenter European registry and there are also plans to extend the clinical experience to a randomized study involving primary lesions. This stent became commercially available as of November 1995.

CONCLUSIONS

This new low-profile flexible stainless steel balloon-expandable stent overcomes some of the shortcomings of existing stent technology. Its main features are good hemodynamic characteristics and excellent conformability, as well as preserved access to side branches. Early clinical results are favorable; however, comparisons with other stents are pending, and antithrombotic coatings are being investigated.

REFERENCES

1. Serruys PW, Juilliere Y, Bertrand ME, Puel J, Rickards AF, Sigwart U. Additional improvement of stenosis geometry in human coronary arteries by stenting after balloon dilatation. Am J Cardiol 1988;61:71G–76G
2. Kaufmann U, Sigwart U. Suppression of residual pressure gradients after angioplasty by stenting. J Interv Cardiol 1989;2:5–8
3. Serruys PW, de Jaegere P, Kiemeneij C et al. A comparison of balloon expandable stent implantation with balloon angioplasty in patients with coronary artery disease (The Benestent study). N Engl J Med 1994;331:489–95
4. Fichman DL, Leon MB, Baim DS et al. A randomized comparison of coronary stent placement and balloon angioplasty in the treatment of coronary artery disease (The STRESS trial). N Engl J Med 1994;331:496–501
5. Sigwart U, Puel J, Mirkovitch V, Joffre F, Kappenberger L. Intravascular stents to prevent occlusion and restenosis after transluminal angioplasty. N Engl J Med 1987;316:701–6
6. Sigwart U, Urban P, Sadeghi H, Kappenberger L. Implantation of 100 intracoronary stent. Learning curve effect on the occurrence of acute complications, abstracted. J Am Coll Cardiol 1989;13:107a
7. Sigwart U. The self expanding stent. pp. 605–27. In Topol E (ed): Textbook of Interventional Cardiology. WB Saunders, Philadelphia, 1990
8. Schatz R. A view of vascular stents. Circulation 1989;79:445–57
9. Schatz RA, Baim DS, Leon M et al. Clinical experience with the Palmaz-Schatz coronary stent. Circulation 1991;83:148–161
10. Roubin GS, Robinson KA, King SB et al. Early and late results of intracoronary arterial stenting after coronary angioplasty in dogs. Circulation 1987;76:891–7
11. de Jaegere PP, Serruys PW, Bertand M et al. Wiktor stent implantation in patients with restenosis following balloon angioplasty of a native coronary artery. Am J Cardiol 1992;69:589–602
12. Reifart N, Langer A, Stoerger H et al. Strecker stent as a bail out device following percutaneous transluminal coronary angioplasty. J Interv Cardiol 1992;5:79–83
13. Ellis SG, Savage MP, Fischman DL et al. Restenosis after placement of Palmaz-Schatz stents in native coronary arteries: initial results of a multi-centre experience. Circulation 1992;86:1836–44
14. Sigwart U. Coronary stents: will they survive? pp. 169–178. In: Sigwart U, Frank G.I. (eds): Coronary Stents. Springer-Verlag, New York, 1992
15. Sigwart U, Khosravi F, Virmani R et al. Bronco: ein neuer, Balloon-expandierbarer flexibler stent. Z Kardiol 1993;82:71
16. Sigwart U, Haber RH, Kowlachuk GJ, Simonton CA, Virmani R. Bronco: a new balloon expandable coronary stent. Eur Heart J 1993

56 Temporary Stenting With the ACS Flow Support Catheter

Simon Gibbs

Ulrich Sigwart

Temporary stents are intended to treat abrupt coronary artery closure following balloon dilation. The first temporary stent was developed by Dr. Phillipe Gaspard in Lyon, in association with ACS, (Santa Clara, CA). Animal experiments began in 1986; the stent was first tested in the rabbit abdominal aorta and later in the coronary artery of the dog.[1,2] Clinical evaluation was undertaken in 1988, and international multicenter evaluation began in 1991.[3]

The aim was to develop an effective perfusion device to restore myocardial perfusion after abrupt vessel closure. The device was intended both as a bridge and to reduce the need for emergency coronary artery surgery. Since the temporary stent would be removed, anticoagulation following the procedure would be unnecessary. Compared with perfusion balloons the temporary stent would perfuse the side branches across which it would expand and would have proven flow characteristics.

MECHANISM OF ACTION

The mechanism of action is shown in Figure 56-1. The collapsed stent is positioned across the area of coronary artery dissection (Fig. 56-1A). A screw action manipulator on the proximal end of the catheter is used to expand the cage to the desired size and collapse it as required (Fig. 56-1B). As the cage expands it shortens. The cage works on the one-size-fits-all principle. It can be expanded up to a maximum diameter of 4 mm and exerts a low radial force (up to 300 mmHg) on the vessel wall. Since the mesh of the cage allows the blood to flow through it, side branches that have been covered by the cage remain perfused. At the end of the procedure the screw action manipulator is used to collapse the cage, which can then be removed.

The temporary stent is used in the event of abrupt vessel closure; an angioplasty guidewire 0.014″ in diameter is positioned across the area of closure. A 10-ml syringe filled with heparinized saline is connected to the side arm of the proximal adapter on the catheter. After the protective sheath from the expandable wire cage is removed, the screw action manipulator is rotated until the cage is fully expanded, while saline is drawn into the barrel of the manipulator. The screw action manipulator is then rotated in the opposite direction to collapse the cage. This action also flushes the catheter. The cage is resheathed with the clear protective sheath, and then the packaging stilette is removed from the distal lumen of the cage. The catheter is then loaded onto the guidewire, which has been positioned in the coronary artery. Only after the guidewire exits from the notch located 30 cm from the tip of the catheter should the protective sheath around the wire cage be removed. The catheter is then advanced along the guidewire through the Y-connector assembly and into the guiding catheter.

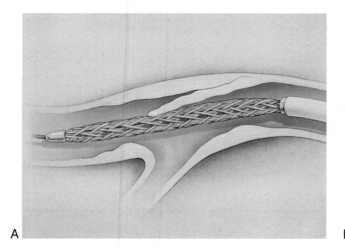
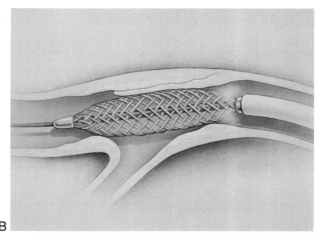
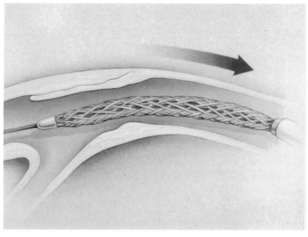

Fig. 56-1. Schematic diagram of the flow support catheter. **(A)** An intimal dissection at the site of a side branch. The collapsed metal cage has been advanced across the site of stenosis. **(B)** The cage has been expanded. Luminal stenosis is reduced, and the side branch can now be perfused. **(C)** The cage is collapsed and can now be withdrawn back into the guide catheter. The dissection flap is adherent to the vessel wall (From Gibbs et al.,[4] with permission.)

PATIENT POPULATION

The stent is appropriate for patients undergoing routine coronary angioplasty in whom there is an acute impairment of coronary blood flow after balloon inflation or a poor angiographic result requiring intervention to prevent impaired blood flow. Patients should be candidates for coronary artery surgery. The temporary stent cannot be used if the vessel size is larger than the maximum size of the cage. The minimum vessel diameter should be about 2.5 mm.

PRETREATMENT

The patient should have received aspirin before the angioplasty procedure and should be heparinized during the procedure to maintain an activated clotting time in the range of 300 to 750 seconds.

OPERATIVE TECHNIQUE AND TIPS

The tip of the catheter is composed of a moderately radiopaque braided wire mesh cage (30 mm long) permanently attached to a 3.7-F catheter. Radiopaque markers are found at each end of the cage.

Care should be taken in advancing the catheter into the coronary artery since the temporary stent is stiffer than a normal angioplasty balloon. The two radiopaque markers at either end of the cage are well seen on fluoroscopy. They should be positioned across the area of vessel closure so that the device is more than half way across the injured area of the vessel. As the cage is expanded it will also shorten. The larger the vessel diameter the greater will be the shortening. The expanded cage should cover branches arising at the site of vessel closure, since this will improve their perfusion. An angiogram should be performed once the temporary stent has been positioned. If the position is at first inadequate, the device is easily collapsed, repositioned, and re-expanded until the optimum position is found.

During device expansion, the blood pressure and electrocardiogram (ECG) should be monitored. If the patient develops chest pain or if ECG changes occur, clotting should be checked and a repeat angiogram performed to ensure that the device is not becoming blocked. Chest pain and ECG changes may occur if the device is not optimally positioned, and in this case repositioning may result in resolution of the problem.

The guidewire must not be withdrawn into the catheter because the stent cage cannot be manipulated unless it is mounted on a guidewire. When the temporary stent is used as a bridge to surgery, the device should be removed after the affected coronary artery has been grafted. The temporary stent should remain in a coronary artery for up to 12 hours. The optimal duration for temporary stenting is still unknown.

POST OPERATIVE MANAGEMENT

Since the temporary stent is completely removed after use, no specific postoperative management is required.

FOLLOW-UP

Follow-up should be conducted according to the outcome of the procedure during which the temporary stent was used. If the temporary stent produced a satisfactory result, follow-up should be the same as for routine balloon angioplasty.

RESULTS

Two clinical trials of the temporary stent as a bail-out procedure have been performed. The trials vary only in a minor protocol difference. Patients were selected on the basis of angiographic evidence of an inadequate result of coronary angioplasty associated with local dissection of the coronary artery, angina, or ECG changes. The temporary stent was placed across the dissection for 30 minutes, after which the stent was collapsed and the result reviewed by the investigator. The investigator then had the option to expand the stent for a further 30 minutes if desired.

Clinical and angiographic variables were collected at baseline during the procedure and at follow-up. This phase I study differed from the second, phase II study in that the two stent expansions were for periods of 60 minutes in the phase II trial.

The results of both trials were similar. Phase I consisted of 56 patients enrolled during 1991 to 1992. The use of the temporary stent following dissection of the coronary artery restored antegrade blood flow, reduced angina, and tended to normalize ECG abnormalities. The average time of cage expansion was 68 minutes. In one case there was an expansion time of 720 minutes and the patient was managed in the coronary care unit over night. After the temporary stent was collapsed, although dissection improved in about three-fourths of the patients, it was resolved in only 16%. As regards in-hospital outcome, over half the patients had a secondary intervention after the use of the temporary stent; coronary artery surgery was required in 31%. Myocardial infarction occurred in 22% of this clinically unstable group. One patient died, but this was not attributed to the device. The device provided good coronary perfusion as a bridge to coronary artery surgery in 73% of the patients in whom this was attempted.

In the phase II study 53 subjects were enrolled during 1992 to 1993. The average cage expansion time was 75 minutes. The dissection grade was improved in half the patients following the use of the temporary stent, and in 33% of patients there was no evidence of the initial dissection at the end of the procedure. In 13% of the subjects a Q-wave myocardial infarction occurred. Coronary artery surgery was required in 24%.

The experience of one center has been published[4]; patients requiring bail-out treatment at the time of balloon angioplasty underwent the insertion of a temporary stent.[4] The device improved coronary blood flow in all cases, with a reduction in luminal stenosis and resolution of symptoms. It was expanded for an average of 85 (range, 300 to 209) minutes. In six patients it was used as a bridge to further treatment (permanent stent in four and coronary artery surgery, in two), and two patients did not need further treatment. The authors emphasize its ease of use for operators with limited or no experience with permanent stents.

The temporary stent easily accessed and crossed target lesions when coronary angioplasty had failed. The expanded stent provided good blood flow to the distal coronary artery and improved angina and ECG changes. Complete resolution of the dissection was achieved in only one-third of patients. The device is an effective bridge to coronary artery surgery, in par-

stent could be deployed by inserting it as a straight wire through a tube with cold saline injection. A similar technique was suggested later for insertion of a nitinol coil stent into the aorta of animals.[12] These techniques involved inserting the straightened stent, which is kept below the transition temperature in the martensitic shape, by ice-saline injections. On delivery to its site, the stent is heated by the blood and resumes it original shape and dimensions. Another type of vascular nitinol prothesis was tested in carotid and iliofemoral applications in dogs.[13] Excellent patency and compatibility with the nitinol material was demonstrated without evidence of inflammation or thrombosis.

The longest clinical experience with vascular nitinol stents comes from Russia for peripheral[14] and renal indications.[15] A nitinol spiral was implanted in peripheral arteries in 121 locations over 5 years. Acute patency was achieved in 93.7%; however, the long-term results were poor for the superficial femoral and popliteal arteries.

Nitinol stents for coronary application have been previously designed and tested in dogs.[16,17] Designed as a dense coil, this stent is tightly wound on a catheter at a temperature below the transition temperature and deployed using high-temperature (70° to 80°) saline injection to regain its memorized deployed configuration. Preliminary work with these stents showed that the spacing between the coils is important to minimize the proliferative process and maintain side branch patency.[18,19]

THE SELF-EXPANDING NITINOL VASCULAR AND CORONARY STENT

Design

A nitinol self-expandable stent with a special restraining mechanism was recently developed and used in extravascular applications.[20] This stent utilizes the material properties of nitinol differently than other nitinol stents. The stent is designed as a coil with two terminal end balls for mounting. An example of the stent mounted on the delivery catheter and in its released configuration is shown in Figure 57-1. The stent is restrained on the catheter at its proximal and distal terminal balls by string ties, which are released by a single metal wire hooked to the pulley-handle at the proximal end of the catheter. The stent is mounted on the catheter, with a densely coiled distal portion and a proximal portion with coil density equal to that of the released stent (Fig. 57-1B), so that the proximal portion of the stent corre-

sponds to the final length of the released stent. To deploy, the release wire is pulled back and sequential releases of the distal and proximal ends of the stent occur. The stent immediately uncoils as it expands, reaching its final dimensions.

Because of its length, the peripheral stent is restrained on the catheter at the two ends as well as in the middle (Fig. 57-2). The loose windings in the middle of the stent, which correspond to the released stent length, are embraced by dense windings on each side. Using two wires, the distal and proximal parts are released first, and the middle restraint of the stent is released last (Fig. 57-2B), ensuring precise centering of the relatively long stent in the stenosis. The metal coverage of the endovascular area ranges between 7 and 15% depending on wire thickness and coil density.

Animal Experiments

A series of experiments in dogs, aimed at testing the safety and performance of the stents and the long-term histologic response of coronary arteries, were performed.[21–23] Stents were implanted in the coronary arteries of 23 dogs. Safety and reliability of stent deployment, full expansion, and patent lumen were proved. However, oversizing the stent to three times the arterial diameter resulted in acute arterial occlusion. Follow-up of up to 12 months for 16 dogs showed 100% patency at follow-up. Histologic studies showed an initial proliferative response starting at 2 weeks, followed by complete stent coverage with neointimal formation at 1 month. Mild-to-moderate intimal hyperplastic process was present at 3 to 6 months (Plate 1) and tended to regress at 12 months. Intimal thickness and the angiographic patency of the stented segment for the group of dogs is shown in Table 57-1. Note that intimal thickness shows a typical increase from 1 week to 3 months. However, after 3 months the intimal thickness did not increase. In summary, the experience in normal coronary arteries in dogs shows that (1) the stent can be safely and reliably implanted in coronary arteries, and (2) a modest intimal proliferative response to the self-expanding nitinol stent is not different from reports for other balloon-expandable metal stents.

Together with earlier reports on the biocompatibility of nitinol, current observations establish the role of nitinol as an important material for intravascular stents.[16,17,24–26]

Experience in Peripheral Arteries in Patients

Stents for peripheral use have so far been implanted in more than 20 patients, most of them in France.[27,28] The clinical protocol includes the following:

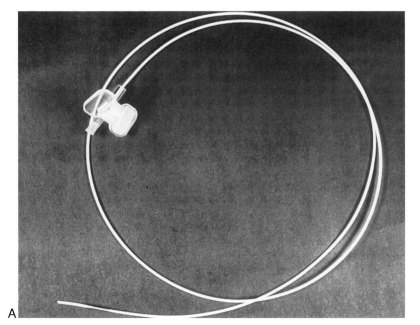

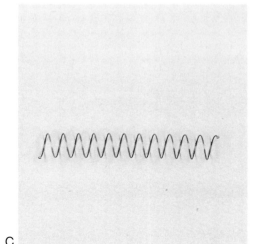

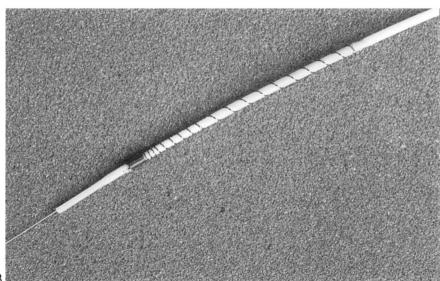

Fig. 57-1. (A) The coil stent mounted on the delivery catheter. **(B)** Note the densely wound distal portion and loosely wound proximal portion of the stent. On release of the distal tip of the stent, the entire stent uncoils as it expands, and the densely wound portion of the stent disappears. Final deployed stent location and length match the loosely wound portion of the mounted stent. **(C)** Released coronary stent.

Table 57-1. Angiographic Dimensions (D) at Follow-up Angiography and Intimal Thickness (IT) of the Stented Segment

Duration	1–2 weeks	1 mo	3 mo	6 mo	12 mo
D (mm)					
Control	2.6	2.9	2.6	2.6	3.0
Follow-up	2.5	2.7	2.6	2.7	3.0
IT (μm)	30 ± 10	141 ± 105	227 ± 104	211 ± 99	170 ± 42

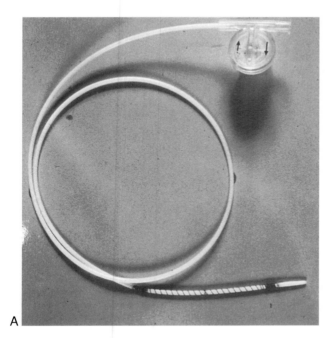

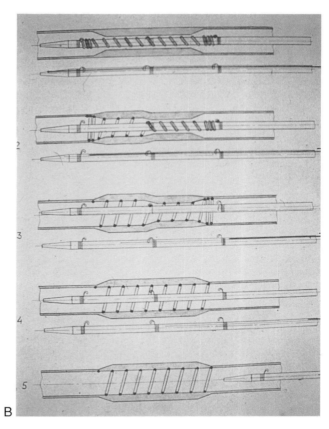

Fig. 57-2. (A) Mounted peripheral stent. Due to its length, it is restrained on the catheter at the two ends as well as in the middle. **(B)** Mechanism of release of the peripheral stent (see text for details).

1. On the day before implantation 100 mg aspirin, 20 mg/8hr nifedipine (or other equivalent calcium channel blocker) is started. An intravenous infusion of 150 mg heparin/24hr is started.
2. At procedure onset an intravenous bolus administration of 10,000 U of heparin and 3 cefamandole given over 30 minutes is started.
3. Subcutaneous heparin is administered twice daily for 2 weeks after the procedure.
4. Long-term treatment includes 100 mg aspirin daily and oral coumadin for 3 months.

Acute angiographic patency was checked by angiography at the time of the procedure. Venous angiography to show patency of the stent was performed the day following the procedure before discharge. Follow-up angiography was performed between 3 and 6 months.

An example of a stent in a femoral graft before and after release is shown in Figure 57-3. Note the two dense partitions at the proximal and distal ends of the stent before release, and the stent after full expansion. As the stent expands, the densely wound portion of the mounted stent disappears, and the

final length of the stent is equal to the central portion of the mounted stent. An angiographic view of the femoral artery before and after release is shown in Figure 57-4. Note the dissection in the artery that is widely tapered to the arterial wall upon stent deployment. Preliminary results show acute patency of 100%. Further dilation of the stent with a balloon was easily achieved without migration of the stent (n = 3). Venous angiography demonstrated patency in all patients within 24 hours of the procedure. Restenosis occurred in two patients. In one of them the stent was removed surgically during a bypass operation; histologic examination showed that the stent did not provoke any inflammatory response.

Initial Experience in Coronary Arteries

The performance of the stent in human coronary arteries is currently under investigation, with encouraging preliminary results. To date, 11 stents have been implanted in five patients (Rambam Medical Center, Haifa, Israel) for an indication of chronic

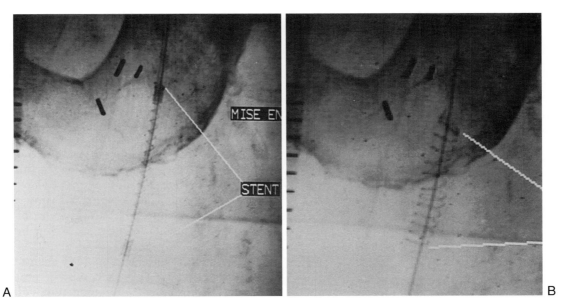

Fig. 57-3. Stent in the femoral graft before release **(A)** and after release **(B)**. (From Bayer et al.[22] with permission.)

total arterial occlusion. It was shown that the nitinol self-expanding stent can provide adequate arterial support in the most difficult cases of diffuse disease and large dissections. The stents can be implanted in sequence to cover a long region of extended dissection, or to prevent recoil. Figure 57-5 shows a case with two stents implanted in the proximal right coronary artery to cover a dissected region 30 mm long.

Potential Clinical Indications

The nitinol vascular stents are an attractive addition to the stents currently available. The self-expanding stent can tack arterial dissections, prevent elastic recoil, and match the local contour of the artery. Therefore, the stent can potentially be used for a variety of indications including reduction of restenosis.

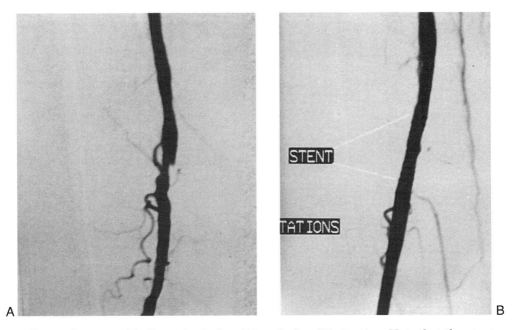

Fig. 57-4. Femoral artery with dissection before **(A)** and after **(B)** stenting. Note that the stent successfully tapers the dissection. (From Beyar et al.,[22] with permission.)

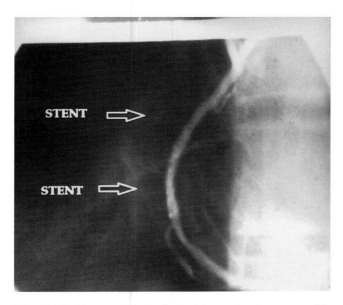

Fig. 57-5. Two stents implanted in series to cover a 30-cm-long dissection in a proximal right coronary artery.

Its longitudinal flexibility is an important feature that offers an advantage over some other stents.

The nitinol coil stent can be used to treat bail-out conditions and to prevent restenosis. In addition, this stent may be indicated for vein graft stenosis. Final recommendations for the use of this stent, compared with other stents, will be determined in the future based on large-scale clinical trials.

This stent has been used successfully for the peripheral ileac, femoral, and popliteal arteries. It is believed that it can be used safely for tacking dissections and prevention of recoil; it can also be safely used over joints because of the combination of longitudinal flexibility and elastic properties, which prevent external compression of the stent.

REMOVABILITY OF NITINOL STENTS AND THE TEMPORARY STENT CONCEPT

Stent deployment is currently an irreversible process in most cases. The need to remove a stent, although rare, may be indicated in the following cases:

1. *Improper placement.* If the stent has been improperly deployed or has migrated acutely, it may, if possible, be removed. Most of the current stents are not removable without major surgery, and a significant problem is presented if the lesion cannot be accessed. While the needs of the removable/temporary stent for this indication are decreasing with increased reliability of stent deployment, the possibility of immediate removal of a stent may facilitate some of the clinical decisions the cardiologist faces.

2. *Use of the stent as a temporary device during acute bail-out conditions.* The stent may be used to maintain vessel patency temporarily until the patient is stable enough to undergo surgery. When the risk of subacute thrombotic complications of a permanent stent is not advisable, this alternative route may be a safe option for stabilizing the patient for a few hours to a day, before performing bypass surgery. By keeping the time of stent presence to less than 24 hours, the risk of thrombotic complications, typically occurring later, is very small.

3. *Use of the stent as a temporary device to maintain vessel patency.* The stent may be employed for a limited period so that, upon removal, the artery will maintain its patency. This is the most attractive indication for a temporary/removable stent. The possibility of tapering a dissection preventing elastic recoil of the artery (or both) by implantation of temporary stents may allow the treatment of bail-out conditions without the need for bypass surgery; the possible later complication of subacute thrombosis may also be avoided. Two questions must still be answered: (a) how traumatic is stent removal; and (b) what is the time frame for stabilizing bail-out conditions (i.e., attaching a dissection to the wall or preventing the elastic recoil of the artery or both)?

Three devices for such indications have been proposed so far:

1. *The flow support catheter.* A basket wire design that can be dilated mechanically and kept in the artery for a limited period has been suggested.[29, 30]

2. *The heat-activated removable temporary stent.* This is a nitinol stent mounted on a balloon. It is deployed by balloon inflation, deforming the stent plastically to its in situ configuration. When removal is indicated, hot saline injections transform the stent to its austenitic collapsed configuration after a removal catheter is placed within the stent. The shrunk stent, caught on the catheter, is then retracted. Animal studies have shown that this stent is removable up to 1 week following implantation.[28]

3. *The self-expanding nitinol coil removable/temporary stent.* The nitinol stents can be removed by pulling the stent as a straight wire through a removal catheter advanced toward the proximal

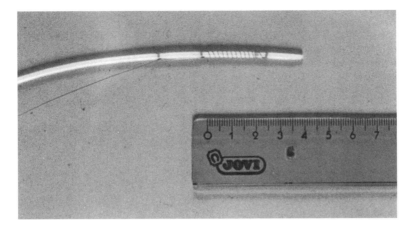

Fig. 57-6. Temporary stent. The coil stent is continuous with a long wire.

end of the stent. By being pulled into the catheter, the stent undergoes "atraumatic uncoiling" (i.e., it uncoils in its own groove in the catheter as it disappears into the catheter). The stent can be removed either by catching its proximal end or by implanting a temporary version of the stent, which is the same stent design continuous with a long wire (Fig. 57-6).

The feasibility of stent removal was tested in a plastic tube arterial simulator and in iliac arteries in dogs.[27] No macroscopic intimal tears or intimal damage could be seen in the iliac arteries after removal of the stents within 24 hours. A misplaced stent could also be removed from an iliac artery in one patient after 3 hours without sequela. The temporary stent has also been implanted in two patients with dissection of peripheral arteries. In both cases placement and removal (after 2 hours) were uneventful, and no damage to the arterial wall was demonstrated.

CONCLUSIONS

The nitinol self-expanding stent has proved to be safe and effective as a permanent stent in peripheral arteries and may be used over tortuous and joint lesions that are difficult or impossible to reach with other, balloon-expandable stents. The experience in coronary arteries is promising and awaits large randomized studies. With the wide acceptance of permanent stents today, the role of temporary stents is still unclear. Some indications for the use of the temporary stent may still exist in regard to local delivery of drugs.[31]

ACKNOWLEDGMENTS

The author would like to thank Dr. M. Henry for providing the pictures of the clinical cases implanted at the Polyclinique D'Essey, Nancy, France.

REFERENCES

1. Dotter CT. Transluminally placed coil spring endarterial tube grafts: long term patency in canine popliteal artery. Invest Radiol 1969;4:329
2. Palmaz CJ, Windeler SA, Garcia F et al. Atherosclerotic rabbit aortas: expandable intraluminal grafting. Radiology 1986;160:723
3. Schatz RA, Baim DS, Leon M et al. Clinical experience with the Palmaz-Schatz coronary stent. Initial results of a multicenter study. Circulation 1991;83:148
4. Roubin GS, Cannon AD, Agrawal SK et al. Intracoronary stenting for acute and threatened closure complicating percutaneous transluminal coronary angioplasty. Circulation 1992;85:916
5. Buchwald A, Unterberg G, Werner G et al. Initial clinical results with the Wiktor stent: a new balloon expandable coronary stent. Clin Cardiol 1991;14:374
6. Reifart N, Langer A, Storger H et al. Strecker stent as a bailout device following percutaneous transluminal coronary angioplasty, J Interv Cardiol 1992;5:79
7. Serruys PW, Straus BH, Beatt KJ et al. Angiographic follow up after placement of a self expanding coronary artery stent. N Engl J Med 1991;324:13
8. Civjan S, Huget EF, Desimon LB. Potential applications of certain nickel-titanium (nitinol) alloys. J Dental Res 1975;54:89-96
9. Duerig TW, Melton KN, Stoekel D, Wayman CM. Engineering Aspects of Shape Memory Alloy. Butterworth & Heinemann, London UK, 1990
10. Simon M, Athanasoulis CA, Kim D et al. Simon nitinol inferior vena cava filter: initial clinical experience. Radiology 1989;172:99
11. Dotter CT, Buschmann RW, McKinney MK, Rosch J. Transluminal expandable nitinol coil stent grafting. Radiology 1983;147:259

12. Cragg AH, Lund G, Rysavy JA et al. Percutaneous arterial grafting. Radiology 1984;150:45
13. Kambic H, Sutton C, Oku T et al. Biological performance of TiNi shape memory alloy vascular ring prosthesis: a two year study. Int J Artif Organs 1988;11:487
14. Rabkin IKH, Germashev VG. 5-yr experience with roentgenologically controlled endovascular nitinol prosthesis (in Russian). Vestn Rentgenol Radiol (in Russian) 1991;2:45–54
15. Rabkin IKh, Shabalin AIa, Natsvlishvili ZG et al. Radioendovascular prosthesis of renal arteries in patients with renovascular hypertension [in Russian]. Kardiologiia 1990;30:11
16. Sutton CS, Oku T, Harasaki H et al. Titanium-nickel intravascular endoprosthesis: a two year study in dogs. Am J Radiol 1988;151:597
17. Sutton CS, Tominaga R, Harasaki H et al. Vascular stenting in normal and atherosclerotic rabbits: studies of the intravascular endoprosthesis of titanium-nickel alloy. Circulation 1990;81:667
18. Tominaga R, Emoto H, Kambic HE et al. Intravascular endoprostheses. Effect of surface geometry on restenosis and side branch patency. ASAIO Trans 1989;35:376
19. Tominaga R, Kambic HE, Emoto H et al. Effects of design geometry of intravascular endoprostheses on stenosis rate in normal rabbits. Am Heart J 1992;123:21
20. Yachia D, Beyar M. Temporarily implanted urethral coil stent for the treatment of recurrent urethral strictures: a preliminary report. J Urol 1991;146:1001
21. Beyar R, Shofti R, Grenedier E et al. Coronary arterial histological response to the self expandable nitinol stent. J Am Coll Cardiol 1993;21:336A
22. Beyar R, Henry M, Shofti R et al. Self expandable nitinol stent for cardiovascular applications: canine and human experience. Cathet Cardiovasc Diagn 1994;32:162
23. Grenedier E, Shofti S, Beyar M et al. Self expandable hyperelastic nitinol stent: immediate and long term results in dogs. Am Heart J 1994;128:870
24. Castleman LS, Motzkin SM, Alicandri FP, Bonawit VL. Bio-compatibility of nitinol alloy as an implant material. J Biomed Mater Res 1976;10:695
25. Prince MR, Salzman EW, Schoen FJ et al. Local intravascular effects of the nitinol wire blood clot filter. Invest Radiol 1988;23:294
26. Putters JL, Kaulesar Sukul DM, de Zeeuw GR et al. Comparative cell culture effects of shape memory metal (nitinol), nickel and titanium: a bio-compatibility estimation. Eur Surg Res 1992;24:378
27. Beyar R, Henry M. Removable self expandable nitinol coil stent: initial report on in-vitro, canine and human results. J Am Coll Cardiol 1993;21:439A
28. Henry M, Beyar R. Initial clinical experience with the InStent nitinol permanent and temporary stents. Circulation 1993;88:I–586
29. Gaspard PE, Didier BP, Delsanti GL. The temporary stent catheter: a nonoperative treatment for acute occlusion during coronary angioplasty. J Am Coll Cardiol 1990;15:118A
30. Khorsandi MJ, Eigler NL, Litvak F et al. Heat activated recoverable temporary stents: histopathological and angiographic observations for implantations of up to six weeks. J Am Coll Cardiol 1993;21:439A
31. Dev V, Lambert T, Shethe S et al. Kinetics of drug delivery to the arterial wall via polyurethane coated removable nitinol stent. Circulation 1993;88:I–310

58 HARTS Removable Stent

Frank Litvack
Ken Mahrer
Vishva Dev
Mehran Khorsandi
Joel Kupfer
James S. Forrester
Neal Eigler

Intracoronary stents have been introduced to deal with critical limitations of coronary angioplasty including abrupt arterial occlusion, suboptimal dilation, and restenosis. Several different permanent stent designs are now in clinical practice that differ in geometry, metallic composition, and technique of deployment. The objective of all stent designs is to provide a widely patent lumen by preventing elastic recoil and controlling endothelial flaps and dissections.[1–6]

LIMITATIONS OF PERMANENT STENTS

Despite the undeniable benefits of permanent stents, their deployment introduces new clinical problems. Stents are thrombogenic, and patients have required an aggressive regime of anticoagulation to minimize coronary thrombosis. Despite this adjunctive pharmacologic intervention, the rate of subacute thrombosis following elective stent implantation is at least 2 to 3%.[7–9] Furthermore, when stents are implanted for emergency angioplasty dissection, the rate of subacute thrombosis may be considerably higher.[10] Subacute thrombosis typically occurs from days 5 to 10 after implantation and usually results in acute myocardial infarction. To limit these complications, stent patients must stay in the hospital 5 to 7 days for regulation of the anticoagulation regimen. This prolonged hospitalization increases the cost of treatment. The vigorous use of anticoagulants results in a 10 to 20% incidence of significant groin hematoma and/or need for transfusion or surgical repair.[10,11] Following discharge, stent patients remain anticoagulated for several weeks. This has the potential of increasing the risk of major bleeding and is a contraindication for patients with bleeding tendencies including peptic ulcer and other gastroenterologic diseases. Finally, placement of a stent within the vessel must be very precise. If it is incorrectly placed, there is no way to remove or reposition the stent, and the patient must remain with the stent in the incorrect position as a permanent prosthesis.

RATIONALE FOR TEMPORARY STENTING

To address the limitations of permanent stents, several research groups are endeavoring to develop temporary or removable stents. The rationale is to attempt to achieve many or all of the benefits of permanent stenting without the need for a permanent endovascular prosthesis and the ensuing risks. These devices fall into three categories: first, metallic, expandable or retractable mesh devices attached to a catheter[12,13]; second, stents made out of biodegradable materials[14]; and third, nonattached, fully removable metallic stents, including the HARTS (heat-activated removable temporary stent) device.[15] The metallic, catheter-attached temporary stents can be left in place for only a few hours. There is no option to leave them in place permanently or even for several days. Biodegradable stents are an intriguing concept, but a suitable material with the correct properties of strength, clot resistance, and uniform degradation without microembolization has not yet been identified. Furthermore, unless a biodegradable device with antithrombotic properties is developed, it is likely that several weeks of anticoagulation will still be required.

HEAT-ACTIVATED REMOVABLE TEMPORARY STENT

The HARTS device relies on the properties of nickel titanium (nitinol), which on heating to a specific transition temperature undergoes a phase change and reassumes the original shape in which it was configured. Although others, including Dotter et al.[16] in the 1960s, have conceived using so-called "shape memory" metals for stenting, they have always envisioned the phase changes as integral to the expansion and deployment of the stent. The unique features of the HARTS device are that it not only uses phase change for expansion and implantation, but also utilizes this property for shrinking and removing the stent.

Nitinol exists in either a martinsite or an austinite crystal phase. At body temperature, the stent is predominantly in the martinsitic phase and is a deformable structure. One of the properties of the metal is that a "memory" state can be "programmed" into it. For the purposes of coronary stenting, the memory shape is the shape of the stent in its collapsed configuration. The stent is deployed, as are most coronary stents, by means of balloon expansion so that the expanded stent diameter approximates that of the artery. The balloon expansion induces an increase in the proportion of certain martinsitic elements in the metal but not the plastic deformation seen with other stents. The balloon is then removed and the stent remains in place. At some later time, a specially designed recovery catheter is inserted into the coronary artery. This recovery catheter is similar to a standard balloon angioplasty catheter but without a balloon. Between two opaque markers located at the distal end of the catheter is the "landing zone." The landing zone of the catheter has multiple small holes connected through to the inner lumen. For recovery, 5 ml of warm crystalloid solution (above the 50° to 60°C transition temperature of the metal) is injected through the recovery catheter so that the fluid exits from the small holes in the landing zone and bathes the stent. As the stent temperature rises above its transition temperature and because it has not been plastically deformed, it will revert to its "memory" shape by transitioning to the austinite phase. As such, the stent will collapse with a significant force and attach itself to the landing zone of the recovery catheter. Once this is achieved, the recovery catheter is removed through the guide catheter and the stent extracted from the body.

The first iteration of the HARTS device described by Eigler et al.[15] was a prototype constructed of multiple segments of nickel titanium alloy wire 0.009" in diameter. The wire segments were connected by stainless steel tubing crimp joints to form a tubular mesh stent. The initial experience with the implantation and recovery of this HARTS design in canine coronary arteries has been reported. Seventy-eight prototype wire stents were deployed by balloon expansion in the coronary arteries of 28 dogs and left in place for up to 6 months. Thirty minutes to 1 week after implantation, 70 stents were recovered by flushing the coronary arteries with 3 to 5 ml of warmed Ringer's lactate solution. All stents were successfully recovered and removed percutaneously. The mean vessel diameter with the stent in place was $12 \pm 6\%$ ($P <0.05$) greater than the baseline diameter. The mean vessel diameter after stent removal remained enlarged $6 \pm 3\%$ ($P <0.05$). There was no angiographic evidence of thrombosis, dissection, embolization, or stent migration.

Implantation and removal of the stent was associated with some evidence of vascular injury at the implantation site. In most instances, this was limited to focal intimal or medial injury beneath the position of the stent struts with preserved intima in the intervening segments. When oversized stents were deployed (>1.4 times normal vessel diameter), there was evidence of disruption of the intima and media with some periadventitial hemorrhage. There did not appear to be any relation between the extent of vascular injury and the duration of stent placement. Histologic sections of arteries following 6 months of stent implantation revealed endothelial ingrowth over the stent struts. In general, the pathologic findings seen following HARTS implantation were consistent with those defined following balloon angioplasty and permanent stenting of normal arteries. There was no gross evidence of thrombus formation. Histologic study revealed microscopic thrombi in one-third of the stented sites, and scanning electron microscopic examination of the recovered stents revealed occasional fibrin, red blood cells, and platelets.

Experiments with the first HARTS design described above revealed elasticity and recoil of the stent following balloon removal. As such, it was believed that the meshed wire designed was suboptimal for clinical application. Significant effort was expended in redesigning the HARTS stent to be fabricated in a slotted tubular design. Nitinol hypotubing was drawn and the stents cut using an electrodiode technique. This process led to the development of the current HARTS design, which is 14.5 mm in length and constructed of two 7.0-mm segments joined by a 0.5-mm bridge. As with the first iteration, the stent is mounted on the balloon and deployed by initiating metallic phase change through balloon expansion. The balloon is then removed and the stent left in place for a variable period of time. At the time of recovery, the recovery catheter is inserted and the stent extracted by the infusion of warm crystalloid and capture of the stent on the landing zone of the catheter.

Preclinical evaluation has demonstrated that the new HARTS design can be deployed and retrieved in a manner initially described for the wire mesh design. Importantly, quantitative angiographic analysis has revealed that stent recoil is less than 10%.

POTENTIAL CLINICAL APPLICATIONS OF THE HARTS DEVICE

Bailout Device

Perfusion balloon catheters currently represent an indispensable component of the interventionalist's armamentarium. Acute occlusion occurs in approximately 6 to 8% of balloon angioplasty procedures.[17]

At present, the standard of care is to use a perfusion balloon to attempt prolonged dilation in most cases of abrupt occlusion that do not respond to prolonged conventional balloon dilation. Temporary stenting may have some advantage over the perfusion balloon in that greater arterial patency and flow is achievable and the device may be left in place for several hours to days. Permanent stents have been successfully applied for treatment of acute occlusion.[10,11] As described above, permanent stent placement for this indication is associated with limitations, including a relatively high rate of subacute thrombosis, vascular complications, and prolonged hospitalization. It is possible that much of the benefit of permanent stenting may be achieved with the use of temporary stents for several hours to a few days. This contention is supported by recent reports of overnight application of perfusion balloons for refractory dissection following balloon angioplasty.[18] This hypothesis will need to be tested in controlled clinical trials.

Suboptimal Angioplasty

Both prolonged balloon dilation and permanent stents have been useful for improving angiographic appearance following suboptimal balloon dilation.[10,11] Clinical experience has demonstrated that prolonged (5 to 30 minutes) balloon inflation can yield acceptable angiographic results in as many as 50% of patients following suboptimal angioplasty. The duration of balloon inflation, even with a perfusion balloon, is limited by thrombogenicity and ischemia. It is possible that the temporary stent will offer significant advantages over the perfusion balloon for this indication because of its ability to optimize flow and provide "stenting" effects for several hours to days. Controlled clinical trials will be necessary to test the hypothesis.

Limitation of Restenosis

Available data with the Johnson & Johnson Palmaz-Schatz stent indicate that this device may reduce angiographic restenosis rates by one-third to one-half compared with conventional balloon angioplasty.[19,20] The two ongoing randomized trials as well as data from the prospective multicenter registry reveal that in selected cases, angiographic restenosis rates of 15 to 25% in native arteries and 25 to 35% of vein grafts may be achieved. If further validated, this indication represents a potential major application for permanent stenting. It appears, however, that only certain permanent stent designs, including the slotted tubes, may provide this advantage. The question arises for permanent stents of whether the costs and risks of prolonged hospitalization, anticoagulation, and the potential for the catastrophic complication of subacute thrombosis will be outweighed by any potential reduction in restenosis rates. Furthermore, the Palmaz-Schatz stent is only applicable in arteries 3 mm or larger in diameter because in smaller arteries, the subacute thrombosis rate appears elevated. The mechanism of restenosis reduction following Palmaz-Schatz stenting results from the creation of the largest possible lumen following the angioplasty procedure. Recent angiographic and intravascular ultrasound data have demonstrated that restenosis occurs as a result of the combination of elastic recoil and intimal ingrowth.[21,22] The contribution of elastic recoil is probably greater than previously recognized. The reduction of restenosis following permanent stenting occurs even though metallic struts stimulate smooth muscle proliferation over weeks to months.[23] Thus, the late loss in lumen diameter following stenting is greater than following balloon angioplasty alone, but the net gain is greater following stenting because of a marked reduction in elastic recoil. It is possible that prolonged (hours to days) mechanical stretching with a removable stent will result in sufficient plastic deformation and stretch to the vessel wall and elastic tissues so that a large diameter may be maintained even following removal of the stent, that is, the elastic recoil seen following conventional angioplasty may be reduced. If this proves true, then temporary stenting may play a role in reducing angiographic restenosis rates. At present this hypothesis is totally unproven.

"Stentoplasty"

Balloon angioplasty works by stretching, tearing, and compressing atherosclerotic plaque, thrombus, and vascular tissue. The acute efficacy of balloon dilation is limited by occasionally unpredictable and excessive tissue tearing and significant early elastic recoil. Routine expansion of the plaque by a stent-covered balloon may result in the development of multiple minute fractures in the fibrous cap of the atheroma, which allows a more predictable expansion of the vessel. This procedure would consist of dilating the vessel with a stent-covered balloon and leaving the temporary stent in place for several hours after the balloon is withdrawn. Hypothetically, this would result in an even expansion of the plaque with sealing off of small dissections. Prolonged stretching and plastic deformation may eliminate or reduce elastic recoil of the vessel. This could yield a larger acute gain and greater minimal luminal diam-

eter and may eliminate so-called suboptimal percutaneous transluminal coronary angioplasty results. This hypothesis will need to be validated or refuted in controlled clinical trials.

Delivery of Pharmaceutical or Other Therapeutic Agents

Inhibition of vascular smooth muscle cell proliferation and deposition of extracellular matrix are the ultimate goals for the prevention of restenosis. If this could be achieved along with minimizing elastic recoil, it is likely that restenosis rates could be significantly reduced. Despite early expectations, none of the new interventional technologies, with the exception of permanent stents in selected settings, have demonstrated significant efficacy at reducing restenosis rates. To date, no systemically delivered pharmacologic agent has shown any reduction of restenosis rates.

Other investigators have developed catheters designed for localized delivery of pharmaceutical agents to atherosclerotic lesions. Several limitations of these devices exist. Drug is delivered by the agents for a brief period during or following the angioplasty injury (for seconds to several minutes). It may be necessary to deliver the inhibitive agent for several days, during which the proliferative processes are initiated. Delivery of a short-acting pharmaceutical agent locally at the time of the acute injury may be ineffective. Finally, some of the devices for drug delivery involve the generation of high-pressure jets that may themselves damage the arterial wall and further stimulate delivery response.

Temporary stents with local drug delivery capabilities may overcome these limitations. Our group has developed polymer coatings placed on the stent that are capable of slowly releasing various drugs.[24,25] We have shown that forskolin, a naturally occurring adenylate cyclase activator, can be delivered in high local concentration off the stent and can be retained in the arterial wall for many hours. At 4 hours after implantation, the concentration of drug in the vascular media was 60 μg/g tissue versus 0.13 μg/g in blood. Release rate from stent into blood averaged 3.7 μg/min, and at 24 hours, media forskolin level was 4.9 μg/g. Furthermore, we have demonstrated that the delivered drug is pharmacologically active and, in the case of forskolin, capable of inhibiting stent thrombosis.[25] We have also delivered derivatives of vitamin A off the stent, achieving a vessel wall-to-blood concentration ratio of 6,000:1. Because of the extreme lipophilic nature of that compound, the drug remains in the arterial wall for several days with relatively slow elution.[24] More clinical research is required to complete and develop the drug delivery systems and to evaluate the effectiveness of various pharmaceutical agents. Pharmaceutical agents including anticoagulant, antithrombin, antiplatelet, and antiproliferative drugs may be eventual candidates for local delivery.

CONCLUSIONS

Preclinical experience has demonstrated the feasibility of implantation and retrieval of the HARTS temporary stent for up to 1 week following delivery. When stents are left in place longer, they become endothelialized, as do other permanently deployed stents. Potential indications for the HARTS device include treatment of acute occlusion and suboptimal postangioplasty results, limitation of restenosis by minimizing elastic recoil, "stentoplasty," and local delivery of pharmaceutical or other bioactive agents. All work to date is preclinical, and the hypothetical indications and applications will need careful testing in controlled clinical trials.

ACKNOWLEDGMENTS

Work supported in part by generous donations from the Cedars-Sinai Grant Foundation and Mr. and Mrs. Irving Cooper.

REFERENCES

1. Serruys PW, Strauss BH, van Beusekom HM et al. Stenting of coronary arteries: has a modern pandora's box been opened? J Am Coll Cardiol 1991;17:143B.
2. Schatz RA, Baim DS, Leon M et al. Clinical experience with the Palmaz-Schatz coronary stent: initial results of a multicenter study. Circulation 1991;83:148.
3. Serruys PW, Strauss BH, Beatt KJ et al. Angiographic follow-up after placement of a self-expanding coronary artery stent. N Engl J Med 1991;324:13.
4. Urban P, Sigwart U, Golf S et al. Intravascular stenting for aortocoronary venous bypass grafts. J Am Coll Cardiol 1989;13:1085.
5. Roubin GS, King SB, Douglas JS et al. Intracoronary stenting during percutaneous transluminal coronary angioplasty, abstracted. Circulation 1990;81:IV 92.
6. Haude M, Erbel R, Straub U et al. Results of intracoronary stents for management of coronary dissection after balloon angioplasty. Am J Cardiol 1991;67:691.
7. Litvack F. Intravascular stenting for prevention of restenosis: in search of the magic bullet. J Am Coll Cardiol 1989;13:1092.
8. Topol EJ. Promises and pitfalls of new devices for coronary artery disease. Circulation 1991;83:689.
9. Hermann HC, Buchbinder M, Clemen MW et al. Emergent use of balloon-expandable coronary artery stenting for failed percutaneous transluminal coronary angioplasty. Circulation 1992;86:812–819.
10. George BS, Voorhees WD III, Roubin GS et al. Multicenter investigation of coronary stenting to treat acute or threatened closure after percutaneous transluminal coronary angioplasty: clinical and angiographic outcomes. J Am Coll Cardiol 1993;22:135.
11. Schatz RA, Baim DS, Leon M et al. Clinical experience with the Palmaz-Schatz coronary stent: initial results of a multicenter study. Circulation 1991;83:148.
12. Clugston R, Oesterle SN, Matthews R et al. Flow support catheter for prolonged maintenance of coronary blood flow. Cathet Cardiovasc Diagn 1991;24:308.
13. Whitlow PL, Gaspard P, Kent K et al. Improvement of coronary dissection with a removable flow support catheter: acute results, abstracted. J Am Coll Cardiol 1992;19:217A.
14. Gammon RS, Chapman GD, Agarwal GM et al. Mechanical features of the Duke biodegradable intravascular stent, abstracted. J Am Coll Cardiol 1991;17:235A.
15. Eigler N, Khorsandi MJ, Forrester JS et al. Implantation and recovery of temporary metallic stents in canine coronary arteries. J Am Coll Cardiol 1993;22:1207.
16. Dotter CT, Buschmann RW, McKinney MK et al. Transluminal expandable nitinol coil stent grafting: preliminary report. Radiology 1983;147:259.
17. Detre KM, Holmes DR, Holubkov R et al. Incidence and consequences of periprocedural occlusion: the 1985–1986 National Heart, Lung and Blood Institute Percutaneous Transluminal Coronary Angioplasty Registry. Circulation 1990;82:739.
18. van der Linden LP, Bakx LM, Sedney MI et al. Prolonged dilation with an autoperfusion balloon catheter for refractory acute occlusion related to percutaneous transluminal coronary angioplasty. J Am Coll Cardiol 1993;22:1016.
19. Serruys PW, Macaya C, de Jaegere P et al. Interim analysis of the Benestent-trial. Circulation 1993;88:3195.
20. Schatz RA, Penn IM, Baim DS et al. STent REStenosis Study (STRESS): analysis of in-hospital results. Circulation 1993;88:3194.
21. Hanet C, Wijns W, Xavier M, Schroderer E. Influence of balloon size and stenosis morphology on immediate and delayed elastic recoil after percutaneous transluminal coronary angioplasty. J Am Coll Cardiol 1991;18:605.
22. Kovach JA, Mintz GS, Kent KM et al. Serial intravascular ultrasound studies indicate that chronic recoils is an important mechanism of restenosis following transcatheter therapy. p. 236. Restenosis Summit V, Cleveland Clinic Foundation, 1993.
23. Karas SP, Gravanis MB, Santoian EC et al. Coronary intimal proliferation after balloon injury and stenting in swine: an animal model of restenosis. J Am Coll Cardiol 1992;20:467.
24. Dev, V, Lambert T, Sheth S et al. Kinetics of drug delivery to the arterial wall via polyurethane coated removable nitinol stent—comparative study of 2 drugs. Circulation 1993;88:1657.
25. Lambert T, Dev, D, Litvack F et al. Localized arterial drug delivery from a polymer coated removable metallic stent: kinetics and bioactivity of Forskolin. Circulation 1993;88:1659.